Cawson's Essentials of
ORAL PATHOLOGY
and ORAL MEDICINE

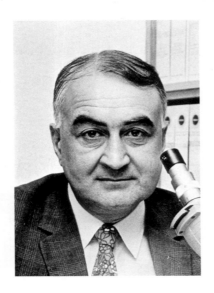

Professor Roderick A. Cawson

BDS, FDSRCS, LMSSA, MB BS, MD, FRCPath
1921–2007

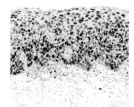

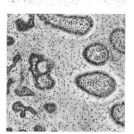

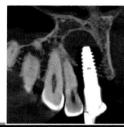

Tenth Edition

Cawson's Essentials of
ORAL PATHOLOGY
and ORAL MEDICINE

Edward W. Odell

BDSRCS MSc PhD FRCPath

Emeritus Professor of Oral Pathology and Medicine,
King's College London
Consultant in Head and Neck Pathology,
Guy's and St Thomas' NHS Foundation Trust, London

ELSEVIER

First edition 1962
Second edition 1968
Third edition 1978
Fourth edition 1984
Fifth edition 1991
Sixth edition 1998
Seventh edition 2002
Eighth edition 2008
Ninth edition 2017

Notices

Practitioners and researchers must always rely on their own experience and knowledge in evaluating and using any information, methods, compounds or experiments described herein. Because of rapid advances in the medical sciences, in particular, independent verification of diagnoses and drug dosages should be made. To the fullest extent of the law, no responsibility is assumed by Elsevier, authors, editors or contributors for any injury and/or damage to persons or property as a matter of products liability, negligence or otherwise, or from any use or operation of any methods, products, instructions, or ideas contained in the material herein.

ISBN: 978-0-323-93549-4
978-0-3239-3573-9

Senior Content Strategist: Alexandra Mortimer
Content Project Manager: Fariha Nadeem
Design: Christian Bilbow
Illustration Manager: Anitha Rajarathnam
Marketing Manager: Deborah Watkins

Printed in India

Last digit is the print number: 9 8 7 6 5 4 3 2 1

Working together
to grow libraries in
developing countries

www.elsevier.com • www.bookaid.org

Contents

Preface

With its tenth edition, this textbook celebrates its 60th anniversary. When the first edition appeared in 1962 the practice of dentistry was very different. The book covered practical surgery and topics such as facial fractures that dental students were expected to know, and possibly use, immediately on qualification. Surgery was a significant part of general practitioner's workload, biopsy was routinely performed and oral conditions were managed without medical support. Constant introduction of new drugs and concerns about interactions in dentistry made pharmacological and general medical knowledge essential.

Advances in restorative care, implants, the ageing of population, and increased demand for cosmetic treatment have contracted dentistry back to management of teeth and periodontium to the extent that some dentists now practice on the edges of the cosmetic industry. The expansion of postgraduate specialties has brought many of the topics in this book into specialist, rather than general, practice. Nevertheless, the undergraduate dental students need to be familiar with many of the conditions included. As noted in the learning guide, the average general practice will have many patients with oral diseases that need to be managed and many of the conditions are seen in primary care, even if only infrequently.

This edition has evolved to meet the changed needs of its readers. Previous editions were written for undergraduates in dentistry, with the emphasis on explanation and fostering understanding of oral disease. However, the last two editions have been used more by postgraduates, who need a reference book with less explanation and more facts. Factual content and additional references have been added to increase the breadth and depth of coverage for this audience". It has been updated in accordance with the 2023 WHO Classifications of Head and Neck Tumours and the 2020 International Classification of Orofacial Pain. More diseases have been added, both well-established entities and new ones, such as Covid-19 and Mpox. A new chapter on cosmetic procedures has been added. However, it retains its key focus on oral and facial disease, the medical aspects of dentistry and differential diagnosis. References to onward reading have been carefully selected to avoid propagation of the misinformation available on the internet. My hope is that whoever reads the book will find it interesting and informative.

My thanks are to Alex Mortimer, Fariha Nadeem and the production staff at Elsevier for maintaining the excellent production standards of previous editions.

I am grateful to colleagues who have helped me by suggesting changes, reading chapters, and providing material, particularly Prof Francis Hughes for Periodontology, Dr Stacey Clough for Special Care Dentistry, and Dr Jackie Brown for Radiology. Most of all, my thanks go to my wonderful wife Wendy for her unconditional support and for maintaining her sense of humour during the year I spent in front of my computer writing this new edition.

References

References to further reading are inserted throughout, immediately adjacent to the relevant text. To make searching for web URLs straightforward, links to the relevant websites can be found at http://sites.elsevier.com/cawsonsessentials. Various types of reference are provided, all designed to be immediately available through the internet. In the electronic version of this book they are direct links:

PubMed ID: These are shown with a few words of description and a number in the format PMID: 25556809. Entering the text PMID and number into an Internet search engine should take the reader direct to the reference. Alternatively, it can be entered direct into the PubMed search box at the top of the main page at the PubMed website at http://www.ncbi.nlm.nih.gov/pubmed/ and this has the advantage of immediately showing the abstract and links to the full text of the article. References have been selected to be open access full text publications where possible, but it may be necessary to log in to publishers' websites or access through an institution library to obtain the full text. Use the references in these papers to direct onward reading.

PubMed Central ID: These are shown similarly, with a few words of description and a number in the format PMCID: PMC4334280. The majority of PubMed Central ID numbers have been changed to PubMed IDs in this edition. If an open access PubMed Central version is available, there will be a link direct to it on the PubMed webpage. Otherwise PMC reference numbers can be resolved in the same way as above. If searching on the PubMed website for a PMC number, do not forget to select PMC in the window to the left of the search box.

ISBN numbers: These are ISBN13 codes to books in the format ISBN-13: 978-0723435938. The numbers can be entered either into a search engine, although a search in the website of an online bookseller or your university library will take you directly to the book title and a copy. Where possible, books available in electronic format have been selected.

Web Uniform Resource Locators URLs or web addresses. These may be entered directly into the address bar of a web browser. Some are long and complex and case sensitive. To avoid this, some are given just as the home page of an organisation with instructions on text words to enter into the search box. These should find the relevant resource more reliably that a complex URL that may change.

DOI: Digital Object Identifiers can be resolved at the DOI website https://www.doi.org/

Principles of investigation, diagnosis and treatment

The principles of patient investigation and diagnosis are summarised in Box 1.1.

TAKING A HISTORY

Taking a history and making a diagnosis are not completely generic skills that can be learned and then applied to any patient. Gaining rapport, listening and questioning skills are common to all complaints, but to ask targeted incisive questions requires the ability to construct a good differential diagnosis. Effective history-taking is therefore founded in clinical and pathological knowledge.

Rapport is critical for gaining trust and eliciting the most useful information, but gaining rapport can be difficult because almost all patients are nervous to a degree, some are inarticulate and others are confused. History-taking needs to be tailored to the individual patient.

Initial questions should allow patients to speak at some length and to gain confidence. It is usually best to start with an 'open' question (Tables 1.1 and 1.2). Medical jargon should be avoided, because even regular hospital attenders who appear to understand medical terminology may use it wrongly and misunderstand. When a patient uses technical jargon, it is wise to check what they mean by it. Leading questions, which suggest a particular answer, should be avoided because patients may feel compelled to agree with the clinician.

It is sometimes difficult to avoid interrupting patients when trying to structure the history for the written record. Structure can only be given after the patient has had time to give the information. Constant note-taking while patients are speaking is undesirable. Notes should be a summary of relevant information only.

Questioning technique is most critical when eliciting any relevant social or psychological history or dealing with embarrassing medical conditions. It may be appropriate to delay asking such questions until after rapport has been gained. Some patients do not consider medical questions to be the concern of the dentist and it is important to be able to give reasons for such questions.

During history-taking, the mental and emotional state of the patient should be assessed. This may have a bearing on some diseases and will also suggest what the patient expects to gain from the consultation and treatment. If the patient's expectations are unreasonable, it is important to try to modify them during the consultation, otherwise no reassurance or treatment may be satisfactory (Box 1.2).

Demographic details

The age, sex, ethnic group and occupation of the patient should be noted routinely; even though apparently trivial, such information is occasionally critical. Increasing age predisposes to malignant neoplasms, autoimmune disease tends to have onset in middle-aged female patients and aphthous stomatitis is often diagnosed in the young. Identifying and recording a patient's heritage or ethnic group can be misconstrued, but it

---

Box 1.1   Principles of investigation and diagnosis
A detailed medical and dental history

- Clinical examination
  - Extraoral
  - Intraoral
- Investigations selected for specific purposes
  - Testing vitality of teeth
  - Radiography or other imaging techniques
  - Biopsy for histopathology (including immunofluorescence, immunocytochemistry, molecular biological tests)
  - Specimens for microbial culture
  - Haematological or biochemical tests

Table 1.1   Types of questions

Type of question	Example
Open	Tell me about the pain.
Closed	What does the pain feel like?
Leading	Does the pain feel like an electric shock?

Table 1.2   Advantages and disadvantages of types of questions

Types of question	Advantages	Disadvantages
Open	Allows patients to use their own words and summarise their view of the problem	Clinicians must listen carefully and avoid interruptions to extract the relevant information
	Allows patients partly to direct the history-taking, gives them confidence and quickly generates rapport	Patients tend to decide what information is relevant
Closed	Elicits specific information quickly	Patients may infer that the clinician is not really interested in their problem if only closed questions are asked
	Useful to fill gaps in the information given in response to open questions	Important information may be lost if not specifically requested
	Prevents vague patients from rambling away from the complaint	Restricts the patient's opportunities to talk

Box 1.2   Essential principles of history-taking

- Introduce yourself and greet the patient by name
- Be culturally aware
- Act courteously and respectfully, maintain professional detachment
- Put patients at their ease, be empathic
- Start with an open question
- Mix open and closed questions
- Avoid leading questions
- Avoid medical and dental jargon and idiomatic expressions
- Listen 'actively'
- Explain the need for specific questions if asked
- Divide the consultation into manageable sections for the patient
- Summarise your findings back to the patient for confirmation of meaning
- Assess the patient's mental health state
- Assess the patient's expectations from treatment

Box 1.3   History of the present complaint

- Record the description of the complaint *in the patient's own words*
- Elicit the exact meaning of those words
- Record the duration and the time course of any changes in symptoms or signs
- Include any relevant facts in the patient's medical history
- Note any temporal relationship between them and the present complaint
- Consider any previous treatments and their effectiveness
- Check previous investigations to avoid their unnecessary repetition

Table 1.3   Features required in a pain history

Characteristic	Informative features
Character	Ache, tenderness, dull pain, throbbing, stabbing, electric shock. These terms are of limited use, but information on the constancy of pain is useful
Severity	Mild – responds to mild analgesics (e.g., aspirin/paracetamol) Moderate – unresponsive to mild analgesics Severe – disturbs sleep
Duration	Time since onset. Duration of pain or attacks
Nature	Continuous, periodic or paroxysmal If not continuous, is pain present between attacks?
Initiating factors	Any potential initiating factors Association with dental treatment, or lack of it, is especially important in eliminating dental causes
Exacerbating and relieving factors	Record all and note especially hot and cold sensitivity or pain on eating as they suggest a dental cause
Localisation	The patient should map out the distribution of pain if possible. Is it well or poorly defined? Does it affect an area supplied by a particular nerve or artery? Is the distribution of the pain consistent with sensory nerve anatomy?
Referred pain	Try to determine whether the pain could be referred
Other neurological features	If the pain suggests a neuralgia, is it accompanied by sensory deficit or paraesthesia and are any motor alterations present?

cannot be avoided for fear of being considered racist. Many diseases have a restricted ethnic distribution that aids diagnosis, such as Paget's disease of bone* or florid cemento-osseous dysplasia.

History of the present complaint

Frequently, a complaint, such as toothache, suggests the diagnosis. In most cases, a detailed history (Box 1.3) is required and sometimes, as in aphthous ulceration, a provisional diagnosis can be made on the history alone.

If earlier treatment has been ineffective, any previous diagnosis must be reconsidered. Many patients' lives have

---

* This book continues to use medical eponyms. Although some would prefer to see all medical eponyms banished, many remain in widespread use. It is generally accepted that the person associated with the condition or anatomical structure was rarely the first person to describe it, but they often produced the most comprehensive description or added significant understanding of the pathogenesis. The original suggestion that eponyms should be discontinued in medical literature (PMID: 46972) did indicate that eponyms should continue if "time-honoured designations unless there is good reason for change".

Unfortunately alternative names are often no better than the eponym and some diseases, such as Parkinson's disease have no good alternative. Eponyms also introduce an interesting element of history into medicine and dentistry.

been shortened by having malignant tumours treated with repeated courses of antibiotics.

Pain is completely subjective and, when physical signs are absent, special care must be taken to detail all its features (Table 1.3). Especially important are features suggesting a dental cause. Pain from a fractured tooth or cusp, dental hypersensitivity or pain on occlusion is easily misdiagnosed.

Causes of pain are discussed in detail in Chapter 39.

Medical history

A medical history is important because it aids the diagnosis of oral manifestations of systemic disease. It also ensures that medical conditions and medications that affect dental or surgical treatment are identified. Such conditions are increasingly frequent in aging populations worldwide.

To ensure that nothing significant is forgotten, a printed questionnaire for patients to complete is valuable and saves time. It also helps to avoid medicolegal problems by providing a written record that the patient's medical background has been considered. Some patients may find it easier to fill in a questionnaire than answer questions. However, a questionnaire alone does not constitute a medical history, and the information must be checked verbally, augmented as necessary and confirmed with the clinician's signature. It is important to

Table 1.4   Questions to be included in a medical history and their relevance*

Question	Subsidiary or follow-up questions	Important features of relevance – not all can be included
Are you taking any medicines, medications or tablets at present?	Including over-the-counter drugs and complementary medicine such as herbal remedies or recreational drugs	Potential interactions with treatment for oral conditions Potential oral adverse effects of drugs, of which there are many Steroid use and risk of steroid collapse, infections in immunosuppression Some herbal preparations interact with sedation drugs
	Include medication taken in the past	Patients may forget past courses of drugs with important effects such as bisphosphonates (risk of osteonecrosis), or gold injections (risk of lichenoid reaction) and others
Have you ever been in hospital for any illnesses or operations?	Any problems with the operation or the anaesthetic?	Hospitalisation usually indicates severe health problems; this general question should reveal information on malignant disease, chemotherapy, radiotherapy and immunosuppression
	… routine recovery, not readmitted, no allergies? How long were you in hospital?	Indicate previous reactions to anaesthetics and possibly bleeding problems or other medical complications
Do you carry any medication cards or MedicAlert, Medi-Tag, Mediband or similar devices?		Provide details of medications, doses and effect, usually anticoagulants, steroids, allergies and significant medical conditions Note that some of these alerts may carry patient-reported diagnoses as well as medically confirmed diagnoses
Do you have, or have you had, any problems with your heart?	Elicit type, particularly valvular disease	Indicates risk of angina, myocardial infarct or other cardiac emergency in the dental surgery Potential anaesthetic problem Possible predisposition to infective endocarditis, depending on defect
Have you ever had rheumatic fever?	Do you have any heart damage as a result?	Possible predisposition to infective endocarditis
Do you have, or have you had, hepatitis or jaundice?	Known or likely type of hepatitis, if unknown clues may be in where and how it was contracted and the clinical course Questions to exclude non-infectious causes of jaundice such as haemolytic anaemias, gall stones, liver failure, alcohol, etc.	Infection control risk for hepatitis B and C Liver damage can cause coagulation defect, and the metabolic defect can contraindicate prescription of some drugs
Have you ever had epilepsy or other fits or faints?	Assess severity of epilepsy, type of seizure, frequency, duration and eliciting factors	Risk of epileptic attack or status epilepticus in the dental surgery Adverse effects of antiepileptic drugs such as phenytoin
	Degree of drug control and date and severity of last seizure	Likelihood and possible severity of future seizure(s)
	If other type of seizure or fit, what cause?	Fits of unknown cause may relate to head and neck neurological complaints and indicate a CNS cause Risk of vasovagal attack in dental surgery
Do you have diabetes?	How is it managed? With insulin, other drugs or diet?	Risk of hypoglycaemic collapse in insulin dependent diabetics, and, less likely, hyperglycaemia
	How well controlled? Ever requiring hospital admission?	Diabetes predisposes to infection, particularly candidal but also bacterial and periodontal disease Dry mouth may result from dehydration
	How is blood glucose monitored? Normal levels and range	
Do you have high blood pressure?	Taking the blood pressure may be required and is a recommendation for dentists in some countries. Hypertension is often asymptomatic and dentists have a role in detecting and referring patients with poorly controlled or undetected hypertension.	May indicate risk of stroke, angina or myocardial infarction in the dental surgery Oral adverse reactions of antihypertensive drugs include dry mouth, gingival hyperplasia, lichenoid reactions, burning mouth and taste loss Risk of interaction with some vasoconstrictors in local anaesthetic Anaesthetic risk Patients may faint from hypotension after rising from a supine position for dental treatment
Have you ever been anaemic?	Do you know the reason?	Anaemia predisposes to numerous oral conditions including aphthous stomatitis, candidosis, glossitis and burning mouth
	Do you or anyone in your family have thalassaemia? For patients of African heritage, do you or anyone in your family have sickle cell anaemia?	Anaesthetic risk for sickle cell anaemia and thalassaemia. Thalassaemia is now so geographically widespread that limiting questioning to people of Mediterranean heritage is too specific

Continued

Table 1.4 Questions to be included in a medical history and their relevance*—cont'd

Question	Subsidiary or follow-up questions	Important features of relevance – not all can be included
Do you have any allergies …	Ask specifically about penicillin and other drugs including local anaesthetic	Reveals atopic patients prone to allergy
… to medicines? … to metals, foods, plasters, etc.?	Ask whether the patient has ever taken penicillin	Allergies to medication potentially prescribed by the dental surgeon, including related drugs Latex allergy and cross-reacting food allergies Identify potential triggers of attack relevant to dentistry
… or asthma, hay fever, rashes, etc.?		Rashes may be cutaneous counterparts of oral disease Potential adverse effects of steroid inhalers used for asthma
Have you ever had any problems stopping bleeding after a cut or surgery?	Does anyone else in your family have problems with bleeding? Have problems followed tooth extraction? Have you ever taken Warfarin or any medicines to 'thin' your blood?	Risk of haemorrhage following extraction, surgery or possibly local anaesthetic If familial, raises possibility of haemophilia and other inherited bleeding conditions Contraindicates prescription of drugs that prolong bleeding such as aspirin Anticoagulants interact with drugs prescribed for oral conditions and prolong bleeding after surgery
Have you ever come into contact with someone with human immunodeficiency virus (HIV) infection or acquired immunodeficiency syndrome (AIDS)? … or any other sexually transmitted infection?	An open question to allow patients to proffer relevant information in this sensitive area. Not usually followed up unless the patient offers that they are or may be HIV positive, in which case minimum information required is the name of the relevant physician and permission to contact them for details of the condition If positive ask about viral load, CD4 count and medication	Infection control risk following blood exposure Oral manifestations of immunosuppression Risk of significant medical complications that may present to the dental surgeon Oral adverse effects of anti-HIV medication and drug interactions Patients at risk should be encouraged to have an HIV test Gives an indication of degree of immunosuppression and infection risk
Do you smoke? Or use smokeless tobacco or betel quid …	Type and amount smoked, expressed in pack years (number of 20-cigarette packs per day multiplied by number of years of smoking). 25 g or 1 oz loose tobacco is equivalent to 50 cigarettes.	Predisposes to oral, nose and sinus and aerodigestive tract carcinoma Predisposes to atheroma, hypertension and cardiac disease Associated with oral red and white lesions and potentially malignant disorders Amenable to cessation advice in the dental setting
… or marijuana, cannabis or other drugs?		Cannabis carries additional health risks over smoking, possibly including oral carcinoma
Do you drink alcohol?	Units consumed per week and type of alcohol	Synergistic effect with smoking for oral potentially malignant disorders and oral cancer
For female patients, is there any chance you might be pregnant …	Stage of pregnancy	Risk from X-ray exposure Pregnancy modulates healing and is association with remission in aphthous stomatitis and predisposes to pyogenic granuloma and gingivitis
… or are trying to become pregnant?		Contraindicates prescription of many drugs
Are you otherwise generally fit and well?		An open question to allow patients to provide information that may not be covered by more specific questions
For parents of child patients – is your child receiving any other therapy or special support?	Type and reason Developmental milestones achieved? Any additional support at school?	A broad question to identify behavioural and developmental conditions that may affect provision of treatment
Do any diseases run in your family?		May reveal haemophilia and other bleeding disorders and a host of other genetic diseases and syndromes
Is there anything else about your health you would like to tell me?		May reveal general malaise, fevers, weight loss, psychiatric problems and reveal attitudes to health and disease not elicited by other questions
Do you experience any mental health conditions?		The stigma attached to mental health and learning difficulty problems requires a subtle approach if this is suspected but nothing has been elicited by previous questioning.

*There is deliberate 'redundancy' in medical history questioning, that is, a point of significance may be covered by questioning from more than one perspective to ensure nothing significant is missed. Thus, even if a patient claims that their heart is healthy, rheumatic fever should be asked about specifically and jaundice and hepatitis both explored independently. Patients may well not recognise medical names and react to one question but not another.
This table groups conditions that are related, but some favour following a systems-based approach, a surgical sieve, various mnemonics or a medical history questionnaire. Clinicians should become adept at using whatever system they prefer and use the same system all the time to avoid inadvertent omissions.
A standardized European medical health questionnaire is available (**PMID:** 18299219). This links to and expands on the American Society of Anaesthesiologists (ASA) Physical Status Classification System. This questionnaire is comprehensive but, like the ASA system, is focused on detecting potential medical complications of dental treatment rather than eliciting medical history for diagnosis of oral disease.

assess whether the patient's reading ability and understanding are sufficient to provide valid answers to the questionnaire.

Medical history questionnaires vary widely in style and the questions asked. All dental surgeons should be able to take a history without the guidance of a questionnaire. The questionnaire itself is less important than understanding exactly why the questions are being asked and what follow-up questions are relevant (see Table 1.4). However, some structure is required to ensure no items are missed, and questionnaires perform a useful function in this regard.

If the patient's history suggests, or examination reveals, any condition beyond the scope of the dentist's experience or clinical knowledge, referral for a specialist medical examination may be necessary.

Medical warning cards may indicate that the patient is, for example, a haemophiliac, on long-term corticosteroid therapy or is allergic to penicillin. It is also worthwhile to leave a final section open for patients to supply any other information that they think might be relevant.

A detailed drug history is essential. Drugs can have oral effects or complicate dental management in important ways (Ch. 16 and Ch. 43).

In the relevant ethnic groups, enquiry should be made about the many potentially carcinogenic habits such as betel quid (pan), khat, hookah or smokeless tobacco use (Ch. 20).

Holistic patient assessment PMID: 24923937

Theory of diagnostic reasoning for dentists PMID: 21094715

Medical history US perspective PMID: 9344272

The European standardized medical risk-related history questionnaire PMID: 18299219

Web URL 1.1 UK good practice guideline for clinical examination and records URL: https://cgdent.uk/clinical-examination-and-record-keeping/ (requires FGDP login)

The dental history

A dental history and examination are obviously essential for the diagnosis of dental pain or to exclude teeth as cause of symptoms in the head and neck region.

Symptoms of toothache are normally recognised as such by patients but are very variable and may masquerade as a variety of conditions from the trivial to the sinister (Box 1.4). The relationship between symptoms and any dental treatment, or lack of it, should be noted.

The family and social history

Whenever a symptom or sign suggests an inherited disorder, such as haemophilia, the family history should be elicited. Ideally, this is recorded as a pedigree diagram noting the proband (presenting case) and all family members for at least three generations. Even when no familial disease is suspected, questions about other family members often lead naturally into questions about home circumstances, relatives and social history which can be revealing if, for example, psychosocial factors are suspected.

Web URL 1.2 Drawing a pedigree chart URL: https://www.genomicseducation.hee.nhs.uk/taking-and-drawing-a-family-history/

Consent

It is imperative to obtain patients' consent for any procedure, including examination. At the very least, any procedures to be used should be explained to the patient and verbal consent obtained. If no more than this is done, the patients'

Box 1.4   Toothache and its mimics

- Toothache
  - Pulpitis
  - Periapical periodontitis
  - Fractured cusp/tooth
  - Dentine hypersensitivity
- Mimics of toothache
  - Prodromal Herpes zoster infection
  - Postherpetic neuralgia
  - Trigeminal neuralgia
  - Neuropathic pain after trauma or central nervous system disease
  - Maxillary sinusitis
  - Temporal arteritis
  - Migrainous neuralgia
  - Otitis media
  - Referred pain of angina pectoris
  - Referred pain of temporomandibular joint myofascial pain dysfunction
  - Atypical odontalgia / facial pain

---

verbal consent should be noted in their records. However, it is better to obtain written consent, and this is now often required for any minor procedure in some countries. Many hospitals now require clinicians to give precise descriptions of treatment plans, however routine, and to obtain written consent. Written treatment plans are also required in dental practice in the UK.

Patients have a right to refuse treatment. Any such refusals may sometimes be due to failure of the clinician to explain the need for a particular procedure, or failure to soothe the patient's fears about possible complications. Some of these fears may be irrational, but all fears are real to the patient. In such cases, even prolonged explanations and persuasion may be unsuccessful, and a patient's signature in the notes may then be required as evidence of their wish not to consent.

When a biopsy is necessary, the patient will consent to the surgical procedure but must also be made aware that their tissue may be retained in the pathology department for many years in case future reference to it is needed. When the biopsy is also to be used for DNA analysis, the patient must be made aware of this, and when there are implications for other family members' health, the consent process may be complex.

In the case of more major surgery, a consent form may need to take into account a general anaesthetic, the nature of the operation and significant complications or risks. This will require knowledge of the pathology of the disease. For example, in the case of an ameloblastoma, it would be necessary to point out the risk of recurrence after a conservative removal versus the complications of a larger excision.

For consent to be legally valid, patients must be given sufficient information about the proposed treatment for them to make their own decision and the clinician must check that the information has been understood. This is formalised in the concept of 'informed consent', although being informed is only one factor required to make consent valid under UK law (Table 1.5). The UK law on consent is complex and often enshrined in case law rather than Acts of Parliament. The Mental Capacity Act 2005 and The Human Tissue Act 2004 both govern some aspects, but consent

Table 1.5 Requirements for consent

Capacity	Not impaired for any reason May differ procedure to procedure Understands information given Able to weigh information to make a decision
Voluntary	Given freely Without pressure or undue influence

Informed	Understands nature and purpose of procedure
	Aware of the operator's training and competence
	No relevant information is withheld
	Told of 'material' or 'significant' risks or
	    unavoidable risks, even if small
	Informed of alternatives to the proposed treatment
	Aware of the risks of not having the treatment
	Aware of how any tissue removed will be
	    treated and stored

Clinician	Informed and trained Able to judge capacity

Timing	Consent is a process, not a single event, and
	    must be checked and revisited
	Consent remains in force until withdrawn
	Consent should be given within a reasonable
	    timeframe of the procedure
	Material changes in any element must be
	    explained

Recorded	The process of obtaining consent must be
	    recorded
	Written consent is required for significant
	    procedures and risks

evolves constantly, and readers need to be aware of the regulations and professional advice (the latter often more stringent) in force where they practice. When a written consent is required, a standardised form should be used to ensure compliance with local requirements.

Particular difficulties in oral medicine and surgery arise with the prescription of drugs because reactions are varied but infrequent. Usually, patients do not clearly distinguish risk and harm and tend to make decisions about treatments based on the magnitude of potential harm. It is difficult to explain to a patient that anaphylactic reactions in persons not known to be allergic to penicillin are exceedingly rare but, nevertheless, potentially fatal.

Patients reading the extensive information leaflets provided with prescription drugs are frequently concerned about the risks of even safe drugs such as aspirin. Since it is estimated that 200 million tablets of it are consumed every year, the chances of a reaction are almost infinitesimally small. The amount of information to be given to the patient is that which would be expected by 'the prudent patient'. However, patients differ, some reading drug information leaflets avidly, whereas others dispose of them unread. The dentist must balance the information given against the patient's expectation. For surgical interventions the patient must be told all 'material facts', specifically including any dangers of the procedure to that particular patient.

Consent is not normally taken from patients for prescription of medications. However, the same principles apply because significant adverse effects can be caused by drugs for dental treatment. It is important to maintain vigilance to reduce risk, for instance by recording allergies and checking before prescribing. Sometimes patients at risk of severe adverse effects can be identified. For example, in the case of azathioprine, patients deficient in the enzyme thiopurine methyltransferase (TPMT) can be excluded from treatment because of their risk of bone marrow toxicity. Fortunately such examples are rare but risks from drugs are unpredictable in type and severity.

It is essential to point out any precautions necessary when taking a particular drug and warn patients to return as soon as they think that there has been an adverse reaction. Adverse reactions should be reported in the UK through the yellow card system.

Web URL 1.3 UK consent (includes separate Scotland advice):

URL: https://www.dentalprotection.org/uk/articles/consent-advice-booklet

CLINICAL EXAMINATION

Extraoral

First, look at the patient, before looking into the patient's mouth. Anaemia, thyroid disease, long-term corticosteroid treatment, parotid swellings or significantly enlarged cervical nodes are just a few conditions that can affect the facial appearance.

Palpate the parotid glands, temporomandibular joints (for clicks, crepitus or deviation), cervical and submandibular lymph nodes and thyroid gland. Lymphadenopathy (Ch. 32) is a common manifestation of infection but may also signify a malignant disease – the cervical lymph nodes are often the first affected by lymphomas. Note the character (site, shape, size, surface texture and consistency) of any enlargement. Always examine the neck from behind the patient and palpate through slack, not taut, skin. Guide the patient's head forward and to one side with one hand to loosen the skin and platysma muscle and move the sternomastoid muscle, below which some nodes lie. Use the flat tips of the fingers with sufficient pressure to feel through overlying tissues. Proper examination of the neck is not possible with the patient supine; the patient should be sitting upright or leaning slightly backward.

Press on the maxilla and frontal bone over the sinuses to elicit tenderness if sinusitis is suspected.

Oral examination

Examination of the oral cavity can be performed adequately only with good light, mirrors and compressed air or other means of drying the teeth. If viscid saliva prevents visualisation of the tissues and teeth, a rinse with a traditional dentists' mouthwash will help. This contains sodium bicarbonate, and the alkaline pH changes the charge on the salivary mucins and makes them more soluble.

Soft tissues

The soft tissues of the mouth should usually be inspected first. Examination should be systematic to include all areas of the mouth. Care should be taken that mirrors or retractors do not obscure lesions. To ensure complete examination of the lateral tongue and posterior floor of mouth, the tongue must be held forward in gauze and gently reflected from side to side.

Abnormal-looking areas of mucosa should be palpated for scarring or induration indicating previous ulceration, inflammation or malignancy. Examination should include deeper tissues accessible to palpation from their oral aspect, including the submandibular glands.

If abnormalities extend close to the gingiva, the gingival crevice or pockets should be probed for any communication. Mucosal nodules, especially those on the gingiva or alveolar mucosa that suggest sinus openings, should be probed to identify any sinus or fistula. Check the openings of the salivary ducts while expressing saliva by gentle pressure. Check that saliva flows freely and equally from all glands and is clear in colour. Do not mistake normal anatomical variations (Table 1.6) for disease.

After examination of the oral mucosa, try to visualise the oropharynx and tonsils.

Retrocuspid papilla PMID: 1065843

Foliate papilla ISBN-13: 978-0723438120

Leukoedema: Review: PMID: 1460680

Teeth

When undertaking a consultation for a complaint apparently unrelated to teeth, dental examination must still be thorough, both for the patient's sake and for medicolegal reasons. As a minimum, the standing teeth with a summary

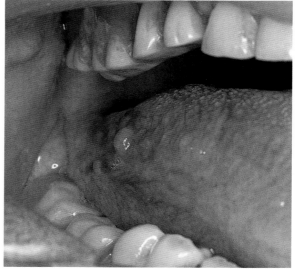

Fig. 1.1 Large foliate papilla or lingual tonsil that may be mistaken for a lesion on the side of the tongue.

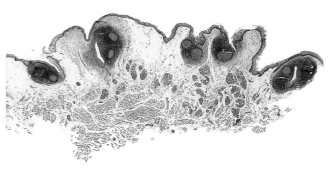

Fig. 1.2 Section showing the nodular surface, small tonsillar crypts and lymphoid follicles in a foliate papilla.

Table 1.6 Some anatomical variants and normal structures often misdiagnosed as abnormalities

Structure	Description
Fordyce's spots	Sebaceous glands lying superficially in the mucosa are visible as white-coloured or cream-coloured spots up to 0.5 mm across. Usually on labial mucosa and buccal mucosa. Occasionally prominent and very numerous (Figs 18.1 and 18.2). Increase in prominence with age
Lingual tonsils	Enlarge with viral infection and occasionally noted by patients. Sometimes large or ectopic and then mistaken for disease (Figs 1.1 and 1.2)
Circumvallate papillae	Readily identifiable but sometimes prominent and misinterpreted by patients or healthcare workers
Retrocuspid papilla	Firm pink nodule 0.5–4 mm diameter on the attached gingiva lingual to the lower canine and lateral incisor, usually bilateral but sometimes unilateral. Prominent in children but regresses with age
Dorsal tongue fur	Furring of the dorsal tongue mucosa is very variable and is heavier when the diet is soft. Even light furring may be regarded as pathological by many patients. When pigmented black by bacteria and with overgrowth of the filiform papillae, the condition is called black hairy tongue (Ch. 17)
Leukoedema	A milky white translucent whitening of the oral mucosa that disappears or fades on stretching. More common Black people (Ch. 18)
Tori	Exostoses in the midline of the palate or in the lingual alveolus in the premolar region are termed tori (Ch. 12). They are present by young adulthood and also arise at other sites, particularly on the maxilla over premolar and canine roots.

of their periodontal health, caries and restorative state and any tooth wear should be recorded. When dental pain is a possibility, full charting, assessment of mobility and percussion of teeth are necessary and further investigations will probably be required.

The vitality of teeth must be checked if they appear to be discoloured or causing symptoms. It is also essential to determine the vitality of teeth in the region of cysts and other radiolucent lesions in the jaws at presentation. The information may be essential for diagnosis and cannot be determined after treatment.

To be absolutely certain, several methods may have to be used. Checking hot and cold sensitivity and electric pulp testing are relatively easily performed (Box 1.5). Unfortunately, it may not be apparent that a pulp test result is misleading. Care must always be taken to avoid causes of false-positive or false-negative results (Table 1.7). Poorly localised pulp pain from teeth of dubious vitality can be difficult to ascribe to an individual tooth. In such circumstances, a diagnostic local anaesthetic injection on a suspect tooth may stop the pain and indicate its source.

Pulp test accuracy PMID: 26789282

MEDICAL EXAMINATION

In practice, it is usual for dental investigations to be performed first, but the dentist should be capable of performing simple

Box 1.5 Precautions for electric pulp testing

- Remember these are sensibility tests of nerve continuity and patient reaction, not direct tests of vitality
- Isolate individual teeth with a small portion of rubber dam if necessary
- No one method is completely reliable; supplement electric methods with hot and cold tests to be certain
- Ensure the correct method is being followed, depending on whether the tester is bipolar or unipolar
- Use an electrically conducting jelly or other agent to ensure good electrical contact
- Always record electric pulp test values in the notes – a progressive change in reading over time may indicate declining vitality
- A definite failure to react or clear vitality are more useful outcomes than the numerical reading on the control
- If results remain uncertain, cut a test cavity or remove suspect restorations without local anaesthetic
- Compare reading with those from control teeth – usually contralateral teeth of the same type
- Use Doppler flowmetry to determine blood flow when pulpal nerve function is compromised, for instance following trauma

Table 1.7 Possible causes of misleading electric pulp test results

Problem	Causes to consider
Pulp by-passed by electric current	Electrical contact with next tooth through touching amalgam restorations, orthodontic appliance or saliva
	Electrical contact with gingival margin through amalgam restoration or saliva film
False positive	Stimulus can be conducted by fluid in necrotic pulp chamber and felt by stimulating nerves in the periodontal ligament
Electrical insulation of the pulp	Large composite or non-conducting restorations
Falsely low reading	Incompletely formed root apex
	Teeth being moved orthodontically
	Operator's gloves can partially insulate the electrical circuit of some testers
Partially vital pulps	Multiple canals
No check on validity of results	No normal teeth for comparison
Patient fails to report accurately	Failure to differentiate pulpal from soft tissue or periodontal ligament sensation

Table 1.8 Useful diagnostic information from examination of the hands

Site	Signs
Flexor surface of wrist	Rash (or history of rash) consisting of purplish papules suggests lichen planus, especially if itchy
Finger morphology	Clubbing may be associated with some chronic respiratory and cardiac conditions (including infective endocarditis), lung cancer, lung abscesses, cardiac disease and other remote malignant neoplasms
	Joint changes may suggest rheumatoid arthritis (joint swelling, ulnar drift) or osteoarthritis (Heberden's nodes)
Abnormal nails	Koilonychia suggests longstanding anaemia.
	Hypoplastic nails may be associated with several inherited disorders of epithelium with oral significance including ectodermal dysplasia and dyskeratosis congenita
Skin of fingers	May be thin, shiny and white in Raynaud's phenomenon (periodic ischaemia resulting from exposure to cold – often associated with autoimmune conditions particularly systemic sclerosis (Fig. 1.3) or Sjögren's syndrome)
	Note any tobacco staining. Is the degree commensurate with the patient's reported tobacco use?
Palmar-plantar keratosis	Associated with several syndromes including Papillon–Lefèvre syndrome (including early-onset periodontitis)

for conjunctivitis or signs of mucous membrane pemphigoid, anaemia or jaundice. Examination of the hands may also reveal relevant information (Table 1.8). Dentists should be able to examine cranial nerve function, but more extensive medical examination by dentists is usually performed only in hospitals.

CLINICAL DIFFERENTIAL DIAGNOSIS

The diagnosis and appropriate treatment may be obvious from the history and examination. More frequently, there are several possible diagnoses, and compiling a differential diagnosis becomes a critical part of the overall diagnostic process. At this stage the clinician must integrate their knowledge of likely diseases and their range of presentations with the findings from one specific patient, thinking broadly but keeping focused. If a good differential diagnosis is compiled, then the process of selecting investigations and narrowing down to the final diagnosis will usually be straightforward. Conversely, if the correct diagnosis is not included in the differential diagnosis, it may never be discovered. Mistakes often follow clinicians simply forgetting to consider a possible diagnosis, and a written differential diagnosis helps even experienced clinicians to organise their thoughts.

A well-crafted differential diagnosis lists possible diagnoses in order of probability, based on their prevalence and the likelihood of causing a specific combination of symptoms

medical examinations of the head and neck. Examination of the skin of the face, hair, scalp and neck may reveal unexpected foci of infection to account for cervical lymphadenopathy or even malignant neoplasms. The eye can readily be inspected

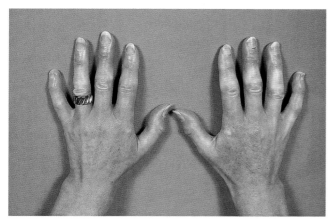

Fig. 1.3 Hands with taut, shiny, pale skin on the tapering fingers, a long-term effect of Raynaud's phenomenon, in this case associated with systemic sclerosis.

and signs. Even if only one diagnosis seems appropriate, it is worthwhile to note the next most likely possibility and any other causes which can be excluded. This ensures that all appropriate investigations are remembered and reduces the possibility of the patient having to return for further investigations. When the patient's complaint or presentation is relatively nonspecific, do not list every possible cause. Too long a list is difficult to convert into a focused investigation strategy, and it may be best to use generic terms such as 'benign neoplasm' or 'odontogenic tumour' to keep the initial list manageable.

When the list includes conditions with significant implications for the patient, such as a malignant neoplasm, it is conventional to put them at the top of the list even though their likelihood may be low. This ensures important diagnoses are not forgotten and that they are investigated and excluded first, before moving on to more likely, but less serious, conditions.

INVESTIGATIONS

Innumerable types of investigation are possible. It may be difficult to refrain from asking for every conceivable investigation so as not to miss something unsuspected and to avoid medicolegal complications. Although it may be tempting to explore every possibility, however remote, this approach may prove counterproductive in that it can produce a plethora of reports that confuse rather than inform. The more investigations performed, the more likely one will produce a spurious result.

The differential diagnosis forms the basis on which investigations are selected and keeping focused on the list ensures that only appropriate investigations are requested. Every investigation must be selected to answer a specific question, and none should be regarded as a 'routine test'. Some investigations carry risks that may need to be balanced against the probability of a useful result, notably those involving X-rays.

In all healthcare systems, investigations are expensive, some exceedingly so, and some can only be performed in specialised centres. It is the duty of every clinician to keep the cost-to-benefit ratio of investigations in mind and order only those that will confirm the differential diagnosis or exclude options from it. Often investigations that specifically exclude diseases are the most valuable.

A few diseases, such as mumps, may be diagnosed on the basis of a single test, but others, such as Sjögren's syndrome*, may require many tests and some difficult interpretation to make the diagnosis.

Any test will occasionally produce an erroneous result. Sometimes this is the result of inappropriate samples or delay in specimen transport. However, for many blood tests, a result may be flagged as 'out of normal range' because the value is in the highest or lowest 5% of the population. This is not necessarily an abnormal result. Unexpected or inexplicable test results are often best repeated before accepting the result, provided the test is easily performed.

Screening and diagnostic tests

This book is primarily concerned with diagnosis, but the difference between screening and diagnostic tests must be appreciated.

To be useful in diagnosis, a test result, whether positive or negative, must indicate a specific disease or condition. This is measured by the parameters of the sensitivity, specificity, positive predictive value and negative predictive value of the test. The definitions of these parameters are shown in Table 1.9.

Sensitivity describes whether a test can correctly identify a condition, and the specificity determines whether it can correctly exclude a condition. However, no test is completely accurate, and there are always false-positive and false-negative (incorrect) results. You can also see from the definitions that the sensitivity and specificity are only measures that relate to a population in which the correct disease status is already known. That is not helpful when using the test in real life, and the value of the test is better described by the positive and negative predictive values. The ideal test would have a high positive and a high negative predictive value.

A further complication is introduced by considering the value of tests when they are performed in different circumstances. Suppose a test is not very accurate, but the disease being tested for is very common. Under these circumstances, the test will perform well enough to be useful because a few false-positive results will be outweighed by the value in detecting the many patients with the disease. However, if the disease were very rare, the majority of the results would be false positive and the test would be useless.

The value of the test therefore depends on how it is used. If a clinician performs many tests on all patients, the positive predictive values will not be as high as if the test were used in a more focused manner. This explains why tests must be used to answer specific questions and not thrown randomly at difficult diagnostic dilemmas.

---

*This book continues to use an apostrophe after many eponyms. It has been suggested that this should be abolished (PMID: 46972) because "the author neither had nor owned the disorder". This idea has been promoted by those who think that the change gives patients 'ownership' of their disease. However, the suggestion is based on a lack of knowledge of grammar. The 's is not a possessive case, as often said, but a synthetic genitive indicating association rather than ownership. Its meaning is the same as in New Year's Eve, replacing the sense of the word *of*. The genitive case in English is complex and can have many meanings apart from ownership. This usage is known as the classifying or descriptive function. Often the 's is essential to the meaning. Moon molars sounds as if they are named because their pitted surface looks like the moon, an understandable misconception, while Moon's molars clearly associates the first description of this manifestation of congenital syphilis to Henry Moon, a dental surgeon at Guy's Hospital in London. This book is called Cawson's Essentials, not because it belonged to Professor Cawson, but because he wrote it. Not using an apostrophe is more common in US usage than elsewhere.
For a detailed discussion see, Dirckx, JH. The synthetic genitive in medical eponyms: Is it doomed to extinction? Panace@. 2001;2(5):15-24.

Table 1.9 Sensitivity, specificity, positive predictive value and negative predictive value

Parameter	Definition
Sensitivity	The proportion of patients known to have the disease who test positive
Specificity	The proportion of patients known to NOT have the disease who test NEGATIVE
Positive predictive value	The proportion of all positive results that are true positives (correct results)
Negative predictive value	The proportion of all negative results that are true negatives (correct results)

Diagnostic tests are required to have high predictive values, and the more significant the diagnosis, the higher the predictive value must be. Conversely, screening tests are used in population screening and are only intended to identify individuals who might have a disease. Screening tests need to be economical and easily performed in great numbers, and a lower predictive value is acceptable. Patients who test positive for the screening test will then be referred for more accurate diagnostic tests.

Tests used for diagnosis in oral disease generally have high predictive values. Dentists need to be aware that many less-than-ethical companies sell tests to general dental practitioners for the diagnosis of diseases such as caries, periodontal disease, oral cancer and oral premalignant diseases. It is not always clear whether these are screening or diagnostic tests. In some countries these tests are marketed direct to patients. When evaluating whether using such a test is likely to be effective and its use ethical, it would be strongly advisable to find out what the predictive values of the test would be when used in your own patient population.

Imaging

The most informative imaging techniques in the head and neck are radiography and cone beam computerised tomography (CBCT), medical computerised tomography (CT), magnetic resonance imaging (MRI) and ultrasound. Their advantages and disadvantages are shown in Table 1.10.

Plain radiography is widely available, and simple additional techniques can add value (Box 1.6). Even simple manoeuvres, such as introducing a gutta percha point or probe into a sinus to trace its origins, may provide critical information. It is also advisable to request a formal radiologist's report on radiographic films whenever the radiographic features appear unusual or beyond the experience of the clinician.

Imaging and diagnosis ISBN-13: 978-0702045998

Histopathology
Value and limitations

Removal of a biopsy specimen for histopathological examination is the mainstay of diagnosis for diseases of the mucosa, soft tissues and bone. In the few conditions in which a biopsy is not helpful, it may still be valuable to exclude other possible causes.

As with all other investigations, biopsy must address a specific question. For instance, recurrent minor aphthae lack specific microscopic features and biopsy is rarely justified. Conversely, a major aphtha may mimic a carcinoma that only microscopy will exclude.

Histological examination is not a 'test' in the same way as a blood investigation. The pathologist will issue a report that describes the macroscopic and histological features seen in the specimen and provide an interpretation, usually specific, sometimes less so (Box 1.7). The interpretation will be based on the clinical information transmitted to the pathologist on the request form, and often this is critical to the reported diagnosis. Pathology reports, and not just the 'bottom line' diagnosis, need to be read and understood because they may contain important caveats about the confidence with which a diagnosis is made or suggestions for further investigations.

Biopsy

Biopsy is the removal and examination of a part or the whole of a lesion.* There are several different biopsy techniques (Box 1.8).

The most important technique is surgical biopsy. Leaving aside medical contraindications, the only important contraindications to biopsy are when the site of disease contains important structures, such as the facial nerve in the parotid gland, or when the biopsy risks seeding a tumour more widely in the tissues. The most common parotid neoplasm (pleomorphic adenoma) has an unusual tendency to spread and recur at a biopsy site because of its gelatinous nature. In such instances, alternatives would be to perform a fine needle aspiration or excise the entire lesion with a margin of surrounding normal tissue and confirm the suspected diagnosis afterwards.

Selecting the biopsy site

If the wrong site is selected for biopsy, the chance of a definitive diagnosis is reduced. Choice of site is often a compromise between ease of access, methods available and removing the ideal tissue sample.

Identifying the ideal tissue should take precedence and requires the clinician to understand the disease process at a microscopic level so that the tissue most likely to show diagnostic features is selected. For large tumours, a central sample is often easiest, but it is often critical to include the margin to assess the growth pattern and possible peripheral invasion. For mucosal disease, ulcers must be avoided because they are inflamed and have no epithelium. For potentially malignant diseases, red and speckled areas are the most important, followed by white areas. For immunobullous disease, the perilesional tissue is best because it is less friable and will not disintegrate on biopsy. However, samples for immunofluorescence should be taken away from the lesion, usually from clinically normal buccal mucosa, because they are used to identify bound autoantibody and not the histopathology of the active disease.

It is often stated that a biopsy should include normal tissue at the margin. However, this is widely misunderstood. The pathologist does not require adjacent tissue for comparison; he or she will be very familiar with the normal histological variation in the mouth. However, there may be better reasons for choosing to include normal tissue in the sample. Cancers and some other lesions can be friable and disintegrate on biopsy so that having some normal tissue at one end helps support the sample and holds the suture more firmly. If a malignant process is suspected, the margin is where invasion of surrounding tissue will be seen. When performing an excision biopsy, a small collar of normal tissue may prevent recurrence of some lesions. When removing a sample of a white lesion, including the edge will aid diagnosis of mild

---

*Biopsy is derived from the Greek words meaning 'to see in life'. Thus, a biopsy specimen is taken from a living patient. Its opposite is necropsy: 'to see in death'; a post-mortem or autopsy.

degrees of dysplasia. However, always try to take the largest sample of lesional tissue and only include normal tissue for a specific reason.

Large lesions and those with areas that look or feel different may well require several biopsies to sample them adequately. Those in which the epithelial thickness is markedly increased, such as verrucous carcinoma and verrucous leukoplakias, may need a sample several millimetres thick. The specimen must extend down to and include the underlying connective tissue to assess whether or not invasion is present.

It can be seen that selecting the correct site can be a challenging intellectual exercise requiring a good differential diagnosis and knowledge of the basic histopathology of the likely disease – just one reason why dental students should know some basic histopathology.

Surgical biopsy methods

Surgical removal of tissue to determine the diagnosis may be undertaken with a scalpel, biopsy punch, cutting laser, electrocautery or a wide cutting needle ('core biopsy'; Trucut biopsy). In general, a scalpel biopsy is almost always preferred for intraoral sampling. The tissue is removed cleanly without damage, and the incision can be shaped to heal by primary intention. Silk sutures are soft and comfortable in the mouth, and an appointment for removal a few days later

Table 1.10   Imaging techniques for lesions of the head and neck

Technique	Advantages	Limitations
Conventional radiography	Widely available and inexpensive Simple, many common lesions may be identified with a high degree of accuracy Panoramic radiographs can show unsuspected lesions	Small X-ray dose unavoidable Difficult to interpret in some areas of the jaws because of the complex anatomy Little information about soft tissue lesions
Computerised tomography (CT)	Good definition of soft tissue structures in any plane Useful for areas of complex anatomy such as maxilla or base of skull Definition further improved by use of contrast media	Expensive Available only in hospitals Frightening for patients. Scanner tunnel can provoke claustrophobia Shadows of dental restorations can obscure part of the image Larger X-ray dose than plain radiographs
Cone beam CT	Low-cost high-resolution CT ideal for the head and neck, oral surgery, implantology and endodontics	As CT but lower dose and higher resolution Has quickly become a routine radiological investigation for head and neck diagnosis Image density not directly proportional to bone density Relatively poor soft tissue resolution
Radiography or CT with contrast medium	Valuable for outlining extent of duct systems, hollow structures such as cysts or blood vessels (angiography), etc.	Requires more expertise than plain radiography
Magnetic resonance imaging (MRI)	Produces clear tomograms in any plane without superimposition Particularly good for soft tissue lesions, better than CT No X-ray dose Clear definition of bones and teeth	Expensive and limited availability Frighteningly noisy. May be refused by claustrophobic patient (as for CT) Slow, sometimes scans take more than 1 hour Possible risk to the foetus (unconfirmed)
Ultrasound	No X-ray dose Shows soft tissue masses and cysts well Useful for salivary gland cysts, Sjögren's syndrome, stones, and for thyroid and neck lesions May be combined with Doppler flow analysis to measure blood flow through a lesion	Limited resolution, requires expertise in interpretation A dynamic technique interpreted live and difficult to record effectively in pictures Overlying bone obscures soft tissue lesions
Scintigraphy	Uses a radioactive isotope to visualise particular types of cells With technetium 99^{m} provides an assessment of function in each salivary gland Can be used if sialography not possible Other isotopes are used for detection of bone metastases	Equipment not always available Small radiation dose but isotope rapidly cleared
Positron emission tomography (PET scanning)	Short-life radioactive isotope used to identify biochemical activity, usually glycolysis, to identify putative tumour size, location or metastasis Good for identifying unsuspected metastases Helps identify neoplasms when post-surgical artefact or inflammation obscure them on CT or MRI Also available as a combined PET-CT and PET-MRI scan, but with reduced CT or MRI resolution	Expensive Intake of radioactive substance Risk of detecting unsuspected abnormalities of minimal or no significance that then require further investigation

Box 1.6 Requirements for useful oral radiographic information

- Always take bitewings when dental pain is suspected. Small carious lesions may be missed in periapical films and poorly localised pain may originate in the opposing arch
- When imaging bony swellings with plain films, always take two views at right angles
- Panoramic tomograms often cannot provide high definition of bony lesions. Only a cross-section of the lesion is in the focal trough and if the bone is greatly expanded, only a small portion will be in focus. To detect internal structure in bony lesions, plain films such as oblique lateral views of the mandible or oblique occlusal films are better. For better localisation where complex anatomical features are superimposed, cone beam computed tomography may be more useful
- Cone beam imaging provides excellent bone imaging but has poor soft tissue contrast
- Radiography of soft tissues is occasionally useful, for instance to detect a foreign body or calcification in lymph nodes

Box 1.7 Possible reasons for failures in histological diagnosis

- Specimen poorly fixed or damaged during removal (e.g., Figs 1.4 and 1.5)
- Specimen unrepresentative of the lesion or too small
- Plane of histological section does not include critical features
- The disease does not have diagnostic histological features, e.g., aphthous ulcers
- The histological features have several possible causes, e.g., granulomatous inflammation
- The histological features are difficult to interpret, e.g., malignant tumours may be so poorly differentiated that their type cannot be determined
- Inflammation may mask the correct diagnosis

Box 1.8 Types of biopsy

- Surgical biopsy (incisional or excisional)
  - Fixed specimen for routine diagnosis
  - Frozen sections for rapid diagnosis
  - Fresh tissue for immunofluorescence, microbiological culture or molecular analysis
- Fine needle aspiration biopsy
- Wide needle/core biopsy

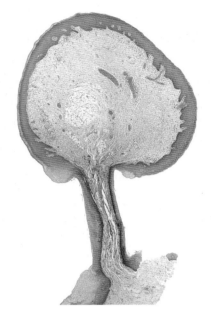

Fig. 1.4 An artefactual polyp produced by grasping normal mucosa with forceps to steady it during biopsy.

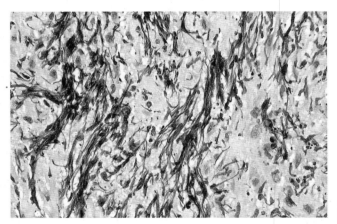

Fig. 1.5 Stringy artefact. This appearance is due to breakage of cells and their nuclei when the specimen is stretched or crushed. It is particularly common in lymphoma and some types of carcinoma.

provides an opportunity to review healing and discuss the diagnosis. Resorbable sutures may be used to avoid a second appointment but are spiky and less comfortable and often persist for many days in the mouth.

Removal of tissue using laser or electrocautery is useful to prevent bleeding, and the coagulated surface requires no sutures. These techniques are most useful to remove excess tissue or excise nodular lesions of the gingiva or mucosa. However, even when properly adjusted, the heat or electrical current will pass through the tissue and denature it, rendering a proportion of the sample unsuitable for diagnosis.

Electrocautery is particularly prone to damage epithelium over a wide area and should never be used for a biopsy to assess dysplasia or other epithelial diseases but is ideal for removal of suspected fibroepithelial polyps.

Cutting needles or core biopsies are useful to remove a core of tissue, usually 1 mm or so in diameter, from deeper structures such as lymph nodes in the neck (Box 1.9).

A biopsy punch is a circular cutting blade designed to excise a circle of skin. These work well on skin because, when the blade penetrates to the subcutaneous fat, a cylinder of skin is mobilised and can be lifted upwards and sliced off. However, punches are badly suited to oral biopsy. The circular blade will only cut taut tissue so that flexible mucosa has to be stretched before cutting. After cutting the sample springs back to its original size, and may then be too small, less than half the punch diameter. The round wound does not lend itself to healing by primary intention or easy closure with sutures. Punch biopsy is often recommended on firm tissue such as the palate and for salivary neoplasms on the palate. At these sites, it is easy to orientate the punch perpendicular to the tissue. Even here it can fail if the deep core of tissue remains fixed to the patient and only a disc of overlying

---

Box 1.9   Core or needle biopsy

- Needle up to 2 mm diameter is used to remove a core of tissue
- Specimen processed as for a surgical biopsy
- Larger sample than fine needle aspiration (FNA), preserves tissue architecture in the specimen
- Definitive diagnosis more likely than with FNA
- Risk of seeding some types of neoplasms into the tissues
- Risk of damaging adjacent anatomical structures, causing haemorrhage or nerve damage
- Useful for inaccessible tumours, e.g., in the pharynx or lymph nodes
- Less used in the head and neck now that FNA is more widely available, but may be the next step if FNA fails

---

Box 1.10   Essential biopsy principles

- Choose the most diagnostic or suspicious area, e.g., red area when potential malignancy is suspected in the oral mucosa
- Avoid ulcers, sloughs or necrotic areas
- Give regional or local anaesthetic – do not inject into the lesion
- Include normal tissue margin if the lesion itself may be friable or malignancy is suspected
- Specimen should preferably be at least 10 x 6 mm and 3 mm deep for mucosal disease, larger for large lesions, smaller on mucoperiosteum
- For mucosal disease, specimen edges should be vertical, not bevelled
- Design the sample shape and incision for easy primary closure
- Before incising, pass a suture through the specimen to control it and prevent it being swallowed or aspirated by the suction
- For large lesions, several areas may need to be sampled
- Include every fragment removed for histological examination
- Never open, incise or divide the specimen, always send it intact
- Suture and control any post-operative bleeding
- Label specimen bottle with patient's name and clinical details
- Warn patient of possible soreness afterward. Give or recommend an analgesic
- Check the histological diagnosis is consistent with the clinical diagnosis and investigations
- Discuss with pathologist or repeat biopsy if diagnosis is unclear or not understood

---

mucosa comes away. Elsewhere a scalpel biopsy is almost always preferred. Despite this, punch biopsy has become popular with dentists because of its speed and simplicity. It is better to take a biopsy with a technique you are happy with than to avoid it, but biopsy punches must be used intelligently.

Surgical biopsy may be incisional or excisional. Incisional biopsy is the removal of part of the lesion for diagnosis only. In excisional biopsy, the whole lesion is removed. The latter is usually performed to confirm a confident clinical diagnosis or when a lesion is too small to require diagnosis and removal in separate steps.

Oral biopsy is a simple procedure that should be within the capability of any dentist. Avoiding or referring for a biopsy in the mistaken belief that the procedure is too unpleasant for general practice is unwarranted. Surveys show that patients rarely complain or suffer adverse consequences from mucosal biopsy, often take no analgesia afterward and much prefer to have their disease properly investigated. Occasionally, sedation or general anaesthesia is required for children or specific patients, and referral is necessary.

The pathology request form should contain all the clinical information used to reach the clinical diagnosis. The purpose is to ensure an accurate diagnosis and not (as some clinicians seem to think) to see whether the pathologist can guess it without the relevant information. If appropriate, give the vitality of teeth associated with the lesion.

The essential principles of biopsy are summarised in Box 1.10.

Patient view: PMID: 11235976

Frozen sections

Frozen section is a laboratory technique that allows a stained slide to be examined within 10 minutes of taking the specimen (Box 1.11). The tissue is sent fresh to the laboratory to be frozen by immersion in liquid nitrogen (–196°C) or dry ice (–78°C), very cold to ensure freezing is near instantaneous and does not allow time for ice crystals to form in the tissue (which would expand and break open the cells). A section is then cut on a refrigerated microtome and stained. The equipment for frozen sections is often in the theatre suite to speed the process even further.

Frozen sections can only be justified if the rapidity of the result will make an immediate difference to the operation in progress because the technique is less slightly accurate than routine histopathology. This low risk of misdiagnosis means that frozen section is used more frequently to assess whether excision margins are free of a cancer during an operation

---

Box 1.11   Advantages and limitations of frozen sections

- Can establish, during an operation, whether or not a tumour is malignant and whether excision needs to be extended
- Can confirm, during an operation, that excision margins are free of tumour
- Microscopic appearances differ from those in fixed tissue
- Freezing artefacts due to poor technique can distort the cellular picture
- Definitive diagnosis sometimes impossible
- Only to be used when the result will alter the immediate surgical plan

---

rather than to make a preoperative diagnosis. If a rapid diagnosis is required in other circumstances, techniques such as fine needle aspiration biopsy or a routine specimen with special rapid laboratory processing are usually preferable.

Fine needle aspiration biopsy

Removing very small numbers of cells by aspiration using a fine needle (FNA), even if not completely conclusive, is often sufficient to distinguish benign from malignant neoplasms, to initiate treatment or to indicate a need for further investigations. FNA should be used as an early step in the diagnosis of salivary neoplasms, lymph nodes in the neck, thyroid lumps and other deep tissues. Among the diagnoses that can be confidently made on FNA are many types of salivary neoplasm, tuberculosis and high-grade lymphomas (Box 1.12).

Brush biopsy and exfoliative cytology

This technique uses a round stiff-bristle brush to collect cells from the surface and subsurface layers of an epithelial lesion by vigorous abrasion and is discussed more fully in Chapter 20. It is an excellent method for taking small samples for experimental analysis, as a screening test or for patient follow-up but has not yet achieved an evidence base for oral diagnosis. The sample removed can be analysed in a variety of ways.

Exfoliative cytology is examination of cells scraped from the surface of a lesion but samples only surface cells and provides no information on deeper layers. It is now rarely used in the mouth, brush biopsy (Box 1.13) having superseded it.

Box 1.12 Principles and uses of fine needle aspiration biopsy

- A narrow (21-gauge) needle is inserted into the lesion and cells aspirated and smeared on a slide
- Rapid and usually effective aid to diagnosis of swellings in lymph nodes and parotid tumours especially
- Cells can be fixed, stained and examined within minutes
- Valuable when surgical biopsy could spread tumour cells (e.g., pleomorphic adenomas)
- For deep lesions, ultrasound or radiological guidance may be used to ensure that the needle enters the lesion
- No significant complications
- Small size of the needle avoids damage to vital structures in the head and neck
- Cells may be pelleted and processed for sections to allow immunocytochemistry and other specialised stains
- Some sample may be sent for microbiological culture
- Small specimen may be unrepresentative; several 'needle passes' often taken
- Definitive diagnosis not always possible (though a differential diagnosis may be very helpful to plan treatment or further investigations)

Box 1.13 Uses and limitations of brush biopsy

- Quick, easy
- Samples all levels in the epithelium, but no deeper
- Local anaesthetic not required
- Useful research technique
- Value depends on the analytical method applied to the sample
- Unreliable for diagnosing cancer. Frequent false-positive and false-negative results

---

Laboratory procedures

Although a clinician does not need to understand the details of laboratory procedures, it is necessary to understand the principles to enable the optimal results to be obtained. Failure to prepare or send the specimen appropriately can prevent diagnosis and necessitate an additional biopsy.

Fixation

Fixation is a key process. Fixation denatures the molecules in the tissue, killing the cells and preventing their enzymes from degrading the tissue, so stabilising it against autolysis.

The surgeon must immerse the specimen in ten times the specimen volume of 10% formal saline immediately on removal. Do not delay. In the absence of proper fixative, it is better to delay the biopsy and obtain the correct solution. Specimens placed in alcohols, saline or other materials commonly available in dental surgeries are frequently useless for diagnosis (Box 1.14). Do not confuse 10% formal saline (formol saline) with normal saline. Formal saline is formaldehyde dissolved in saline and kills and fixes tissue to prevent autolysis. Normal saline is isotonic saline, not a fixative.

Special types of fixative are required for electron microscopy and for urgent specimens. Whenever microbiological culture is required, the specimen should be sent fresh to the laboratory or a separate specimen taken because fixation will kill any micro-organisms.

All fixatives take time to diffuse through the tissue and fix it, many hours for large surgical resections.

Tissue processing

The fixed tissue is dehydrated by immersion in a series of solvents and impregnated with paraffin wax. The wax block is mounted on a slicing machine called a microtome and sections, usually 4 μm thick, are cut and mounted on glass microscope slides for staining. It takes 24–48 hours to fix, process, section and stain a specimen before the pathologist can report on it. In many laboratories the stained section is digitised and the pathologist can examine the tissue on a computer screen rather than a microscope, allowing measurements and facilitating automated counting and artificial intelligence diagnostic aids.

Box 1.14 Essential points about specimen fixation

- Fixation is a critical step to prevent autolysis and degradation of the microscopic structure of the specimen
- The usual, routine fixative is 10% formal saline (formaldehyde solution in saline or, ideally, in a neutral pH saline buffer)
- Fixation must be complete before the specimen can be processed
- Fixative must diffuse throughout the specimen–fixation is a slow process
- Small surgical specimens fix overnight, but large specimens take 24 hours or longer
- Chemical reaction with the tissue causes the fixative to become weaker as fixation proceeds. Therefore, specimens should generally be put in at least ten times their own volume of fixative
- Never fix specimens for microbiological culture or immunofluorescence; take these fresh to the laboratory immediately on removal or use special transport media

Table 1.11 Examples of haematoxylin and eosin staining of various tissues

Eosin (acidic, red)	Haematoxylin (basic, blue)
Cytoplasm of most cells*	Nuclei (DNA and RNA)
Keratin	Mucopolysaccharide-rich ground substance
Muscle cytoplasm	Reversal lines in decalcified bone
Bone (decalcified only)	
Collagen	

*The cytoplasm of some cells (such as oncocytes in some salivary gland tumours) is intensely eosinophilic. In others such as plasma cells it is basophilic or intermediate (amphophilic).

Some common stains used for microscopy

The combination of haematoxylin and eosin (H&E) is the most common routine histological stain. Haematoxylin is a blue-black basic dye; eosin is a red acid dye. Their typical staining patterns are shown in Table 1.11.

Periodic acid–Schiff (PAS) stain is probably the second most frequently used stain. It stains sugar residues in carbohydrates and glycosaminoglycans pink. This is useful to identify salivary and other mucins, glycogen and candidal hyphae in sections. Alcian blue is a turquoise stain for proteoglycans with negatively charged sugars, such as the sialic acid containing salivary mucins. Salivary mucins therefore stain with both PAS and Alcian blue, whereas ground substance in connective tissue stains only with Alcian blue.

Decalcified and ground (undecalcified) sections

Specimens containing bone and teeth need to be softened by decalcifying in acid to allow a thin section to be cut. This delays the diagnosis by days or weeks according to the size of the specimen and technique used.

Decalcification must be avoided if examination of dental enamel is required, for instance to aid diagnosis of amelogenesis imperfecta, because the heavily mineralised enamel is almost completely dissolved away. In such cases, a ground section is prepared by sawing and grinding using special saws and abrasives.

Immunofluorescent and immunohistochemical staining

Immunostaining methods make use of the highly specific binding between antibodies and antigens to stain specific molecules in the tissues.

Antibodies that bind to specific antigens of interest can be purchased. They are produced either by immunising animals with the purified target molecule and then separating the resulting antibodies from serum, or generated *in vitro* (monoclonal antibodies). The staining process is shown in Figs 1.6–1.8. The antibody binds extremely specifically to the target molecule, and the combination is made visible, either by binding a fluorescent molecule that can be seen in an ultraviolet microscope or an enzyme such as peroxidase that can react with a soluble substrate to form a visible red or brown deposit. Immunofluorescence is the more sensitive technique but is usually performed only on frozen sections.

Immunostaining has revolutionised histological diagnosis. Antibodies are available to stain many cell components and are widely used to identify epithelium (by staining cytokeratin molecules), lymphocyte subtypes (by staining T cell and B cell membrane antigens), viruses (by staining their surface antigens) and cell proliferation (by staining molecules involved in the cell cycle). In most laboratories, immunostaining is a relatively low-cost automated process.

It is important to know when immunostaining is required because fixation or decalcification may denature the antigens in the tissue and so prevent the antibody binding. Specimens for immunofluorescence must not be fixed in formalin but immediately be sent to the laboratory or sent in special transport medium.

The main circumstances in which diagnosis depends on immunostaining are shown in Table 1.12.

Molecular biological tests

Molecular diagnostic tests have revolutionised medical diagnosis, particularly in screening for and identifying genetic abnormalities and for rapid identification of tumours, bacteria and viruses. Techniques are evolving rapidly, and only principles will be illustrated. DNA sequencing and techniques for detecting messenger RNA expression are now rapid and inexpensive, and many medical tests based on single-sequence targets are being replaced by targeted sequencing of multiple specific genes or even whole-genome sequencing.

These methods are not yet widespread in dentistry but are available in most large hospitals and increasingly used for cancer diagnosis. When confronted with a difficult diagnosis, it is sensible to discuss the case with the pathologist or microbiologist before biopsy, to ensure that appropriate samples are available for these specialised tests.

In addition to its role in diagnosis, molecular analysis is increasingly used to select appropriate treatments. Examples include drugs targeting specific chromosomal fusions in salivary and soft tissue tumours and treatments targeting individual mutations, such as the *BRAF* p.V600E mutation found in ameloblastoma.

Polymerase chain reaction and quantitative polymerase chain reaction analysis

When a known DNA or RNA sequence is associated with a specific disease, it can be detected by polymerase chain reaction (PCR). In this test, the clinical sample is solubilized, and the nucleic acids within it hybridised with probes complementary to the target sequence. If, and only if, the target sequence is present, PCR will copy the nucleic acid repeatedly until enough is synthesised to be detected, either in an electrophoresis gel (Fig. 1.9) or by another laboratory method. PCR is rapid and can be automated on robotic analysers.

Common applications of PCR are detecting pathogens or mutations in genes. Identification of mycobacteria is a good example of the value of this type of test. Previously, identification of mycobacterial infection required approximately 6 weeks to culture the sample. PCR can be performed in 48 hours, is more sensitive and differentiates different types of mycobacteria with a high degree of precision. PCR is also used to detect the causative mutation of fibrous dysplasia and to detect micrometastases in sentinel node biopsy.

PCR is extremely sensitive. It can detect a single copy of a nucleic acid sequence in a sample, but this high sensitivity makes it prone to false-positive results. Quantitative PCR (qPCR) is an automated process that detects the PCR product while the amplification is in progress and uses the rate of amplification to measure how many copies of the target

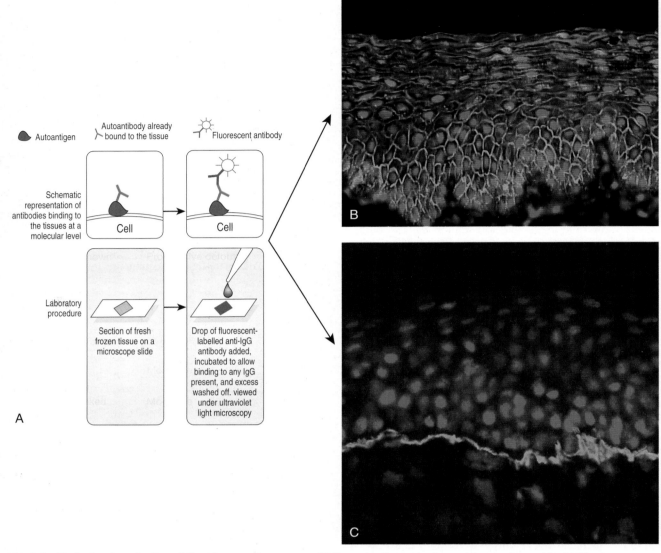

Fig. 1.6 Method and application of direct immunofluorescence. (A) Example: diagnosis of pemphigus and pemphigoid. Aim: to detect the site of the immunoglobulin (IgG) autoantibody already bound to the tissues in a biopsy. All tissues contain a small amount of immunoglobulin from serum, but this is not bound and so is washed away in the process. Green fluorescence indicates site of antibody binding; red fluorescence is a stain for cell nuclei to make the tissue structure more easily interpreted. (B) In pemphigus, green fluorescence reveals IgG autoantibody bound around the surface of the prickle cells in the epithelium (see Fig. 16.28). (C) In pemphigoid, green fluorescence reveals IgG autoantibody bound along the basement membrane (see Fig. 16.33). *(Courtesy Dr B Bhogal.)*

sequence were originally present in the sample. This allows threshold values for a true positive result to be defined and adds a further level of confidence in the result.

The high sensitivity may not always be advantageous. During the COVID-19 pandemic, PCR tests were widely used as the most sensitive test, but gave a positive result from tiny quantities of viral RNA and RNA fragments after recovery from disease, long after the patient was no longer infectious.

In situ hybridisation and fluorescent in situ hybridisation analysis

Known DNA and RNA sequences can also be detected by in situ hybridisation (ISH) or fluorescent in situ hybridisation (FISH). As in PCR, the sequence of interest is detected by hybridising with a complementary probe, but the hybridisation is performed on tissue sections instead of on solubilised tissue. As in PCR, the probe will only bind if

the target sequence is present. Once bound, the probe can be rendered visible by a fluorescent marker or enzyme reaction in the same way that bound antibodies are visualised in immunohistochemistry. In situ hybridisation is less sensitive than PCR but has the advantage that the location of the target sequence can be seen in the tissue, so that it can be confirmed it is in the expected place, nucleus or cytoplasm, and in the correct tissue. This adds an additional level of confidence that the test is detecting the correct target and makes it popular for tumour diagnosis. PCR, being performed on solubilised tissue, cannot demonstrate this.

In situ hybridisation is an automated staining process in many laboratories and often used to detect viruses in tissues. Epstein Barr virus and HPV type 16 genes integrated in oropharyngeal carcinoma are common applications in dentistry.

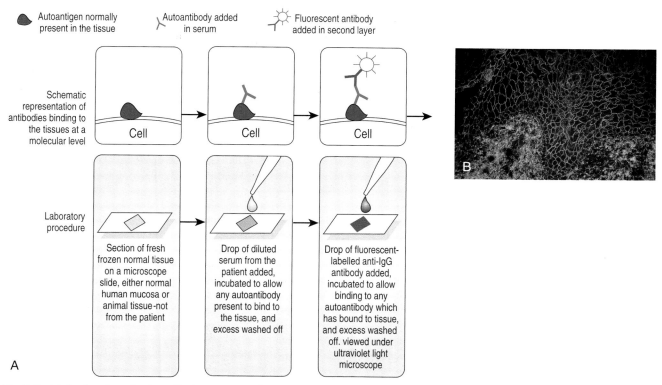

Fig. 1.7 Method and application of indirect immunofluorescence. (A) Example: diagnosis and control of treatment for pemphigus. Aim: to detect circulating autoantibody in the serum of patients with pemphigus. (B) If present, serum autoantibody binds around the surface of the prickle cells in the epithelium and is revealed by the binding to it of the green fluorescent antibody. Non-binding irrelevant immunoglobulins wash away. In this example the nuclei are not counterstained red.

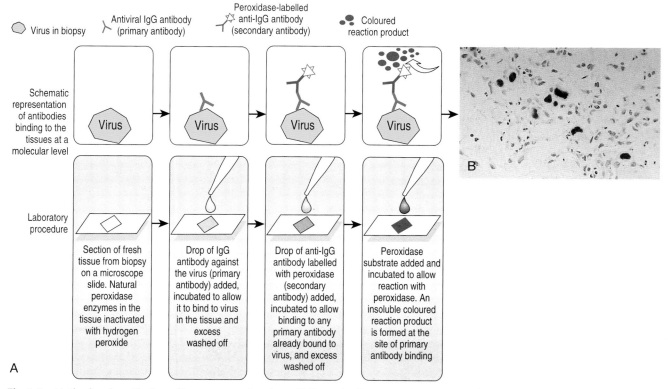

Fig. 1.8 Method and application of immunocytochemistry. (A) Example: diagnosis of viral infection. Aim: to detect viral antigens in infected cells. (B) In this example, brown reaction product identifies cells infected with cytomegalovirus.

Table 1.12 Important uses of immunostaining techniques

Disease	Molecule detected	Significance
Infections	Specific pathogens	Epstein Barr virus in epithelial cells in oral hairy leukoplakia, *Treponema pallidum* in ulcers indicates syphilis
Pemphigus	Autoantibody bound to epithelial desmosomes (desmoglein 3)	Indicates pemphigus
Pemphigoid	Autoantibody and/ or complement C3 bound to basement membrane	Indicates pemphigoid
Myeloma or B-cell lymphoma	Monoclonal production of kappa or lambda light chains of immunoglobulin	Monoclonal production (production of only one isotype of light chain) indicates a neoplastic process. Production of both types indicates a polyclonal infiltrate that is inflammatory in nature
Lymphomas	Cell surface markers specific for different types of T and B cells	Indicates whether a lymphoma is of B- or T-cell origin and its type, essential for treatment
Undifferentiated tumours	Intermediate filaments (components of the cytoskeleton)	Presence of cytokeratins indicates an epithelial neoplasm, vimentin a mesenchymal neoplasm and desmin or myogenin a muscle neoplasm

NB Positive reactions, in themselves, are not necessarily diagnostic of disease and must be interpreted in the light of other histological and clinical findings.

It is also the method of choice to detect the fusion genes that result from chromosomal translocations, which are often specific to individual types of salivary neoplasms (Ch. 23). The break points in the chromosomes are known, and two probes labelled with different colour fluorescence markers are designed to bind on each side of the break point. In a normal cell the probes bind close together, one on each side of the potential break point, and can be seen down a microscope as four spots of colour in each nucleus (because there are two copies of each gene in a normal cell). Both colours are visible close together. If one of the gene copies is rearranged (the gene is broken), one pair of markers binding to the normal chromosome will show the normal pattern. The fluorescent markers on each side of the broken gene no longer bind close together and are seen as two widely separated spots of colour in the nucleus.

The application of in situ hybridisation is shown in Figs 1.10 and 1.11.

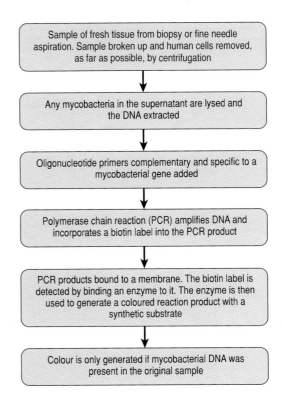

Fig. 1.9 Example application for the technique of polymerase chain reaction for identification of mycobacterial infection.

Haematology, clinical chemistry and serology

Blood investigations are clearly essential for the diagnosis of diseases such as leukaemias, myelomas or leukopenias which have oral manifestations, or for defects of haemostasis that can greatly affect management. Blood investigations are also helpful in the diagnosis of other conditions such as some infections and sore tongues or recurrent aphthae that are sometimes associated with anaemia.

As noted earlier, tests should address specific questions (Table 1.13). The request form should always be completed with sufficient clinical detail to allow the haematologist or clinical chemist to check that the appropriate tests have been ordered and to allow the interpretation of the results. It is important to include details of any drug treatment on blood test request forms. Always put the blood into the appropriate tube because some anticoagulants are incompatible with certain tests. A haematologist will not be impressed by a request for assessment of clotting function on a specimen of coagulated blood.

Microbiology

Despite the most common oral diseases being infectious, traditional microbiological culture of organisms is surprisingly rarely of practical diagnostic value in dentistry (Table 1.14, Box 1.15). Direct Gram-stained smears will quickly confirm the diagnosis of thrush or acute ulcerative gingivitis, and H&E-stained smears can show the distorted, virally infected epithelial cells in herpetic infections more easily than microbiological tests for the organisms themselves.

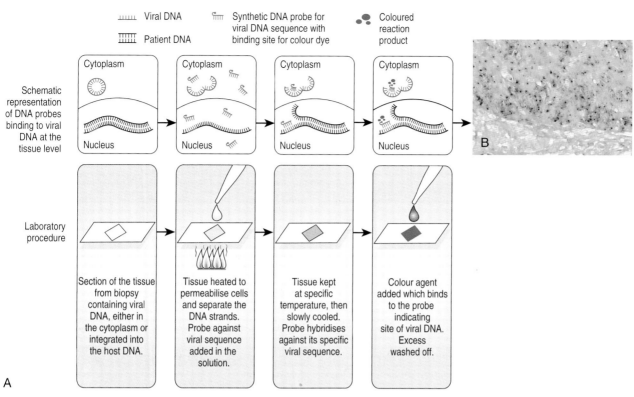

Fig. 1.10 (A) Method and application of in situ hybridisation to detect viral DNA in tissues. (B) In this carcinoma, blue colour reaction product indicates the site of human papillomavirus DNA.

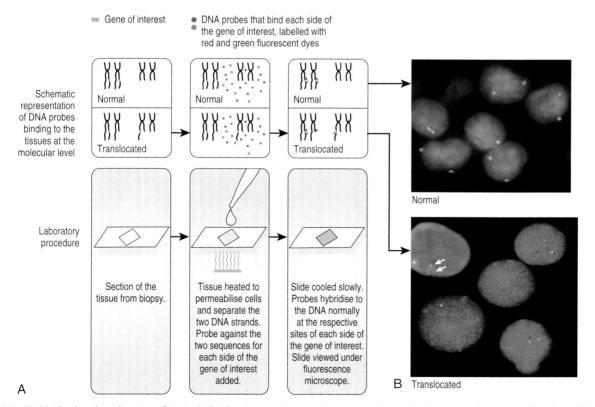

Fig. 1.11 (A) Method and application of in situ hybridisation to detect a chromosomal translocation using 'break apart' probes. (B) In this salivary carcinoma, the *myb* gene (blue) is translocated to another chromosome. In the normal cell the red and green probes are seen to bind to the DNA close together, each side of the *myb* gene. In the cell with the translocation, one copy of the gene is normal, but the other shows 'break apart' of the red and green probes, indicating a translocation involving a break point between the binding sites of the two probes within or close to the gene of interest. For the *myb* gene, this indicates that the carcinoma is an adenoid cystic carcinoma. When the red and green fluorescent spots are very close, the red and green colours merge to produce yellow. The background blue is a DNA-binding dye to show the nuclei.

Table 1.13 Types of blood test useful in oral diagnosis (see also Appendix 1.1)

Test	Main uses
'Full blood picture' usually includes erythrocyte number, size and haemoglobin indices and differential white cell count	Anaemia and the effects of sideropaenia and vitamin B_{12} deficiency associated with several common oral disorders. Leukaemias
Blood film	Leukaemias, infectious mononucleosis, anaemias
Erythrocyte sedimentation rate	Raised in systemic inflammatory and autoimmune disorders Particularly important in giant cell arteritis and Wegener's granulomatosis
Serum iron and total iron-binding capacity	Iron deficiency associated with several common oral disorders
Serum ferritin	A more sensitive indicator of body stores of iron than serum iron and total iron-binding capacity but not available in all laboratories
Red cell folate level	Folic acid deficiency is sometimes associated with recurrent aphthous ulceration and recurrent candidosis
Vitamin B_{12} level	Vitamin B_{12} deficiency is sometimes associated with recurrent aphthous ulceration and recurrent candidosis
Autoantibodies (e.g., rheumatoid factor, antinuclear factor, DNA-binding antibodies, SS-A, SS-B)	Raised in autoimmune diseases. Specific autoantibody levels suggest certain diseases
Viral antibody titres (e.g., Herpes simplex, Varicella zoster, mumps virus)	A rising titre of specific antibody indicates active infection by the virus
Paul–Bunnell or monospot test	Infectious mononucleosis
Syphilis serology	Syphilis
Complement component levels	Occasionally useful in diagnosis of systemic lupus erythematosus or familial angio-oedema
Serum angiotensin-converting enzyme	Sarcoidosis
Serum calcium, phosphate and parathormone levels	Paget's disease and hyperparathyroidism
Human immunodeficiency virus (HIV) test	HIV infection
Skeletal serum alkaline phosphatase	Raised in conditions with increased bone turnover, e.g., Paget's disease and hyperparathyroidism Lowered in hypophosphatasia
Serum IgG4 level	Often raised in IgG4-related disease, but predictive value is not high

Table 1.14 Microbiological tests useful in oral diagnosis

Test	Main uses
Culture and antibiotic sensitivity	Detect unusual pathogens, e.g., actinomyces in soft tissue infection Antibiotic sensitivity for all infections, particularly osteomyelitis and acute facial soft tissue infection
Smear for candida	Candidosis
Viral culture or antigen screen	Viral culture identifies many viruses but requires considerable time Screening for viral antigen by ELISA or similar immunological methods is faster but detects a more limited range of viruses

A key microbiological investigation is culture and sensitivity of pus organisms. Whenever pus is obtained from a soft tissue or bone infection, it should be sent for culture and determination of antibiotic sensitivity of the causative microbes. Those of osteomyelitis, cellulitis, acute parotitis or other severe infections need to be identified if appropriate antimicrobial treatment is to be given. However, treatment has usually to be started empirically without waiting for the result, which takes a few days; the sensitivity test may dictate a change of treatment later.

Soft tissue infections of the head and neck are often treated without microbiological diagnosis. This is partly because the flora is complex and mixed with many anaerobes and organisms that are difficult to culture. The anaerobes do not survive ordinary sample-taking procedures. Culture results are usually a poor reflection of the actual flora unless specialised anaerobic sampling and culture are performed. When antibiotic treatment fails, advice should be sought from a microbiologist as to whether this type of sampling may help.

Viral identification is rarely required for oral diseases because many oral viral infections are clinically typical and indicate the causative virus. A smear alone may show the nuclear changes of herpetic infection in epithelial cells from the margins of mucosal ulcers. A more sensitive and almost as rapid result may be obtained by sending a swab for virus detection using ELISA (enzyme-linked immunosorbent assay) or PCR analysis.

Key reminders for microbiological investigations are in Box 1.15.

> **Box 1.15   Reminders for microbiological investigation**
> - Always take a sample of pus for culture and antibiotic sensitivity from bone and soft tissue infections *before* giving an antibiotic
> - Always take the temperature of any patient with a swollen face, enlarged lymph nodes, malaise or other symptom or sign that might indicate infection
> - Culture of *Candida* from the mouth does not necessarily indicate infection because this is a commensal organism. Demonstration of hyphae in a scraping of epithelial cells indicates active infection.

Other clinical tests

Urine tests are valuable for the diagnosis of diabetes (suggested by repeated candidal or periodontal infection), kidney damage which can have resulted from autoimmune disorders such as granulomatosis with polyangiitis (Wegener's granulomatosis) and for the detection of Bence-Jones protein in myeloma.

Taking the patient's temperature is an easily forgotten investigation. The temperature should be noted whenever bone or soft tissue infections are suspected. It helps distinguish facial inflammatory oedema from cellulitis and indicates systemic effects of infections and the need for more aggressive therapy.

Interpreting investigations and making a diagnosis and treatment plan

Check that the results of each investigation are compatible with the proposed diagnosis. If a result appears at odds with other information, take into account the normal variation, perhaps with age or diurnal variation, and consider the possibility of false-positive and false-negative results. A common cause of unusual blood test results is a delay in transporting blood samples to the laboratory.

Further advice and specialised tests may be appropriate, but more extensive investigations, those carrying risks or radiation dose, are best organised through other medical specialties. In referrals, it is important to state whether the dentist is requesting the medical specialist to exclude a condition and refer the patient back, or to take over the investigation. If the latter, it is essential that dental causes have been completely eliminated as the cause of the problem.

Finally, ensure that the patient's notes include a complete record of the consultation and investigation results. This must be correctly dated, legible, limited to relevant facts and include a clear complaint history, list of clinical findings, test results and plan of treatment organised in a suitable form for quick reappraisal. It must be signed by the clinician and, in addition, the name should be printed below. It should be possible for another person to continue to investigate or treat the patient without difficulty on the basis of the clinical record.

Photography or computerised video imaging is a very valuable adjunct to the clinical record. Pictures are especially useful in monitoring lesions that vary in the course of a long follow-up, for instance, white patches. It is useful to include teeth or a scale in the frame to allow accurate assessment of small changes in size. Photographs may also be helpful in explaining to patients about their condition and to show the effects of treatment, but consent for the intended uses of the photographs must be obtained first, and digital image files must be stored securely in the same way as other patient-identifiable digital files.

Appendix 1.1

Normal haematological values

Red cells

Haemoglobin (adults)	Males 130–170 g/L	Females 115–165 g/L
Haematocrit (packed cell volume – PCV)	Males 0.40–0.54%	Females 0.36–0.47%
Mean cell volume (MCV)	80–100 fL	
Mean cell haemoglobin concentration (MCHC)	300–370 g/L	
Mean cell haemoglobin	27–32 pg	
Red cell count	Males 4.5–6.5×10^{12}/L	Females 3.8–5.8×10^{12}/L
Erythrocyte sedimentation rate (ESR)	Males 1–10 mm/h	Females 3–15 mm/h

White cells

Total count	3.6–11×10^9/L
Neutrophils	1.8–7.5×10^9/L
Lymphocytes	1–4×10^9/L
Monocytes	0.2–0.8×10^9/L
Eosinophils	0.1–0.4×10^9/L

Platelets

140–400×10^9/L

Note. These reference ranges are for adults and are calculated assuming a normal distribution of results and excluding the upper and lower 2.5% of the range as abnormal. Therefore, approximately 5% of healthy persons have values outside the figures quoted above. These are average values and vary slightly between laboratories, and you should always check normal values with the testing laboratory. Reference ranges for some tests may vary between different ethnic groups.

Disorders of tooth development | 2

Development of an ideal dentition depends on many factors (Box 2.1).

Significant structural defects of teeth are much less common than irregularities of alignment of the teeth and abnormal relationship of the arches. The main groups of disorders affecting development of the dentition are summarised in Table 2.1 and Summary chart 2.1 and Summary chart 2.2.

ABNORMALITIES IN THE NUMBER OF TEETH

Anodontia

Total failure of development of a complete dentition (anodontia) is exceedingly rare. If the permanent dentition fails to form, the deciduous dentition is retained for many years. If the teeth survive caries, attrition will eventually destroy the crowns. Lack of alveolar bone growth may make implant placement difficult.

Isolated oligodontia

Oligodontia, often referred to as hypodontia, means few teeth. Failure of development of one or two teeth is relatively common and often hereditary. The teeth most frequently missing are third molars, second premolars or maxillary second incisors (Fig. 2.1), the last teeth in each series. Absence of third molars can be a disadvantage if first or second molars, or both, have been lost; otherwise, orthodontic problems of alignment and space loss are the only effects.

Absence of lateral incisors can sometimes be conspicuous because the large, pointed canines erupt in the front of the mouth beside the central incisors. It is often impossible to prevent loss of space, even if the patient is seen early. It is also difficult and time consuming to make space by orthodontic means to replace the laterals, so combined procedures with prosthodontic replacement are often used. Disguising the shape of the canines is destructive of the tooth, usually unconvincing cosmetically and produces a poor contact.

Oligodontia without a syndromic association or systemic disease can be caused by alterations in over 15 genes, most commonly *WNT10*, *AXIN2* or *LRP6* in the WNT signalling pathway and *MSX1* in the transforming growth factor beta pathway. These are the same genes that are often altered in the syndromes with oligodontia.

General review PMID: 24124058

Genetic causes PMID: 25910507 and 29969831

Oligodontia or anodontia with systemic defects
Anhidrotic (hereditary) ectodermal dysplasia

Ectodermal dysplasia has several forms. The most common is the type 1 or X-linked hypohidrotic form described here, but there are other modes of inheritance and clinical variations. Ectodermal dysplasia 1 is caused by mutation in the

Box 2.1 Requirements for development of an ideal dentition

- Formation of a full complement of teeth
- Normal structural development of the dental tissues
- Eruption of each group of teeth at the appropriate time into an adequate space
- Normal development of jaw size and relationship
- Eruption of teeth into correct relationship to occlude with their opposite numbers
- Maintenance of tooth position by normal soft tissue size and pressure

Table 2.1 Disorders of development of teeth

Abnormality	Examples
Number	Anodontia
	Oligodontia (hypodontia)
	Additional teeth (supernumerary and supplemental)
Eruption	Delayed eruption
	Primary eruption failure
	Natal teeth
	Cleidocranial dysplasia
Enamel	Amelogenesis imperfecta
	Chronological hypoplasia
	Molar-incisor hypomineralisation
	Fluorosis
Dentine	Dentinogenesis imperfecta
	Dentinal dysplasia
	Vitamin D-resistant rickets
Cementum	Hypophosphatasia
All dental hard tissues	Regional odontodysplasia
Dental hard tissues and bone	Segmental odontomaxillary dysplasia
Pigmentation	Tetracycline pigmentation
	Rhesus incompatibility and jaundice
	Porphyria
Effects of systemic disease	Congenital syphilis
	Developmental arrest or delay
Minor tooth anomalies and abnormal tooth shape	Geminated (double) teeth
	Macrodontia
	Microdontia
	Dens invaginatus and evaginatus
	Talon cusp
	Additional roots or cusps
	Enamel pearls

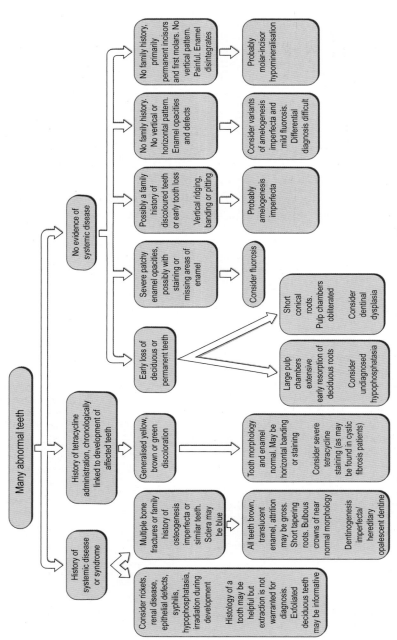

Summary chart 2.1   Differential diagnosis of developmental defects of the teeth.

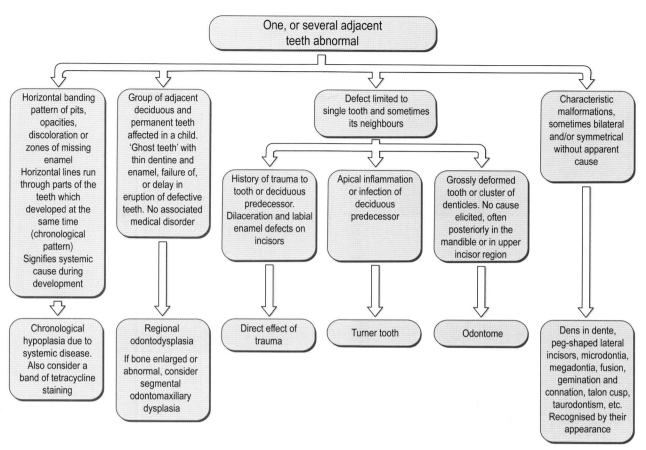

Summary chart 2.2 Differential diagnosis of developmental and acquired abnormalities of one or a group of teeth.

EDA or ectodysplasin-A gene on the X chromosome. Female carriers have minimal features, sometimes only peg-shaped upper lateral incisors.

The main features are summarised in Box 2.2. In severe cases, no teeth form. More often, most of the deciduous teeth form, but there are few or no permanent teeth. The teeth are usually peg-shaped or conical (Fig. 2.2).

When there is anodontia, the alveolar process, without teeth to support, fails to develop and has too little bone to support standard implants without surgical bone augmentation. The profile then resembles that of an older person because of the gross loss of vertical dimension. The hair is fine and sparse (Fig. 2.3), particularly in the tonsural region. The skin is smooth, shiny and dry due to absence of sweat glands. Heat is therefore poorly tolerated. The fingernails are usually also defective. As a temporary measure, composite restorations can disguise peg-shaped teeth and dentures or overdentures are usually well tolerated by children. Implants cannot be placed in the maxilla during growth, but it may be possible to use mini-implants or implants in the anterior mandible from a young age because, without teeth to erupt, alveolar growth is complete. Ultimately, a tooth-supported fixed partial denture or implant-supported overdenture is often a good solution.

Web URL 2.1 Ectodermal dysplasia URL: http://rarediseases.org/rare-diseases/hypohidrotic-ectodermal-dysplasia/

Other conditions associated with oligodontia

There are over 100 rare syndromes in which oligodontia is a feature, but the only common one is Down's syndrome (Ch. 40). One or more third molars are absent in more than 90% of patients with the syndrome, and absence of individual teeth is also common. Very rarely anodontia occurs. Less frequent disorders with oligodontia include cleft lip and palate, chondroectodermal dysplasia and oro-facial-digital syndrome.

Additional teeth: hyperdontia

Additional teeth are relatively common in the permanent dentition, affecting 1%–3% of the population, more frequently males. The teeth are usually of simple conical shape and less frequently resemble teeth of the normal series. These are the results of organised development and maturation under genetic control, not simple excessive growth of the dental lamina.

Supernumerary teeth are any additional teeth (Fig. 2.4). Conical or more seriously malformed additional teeth form most frequently in the incisor or molar region and, very occasionally, in the midline of the maxilla (mesiodens, Fig. 2.5).

Supplemental teeth are supernumerary teeth with a normal morphology, and they are usually an extra tooth at the end of the incisor, premolar or molar series (also seen in Fig. 2.5). Most supernumerary teeth in the deciduous dentition are supplemental.

Effects and treatment

Additional teeth usually erupt in abnormal positions, labial or buccal to the arch, creating stagnation areas and greater susceptibility to caries, gingivitis and periodontitis. Alternatively, a supernumerary tooth may prevent a normal tooth

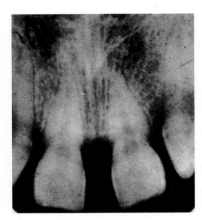

Fig. 2.1 Congenital absence of lateral incisors with spacing of the anterior teeth.

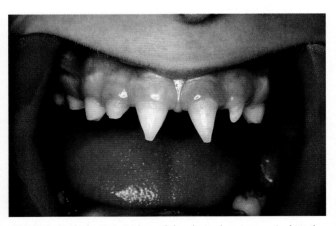

Fig. 2.2 Anhidrotic ectodermal dysplasia showing conical teeth.

from erupting, resorb roots of adjacent teeth or cause crowding and malalignment. These additional teeth are usually best extracted.

Review PMID: 24124058

Syndromes associated with hyperdontia

These syndromes are all rare, but probably the best known are cleidocranial dysplasia (Ch. 13), in which many additional teeth develop but fail to erupt, and the Gardner variant of familial adenomatous polyposis (Ch. 12).

DEFECTIVE ENAMEL FORMATION

Structural defects of the enamel, such as pitting, discoloration or failure to form can only arise during development.

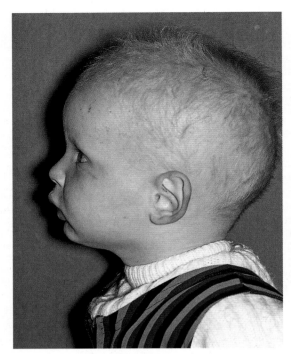

Fig. 2.3 Anhidrotic ectodermal dysplasia showing typical fine and scanty hair and loss of support for the facial soft tissues.

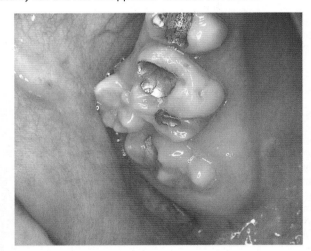

Fig. 2.4 A paramolar, a buccally placed supernumerary molar tooth.

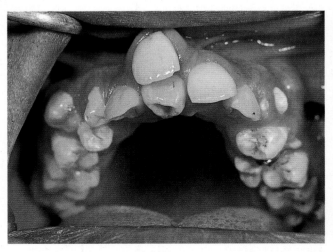

Fig. 2.5 Maleruption of a midline tuberculate supernumerary and two supplemental premolars causing ectopic eruption of adjacent teeth through gross crowding.

Hypoplasia of enamel is not an important contributory cause of dental caries. Only normally formed enamel can become carious, and hypoplasia due to fluorosis is associated with enhanced resistance. Diagnosis of developmental defects can be challenging and molecular diagnosis is becoming available for indeterminate cases.

Molecular diagnosis PMID: 26502894

Defects of deciduous teeth

Calcification of deciduous teeth begins at approximately the fourth month of intrauterine life. Disturbances of metabolism or infections that affect the foetus at this early stage without causing abortion are rare. Defective structure of the deciduous teeth is therefore uncommon but, in a few places, such as parts of India, where the fluoride content of the water is very high, the deciduous teeth may be mottled.

The deciduous teeth may be discoloured by abnormal pigments circulating in the blood. Severe neonatal jaundice may cause the teeth to become yellow, or there may be bands of greenish discoloration. In congenital porphyria, a rare disorder of haemoglobin metabolism, the teeth are red or purple. Tetracycline given during dental development, contrary to guidelines, is now a rare cause of permanent discoloration. These conditions usually also affect the permanent teeth and are discussed later in this chapter.

Defects of permanent teeth

Single permanent teeth may be malformed as a result of local causes such as periapical infection of a predecessor ('Turner tooth' – Fig. 2.6), or trauma from intubation while a preterm neonate (Fig. 2.7). Defects of multiple teeth usually indicate previous systemic disease as summarised in Box 2.3.

Amelogenesis imperfecta

➜ Summary chart 2.1 p. 24

Amelogenesis imperfecta is a group of conditions caused by defects in the genes that encode enamel matrix proteins or other proteins or enzymes required to process or mineralise the matrix. Classification is complex and based on pattern of inheritance, type of defect (enamel hypoplasia, hypomineralisation or hypomaturation) and appearance (smooth, rough or pitted). At least 16 presentations have been recognised on clinical grounds, but some are the same genetic condition with differing severity, and the classification is contentious.

Inheritance can be autosomal dominant, recessive or X-linked and occasional cases are sporadic. However, the most common types have an autosomal inheritance and are thought to be caused by mutations in the genes for ameloblastin (C4), enamelin (C4) or tuftelin (C1). In the case of the autosomal dominant type of amelogenesis imperfecta, the defective gene is enamelin (C4).

The less common X-linked types are caused by a variety of defects in the *AMELX* gene encoding amelogenin, located on the X and Y chromosomes (the copy on the Y gene being inactive) and, confusingly, it seems the same mutation can sometimes cause hypoplasia, hypomineralisation or hypomaturation in different patients.

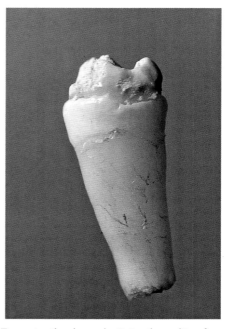

Fig. 2.6 Turner tooth, a hypoplastic tooth resulting from periapical infection, usually of a deciduous predecessor.

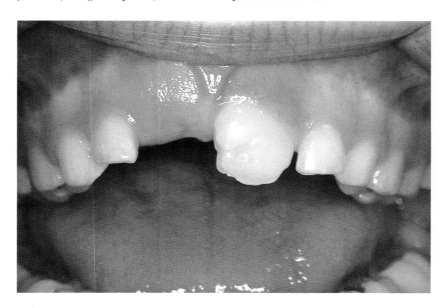

Fig. 2.7 Localised dental disturbance caused by prolonged intubation during tooth development. The upper left central incisor shows enamel pitting incisally, and the upper right central incisor is deformed and has failed to erupt.

Genetic factors act throughout the whole duration of amelogenesis. Characteristically, therefore, all teeth are affected, and defects involve the whole enamel or randomly distributed patches of it. By contrast, exogenous factors affecting enamel formation (with the important exception of fluorosis) tend to act for a relatively brief period and produce defects related to that period of enamel formation (a chronological pattern).

Until there is a better understanding, dentists should at least be able to identify the three clinical types of hypoplasia, hypocalcification and hypomaturation and take a family history, which may reveal an inheritance pattern.

Review types and causes PMID: 16838342

Detailed molecular mechanisms PMID: 28694781

Hypoplastic amelogenesis imperfecta

The main defect in this type is deficient formation of matrix, so that the amount of enamel is reduced but normally mineralised. The enamel is either randomly pitted, grooved or uniformly very thin, but hard and translucent (Fig. 2.8). The defects tend to become stained, but the teeth are not especially susceptible to caries unless the enamel is scanty and fractures to expose dentine.

The main patterns of inheritance are autosomal dominant and recessive, X-linked and (a genetic rarity) an X-linked dominant type. In the last type, there is almost complete failure of enamel formation in affected males, whereas in females the enamel is vertically ridged (Figs 2.9–2.11). Tooth eruption can be delayed and some types are associated with anterior or lateral open bite. The irregular enamel outline but normal mineralization allow diagnosis before eruption radiographically (Figs 2.12-13). Occasionally, cases are difficult to classify (Fig. 2.14).

Hypomaturation amelogenesis imperfecta

The enamel is normal in thickness on eruption but with opaque, white to brownish-yellow patches caused by failure of maturation, a process of matrix removal and increasing mineralisation that is partly developmental and partly post-eruptive. The appearance can mimic fluorotic mottling if the spots are small (Figs 2.15 and 2.16). However, affected enamel is soft and vulnerable to attrition, though not as severely as the hypocalcified type.

There are several variants of hypomaturation defects such as a more severe, autosomal dominant type combined with hypoplasia and milder forms limited to only some tooth surfaces.

Box 2.3   Multiple malformed permanent teeth: important causes

Genetic
- Amelogenesis imperfecta
  - Hypoplastic
  - Hypomaturation
  - Hypocalcified
- Chronological hypoplasia
- Molar-incisor hypomineralisation
- Dentinogenesis imperfecta
- Dentinal dysplasia
- Regional odontodysplasia
- Segmental odontomaxillary dysplasia
- Multisystem disorders with associated dental defects
- Hypophosphatasia

Infective
- Congenital syphilis

Metabolic
- Rickets
- Hypoparathyroidism

Drugs
- Tetracycline pigmentation
- Cytotoxic chemotherapy

Fluorosis

Other acquired developmental anomalies
- Fetal alcohol syndrome
- Radiotherapy

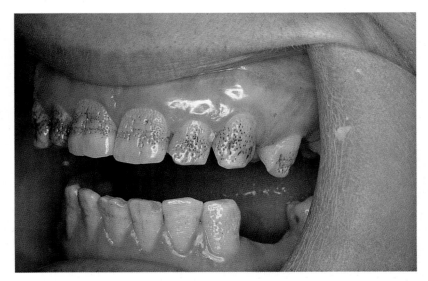

Fig. 2.8   Amelogenesis imperfecta, hypoplastic pitted type. Enamel between pits appears normal.

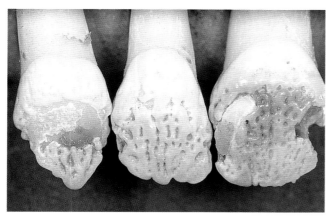

Fig. 2.9 Close-up of X-linked dominant hypoplastic type amelogenesis imperfecta. These teeth, from an affected female, show the typical vertical ridged pattern of normal and abnormal enamel as a result of Lyonisation.

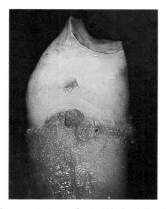

Fig. 2.10 Amelogenesis imperfecta X-linked dominant hypoplastic form in a male. This premolar has a cap of enamel so thin that the shape of the crown is virtually that of the dentine core.

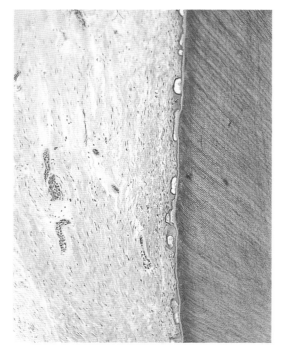

Fig. 2.11 Amelogenesis imperfecta X-linked dominant hypoplastic type in a male showing a thin translucent layer of defective enamel on the dentine surface (dentine right).

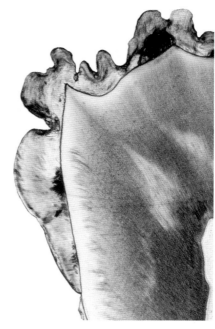

Fig. 2.12 Amelogenesis imperfecta, hypoplastic type. In this pitted hypoplastic type, the pits are seen to be focal areas of reduced enamel formation with incremental lines diverted around them. No enamel has been lost from the pit, it has developed this shape.

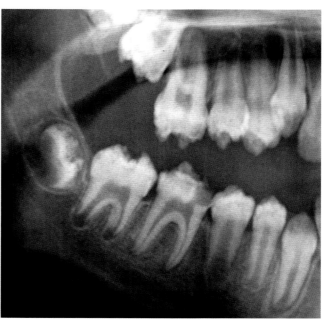

Fig. 2.13 Radiographic appearance of amelogenesis imperfecta hypoplastic pitted type, from the same patient as in Fig. 2.12. The irregular outline is visible. Note the normal enamel radiodensity where enamel is continuous enough to assess it.

Hypocalcified amelogenesis imperfecta

Enamel matrix is formed in normal quantity but is poorly calcified. When newly erupted, the enamel is normal in thickness and form, but weak, chalky and opaque in appearance.

The teeth tend to become stained, and enamel is relatively rapidly worn away. The upper incisors may acquire a shoulder due to the chipping away of the thin, soft enamel of the

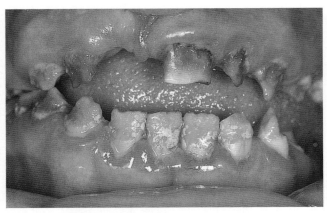

Fig. 2.14 Amelogenesis imperfecta, indeterminate type. Some cases, such as this, are difficult to classify but are clearly inherited, as shown by their long family history.

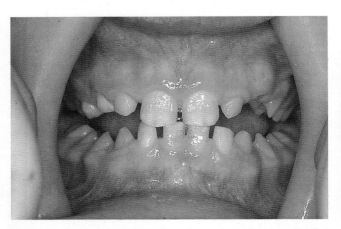

Fig. 2.15 Amelogenesis imperfecta, hypomaturation type. Tooth morphology is normal, but there are opaque white and discoloured patches.

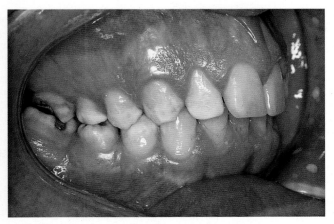

Fig. 2.16 Amelogenesis imperfecta, one of the several hypomaturation types. In this form there are opaque white flecks and patches affecting the occlusal half of the tooth surface.

incisal edges (Fig. 2.17). There are dominant and recessive patterns of inheritance.

Chronological hypoplasia

➔ Summary chart 2.1 p. 24

Any severe disturbance of metabolism can halt enamel formation. Dentine formation is less sensitive to insult,

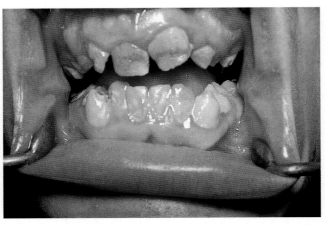

Fig. 2.17 Amelogenesis imperfecta, hypocalcified type. The soft chalky enamel was virtually of normal thickness and form but has chipped away during mastication leaving a characteristic shoulder, seen best on the upper left central incisor.

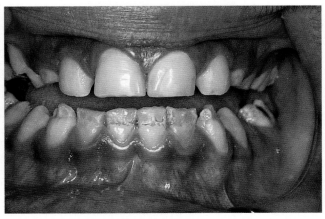

Fig. 2.18 Chronological hypoplasia due to metabolic upset. Defects are linear and run horizontally across the crown corresponding to the level of enamel forming during a severe illness.

so tooth formation will usually continue to produce a normally shaped tooth with only a band of enamel missing. The usual causes are the childhood fevers or severe infantile gastroenteritis. Measles with severe secondary bacterial infection was the most common cause of chronological hypoplasia but is rare since measles vaccination.

Unlike inherited forms of hypoplasia, only a restricted area of enamel is missing, corresponding to the sites of development at the time of the illness. Since enamel forms progressively from the incisal edges and cusp tips, the hypoplasia is characterised by a pattern of horizontal defects, either pits, grooves or a completely missing band of enamel across the crowns of the teeth.

Defects are usually in the incisal third of incisors, suggesting that the disorder had its effect during the first year or two of life, when such infections cause the most severe systemic upset (Fig. 2.18). Metabolic disturbance *in utero* or around birth affects the primary teeth in addition (Fig. 2.19). The horizontal pattern is important in distinguishing chronological hypoplasia from genetic causes of hypoplasia and determining the timing of the systemic disease (Fig. 2.20).

Molar-incisor hypomineralisation

→ Summary chart 2.1 p. 24

Molar incisor hypomineralisation is an unexplained, apparently recently recognised and increasingly frequent condition defined by hypomineralisation of some or all first permanent molars and incisors (Fig. 2.21). The teeth erupt normally and have patchy opaque and yellow-brown patches on the enamel of the occlusal third of the crowns. The enamel surface is hard, but the underlying enamel is soft and breaks down, leaving a stained rough and soft surface that is prone to caries. The defects are sharply demarcated. Cervical enamel is usually normal and the pattern may mimic the appearance of a chronological horizontal defect.

The cause is probably failure of enamel maturation, but the presentation and family history are distinct from amelogenesis imperfecta and chronological hypoplasia. It appears that many cases are similar to chronological hypoplasia in aetiology, but the systemic upset is milder and insufficient to cause the more severe defect of hypoplasia. A very wide range of types of illness appear to be able to cause hypomineralisation.

Molars are usually affected more severely than incisors. The affected teeth are characteristically hypersensitive and difficult to anaesthetise. Restorations often fail, partly due

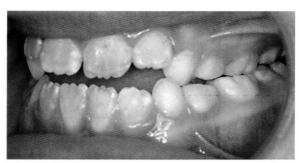

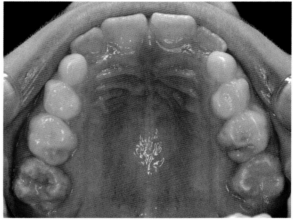

Fig. 2.21 Molar-incisor hypomineralisation. Typical appearance with discolouration and breakdown of enamel almost exclusively on permanent incisors and first molars.

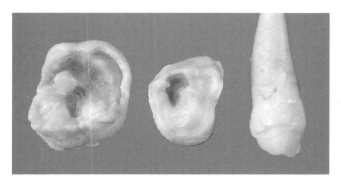

Fig. 2.19 Chronological hypoplasia with loss of primary molar occlusal enamel and a horizontal ridge on the upper canine.

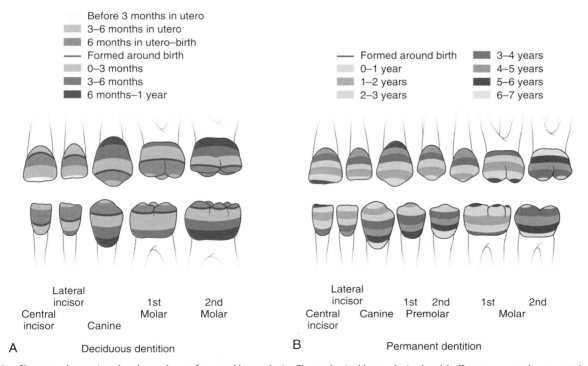

Before 3 months in utero
3–6 months in utero
6 months in utero–birth
— Formed around birth
0–3 months
3–6 months
6 months–1 year

— Formed around birth
0–1 year
1–2 years
2–3 years
3–4 years
4–5 years
5–6 years
6–7 years

Lateral
incisor   1st   2nd
Central   Molar   Molar
incisor   Canine

A   Deciduous dentition

Lateral
incisor   1st   2nd   1st   2nd
Central   Canine Premolar   Molar
incisor

B   Permanent dentition

Fig. 2.20 Charts to determine the chronology of enamel hypoplasia. Chronological hypoplasia should affect many teeth symmetrically consistent with the time of illness.

to the adverse crown shape and partly because the enamel is not amenable to use of adhesive materials, even away from the clinically detectable defects. This makes treatment difficult, and after a period of preventive care to remineralise the molars and preserve them as space maintainers, extraction is often the best course of action. Otherwise, full coverage restorations are required. Microabrasion is not sufficient to restore most affected incisors because the soft enamel extends deeply, and restorations or veneers are usually required.

Aetiology PMID: 27121068

Treatment PMID: 16805354, 26856002 and 23410530

Nature of enamel defect PMID: 23685033

Localised enamel defects

Localised enamel opacities and foci of hypoplasia or discolouration are very common and have been linked to locally acting causes such as trauma, infection, extraction of deciduous predecessors, prolonged neonatal intubation and periodontal ligament injection.

DEFECTIVE DENTINE FORMATION

➜ Summary chart 2.1 p. 24

The classification of hereditary dentine defects is unsatisfactory. As in amelogenesis imperfecta, the genetic findings do not correlate well with clinical presentation, and terminology is used inconsistently. The previous widely used classifications (of Witkop and of Shields) are now considered redundant, but no replacement is yet established.

The term *osteogenesis imperfecta* is used when abnormal teeth are associated with bone defects, replacing the term *dentinogenesis imperfecta* (type I). The term *dentinogenesis imperfecta* is used when only the teeth are involved, replacing the term *hereditary opalescent dentine*. Abnormal dentine is referred to as dysplastic, meaning abnormally formed, rather than hypoplastic as used for enamel.

Osteogenesis imperfecta with opalescent teeth ➜ Summary chart 2.1 p. 24

This uncommon defect of collagen formation disturbs formation of both bone and dentine. Many forms are known, and the condition is described in Chapter 13. Types III and IV are those most frequently associated with dentine defects. Both are autosomal dominant traits with mutation in the genes *COL1A1* and *COL1A2* that prevent the procollagen alpha helix polymerising into normal type 1 collagen. The dentine is soft and has abnormally high water content.

In both these types, opalescent teeth are present in over 80% of patients in the primary dentition. Tooth discoloration and attrition is often most striking in the deciduous dentition. Class III malocclusion is associated in over 70% of patients. In type III disease, dental development is delayed in 20% but, in type IV disease, it is accelerated in over 20% of patients.

Dentinogenesis imperfecta

➜ Summary chart 2.1 p. 24

This condition produces identical changes in appearance and structure of the teeth to those in osteogenesis imperfecta but is caused by mutations in the *DSPP* gene that encodes dentine sialoprotein, a dentine matrix protein, rather than collagen

genes. However, the condition may be heterogeneous and other mutated genes have been found. Previously there were thought to be two types (types II and III), but the condition of shell teeth, or type III, is now thought to be just a more severe presentation of type II caused by defects in the same gene. Dentinogenesis imperfecta can be associated with developmental hearing loss.

Clinical features

The teeth are normal in shape but uniformly brownish or purplish and abnormally translucent (Fig. 2.22), giving an opal-like appearance that leads to the clinical description of 'hereditary opalescent dentine'. The appearance is caused by the dark dentine being visible through the enamel, which is usually normal but may have hypoplastic defects in a minority of patients. The shape and size of the crowns is essentially normal, but the roots are slender and stunted, giving the tooth a cervical constriction and bulbous outline radiographically (Fig. 2.23). Dentine formation progresses to obliterate the pulp chamber at an early age. The mantle dentine is relatively normal but below the thin mantle the dentine is poorly formed, so that there is a weak zone in the

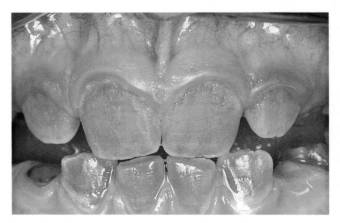

Fig. 2.22 Dentinogenesis imperfecta. Showing the grey-brown translucent appearance of the teeth which are of normal morphology.

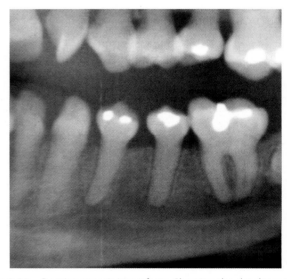

Fig. 2.23 Dentinogenesis imperfecta. Showing the slender roots and bulbous crowns of the 'tulip-shaped' teeth.

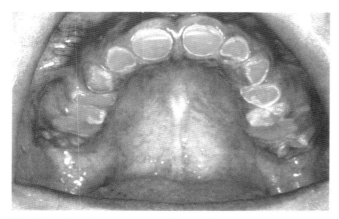

Fig. 2.24 Dentinogenesis imperfecta. In this 14-year-old, the teeth have worn down to gingival level, but the pulp chambers have become obliterated as part of the disease process. A rim of enamel remains around the necks of the teeth.

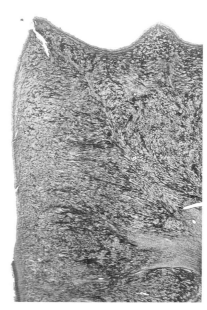

Fig. 2.26 Microscopic appearance of dentinogenesis imperfecta. Two cusps and part of the crown of a molar showing the grossly disorganised tubular structure with inclusions of pulp in the dentine and obliteration of the pulp cavity.

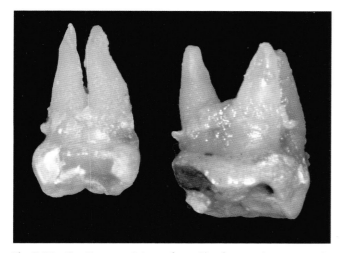

Fig. 2.25 Dentinogenesis imperfecta. Slender tapering roots and loss of enamel through fracturing.

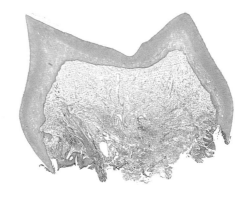

Fig. 2.27 Shell tooth. In this severe form of dentinogenesis imperfecta, only a thin mantle of dentine is formed, and no root develops.

dentine just below the amelodental junction. The lack of resilient dentine to support the enamel allows enamel to chip away, exposing the dentine, which is soft and rapidly wears away, eventually to the gingival level (Figs 2.24 and 2.25). In some patients, only a few teeth are severely affected, whereas the remainder appear normal.

Treatment aims to preserve vertical dimension, avoid extractions to prevent space loss and allow normal alveolar bone growth for implants later. Early application of occlusal composite onlays and preformed metal crowns on molars reduce wear. Worn roots may be used as temporary overdenture abutments but are too soft to survive long.

Severely affected patients may have shell teeth, with only a thin outer mantle layer of dentine tissue surrounding overlarge pulp chambers. Shell teeth are very difficult or impossible to manage conservatively.

Tooth structure

The earliest-formed mantle dentine under the amelodental junction usually appears normal. There is a sharp junction with the deeper defective dentine. This has few tubules, and they run in disorganised patterns. The uniform structure of dentine is absent; extensions of the pulp penetrate

the dentine almost to the enamel (Fig. 2.26) and can be exposed by attrition to devitalise the teeth. Calcification is incomplete and the dentine soft.

The pulp chamber becomes obliterated early, and odontoblasts degenerate. Cellular inclusions in the dentine are common. In shell teeth, the dentine layer is very thin (Fig. 2.27).

Review PMID: 19021896

Classification and types PMID: 25118030

Dentinal dysplasia ('rootless' teeth)

➜ Summary chart 2.1 p. 24

Dentinal dysplasia

This rare disorder was previously called dentinal dysplasia type 1 but is now the only type recognised. The crowns are of normal shape and size, but the roots are either absent or very short and conical. The pulp chambers are obliterated by multiple nodules of poorly organised dentine containing tubules running in sheaves. A range of pulp shapes can result from differing severity, with almost complete obliteration producing crescent-shaped pulps at the level of the floor of the normal chamber. In the worst affected teeth, roots are absent. Teeth tend to be lost early in life (Fig. 2.28). There are pulp extensions through dentine to the enamel, and vitality is lost quickly; otherwise the lack of roots predisposes to early loss through periodontitis.

The coronal dentine and enamel are normal or almost so, but dentinal tubule patterns in the root are abnormal (Fig. 2.29). Both dentitions are affected, the deciduous more severely.

Dentinal dysplasia 'type 2'

The defect in this rare disorder is in the dentine sialoprotein gene, so this disorder is now classified as a severe form of dentinogenesis imperfecta. The tooth crowns have the same opalescent appearance as dentinogenesis imperfecta in the

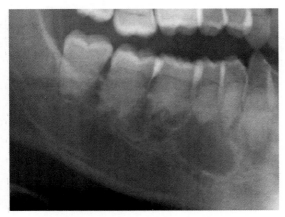

Fig. 2.28 Dentinal dysplasia type 1. Radiograph showing short roots, spontaneous pulp necrosis with apical areas, and obliterated crescent-shaped pulps.

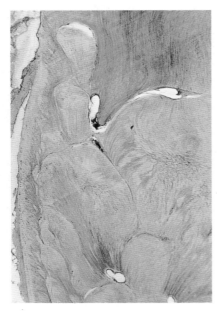

Fig. 2.29 Dentinal dysplasia. The pulp chamber in the short, broad root is obliterated by nodules of dentine with swirling patterns of tubules.

deciduous dentition. The permanent dentition appears normal or nearly normal in colour, but the pulps are larger than normal. A tall, wide coronal pulp extends high into the crown (thistle pulp), sometimes with pulp stones, and more marked in the permanent dentition (Fig. 2.30).

Review PMID: 19021896

DEFECTS OF ENAMEL AND DENTINE

→ Summary chart 2.1 p. 24

Regional odontodysplasia (ghost teeth)

→ Summary chart 2.2 p. 24

This localised disorder of development affects a group of teeth in which there are severe abnormalities of enamel, dentine and pulp. The disorder is not hereditary and a somatic mutation appears to be a likely cause. Although the aetiology is unknown, mutations in *PAX9* and *PIK3CA* have been detected in a few cases and a relationship to segmental odontomaxillary dysplasia proposed. A few cases are associated with facial vascular naevi or abnormalities such as hydrocephalus. There is no sex or racial predilection.

Clinically, regional odontodysplasia may be recognisable at the time of eruption of the deciduous teeth (2–4 years) or of the permanent teeth (7–11 years). The maxillary teeth are most frequently affected. Either or both dentitions, and one or, at most, two quadrants may be affected. The abnormal teeth frequently fail to erupt but, if they do, show yellowish deformed crowns with a rough surface.

Affected teeth have very thin enamel and dentine surrounding a greatly enlarged pulp chamber. In radiographs, the teeth appear crumpled and abnormally radiolucent or hazy, due to poor mineralisation, explaining the term 'ghost teeth' (Figs 2.31 - 2.33).

Histologically, the enamel thickness is highly irregular and lacks a well-defined prismatic structure. The dentine, which has a disorganised tubular structure, contains clefts and interglobular dentine mixed with amorphous mineralised tissue. The surrounding follicle soft tissue may contain numerous small calcifications, many of which are mineralized residues of enamel epithelium (Figs 2.34–2.35).

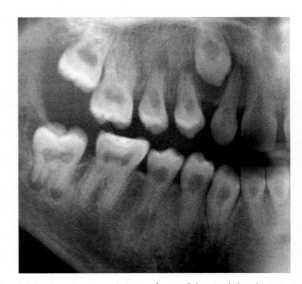

Fig. 2.30 Dentinogenesis imperfecta of dentinal dysplasia type 2 presentation. The pulp chambers are rounded, tall and wide in the developing dentition. The classical 'thistle-shaped' pulp appearance is seen in the lower canine and premolars.

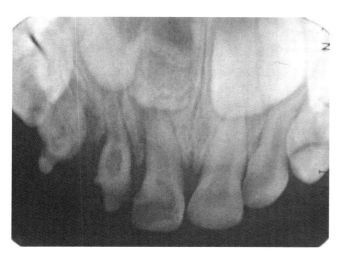

Fig. 2.31 Radiographic appearance of regional odontodysplasia. In the anterior regions the condition usually stops at the midline.

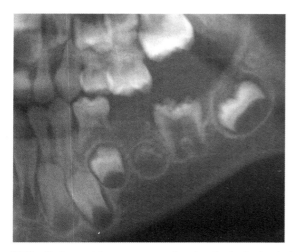

Fig. 2.32 Radiographic appearance of regional odontodysplasia. The lower left 5 and 6 are affected. Note their abnormal outline and radiodensity by comparison with the 4 and 7.

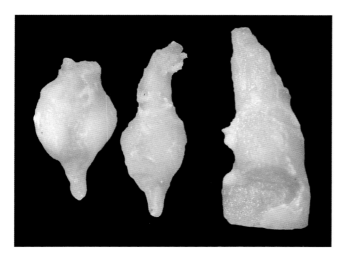

Fig. 2.33 Regional odontodysplasia. Distorted and hypoplastic teeth from the case shown in Fig. 2.31.

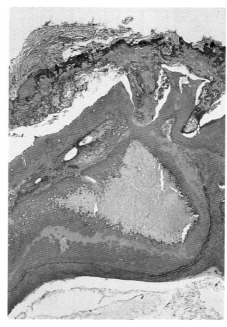

Fig. 2.34 Regional odontodysplasia. Both enamel and dentine are deformed, and there is calcification of the reduced enamel epithelium seen as a dark blue line at the top of the image.

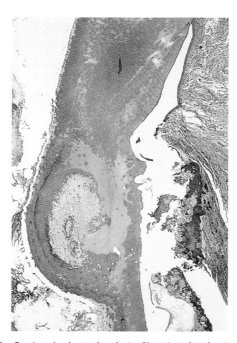

Fig. 2.35 Regional odontodysplasia. Showing dysplastic dentine with a disorganised tubule structure, an irregular enamel space and mineralised enamel epithelium.

If they erupt, the teeth are susceptible to caries and fracture. If they can be preserved and restored, crown and root dentine continue to form, and the teeth may survive long enough to allow normal development of the alveolar ridge and occlusion. However, extractions are often required eventually. This should not be done until it is certain that eruption has completely failed or the defects are too severe to be treatable. Unerupted teeth may be left in situ to preserve alveolar bone.

Review and cases PMID: 2549236

Cases PMID: 14714196

Natural history and treatment PMID: 17613259

Segmental odontomaxillary dysplasia

This rare disorder is frequently mistaken for fibrous dysplasia or regional odontodysplasia.

Segmental odontomaxillary dysplasia causes unilateral expansion of the alveolar process of the maxilla in a child in the deciduous or mixed dentition. One premolar and molar region is most frequently affected. Enlargement is due to both fibrous enlargement of the gingiva and of the alveolar bone. The antrum is small, and the maxilla is distorted, although only rarely to the extent of causing facial asymmetry. Eruption of teeth in the affected area is delayed, and they are hypoplastic to varying degrees, with enlargement of the pulps, thin pitted enamel, an irregular pulp-dentine interface and many pseudoinclusions in poorly organised dentine, and pulp stones. Permanent successors, particularly the premolars, may be absent.

Some patients have facial vascular or epidermal naevi and the combination of **H**emimaxillary enlargement, **A**symmetry of the face, **T**ooth abnormalities, and **S**kin abnormalities has been referred to as HATS syndrome. The cause of segmental odontomaxillary dysplasia is probably a somatic mutation and mosaicism of the *PIK3CA* gene, though the *ACTB* gene has also been implicated. *PIK3CA* encodes a signalling protein and *ACTB* the cytoskeletal protein actin. Similar mutations are known to cause local tissue overgrowth including epidermal naevi, explaining these apparently unconnected features. Since the cause is a somatic mutation, the condition is not inherited.

Radiographically, there is a zone of bone sclerosis with a coarse, often vertically-orientated, trabecular pattern and loss of the cortex and missing and distorted teeth (Fig. 2.36). Histologically, the sclerotic zone consists of woven bone trabeculae in bland fibrous tissue and appears superficially similar to the regressing stage of fibrous dysplasia. Both radiographs and histology are therefore necessary for diagnosis.

Case series PMID: 21684782 and 29389339

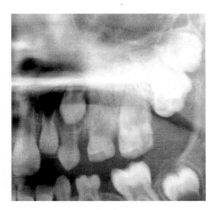

Fig. 2.36 Segmental odontomaxillary dysplasia. Showing abnormal upper primary molars that are indistinct against a background of even, coarsely trabecular bone. Permanent successors are absent.

OTHER SYSTEMIC DISEASES AFFECTING TEETH

Other metabolic disturbances

Rickets can cause hypocalcification of the teeth, but only if unusually severe (see Ch. 13).

Early-onset idiopathic hypoparathyroidism is rare. Ectodermal effects are associated. The teeth may therefore be hypoplastic with ridged enamel, short blunt roots and persistently open apices (Fig. 2.37). The nails may be defective, and there may be complete absence of hair. Patients with early-onset idiopathic hypoparathyroidism may later develop other endocrine deficiencies (polyendocrinopathy syndrome), and chronic oral candidosis may be the first sign (Ch. 15).

Hypophosphatasia. This rare genetic disorder can have severe skeletal effects as a result of failure of development of mature bone. There may also be failure of cementum formation causing early loss of teeth (Fig. 2.38). In milder forms, premature loss of the deciduous incisors is characteristic and occasionally the only overt manifestation of the disease.

Hypophosphatasia dental effects PMID: 19232125

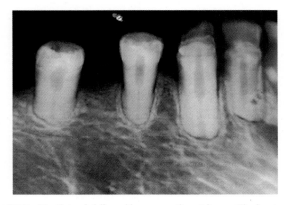

Fig. 2.37 Teeth in childhood hypoparathyroidism with short blunt roots, open apices and large pulp chambers.

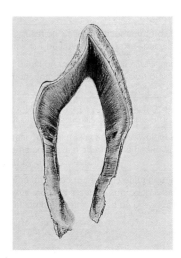

Fig. 2.38 Unstained ground section of a tooth in hypophosphatasia showing the enlarged pulp chamber and absence of cementum.

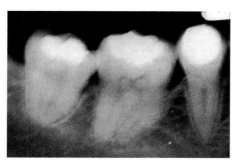

Fig. 2.39 Multiple pulp stones in a case of Ehlers–Danlos syndrome.

Ehlers–Danlos syndromes

This group of collagen disorders is characterised (to varying degrees) by hypermobile joints, loose hyperextensible skin, fragile oral mucosa and, in type VIII, early-onset periodontitis. There may also be temporomandibular joint symptoms such as recurrent dislocation (see main section in Ch. 14).

The main dental abnormalities are small teeth with short roots and multiple pulp stones (Fig. 2.39).

Gardner's syndrome (familial adenomatous polyposis)

The Gardner variant of familial adenomatous polyposis (often referred to as Gardner's syndrome) is characterised by multiple osteomas, especially of the jaws, colonic polyps and skin tumours. The majority of patients have dental abnormalities. These include impacted teeth other than third molars, supernumerary or missing teeth and abnormal root formation (Fig. 2.40). This syndrome is discussed and illustrated further in Chapter 12.

Colon carcinoma develops in almost all patients by middle age, and the mortality is high. The dental abnormalities can be detected in childhood or adolescence, and recognition of this syndrome may be life saving.

Epidermolysis bullosa

Epidermolysis bullosa is a genetic blistering disease of skin and mucosae (Ch. 16). Dental abnormalities include fine or coarse pitting defects, or thin and uneven enamel, which may also lack prismatic structure. The amelodentinal junction may be smooth. Dental defects vary in the different subtypes of the disease but are most frequent in the autosomal recessive, scarring type of epidermolysis bullosa in which there may be delayed, or failure of, eruption. The defects result from poor adhesion between ameloblasts during development.

Congenital syphilis → Summary chart 2.1 p. 24

Prenatal syphilis, the result of maternal infection, can cause a characteristic dental deformity, described by Hutchinson in 1858.

If the fetus becomes infected at a very early stage, abortion follows. Infants born with stigmata of congenital syphilis result from later fetal infection, and only the permanent teeth are affected. The characteristic defects are usually seen in the upper central incisors.

The incisors (Hutchinson's incisors) are small, barrel-shaped and taper toward the tip (Fig. 2.41). The incisal edge sometimes shows a crescentic notch or deep fissure which forms before eruption and can be seen radiographically. An anterior open bite is also characteristic. The first molars may be dome-shaped (Moon's molars) or may have a rough

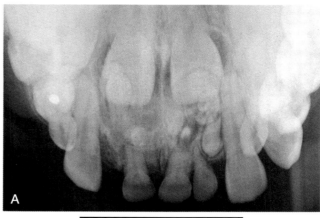

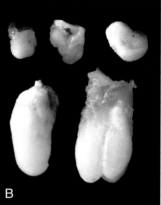

Fig. 2.40 Gardner's syndrome. Multiple unerupted abnormally formed supernumerary teeth. See also Fig. 12.8.

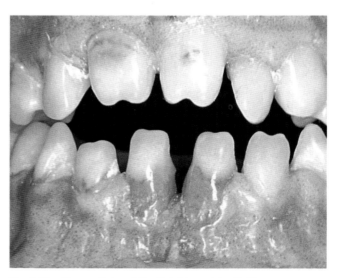

Fig. 2.41 Congenital syphilis: Hutchinson's teeth. The characteristics are the notched incisal edge and the peg shape tapering from neck to tip. *(From Cawson RA et al, 2001. Oral disease. 3rd ed. St Louis: Mosby.)*

pitted occlusal surface with compressed nodules instead of cusps (mulberry molars) (Fig. 2.42). These defects are often thought largely of historical interest, but congenital syphilis has reappeared in developed countries including the UK. Several hundred cases of congenital syphilis occur every year in the United States, and worldwide half a million infants die from it every year.

The effects are due to infection of the dental follicle by *Treponema pallidum*. The postulated consequences are chronic inflammation, fibrosis of the tooth sac, compression of the developing tooth and distortion of the ameloblast layer. *T. pallidum* and inflammation are proposed to cause proliferation of the odontogenic epithelium, which bulges and kinks into the dentine papilla, causing the characteristic central notch.

Vitamin D-resistant rickets

This term is given to familial hypophosphataemia, a rare X-linked dominant disease that causes phosphate loss in the kidneys, and consequent rickets that does not respond to vitamin D. Patients have short legs, wide skull sutures and kyphosis develops during adulthood.

The teeth have abnormally large pulp chambers with fine extensions of the pulp horns to the tips of the cuspal dentine (Fig. 2.43). These are prone to exposure by attrition or fracture and are often invisible radiographically. A periapical granuloma on an apparently normal tooth is a common presentation.

Calcification of dentine is defective. The typical inter-globular mineralisation of rickets is seen throughout the dentine.

EXTRINSIC AGENTS AFFECTING TEETH

➔ Summary chart 2.1 p. 24

Drugs

Tetracycline pigmentation

Tetracycline is taken up by calcifying tissues, and the band of tetracycline-stained bone, dentine or enamel fluoresces bright yellow under ultraviolet light.

The teeth become stained only when tetracycline is given during their development, and it can cross the placenta to stain the developing teeth of the fetus. More frequently, permanent teeth are stained by tetracycline given during infancy. Tetracycline is deposited along the incremental lines of the dentine and, to a lesser extent, of the enamel.

The more prolonged the course of treatment, the broader the band of stain and the deeper the discoloration. The teeth are at first bright yellow but become a dirty brown or grey (Figs 2.44 and 2.45). The stain is permanent, and when the permanent incisors are affected, the dark appearance can only be disguised. When the history is vague, the brownish colour of tetracycline-stained teeth must be distinguished from dentinogenesis imperfecta. In dentinogenesis imperfecta, the teeth are obviously more translucent than normal and, in many cases, chipping of the enamel from the dentine can be seen. In tetracycline-induced defects, the enamel is not abnormally translucent and is firmly attached to dentine. In very severe cases, intact teeth may fluoresce under ultraviolet light. Otherwise, the diagnosis can only be confirmed by linking the developmental age of the affected teeth to timing of exposure or after a tooth has been extracted. In an undecalcified section, the yellow fluorescence of the

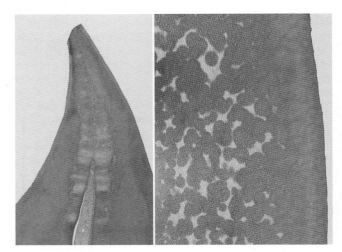

Fig. 2.43 Vitamin D-resistant rickets. A fine pulp extension into the incisal tip dentine is just visible on the left. Right, at higher power, there is prominent globular mineralisation of dentine.

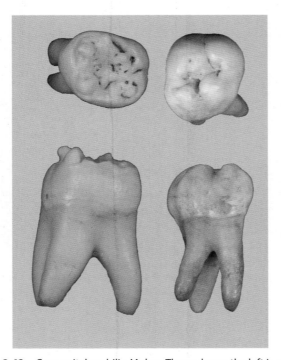

Fig. 2.42 Congenital syphilis: Molars. The molar on the left is a mulberry or Fournier molar with cusps surrounded by a hypoplastic groove producing a knobbly surface. That on the right is a Moon's molar, with a smooth rounded crown that tapers toward the occlusal surface. *(Copyright Museums at the Royal College of Surgeons.)*

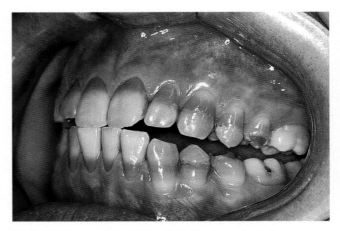

Fig. 2.44 Tetracycline staining. Note the chronological distribution of the dark-brown intrinsic stain.

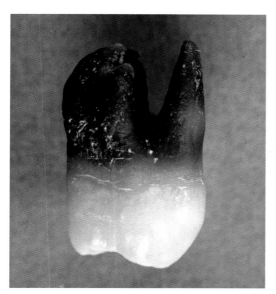

Fig. 2.45 Minocycline staining. Now one of the commoner forms of tetracycline staining since administration in childhood is controlled, limited to third molar roots from use of minocycline for acne during adolescence.

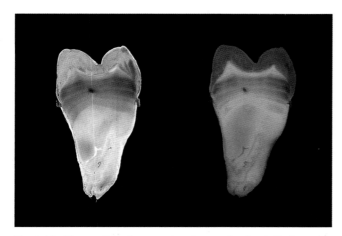

Fig. 2.46 Tetracycline pigmentation. Ground (undecalcified) section (*left*) shows the broad bands of tetracycline deposited along the incremental lines of the dentine; (*right*) same section viewed under ultraviolet light shows fluorescence of the bands of tetracycline.

tetracycline deposited along the incremental lines can be easily seen (Fig. 2.46).

It is no longer necessary to give tetracycline during dental development. There are equally effective alternatives, and it should be avoided from approximately the fourth month to at least the 12th year of childhood, ideally the 16th year. Nevertheless, tetracycline staining is still seen.

Tetracyclines that achieve a high blood level may still stain apparently fully formed teeth, for example minocycline may darken teeth in which there is reactionary dentine formation following trauma.

Minocycline stain PMID: teeth 23887527 and bone 7614206

Cytotoxic chemotherapy

Increasing numbers of children are surviving malignant disease, particularly acute leukaemia, as a result of cytotoxic chemotherapy.

> **Box 2.4 Dental fluorosis: distinctive features**
> - Clinically evident fluorosis limited to areas where fluorides in water exceed approximately 2 parts per million
> - Only those who have lived in a high-fluoride area during dental development show mottling
> - The defect is not acquired by older visitors to the area
> - Permanent teeth are affected; mottling of deciduous teeth is rare
> - Mottled teeth are less susceptible to caries than normal teeth from low-fluoride areas
> - A typical effect is spotty paper-white enamel opacities
> - Brown extrinsic staining of these patches may be acquired after eruption

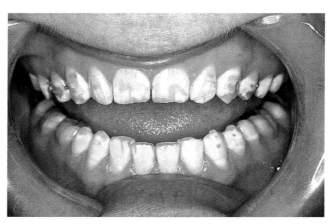

Fig. 2.47 Fluoride mottling. In this case, from an area of endemic fluorosis, there is generalised opaque white mottling with patchy enamel hypoplasia. Note the resemblance to the hypomaturation type of amelogenesis imperfecta.

Among survivors, teeth that develop during treatment may have short roots, hypoplasia of the crowns and enamel defects. Microscopically, incremental lines may be more prominent, corresponding to growth arrest or delay during the period of chemotherapy. In extreme cases, tooth formation may be aborted so that oligodontia results.

Fluorosis → Summary chart 2.1 p. 24

Mottled enamel is the most frequently seen and most reliable sign of excess fluoride in the drinking water. It has distinctive features (Box 2.4). The highest fluoride levels completely disrupt amelogenesis, producing hypoplastic patches. Lower levels inhibit mineralisation and prevent enamel maturation.

Clinical features

Mottling ranges from paper-white matt patches to opaque, brown, pitted and brittle enamel. Clinically, it may be difficult to distinguish fluorotic defects from amelogenesis imperfecta when the degree of exposure to fluoride is unknown (Figs 2.47–2.49).

There is considerable individual variation in the effects of fluorides. A few patients acquire mottling after exposure to relatively low concentrations (Fig. 2.50), while others exposed to higher concentrations appear unaffected. Being a systemic effect, fluorosis is bilateral and usually affects all teeth, though a chronological pattern could result from a

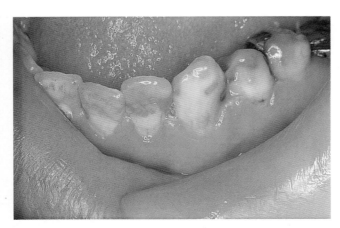

Fig. 2.48 Fluorosis. Moderate effects from an area of endemic fluorosis. Irregular patchy discoloration.

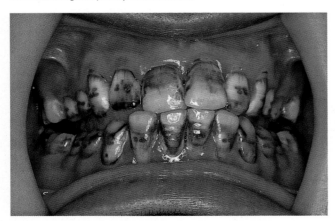

Fig. 2.49 Fluorosis. Severe effects from an area of endemic fluorosis. Closer view showing irregular depressions caused by hypoplasia and white opaque flecks and patches.

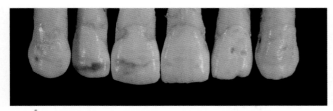

Fig. 2.50 Fluorosis from an area of previous endemic natural fluorosis in Gloucestershire, UK.

limited period of exposure. The perikymata are enhanced and visible clinically in severe cases, producing what appear to be horizontal lines, which misleadingly suggest chronological hypoplasia.

Changes due to mottling are graded as shown in Box 2.5.

Pathology

Fluoride exerts its effects through inhibition of ameloblasts. At intermediate levels (2–6 ppm), the enamel matrix is normal in structure and quantity. The form of the tooth is unaffected, but there are patches of incomplete enamel calcification beneath the surface layer. These appear as opacities because of high organic and water content that cause light reflection. Where there are high concentrations of fluorides (higher than 6 ppm), the enamel is pitted and brittle, with severe and widespread staining. Deciduous teeth are rarely mottled because excess fluoride is taken up

Box 2.5   Grading of mottled enamel

- Very mild. Small paper-white areas involve less than 25% of surface
- Mild. Opaque areas involve as much as 50% of surface
- Moderate. The whole of the enamel surface may be affected with paper-white or brownish areas or both (Fig. 2.47)
- Severe. The enamel is grossly defective, opaque, pitted, stained brown and brittle (Fig. 2.48)
- There are several different indices for measuring fluorosis, with increasing grades based on the area of white opacity, staining, discrete and, in the most severe, confluent pitting and missing enamel. All scoring is subjective and the mildest degrees of mottling may not necessarily be the result of fluorosis.

PMID: 7993559

by the maternal skeleton. However, when fluoride levels are excessively high (higher than 8 ppm), as in parts of India, North and central Africa and Brazil, mottling of deciduous teeth may be seen.

With severe mottling of the enamel, other effects of excessive fluoride intake, especially sclerosis of the skeleton, may develop. Radiographically, increased density of the skeleton may be seen in areas where the fluoride content of the water exceeds 8 ppm.

The severity of defects in relation to fluoride concentrations is shown in Table 2.2, and its relationship to caries prevalence in Fig. 2.51.

Mild dental fluorosis is not readily distinguishable from non-fluoride defects, and non-specific defects are more common in areas where the water contains less than 1 ppm of fluoride. Minimal mottling is associated with levels of 1 ppm fluoride in temperate climates and 0.7 ppm in hotter countries.

Mild enamel mottling has many causes that cannot usually be distinguished, even by analysis of an extracted or exfoliated tooth but this mild degree is not normally noticed by patients.

Fluorosis prevention in areas where fluoride is not controlled in drinking water relies on selecting appropriate supplementation measures and ensuring no additional sources of fluoride are being used, even inadvertently. Fluoride toothpastes must be used and stored carefully, and their use monitored to avoid overdose.

Pathology of fluorosis PMID: 21701193

Treatment of opacities PMID: 26856002

Other acquired developmental anomalies
Dilaceration

Trauma to a developing tooth can rotate it and cause the root to form at an angle to the normal axis of the tooth – a deformity known as *dilaceration*. The sudden disturbance to odontogenesis may cause the formation of highly irregular dentine at the bend, but the angulated root that develops after trauma is often of normal tubular dentine. The hook-shaped tooth is likely to be difficult to extract (Figs 2.52 and 2.53).

Fetal alcohol syndrome

Maternal alcoholism may cause developmental defects in the fetus. The eyes typically slant laterally, the lower half

Table 2.2   Effects on enamel of fluoride levels in drinking water

Fluoride concentration	Effects	Clinical appearance
Less than 0.5 ppm	Very mild or mild defects in as many as 6% of patients	Inconspicuous
0.5 to 1.5 ppm	At the upper limit, 22% show very mild defects	
2.5 ppm	Very mild or mild defects in more than 50% Moderate or severe defects in nearly 10%	Noticeable
4.5 ppm	Nearly all patients affected to some degree; 46% have 'moderate' and 18% 'severe' defects	Disfiguring
6.0 ppm and more	All patients affected; 50% severely disfiguring	

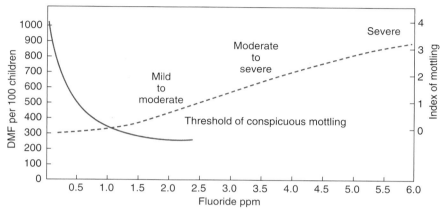

Fig. 2.51   Caries prevalence and mottling. The general relationship between the prevalence of caries (*continuous line*) and the severity of mottling (*broken line*) in persons continuously exposed to various levels of fluoride in the water during dental development. The optimum level of fluoride can be seen to be approximately 1 part per million. Higher concentrations of fluoride cause increasing incidence and severity of mottling without a comparable improvement in resistance to caries. The index of mottling is obtained by giving an arbitrary value for each degree of mottling and relating the numbers of patients with each grade to the total number examined.

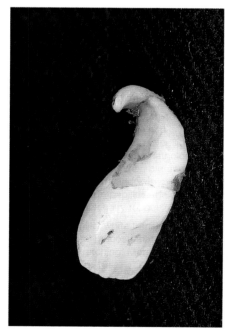

Fig. 2.52   A dilacerated upper central incisor. There has been an abrupt change in the direction of root growth after approximately half of the root was formed.

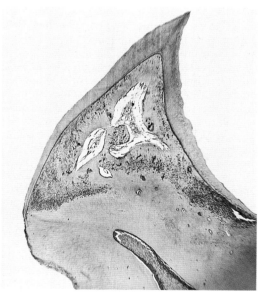

Fig. 2.53   Another dilacerated tooth showing, in addition to the deflected root, a change in enamel contour and disorganised coronal dentine formed after the causative trauma. The junction between dentine formed before and after trauma is clearly seen.

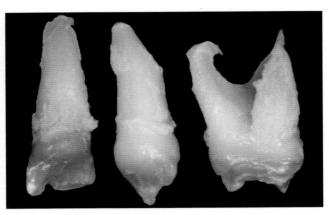

Fig. 2.54 Rhesus incompatibility. Deciduous teeth from a patient who suffered haemolytic anaemia from rhesus incompatibility. There is greenish discolouration of the dentine and enamel formed before birth.

of the face is elongated and there is learning disability. Dental development may be delayed, and there may be enamel defects, such as mottled opacities in the enamel near the incisal margins, but elsewhere abnormal enamel translucency.

Rhesus incompatibility

Maternal-fetal rhesus blood group incompatibility causes haemolytic disease of the newborn, in which maternal anti-rhesus antibodies cross the placenta and cause haemolytic anaemia in a fetus with a rhesus-positive blood group ('Rh disease'). If jaundice is severe, bilirubin can bind to the developing teeth, causing green or grey-yellow discolouration (Fig. 2.54).

ODONTOMES AND MINOR TOOTH ANOMALIES

There is a spectrum of abnormal tooth formation ranging from slight malformations, such as an exaggerated cingulum or extra roots or cusps on otherwise normal teeth to disorganised masses of dental hard tissues called odontomes (or odontomas). Odontomes are hamartomas and described with the odontogenic tumours (Ch.11).

Dens invaginatus is an exaggeration of the process of formation of a cingulum pit and usually affects permanent upper lateral incisors, occasionally canines or central incisors, in males. Dentine and enamel-forming tissue invaginate into the pulp to appear radiographically as a tooth-within-a-tooth (*dens in dente,* Fig. 2.55). In the most extreme form, dens invaginatus, also known as an invaginated or dilated odontome, the invagination extends the whole length of the root and sometimes extends through a widely dilated apex (Fig. 2.56). Often the invagination has incomplete walls allowing the exterior to communicate with the pulp and devitalise it. Alternatively, food debris lodges in the cavity to cause caries which rapidly penetrates the superficially located pulp chamber.

Dens evaginatus is the opposite, an enamel- and dentine-covered spur extending outward from the occlusal surface of a premolar or molar, usually in the lower arch and frequently forming bilaterally and symmetrically (Fig. 2.57). Fracture exposes the internal pulp horn present in about half of cases. Dens evaginatus affects the permanent dentition almost exclusively and is usually found in patients of Asian heritage.

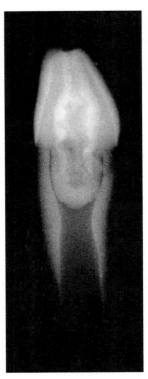

Fig. 2.55 Dens in dente or mild invaginated odontome. In this radiograph, the enamel-lined invagination and its communication with the exterior at the incisal tip are clearly seen. The pulp is compressed to the periphery.

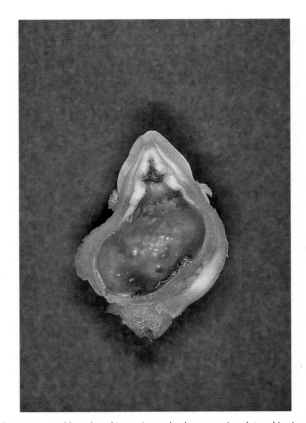

Fig. 2.56 A dilated and invaginated odontome in a lateral incisor, sectioned vertically. The central cavity communicates with the exterior through an invagination in the cusp tip.

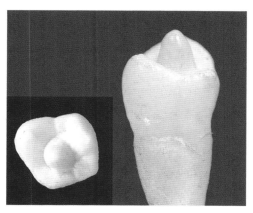

Fig. 2.57 Dens evaginatus from a lower premolar, occlusal surface inset.

Geminated teeth, meaning double or twinned teeth, are most common in the maxillary incisor region. One very wide crown is present, appearing to result from fusion of two adjacent teeth, though the adjacent tooth may be present or absent. The tooth may have two pulp chambers that are entirely separate, joined in the middle of the tooth or branched, with the pulp chambers of separated crowns sharing a common root canal. The crowns may be entirely separate or divided only by a shallow groove. The roots may be single or double. This malformation is commoner in the deciduous dentition. Trying to decide whether such teeth arise by fusion of two tooth germs or partial splitting of a single germ is pointless, and it seems likely that the condition is genetic; it is often bilateral and does not arise from excessive crowding.

These malformed teeth usually need to be removed before they obstruct the eruption of other teeth or become infected, or for cosmetic reasons. Endodontic treatment may be possible in some cases.

Enamel pearls are uncommon, minor abnormalities that are formed on otherwise normal teeth by ameloblasts that differentiate in Hertwig's root sheath to form a small nodule of enamel below the amelocemental junction. The pearls are usually round, a 1–2 millimetres in diameter and often form at the bifurcation of upper permanent second and third molars (Figs 2.58 and 2.59). Many are chance findings on cone-beam computed tomography (CT).

Enamel pearls may consist of only a nodule of enamel attached to the root surface or may have a core of dentine containing a horn of the pulp. If near the gingival margin, they may cause a stagnation area and local periodontitis. If they contain pulp, this will be exposed if the pearl is removed. The enamel and dentine are normal histologically.

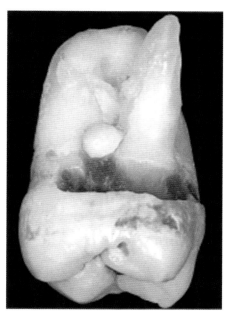

Fig. 2.58 Enamel pearl. There is a small mass of enamel at the root bifurcation of this maxillary molar.

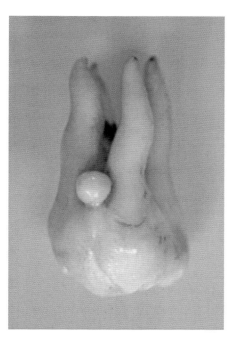

Fig. 2.59 Enamel pearl associated with a spur of enamel joining the crown to the pearl.

DISORDERS OF ERUPTION

Normal eruption

Eighteenth-century parish registers are replete with the names of infants who died as a result of teething. Although this is now considered impossible, other myths about tooth eruption abound.

Teething coincides with a period of naturally low resistance to infection and declining maternal passive immunity during which viral infections are common. Eruption is associated with a very slight rise in temperature (not a fever), mild discomfort locally, reflex salivation causing drooling and, sometimes, reddening of cheeks. Systemic symptoms during teething should therefore be investigated because, if significant, they are more likely to be caused by primary herpetic gingivostomatitis or other treatable infection. In many infants teething passes unnoticed (Box 2.6). The signs and symptoms are not specific and are also seen in those of similar age not teething, in whom they pass unremarked. Despite this and lack of effect, teething ointments, gels and products remain available, but often contain undesirable ingredients such as benzocaine, lidocaine, alcohol or sugar.

Fusion of the enamel epithelium with the oral epithelium allows eruption without bleeding, but the urge to chew during teething is strong, and trauma to the mucosa may cause haemorrhage into the follicle over an erupting tooth before it reaches the surface ('eruption haematoma', Fig. 10.24).

Very occasionally eruption of permanent molars is associated with painless loss of a small sequestrum. Bone lying in the concavity of the crown can be resorbed around the periphery while the cusps erupt, cutting off its blood supply from adjacent tissues ('eruption sequestrum'). Lower first permanent molars are the most frequently affected teeth. Similar calcified nodules can also arise from microscopic odontogenic hamartomas in the follicle, composed of dentine, enamel or amorphous mineralised tissue.

Symptoms of teething PMID 10742315

Natal and neonatal teeth

Teeth present at birth (*natal teeth*) or within 30 days of birth (*neonatal teeth*) are almost always normal deciduous lower incisors that erupt prematurely. Occasionally they may be supernumerary teeth, though deciding this can be difficult as radiographs are difficult to take at such a young age. At birth the crown of lower incisors is almost complete and the lack of root makes them very mobile. Such teeth interfere with feeding and may be displaced and inhaled, but they are best retained if possible.

Gingival cysts in infants (*Bohn's nodules*) may be mistaken for erupting teeth in neonates (Ch. 10).

Natal teeth are seen in some rare developmental disorders; pachyonychia congenita, Ellis-van Creveld and Hallermann-Streiff syndromes.

Box 2.6   Normal teething

One-third of infants have no signs or symptoms. Many only have a few.

- Effects are limited to a few days each side of the day of eruption
- Increased biting and rubbing the gingiva
- Reflex salivation and drooling
- Irritability and sleep disturbance
- Rubbing of face and ears
- Facial reddening of the cheek
- Decreased appetite
- Mild temperature increase

Delayed eruption

Eruption of deciduous teeth starts at approximately 6 months, usually with the appearance of the lower incisors, and is complete by approximately 2 years, earlier in females and with considerable individual variation in timing. Mass failure of eruption is very rare despite the biological complexity of the process. More often eruption delay has local causes and affects one or a few teeth.

Failure of a single tooth or adjacent teeth to appear in the mouth within a few months of the contralateral equivalent should trigger radiographic assessment to check for its presence and location. However, delayed appearance of the deciduous dentition in the absence of a cause does not warrant concern until it is delayed for 1 year provided no mechanical cause is evident, as eruption times are so variable.

In generalised delay caused by systemic illness, for instance in preterm infants, recovery normally allows eruption to proceed and after a few years eruption catches up with the normal timetable. Systemic diseases that cause delayed eruption are all rare. Eruption is complex, and many diseases can interfere with it. Both chemotherapy and radiotherapy arrest or interrupt eruption as well as tooth formation.

Single tooth failure of eruption is almost always due to a mechanical obstruction or ankylosis.

Primary eruption failure is a rare condition. Usually some teeth erupt, but then all teeth distally in the quadrant, sometimes all, remain unerupted and may eventually ankylose (Fig. 2.60). Half of cases are familial, and some are associated with mutation of the parathyroid hormone receptor gene. A common mild presentation is failure of eruption of only permanent molars, and the first permanent molars are almost always involved. There may be bilateral involvement, a Class 3 skeletal pattern and oligodontia associated. This condition does not cause delayed eruption of single teeth. Teeth in primary eruption failure do not respond to orthodontic traction, and treatment usually requires extraction. Restoration is then difficult due to lack of alveolar bone growth.

Causes of delayed eruption are shown in Box 2.7.

Primary eruption failure PMID: 17482073

Submerged primary molars

Submerged or infraoccluded primary molars are molars that lie below the occlusal level of adjacent teeth. This may result from delayed eruption or follow full eruption of the tooth. In the latter situation the infraoccluded molar is thought

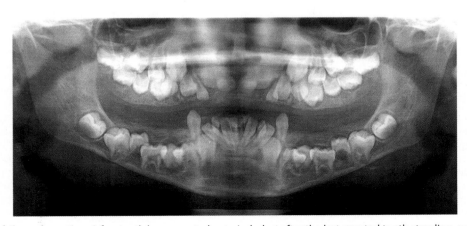

Fig. 2.60   Primary failure of eruption. A few teeth have erupted anteriorly, but after the last erupted tooth standing, none have erupted.

Box 2.7   Causes of delayed eruption of permanent teeth

Localised

- Impaction, usually last teeth in any series
- Insufficient space in the arch, crowding, supernumerary teeth
- Retention of a deciduous predecessor, ankylosis
- Premature loss of a deciduous predecessor, before half of the successor root is formed
- Malposition
- Local pathological process
  - Odontogenic cysts and tumours
  - Cherubism
- Defects of the teeth
  - Dilaceration
  - Connate teeth
  - Turner teeth
  - Regional odontodysplasia
  - Segmental odontomaxillary dysplasia

Generalised

- Delayed development
  - Malnutrition
  - Down's syndrome (Ch. 40)

- Hypothyroidism (Ch. 37)
- Hypoparathyroidism and pseudohypoparathyroidism
- Hypopituitarism
- Sickle cell anaemia
- Metabolic disease with delayed growth
  - Rickets (Ch. 13)
  - Infants with premature birth
  - Human immunodeficiency virus infection in infancy (Ch. 30)
- Increased resistance of overlying mucosa
  - Scarring
  - Hereditary gingival fibromatosis (Ch. 7)
  - Drug-induced gingival enlargement (Ch. 7)
- Iatrogenic
  - Chemotherapy for malignant neoplasms
  - Radiotherapy to the jaws
- Increased resistance of bone or reduced bone turnover
  - Osteopetrosis
  - Gaucher's disease

Complete or near complete failure of eruption

- Cleidocranial dysplasia (Ch. 13)
- Idiopathic or primary eruption failure

to be ankylosed after initial eruption and then overtaken by growth of the surrounding alveolus and eruption of adjacent teeth. This is a relatively common finding in the deciduous dentition, affecting around 1 in 5 children if mild infraocclusion is recognised. It is almost always mandibular molars that submerge.

Diagnosis and prevalence PMID: 26174549

Changes affecting buried teeth

Teeth may occasionally remain unerupted in the jaws for many years without complications or may undergo varying degrees of hypercementosis or resorption (Ch. 6 and Fig. 4.32). Alternatively, dentigerous cysts may develop (Ch. 10), as often happens in cleidocranial dysplasia.

Disorders of development 3

Important developmental disorders of the jaws are summarised in Box 3.1, and some are discussed more fully in other chapters.

CLEFTS OF LIP OR PALATE

Clefts of the palate alone and those of the lip, with or without cleft palate, are genetically distinct conditions. The embryology of the lower face and mechanisms of closure of the palatal shelves and fusion of the soft tissue processes to form the upper lip are very complex. Until around 6 weeks of development, the mouth and future nasal cavity are one. Then fusion of the median nasal process and maxillary processes of the first branchial arch forms the midline alveolar ridge and anterior palate, or primary palate. By the end of week 9, the secondary palate has formed by growth of the palatal shelves, their rotation and fusion. Formation of a complete palate therefore requires growth and migration of tissues, breakdown of epithelium to allow fusion of the opposite palatal shelves and growth of the mandible to allow the tongue to drop out of the way. The process takes slightly longer in females, and the longer period of development makes them more prone to palatal clefts than males. Many genes are involved, and there is a relatively long period during which an environmental insult could interfere with the process. Approximately 1 in 700 babies have clefts of lip and/or palate. Mechanisms are summarised in Figs 3.1 and 3.2.

The sites of clefts vary because the lip and anterior palate (the primary palate) develop independently and before the hard and soft palates (the secondary palate). Isolated cleft lip is therefore the result of an early developmental disorder, whereas isolated cleft palate results from influences acting later, after the primary palate has closed. By contrast, a prolonged disorder of development can prevent both primary and secondary palates from closing and leaves a severe combined cleft (Figs 3.3 and 3.4).

Clefts of both lip and palate form because of failure of growth and migration of mesenchyme to form the alveolus and lip, not because an embryological line of fusion fails to close. This growth deficiency is not necessarily localised to the jaws alone and may affect other sites including arches of cervical vertebrae. In contrast, cleft palate develops because of failure to close the cleft during development.

The main types of clefts are summarised in Box 3.2. A complete cleft of the lip is one that extends into the nose, completely separating the lip into two portions. Incomplete clefts are limited to the lip or lip and alveolus, and there is some continuity between the segments to stabilise the tissues.

Cleft lip and cleft palate

Cleft lip (with or without a palatal cleft) is a single condition that presents with varying degrees of severity. It is the most common craniofacial anomaly and affects approximately 1–2 per 1000 live births, roughly half of whom have a cleft lip alone and half of whom have cleft lip with a cleft palate. Twice as many males as females are affected, and the right side is twice as frequently involved. Native American and Asian populations have the highest incidence.

There is a strong genetic background to cleft lip and palate, but the aetiology is complex. Either dominant or recessive inheritance can be found in familial cases, whereas others appear multifactorial. The risk is considerably greater if one, and particularly if both, of the parents are affected or

---

Box 3.1   Developmental disorders of the jaws, mouth and face

Disorders of the jaws

- Clefts of the palate and/or lip
- Cleidocranial dysplasia (Ch. 13)
- Cherubism (Ch. 13)
- Basal cell naevus syndrome (Ch. 10)
- Gardner's syndrome (Ch. 12)
- Osteogenesis imperfecta (Ch. 13)
- Craniofacial anomalies
- Hereditary prognathism

Disorders of the soft tissues

- Ankyloglossia
- Cowden's syndrome
- Ehlers-Danlos syndrome (Ch. 14)
- Branchial and thyroglossal cysts (Ch. 10)
- Lingual thyroid (Ch. 37)
- White sponge naevus (Ch. 18)
- Some pigmented lesions (Ch. 26)

Disorders of the teeth (Ch. 2)

Box 3.2   Clefts of lip and/or palate

Cleft lip

- Unilateral (usually on the left side), with or without an anterior alveolar ridge cleft
- Bilateral, with or without alveolar ridge clefts
- Unilateral and bilateral clefts may be complete or incomplete

Combined lip and palatal cleft

- Unilateral
- Cleft palate with bilateral cleft lip
- Unilateral and bilateral clefts may be complete or incomplete

Palatal clefts

- Both hard and soft palate
- Soft palate only
- Bifid uvula and submucous cleft

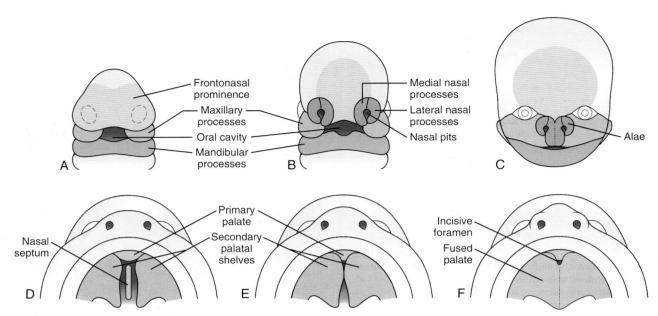

Fig. 3.1 Development of the lip and palate. Schematic diagrams of the development of the lip and palate in humans. (A) The developing frontonasal prominence, paired maxillary processes and paired mandibular processes surround the primitive oral cavity by the fourth week of embryonic development. (B) By the fifth week, the nasal pits have formed, which leads to formation of the paired medial and lateral nasal processes. (C) The medial nasal processes have merged with the maxillary processes to form the upper lip and primary palate by the end of the sixth week. The lateral nasal processes form the nasal alae. Similarly, the mandibular processes fuse to form the lower jaw. (D) During the sixth week of embryogenesis, the secondary palate develops in the form of bilateral outgrowths from the maxillary processes, which grow vertically down the side of the tongue. (E) Subsequently, the palatal shelves elevate to a horizontal position above the tongue, contact one another and commence fusion. (F) Fusion of the palatal shelves ultimately divides the oronasal space into separate oral and nasal cavities. *(From Dixon, M.J., Marazita, M.L., Beaty, T.H., et al. 2011. Cleft lip and palate: understanding genetic and environmental influences. Nat Rev Genet. 12(3), pp. 167–178.)* *PMID: 21331089*

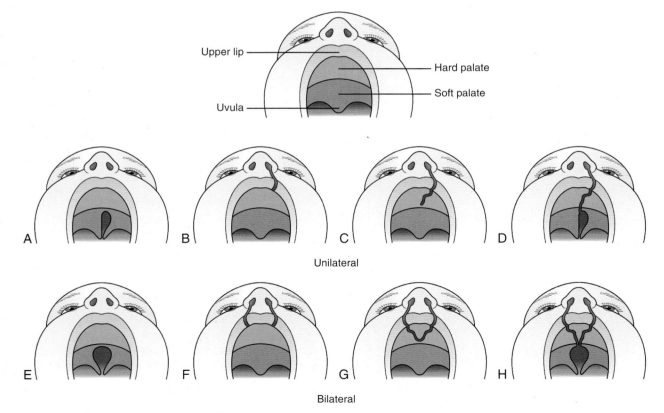

Fig. 3.2 Cleft lip and palate types. A set of illustrative drawings of cleft lip and palate types. A and E show unilateral and bilateral clefts of the soft palate; B, C and D show degrees of unilateral cleft lip and palate; and F, G and H show degrees of bilateral cleft lip and palate.
(From Dixon, M.J., Marazita M.L., Beaty, T.H., et al. 2011. Cleft lip and palate: understanding genetic and environmental influences. Nat Rev Genet. 12(3), pp. 167–178.) *PMID: 21331089*

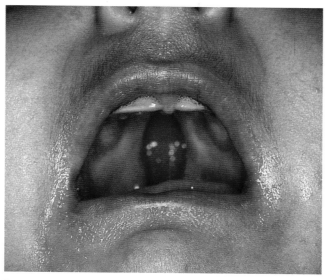

Fig. 3.3 **Cleft palate.** A broad midline cleft is present. *(Courtesy Mrs E Horrocks.)*

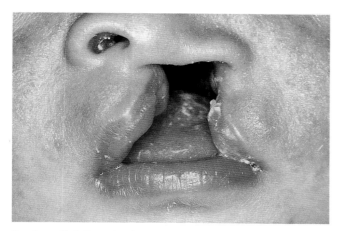

Fig. 3.4 **Cleft lip and palate.** Complete unilateral cleft of palate, alveolar bone and lip joining the oral and nasal cavities. *(Courtesy Mrs E Horrocks.)*

Box 3.3   Management of clefts: important considerations

- Psychological support for the family and later the patient
- Provision for feeding in infancy when palatal clefts are severe
- Prevention of movement of the two halves of the maxilla or premaxilla pending surgery
- Measures to counteract altered speech
- Cosmetic repair of cleft lips
- Later closure of palate
- Monitoring for hearing loss
- Speech and language therapy
- Aggressive dental prevention regime
- Restoration of anterior teeth
- Genetic counselling if syndromic

---

if a parent's cleft is severe. There are many candidate genes affecting different stages of palate development. Hedgehog pathway and *PTCH* gene variants affect growth and patterning, and TGF beta is involved in fusion. Many other genes have been implicated. *IRF6* (interferon regulatory factor 6), *FGFR2* (fibroblast growth factor receptor 2), *MSX1* (Msh homeobox1), fibroblast growth factors (*FGF1* and *FGF8*) and *BMP4* (bone morphogenetic protein 4) are the most likely.

Environmental causes are also recognised and include maternal diabetes, smoking and alcohol, and anti-epileptic, retinoid and other drugs. These environmental causes usually cause clefts combined with other developmental alterations.

Review PMID: 21331089

Management

The birth of a baby with a cleft lip triggers very early involvement of a multidisciplinary team that should include a dentist. Important considerations are summarised in Box 3.3. Immediate considerations are psychological support for the family, both for the initial shock and during many years

of treatment to follow. It is important to establish feeding as soon as possible. Cleft lip alone causes few problems, but a cleft palate prevents suckling, and either a feeding plate to close the opening or specially designed feeding bottles may be required.

Cleft lip is closed surgically, eliminating the cleft, repairing the continuity of the lip muscle and recontouring the philtrum and nasal aperture. Early surgery has the best results with least subsequent scarring and distortion, so repair is usually performed at approximately 3 months of age, but earlier in some centres. Prior to surgery, and ideally starting soon after birth, the contour of displaced tissue can be aligned using pressure from orthodontic-like appliances with extraoral tapes. However, this is complex and may not improve the final outcome.

The palatal cleft is treated initially by an obturator plate that must be replaced regularly as the child grows. Surgery is performed between 9 and 12 months of age, and a bone graft may be required for wide clefts. Surgery aims to not only close the opening but reconstruct the normal muscle attachments of the soft palate. Palatal surgery leads to scarring that inhibits maxillary growth and contributes to the

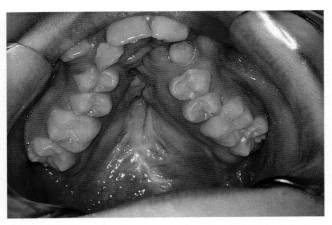

Fig. 3.5 Collapsed maxilla resulting from poorly timed surgical repair of cleft palate. Scarring and growth disturbance produce a distorted narrow maxilla. *(Courtesy Mrs E Horrocks.)*

class III appearance of the face in later life. This is reduced if surgery is performed later, but this compromises speech development. Re-operation may be necessary to lessen the deformity (Fig. 3.5).

Between the ages of 1 and 5 years, attention needs to be paid to hearing, for which ear grommets may be necessary to prevent otitis media and hearing loss. The distorted soft palate musculature fails to open the pharyngeal end of the Eustachian tube, predisposing to glue ear and infection. Poor hearing may interfere with development of speech, already compromised by the inability of the soft palate to effectively seal off the nose when plosive sounds (such as 'p' or 'b') are made. Speech therapy and sometimes soft palate surgery may be undertaken between the ages of 3 and 8 for these reasons. At approximately the age of 8 years orthodontic treatment may start, depending on need, and this and further possible surgery to reconstruct the anterior alveolus or palatal cleft may continue for several years. Thereafter, up to late teenage years, final measures are to improve appearance include excision of scars, rhinoplasty and orthognathic surgery.

More recently, observation of untreated clefts has shown that the growth potential of these tissues is virtually normal. In some centres, therefore, a soft palate cleft is repaired early, but hard palate repair is delayed until 8 or 9 years after temporary closure with an obturator. The results are good facial growth and occlusion, but speech may be impaired to some degree.

The forward rotation of the premaxilla in bilateral clefts can be managed by repositioning of this segment with bilateral bone grafts. Severe maxillary deficiency may be managed by Le Fort I internal distraction to remedy malocclusion and speech.

Despite several large clinical trials, controversies remain about the timing of these operations and the optimum approach.

Treatment review PMCID: 2884751

Surgical treatment PMID: 30851748

Dental effects

However effective the treatment, patients with clefts tend to have poor oral hygiene, gingivitis and dental caries necessitating regular preventive care.

Teeth in the region of the cleft are typically absent, malformed or have hypoplastic enamel. Dental development and eruption are delayed on the cleft side. Severe clefts are associated with absent teeth. Milder alterations are peg-shaped lateral incisors and, sometimes, development of a diminutive lateral incisor on each side of the cleft. Both deciduous and permanent dentitions are affected.

Patient experience PMID: 30072784

Isolated cleft palate

Clefts of the hard palate alone arise when the primary palate and lip form, but the palatal shelves fail to fuse posteriorly. The cleft is wider posteriorly and narrow anteriorly because the shelves fuse from front to back starting at the incisive foramen.

Isolated cleft palate affects approximately 1 in 2000 births and is approximately twice as common in females. Only occasional cases are inherited, but there is a risk of approximately 2% that a second child will be affected.

Extensive review PMID: 26973535

Submucous cleft palate

Submucous clefts are clefts of the bone or muscle covered by intact mucosa, and they are thus usually visible only as a translucent area along the midline of the soft palate. They are present in approximately 1 in 1200 births but are frequently missed. A bifid uvula is a frequent sign of a submucous cleft.

On palpation the bony cleft and a notched posterior nasal spine may be felt, and the diagnosis can be confirmed by imaging. Submucous clefts cause problems through the distortion of the attachment of the muscles of the soft palate. The chief effects are slowness in feeding and nasal regurgitation. Middle ear infections and altered speech result from the changes in muscle attachments and Eustachian tube function, as in overt clefts. Some symptoms are present in 90% of cases.

Diagnosis, and therefore operation to repair the muscle attachments is usually delayed. Earlier surgery provides better speech outcomes.

Case bifid uvula PMID: 26076543

Management

Isolated cleft palate may be missed at birth but almost immediately comes to light by causing feeding difficulties. Isolated cleft palate is treated in the same way as those associated with cleft lip.

Syndromic cleft lip and palate

Approximately 30% of all cases of cleft lip and palate and 50% of cases of cleft palate arise as part of a recognised syndrome. The most common of these is Down's syndrome, in which cleft lip or palate is present in approximately 1 in 200 patients (Ch. 40). Other syndromes with clefts are single gene disorders, and the genes involved are often the same as those implicated in non-syndromic clefts. Different mutations, polymorphisms, variable penetrance or gene control probably account for the different presentations.

Note that a cleft can be the most prominent sign of a syndrome, and also that these syndromes are often associated with other features that affect dental treatment, such as cardiac abnormalities, learning disability and dental anomalies.

Van der Woude syndrome comprises cleft lip and cleft primary and secondary palate (usually a rare combination), lower lip pits, oligodontia, a high arched palate, ankyloglossia and other features. The syndrome is inherited in an autosomal dominant pattern caused by one of several genes, but usually

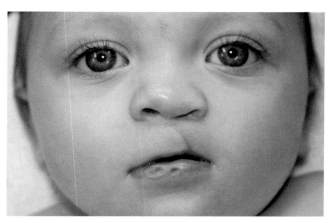

Fig. 3.6 van der Woude syndrome. Cleft lip and lower lip pits.
(From Hartzell L.D., Kilpatrick L.A., 2014. Diagnosis and management of patients with clefts: a comprehensive and interdisciplinary approach. Otolaryngol Clin North Am, 47, pp. 821-852.)

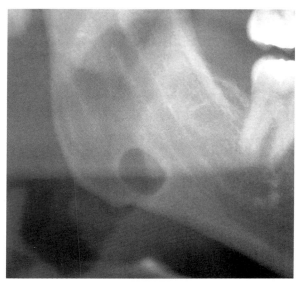

Fig. 3.8 Stafne idiopathic bone cavity. Note the characteristic site.

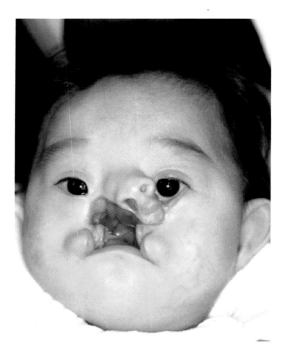

Fig. 3.7 Lateral facial cleft, a severe lateral cleft and severe bilateral cleft lip and palate. *(From Journal of Cranio-Maxillo-Facial Surgery 42 (2014) 1985e1989 42:1985-9.)*

IRF6. The lip pits are characteristic, usually one on each side of the midline and occasionally at the commissures or in the midline of the upper lip (Fig. 3.6). The pits extend several millimetres deep into the lip and may communicate with labial glands, but are not dilated minor gland ducts, rather a developmental groove between growth centres in the embryonic lip. Lip pits may also be seen in other syndromes but less frequently.

OTHER FACIAL CLEFTS

There are more extensive clefts that can develop along the lines of fusion of the maxillary and frontonasal processes (Fig. 3.7), often involving the eye and sometimes the cranium. More rarely they are in the midline. These are associated with severe distortion of the face, often with major tissue deficiency. Such facial clefts are usually continuous with a cleft lip and palate at their inferior end. Surgical correction of the clefts is extremely difficult.

STAFNE'S IDIOPATHIC BONE CAVITY

This is a relatively common developmental anomaly caused by a lobe of the submandibular gland indenting the lingual aspect of the mandible, below the level of the inferior dental nerve canal. The cortex is invaginated into the medullary space. In a panoramic or oblique lateral radiograph the concavity appears to be a circumscribed cyst in the mandible, surrounded by a layer of cortical bone.

Very occasionally one of these cavities arises in the anterior mandible, caused by inclusion of part of the sublingual gland, or ectopic salivary gland.

This condition should be diagnosed radiographically (Fig. 3.8). The cavity has a smooth rounded outline and thick even cortication and does not enlarge. Almost all are unilateral, and most patients are male. Although developmental, it appears that the cavity develops slowly in the second or third decades. Cone beam or other tomographic techniques can confirm that the mandible is indented, rather than containing a cavity. Once diagnosed, no treatment is required, and the change appears to be of no significance.

HEREDITARY PROGNATHISM

The extreme genetic form is often called 'Habsburg jaw'* and is probably a single gene disorder inherited as autosomal dominant. Although this severe inherited form is still occasionally found, most families with a protruding mandible may simply be at one end of the spectrum of normal variation,

---

* Hereditary prognathism has been associated with the Habsburg dynasty. Originally a Swiss family, the Habsburgs ruled many European countries between the 11th and 18th centuries. The trait persisted for generations through interbreeding between European royal families, particularly in the Spanish branch. However, recent evaluation of portraits suggests that the family's striking appearance was caused in part by additional hypoplasia of the maxilla, accentuating the appearance.

PMID: 24942320

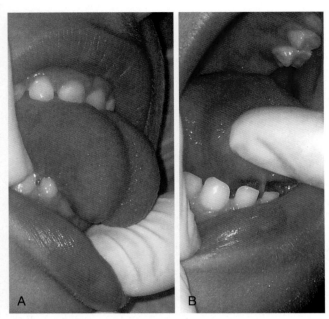

Fig. 3.9 **Ankyloglossia.** On the left the patient has been asked to protrude the tongue, but the tip is tethered to the lingual gingiva and the dorsum furrows along the midline. The tongue has to be displaced to see the tight lingual fraenum (right).

and result from polygenic inheritance. Marked prognathism can also be seen as an acquired condition in acromegaly.

ANKYLOGLOSSIA

Ankyloglossia, or tongue tie, is caused by tethering of the tongue tip to the floor of mouth, lingual alveolar mucosa or gingiva by a short lingual fraenum (Fig. 3.9). In severe cases a broad thick fraenum effectively fuses the anterior tongue to the floor of mouth. The cause is unclear but has been associated with several genes known to cause cleft palate and clefting syndromes. However, most cases are solitary abnormalities and often have a family history suggesting an autosomal dominant inheritance. Nearly half of affected individuals will have an affected first-degree relative. When there is no family history, males are usually affected. The incidence is approximately 3%.

Reduced lingual mobility can affect feeding in the neonatal period and development of an adult pattern swallow, disturbing the soft tissue guidance for tooth position. A frenal attachment high on the attached gingiva may cause a midline diastema. Speech can be affected when the tongue tip cannot contact the upper incisors. Patients develop compensatory speech and swallowing mechanisms, and the condition often regresses slightly during early childhood, so there may be no significant long-term consequences. However, the inability to sweep food debris from the mouth, protrude the tongue or eat ice cream from a cone may drive adults to seek treatment.

Routine surgical treatment is therefore controversial. The fraenum is easily divided, and if there are feeding difficulties, this is appropriate and much more easily performed shortly after birth than in an older child or adult. It is also likely to be most effective before speech and swallowing are established. In general, if a fraenum is attached to the ridge rather than the floor of mouth or within 10 mm of the tongue tip and is not elastic, it is likely to cause problems.

Not all functional tongue tie is associated with an obvious fraenum. The so-called *posterior tongue tie* is a fibrous band below the mucosa tethering the centre of the tongue. It is posterior to the usual site, but still in the anterior tongue, and best thought of as a *deep tongue tie*. The band may only be palpable or noticed because the tongue dimples centrally on movement or will not protrude. Posterior ties also cause feeding difficulties.

Ankyloglossia can develop in adults as a result of scarring diseases, typically severe forms of epidermolysis bullosa, in which the sulci become gradually obliterated by fibrosis, and the tongue is fused to the lower alveolus.

Feeding problems PMID: 12415069

Diagnosis and treatment PMID: 15839394

COWDEN'S SYNDROME

Multiple hamartoma or Cowden's syndrome* is a genetically diverse condition in which patients have mucosal polyps in the gastrointestinal tract, multiple skin and oral nodules and a high risk of developing malignant neoplasms. Mutations are classically in the *PTEN* gene (a tumour suppressor gene that normally acts to inhibit the PI3K and MAPK signalling pathways), although many variants associated with other genes exist.

Inheritance is usually autosomal dominant and skin and mucosal lesions develop in the second decade. Skin lesions are more obvious, with multiple nodules 1 or 2 mm in diameter around the nose and mouth particularly (Fig. 3.10). Histologically the nodules can be found to be caused by a variety of hamartomas including trichilemmomas and neuromas. Multiple oral nodules develop on the dorsum of the tongue, gingiva and buccal mucosa. The appearance is often referred to as *papillomatosis* because of its shape, but viral papillomas are not a feature. All these nodules are benign.

Diagnosis is largely clinical because the oral lesions appear like fibroepithelial polyps on biopsy and have no specific features. Suspected cases need urgent investigation because

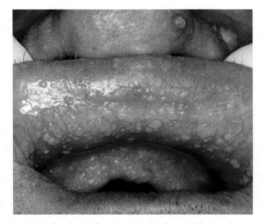

Fig. 3.10 **Cowden's syndrome.** Multiple nodules and papillomatous appearance on labial mucosa and alveolar ridge.
(From Flores, I.L., Romo, S.A., Tejeda Nava, F.J., et al. 2014. Oral presentation of 10 patients with Cowden syndrome. Oral Surg Oral Med Oral Pathol Oral Radiol, 117[4], pp. e301-e310.) PMID: 24560406

---

*Cowden's syndrome is one of the few syndromes named after the patient, rather than the person who first described it.

the risk of breast and thyroid carcinomas in later life is so high.

Web URL 3.1 Review: http://emedicine.medscape.com/article/1093383-overview

Web URL 3.2 Online risk assessor: http://www.lerner.ccf.org/gmi/ccscore/

OTHER CRANIOFACIAL MALFORMATIONS

There are many rare syndromes and diseases with characteristic craniofacial changes. Key features are shown in Table 3.1. The craniosynostoses are caused by early fusion of sutures, distorting the shape of the skull while it grows.

Table 3.1 Other craniofacial malformations

Disorder	Type/cause	Dental and oral signs	Other features
Crouzon syndrome (craniofacial dysostosis)	Cranial synostosis resulting from mutation in fibroblast growth factor 2 gene. Autosomal dominant or sporadic mutations	Small maxilla, dental crowding, high narrow palate, anterior open bite	Varied abnormal skull shape, proptosis and hypertelorism, increased intracranial pressure, hearing loss. Normal intelligence. Epilepsy in 10%
Apert syndrome	As Crouzon syndrome, this is an allelic disorder sharing many features	As Crouzon syndrome, soft palate cleft in one-third of cases, progressive enlargement of posterior alveolus soft tissue. Delayed tooth eruption	As Crouzon syndrome with additional syndactyly and other hand and foot malformations. Learning disability, which can be reduced by early surgery
Treacher-Collins syndrome (mandibulofacial dysostosis)	Developmental anomaly of the first and second branchial arches, autosomal dominant and frequent sporadic mutations in one of three known causative genes affecting neural crest development	High arched palate and crowding. Small mandible with small coronoid process, cleft palate in one-third of cases, severe lateral facial clefts and absent parotid glands occasionally	Characteristic narrow face with small zygoma and outward slanting eyelids. Colobomas (notches) on lower eyelid and absent eyelashes, deformed outer and middle ear, deafness
Hemifacial microsomia (Goldenhaar syndrome)	A unilateral developmental anomaly of the first and second branchial arches	Cleft palate and facial clefts occasionally	Cardiac, vertebral and central nervous alterations. Deformed outer and middle ear, deafness, colobomas on upper eyelids, accessory auricles in front of ears. Very variable presentation, similar to Treacher-Collins but usually unilateral

Dental caries | 4

Quote: 'For sweetness and decay are of one root and sweetness ever riots to decay'.

Ou-Yang Hsiu of Lu-ling (AD 1007–1072)

Dental caries is a disease characterised initially by intermittent subsurface demineralisation of teeth by acids, created by bacterial metabolism of dietary refined sugars. Untreated dental caries is the most common of all diseases worldwide and still a major cause of loss of teeth despite being completely preventable.

The ultimate effect of the caries process is to cause breakdown of enamel and dentine and thus open a path for bacteria to reach the pulp. The consequences of the caries process, even from its earliest stages, include inflammation of the pulp and, later, of the periapical tissues. Acute pulpitis and apical periodontitis caused in this way are the most common causes of toothache. Infection can spread from the periapical region to the jaw and beyond. Although this is nowadays extremely rare in the UK, people in other countries occasionally die from this cause.

Global burden caries PMID: 23720570

Extensive general review PMID: 28540937

AETIOLOGY

In 1890, W. D. Miller showed that lesions similar to dental caries could be produced by incubating teeth in saliva when carbohydrates were added. Miller concluded that caries could result from decalcification caused by bacterial acid production. Miller's basic hypothesis was confirmed in 1954, when Orland and his associates in the United States showed that caries did not develop in germ-free animals.

It has become conventional to consider caries to be multifactorial (Fig. 4.1 and Box 4.1). However, although the multifactorial concept aids understanding, it is critical to realise that caries is caused by dietary sugar intake. All other factors are dependent on that or only modify its effect. The cause of caries is eating refined sugars.

Primary role sugar PMID: 24892213

Diet and caries PMID: 26261186

BACTERIAL PLAQUE

Plaque is an adherent deposit that forms on tooth surfaces. It consists of an organic matrix containing a dense concentration of bacteria (Figs 4.2–4.3). Plaque is further discussed in chapter 7.

In microbiological terms, plaque is a biofilm of bacteria embedded in an extracellular polysaccharide matrix. In the protected environment in a biofilm, conditions are very different from those on a clean tooth surface or in saliva. Bacteria in biofilms can exhibit cooperative activity and behave differently from the same species in isolation in a laboratory culture medium. As a consequence, a biofilm may

be resistant to antimicrobials or to immunological defences to which the individual bacterial species are normally sensitive. The biofilm traps and concentrates bacterial products, favouring survival and interactions between species. Bacterial plaque must therefore be regarded as a living ecosystem and not as a mere collection of bacteria. Plaque is not necessarily pathogenic. It is normal and it is not sensible to try to eradicate it. Plaque concentrates fluoride and has mild protective effect against erosion caused by extrinsic acids. However, in terms of disease, its key feature is the ability to produce, concentrate and retain acid.

Clinically, bacterial plaque is a tenaciously adherent deposit on the teeth. It resists the friction of food during mastication and can only be readily removed by toothbrushing. However, neither toothbrushing nor fibrous foods will remove plaque from inaccessible surfaces or pits ('plaque traps' or 'stagnation areas'; see Fig. 4.4). This tenacious adherence is mediated by the matrix polysaccharides.

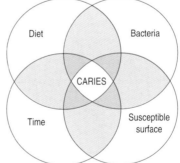

Possible interventions
- Reduce intake of cariogenic sugars, particularly sucrose

Possible interventions
- Reduce *Streptococcus mutans* numbers by reduction in sugar intake
  Active or passive immunisation

Diet   Bacteria

CARIES

Time   Susceptible surface

Possible interventions
- Avoid frequent sucrose intake ('snacking')
- Stimulate salivary flow and sugar clearance

Possible interventions
- Water and other types of fluoridation
- Prevention during post-eruptive maturation
- Fissure sealing
- Remineralising solutions
- Properly contoured restorations

Fig. 4.1 The causes of dental caries.

Box 4.1   Essential requirements for development of dental caries

- Bacterial plaque biofilm
- Cariogenic (acidogenic) bacteria
- Plaque biofilm stagnation sites
- Fermentable bacterial substrate (sugar)
- Susceptible tooth surface
- Time

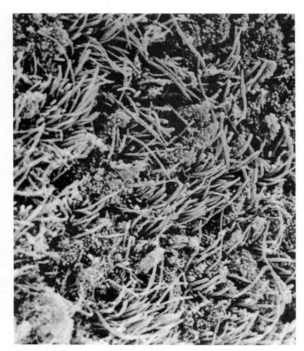

Fig. 4.2 This scanning electron micrograph of plaque shows the large number of filamentous organisms and, in addition, many cocci clustered amongst them. *(Courtesy Dr SJ Jones.)*

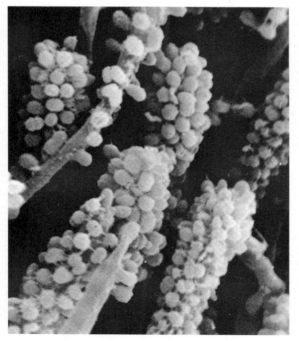

Fig. 4.3 This scanning electron micrograph at higher power shows cocci attached to filamentous organisms to produce the corn-cob type of arrangement sometimes seen in plaque. *(Courtesy Dr SJ Jones.)*

Plaque becomes visible, particularly on the labial surfaces of the incisors, when toothbrushing is stopped for 12–24 hours. It appears as a translucent film with a matt surface that dulls the otherwise smooth and shiny enamel. It can be made obvious by staining with disclosing agents. Little plaque forms under conditions of starvation, but it forms rapidly and abundantly on a high-sucrose diet.

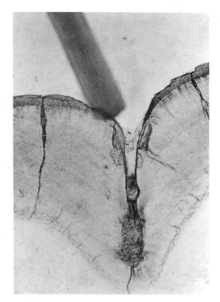

Fig. 4.4 The stagnation area in an occlusal fissure. A ground section of a molar showing the size of the stagnation area in comparison with a toothbrush bristle placed above it. The complete inaccessibility of the fissure to cleaning is obvious.

Box 4.2 Stages of plaque formation

- Deposition of structureless cell-free, pellicle of salivary glycoprotein
- Colonisation of the cell-free layer by bacteria, particularly by *Streptococcus sanguis* and *Streptococcus mutans* strains within 24 hours
- Progressive build-up of plaque biofilm by bacterial polysaccharides and bacterial growth
- Sequential recruitment of different species
- Proliferation of filamentous and anaerobic species as the plaque thickens and matures
- Establishment of a stable bacterial ecosystem

In areas where plaque is undisturbed, growth of bacteria and secretion of matrix thicken the plaque. If sugars are available, they are metabolised to the acid that causes dental caries.

Stages of formation of bacterial plaque

If teeth are thoroughly cleaned by polishing with an abrasive, plaque quickly re-forms (Box 4.2), initially as a pellicle of salivary glycoprotein that gradually thickens and becomes colonized by bacteria from saliva.

MICROBIOLOGY

Substantial evidence indicates that streptococci are associated with the development of caries, particularly of smooth (interstitial) surfaces. These include viridans streptococci, which are a heterogeneous group including *Streptococcus mutans*, *Streptococcus sobrinus*, *Streptococcus salivarius*, *Streptococcus mitior* and *Streptococcus sanguis*. These have the ability to partially lyse blood in laboratory agar culture plates to a green colour (α-haemolysis), hence the name viridans, meaning green.

Viridans streptococci vary in their ability to attach to different types of tissues, their ability to ferment sugars (particularly sucrose) and the concentrations of acid thus produced. They also differ in the types of extracellular polysaccharides that they form.

Certain species, S. mutans and S. sobrinus (together forming the 'mutans group' streptococci) are strongly acidogenic; at low pH, with freely available sucrose, they also store an intracellular, glycogen-like, reserve polysaccharide. When the supply of external substrate dries up, the reserve is metabolised to continue acid production for a time. Drastic reduction in dietary sucrose intake is followed by virtual elimination of S. mutans from plaque and reduces or abolishes caries activity. When sucrose is made freely available again, S. mutans rapidly re-colonises the plaque.

Completely germ-free animals do not develop dental caries when fed a sucrose-rich diet. Experiments using animals known to be colonised by only known species (gnotobiotes) have shown that the most potent causes of dental caries are a limited number of strains of the S. mutans group. Other species are cariogenic, but more weakly, including lactobacilli, bifidobacteria, and less frequent species Atopobium sp. and Slackia sp.

S. mutans and S. sobrinus strains are a major component of plaque in human mouths, particularly in persons with a high dietary sucrose intake and high caries activity (Fig. 4.5). S. mutans isolated from such mouths are virulently cariogenic when introduced into the mouths of animals.

Many other species of micro-organisms can also be found in plaque. However, few others are capable of causing caries in animal models and no others are as virulent. However, the complex ecosystem of plaque includes other species that may interact with and contribute to the cariogenic species being able to persist in plaque when substrate is sparse and to maintain a plaque community that allows them to exert their cariogenic effect.

Caries lesions tend to develop at specific sites, usually approximally or in occlusal pits and fissures, and the cariogenic bacteria are found in the plaque overlying the caries, not floating free in the saliva. These sites tend to be plaque biofilm stagnation areas that are difficult for the patient to clean (Fig. 4.4).

Plaque microbiology ISBN-13: 978-0443101441

The ecological and dysbiotic plaque hypotheses

Although much evidence points to S. mutans and S. sobrinus as the cause of caries, it is possible to have high S. mutans levels in plaque but no caries, and the proportion of S. mutans found in carious lesion flora by nucleic acid sequencing is usually low. This low frequency does not suggest low importance. Current research suggests that S. mutans can only cause caries when it is a component of a mixed plaque that fosters its virulence. S. mutans survives best in acidic plaque at high sucrose levels but requires other organisms to reduce the plaque pH if no sucrose is available, and to provide a supportive ecosystem that allows it to survive. These other organisms may well benefit from the presence of S. mutans, so the whole plaque ecology must be seen as interdependent and cariogenic. The ecological plaque hypothesis suggests that a plaque containing other acid producing and acid resistant bacteria is important to modulate the virulence of S. mutans. Such other species include *Streptococcus mitis*, *Streptococcus oralis*, S. salivarius and *Streptococcus anginosus*, *Lactobacilli sp.*, *Scardovia wiggsiae* (particularly in early childhood caries) and these species are often major constituents of plaque and their roles remain to be clarified. Thus S. mutans should not be blamed as the sole cause of caries. The cariogenic flora revealed by nucleic acid sequencing contains many species and varies between individuals.

Plaque can thus exist in a non-pathogenic commensal state in which the flora either loses or constrains the pathogenic species. Caries is associated with a 'dysbiotic shift' in which supply of refined sugars alters the ecology of the plaque to favour pathogenic species and strains. Time is required for the pathogenic plaque to cause disease, and reversal of the shift within a few months re-establishes the benign flora and may prevent disease. In addition, the flora may be different in different carious lesions in the same mouth.

This explains why caries prediction tests based on S. mutans levels alone are poorly predictive in individual patients. It suggests that properties shared by a group of bacteria are more important (Box 4.3). The hypothesis is very similar to the current view of how periodontitis is caused by a dysbiotic plaque (Ch. 7).

Ecological plaque hypothesis PMID: 20924061 and 12624191

Complexity in microbiology of caries PMID: 28266108

Bacterial polysaccharides

The ability of S. mutans and S. sobrinus to initiate smooth surface caries and form large amounts of adherent plaque depends on its ability to polymerise sucrose into high molecular weight, sticky, insoluble extracellular polysaccharides (glucans). Their cariogenicity depends as much on ability to

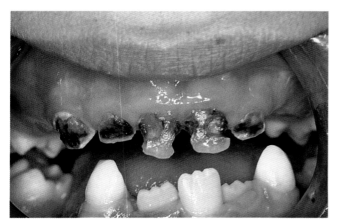

Fig. 4.5 Extensive caries of deciduous incisors and canines. This pattern of caries is particularly associated with the use of sweetened dummies and sweetened infant drinks.

Box 4.3   Essential properties of cariogenic bacteria
• Acidogenic, usually producing lactic acid
• Able to produce a pH low enough (usually pH 5) to decalcify enamel
• Able to survive and continue to produce acid at any pH
• Possess attachment mechanisms for adhesion to salivary glycoprotein in pellicle and plaque matrix
• Able to produce extracellular adhesive, insoluble plaque polysaccharides (glucans)
• Able to produce intracellular polysaccharide nutrient reserve
• Able to survive in the competitive bacterial environment of plaque

form large amounts of insoluble extracellular glucans as on ability to produce acid.

Glucans enable streptococci to adhere to one another and to stick to and colonise the tooth surface, via specific receptors on the bacteria. In this way, mutans group streptococci can colonise freshly cleaned sites, spread from site to site and enable a critical thickness of plaque to build up. The cariogenicity of different *S. mutans* strains is strongly related to production of sticky, insoluble, extracellular glucan. The proportions of the different types of polysaccharide, and the overall amounts formed, depend both on the strains of bacteria present and the different sugars in the diet.

The importance of sucrose in this activity is explained by the high energy of its glucose–fructose bond, which allows the synthesis of polysaccharides by glucosyltransferase without any other external source of energy. Sucrose is thus the main substrate used to make such polysaccharides. On a sucrose-rich diet, the main extracellular polysaccharides are glucans, glucose polymers. Other sugars are, to varying degrees, less cariogenic (in the absence of preformed plaque), partly because they are less readily formed into cariogenic glucans. Fructans formed from fructose are more soluble, produced in smaller amounts and less important in caries.

Acid-producing micro-organisms that do not produce insoluble polysaccharides do not appear to be able to cause caries of smooth surfaces. Even *S. mutans* becomes non-cariogenic when mutations cause it to produce soluble rather than insoluble polysaccharides. Polysaccharides thus contribute to the adhesiveness, bulk and resistance to solubilisation of plaque by saliva.

Although the bacteria produce the acid that demineralises the teeth, polysaccharide is critically important to build up the thick plaque in which the acid can persist, protected from the washing and buffering action of saliva (Fig. 4.6).

Important points about microbiological aspects of dental caries are summarised in Box 4.4.

Plaque matrix PMID: 24045647

S. mutans PMID: 14977543 and 30064426

Acid production in plaque

Sucrose diffuses rapidly into plaque, and acid production quickly follows. These changes can be measured directly in the human mouth by using microelectrodes in direct contact with plaque. It has been shown by this means that, after rinsing the mouth with a 10% glucose solution, the pH falls within 2–5 minutes, often to a level sufficient to decalcify enamel. Even though no more sucrose may be taken and the surplus is washed away by the saliva, the pH level remains at a low level for approximately 15–20 minutes; it returns only gradually to the resting level after approximately an hour. These changes (plotted in the so-called *Stephan curve*) are shown diagrammatically in Fig. 4.7. The rapidity with which the pH falls reflects the speed with which sucrose can diffuse into plaque and the activity of the enzymes produced by the great numbers of bacteria in the plaque. The slow rate of recovery to the resting pH – a critical factor in caries production – depends mainly on factors summarised in Box 4.5.

Acid production, mainly lactic acid, is responsible for caries lesions. When plaque is sampled after exposure to sucrose, lactic acid is the quantitatively predominant acid,

> **Box 4.4   Microbiological aspects of dental caries**
>
> - Dental caries is a bacterial disease
> - The organisms mainly associated with caries are the members of the mutans streptococci group, *Streptococcus mutans* and *Streptococcus sobrinus*
> - The cariogenicity of *S. mutans* has been established by inoculating it into the mouths of otherwise germ-free animals (gnotobiotes)
> - The presence of *S. mutans* in the human mouth is associated with caries activity
> - Other bacteria such as lactobacilli and bifidobacteria contribute to caries, but are relatively weakly cariogenic
> - Plaque cannot be eradicated by antibiotic or antibacterial agents
> - Plaque can be commensal and non-pathogenic
> - A 'dysbiotic shift' to pathogenic plaque is triggered by availability of nutrient sugars

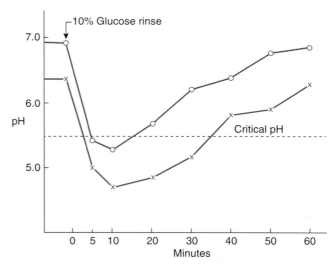

Fig. 4.7 Stephan curves showing the pH in plaque after a sucrose rinse. When the pH falls below the critical level, enamel is at risk of demineralisation. Patients with active caries tend to show a lower fall in pH, as in the lower curve because they have a more cariogenic acidogenic plaque. Note the very rapid fall in pH and the slow recovery to the normal level in spite of the very short time the sugar is in the mouth. Carbohydrates which stick to the teeth have a more prolonged effect.

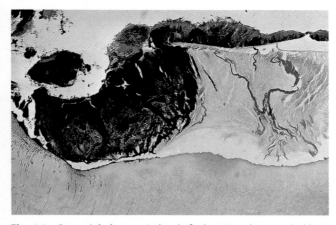

Fig. 4.6   Bacterial plaque. A decalcified section showing darkly staining plaque lying on enamel and within a carious cavity, dentine below. The strongly adhesive nature of plaque is demonstrated by the fact that it has remained intact during tooth extraction and all the processes required to make a section.

particularly during the trough of the Stephan curve. Lactic acid has a lower pK constant and causes a greater fall in pH than equimolar solutions of acetic or propionic acids that may also be detected in plaque.

Stephan curve PMID: 23224410

Plaque minerals

In addition to bacteria and their polysaccharides, salivary glycoproteins, proteins and other components also contribute to the plaque matrix. Calcium, phosphate ions and, often, fluorides are present in significant amounts. There is some evidence of an inverse relationship between calcium and phosphate levels in plaque and caries activity or sucrose intake. The ability of plaque to concentrate calcium and phosphorus is an important factor in the mechanism of caries prevention by mineralising mouthwashes. The level of fluoride in plaque may be high, ranging from 15–75 ppm or more, and is largely dependent on the fluoride level in the drinking water and diet. This fluoride is probably mostly bound to organic material in the plaque but, at low pH levels may become unbound and active in ionic form.

SUCROSE

Ingestion of sucrose leads to a burst of metabolic activity in the plaque, the acid reducing the pH before slowly returning to the resting level. The frequency with which substrate is made available to the plaque is therefore important. When sucrose is taken as a sweet drink, any surplus beyond the capacity of the organisms in the plaque to metabolise it at the time is washed away. If sucrose-containing drinks are taken repeatedly at short intervals, the supply of substrate to the bacteria can be sufficiently frequently renewed to cause acid in the plaque to remain persistently at a destructive level.

A similar effect may be caused by carbohydrate in sticky form, such as a caramel, which clings to the teeth and is slowly dissolved, releasing substrate over a long period. A given amount of sucrose is more cariogenic when fed to animals in small increments at intervals than when the same total amount is fed as a single dose.

In addition to acid production, providing sucrose leads to a significant increase in synthesis of bacterial extracellular polysaccharide. This thickens plaque and prevents acid from diffusing away and being neutralised by saliva.

Colonisation by cariogenic bacteria, especially *S. mutans*, is highly dependent on the sucrose content of the diet. Sucrose is required for initial colonisation, and increasing

availability increases the number of *S. mutans* in plaque. Conversely, severe reduction in dietary sucrose causes *S. mutans* to decline in numbers or disappear from plaque.

Essential features of sucrose incriminating it as the most cariogenic substrate are summarised in Box 4.6.

Primary role sugar PMID: 24892213

Diet and caries PMID: 26261186

Epidemiological studies

The importance of sucrose in human caries is seen in epidemiological studies and a few interventional studies, as summarised in Box 4.7.

Dental caries has been most prevalent in well-nourished, Westernised communities with sucrose-rich diets. Communities living on traditional diets with little or no sucrose had a low prevalence of caries, as seen, for example, in studies of parts of China and of Africa, the Seychelles, Tristan da Cunha, Alaska and Greenland. Many studies were carried out on Inuit races who were caries-free when consuming their traditional diet of seal or whale meat and fish. These non-cariogenic diets vary widely in their composition. The one common feature, and one differentiating them sharply from Westernised diets, is low or negligible consumption of refined sugar, particularly sucrose. Unfortunately, the low cost of sucrose, its near addictive properties and globalization have spread caries to these previously caries-free populations.

Britain is an example of a country where consumption of sucrose has been exceptionally high, though it has recently started to fall. In Britain and other countries, the incidence of caries has risen roughly parallel with rising consumption of sucrose. Food shortages during the 1939–1945 war largely abolished sucrose from the diet and in Britain, Norway and Japan and caries rates fell dramatically (Fig. 4.8). When sucrose became plentiful at the end of the war, caries prevalence rose progressively. Public health measures and fluoridated toothpaste are considered the main reasons for dramatic falls in prevalence over the last decades.

In the UK in 1973, 6% of 12-year-olds had caries, with a mean DMFT (decayed, missing or filled teeth) of 5 teeth. By 2010, the percentage had dropped to 2% and the DMFT to 2. However, prevalence in the deciduous dentition remains high, and in 2013 (the most recent UK survey), 27% of 5-year-olds had decayed teeth and caries is becoming a disease of disadvantaged groups.

Sugar changed history ISBN-13: 978-0140092332

Development of caries and 'Westernisation' of the diet are closely linked. Many countries with a previously low caries incidence still have older adults who are caries-free, but the prevalence of dental caries among children and young people has risen rapidly caused by sweet-eating habits and processed foods with 'hidden' sugars. This effect has also been strikingly well documented in the population of Tristan da Cunha who, until the late 1930s, lived on a simple meat, fish and vegetable diet with a minimal sucrose content and had a very low caries prevalence. With the adoption of Westernised diet, the caries prevalence had risen to eightfold in some age groups by the mid-1960s, after the entire population was temporarily evacuated to the UK.

International increase caries PMID: 19281105

Web URL 4.1 USA caries epidemiology: http://www.nidcr.nih.gov/DataStatistics/FindDataByTopic/DentalCaries/

Web URL 4.2 US caries epidemiology: https://www.cdc.gov/nchs/fastats/dental.htm

Web URL 4.3 UK child caries survey: https://digital.nhs.uk/data-and-information/publications/statistical/children-s-dental-health-survey/child-dental-health-survey-2013-england-wales-and-northern-ireland

Caries has become epidemic only in relatively recent decades while sucrose has become cheaper and widely available. In Britain, there was a sudden, widespread rise in sucrose consumption in the middle of the 19th century. This resulted both from the falling cost of production and, in 1861, the abolition of a tax on sugar. Evidence from exhumed skulls confirms the low prevalence of caries before sucrose became widely available and the steady rise in prevalence thereafter.

Patients unable to metabolise fructose because of an enzyme deficiency (hereditary fructose intolerance) cannot tolerate sucrose (a glucose-fructose disaccharide). These children avoid all sucrose-containing foods and have a comparatively low incidence of caries.

Experimental studies on humans

In the Vipeholm study, more than 400 adult patients were studied in a closed institution for people with learning disability. This was the first controlled study in humans

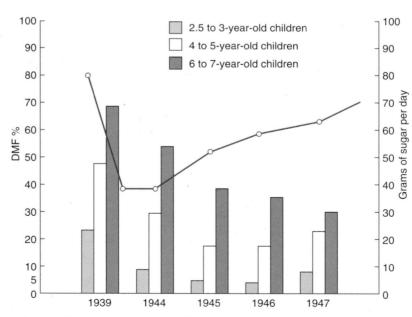

Fig. 4.8 The wartime restrictions on diet and caries in Norway. The continuous line shows an estimate of the individual daily sugar consumption during and after the war. The heights of the columns show the incidence of caries in children of various ages. Rationing of sugar started in 1938, but it is apparent that the incidence of caries declined slowly and continued for a short time after sugar became freely available. The greatest reduction in caries was in the youngest group of children whose teeth were exposed to the wartime diet for the shortest periods. *(From Toverud, G. 1949. Decrease in caries frequency in Norwegian children during World War 2. J Am Dent Assoc 39, p. 127.)*

to demonstrate the cariogenicity of sugars, but its funding and design would now be unethical. Subjects received a basic low-carbohydrate diet to establish a baseline of caries activity for each group. They were then divided into seven groups that were each allocated a different diet. A control group received the basic diet made up to an adequate calorie intake with margarine. Two groups received supplements of sucrose at mealtimes, either in solution or as sweetened bread. The four remaining groups received sweets (toffees, caramels or chocolate), which were eaten between meals.

The effects of sucrose in different quantities and of different degrees of adhesiveness, and of eating sucrose at different times, were thus tested over a period of 5 years. Caries activity was greatly enhanced by the eating of sticky sweets between meals (toffees and caramels) that were retained on the teeth. Sucrose at mealtimes only had little effect (Fig. 4.9). The incidence of caries fell to its original low level when toffees or caramels were no longer given, and caries activity was very slight in the control group having the low-carbohydrate diet.

Vipeholm original paper PMID: 13196991

Vipeholm revisited PMID: 2704974

In another large-scale clinical experiment in Turku (Finland), an experimental group was allowed a wide range of foods sweetened with xylitol (a sugar alcohol) but no sucrose. The control group was allowed as much sugary (sucrose-containing) foods as desired. After 2 years, the experimental group showed 90% less caries than those who had been allowed sucrose.

These two studies, though classics in their time and historically important, describe caries produced by a grossly cariogenic diet. Evidence from these studies has been important in linking frequency of intake to caries, and this has become a fundamental underlying principle of caries prevention. However, in a more normal diet, the amount of sugar consumed may be as important as the frequency, and current evidence suggests no level of refined sugar intake can be considered safe.

Use of sugar substitutes (artificial sweeteners) in place of sucrose greatly reduces caries activity. The cariogenicity of sugars and artificial sweeteners is summarised in Table 4.1.

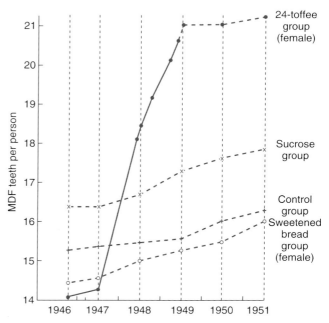

Fig. 4.9   The Vipeholm dental caries study. A simplified diagram showing the results in some of the groups of patients and, in particular, the striking effect on caries activity of sticky sweets eaten between meals when compared with the eating of sugars at mealtimes. The broken lines indicate patients who consumed sugar only at meals; the continuous line shows patients who consumed sugar both at and between meals. *(From Gustafsson, B.E., Quensel, C.E., Lanke, L.S., Lundqvist, C., Grahnen, H., Bonow, B.E., et al. 1954. The Vipeholm dental caries study; the effect of different levels of carbohydrate intake on caries activity in 436 individuals observed for five years. Acta Odontol.Scandi. 11, p. 232.)*

Table 4.1   Sugars and some non-sugar sweeteners*

Compound	Nature and uses	Cariogenicity
Sucrose	A disaccharide sugar (β1–4-linked glucose–fructose)	Highest of all sugars
Glucose, fructose	Monosaccharide sugars	Less cariogenic than sucrose
Lactose and galactose	Monosaccharide (lactose) and disaccharide (galactose) sugars	Less cariogenic than sucrose
Glucose syrups and maltodextrins	Hydrolysis products of starch used as bulk sweeteners	Less cariogenic than all sugars
Hydrogenated glucose syrup and lycasins	Hydrolysis products of starch which are then hydrogenated, used as bulk sweeteners	Less cariogenic than all sugars
Isomalt	Mixture of two unusual 12-carbon sugars	Low cariogenicity
Allulose	Similar to fructose but not metabolised as a sugar	Non-cariogenic
Sucralose	Chlorinated disaccharide of fructose and galactose, intensely sweet, used as bulk sweetener	Non-cariogenic
Xylitol, sorbitol, mannitol, lactitol etc.	Sugar alcohols (polyols) sometimes used as bulk sweeteners	Non-cariogenic
Saccharin, aspartame, thaumatin, acesulfame K and cyclamate, Stevia glycoside (rebaudioside A), Monellin, Brazzein	Non-sugar intense sweeteners	Non-cariogenic
Mogrosides	Natural intense sweetener from melons and gourds, a glycoside polycarbon compound	Insufficient data, likely very low cariogenicity

*Many new medium potency natural sweeteners are known and starting to be used.

The Turku studies PMID: 795260

Cochrane review sugar & caries PMID: 24323509

Primary role sugar PMID: 24892213

SUSCEPTIBILITY OF TEETH TO CARIES

Teeth may be resistant to decay because of factors affecting the structure of the tooth during formation. In the past it was thought that hypocalcification of the teeth or lack of calcium or vitamin D predisposed to caries. This ignored the extensive epidemiological findings that the best-nourished populations had the worst record for dental disease but is still a common belief among patients. Hereditary hypoplasia or hypocalcification of the teeth, aside from molar-incisor hypomineralisation, do not render teeth susceptible to caries. However, newly erupted teeth are generally caries susceptible until post-eruptive maturation is complete.

Effects of fluorides

Fluorides from drinking water and other sources are taken up by calcifying tissues during and after development. When the fluoride content of the water is 1 ppm or more, the incidence of caries declines substantially. Fluoride may affect caries activity by a variety of mechanisms (Box 4.8). High doses of fluoride during dental development do affect the structure of the developing teeth, as shown by mottling of the enamel. However, the lower incidence of dental caries where water is fluoridated at low level is due to its environmental effect on the teeth after eruption. This topical effect reduces solubility of the enamel and promotes remineralisation after phases of acid attack.

Although the intake of fluoride can be supplemented in many ways, water, milk, salt, toothpastes, rinses and varnish to name a few, water fluoridation is considered the most cost effective and the US Centers for Disease Control considers water fluoridation to be one of the ten most important public health measures of the 20th century.

Fluoride is the only nutrient that has been proven to have this protective action, and fluoride in water and toothpastes has had a major impact on caries prevalence. Combined with a much more recent general reduction in sucrose consumption, these factors have made caries in young people largely a disease of the disadvantaged.

Review fluoride and dental health PMID: 27352462 and 31282846

Web URL 4.4 ADA guidelines: https://www.ada.org/ then search 'fluoride clinical guidelines'

Box 4.8 Actions of fluoride on dental caries

- Fluoride is incorporated into the teeth during development (minor effect)
- Topical fluoride agents raise enamel fluoride concentration most when applied post-eruption during enamel maturation, smaller amounts are taken up my mature enamel
- Fluoride acts mainly after eruption in early lesions by reducing enamel solubility and favouring remineralisation
- A constant supply of small amounts of fluoride is most effective in reducing dental caries
- Fluoride may reduce acid generation in plaque

Web URL 4.5 UK recommendations: Perform a web search for 'delivering better oral health evidence toolkit'

Web URL 4.6 Water fluoridation policy in the UK: https://post.parliament.uk/; then search 'water fluoridation dental health'

Role of dentist in water fluoridation PMID: 23283928

Cochrane review water fluoridation PMID: 26092033

Problems with Cochrane review fluoridation PMID: 27056513

SALIVA AND DENTAL CARIES

Saliva is critical in caries. It provides natural buffers to neutralise the acids in plaque, delivers antibacterial compounds and washes sucrose and bacterial products away. However, its effectiveness is severely limited by the plaque matrix, which prevents diffusion of saliva into the plaque.

In animals, removal or inactivation of major salivary glands leads to increased caries activity roughly in proportion to the reduction in saliva production. Dental caries may also become extensive in humans with xerostomia (Ch. 22).

Buffering power

The buffering power of saliva depends mainly on its bicarbonate content and is increased at high rates of flow. The buffering power of the saliva does increase the pH of plaque to a degree and prevents the pH from falling to very low levels. A rapid flow rate, with the greater salivary buffering power that is associated, has been found to be associated with low caries activity.

Inorganic components and enamel maturation

Calcium and phosphate ions can diffuse in soluble form between the enamel surface, plaque and saliva, and concentrations at these three sites are in a dynamic equilibrium. Newly erupted teeth are more susceptible to caries than adult teeth. Radioactive tracer studies show that newly erupted teeth can incorporate 10–20 times as much calcium and phosphate as adult teeth while they undergo post-eruptive maturation. During this process, saliva can provide fluoride for incorporation into the enamel.

Antibacterial activities

Saliva contains thiocyanates, a lysozyme-like substance, the peroxidase system and other theoretically antibacterial peptides and substances. Nevertheless, the mouth teems with bacteria, and there is no evidence that non-specific antibacterial substances in saliva have any significant effect on caries activity.

Immunological defences

Immunological defences against *S. mutans* appear to be the main physiological mechanisms conferring caries resistance on some individuals. Immunological defences could be mediated by immunoglobulin (Ig)A in saliva or IgG in crevicular fluid. The IgG responses are the most important in natural resistance, but the immunity level varies widely between individuals. Protection is not that strong, as demonstrated by the fact that immunodeficiency does not predispose to dental caries. These defence mechanisms are easily overwhelmed if the diet is high in sucrose.

It has been shown that dripping a solution of monoclonal antibody against *S. mutans* onto the teeth prevents recolonisation by *S. mutans* in humans. For this to be effective, plaque must be removed before treatment by using chlorhexidine and effective oral hygiene. The effect of antibody lasts for several months after applications, and this 'passive immunisation' has the potential to reduce caries activity significantly. The effects are probably not mediated by traditional immune mechanisms but rather by binding to the bacteria and preventing adhesion to the forming new plaque. Once new plaque is established without *S. mutans,* the stable biofilm ecosystem prevents recolonisation long after the antibody has been washed away.

Key effects of saliva on plaque activity are summarised in Box 4.9.

Protective effects saliva PMID: 11842922

PATHOLOGY OF ENAMEL CARIES

Enamel, the hardest and densest tissue in the body, consists almost entirely of calcium hydroxyapatite with only a minute organic content. It forms a formidable barrier to bacterial attack. However, once enamel has been breached, infection of dentine can spread relatively easily. Preventive measures must therefore be aimed primarily at stopping the initial attack or at making enamel more resistant.

Enamel is rendered carious by acid diffusing into it and dissolving it. The crystalline lattice of calcium hydroxyapatite crystals is relatively impermeable, but the organic matrix around the apatite crystals and in prism sheaths is permeable to hydrogen ions.

Caries is not a simple solubilisation of enamel, but a dynamic process of alternating phases of demineralisation and remineralisation. This produces the defining characteristic of enamel caries, that initially the solubilisation of enamel is a subsurface process.

Enamel caries develops in four main phases (Box 4.10). These stages of enamel caries are distinguishable microscopically and are also clinically significant. In particular, the incipient or early (white spot) lesion is potentially reversible, but cavity

formation is irreversible and may require operative restorative measures to prevent progression and replace the lost tissues.

The early caries lesion

The earliest visible changes are seen as a white opaque spot that forms most frequently just below a contact point or in a fissure. Despite the chalky appearance, the enamel is hard and smooth to the probe (Fig. 4.10). The microscopic changes under this early white spot lesion can only be seen by using polarised light microscopy or microradiography.

The initial lesion is conical in shape with its apex toward the dentine and a series of four zones of differing translucency can be discerned. Working back from the deepest, advancing edge of the lesion, these zones consist first of a translucent zone; immediately within this is a second dark zone; the third is the body of the lesion and the fourth is the surface zone (Fig. 4.11). These changes are not

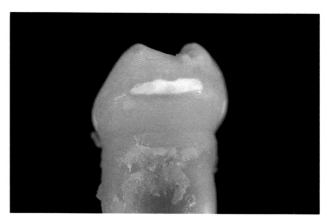

Fig. 4.10 Early enamel caries, a white spot lesion, in a deciduous molar. The lesion forms below the contact point, and is much broader than an interproximal lesion in a permanent tooth.

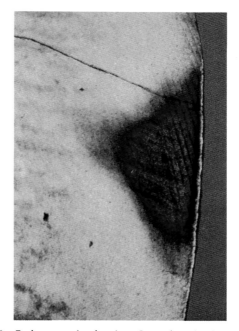

Fig. 4.11 Early approximal caries. Ground section in water viewed by polarised light. The body of the lesion and the intact surface layer are visible. The translucent and dark zones are not seen until the section is viewed immersed in quinoline.

Box 4.9 Key effects of saliva on plaque activity

- Salivary components contribute to plaque formation and form much of its matrix
- Sucrose dissolves in saliva and is actively taken up by plaque
- The buffering power of saliva may limit the fall in pH caused by acid formed in plaque
- The buffering power of saliva is related to the rate of secretion. High flow rates may be associated with lower caries activity
- Reduction in salivary secretion leads to increased caries activity when a cariogenic diet is eaten
- Immunoglobulin A is present in saliva but has little effect on caries activity; it may delay bacterial species from recolonising plaque after cleaning

---

Box 4.10 Stages of enamel caries

- White spot enamel lesion
- A white spot lesion may arrest as a brown spot lesion, or progress to…
- Cavitation
- Dentine and amelodentinal junction spread

Table 4.2 Key features of the zones of enamel caries preceding cavity formation

Zone	Key features	Comments
Translucent zone	1% mineral loss. Earliest and deepest demineralisation	Broader in progressing caries, narrow or absent in arrested or remineralised lesions
Dark zone	2%–4% mineral loss overall but a zone of remineralisation just behind the advancing front	Broader in arrested or remineralised lesions, narrow in advancing lesions
Body	5%–25% mineral loss	Broader in progressing caries, replaced by a broad dark zone in arrested or remineralised lesions
Surface zone	1% mineral loss. A zone of remineralisation resulting from the diffusion barrier and mineral content of plaque. Cavitation is loss of this layer, allowing bacteria to enter the lesion	Relatively constant width, a little thicker in arrested or remineralising lesions

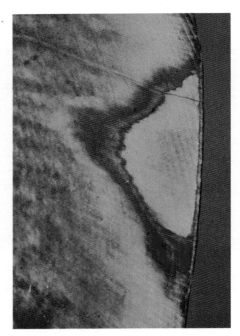

Fig. 4.12 Early approximal caries. Ground section viewed by polarised light after immersion in quinoline. Quinoline has filled the larger pores, causing most of the fine detail in the body of the lesion to disappear (Fig. 4.11), but the dark zone with its smaller pores is accentuated.

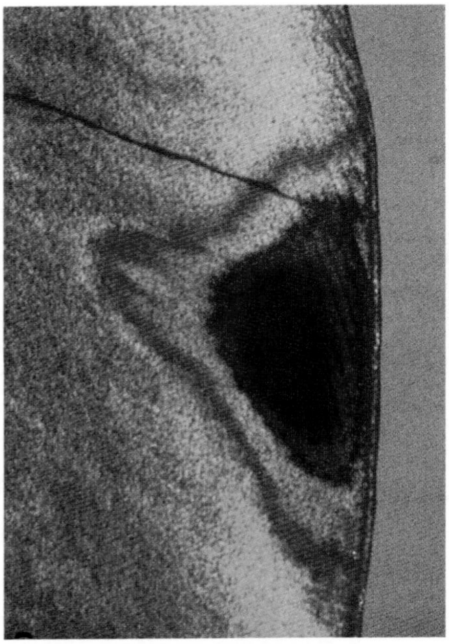

Fig. 4.13 The same lesion (Figs 4.11 and 4.12) viewed dry under polarised light to show the full extent of demineralisation. (Figs 4.11–4.13). *(by Silverstone, L.M., 1983. Remineralisation and enamel caries. New concepts. Dental Update 10, 261–273.)*

due to bacterial invasion, but due to demineralisation and remineralisation in the enamel. The surface remains intact and bacterial cannot enter the lesion. The features of these zones are summarised in Table 4.2.

The translucent zone is the deepest zone. The appearance of the translucent zone results from formation of sub-microscopic spaces or pores where acid has dissolved apatite crystals located at prism boundaries and other areas of high organic content such as the striae of Retzius. The translucent zone is so-called because of its appearance when the section is viewed in polarised light and mounted in quinoline, a compound with the same refractive index as enamel used in experiments on caries in vitro (Fig. 4.12).

The dark zone is fractionally superficial to the translucent zone and shows a greater degree of demineralisation and pores, reflecting lost solubilized apatite, amounting to 2%–4% of the enamel volume. The dark zone is so-called because the quinoline technique reveals additional small pores too small to be filled by quinolone. These contain air and do not transmit light, therefore appearing dark under the microscope. These small pores are caused by remineralisation shrinking larger pores, evidence that caries has phases of repeated demineralisation and remineralisation. Caries lesions that are very slowly progressing or arrested have much wider dark zones and a smaller translucent zone and body, reflecting a greater degree of remineralisation.

The body of the lesion forms the bulk of the lesion and extends from just beneath the surface zone to the dark zone. The body is predominantly a zone of demineralisation. Within it, the striae of Retzius appear enhanced, particularly when mounted in quinoline and viewed under polarised light. Polarised light examination (Fig. 4.13) also shows that apatite loss, as judged by the pore volume, is 5% at the junction with the dark zone, but increases to at least 25% in the centre. Microradiography, which will detect demineralisation in excess of 5%, reveals radiolucent lesions that correspond closely with the size and shape of the body of the lesion (Fig. 4.14). Alternating radiopaque and radiolucent lines, approximately 30 µm apart, can also be seen passing

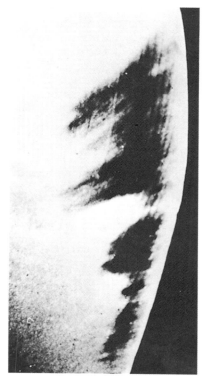

Fig. 4.14 Early approximal caries. A microradiograph of the same section as in Figs 4.11–4.13, showing radiolucency following the same pattern, the intact surface zone and showing spread selectively along the striae of Retzius. *(Courtesy Professor AI Darling.)*

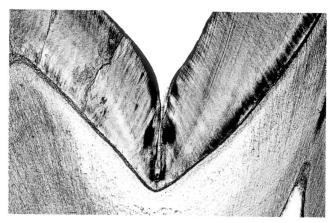

Fig. 4.15 Undecalcified section showing early enamel lesions, seen as dark patches, on each side and around the end of an occlusal fissure.

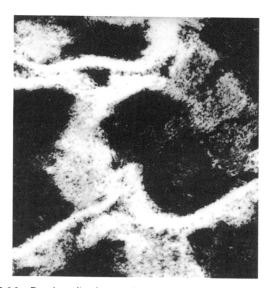

Fig. 4.16 Demineralised enamel. An electron photomicrograph of enamel produced after the action of very dilute acid. The crystallites of calcium salts remain intact in the prism sheaths, while the prism cores and some of the interprismatic substance have been destroyed. The same appearance is seen in early caries. *(Courtesy Dr K Little.)*

obliquely through the subsurface region. These are produced by preferential demineralisation along the striae of Retzius.

The surface zone is the most important zone in terms of prevention and management of the disease. It shows the paradoxical feature that it is much more heavily mineralised than the body and dark zones below it. It remains intact during demineralisation of the subsurface enamel and has a pore volume of only 1%. The explanation is that the surface zone is formed by remineralisation. In vitro, if the surface zone is removed and the enamel is exposed to an acid buffer, the more highly mineralised surface zone forms again by remineralisation using calcium and phosphate from the plaque or diffusing out from the deeper demineralised zones. The thin plaque layer on the surface acts as a diffusion barrier slowing the outward movement of calcium and phosphate, which therefore concentrate near the surface and reprecipitate.

In pit and fissure caries, the same changes take place, but separate lesions form back-to-back on the opposite lateral walls of the fissure. In a two-dimensional sectional view, the same zones as in smooth surface caries are seen on either side of the fissure (Fig. 4.15).

As noted earlier, the initial attack on enamel appears to be by highly mobile hydrogen ions permeating the organic matrix to attack the surface of the apatite crystals (Figs 4.16). The apatite crystals become progressively smaller, reducing from the normal diameter of 35–40 nm to 25–30 nm and in the body of the lesion to 10–30 nm. In the dark zone, by contrast, enamel crystals appeared to have grown to 50–100 nm and in the surface zone to 35–40 nm. These findings confirm that both demineralisation and remineralisation occur in caries lesions. This changes once cavitation develops

and demineralisation comes to dominate the process. Until then, bacteria cannot physically penetrate enamel because of the intact surface layer.

Structure of carious lesions PMID: 15286119

Chemistry of dissolution PMID: 11132767

Cavitation: cavity formation

While the surface layer is intact, bacteria cannot enter the enamel and caries can only progress by diffusion of acid through plaque and into the enamel. If acid attack reaches a critical level or frequency, demineralisation overwhelms the remineralising process that maintains the surface zone, and it breaks down to form a cavity ('cavitation') (Fig. 4.17). Once bacteria can enter the lesion, demineralisation is favoured, and the caries progresses toward the dentine more quickly.

Caries first reaches the enamel-dentine junction at a small area below the centre of the lesion because of the conical shape of the enamel lesion. It then spreads laterally to undermine the

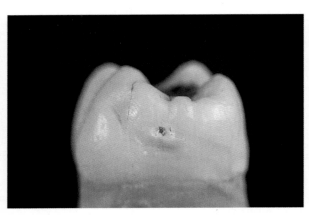

Fig. 4.17   Early cavitation in enamel caries. The surface layer of the white spot lesion has broken down, allowing plaque bacteria into the enamel.

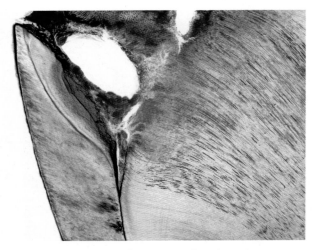

Fig. 4.18 Low-power view of caries spreading along the amelodentinal junction. Enamel, left, with cavity at the top and dentine, right. Bacteria stained dark blue fill the cavity and extend along dentinal tubules and along the amelodentinal junction. Note how caries spreads only a small distance along the amelodentinal junction in advance of caries in dentine. The amelodentinal junction is only a little more susceptible to carious spread than dentine.

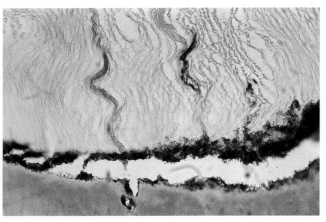

Fig. 4.19 Caries spread along the amelodentinal junction at higher power. Enamel, top, is decalcified to make the section with only matrix remaining, and dentine, below, with the bulk of the carious lesion to the right side. The greater porosity and organic content here allows caries to spread preferentially laterally, though it only spreads to match the lateral extent of the surface caries, until a late stage.

Box 4.11   Process of enamel caries

- Permeation of enamel by hydrogen ions through its organic matrix
- Demineralisation and reduced crystallite size allows acid to penetrate more deeply
- Surface zone formed by remineralisation as calcium and phosphate exiting the lesion are delayed at the surface by the plaque diffusion barrier
- There is alternating demineralisation and remineralisation
- When demineralisation is predominant, cavity formation progresses
- Just behind the advancing front there is a further zone of remineralisation, narrow in advancing lesions, broad in quiescent or arrested lesions (dark zone)
- When remineralisation is predominant, caries arrests but normal enamel cannot reform
- Bacteria cannot invade enamel until cavitation

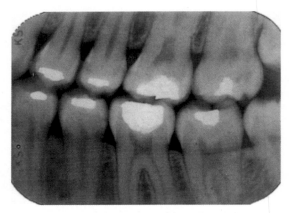

Fig. 4.20   Early enamel caries. Bitewing radiograph showing several approximal lesions, just visible, most clearly in the distal surface of the upper second premolar and mesial surface of the upper first molar. No dentine changes are seen, but they would be present microscopically.

enamel (Figs 4.18 and 4.19). This has two major effects. First, the enamel loses the support of the dentine and is therefore greatly weakened. Second, it is attacked from beneath as well as the side. Lateral spread along the amelodentinal junction is relatively limited and extends only to the widest extent of the enamel lesion at the surface, which determines the area of the initial attack on the dentine.

Once dentine is destroyed and the crown weakened, enamel starts to collapse under the stress of mastication and to fragment around the edge of the cavity, which is by then obvious clinically. By this stage, bacterial damage to the dentine is extensive.

The process of enamel caries is summarised in Box 4.11.

Natural rates cavitation PMID: 22821238

Clinical relevance ISBN: 978-1118935828

PATHOLOGY OF DENTINE CARIES

The earliest stage of dentine caries starts deep to a carious enamel lesion *before* any clinical evidence of cavitation. At the earliest detectable stage of enamel caries radiographically (Fig. 4.20), the dentine changes cannot be seen. Diffusion

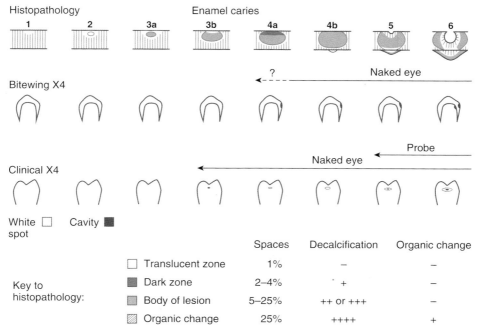

Key to histopathology:

		Spaces	Decalcification	Organic change
☐	Translucent zone	1%	−	−
■	Dark zone	2–4%	+	−
▨	Body of lesion	5–25%	++ or +++	−
▨	Organic change	25%	++++	+

Fig. 4.21 This diagram summarises the sequential changes in enamel from the stage of the initial lesion to early cavity formation and relates the different stages in the development of the lesion with the radiographic appearances and clinical findings. *(By courtesy of Darling, A.I. (Ed.), 1959. The pathology and prevention of caries. Darling. Br. Dent. J. 107, 287–302.)*

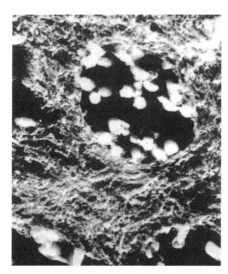

Fig. 4.22 Infection of the dentinal tubules. This electron photomicrograph shows bacteria in the lumen of the tubules. Between the tubules is the collagenous matrix of the dentine. *(Courtesy Dr K Little.)*

of acid from the enamel lesion into the dentine causes demineralisation of the mineral component but leaves the collagenous dentine matrix intact. However, once cavitation occurs and bacteria have penetrated the enamel, acid attacks the dentine over a wide area. The shape of a dentine lesion is therefore conical with a broad base at the enamel junction and its apex toward the pulp (Fig. 4.21).

Infection of dentine is facilitated by the dentine tubules, which form a pathway open to bacteria (Fig. 4.22) once they have been slightly widened by acid attack. After demineralisation, the dentine matrix is progressively destroyed by proteolytic enzymes secreted by bacteria.

The bacteria present at the advancing front of dentine caries form a diverse flora of facultative anaerobes and anaerobes. Commonly isolated species include lactobacilli, *Actinomyces*, *Bifidobacterium* and *Eubacterium*, *Atopobium sp.*, *Propionibacterium sp.* with *S. mutans* in variable amounts, the last contributing to more rapid progression. The flora is proteolytic and more dependent on the dentine matrix for nutrient than dietary sugars.

At first, the decalcified dentine retains its normal structure. Once bacteria have reached the amelodentinal junction, they extend down the tubules, soon fill them and spread along any lateral branches. The tubules become distended by the expanding masses of bacteria and their products, which the softened matrix cannot confine. Later, the intervening tubule walls are destroyed, and collections of bacteria in adjacent tubules coalesce to form irregular liquefaction foci. These, in turn, coalesce to induce progressively more widespread tissue destruction (Fig. 4.23). Eventually, the dentine is completely destroyed. In some areas, bacteria-filled clefts form at right angles to the general direction of the tubules. Clinically, these clefts may allow carious dentine to be excavated in flakes in a plane parallel to the surface (Fig. 4.24).

Caries in dentine thus has zones of demineralisation at the advancing front, bacterial penetration centrally and dentine destruction towards the surface. The degree of destruction of the dentine is critical to restorative treatment. Even in the zone of bacterial penetration, much of the dentine structure is intact and can remineralise. It is therefore possible to restore a tooth, leaving caries and bacteria below the restoration, provided the restoration is of high quality and achieves an adequate adhesive peripheral seal. No nutrients can then reach the bacteria, the caries process halts, and dentine can remineralise.

For clinical purposes, dentine caries is therefore divided into the caries-affected and caries-infected zones (Fig. 4.25). Caries-affected dentine is demineralised and its matrix only partly degraded; some of the tubular structure still remains,

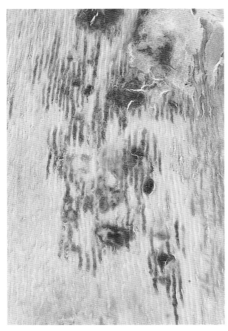

Fig. 4.23 Caries of dentine. Demineralisation has widened the tubules and bacteria, stained dark red, extend along them, further digesting dentine and spreading outwards to form rounded masses.

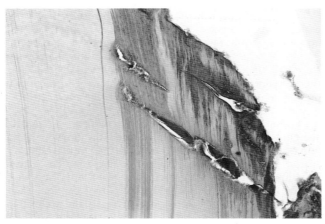

Fig. 4.24 Clefts in carious dentine. Infection is tracking down the tubules from the caries above but has also spread across the tubules, forming heavily infected clefts.

and bacterial numbers are low. In contrast the caries-infected zone, clinically identifiable as soft, wet and brown, is largely demineralised, has no residual intact matrix to remineralise, no tubules and high numbers of bacteria. The caries-infected zone cannot remineralise effectively and provides poor support for a restoration. It usually has to be removed.

The main events in dentine caries are summarised in Box 4.12.

Infected dentine relevance PMID: 26749788

Protective reactions of dentine and pulp under caries

The extension of caries into dentine is significantly slowed by a series of defence reactions mounted by vital dentine and pulp and mediated by odontoblast activity. These reactions are not specific and may be provoked by other irritants such as attrition, erosion, abrasion and restorative procedures. Changes in dentine start even before cavity formation in enamel, but take time to develop and so are more prominent under slowly

Box 4.12 Key events in the development of dentine caries
• Acid permeates to dentine even before cavitation
• Acid permeates through the organic matrix and demineralises dentine
• After enamel cavitation dentine caries accelerates
• Widening of tubules by demineralisation
• Pulp/dentine complex defence reactions start early but are variable and more marked under slowly progressing caries
• Migration of pioneer bacteria along tubules
• Development of a mixed proteolytic bacterial flora in the dentine
• Distortion of tubules by expanding masses of bacteria and breakdown of intervening matrix
• Progressive disintegration of remaining matrix tissue
• There is alternating demineralisation and remineralisation
• Remineralisation cannot reform dentine, but caries can arrest
• Pulp devitalized by acid, inflammation or bacterial extension into the pulp cavity

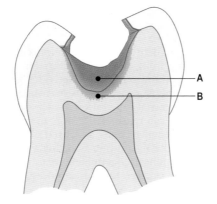
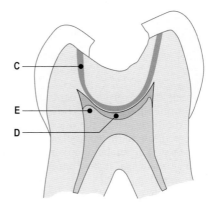

Fig. 4.25 The zones of dentine caries and pulp-dentine defence reactions. Left panel, zones of dentine caries: A, infected dentine, includes both destroyed zones and areas of bacterial penetration; B, affected dentine, demineralised dentine, with sparse bacteria only. Right panel, defence reactions: C, translucent dentine produced by peritubular sclerosis surrounds the lesion; D, regular reactionary dentine reduces the size of the pulp and protects it; E, pulpitis, the immunological and inflammatory reactions triggered by odontoblast damage does not help resistance to caries. *(Fig 9.4 p46, in Case 9 A large carious lesion. Banerjee A in Clinical Problem Solving in Dentistry 3rd edn 2010 Ed Odell E, Churchill Livingstone, Edinburgh.)*

progressing caries. Reactionary dentine is laid down by the original odontoblasts, either as peritubular dentine or in the pulp. Once the odontoblasts die, defence reactions within the dentine cannot occur, but reactive dentine can form at the pulpal surface. This is a more rapid response by odontoblast-like cells that differentiate from pulp cells. Pulpal reactions remain possible until the pulp is devitalised.

Changes in dentine in response to caries are summarised in Table 4.3.

These changes start to develop early but at best can only slow the advance of dental caries. Even the densely mineralised translucent dentine is vulnerable to bacterial acid and proteolysis, and once bacteria have penetrated the normal dentine, they can invade reactionary and reparative dentine to reach the pulp (Figs 4.26–4.30).

CLINICAL ASPECTS OF CARIES PATHOLOGY

Clinical relevance ISBN: 978-1118935828 and PMID: 27099358

Cochrane caries removal PMID: 23543523 and 34280957

Table 4.3   Reactionary changes in dentine and pulp

Response	Key facts
Translucent dentine	A form of reactionary dentine laid down within tubules, peritubular dentine. This reduces the diameter of the dentinal tubules, preventing bacterial penetration and generates a more heavily mineralised dentine by 'tubular sclerosis'. Translucent dentine usually forms in a band approximately halfway between the pulp and amelodentinal junction and along the sides of the carious lesion. It forms a hard more mineralised zone, that may be visible radiographically and is detectable with hand instruments when excavating caries.
Regular reactionary dentine	Forms at the pulp–dentine interface and retains the tubular structure of dentine. Forms in response to mild stimuli and may obliterate pulp horns, increasing the dentine thickness between caries and pulp. Unfortunately, it often forms most on the floor and sides of the pulp chamber where it is of little value in defence against caries. Formed by odontoblasts
Irregular reparative dentine	Forms in response to moderate or severe insult by caries and correspondingly ranges from dentine with irregular tubules to a disorganised bone-like mineralised tissue. Laid down by newly differentiated cells from the pulp rather than odontoblasts.
Dead tracts	Formed when odontoblasts die and their tubules become sealed off. If peritubular dentine formation was extensive before odontoblast death, the dead tract may be sclerotic and inhibit advance of caries. If not, it may allow more rapid progress.

Arrested caries and remineralisation

Pre-cavitation, or 'white spot' caries lesions, may become arrested when the balance between demineralisation and remineralisation is altered in favour of remineralisation. This might follow sucrose restriction, fluoride application or loss of one tooth adjacent to an approximal lesion, the last

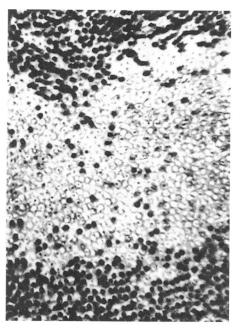

Fig. 4.26   Translucent dentine in dentine caries. The dentinal tubules are seen in cross-section. Those in the centre of the picture have become obliterated by peritubular dentine; only the original outline of the tubules remains visible or occasionally a small central dot of much reduced diameter, and the zone appears translucent to transmitted light. On either side are patent tubules filled with stain. *(Kindly lent by Dr GC Blake and reproduced by courtesy of the Honorary Editors, Blake, G.C., 1958. An experimental investigation into the permeability of enamel and dentine. Proceedings of the Royal Society of Medicine. 51, 678–686.)*

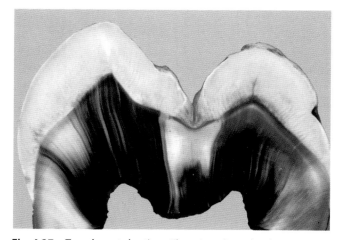

Fig. 4.27   Translucent dentine. There is early occlusal caries in the fissure, and below it peritubular dentine has sealed off the pathway to the pulp to produce a zone of translucent dentine that is less permeable to bacteria and acid. The zone has been made more visible by putting blue dye into the pulp chamber; it cannot pass along the tubules in the translucent dentine as it does elsewhere. *(From Cawson, R.H., Binnie, W.H., a Barrett, A.W., et al. 2001. Oral disease. 3rd ed. St. Louis: Mosby.)*

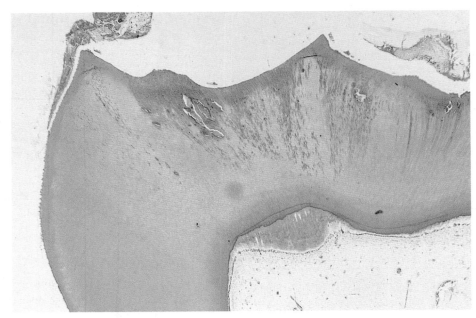

Fig. 4.28 Regular reactionary dentine below occlusal caries. The enamel has been demineralised to make the section and only dentine and pulp remain. Bacteria extend more than half the distance from the amelodentinal junction to the pulp, and the underlying pulp horn has been obliterated by reactionary dentine. The reactionary dentine bulges into the pulp. Note the lack of inflammation in the pulp, relatively well-organised tubular structure and odontoblast layer, reflecting the fact that this reactionary dentine has formed slowly.

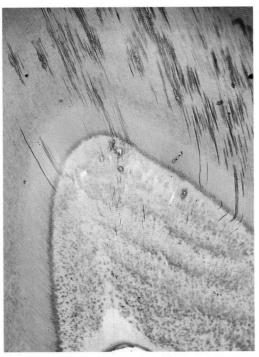

Fig. 4.29 High power view of a pulp horn obliterated by regular reactionary dentine. The occlusal caries lies at the top with bacterial penetrating down tubules to the level of the original pulp outline, seen as a darker stained line. Below this, regular, tubular, secondary dentine has formed and bacteria spreading down the tubules just extend into the tubules of the reactionary dentine. Note how the tubules change direction sharply at the interface with the normal dentine.

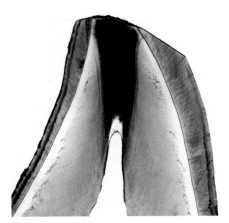

Fig. 4.30 A dead tract. The dentine below the incisal tip is 'dead'; it has no viable osteoblast processes, and dye applied to the incisal edge penetrates the tubules so that the 'dead tract' appears dark. At the proximal end of the tubules, the dead tract has been sealed off by impermeable reactionary dentine through which the stain cannot penetrate. The pulp is thus protected from irritants penetrating along the dentinal tubules, but less effectively than by translucent dentine which is more densely sclerotic and extends over a broader area. Note that the dye in this figure and Fig. 4.27 has been applied to opposite ends of the tubules.

uncovering a stagnation area and permitting adequate oral hygiene procedures. The source of calcium and phosphate to remineralise the lesion is saliva and plaque.

Caries progresses slowly, and under normal conditions, approximately 50% of approximal enamel lesions may not progress radiographically for 3 years, showing that little change may be required to favour reversal of the process. Although remineralisation may return the mineral content of an enamel lesion to close to that of the original enamel, the deposition is irregular, of a variety of different calcium phosphate salts and disorganised at the level of individual crystals. The original enamel structure cannot be regained. Despite this, remineralised lesions that have fluoride incorporated can be less prone to carious attack than intact enamel.

Arrested enamel caries may remain opaque and white or more often becomes discoloured by incorporation of extrinsic stain – the so-called *inactive* or *brown spot lesion*.

Dentine caries may also become arrested. This may result from preventive intervention or follow collapse of overlying enamel, exposing the dentine to saliva and cleaning. Dentine caries below a completely sealed restoration will also arrest and remineralise by using mineral ions that diffuse from the pulp. Remineralisation in dentine does not produce a hard material. The regrowth of crystals is less than in enamel, and the arrest process comprises cessation of demineralisation at the advancing front, cessation of dentine proteolysis by death or inhibition of bacteria in the dentine and deposition of new mineral. Remineralised arrested dentine caries does not feel like normal dentine to the probe, but is nevertheless leathery, hard, and dry, and not soft and wet like active caries.

The much greater natural porosity of dentine caries allows extrinsic stain to be incorporated into arrested caries, and this and bacterial products and reactions between acids and the matrix produce a dark brown colour to arrested dentine caries. If the pulp is vital, arrest of caries allows time for pulp defence reactions to produce peritubular dentine and translucent zones. These increase the mineral density of dentine below the lesion to slow its advance should the caries reactivate. Even the largest carious lesions can arrest if deprived of sucrose and exposed to saliva; caries below leaking restorations usually does not.

Preventive treatment to arrest and remineralise caries has become the paradigm of modern caries management, both for untreated caries and in placing restorations. This makes it important to be able to detect active and arrested caries clinically and indices originally developed for research are often used in clinical practice, notably the International Caries Detection and Assessment System (ICDAS II).

ICDAS II caries assessment PMID: 28955548

Caries in deciduous teeth

In adults, caries usually progresses slowly, and a small cavity may take several months to develop and several years to penetrate the enamel. By contrast, caries in children progresses quickly. Much of this can be accounted for by high sugar diet but, compared with permanent teeth, deciduous teeth have thinner enamel and dentine, wider flatter contact areas producing larger approximal lesions and wider dentinal tubules allowing earlier bacterial penetration.

In addition, young children develop their plaque flora in the first three or four years of life. The mouth is initially sterile and bacterial species gradually colonise the plaque by transfer from the environment and from family members. If the diet is rich in sugar, colonization by pathogenic species is favoured and once established, they become part of a stable plaque ecosystem.

Early childhood caries

Early childhood caries is defined clinically as one or more carious, missing or filled teeth in a child under 6 years. Caries in childhood is no different in its causes or pathology but has some distinctive features. It is increasing in prevalence, affecting approximately 17% of 1-year-old and 55% of 4-year-old children worldwide. Previously the term nursing bottle caries was used, as use of sweetened bottle feeds or dummies was a common cause, but any source of sugars will cause the condition, including lactose from prolonged breastfeeding (Fig. 4.31).

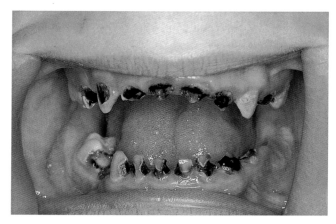

Fig. 4.31 Extensive caries in a child caused by sweetened medication but arrested by treatment and thus appearing darker than active caries.

The pattern of early childhood caries is distinctive, with rapid progression and an unusual distribution of extensive lesions on smooth surfaces of anterior teeth. Lower first deciduous molars are next affected. This pattern is probably accounted for by the mechanism of sugar intake, sugar consistency, prolonged or repeated exposure, and poor oral hygiene.

Childhood caries treatment recommendations PMID: 32610317

Hidden caries

'Occult' or hidden caries describes the situation in which caries starts in an occlusal fissure and forms a very large lesion, often sufficient to destroy much of the coronal dentine and involve the pulp, despite the fact that the enamel remains reasonably intact clinically and the patient suffers minor or no symptoms. Lower permanent molars are the teeth most usually affected, and the presentation is usually seen in children or young adults.

Lack of surface changes means that such lesions are often discovered radiographically, otherwise the true extent may not be revealed until the fissure is opened for exploration or to place a preventive resin restoration. However, these lesions are not truly hidden and careful examination, and transillumination will usually reveal fissure staining or subtle discolouration.

The processes of occult caries are not different from typical caries. The presentation has only become common in the UK in the last 20–30 years and may reflect increasing use of fluoride. This produces a harder more resistant enamel less likely to collapse under occlusal stress, and also more likely to remineralise using calcium and phosphate released from the underlying dentine caries.

Hidden caries must be distinguished from pre-eruptive resorption of intracoronal dentine, a rare condition with very similar radiographic appearance, that can be difficult to distinguish once the tooth has erupted (Fig. 4.32).

Hidden caries PMID: 9448806

Pre-eruptive intracoronal resorption PMID: 31414395

Root surface caries

Caries of the root surface is increasing in incidence as the ageing population retain more teeth. After recession of the gingival margin, cementum and root dentine are accessible to plaque. Root caries only develops on exposed root surface and not below the gingival margin in pockets.

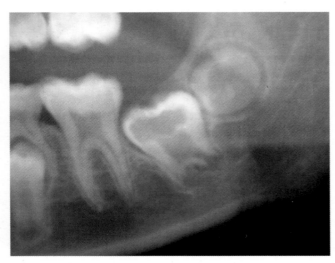

Fig. 4.32 Pre-eruptive coronal resorption has hollowed out the crown, producing an appearance very similar to extensive occlusal 'hidden' or 'occult' caries. Differentiating these two conditions after eruption would be difficult once bacteria have entered the crown.

Cementum is readily decalcified and presents little barrier to caries. Cervical cementum is very thin and invaded along the direction of Sharpey's fibres. Infection spreads between the lamellae along the incremental lines, and underlying dentine is involved almost immediately.

The causative microbial flora includes *S. mutans*, lactobacilli, *Actinomyces viscosus*, *Propionibacterium acidifaciens* and several other species of *Actinomyces*. Organisms such as *Actinomyces sp.* that are unable to cause enamel caries in animal models are capable of causing root caries, but the plaque over root surface lesions is very mixed and contains many putative anaerobic periodontal pathogens too. Once the caries has invaded into dentine, the flora probably matures to one similar to coronal dentine caries.

Like enamel caries, root caries has a surface zone of remineralisation, but it is porous, and bacteria enter the tissues earlier than in enamel caries. Like coronal dentine caries, root caries may be active or inactive and inactive lesions may be managed conservatively.

Root surface caries causes reactionary dentine on the pulp surface apical to the lesion because of the curvature of the dentinal tubules. This allows slowly progressing lesions to eventually penetrate to the coronal pulp without devitalising the apical pulp, which becomes closed off by the reactionary dentine.

Root surface caries is particularly seen in people with a dry mouth and those with poor oral hygiene.

Root caries review PMID: 33236462

Prevention root caries PMID: 23600985

Clinical aspects and prevention of caries

The pathology of dental caries may seem complex and largely irrelevant to clinical dentistry but forms the foundation for effective prevention and restorative strategies. Interventions based on the aetiological factors are shown in figure 4.1. In addition to these interventions that can be applied at the individual patient level, there is a view that caries also has social aspects and should be addressed at a population level in the same way as obesity and diabetes, other diseases caused by refined sugars.

The mechanistic methods of tooth restoration used in the 20th century could be applied without reference to the underlying biology of disease, but modern minimum intervention or minimally invasive dentistry is entirely founded on a good understanding of the pathology of dental caries.

Examples of the clinical relevance of caries pathology are shown in Table 4.4.

Prevention of caries as a non-communicable disease PMID: 30178558

Minimally invasive dentistry ISBN-13: 978-0198712091

Operative treatment and caries activity PMID: 28798430 and 27099358

Cochrane review treatment dentine caries PMID: 34280957

Table 4.4 The pathology of dental caries and its relevance to caries progression, treatment and prevention

Feature	Significance
Plaque flora is a stable ecosystem	The bacterial flora is influenced by its environment, but the ecosystem will resist change in the short term. Denial of cariogenic substrate by dietary control will reduce the number of cariogenic species, but dietary change must be maintained to be effective
The early caries lesion begins as a subsurface process	Bacteria cannot enter the enamel until the surface layer is destroyed and until then can be removed by cleaning. Until cavitation, complete repair by remineralisation is possible and prevention of cavitation is critical
Enamel is permeable, pores between crystallites account for 0.1% of its volume	Acids diffuse in readily to initiate caries and diffuse to dentine to trigger pulp defence reactions early in the lesion's lifespan, well before a lesion cavitates
Odontoblast processes extend to the enamel–dentine junction	
The translucent zone in enamel caries is present in only approximately half of caries lesions examined	The translucent zone indicates progression. Many lesions are not active much of the time
The dark zone of enamel caries is seen in almost all lesions	The dark zone indicates remineralisation. Therefore, almost all lesions undergo periodic phases of remineralisation.
Caries lesions undergo rapid phases of demineralisation and remineralisation. Activity or arrest may be the outcome depending on the relative proportion of each	Caries may remineralise, arrest or progress only very slowly so that, initially, observation or preventive intervention rather than restoration is appropriate for most enamel lesions
The surface zone of an enamel lesion is only 30 μm thick and porous	Pressure from probing may cavitate lesions, converting an arrested or slowly progressing lesion into an active lesion. Diagnosis should not attempt to indent the surface to judge 'stickiness', only to remove plaque and feel the surface texture
	Fluoride and other remineralising agents may enter the lesion easily
	Porous enamel takes up exogenous pigments so that longstanding lesions become 'brown spot' lesions
Fissure caries spreads laterally into the walls of a fissure, more than down from its base	The surface layer of occlusal enamel becomes undermined but is not initially directly involved. It may not fracture or appear abnormal until the underlying lesion is large
The shape of the enlarging occlusal lesion is guided inwards and laterally by the prism direction	An occlusal lesion involves a much greater area of dentine than a comparably-sized smooth surface lesion
The shape of the advancing front of a caries lesion in dentine is smooth and rounded	To conserve tooth structure, cavities should have smooth rounded outlines and no sharp internal angles
Caries spreads laterally along the amelodentinal junction	Lateral extension of a cavity is often determined by clearing caries from the amelodentinal junction (ADJ). However, caries usually only spreads laterally to approximately the extent of the lesion at the enamel surface and in underlying dentine. Although leaving caries at the junction is undesirable because it leaves enamel poorly supported, removal of ADJ caries can be undertaken conservatively
Cavitation develops unpredictably in relation to the size and extent of an approximal lesion on a radiograph	Some assessment of the patient's caries risk involving dietary analysis, fluoride and other factors is required before deciding that any lesion requires operative intervention. Lesions in a high-risk patient cavitate earlier than in a low-risk patient
The pulp–dentine complex responds to caries. The dentine just before the advancing front of a caries lesion is relatively impermeable as a result of remineralisation and tubular infill	The pulp–dentine defence reactions should be preserved, and this is best achieved by non-operative intervention rather than restoration. Minimal dentine should be removed in cavity preparation. In deep lesions, removal of all softened dentine over the pulp should be avoided
Dentine caries may be divided into zones of demineralisation, penetration and destruction or into zones of infected and affected dentine	Traditionally, cavity preparation involved removal of all softened dentine. However, it is not necessary to remove all infected dentine to provide a successful restoration. The correct amount to remove is usually judged by the degree of softening. Discoloration is a less effective indicator. Discoloured but 'reasonably firm' (not hard) dentine may be left in situ. These zones are of little significance beyond understanding the disease process, and none can be reliably identified clinically
Peritubular dentine and remineralisation form a translucent dentine zone that walls off the lesion	Lateral spread is slowed as caries penetrates dentine. When removing softened dentine with hand instruments or a slowly revolving bur, sclerotic dentine may be felt to be harder than adjacent dentine and should be preserved if possible

Continued

Table 4.4   The pathology of dental caries and its relevance to caries progression, treatment and prevention—cont'd

Feature	Significance
Peritubular dentine forms slowly	Only slowly advancing lesions are delayed by this defence reaction. A sclerotic zone visible radiographically indicates a slowly progressing or arrested lesion
Dentine tubules peripherally in mature teeth are slightly smaller than bacterial cocci	Bacterial penetration of dentine toward the pulp can only take place after some dentine demineralisation
Demineralisation precedes bacterial invasion in dentine by a small and variable distance	Not all softened dentine must be removed during cavity preparation
The advancing front of bacterial penetration into dentine is irregular at a microscopic level	The relatively large mechanical instruments used to remove softened dentine will always leave some infected dentine behind. However, if sealed effectively below restorations, these bacteria will be rendered inert
Superficial infected dentine is denatured and cannot remineralise. Deeper affected dentine will remineralise even though it contains bacteria	It is not necessary to remove all infected dentine to place a restoration, only the dentine that cannot remineralise if sealed below the restoration. Therefore, caries removal can be more conservative / minimally invasive below a well-sealed adhesive restoration
Dentine matrix is denatured by bacteria in the superficial layers of the zone of destruction	This renders the dentine susceptible to chemomechanical caries removal using proprietary mixtures of sodium hypochlorite. This procedure removes only the most damaged carious dentine, a conservative approach that preserves the deeper layers that can remineralise
Dentine splits transversely along incremental lines of growth in the zone of destruction	Dentine caries in the outer zone of destruction is easily removed in large flakes with hand instruments
Caries indicator dyes stain softened as well as infected dentine They stain collagen	Adhering strictly to the dye protocol will remove remineralisable dentine that should be left in situ. Caries indicator dyes promote overcutting
Reactionary dentine forms slowly and varies markedly in amount, quality and permeability and is found below only half the lesions in permanent teeth (more frequent in primary teeth)	Reactionary dentine provides little protection below rapidly progressing lesions
Formation of reactionary dentine requires a good blood supply and healthy pulp	Less is formed in older individuals. Once the pulp is inflamed, the quality of any reactionary dentine is poor and it is unlikely to be of much benefit
Symptoms of pulpitis do not correlate well with caries activity, lesion size, pulpal inflammation or even direct pulp involvement	Pulp vitality may be lost without symptoms or with only mild symptoms. An assessment of the state of a pulp is desirable to plan restoration of a deep carious lesion but, if based on symptoms alone, is unlikely to be accurate
Lesions of root caries also have a surface remineralised layer	Avoid hard probing of apparently intact though discoloured surfaces, as for enamel caries
Bacteria penetrate dentine early in root caries lesions but are accessible to non-operative preventive measures	Removal of infected dentine is not always necessary to treat early root caries
Deciduous teeth have approximately half the thickness of enamel of permanent teeth, larger pulps, longer pulp horns and, at least initially, larger dentinal tubules	Caries progresses faster in primary teeth than in permanent teeth

Pulpitis and apical periodontitis 5

PULPITIS ➜ Summary charts 5.1 and 5.2, pp. 81, 82

Pulpitis, inflammation of the dental pulp, is the most common reason for dental pain. The usual cause is caries penetrating the dentine, but there are other possibilities (Box 5.1). Exposure during cavity preparation allows bacteria to enter the pulp and also damages it mechanically (Fig. 5.1). Fracture may either open the pulp chamber or leave so thin a covering of dentine that bacteria can enter through the dentinal tubules. A tooth may crack from masticatory stress, usually after weakening by restoration, and bacteria penetrate along the crack (Fig. 5.2). Thermal damage can trigger pulpitis following cavity cutting with insufficient cooling or following intermittent low-grade thermal stimuli conducted to the pulp by large unlined metal restorations. Chemical damage can result from older types of acidic restoration materials used without a cavity lining.

Pulpitis, if untreated, may persist causing mild intermittent pain for years but is often followed by death of the pulp and spread of inflammatory debris or infection through the apical foramen into the periapical tissues. This inflammation of the periodontal ligament around the apex is called periapical periodontitis.

Clinical features

Pain from dental pulp is transmitted by A-delta and C-fibres. The pulps of individual teeth are not precisely represented on the sensory cortex. Pain from the pulp is therefore poorly localized and may be felt in any of the teeth of the upper or lower jaw of the affected side. Rarely, pain may be referred to a more distant site such as the ear. In early pulpitis, A-delta fibre transmission is associated with better localization, but these fibres are progressively impaired by inflammation and pressure, leaving C-fibre mediated pain, which is poorly localized and often interpreted as referred pain.

Pulp pain is not provoked by pressure on the tooth. The patient can chew in comfort unless there is a large open cavity allowing food to distort or stimulate the dentine thermally or osmotically.

Acute pulpitis. In the early stages the tooth is hypersensitive. Very cold or hot food causes a stab of pain that stops as soon as the irritant is removed. While inflammation progresses, pain becomes more persistent after the stimulus, and there may be prolonged attacks of toothache. The pain may start spontaneously, often when the patient is trying to get to sleep.

The pain is partly due to the pressure on the irritated nerve endings from oedema within the rigid pulp chamber and partly due to release of pain-producing mediators from

---

Box 5.1   Causes of pulpitis

- Dental caries
- Traumatic exposure of the pulp
- Fracture of a crown or cusp
- Cracked tooth
- Thermal or chemical irritation

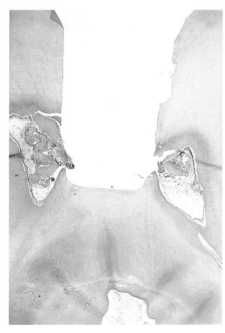

Fig. 5.1   Traumatic exposure. The pulp has been exposed during cavity preparation, and dentine bur debris and larger fragments have been driven into the pulp. The tooth was extracted before a strong inflammatory reaction has had time to develop, but it is clear that some inflammatory cells have already localised around the debris, which will have introduced many bacteria to the pulp.

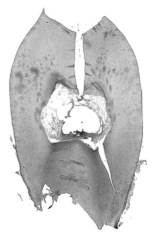

Fig. 5.2   Cracked tooth. The pulp died beneath this crack, which was undetected clinically. Decalcification of the tooth and shrinkage on preparation of a section have revealed the crack.

Table 5.1 Features of 'reversible' and 'irreversible' pulpitis

Reversible pulpitis	Irreversible pulpitis
Pain in short, sharp stabs	Constant throbbing pain with sharp exacerbations
Stimulated by hot and cold or osmotic (sweet) stimuli	Spontaneous exacerbations, as well as hot and cold or osmotic (sweet) stimuli. In late stages cold may relieve the pain
Pain resolves after stimulus removed in seconds or a few minutes	Pain persists several minutes or hours after an exacerbating stimulus
	Exaggerated response to electric pulp testing
	May disturb sleep

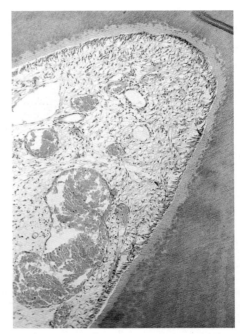

Fig. 5.3 Pulpal hyperaemia. While bacteria are still some distance from the pulp, acid permeating along the dentinal tubules gives rise to dilation of the blood vessels, oedema and a light cellular inflammatory infiltrate in the pulp.

the damaged tissue and inflammatory cells. The pain at its worst is excruciatingly severe, sharp and stabbing in character. It is little affected by simple analgesics.

The outcome of acute pulpitis is unpredictable. Acute pulpitis may be deemed irreversible on the basis of various features (see Table 5.1), but even then the pulp may sometimes survive. Although pulp death is the likely outcome, acute pulpitis may progress to chronic pulpitis, and early treatment can still preserve pulp vitality. A diagnosis of irreversible pulpitis is considered an indication for extirpation of the pulp, but it must be recognised that the diagnostic criteria are poorly defined.

Chronic pulpitis may develop with or without episodes of acute pulpitis. Symptoms of chronic pulpitis are very variable, usually there are bouts of dull pain, brought on by hot or cold stimuli or occurring spontaneously. There are often prolonged remissions, and there may be recurrent acute exacerbations. Unfortunately, many pulps under large carious cavities or restorations die painlessly. The first indication is then development of periapical periodontitis, either with pain of periodontal ligament origin or a periapical radiolucency seen by chance in a radiograph.

Pathology

Pulpitis caused by early caries results from penetration of acid and bacterial products through the dentine, and later from a mixed bacterial infection penetrating to the pulp. There is no relationship between the severity or type of pain and the histological features in the pulp or the extent of caries. Histology shows all degrees of inflammation and even progression to pulpal necrosis regardless of pain.

Acute closed pulpitis. Closed pulpitis refers to inflammation inside an intact closed pulp chamber. Histologically, there is initial hyperaemia limited to the area immediately beneath the irritant (Fig. 5.3). Infiltration by inflammatory cells and destruction of odontoblasts and adjacent pulp follow. A limited area of necrosis may result in formation of an abscess, localised by granulation tissue (Figs 5.4–5.7). Later, inflammation spreads until the pulp is obliterated by dilated blood vessels and acute inflammatory cells (Fig. 5.8). Necrosis follows when pressure occludes the apical vessels.

Chronic closed pulpitis. The main features are a predominantly mononuclear cell infiltrate and inflammation more limited in extent. A small area of pulpal necrosis and pus formation may be localised by a well-defined wall of granulation tissue, and a minute abscess may thus form. The remainder of the pulp may still appear normal.

Given time for the pulp to mount a reaction, as for instance beneath a relatively uncontaminated exposure, inflammation may become well localised. A partial calcific

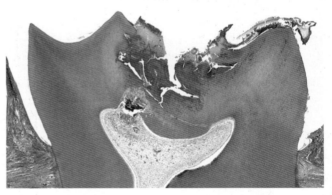

Fig. 5.4 Acute pulpitis. Low-power view showing occlusal caries penetrating to the pulp through a layer of reactionary dentine. There is a focus of acute inflammatory cells beneath the carious exposure in the pulp horn but the remaining pulp is uninflamed.

barrier may wall off the exposure with reactionary dentine around the margins, as seen following pulp capping. Calcific barriers can be seen radiographically as 'dentine bridges' and may also form apically following use of calcium hydroxide to induce apex closure. Unfortunately, the calcified layer is frequently incomplete and forms less of a barrier than might be thought (Figs 5.9 and 5.10). However, in successful cases, induction of a complete barrier of tubular reactionary dentine by pulp capping may allow preservation of the remainder of the pulp.

The chief factor hampering pulpal survival is its enclosure within the rigid walls of the pulp chamber and, in fully formed teeth, the limited aperture for the apical vessels. In acute inflammation, these vessels can readily be compressed by inflammatory oedema and thrombose. The pulp thus has its blood supply cut off and it dies. This may be rapid in the case of acute pulpitis or delayed in chronic lesions. The relatively prolonged survival of chronically inflamed pulps is shown by the persistence of symptoms during a long

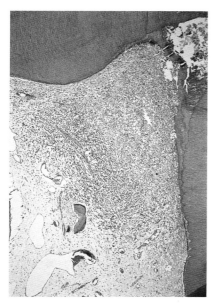

Fig. 5.5 **Acute pulpitis.** Beneath the carious exposure (top right) a dense inflammatory infiltrate is accumulating but there is not yet abscess formation. More deeply, lower left, the pulp is hyperaemic, with dilated blood vessels.

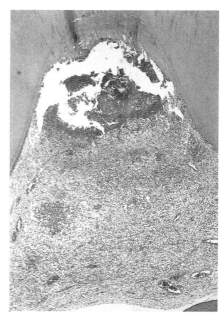

Fig. 5.7 **Acute caries and pulpitis.** Infection has penetrated to the pulp. Part of the pulp has been destroyed, and an abscess has formed, containing a bead of pus.

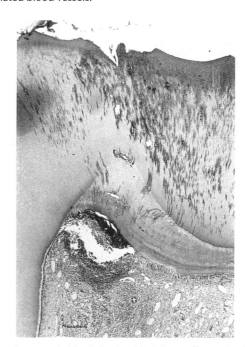

Fig. 5.6 **Acute pulpitis.** Infection (dark lines of bacteria along tubules) has penetrated a thin layer of reactionary dentine on the roof of the pulp chamber causing inflammation throughout the pulp and pus to form in the pulp horn.

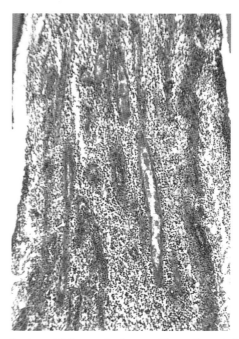

Fig. 5.8 **Acute pulpitis: terminal stage.** The entire pulp has been destroyed and replaced by inflammatory cells and dilated vessels.

period. However, pulp death is usually the end result unless treatment is provided.

Open pulpitis. Necrosis of the pulp from oedema compressing the blood supply is less likely when the walls of the chamber are open to allow pressure to dissipate. When there is a wide coronal pulp exposure, or when there are incompletely formed open apices or multiple apices, the balance is tipped in favour of host defences. A chronically inflamed pulp can then survive despite being open to the oral cavity and heavily infected (Fig. 5.11).

Chronic hyperplastic pulpitis (pulp polyp). In this rare condition, despite wide pulpal exposure, the pulp not merely survives but proliferates through the opening to form a pulp polyp.

A pulp polyp appears as a dusky red or pinkish soft nodule protruding from the pulp to fill a carious cavity. It is painless but may be tender and bleed on probing. It should be distinguished from proliferating gingival tissue extending over the edge of the cavity by tracing its attachment (Fig. 5.12). When a pulp polyp forms, the pulp itself becomes replaced by granulation tissue (Fig. 5.13). The surface of the polyp eventually becomes epithelialised and covered by a layer of well-formed stratified squamous epithelium. This protects the granulation tissue and allows inflammation to subside

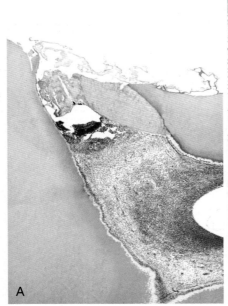

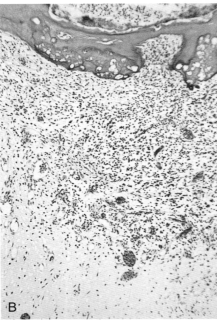

Fig. 5.9   Calcific barriers. (A) Pulpitis with formation of a barrier of thick reactionary dentine in the pulp horn, but with an abscess immediately below it. The rest of the pulp is inflamed. (B) Higher-power view of a calcific barrier induced by calcium hydroxide direct pulp capping. In this case the barrier is thin, inflammation in the underlying pulp has not subsided and the pulp cap has failed.

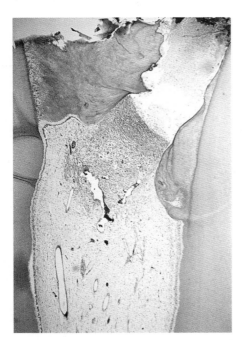

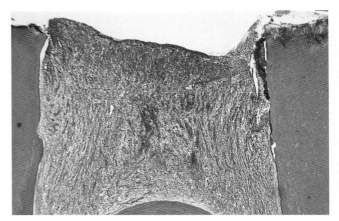

Fig. 5.11   Open pulpitis. Beneath the wide exposure the pulp has survived in the form of granulation tissue, with the densest inflammatory infiltrate immediately beneath the open surface.

Fig. 5.10   Pulp capping. This pulp capping has induced a thick layer of reactionary dentine (with regular tubules, best seen on the left side of the pulp chamber wall coronally) and reparative dentine with a more irregular structure (on the right of the pulp wall). Unfortunately these reactions do not produce a complete barrier, and failure of the procedure is indicated by the inflammatory cells concentrated below a gap in the barrier.

and the granulation tissue to mature into fibrous tissue. The same degree of pulpal proliferation can occasionally be seen in teeth with fully formed roots (Fig. 5.14) but is most common in children. As in open pulpits, this is because open apices provide a better blood supply and prevent the pulp from dying as a result of pulpal oedema.

Management

The chances of an inflamed pulp surviving are poor, and treatment options are limited (Box 5.2). As noted previously,

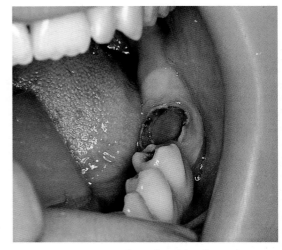

Fig. 5.12   Pulp polyp. An inflamed nodule of granulation tissue can be seen growing from the pulp chamber of this broken down first permanent molar.

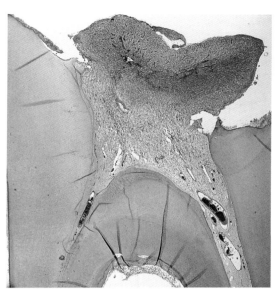

Fig. 5.13 Pulp polyp, early stage. A hyperplastic nodule of granulation tissue is growing out through a wide exposure of the pulp. The surface is ulcerated, and the loose pulp has been replaced by the proliferation of fibrous tissue and vessels with inflammatory cells.

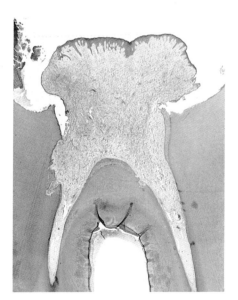

Fig. 5.14 Pulp polyp, late stage. In this broken-down molar, the granulation tissue proliferating from the pulp cavity has acquired an epithelial covering over much of its surface, seeded by shed epithelial cells from the mucosa adhering to the surface. As a result inflammation has subsided and the polyp is maturing to a more fibrous tissue. Note also the internal resorption of the coronal pulp chamber (left) as a result of pulpal inflammation.

the concept of irreversible pulpitis is considered useful for treatment planning, but criteria are poorly defined. Antibiotics have no effect on pulpitis, which is not a conventional infection.

Open pulpitis is usually associated with gross cavity formation, and it is rarely possible to save the tooth, despite the vitality of the pulp.

Key features of pulpitis are summarised in Box 5.3, and the sequelae of pulpitis are shown in Summary chart 5.1.

Pulpitis diagnosis PMID: 33818812

Box 5.2   Treatment options for pulpitis

- If fractured or cracked, stabilise fracture and seal pulp temporarily
- Removal of caries, obtundent or steroid dressing
- Removal of caries and pulp capping
- Pulpotomy, conservative pulp therapy or pulp capping
- Pulp extirpation and endodontic treatment
- Extraction
- Analgesics are largely ineffective
- Antibiotics have no value

Box 5.3   Key features of pulpitis

- Pulpitis is caused by infection or irritation of the pulp, usually by caries
- Pulp pain is poorly localised
- Chronic pulpitis is often symptomless
- Untreated pulpitis usually leads to death of the pulp and spread of inflammation to the periapical tissues
- The distinction between reversible and irreversible pulpitis can be difficult to make

---

PULP CALCIFICATIONS

Pulp stones, rounded masses of dentine that form within the pulp, can be seen in radiographs as small opacities. In the past, they were thought to cause symptoms but do not. They are common in normal teeth but have an increased frequency in teeth affected by caries, trauma, orthodontic movement and other potential irritants.

For unknown reasons, they are common in the teeth of patients with Ehlers-Danlos syndrome (Ch. 14), dentinal dysplasia type II (Ch. 2) and the rare disease tumoral calcinosis.

Histologically, pulp stones consist of dentine with normal or incomplete tubule formation (Fig. 5.15). A distinction used to be drawn between pulp stones that lie free in the pulp and those attached to the pulp chamber wall as seen on microscope slides. However, this is frequently an illusion caused by a plane of section that fails to pass through the connection between the pulp stone and the pulp wall and the difference is of no significance. Most are large rounded irregular calcifications, often based on a central nidus of unknown material. Others, referred to as diffuse calcifications, lie parallel with the pulp wall and are thought to be an age-related degenerative change.

Pulp stones and diffuse calcification are of no clinical significance except insofar as they may obstruct endodontic treatment.

PERIAPICAL PERIODONTITIS, ABSCESS AND GRANULOMA → Summary chart 5.2, p. 82

Once the pulp is necrotic, inflammation and infection, bacterial products or other irritants spread through the apex into the periodontal ligament . The key diagnostic feature is tenderness of the tooth in its socket as movement compresses the inflamed periodontal ligament. Pulpal infection following caries is by far the most common cause (see Summary chart 5.2).

Sometimes, a necrotic pulp is sterile, as for instance following trauma that damages the apical vessels or devitalization by electrocautery. In such cases, periapical periodontitis results

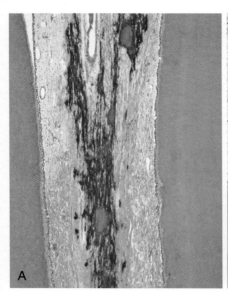

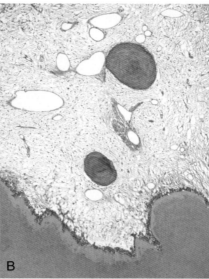

Fig. 5.15 Pulp stones. (A) The dystrophic or diffuse pulp mineralisations often found as an age change. (B) Rounded nodules of calcified tissue, in this case resembling bone rather than dentine.

from irritants and mediators from the necrotic tissue rather than bacteria.

Endodontic procedures can trigger periapical inflammation by perforation or pushing infected material or irritants such as hypochlorite through the apex. Provided the canal is clean and sealed, such acute episodes usually resolve quickly, unless large amounts of filling material remain beyond the apex.

Occlusal trauma from an over-contoured restoration will also cause an acute but usually transient sterile apical periodontitis. This will subside as the periodontal ligament remodels to accommodate the changed position of the tooth and the occlusal forces cause orthodontic movement of the tooth.

The diagnosis of pulpal, periodontal and other pain in the teeth and alveolus is summarised in Summary chart 5.2.

ACUTE APICAL PERIODONTITIS

→ Summary chart 5.1, p. 81

Spread of infection through the apex brings the causative bacteria from a protected site into an environment where the host can mount an effective response. Acute inflammation and an immune reaction are triggered.

Clinical features

The patient may give a history of pain due to previous pulpitis, and the associated tooth may be carious, restored or discoloured due to death of the pulp. Formation of inflammatory exudate in the periodontal ligament causes the tooth to be extruded by a minute amount and the bite to fall more heavily on it. The tooth is at first uncomfortable, then increasingly tender, even to mere touch. Hot or cold substances do not cause pain in the tooth unless some viable pulp remains, as it may in a multirooted tooth.

Unlike pulpitis, apical periodontitis is accurately localized by pain fibres and proprioception in the periodontal ligament, and the patient will usually point correctly to the causative tooth.

Radiographs give little information because bony changes take time to develop. Immediately around the apex, the lamina dura may appear slightly hazy and the periodontal space may be slightly widened. When acute periodontitis is due to an acute exacerbation in a periapical granuloma (see later in this chapter), the granuloma can be seen as an area of radiolucency at the apex.

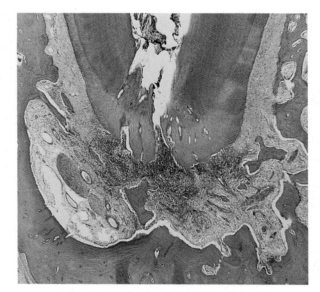

Fig. 5.16 Acute apical periodontitis. In this early acute lesion, inflammatory cells, mainly neutrophil polymorphonuclear leucocytes, are seen clustered around the apex of a non-vital tooth. The inflammatory cells are spreading into bone, and there has only been time for a small amount of bone resorption to develop. This would be seen radiographically only as slight fuzziness of the apical lamina dura.

While apical periodontitis remains a localised apical inflammatory change, no facial oedema or alveolar tenderness or other reactions develop. Their onset indicates progression to apical infection.

Pathology and sequelae

Acute apical periodontitis is a typical acute inflammatory reaction with engorged blood vessels and packing of the tissue with neutrophils (Fig. 5.16). These changes are initially localised to the immediate vicinity of the apex.

At this stage periapical periodontitis is usually treated, triggered by the severe toothache. Extraction of the causative tooth or extirpation of the pulp and root filling eliminates the source of infection and drains the exudate. These are the simplest and most effective treatments. Antibiotics should not be given for simple acute periodontitis if immediate dental treatment is available.

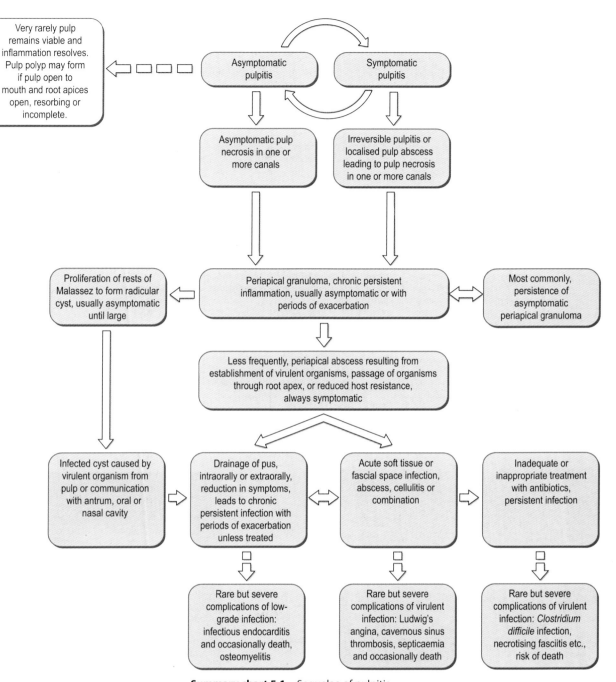

Summary chart 5.1   Sequelae of pulpitis.

If untreated, there are two possible outcomes depending on the balance between the virulence of the bacteria and the host defences. The usual outcome is that a chronic periapical granuloma forms (later in this chapter). However, if the bacterial load is high, species are virulent or host response is inadequate, the infection will progress to an apical (or dentoalveolar) abscess (Box 5.4).

> **Box 5.4   Possible complications of acute apical periodontitis**
>
> • Apical abscess formation
> • Regional lymphadenopathy
> • Spreading infection

ACUTE APICAL (DENTOALVEOLAR) ABSCESS

The bacterial flora in the pulp chamber includes potentially virulent species, mostly anaerobic, but can only induce an abscess if sufficient bacteria pass through the apex. The bacteria trigger acute inflammation, pus starts to form and pain becomes intense and throbbing in character. At this stage, the gingiva over the root is red and tender, but there is no swelling while inflammation is confined within the bone. Like apical periodontitis, the pain of an apical abscess is accurately localised by the patient because periodontal ligament pain and proprioceptors are triggered.

Toothache or pain felt in teeth or alveolus							
Pain of pulpal origin Sensitivity to sweet, hot or cold, poorly localised			Pain of periodontal ligament origin Pain on biting or pressure on tooth, usually well localised to one or more teeth			Neurological or vascular pain	Neuralgic or psychogenic pain
Dentine hypersentivity	Pulpitis Tooth is vital or partially vital and may be hypersensitive to testing		Cracked tooth or cusp	Periapical periodontitis	Periodontal abscess	Maxillary sinusitis		
Pain of short duration more or less limited to period of stimulus, particularly cold	Reversible pulpitis Symptoms may be limited to duration of stimulus or persist for varying period afterward, caries or other cause may be evident	Irreversible pulpitis Poorly defined entity, usually identified by severe continuous or spontaneous pain	Shooting or electric shock-like pain on biting, often only on one cusp or in one direction, also when a fracture line involves periodontal ligament	Pain on pressure to single tooth, caries or other cause of pre-existing pulpitis may be present, periapical, lateral canal or furcation radiolucency only in longstanding cases	Pain on pressure to single tooth, tooth vital, abscess in ligament visible or revealed by probing furcation or deep pocket	Tenderness on pressure to teeth with apices near sinus, usually concurrent or recent nasal or sinus symptoms, not usually severe pain	Teeth vital unless previously devitalised for other reasons	Unusual localisation trigger or perceived cause, associated with depression, anxiety or delusional states, teeth vital unless previously devitalised for other reasons
Confirm diagnosis by identifying exposed dentine or tooth wear and applying appropriate treatment	May resolve on treating cause but once established may progress to irreversible pulpitis, even after an asymptomatic period	Responds most reliably to extirpation of pulp or extraction	Confirm by identifying crack	Resolves on drainage or extirpation of pulp or extraction	Resolves on drainage and local treatment or extraction	Resolves on treatment of sinusitis	Consider mimics of pulpitis such as trigeminal neuralgia and the prodromal symptoms of facial Herpes zoster infection	Consider atypical odontalgia, atypical facial pain, 'phantom tooth' etc., but only after excluding organic causes

Summary chart 5.2   Pulpal, periodontal and other pain felt by patient as 'toothache'.

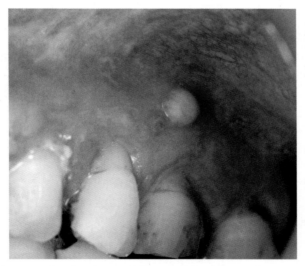

Fig 5.17   Alveolar abscess with a sinus from the premolar apex to the overlying alveolar mucosa, where a small bead of pus is visible through the distended mucosa (a 'pointing' sinus). Once this bursts and the sinus drains, the opening will become much less obvious.

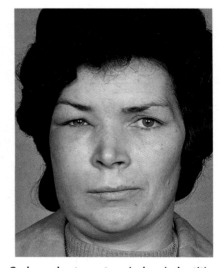

Fig. 5.18   **Oedema due to acute apical periodontitis.** An acute periapical infection of a canine has perforated the buccal plate of bone causing oedema of the face; this quickly subsided when the infection was treated.

An established abscess will usually either drain through a sinus and become chronic or, much more rarely, progress to osteomyelitis or cellulitis. Usually, pus and exudate will burrow a sinus tract to the closest alveolar mucosa (Fig 5.17), unless an adjacent pocket or the nearby skin provide a path of less resistance. Once infection escapes into the medullary cavity of the bone, oedema may develop in the soft tissues of the face (Fig. 5.18).

Escape of pus to the skin is not common, but a classical presentation is the tracking of a sinus onto the skin near the chin as a result of a traumatically devitalised lower incisor (Figs 5.19–5.20). The regional lymph nodes may be enlarged and tender, but systemic symptoms are usually slight or absent.

Escape of pus takes a few days after the onset of pain; this relieves the pressure and pain quickly abates. If the exudate cannot escape, it may distend the soft tissues elsewhere to form a soft tissue abscess or cellulitis as described in Chapter 9.

Apical abscesses are polymicrobial infections and numerous pathogenic species are present, including *Bacteroides sp.*, *Prevotella sp.*, spirochaetes, *Porphyromonas sp.*, *Streptococcus*

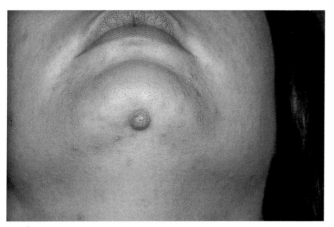

Fig. 5.19 A persistent skin sinus from a lower incisor rendered non-vital by a blow some time previously. This young woman was seen and treated unsuccessfully for 2 years by her doctor, surgeons and dermatologists before anyone looked at her teeth.

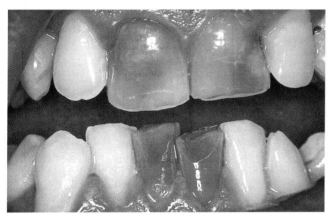

Fig. 5.20 Non-vital incisor teeth, in this case as a result of trauma. Haemorrhage and products of autolysis of the pulp discolour the dentine and darken the teeth.

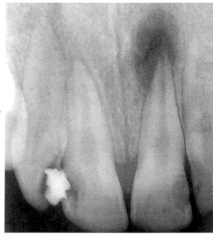

Fig. 5.21 Chronic apical abscess. Periapical bone resorption has developed as a result of inflammation. The area of radiolucency corresponds with the histological changes seen in figure 5.22.

sp., Fusobacterium sp. and *Actinomyces sp.* No particular species can be identified that are particularly responsible for symptoms or progression. Despite the mixed nature of the infection, penicillins remain the most effective antibiotics, with metronidazole reserved for patients allergic to penicillin. However, an apical abscess cannot be treated by antibiotics alone; the causative tooth or its pulp must be dealt with because bacteria in the pulp chamber are inaccessible to the drug.

Symptoms and antibiotic treatment PMID: 16457000

US guideline antibiotic treatment PMID: 31668170

Fatal outcome PMID: 8105884

CHRONIC APICAL PERIODONTITIS AND PERIAPICAL GRANULOMA

→ Summary chart 5.1, p. 79

Most necrotic pulps do not progress to abscess, but form a chronic periapical granuloma, a focus of chronic inflammation at the root apex. Most develop without symptoms, but they can also arise after acute apical periodontitis, particularly when it has been inadequately treated and resolved incompletely.

A periapical granuloma is caused by frustrated healing. The granuloma itself is sterile in almost all cases, but bacteria and irritants from necrotic tissue remain in the pulp chamber, inaccessible to the host response. Small numbers of bacteria may occasionally pass through the apex but are quickly eliminated by the host defences. However, the continual trickle of irritants from the persistent reservoir of infection in the root canal into the periapical region prevents healing.

Clinical features

The tooth is non-vital and may be slightly tender to percussion, but otherwise, symptoms may be minimal and are often completely absent.

Many periapical granulomas are first recognised as chance findings in a radiograph (Fig. 5.21). The granuloma forms a 'periapical area' of radiolucency a few millimetres in diameter with loss of continuity of the lamina dura around the apex. In longstanding lesions there may be hypercementosis on the adjacent root or slight superficial root resorption. The margins of the radiolucency may appear fuzzy when inflammation or infection are active, but are usually well defined and appear sharp, sharper in larger lesions. Good demarcation and size alone are not evidence of radicular cyst formation (Ch. 10).

Pathology

A periapical granuloma is a typical focus of chronic inflammation characterised by lymphocytes, macrophages and plasma cells in granulation tissue. It is important to recognise that a periapical granuloma does not contain true granulomas histologically. The term granuloma is a historic description for granulation tissue, in the same way that the word is used in pyogenic granuloma.

Inflammation is densest in the centre, close to the root apex, and there is an uninflamed layer of fibrous tissue around the periphery separating the inflamed tissue from the bone. Osteoclasts resorb the bone peripherally to make space for the granuloma. There may be a central cavity with a few neutrophils, but no pus and no infection (Figs 5.22 and 5.23).

Inflammation may trigger epithelial rests of Malassez in the adjacent periodontal ligament to proliferate (Fig. 5.24), and this is the mechanism by which radicular cysts occasionally develop (Ch. 10).

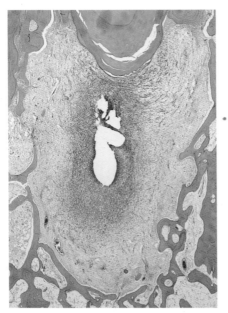

Fig. 5.22   Chronic periapical abscess. At the apex of the non-vital tooth (top centre of picture) is an abscess cavity surrounded by a thick fibrous wall densely infiltrated by inflammatory cells, predominantly neutrophils. Periapical bone has been resorbed and the trabeculae reorientated around the mass.

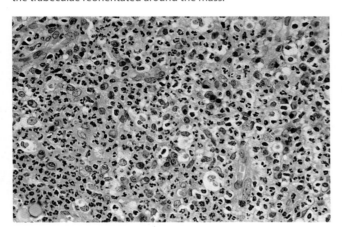

Fig. 5.23   High-power view of an apical granuloma showing neutrophils, lymphocytes and plasma cells in loose oedematous fibrous tissue.

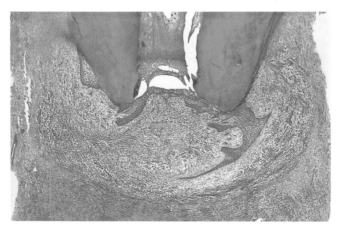

Fig. 5.24   Epithelial proliferation in an apical granuloma. Inflammation induces proliferation of odontogenic epithelium in rests of Malassez in the periodontal ligament. This change may lead to cyst formation (Ch. 10).

Treatment and sequelae

A periapical granuloma will resolve if the causative necrotic pulp is removed, so extraction or endodontic treatment are the two options. Persistence after root canal treatment indicates treatment failure and retreatment or apicectomy may be required (Fig. 5.25).

Without treatment, the most likely outcome for a periapical granuloma is that it will persist largely unchanged. There may be acute inflammatory exacerbations with symptoms from time to time, often insufficient to cause a patient to seek treatment.

The risk of leaving an untreated periapical granuloma is that it will develop into an acute periapical abscess. This is unpredictable, and granulomas that have been asymptomatic for decades may suddenly develop into an abscess. During any of these acute abscess exacerbations, a sinus may form. Sinus formation reduces pressure and usually allows the infection to persist as a chronic low-grade infection. Sinuses will normally heal when the cause is treated and do not require excision. Otherwise, they may drain intermittently and heal after each acute exacerbation.

Successful treatment is followed by resolution of inflammation, reforming of the lamina dura and periodontal ligament and bone around the apex. In rare cases, there is healing only by fibrosis. This is more frequent in the maxilla than mandible and when inflammation has resorbed the

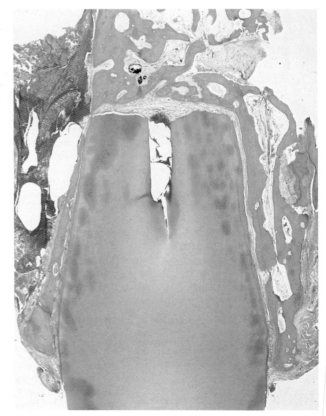

Fig. 5.25   Low-power to show the effects of successful apicectomy. The chronic inflammatory reaction has entirely cleared. New bone has formed to replace the excised apex with a new continuous periodontal ligament and lamina dura. The root filling material in the canal has been lost in preparing the section because it is too hard to cut. A few fragments of the reverse root filling material left in the surgical cavity have been incorporated into the medullary bone, seen as dark specks above the end of the sectioned root. These have been incorporated into the tissue without inducing inflammation.

Box 5.5 Reasons for persistence of chronic apical periodontitis after root canal treatment

- Periapical granuloma persistence
  - Bacterial flora remaining in canal(s) without good apical seal
  - Extraradicular infection
  - Foreign body reaction
    - extruded endodontic materials
    - food material impacted through open canal
    - cholesterol crystals from haemorrhage
- Healing by scar formation
- Radicular cyst formation

overlying cortical bone. Fibrous healing to produce an apical scar is seen radiographically and appears similar to a persisting granuloma, causing a potential problem in diagnosis and when assessing the success of root canal therapy.

Persistence of a periapical granuloma following root treatment is very occasionally due to the presence of bacteria within the granuloma. Although most periapical granulomas are sterile, the bacteria being limited to the pulp, in a very small number of cases *Actinomyces* or other organisms can form a biofilm on the outer root surface or free-floating colonies in the centre of the granuloma. This must be distinguished from an acute periapical abscess. The organisms in 'extraradicular infection' are of low virulence and remain localised, cause persistent low-grade inflammation but do not form much pus or cause a spreading infection. Extraradicular infection usually has to be eliminated by apicectomy or extraction.

Failure to heal after treatment requires investigation. Reasons include inadequate root canal treatment, extraradicular infection and an apical foreign body reaction to food components forced through the apex when the coronal pulp chamber is exposed by caries or left open to drain to too long ('pulse' granuloma). Occasionally what appears clinically as a periapical granuloma is a radicular or other cyst (Ch. 10), cemento-osseous dysplasia (Ch. 11), odontogenic tumour (Ch. 11.) or other completely unexpected disease.

Causes of treatment failure are summarised in Box 5.5 and Summary chart 5.1.

Causes of failed treatment PMID: 16584489

Tooth wear, resorption, hypercementosis and osseointegration

6

TOOTH WEAR

Tooth wear is a widely used although rather non-specific and somewhat misleading term that includes the processes of non-carious tooth damage or 'tooth surface loss' – attrition, abrasion and erosion. In any one affected patient, more than one of these processes is often active.

Tooth wear is common worldwide and a moderate degree affects up to half of many populations. Incidence increases with age, though attrition is normal in the deciduous dentition.

Multifactorial aetiology PMID: 24993256

Review PMID: 33350551

Attrition

Attrition is wear from tooth-to-tooth contact and affects the tips of cusps and incisal edges most severely (Fig. 6.1). Attrition is a normal physiological process, and wear increases with age. Mamelons are soon lost from incisors, and by middle age attrition will have worn through the enamel on many male individuals' incisal edges and canine cusp tips. Attrition is increased when fewer teeth take the masticatory load or when the enamel is malformed. Attrition is enhanced in people with bruxism and on teeth in premature occlusion.

Attrition is often said to be worse with a coarse diet, but if the diet itself is abrasive, the effect is mixture of attrition and abrasion.

Reactionary dentine forms in response to this slow process and protects the pulp (Figs 4.28 and 4.29). Dentinal tubular sclerosis prevents dentine hypersensitivity resulting from pure attrition.

Pure attrition almost never needs treatment; if wear is significant, an additional component of abrasion or erosion should be suspected.

Abrasion

Abrasion is wear of the teeth by an abrasive external agent. The most common form is occlusal wear from an abrasive diet and is frequent in less developed countries and in ancient skulls.

Abrasion of the necks of the teeth buccally is seen mainly in older people as a consequence of overly vigorous tooth brushing or use of too abrasive a dentifrice. A horizontal brushing action is often blamed, but the evidence is slim, and once a groove develops, the brush bristles are deflected into it regardless of technique. Abrasion affects both enamel and root dentine, but the softer dentine is abraded more easily. The exposed dentine is shiny and smooth, polished by the abrasive. Eventually, grooves worn into the necks of the teeth can be so deep as to extend into the site of the original pulp chamber, by then obliterated by reactionary dentine to protect the pulp (Figs 6.2 and 6.3). The crown of the tooth may even break off without exposing the pulp. Cervical abrasion can hamper endodontic treatment by causing pulpal obliteration just below cervical level. A switch to a minimally abrasive toothpaste is essential.

A variety of habits may also cause localised abrasion such as pipe smoking and opening hairpins or holding pins (Fig. 6.4). These take years to develop because such items are not very abrasive.

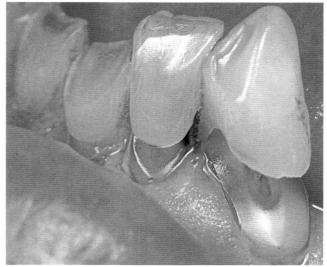

Fig. 6.2 Attrition and abrasion. Chronic physical trauma to the teeth produced by chewing and over-vigorous use of a toothbrush. The incisal edges of the teeth have worn into polished facets, in the centres of which the yellowish dentine is visible. The necks of the two nearest teeth have been deeply incised by tooth brushing, also exposing dentine. The pulp has been obliterated by secondary dentine formation, but its original site can be seen in the centre of the exposed dentine.

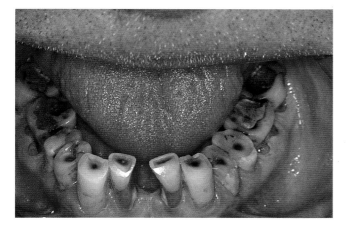

Fig. 6.1 Attrition. Excessive wear of the occlusal surfaces of the teeth, as a result of an abrasive diet. The site of the pulp of several teeth is marked by reactionary dentine which, being relatively porous, has become stained. Teeth remain vital.

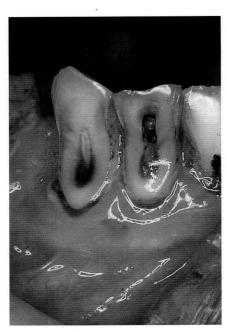

Fig. 6.3   Mixed pattern tooth loss. In this case, elements of erosion and abrasion are present. Note the shiny polished surface produced by abrasion.

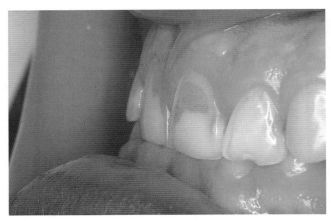

Fig. 6.5   Erosion. Saucer-shaped defects on the labial enamel resulting from acid drinks being trapped between the upper lip and teeth. See also Fig. 35.1.

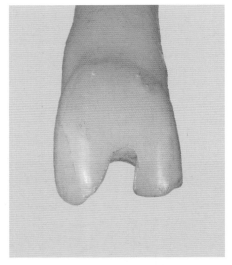

Fig. 6.4   Localised abrasion caused by opening hair grips.

When abrasion appears extensive, it is important to ensure that there is not an element of erosion.

Erosion

Erosion is progressive solubilisation of tooth substance by exposure to acid. Enamel is completely dissolved and dentine demineralised, softened and rendered prone to abrasion and attrition. Erosion is an increasing problem, and when tooth wear is severe, there is usually a significant erosive component.

The most common cause is dietary acids from consumption of carbonated soft drinks or fruit juices, or both (Fig. 6.5). Carbonated drinks are buffered to maintain their acidity, and this enhances the solubilisation effect. Cola-type drinks and red wine have a pH of approximately 2.5, and fruit juices approximately 3.5. Carbonated water is acidic but with minimal buffering capacity and so is not damaging. Health

concerns are reducing consumption of these drinks, but the focus is on calorie and sugar content rather than acidity. The average UK citizen drinks around 80 litres of such drinks a year and consumption is falling only slowly. Erosion tends to be in those with high consumption, but there is concern about erosion in children and the effects of lifelong low-level exposure. Approximately half of the fruit juice in the UK is drunk by children, and a third of 6-year-olds and a quarter of 12-year-olds have some degree of erosive tooth wear. In the United States, consumption of carbonated drinks has declined 25% since 2000 while consumers switch to fruit juices for health reasons, but these in excess can be even more damaging.

Chronic regurgitation of gastric secretions, typically as a consequence of chronic pyloric stenosis, is a potent erosive challenge. The affected tooth surfaces are often, but not always, the palatal surfaces of the upper teeth (see Fig. 35.1). Similar damage can result from self-induced vomiting. The latter is characteristic of bulimia (see Ch. 41).

In the past, industrial exposure to corrosive chemicals was a significant cause of dental erosion. This is now of only historical interest, but exposure to wine in wine tasters and acidic swimming pool water can all induce erosion as an occupational hazard. Some tooth-whitening products have an acidic pH (most are alkaline) and are best avoided because prolonged application in trays can be very damaging.

Saliva has a protective effect, and dry mouth increases the risk of erosion. Patients should not brush their teeth until 1 hour after an acid exposure to avoid abrasion contributing to the tooth wear.

Erosion is worse on maxillary teeth, on occlusal, palatal and labial surfaces. Minor degrees are easily missed. Cusp tips are lost and become dimpled; the curvature of buccal and palatal surfaces is flattened and then rendered concave. Palatal enamel loss leaves the incisal labial enamel as a thin, sharp ridge with abnormal translucency and colour and a tendency to chip away in small fragments.

Once enamel is lost, the exposed dentine wears away much faster by the combination of erosion and abrasion. Eventually the clinical crowns of all teeth are short, and vertical dimension is reduced.

Treatment should be conservative. Identifying the cause and instituting a preventive regime through diet analysis and medical history determines the intervention. Wear is slow. Study models, photographs and follow up can be used to assess treatment effect, and restorative intervention may only be required for cosmetic reasons. Dentinal hypersensitivity is a common finding because erosion opens exposed dentinal tubules. This is reduced by fluorides and removal of the cause. If patients cannot stop acid drinks, a reduced intake can be rendered safer by dilution or drinking through a straw. If interocclusal space is reduced, a Dahl-type appliance may generate space required for restorations when wear is very severe. Patients with regurgitation or bulimia need medical referral.

Diagnosis and treatment PMIDs: 22240686, 22281629, 22322760, 22361546

Erosion intrinsic causes PMID: 24993266 and 29389338

Abfraction

Abfraction is a theoretical concept that has never been proven to apply to human teeth in normal function. The hypothesis is that occlusal stress is concentrated around the cervical region of the tooth, flexing and microfracturing the cervical enamel. The enamel is supposed to be weakened as a result, prone to fracture, and predisposed to abrasion.

Abfraction PMID: 24250083 and 19228125

BRUXISM

Bruxism is the term given to periodic repetitive clenching or rhythmic forceful grinding of the teeth. Some 10–20% of the population report the habit, but the incidence rises to 90% when intermittent subconscious grinding is included. Bruxism has an equal sex incidence, is more common in children and young adults and uncommon after middle age. The aetiology is unknown but probably multifactorial. Bruxism is also common in people with various disabilities (Ch. 40). Grinding the teeth is sometimes a subconscious response to frustration and, although usually brief, may be acquired as a more prolonged habit and damage the teeth.

Bruxism is divided into nocturnal and daytime types. In nocturnal bruxism, the teeth are clenched or ground many times each night but for only a few seconds at a time. Bruxism is performed during light sleep, and the movement is a grinding movement that can be heard by a bystander. The forces exerted and the total time of occlusal contact are much longer than physiological occlusal contact.

People who brux during the day may grind, clench, or perform other parafunctional habits such as cheek, tongue or nail biting or tongue thrusting in addition. The last of these can be seen to cause a crenellated lateral border of the tongue. The daytime bruxing movement tends to be clenching rather than grinding and is not usually audible. Muscle symptoms, if any, worsen as the day progresses. Daytime bruxism is seen more frequently in females. Whether it is a response to stress is controversial.

Bruxing is often performed in a protrusive or lateral excursion so that the forces are borne on few teeth and in an unfavourable direction. The resulting attrition can be deeply destructive, particularly in a Class II division 2 incisor relationship. The signs of bruxism are shown in Box 6.1.

Only the grinding itself is diagnostic and may be unknown to the patient. The attrition caused could look like that of physiological wear. Bruxism is variably associated with muscle pain and headaches. The muscle pain of night bruxism is felt in the morning and is the same as muscle pain felt in other muscles after exercise. However, most 'bruxists' experience

Box 6.1   Features and effects of bruxism
• Noise during grinding (nocturnal bruxism)
• Attrition, wear facets but rarely dentine sensitivity
• Fracture of cusps and restorations
• Increased (adaptive) mobility of teeth
• Hypertrophy of masseter and anterior temporalis muscles
• Sometimes, although rarely, myalgia and limitation of jaw movement
• Sometimes, although rarely, tenderness on palpation of masticatory muscles

no pain, and pain does not correlate with the severity of the grinding or clenching.

Bruxism is often considered to be linked to temporomandibular pain dysfunction syndrome, but the association is not strong (Ch. 14). It has also been suggested that bruxism may result from occlusal interference, but bruxism may even be carried out with complete dentures.

Bruxism has been linked to several medical conditions. It is common in people with learning disability, Down's syndrome, cerebral palsy, Parkinson's disease and autism spectrum disorders, but causative associations are difficult to prove in such a common condition. A number of drugs are associated with bruxism including selective serotonin reuptake inhibitors, tricyclic antidepressants, amphetamines, caffeine and drugs of abuse, particularly 'ecstasy' (methylenedioxymethamphetamine or MDMA). Others such as dopamine antagonists cause repetitive mandibular movements rather than bruxism.

Management

Bruxism should be treated conservatively, and any intervention should be reversible. Reassurance and explanation are often all that are required, and stress management such as relaxation, hypnosis or sleep advice may be tried.

Any restorative or implant treatment must be planned taking the extra occlusal load into account because bruxism is associated with high failure rates of restorations such as veneers and also predisposes to cusp fractures.

Appliances are widely prescribed, but there is no firm evidence to support their use. Claims that appliances act by changing the vertical dimension, relieving occlusal interference, repositioning the condyles, changing mandibular posture or preventing periodontal ligament proprioception are unproven, and their mechanisms of action are unknown. Nevertheless, appliances frequently appear to be effective, and they can be useful to protect against severe attrition. Appliances may be attached to upper or lower arches, including flat posterior bite planes and various types of occlusal splints. All should be worn at night only and initially for 1 month. If there is no improvement, treatment should be discontinued to prevent adverse effects on the soft tissues and occlusion.

If effective, the appliances may be worn intermittently during exacerbations. Soft vacuum-formed appliances are inexpensive and readily fitted as a short-term diagnostic aid but are quickly worn out by a determined bruxist. Any type of appliance can occasionally worsen bruxism. If bruxism appears in relation to anxiety, a short course of an anxiolytic may help break the habit. Occlusal adjustment has been shown to be ineffective and should be avoided.

Appliances probably do not help daytime bruxism.

In severe bruxism, injection of botulinum toxin type A is shown to reduce the frequency of bruxism episodes and muscle tenderness but accepted protocols are not yet defined (Ch. 27).

Sleep bruxism PMID: 26758348

Awake bruxism PMID: 28550845

RESORPTION OF TEETH

Teeth can be resorbed by osteoclasts in the same way as bone. The cells are often referred to as *odontoclasts*, although they develop from the same precursors as osteoclasts and are differentiated only because they resorb teeth and are slightly smaller. Precursor cells are present in the periodontal ligament and in the dental pulp and can be triggered to migrate to the tooth surface and differentiate into odontoclasts by specific mediators.

Odontoclasts resorb and remove dentine by the same mechanisms as osteoclasts resorb bone (Fig. 6.6), excavating Howship's lacunae along the resorbed surface. Resorption is intermittent, and odontoclasts may not always be present as they disappear during inactive periods. Whenever resorption takes place, there is usually some attempt at repair by apposition of cementum or bone and resorption and repair follow a cyclical progression.

The pattern of intermittent resorption and repair can occasionally lead to ankylosis, in which a tooth becomes fused to the surrounding bone. This may be seen in both permanent and deciduous teeth but causes more problems in the deciduous dentition because the jaw is still growing. Ankylosis will markedly delay shedding of the tooth and eruption of the permanent successor. The ankylosed tooth submerges as the alveolus grows around it, and there may be space loss as distal teeth tip into the space. Submerged teeth usually need to be removed surgically. Ankylosis in the permanent dentition is often associated with replacement resorption, leading to eventual loss of the tooth.

Resorption of deciduous teeth

The deciduous teeth are progressively loosened and ultimately shed by resorption as a physiological process. The cyclical nature of resorption causes the looseness of the teeth to vary before they are shed. It used to be thought that pressure from the permanent successor induced resorption, but it is now known that the follicle of the permanent successor produces soluble factors that control the resorption of both the bone and deciduous tooth root in the path of eruption. When a permanent successor is absent, resorption of deciduous tooth root starts later than normal and progresses much more slowly. However, it does usually progress until eventually the tooth is lost.

The main complication of resorption of deciduous teeth is ankylosis and submergence (see previous section). Occasionally resorption from the lateral aspect of the root cuts off a fragment that remains buried. This can either be resorbed or may eventually exfoliate like a small sequestrum of bone.

Resorption of permanent teeth

All teeth have microscopic areas of resorption and repair of no significance on their root surface, but more extensive resorption of permanent teeth is pathological. There are various causes (Box 6.2). The most common are inflammation and pressure from malpositioned teeth (Fig. 6.7). A minor degree of inflammatory resorption is common on root apices associated with periapical granulomas. Occasionally, this is a prominent feature radiologically leading to concern over the diagnosis (Fig. 6.8).

Resorption of tooth roots by lesions such as tumours and cysts is often said to indicate malignancy. However, resorption can result from simple pressure, and benign cysts and neoplasms may cause resorption if they are present for sufficient time. The quality of the resorption is more important in defining a possible malignant neoplasm. Resorption by malignant neoplasms is typically rapid, irregular and described as 'moth-eaten' radiographically. Resorption by benign cysts and tumours has a sharper more regular outline ('knife edge' resorption).

Cementum is most readily resorbed, whereas enamel is the most resistant tissue, but sometimes the crown of an impacted tooth may be completely destroyed, although this takes many years (Fig. 6.9). Immature permanent teeth are resorbed more quickly because the dentine is less heavily mineralised and the dentine around open apices is very thin.

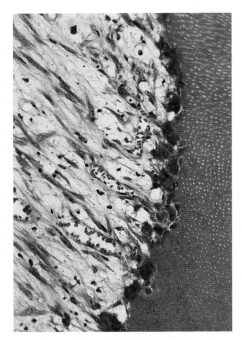

Fig. 6.6 Resorption during periapical periodontitis. Active osteoclastic resorption of dentine is continuing in the presence of inflammatory exudate. This is a common change but usually minor in extent.

Box 6.2	**Important causes of resorption of permanent teeth**

- Periapical periodontitis. The most common cause, but is usually slight
- Impacted teeth pressing on the root of an adjacent tooth
- Unerupted teeth. Over many years these may undergo resorption or hypercementosis, or both
- Replanted teeth. These are sometimes rapidly and grossly resorbed
- Excessive orthodontic force
- Pressure from cysts and neoplasms
- Idiopathic resorption, external or internal

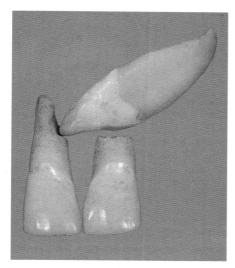

Fig. 6.7 Gross root resorption of two upper central incisors induced by an unerupted canine that has migrated across the midline.

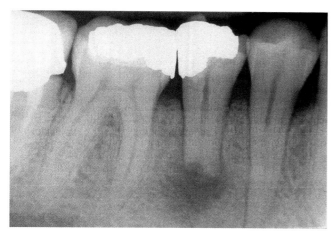

Fig. 6.8 Inflammatory resorption of the root apex induced by periapical periodontitis resulting from the non-vital pulp.

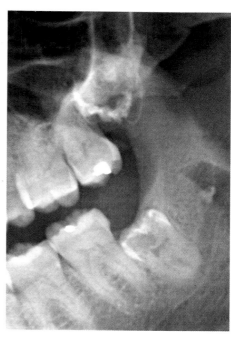

Fig. 6.9 Resorption of unerupted third molars. The crowns are hollowed out, and little more than the enamel of the upper molar remains. *(Courtesy Mrs J Brown.)*

Idiopathic resorption

Idiopathic resorption of permanent teeth may start from the pulpal surface or the external surface. Either can produce the clinical feature of 'pink spot', a rounded pink area where the vascular resorbing tissue has become visible through the enamel overlying the resorbed dentine. A pink spot centrally in the crown suggests internal resorption, and one close to the gingival margin suggests external resorption. Idiopathic resorption often affects several teeth, sometimes many, and additional lesions should be sought radiographically when one is found.

Mechanisms and diseases PMID: 20659257

Internal resorption

Internal idiopathic resorption is an uncommon condition in which dentine is resorbed from within the pulp. Resorption tends to be localised, producing the characteristic sign of a well-defined rounded area of radiolucency in the crown or midroot (Fig. 6.10 and 6.11). Resorption is often detected by chance on a radiograph.

The cause is unknown, but it may occasionally follow trauma, caries or restoration. Inflammation is often present

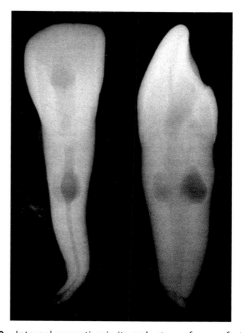

Fig. 6.10 Internal resorption in its early stages forms a fusiform expansion of the pulp chamber, as seen on the left. A radiograph at right angles shows the resorption has burrowed out to perforate the root surface.

in the pulp, and some consider this presentation a type of inflammatory resorption.

Treatment involves removing the pulp and filling the root before too much dentine is lost, the root is perforated or the crown fractures off.

Internal resorption review PMID: 20630282

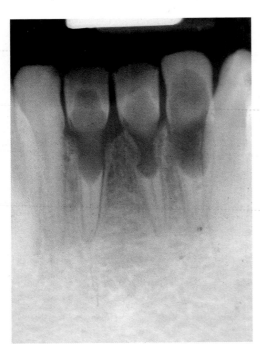

Fig. 6.11   Idiopathic internal resorption. In this unusually severe example, resorption affects the roots of three lower incisors. Note the smooth outline and process centred on the pulp.

External resorption

Idiopathic resorption starting externally may be localised to one tooth or generalised, the latter often affecting a group of teeth but sometimes the whole dentition. The cause is unknown, although a mild degree of inflammation is often suspected. Usually, a limited area of the root is attacked from its external surface near the amelocemental junction (Figs 6.12-6.14) and resorption penetrates almost to the pulp. A very thin band of circumpulpal dentine is preserved, at least initially, and the resorption tends to burrow up and down around the pulp. Once this barrier is lost, and if the resorption defect communicates with a pocket or the crevice, bacteria may enter the pulp. Resorption in the crown (Fig. 6.14), may produce a pink spot (Fig. 6.15). Accessible defects may be amenable to restoration with mineral trioxide or other materials, but long-term success is unpredictable.

Generalised resorption usually starts either at the amelo-dentinal junction or near the apex. Over the course of years, the roots of multiple teeth may be destroyed (Fig. 6.16). The lost tissue is partially repaired by bonelike tissue, but eventually lost. Devitalising of teeth does not slow progress, and no treatment is effective.

A minor degree of external resorption is common around the apex of incisors following orthodontic treatment, particularly apically when fixed appliances are used to move the root apex or if high forces are used.

External cervical resorption review PMID: 29704466 and 29737544

Replacement resorption

Replacement resorption is a form of slow progressive external resorption in which the tooth is gradually replaced by bone, rather than leaving a defect filled by soft tissue. Replacement resorption follows ankylosis and is therefore a complication of luxation injuries, avulsion and re-implantation. Following injury there is a short period of inflammatory resorption

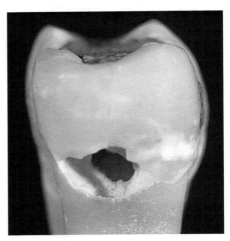

Fig. 6.12   Idiopathic external resorption. Resorption frequently starts at the amelocemental junction. In this case, the pulp is exposed.

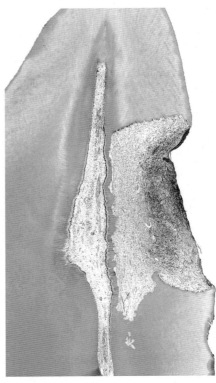

Fig. 6.13   Idiopathic external resorption. A localised area of destruction of dentine produced by osteoclastic activity. The cavity is filled with fibrous tissue containing some inflammatory cells superficially. The pulp shows no reaction, and the sparing of the circumpulpal dentine until a late stage is a characteristic feature of external resorption.

proportional to the severity of the injury. This can often be treated by using calcium hydroxide dressings in the root canal if the resorption is apical. However, when the injury to the periodontal ligament is severe, healing occurs by recruitment of precursor cells from the adjacent bone marrow, causing bony repair and ankylosis. If more than a small area of the root surface is involved by the ankylosis, the tooth effectively becomes part of the bone, and the normal physiological mechanisms of continuous bone turnover lead to progressive replacement of dentine by bone. The resorption progresses

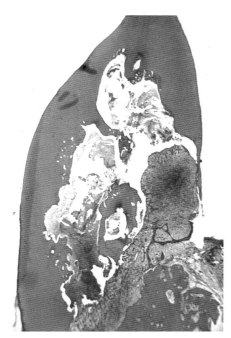

Fig. 6.14   Idiopathic resorption, late stage. A grossly resorbed central incisor with a widely perforated pulp wall. Granulation tissue is growing into the pulp from the gingival margin, and bony repair tissue has been laid down more deeply.

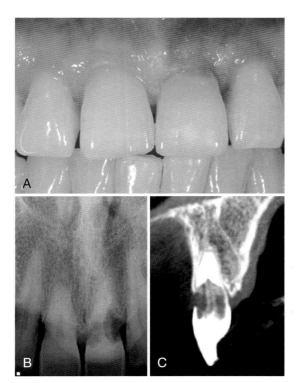

Fig. 6.15 Pink spot. A, External resorption has extended up into the upper left central incisor crown and is visible as a subtle pink colour in the gingival third of the crown. B, A periapical radiograph revealed ragged radiolucent defects mesially and distally with communication to the gingiva near the amelocemental junction. C, A reconstructed coronal cone beam computed tomography slice reveals the true extent of the resorption. Note the typical preservation of a thin layer of circumpulpal dentine. *(Source: Bakhsh AA, Durack C, Ricucci D et al. Root resorption. In Berman LH, Kenneth MH, Rotstein I [eds], Cohen's Pathways of the Pulp, 12th Edition [2021], St. Louis, Elsevier Inc)*

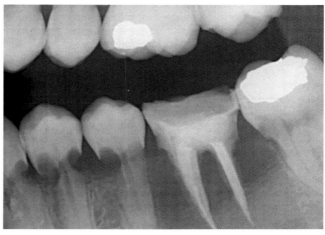

Fig. 6.16 Generalised external resorption, with all lower teeth in this image affected. Resorption in a similar pattern affected all lower incisors. The first molar root is almost completely lost. The preserved circumpulpal dentine is visible in the premolars.

Box 6.3   Causes of hypercementosis

- Ageing
- Increased occlusal load
- Over-erupted teeth
- Periapical periodontitis. A common cause but minor in amount. Close to the apex there is usually a little resorption, but coronally cementum is laid down, forming a shoulder
- Functionless and unerupted teeth. Hypercementosis and resorption may both be present
- Paget's disease. May cause an irregular mass of cementum on the root with a histological 'mosaic' pattern of enhanced resorption and deposition (Ch. 13)
- Cementoblastoma (Ch. 11) and cemento-osseous dysplasia are distinct diseases (Ch. 12)

---

relentlessly and traumatised incisors in children can be completely lost in less than 5 years. In adults the process is slower but still essentially irreversible.

Replacement resorption is always associated with ankylosis. Teeth have an abnormal percussive note, no mobility and loss of lamina dura and periodontal ligament radiographically.

After trauma PMID: 7641622

HYPERCEMENTOSIS

Cellular cementum has a low turnover rate to maintain the fibre attachments of the periodontal ligament. Cementoblast precursor cells lie in the periodontal ligament and are recruited for normal turnover and to repair root fractures or resorption defects. New cementum is added to the surface without significant resorption so that the normal thickness of the cementum increases slightly with age.

Cementum is essentially bone, but unlike bone has no internal vascular supply and no innervation because it has no medullary spaces.

Deposition of excessive amounts of cementum is not uncommon and has several possible causes (Box 6.3), of which inflammation is probably the commonest pathological

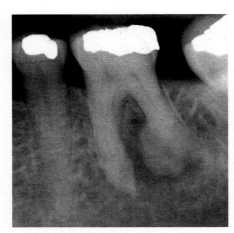

Fig. 6.17 Hypercementosis as a result of apical inflammation.

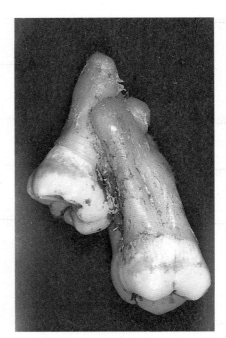

Fig. 6.19 **Concrescence.** Two upper molars fused together by cementum.

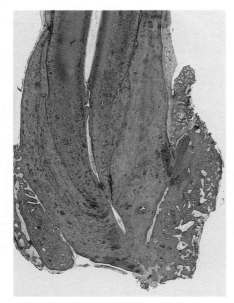

Fig. 6.18 **Hypercementosis in Paget's disease.** An irregular craggy mass of bonelike cementum has been formed over thickened regular and acellular cementum.

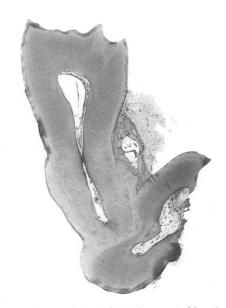

Fig. 6.20 **Concrescence.** Histological section of fused teeth reveals that the teeth are joined by cementum and not dentine.

cause (Fig. 6.17). Acromegaly and calcinosis are also reported to cause hypercementosis, but the effect is rare and not significant.

Hypercementosis is often noted radiographically, with widening of roots, usually in their apical third to produce a blunt root tip. The periodontal ligament space and lamina dura is intact around the cementum. Hypercementosis is not associated with ankylosis.

Increased thickness of cementum is not itself a disease, and no treatment is necessary. If hypercementosis is gross, as in Paget's disease, extractions become difficult (Fig. 6.18). The cementoblastoma (Ch. 11) is a benign neoplasm of cementoblasts that can appear like hypercementosis radiographically, but there is root resorption and a characteristic presentation. Cemento-osseous dysplasia (Ch. 11) is also a distinct condition easily confused with hypercementosis.

The lesions previously called cementomas are dealt with in Chapter 12.

Concrescence is hypercementosis that causes fusion of the roots of adjacent teeth (Figs 6.19 and 6.20). It is rarely noticed until an attempt is made to extract one of the teeth. The two teeth are then found to move together and surgical intervention becomes necessary.

Cemental tear

A cemental tear is a rare condition in which a piece of cementum becomes fractured from the root. The fragment may be small or an extensive strip of cementum.

Cemental tears usually affect male patients, people aged over 60 years and single rooted teeth, most commonly

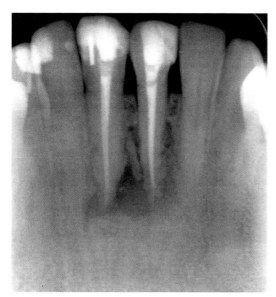

Fig. 6.21 Cemental tear affecting the patient's lower left central incisor producing a long flake of separated cementum lying in an inflammatory mass of granulation tissue with loss of surrounding lamina dura.

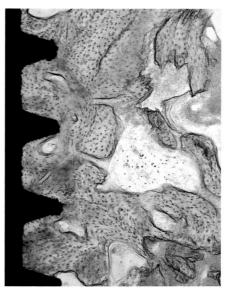

Fig. 6.22 Successful osseointegration. Bone (*unstained right*) in contact with implant thread (*left*). The tiny gap between the two is not appreciated with light microscopy.

maxillary incisors. The cementum may fracture at the dentine interface or internally along its incremental lines.

The cause is unknown but acute trauma, occlusal overloading, aging and possibly hypercementosis may contribute. Endodontic lateral perforation of a root or instrumentation beyond the apex may also occasionally dislodge a fragment of cementum. Most cemental tears affect the middle or cervical third of the root.

The effects depend on the size and level of the fragment. Those in the middle and cervical thirds of the root are associated with inflammation, resorption of the lamina dura and, once this communicates with a pocket, a rapidly progressing localised periodontitis. Radiologically this appears as a localised infrabony pocket containing a radiopaque foreign body and this is a common presentation. In such cases a periodontal-endodontic lesion or vertical root fracture need to be excluded. Those lying more apically produce periapical or periradicular radiolucency without loss of tooth vitality (Fig. 6.21).

Treatment relies on removing the fragment where possible, by nonsurgical periodontal therapy or localised flap surgery, though severe localised periodontal destruction may require extraction or combined endodontic treatment. Apical cemental tears are more difficult to treat.

Review PMID: 22794205 and 31447326

Treatment PMID: 34403513

PATHOLOGY OF OSSEOINTEGRATION

Osseointegrated implants have revolutionised dentistry and are also used to retain facial prostheses, obturators and bone-conduction hearing aids.

Osseointegration is defined as a direct structural and functional connection between viable bone and the surface of a load-bearing implant. This is possible only by using implants made from a limited number of metals, principally titanium, niobium and some of their alloys. The correct implant shape is also necessary to provide maximum surface area and transmit load effectively to the bone.

Successful osseointegration is achieved by bone growing to contact or to almost contact the implant. No periodontal ligament is present, and the implant is held tightly by friction and a thin layer of collagen and proteoglycan bone matrix about 100 nm thick (Fig. 6.22). The implant surface does not itself induce bone formation but, in medullary bone, both trabeculae of bone and marrow spaces may contact the implant and the bone and implant become chemically bonded together.

When an implant is placed into bone, much of the initial resistance to movement comes from tight apposition of the thread coronally in the cortical bone and stabilization by bone around its apex. In the medullary bone the implant is surrounded by blood and platelets are activated as in a normal healing response. The healing response recruits new osteoblasts from the surrounding bone and marrow and new blood vessels from the marrow. These form woven bone from the edge of the trephine hole toward the implant (distance osteogenesis), stopping just short of the implant. Bone precursors also attach to the implant, lay down bone matrix on it and form bone in direct contact with it (contact osteogenesis). Both types of healing occur around any one implant, but it is considered that the greater the area of contact osteogenesis, the better. Contact osteogenesis requires migration of the bone precursor cells through the organising clot to the implant surface, and fibrin adhesion to the implant is critical for this process. Once bone is formed, it undergoes a process of slow remodelling and increases the bonding of bone to the implant. The cortical bone support is important to stabilise the implant through the early healing phase, and it is helpful that this bone remodels very slowly. The force required to remove implants increases over several months after placement as healing and remodelling progress.

Because there is no periodontal ligament, there are no proprioceptive or pain fibres. There is no possibility of implant movement to cushion acute impact or to allow movements to adapt to functional forces. Thus, implants placed in growing jaws submerge like ankylosed teeth or move unpredictably. Orthodontic movement is not possible so that mini-implants make excellent anchorage for orthodontics. However, bone trabeculae do remodel around an implant in response to stress transmitted directly to the bone.

Bacteria are unable to penetrate between the mucosa and implant because a periodontal cuff develops that bears some similarity to the normal gingiva. As more apically, there are no collagen fibres joining the soft tissue to the implant. Instead, the collagen fibres in the cuff run circumferentially around the implant or its abutment. A non-keratinised junctional epithelium forms against the titanium surface, and a gingival sulcus of variable depth may be present. This epithelium is derived from the surrounding mucosa and adheres to the implant through hemidesmosomes in the same way as normal junctional epithelium adheres to tooth.

There are said to be no absolute contraindications to implant placement, but the factors listed in Box 6.4 should be considered potential problems because they are associated with a higher rate of implant failure. The infective endocarditis risk is unknown. Implant placement is a sterile procedure of lower risk than manipulating teeth and, provided the implants are well maintained, the risk of infection is very low.

Review osseointegration PMID: 12959168 and 28000277

Implant failure and peri-implantitis

Failure of implants is defined by progressive bone loss and increasing mobility and usually manifests shortly after placement or initial loading. Increased probing depths are often also present. Failure of integration during the healing period may be caused by movement, such as from that from early loading, or implant extending outside the cortex because of perforation or dehiscence.

Failure in the longer term is principally from bone loss caused by excessive loading or peri-implantitis.

Excessive loading may result from bruxism, non-axial forces from poorly designed superstructures or having too few implants to resist normal occlusal forces. Excessive loading tends to cause deep angular bone loss around the implant. The mechanisms are unclear but may involve microfractures of the superficial bone around the implant. Fracture of the implant itself is rare.

Plaque-induced inflammation around implants is called *peri-implant mucositis*, analogous to gingivitis and, if bone loss develops, *peri-implantitis*, and the microbial flora and host responses are similar to those in gingivitis and periodontitis. Peri-implantitis is preceded by mucositis, which is considered reversible if oral hygiene is improved. In peri-implantitis, infrabony pockets do not develop because there are no contact points or interdental papillae to form a local plaque trap. Bone loss is horizontal or forms a broad saucer-shaped defect that affects the entire implant circumference (Fig. 6.23). Peri-implant disease affects approximately 6% of all implants placed, rising to 20% after 10 years. Some degree of mucositis is found in 80% of individuals with implants, but in most patients this does not progress to bone loss.

If osseointegration fails, early peri-implantitis can develop quickly by extension of plaque biofilm along the implant

---

Box 6.4 Factors associated with implant failure and relative contraindications to implant placement

- Incomplete facial growth
- Uncontrolled diabetes
- Contraindications to surgery, such as bleeding tendencies
- Smoking
- Patients prone to osteomyelitis
  - Sclerotic bone or bone disease at site
  - Previous radiotherapy to the jaws
  - Previous intravenous bisphosphonate treatment
- Poor quality bone at site
  - Thin cortex
  - Sparse trabeculation
  - Osteoporosis
- Active periodontal disease or poor oral hygiene
- Mucosal disease
- Possibly, high-risk patient for infective endocarditis?

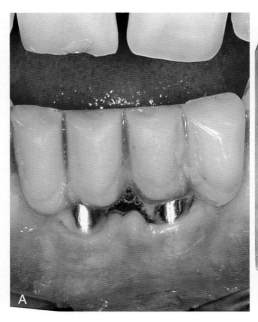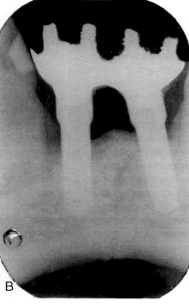

Fig. 6.23 Peri-implantitis. There is pocketing with a bead of pus exuding onto the gingival margin and a broad ring of bone loss evident radiographically. These older cylindrical coated implants were prone to peri-implantitis. *(Courtesy Professor R Palmer.)*

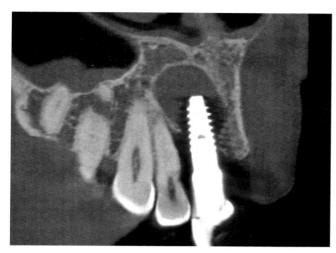

Fig 6.24 Apical implantitis. A well-defined corticated radiolucency around the implant apically that had an epithelial lining, resembling a radicular cyst. *(Courtesy Dr G Barwell)*

surface without developing angular bone defects. This is seen as a fine radiolucent zone around the implant, a much more subtle radiographic change that in more chronic peri-implantitis.

It is also possible, although much rarer, for implants to develop an apical peri-implantitis. This affects approximately 1%–2% of all implants placed, more commonly in the mandible. It presents as an apical radiolucency similar to a periapical granuloma, sometimes with pain, swelling and a sinus tract. The likely cause is persistence of apical inflammation from the pre-existing tooth. Even more rarely, the equivalent of a radicular cyst (Ch. 10) may form at the implant apex (Fig 6.24). Rests of Malassez from the original periodontal ligament and inflammation may persist after placement or an implant may be placed inadvertently into a pre-existing radicular cyst.

Other causes of failure are listed in Box 6.4 and complications of implant placement in Box 6.5. In addition, implants are more likely to fail in the maxilla than the mandible, if there is movement during healing, or if the bone is overheated by the drill during placement. Poor quality bone is often blamed for failure, often on grounds of minimal cortical thickness. However, implants can be successful in medullary bone with little cortex. Relatively avascular or sclerotic bone that heals poorly is probably a greater risk.

The question of whether it is possible to mount a true allergic reaction to titanium dental implants is a controversial issue. Implants are made of alloys containing aluminium, vanadium or other metals to increase the strength. Cases of implants being associated with skin reactions and a peri-implantitis like inflammation are recorded, but the mechanisms are unclear. Titanium, in pure form, appears an unlikely allergen and various tests to detect hypersensitivity are not yet of proven benefit.

A further question that is unanswered is whether wear debris and tiny titanium metal particles eroded from the implant surface have any effects. Such particles can be generated by microscopic movements between the implant and abutments, or generated by inflamed tissue abutting the implant and can be found in the gingiva around implants

---

Box 6.5   Complications of implant placement

General surgical complications

- Bleeding, haematoma in floor of mouth or into antrum
- Tissue emphysema
- Acute infection
- Devitalisation of bone from high torque or trephine speed
- Aspiration or ingestion of implant or instrument

Damage to adjacent structures

- Lingual and inferior alveolar and mental nerves
- Sublingual and submental arteries
- Sinus or nasal floor
- Canalis sinuosus
- Tooth roots

Misalignment or incorrect placement

Unstable implant

Fracture of atrophic mandible

Apical implantitis (retrograde peri-implantitis)

Complications of sinus lift and ridge augmentation

Perforation into sinus

Sinusitis

Implant loss

- Early loss
  - Persistent inflammation
  - Mobility on placement
- Late loss
  - Plaque induced peri-implantitis
  - Overloading and loss of integration

---

with peri-implantitis, in epithelial cells, in macrophages in the gingiva and possibly more widely in the body.

A number of cases are reported in which squamous carcinoma appears to have developed in close association with implants. This appears a chance association and in some cases the implants have been placed into mucosa with potentially malignant changes. There is no evidence that implants exert a carcinogenic effect. When a carcinoma does develop close to an implant, it does not appear to grow along the interface so that healthy implants do not provide an easy path for carcinoma to penetrate into the medullary cavity (though removal of the implant would).

Occasionally, patients are seen with non-osseointegrated implants such as blade implants or pins of various metals. These historic types of implant usually failed rapidly as a result of infection (Fig. 6.25).

Allergy to titanium PMID: 27027398

Titanium allery tests PMID: 35819566

Treatment of peri-implantitis PMID: 35899987 and 35103327 and other papers in this issue.

Implant corrosion PMID: 28612506 and 30892769

Implants and oral carcinoma PMID: 35338331

Classification peri-implant inflammation PMID: 29926489

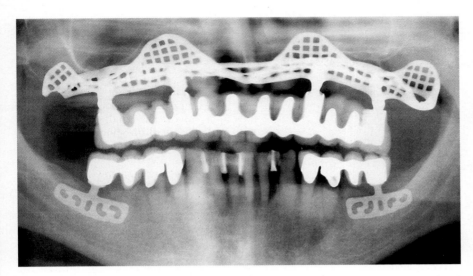

Fig. 6.25 Gross infection around an old type of implant. There is a subperiosteal cast metal implant in contact with almost all the maxillary alveolus. Note the extensive bone loss below it, visible most clearly at the left tuberosity. There are two blade implants in the mandible, both with bone loss extending down the stem to involve the blade. The patient is at risk from severe infection and continued bone destruction until the implants are removed. *(Courtesy Professor R Palmer.)*

Periodontal diseases | 7

THE NORMAL PERIODONTAL TISSUES

The periodontal tissues have a complex anatomy specialised to resist masticatory forces and seal around the teeth (Box 7.1).

The oral outer epithelium of the free and attached gingiva is stratified squamous and thinly parakeratinised. Opposing the teeth, the *epithelial attachment* is made by the junctional epithelium adhering to enamel (Fig. 7.1), achieved by the cells secreting a basement membrane onto the enamel and attaching to it by hemidesmosomes. The attachment to the enamel appears histologically as a clear cuticle (Fig. 7.2). It forms an effective seal, protecting the underlying connective tissues. The epithelial attachment is so firmly adherent to the tooth surface that tension, during histological preparation or tooth extraction, tears through the epithelium itself rather than pulling the epithelium from the tooth (see Fig. 7.2). Junctional epithelium has a high turnover rate, fewer intercellular attachments and more intercellular space than mucosal epithelium. This results in higher permeability than other parts of the gingiva, potentially allowing the passage of molecules from the gingival crevice to the connective tissues. The epithelial attachment is constantly reformed as the basal cells divide, mature and move upward to be shed in the crevice.

When periodontitis develops, the attachment migrates apically but remains firmly attached to the tooth surface cementum by the same mechanisms. The junctional epithelial cells are then believed to have an important role in regulating

> ### Box 7.1 Anatomical regions of normal healthy gingival tissue
>
> - *Junctional epithelium.* Extends from the amelocemental junction to the floor of the gingival sulcus and forms the epithelial attachment to the tooth surface
> - *Sulcular epithelium.* Lines the gingival sulcus and joins the epithelial attachment to the gingival epithelium
> - *Free gingiva.* Coronal to the amelocemental junction and attached gingiva and includes the tips of the interdental papillae, forms the soft tissue wall of the crevice
> - *Attached gingiva.* Extends from the gingival crest to the mucogingival junction and is bound down to the superficial periodontal fibres and periosteum to form a mucoperiosteum

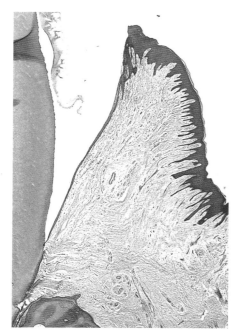

Fig. 7.1 Gingival sulcus and epithelial attachment. This sagittal section shows the normal appearances. Enamel removed by decalcification of the specimen has left the triangular space between tooth and soft tissue. The epithelial attachment runs along the enamel surface, seen as a thin line of epithelium from the top of the papilla to the amelocemental junction. The gingival sulcus, minute in extent, is formed where the papilla curves away from the line of the enamel surface. There is hardly any inflammatory infiltrate, just some epithelial rete hyperplasia in the free gingiva to indicate that a small amount of inflammation is present.

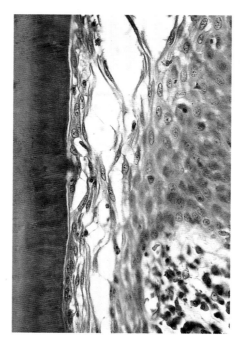

Fig. 7.2 The strength of the epithelial attachment. On this tooth the epithelial attachment has migrated on to the surface of the cementum as a result of periodontal disease. The epithelium has been torn away from the tooth, but the tear is within the junctional epithelium, leaving some of its cells still adherent to the cementum and attached by a clear cuticle. A similar strength is seen when the junctional epithelium is attached to enamel.

Box 7.2   Principal fibres of the periodontal ligament
- *Oblique fibres* form a suspensory ligament from the lamina dura of the socket to the root surface, inclined in an apical direction
- *Horizontal fibres* form a dense group attaching neck of tooth to rim of socket
- *Transeptal fibres* of the horizontal group are not attached to alveolar bone but pass superficial to it and join adjacent teeth together. They protect the inter-dental gingiva by resisting forces that would otherwise separate the teeth and open the contact points
- *Gingival fibres* form a cuff round the neck of the tooth supporting the soft tissues and protecting the epithelial attachment. They resist separation of the gingivae from the tooth

and modulating local immunological and inflammatory responses though cytokine production.

The *attached gingiva* is firmly bound down to the underlying bone to form a tough mucoperiosteum. Its stippled appearance is due to the intersections of its underlying epithelial rete ridges and the bundles of collagen inserted into the connective tissue papillae.

The *alveolar mucosa* is the thin mucosa extending from the sharply demarcated mucogingival junction into the sulcus. It has a smooth surface, darker colour and overlies loose mobile fibrous tissue. Underlying blood vessels can often be seen through the epithelial layer. It should not be confused with *alveolar ridge mucosa*, the mucoperiosteum of an edentulous ridge.

Classic description anatomy PMID: 5005682

Anatomy of periodontium ISBN-13: 978-0723438120

Gingival and periodontal fibres

The periodontal ligament comprises densely packed bundles of collagen fibres running from tooth to bone interspersed by loose connective tissue containing wide blood vessels and nerves. Compression of the ligament forces blood out through channels in the lamina dura into adjacent medullary bone, producing a viscoelastic cushion against compression and tension. The normal thickness of the periodontal ligament is approximately 0.1–0.3 mm.

The principal fibres are arranged in a series of fairly well-defined groups (Box 7.2).

The periodontal ligament fibres are embedded in cementum at their inner ends and in the lamina dura at their outer ends. New fibres replacing those that have aged, or forming in response to new functional stresses, are attached by apposition of further layers of cellular cementum, which becomes gradually thicker with age. The lamina dura is a layer of cortical bone continuous, at the margin of the sockets, with the cortical bone of the alveolus.

The cell rests of Malassez, remnants of Hertwig's root sheath, lie in the mid and apical thirds of the ligament forming a meshwork that may contribute to maintenance of the ligament. They are important for cyst formation (Ch. 10) but are not thought to play a role in periodontitis.

Gingival crevicular fluid (exudate)

In health, a minute amount of fluid can be collected from the gingival margins. This crevicular fluid is a transudate in health, passing through the permeable junctional epithelium.

Table 7.1   Classification of Periodontal Diseases and Conditions

The periodontal disease status of an individual is defined by one of the mutually exclusive diagnoses in items 1, 2, 4, 5, or 6. In addition, any of items 2, 7, 8, 9 and 10 can co-exist with this periodontal disease status.

1. Health:
   intact periodontium
   reduced periodontium
2. Plaque-induced gingivitis: (localised /generalised gingivitis)
   intact periodontium
   reduced periodontium
3. Non plaque-induced gingival diseases and conditions
4. Periodontitis:
   localised (< 30% teeth)
   generalised (> 30% teeth)
   molar-incisor pattern
5. Necrotising periodontal diseases
6. Periodontitis as a manifestation of systemic disease
7. Systemic diseases or conditions affecting the periodontal tissues
8. Periodontal abscesses
9. Periodontal-endodontic lesions
10. Mucogingival deformities and conditions

When inflammation develops, it becomes an inflammatory exudate and the amount increases greatly with the degree of inflammation. Its composition changes while inflammation develops, and in established inflammation it contains immunoglobulin (Ig), other serum proteins and migrating neutrophils and macrophages. Crevicular fluid is not a secretion (there are no glands in this region).

Even in apparent health, there are always a few inflammatory cells in the gingiva and a very minor degree of inflammation.

CLASSIFICATION OF PERIODONTAL DISEASES

The terms *gingivitis* and *periodontitis* usually refer only to plaque-related inflammatory disease. However, there are also diseases that predispose to periodontitis and conditions that, though not induced by plaque, are worsened by it. Other diseases as diverse as tuberculosis or lichen planus may affect the gingivae occasionally. Currently, the internationally accepted 2018 classification of periodontal diseases is that arising from the 2017 World Workshop for a Classification of Periodontal Diseases, a simplified version of which is shown in Table 7.1.

Classification PMID: 29926952 and corrections 29926495

Classification changes explained PMID: 29926489

Application to diagnosis Web URL 7.1 https://www.bsperio.org.uk/assets/downloads/BSP_BPE_Guidelines_2019.pdf

GINGIVITIS

Gingivitis is a largely asymptomatic, low-grade inflammation of the gingivae, induced by bacterial plaque growing on the teeth along the gingival margin. The cause is inadequate oral hygiene, sometimes exacerbated by local plaque traps (Figs 7.3 and 7.4).

Gingivitis always precedes development of periodontitis, but not all gingivitis will progress to involve deeper tissues. The features distinguishing periodontitis from gingivitis

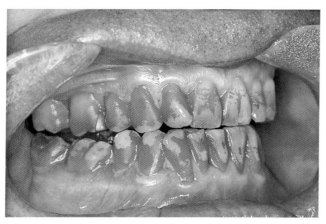

Fig. 7.3   Accumulation of plaque stained by disclosing solution after 24 hours without oral hygiene measures.

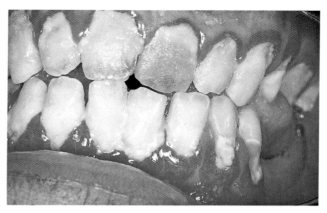

Fig. 7.5   Severe gingivitis. A florid, bright-red band of gingival inflammation results from very poor oral hygiene. The gingival margin is thickened and rounded by oedema and has lost its smooth sharply defined anatomy. Thick accumulations of plaque are visible on all tooth surfaces.

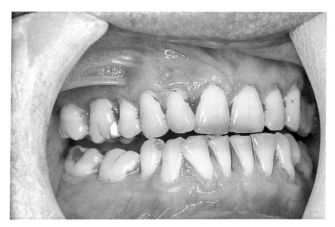

Fig. 7.4   The effects of tooth brushing in the same patient. Plaque remains interdentally in most areas, explaining why gingivitis is often localised here.

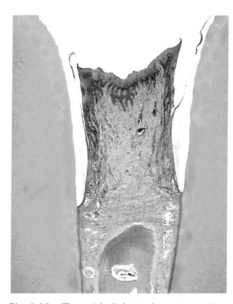

Fig. 7.6   Gingivitis. The epithelial attachment remains on enamel in the lower half of its length and extends down to finish at the level of the amelocemental junction. Inflammatory cells are concentrated along and just below the junctional epithelium and extend into the deeper gingiva, around the interradicular fibres. The alveolar crest is not resorbed. There is a small pocket or deepened crevice, the extent of which can be identified by the junctional epithelium rete hyperplasia.

are loss of bone at the alveolar crest, apical migration of the junctional epithelial attachment, and loss of marginal periodontal ligament. Until this happens, and probably for a short period afterward, gingivitis can generally be cured by plaque control. By contrast, loss of bone in periodontitis is essentially irreversible.

Clinical features

The gingivae become red and slightly swollen with oedema along the gingival margin (Fig. 7.5). *Hyperplastic gingivitis* is a term sometimes given to gingivitis in which the gingiva appears to enlarge. This is a result of inflammatory oedema rather than genuine tissue hyperplasia and largely resolves with treatment.

Pathology

By definition, inflammation in gingivitis is restricted to the gingival margins and does not affect the periodontal ligament or bone (Fig. 7.6).

The development of gingivitis has been arbitrarily divided histologically into 'initial', 'early' and 'established' phases (Table 7.2), whereas the fourth 'advanced' stage refers to periodontitis. It must be appreciated that these stages are artificially distinguished, being largely based on animal studies and experimental gingivitis studies in humans. They simply

reflect the stages of development of chronic inflammation as would be seen in any tissue. By the standard of the very slow rate of disease progression in a patient, all these stages are very rapid early events, probably within the first few weeks of disease initiation. The more important pathological processes in gingivitis and periodontitis are those of long-term chronic inflammation.

Traditional 'stages' PMID: classic study 765622 and updated 28758305

Microbiology

Although gingivitis and periodontitis are caused primarily by microbial plaque, these diseases are not simple infections. In a classical bacterial tissue infection, a pathogenic species grows to become numerically dominant and produces

Table 7.2   The classical stages of gingivitis and periodontitis as described by Page and Schroeder in 1976.

Initial lesion gingivitis	Early lesion gingivitis	Established lesion gingivitis	Advanced lesion periodontitis
Develops within 24–48 hours of exposure to plaque	Develops after approximately 7 days	Develops after 2–3 weeks	Extension of plaque into the crevice
Plaque related to gingival sulcus	Tissue contains inflammatory infiltrate of neutrophils and lymphocytes	Dense, predominantly plasmacytic infiltrate around the crevice	Pocket formation
Vasodilatation	Vascular proliferation	Infiltrate fills but is limited to interdental papillae	Loss of attachment
Infiltration by neutrophils and fewer macrophages	Epithelial hyperplasia in the crevice wall	Destruction of superficial connective tissue fibres	Bone loss
Crevicular fluid flow increases	Deepened crevice.	Deepened gingival crevice	
Clinically gingiva appears healthy	Inflammation is visible clinically	More prominent vascular exudation	
		Epithelial attachment remains at or near amelocemental junction	
		Alveolar bone and periodontal ligament remain intact	
		Can remain stable	

disease through specific virulence factors. In gingivitis and periodontitis the causative organisms remain outside the tissues and induce inflammation by soluble factors, triggering immune responses and interfering with host defences. There is a complex host-microbial balance in which the bacteria survive but have their growth limited by the host response. Traditionally, plaque was investigated by microbiological culture, but many organisms in plaque are not cultivable. Current understanding is based on molecular methods, identifying species by nucleic acid sequencing. This has revealed a much greater complexity than was appreciated by even the most careful culture techniques, defining about 500 different species in plaque, many still uncharacterised and uncultivable.

The structure of plaque is analogous to an ecosystem, with bacterial species interdependent on one another for their survival. Interactions between species include providing growth factors and nutrients, signalling, adhesion, protection from oxygen and host defences and even transfer of genetic material. Such interactions may be competitive or cooperative. Cooperative interactions are reflected in spatial organization into 'consortia' of interdependent species forming structures in plaque, such as 'corn on the cob' (Fig. 4.3) or 'hedgehog' structures. The biofilm of plaque has been considered by some to be the equivalent of one enormous organism; it is more than the sum of many individual bacterial species stuck together in a biofilm.

The key pathogenic features of dental plaque are shown in Box 7.3.

Biofilm ecology PMID: 26120510

Structural organization of plaque PMID: 26811460

Plaque bacterial communities PMID: 30301974

Not all plaque is pathogenic. Small amounts are present in all mouths between cleaning, cleaning does not remove it all and inflammation does not develop for a few days after cleaning stops. Even in established gingivitis, there is not necessarily progression to periodontitis. Thus, there is a truly commensal plaque that can be associated with gingival health, plaque that causes only mild inflammation without progression, and a truly pathogenic plaque associated with tissue damage. Something tips a balance between the host

> **Box 7.3   Key features of dental plaque**
> - Is an insoluble strongly adherent biofilm
> - Matrix protects constituent bacteria from host and environmental change
> - Is outside the tissues, in the crevice or a pocket
> - Contains many species in a stable ecology
> - Many species are obligate or facultative anaerobes
> - Has a structure based on physical aggregation of consortia of interdependent microbial species
> - Comprises different flora in small adjacent sites adapted to local environment
> - Adapts to external stimuli, is dynamic
> - Supragingivally, much more extracellular polysaccharide matrix is formed

and the flora to trigger disease development and progression. Whether this is the host response to the bacteria or ecological changes in plaque remains contentious, but evidence suggests that the primary cause is changes in the plaque constituent species and metabolism.

Over the decades, theories of how plaque causes disease have evolved. Initially, the **non-specific plaque hypothesis** blamed the plaque bulk and proposed that the total volume was more important that the constituent species, differences in disease being primarily determined by patient susceptibility. Later, the **specific plaque hypothesis** proposed that there were individual pathogenic species that could be identified by virulence factors (Table 7.3) and association with diseased tissue sites. Many potential specific pathogens with impressive virulence factors were identified, but it became clear that some sites were inflamed in their absence and that these bacteria were often not numerically significant. The **bacterial complex theory** identified bacterial species that tended to be found together, and suggested that combinations, such as the 'red complex' of *Treponema denticola*, *Porphyromonas gingivalis*, *Tannerella forsythia*, were important. The **ecological plaque hypothesis** built on knowledge of plaque as an interdependent community of cooperating species. It proposed that the interdependence of species enabled evolution of a pathogenic flora that could better resist host defences through their cooperative interdependence.

Table 7.3 Possible virulence factors of plaque bacteria

Type of factor	Function and examples
Anaerobic tolerance	Many are obligate or facultative anaerobes that can survive at low oxygen tension and low pH in the pocket
Metabolically adapted	Able to metabolise host derived compounds to extract iron, peptides and other nutrients, either alone or in co-operative consortia of species
Enzymes	Collagenase, trypsin, fibrinolysin, hyaluronidase, chondroitin sulphatase, heparinase, ribonuclease and deoxyribonuclease. Immunoglobulin proteases. *P. gingivalis* gingipain, provides nutrients and iron, acts as adhesion factor
Cytotoxic metabolic products	Indole, ammonia and hydrogen sulphide, reducing agents
Specific toxins	Powerful leukotoxins (particularly that of *Aggregatibacter actinomycetemcomitans*), epitheliotoxins (*Porphyromonas gingivalis* and *Prevotella intermedius*)
Endotoxin	From all Gram-negative bacteria, more potent from some species than others
Capsular polysaccharides	Complement resistance and host defence evasion in many species
Fimbriae	Adhesion factors in many species. *P. gingivalis* fimbriae mediate invasion of host cells
Bone-resorbing factors	*Actinomyces viscosus* bone-resorbing factor

Table 7.4 Bacterial species in plaque associated with health and disease

Species in plaque associated with gingival health	Species unchanged in health and disease ('core species')	Species in plaque associated with periodontitis
Actinomyces naeslundii	*Campylobacter gracilis*	*Bacteroides* sp.
Other *Actinomyces* sp.	*Fusobacterium nucleatum*	*Desulfobulbus* sp.
Rothia aeria		*Eubacterium saphenum*
Rothia dentocariosa		*Fretibacterium* sp.
Streptococcus sanguinis		*Porphyromonas endodontalis*
		Porphyromonas gingivalis
		Prevotella intermedia
		Selenomonas sputigena
		Tannerella forsythia
		Treponema denticola
		Other *Treponema* sp.

Adapted from PMID 32385883

Changes in the stable healthy plaque ecology were thought to be driven by environmental factors such as thick plaque producing anaerobic environments, inflammation and changes in nutrients.

Current understanding is encompassed by the **dysbiotic plaque hypothesis** and the **'keystone pathogen'* hypothesis**. In this refinement of the ecological hypothesis, the entire plaque ecology undergoes a shift from a symbiotic flora, structure and metabolism to a dysbiotic disease-producing state, driven by interdependent reactions between host and bacterial factors. Keystone pathogens are bacterial species that, though present in only low numbers, exert a disproportionate effect on the ecology of the plaque, not only influencing its constituent species but inducing apparently benign bacterial species to shift into a pathogenic metabolic pattern. In this model the distinction between commensal and pathogenic species is blurred. Species proposed as keystone pathogens are often the same species considered pathogens under previous theories. The best understood keystone pathogen in gingivitis and periodontitis is *Porphyromonas gingivalis*. This has numerous virulence factors but is unable to cause periodontitis as a pure infection in animals even though it is

a powerful promoter of severe disease in combination with other organisms.

Plaque is often studied in experimental gingivitis models in which tooth cleaning is stopped and plaque sampled at different time periods.

Healthy (uninflamed) gingivae. The plaque is supragingival and thin (10–20 cells thick). Gram-positive bacteria predominate and include *Actinomyces* species, *Rothia*, viridans streptococci and *Streptococcus epidermidis*. In older people in periodontal health, Gram-positive bacteria, particularly streptococci, form the largest single group (50% of the predominant cultivable flora). These organisms are colonisers, able to adhere to pellicle. Gram-negative bacteria are present, but in smaller proportions and include *Porphyromonas sp.* and *Fusobacterium sp.*

Early (and experimental) gingivitis. If toothbrushing is neglected for several days, plaque grows in thickness and is typically 100–300 cells thick. In the earliest stages, bacteria proliferate, but the plaque remains Gram positive in character, and *Actinomyces* species become predominant.

Gingivitis. With time, Gram-negative organisms become increasingly prominent and the plaque becomes more anaerobic. *Veillonella*, *Fusobacterium* and *Campylobacter* species become more conspicuous, and the Gram-negative anaerobes normally considered to be associated with disease appear.

Some species, such as *Fusobacterium nucleatum* and *Campylobacter sp.* are found in both health and disease ('core species').

Bacterial species associated with health and disease are shown in Table 7.4.

Oral microbiome PMID: 27857087

Ecological plaque hypothesis PMID: 12624191

The Keystone pathogen hypothesis PMID: 22941505

Role of the bacterial flora PMID: 32385883

Calculus is calcified plaque. The calcification is less significant than the adherent biofilm of plaque on its surface. However, calculus distorts the gingival crevice and, by extending the stagnation area, promotes retention of greater amounts of plaque (Fig. 7.7). In gingival health and gingivitis, calculus is almost exclusively supragingival and forms opposite the orifices

---

* The concept of a keystone pathogen is based on the keystone, the wedge-shaped stone at the centre of a stone arch. The keystone is a single minor component but structurally essential, without it the arch collapses. Similarly, keystone pathogens are thought to support and control the structure of plaque despite their small numbers.

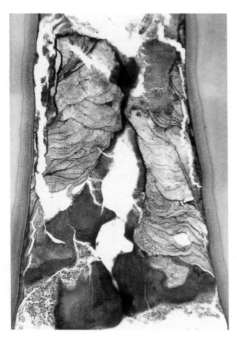

Fig. 7.7 **Large deposits of subgingival calculus,** showing the layered structure resulting from incremental deposition, adhering to the tooth roots on each side of the picture. The calculus has a brown colour from blood and bacterial pigment within it. A thick layer of plaque, stained dark blue, adheres to the calculus and large amounts are trapped below the deep surface of the calculus (at the bottom of the image).

of the major salivary glands in the lower incisor and upper first molar areas. It cannot be removed by the patient and provides a rough, plaque-retentive surface. Several compounds, such as pyrophosphates, added to dentifrices have been shown to reduce calculus formation to variable degrees.

Management

Gingivitis is readily recognisable from the clinical features already described, supported by probing to assess bleeding and exclude loss of attachment. Radiographs show intact crestal alveolar bone. The diagnosis is confirmed by resolution of gingivitis when effective oral hygiene measures become established. Calculus and any local exacerbating factors must be dealt with if possible.

Systemic predisposing factors

There are several predisposing factors to gingivitis, notably diabetes and pregnancy. These also predispose to periodontitis and are discussed later in the chapter (Box 7.6).

PERIODONTITIS

Periodontitis is present once inflammation extends beyond the gingiva to involve the periodontal ligament and resorb the crestal bone. Periodontitis is always preceded by gingivitis, and gingivitis persists in the presence of periodontitis.

Periodontitis is the chief cause of tooth loss in later adult life, but symptoms are typically minimal. Many patients remain unaware of the disease until teeth become loose. Despite generally improving oral health, severe periodontitis still affects 10%–15%, and moderate periodontitis affects approximately half of the adult population in the UK.

Clinical features

Periodontitis is often largely asymptomatic. In the early stages patients may complain only of gingival bleeding or an unpleasant taste. Periodontitis is a potent and common cause of halitosis.

The clinical appearance of periodontitis can vary greatly from modest signs of gingival inflammation to marked swelling and redness of the gingival margins. This variation in the appearance of the gingiva depends on the level of plaque control, risk factors such as smoking (which reduces inflammation), pregnancy and diabetes (which increase inflammation) and individual variation in the inflammatory response. The gingival appearance does not correlate well with the amount of deeper destruction of the periodontal tissues.

Loss of attachment leads to pocketing so that a probe can be passed between teeth and gingiva. In untreated or severe disease, the interdental papillae detach from the teeth. As pockets deepen, the papillae are destroyed and the gingival margin tends to become straight with a swollen, rounded edge. Calculus forms in pockets, trapping more plaque, and bone loss renders the teeth mobile. Teeth tend to drift out of alignment and are dull to percussion and eventually become increasingly loose. In a florid untreated case, bleeding follows minimal pressure, pus may be expressed from pockets and teeth may eventually exfoliate spontaneously.

In some patients, recession is the predominant sign, especially where the gingival tissues are thin. Pocket formation may be limited, but the gingival margin migrates apically with loss of attachment, reducing tooth support and resulting in a similar outcome.

Radiology

The earliest change is loss of definition and blunting of the tips of the alveolar crests. Bone resorption usually progresses in a predictable manner. In early periodontitis bone levels remain the same along a row of teeth (horizontal bone loss; Fig. 7.8). Later complex patterns of bone loss may develop as more bone is lost at sites of pockets and greater inflammation. These sites of destruction are determined by the underlying anatomical features of teeth and bone, local plaque traps and calculus and consequent changes in the plaque composition and metabolism locally.

Aetiology

The aetiology of periodontitis is primarily the long-term presence of dental plaque. However, there is wide individual variation in susceptibility to periodontitis due to the effects of risk factors discussed later. In the presence of plaque, persistence of inflammation leads to a vicious cycle in which swelling and false pocketing promote plaque retention, and the more protected subgingival environment fosters development of a more anaerobic dysbiotic plaque. As more of the gingival soft tissues become inflamed, the inflammation extends close to the crestal bone, causing bone loss and migration of the epithelial attachment onto cementum. Periodontitis, once established, is generally irreversible and self-perpetuating in the absence of adequate treatment, though it may remain stable for many years.

The main features of the pathology of periodontitis are summarised in Box 7.4.

Microbiology

The dysbiotic plaque hypothesis discussed under gingivitis also applies to periodontitis. As noted previously, the microbial

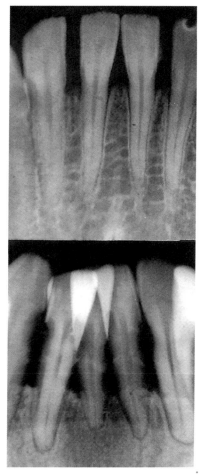

Fig. 7.8 Early and severe horizontal bone loss in advanced periodontitis.

flora in gingivitis is a highly complex and stable ecosystem of interdependent bacterial species in a matrix of polysaccharides, forming an adherent biofilm, which has undergone a dysbiotic shift to cause inflammation. Compared to supragingival sites, the environment in a pocket has a lower oxygen concentration and fewer salivary nutrients and cannot be colonised by many of the aerobic bacterial species in supragingival plaque. The pocket is first colonised by facultative anaerobic Gram-positive organisms, cocci, then rods and filaments that can adhere to the tooth. Once these are established, Gram-negative organisms and true anaerobes, which are less adherent to tooth, but adhere to other species, can colonise the plaque. Eventually a community of organisms is established, adapted to anaerobic conditions and nutrients from the pocket exudate. This takes months or years.

Plaque related to the pocket wall is less densely packed than supragingival plaque and the many Gram-negative bacteria, including anaerobes and, are arranged in complex structures of interdependent consortia of species. As disease is established the number of different species in plaque increases dramatically and this more diverse plaque flora is more effective at metabolizing a broader range of nutrients, and probably also provides enhanced protection against the host defences. Some of these species have been considered pathogenic on the basis of their association with bleeding and progressing destruction (Box 7.5).

Many of the disease-associated bacterial species shown in Box 7.5 and Table 7.4 have potential virulence factors (Table 7.3) including enzymes, toxins and bone-resorbing factors. Although disease is often associated with these species, which overall increase from a few percent to constitute half of the plaque, they are not always present and their virulence is considered to be controlled by a small number of keystone pathogens. Dysbiotic plaque shows increased gene expression for motility, nutrient and iron metabolism, lipopolysaccharide synthesis and probably other virulence factors. When molecular techniques are used to search for expression of possible virulence factors in disease-associated plaque it is found that many are produced by species normally considered commensal or of minor significance. The entire plaque has become dysbiotic. In addition, the total bulk of plaque is increased in disease, including the presence of additional numbers of species associated with health and core species. There are 1000 times more bacteria in diseased sites than healthy sites, but the number appears to still be less important that the nature of the plaque.

One important implication of this understanding is that plaque might be returned to a non-pathogenic form by treatment targeted at specific keystone species.

Porphyromonas gingivalis PMID: 24741603

Aggregatibacter actinomycetemcomitans PMID: 20712635

Keystone pathogen hypothesis PMID: 22941505

Role of the bacterial flora PMID: 32385883

Interestingly, plaque also contains viruses, fungi and archaea. Viral infections can synergise with the bacterial flora in other diseases, as seen in sinusitis following viral infection. Some viruses produce cytokine analogues and viruses can interfere with neutrophil, macrophage and complement activity. Epstein–Barr virus, cytomegalovirus and other herpesviruses have been particularly associated with severe periodontitis and necrotising periodontitis. Some may be infecting lymphocytes in the gingiva (being latent after prior systemic infection) or the epithelium, but viruses are also found free within the subgingival plaque. Although their role is controversial and evidence for their importance in periodontitis is circumstantial at best, possible mechanisms by which viral infection of lymphocytes could alter inflammatory processes are known.

Candida albicans is also found in plaque but is associated with health and numbers reduce as disease develops.

Viruses in periodontitis PMID: 26980964

Pathology

A number of pathological principles are important in understanding periodontitis and its treatment. Periodontitis is a classic chronic inflammatory condition with persisting inflammation together with concurrent attempts at repair. In periodontitis the chronicity is caused by the persistence of bacterial plaque, which is difficult to remove and reforms constantly. Although many bacterial virulence factors have the potential to cause tissue damage directly, the damage that occurs is largely the result of the action of host defence mechanisms.

Bacteria remain largely in the pocket. The vast majority of the bacteria in periodontitis and gingivitis are in the subgingival plaque, forming an organized biofilm adherent to the root surface. This provides the organisms with a relatively protected environment outside the body, plentiful nutrients and a protective plaque ecosystem of interdependent species.

Subgingival calculus. Calcification of plaque in a pocket produces subgingival calculus. The deposits are thin, more widely distributed, harder, darker and more firmly attached than supragingival calculus. Calculus appears laminated histologically, reflecting incremental mineralisation. The colour is caused by incorporation of blood breakdown products in the plaque before calcification. Subgingival calculus perpetuates periodontitis. It acts as a plaque trap by retaining a reservoir of bacteria adherent to its surface and acts as a physical barrier to healing. Effective removal also acts as a surrogate marker for thorough root surface cleaning and is important in achieving good treatment outcomes.

Chronic inflammation. The chronic inflammatory response to plaque accumulation results from bacterial virulence factors triggering non-specific innate and adaptive immune mechanisms though the action of a complex network of regulatory cytokines. Cytokine actions can be both pro- and anti-inflammatory and mediate the mechanisms of tissue breakdown.

Neutrophils migrate continually into pockets though junctional epithelium, probably rendering it permeable to bacterial products as a result. Plasma cells typically predominate in the tissues, accompanied by lymphocytes. These inflammatory cells infiltrate the gingival connective tissue and spread between the bundles of collagen fibres (Fig 7.9). Dense sheets of these cells accumulate, especially under the pocket lining epithelium, close to the plaque and calculus. The pocket lining epithelium and fibroblasts in the pocket wall are recruited to perform inflammatory functions, secreting cytokines.

Pocketing depends on the thickness of the gingival tissues. When plaque extends along the tooth surface and the overlying gingiva is thin, the gingiva is lost, producing recession. Thick gingiva is more resilient and becomes undermined by the destruction extending down the root, producing pocketing (Fig. 7.10 and 7.11). Pockets protect the plaque from removal by abrasion or tooth cleaning and expose a large surface area of tissue to irritation by bacteria and their products. Pockets also favour the growth of anaerobic bacteria.

Pockets may be deep and narrow or surround a tooth (Fig 7.12). The pocket lining epithelium is continuous with the gingival epithelium at the pocket mouth and is often hyperplastic but very thin. At the base of the pocket the epithelium forms the epithelial attachment. **Ulceration** of the lining is often described but rarely seen histologically. If it develops, it seems likely that it heals rapidly.

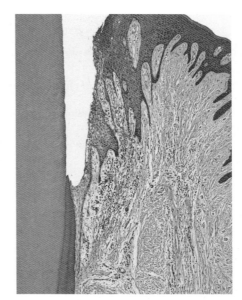

Fig. 7.9 Transition from gingivitis to periodontitis. No pocket has yet formed, but the epithelial attachment has extended on to the cementum and inflammation has induced epithelial hyperplasia, as evidenced by development of rete processes, normally absent in junctional epithelium. Inflammatory cells (blue in colour) are localized around the crevice filling and expanding the spaces between the red-stained collagen fibres.

Epithelial migration. The epithelial attachment migrates from enamel on to cementum, forming the floor of the pocket (Figs 7.9, 7.13 and 7.14). The attachment to cementum is strong, and a clear refractile cuticle formed by the epithelium can sometimes be seen joining the epithelium to the root

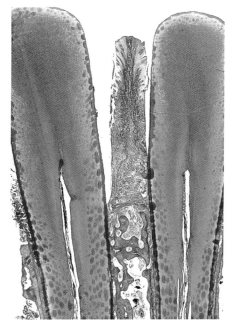

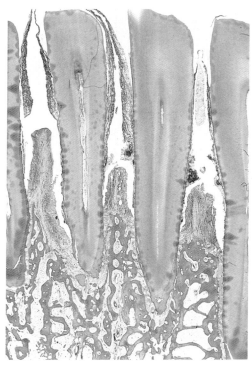

Fig. 7.12 Severe bone loss. Extensive bone loss with insufficient bone support for effective treatment. The tooth to the left of centre has infrabony pocketing extending almost to the apex on the left side of the image, though the pulp remains vital. The teeth on the left both have deep pocketing and between the two on the right there is both pocketing and recession.

Fig. 7.10 **Established periodontitis.** In this woman of 33 years, periodontal pockets have extended onto cementum and inflammatory cells fill the interdental gingiva.

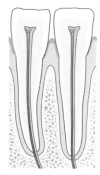

Normal supporting tissues

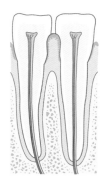

False pocket

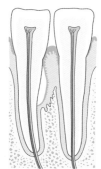

Infrabony pocket
(vertical or angular bone loss)

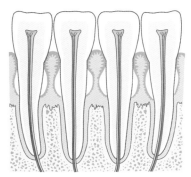

Suprabony pocketing
(horizontal bone loss)

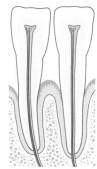

Gingival recession

Fig. 7.11 **Pocket formation in periodontal disease.** A simplified diagram to show the relationship between periodontal soft tissues and alveolar bone in the different presentations of periodontal disease.

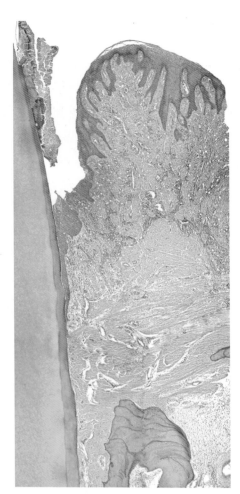

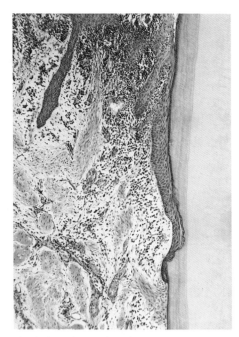

Fig. 7.14   Periodontitis. Higher-power view showing the epithelial attachment lying against cementum. Note how collagen has been lost from the areas containing inflammatory cells, which seem to be floating in space.

Fig. 7.13   Periodontitis. The amelocemental junction lies at the top of the picture covered by plaque and calculus that extend into the upper pocket. The epithelium of the pocket wall is hyperplastic and has developed rete processes, but at the base of the pocket, the lining epithelium forms an epithelial attachment tightly apposed to the cementum. The alveolar bone crest shows resting and reversal lines indicating remodelling during phases of bone loss and quiescence. A broad band of uninflamed densely fibrous tissue, almost scar tissue, separates the bone from the inflamed tissue.

surface (see Fig. 7.2). The length of the epithelial attachment is variable but may extend over several millimetres.

Destruction of periodontal fibres. Collagen fibres in gingiva and periodontal ligament are destroyed progressively from the gingival margin down to the level of the floor of the pocket, but only in a localised zone around the pocket (Fig. 7.14). Beyond this, there is fibrosis resulting from inflammation, but the extra collagen is not organised into functional bundles to support the tooth or gingiva. Fibroblasts in the inflamed tissue are recruited to an inflammatory function, removing collagen to allow other inflammatory cells to accumulate and move and producing cytokines.

Destruction of alveolar bone starts at the alveolar crest. The bone crest recedes just in advance of the floor of the pocket. The zone of inflammation in the gingiva or around the pocket is invariably separated from the underlying bone by a thin zone of uninflamed fibrous tissue (see Fig. 7.13). Inflammatory cells never appear to be in direct contact with the bone but resorb it remotely by activation of osteoclastic resorption. Osteoclasts

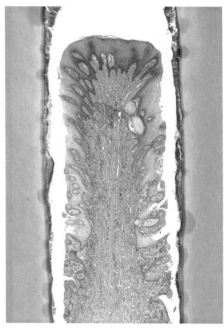

Fig. 7.15   Advanced periodontitis. The cementum on the pocket walls is covered with a thin layer of plaque. The epithelium of the pocket lining is hyperplastic and irregular, and the pocket extends beyond the lower edge of the picture.

are rarely seen histologically, probably because their action is intermittent and the rate of bone destruction is extremely slow. Bone loss occurs in parallel with loss of attachment and allows the pocket base to extend apically (Fig. 7.15).

Innate immune mechanisms are thought to be critically important as defence mechanisms, particularly the non-specific responses of neutrophils and macrophages to bacteria. These are probably responsible for preventing bacterial invasion of the tissues, and their importance is seen in the rapid periodontal destruction associated with almost all conditions where neutrophil function is impaired or deficient, such as diabetes mellitus, smoking, and rare diseases such as Papillon-Lefèvre syndrome and leukocyte adhesion deficiency.

Neutrophils are seen at all stages of disease and their numbers increase with disease severity. Migration through the junctional epithelium probably increases its permeability. In the pocket, neutrophils are almost the only functional host defence cells and a layer of neutrophils covers the plaque surface, walling it off from the tissues. Neutrophils phagocytose and kill bacteria and their antibacterial compounds and enzymes can damage host tissues as well. These are secreted extracellularly in the pocket often as 'neutrophil extracellular traps', complexed with DNA. Neutrophils also secrete pro-inflammatory cytokines and recruit other cells to the inflamed tissue.

The complement system is activated in periodontal inflammation, probably by multiple mechanisms including cleavage by bacterial proteases and lipopolysaccharides. It can opsonise bacteria directly to enhance phagocytosis and killing by neutrophils in the crevice. However, this protective role is probably small and few periodontal bacterial species are susceptible to lysis by complement. However, it exerts other, probably more important, effects generating chemotactic factors to recruit neutrophils and macrophages and activating inflammatory and immune cells to promote the inflammatory process. In animal models, complement inhibition reduces inflammation and bone loss.

Adaptive immune mechanisms are involved in periodontal disease, as they are in every microbial disease. However, effective antibody responses are hampered by the fact that the target bacteria lie outside the body in the pocket, where the environment is controlled by the bacteria and not the host. Antibodies produced against plaque bacteria may mediate opsonisation and killing of bacteria by neutrophils and macrophages in the pocket and can also activate complement in the pocket, though probably with little protective effect. The bacteria in the biofilm on the tooth are protected by the matrix but unattached bacteria near the pocket wall may be more susceptible.

While humoral responses might kill bacteria directly, cell-mediated immunity plays a critical role maintaining and controlling inflammation. T helper cell subsets including Th1, Th2, Th17 and Treg cells each secrete specific profiles of cytokines and the balance between these cell types may influence progression.

Bacteria very rarely penetrate the tissues. Although bacteria can penetrate the tissues, as demonstrated by the bacteraemias associated with toothbrushing and tooth movement, the significance to periodontitis is unclear. Some bacterial species have the ability to invade the tissues, including *P. gingivalis*, *T. forsythia*, *F. nucleatum*, *A. actinomycetemcomitans* and *T. denticola* but do so only in small numbers. It is likely that invasion happens only from time to time and its importance is unclear.

Mechanisms of tissue damage
A degree of tissue damage always accompanies inflammation and is often prominent in bacterial diseases. This damage is not a 'bystander effect' but an integral function of inflammation, which must remove tissue components such as collagen to allow inflammatory cell migration, accumulation and function. Overall, damage by host mechanisms is minor and constrained by control mechanisms, so that disease progression in periodontitis is very slow; inflammation and immunity are overall protective.

The cytokine networks regulating the inflammatory response have a high degree of redundancy, meaning that a complex network of pathways is active, each with overlapping and complementary effects. Cytokines regulate tissue damage through the action of specific effector mechanisms. Connective tissue breakdown is mediated largely by the matrix metalloproteinase enzymes (MMPs) that normally mediate tissue turnover but are upregulated in periodontal (and many other) diseases. MMPs are produced by activated macrophages and fibroblasts in the gingiva to degrade collagen, laminin, fibronectin, fibrin and other connective tissue matrix components.

Bone resorption is entirely dependent on osteoclasts. Osteoclasts are short-lived cells which form by fusion of pro-monocyte cells specifically under the control of the osteoclast activator RANKL. In inflamed periodontium, RANKL is expressed by T helper cells, macrophages and fibroblasts induced by inflammatory cytokines.

Overall, it is clear that the inflammatory and immunological reactions in periodontitis are protective. The importance of inflammation is seen in the susceptibility to disease in people who smoke or have diabetes and the importance of immunity in the necrotizing periodontal diseases seen in HIV infection.

Episodic and chronic nature of destruction. Like many other chronic diseases, periodontitis progresses very slowly in an episodic pattern with long periods of stability despite the presence of huge numbers of bacteria in periodontal pockets. In an otherwise healthy person, it is not uncommon for half a century to pass before 1 cm of alveolar bone is lost. Although overall slow, destruction occurs in rapid spurts. These may be triggered by reduction in host defences or perhaps by poorly understood ecological and dysbiotic changes in the plaque flora driven by changes in the subgingival environment.

Neutrophil NETs PMID: 26442948

Review role neutrophils PMID: 34899756 and in detail 31850633

Bone loss mechanisms PMID: 33884712

Pocket epithelial role PMID: 30837987

Role of fibroblasts PMID: 36359741

Humoral immune responses PMID: 29476652

Periodontal disease susceptibility

As noted earlier, there is a wide variation in susceptibility to periodontal disease, which is largely independent of level of plaque control. Thus, the presence of microbial plaque is required for progressive periodontitis to develop but host-mediated tissue damage is also required for disease to progress. Various risk factors have been identified that may determine disease susceptibility and the major ones include smoking, some systemic diseases, genetic and psychosocial factors. There is some evidence that diet may influence disease susceptibility. In addition, colonization of plaque by specific bacteria may also markedly influence disease progression.

Both local and systemic factors can exacerbate gingivitis and periodontitis (Box 7.6).

Smoking

Smoking is probably the single most important risk factor for periodontitis. Regular smoking increases risk of periodontitis by between 3-fold to 5-fold, increases the rate of disease progression and also markedly impairs responses to periodontal treatment. The effects of smoking are cumulative and dose dependent. There is evidence that the effects of smoking are gradually reduced following smoking cessation.

Clinically, smokers often exhibit reduced signs of inflammation such as swelling and bleeding. Smoking is known to interfere with inflammatory and immune reactions, probably by activating endothelial and inflammatory cells in the lungs and circulation, and by inducing them to secrete cytokines and other compounds inappropriately. Reduced neutrophil numbers are seen in periodontal pockets. All forms of tobacco smoking have the effect. Smokeless tobacco use also promotes periodontal destruction but by direct vascular and abrasive effects. There is not yet data on the effects of vaping (e-cigarette use) on periodontal risk.

Smoking and periodontitis PMID: 35950749

Diabetes mellitus

Diabetes increases the risk of periodontitis by up to 3-fold. Disease severity is directly related to hyperglycaemia and patients with poorly controlled diabetes, particularly if glycosylated haemoglobin levels are above 9%, are worst affected. In well-controlled diabetes, acceleration of periodontal disease may not be noticeable. Both type 1 and type 2 diabetes predispose; there is a well described global epidemic of type 2 diabetes which accounts for around 95 % of all cases and makes diabetes one of the most common risk factors for periodontitis. The links between periodontitis and diabetes are probably explained by a reduction in neutrophil function and excessive cytokine responses by macrophages caused by interaction with advanced glycation end products.

In recent years, it has become clear that people with diabetes and periodontitis are more at risk of other diabetic complications such as nephropathy and ischaemic heart disease. It has been suggested that periodontal inflammation or pathogenic bacteria may account for these links, and it has been shown that periodontitis can predict the other complications. Several studies have shown that effective periodontal disease treatment can improve diabetic control, though the effect is relatively small.

There is a role for dental practitioners to identify patients with undiagnosed diabetes on the basis of their periodontitis and refer them for diagnosis.

Diabetes and periodontitis PMID: 35913467

Effects of treatment on diabetes PMID: 35612801

Pregnancy

Pre-existing gingivitis may become more severe from the first 2 months of pregnancy (see Fig. 37.8). If oral hygiene is poor, inflammatory erythema, bleeding and oedema can be very florid. Swelling accentuates false pocketing. These changes are considered to result from the effects of oestrogens and progesterone on gingival vessels, but there is also evidence of an altered bacterial flora, probably due to these and other pregnancy-related compounds being bacterial nutrients. Pregnancy gingivitis can be much ameliorated or abolished by a strict oral hygiene regimen and improves after parturition.

The most florid presentation is a localised pyogenic granuloma (see Fig. 37.9) or 'pregnancy epulis'. These develop and grow very rapidly but respond to simple excision after parturition. A pregnancy epulis always develops in a background of pregnancy gingivitis.

There is no evidence that pregnancy influences progression of periodontitis *per se.*

Genetic Factors

Studies of twins, family studies and gene association studies all provide compelling evidence of an important role for genetic factors in determining periodontal disease susceptibility, particularly in younger adults with severe disease. Apart from the very rare syndromic conditions discussed later, this appears to be the result of the action of many normal variants of genes (polymorphisms). These may have very little effect individually but when combined may significantly affect susceptibility. Genome-wide association studies and simple gene association studies have provided a variable list of potential candidate genes involved, but no clear consensus on the role of specific genetic polymorphisms has emerged to date.

Psychosocial Factors

Psychosocial factors, which include stress, coping and emotional intelligence, have been found to influence periodontal disease susceptibility. Stress and other psychological constructs have long been known to influence biological responses such as cortisol secretion and inflammatory responses and carry increased risk for diseases such as cardiovascular disease. Psychosocial factors may also have an indirect effect on susceptibility through poor plaque control and smoking. The overall size of the effect is probably small but up to a 2-fold increased risk has been reported.

Other Systemic Risk Factors

Other systemic conditions can predispose to severe progressive periodontitis. Many of these are the result of specific genetically determined conditions, often affecting neutrophil function and generally are rare. These are considered later in this chapter.

Principles of management

Details of treatment are beyond the scope of this text, but principles will be given as they relate to the pathology. The main principles are summarised in Box 7.7.

Plaque must be removed, by time-honoured, manual methods of plaque control. Professional input includes education, mechanical plaque and calculus removal and removal of restoration overhangs and other plaque traps. As plaque is the primary causative factor, this alone reduces inflammation, and may resolve gingivitis.

When pockets are present, plaque removal requires professional assistance and the aim of subgingival scaling or root debridement is to remove all (or almost all) plaque and calculus from any root surface irregularities. Root debridement cannot remove subgingival plaque entirely or prevent it reforming, but it reduces bacterial bulk, disturbs the plaque environment, renders the pocket more aerobic and favours the return of the plaque flora a symbiotic state. This tips the balance in favour of healing, inflammation reduces, the tissues shrink and the pocket lining junctional epithelium reattaches to the cementum and enamel surface to produce a 'long epithelial attachment' extending from the level of the old pocket floor to

Box 7.7   **General principles of management of periodontal disease**
- Prevention is most effective
- Control of supragingival bacterial plaque by oral hygiene
- Establishment of healthy tooth and gingival contour accessible to plaque control
- Prevent food packing due to poor contact points
- Removal of subgingival plaque and calculus, root debridement, by professional cleaning
- Use of antibiotics in selected cases
- Mucogingival surgery in selected cases
- Extraction of teeth with poor prognosis to preserve bone
- Maintenance long-term

Box 7.8   **Potential complications of periodontitis**
Local
- Periodontal abscess and spread of infection
- Tooth mobility and drifting
- Tooth loss through exfoliation

Systemic
- Infective endocarditis
- Atherosclerosis and cardiovascular disease
- Poor diabetic control
- Preterm birth

the gingival margin. The long epithelial attachment is firm, shallower probing depths result, and it is sufficiently robust to remain in place for the life of the patient provided supragingival plaque is controlled. However, reattachment of connective tissue to the tooth with a reformed periodontal ligament cannot be expected with these treatments. Bone loss will remain, periodontal ligament fibres will not reattach to cementum and the functional periodontal ligament remains reduced in length. Some recession also usually results from reduction of gingival inflammation, reducing pocket depth from the coronal end. These procedures can be expected to be successful if the initial pocket was less than 5 mm in depth.

Deeper pockets are less likely to respond for several reasons. They are more difficult to debride as the more apical root morphology of many teeth is unfavourable, with concavities and furcations, the depth maintains low oxygen tension and pH that favours recolonization by anaerobes. In addition, patients who have deep pockets are more likely to have risk factors that may compromise healing. Deeper pockets may require flap surgery to facilitate cleaning of the roots.

The ultimate goal of treatment would be to reconstitute the periodontal ligament and alveolar bone, regain tooth support and reduce any residual pocket to the normal crevicular depth. Unfortunately, such reattachment is usually impossible to achieve, and may not be necessary since the long epithelial attachment effectively eliminates the pocket and prevents progression. However, reattachment can be attempted in selected cases by controlling the healing process so that only cells from the remaining healthy periodontal ligament repopulate the root surface after surgery. These have the capacity to form new functional periodontal ligament but can only do so slowly and the more rapid tissue ingrowth from the surface must be prevented by inserting a barrier membrane between the flap and root surface ('guided tissue regeneration'). Though this can be successful, it is unpredictable and only small amounts of reattachment can be expected.

The prognosis after treatment is highly dependent on maintaining good oral hygiene, though factors that predispose to disease also reduce effectiveness of treatment (Box 7.6). Most teeth that are lost are extracted in the 5 years after treatment, and these are usually teeth that had adverse features at initiation of treatment. Once pocketing has extended beyond the point where treatment can be beneficial, the teeth should be extracted. Deep pockets are a source of sepsis that may have remote effects such as infective endocarditis. Making an early

planned decision to extract teeth preserves bone for implants or dentures.

Role of antibiotics

While it might seem that antibiotics would be effective in periodontitis, they are rarely used. The biofilm is mostly dead bacteria and matrix that would be unaffected. Bacteria in a biofilm resist antibiotics better, and individual species are increasingly showing antibiotic resistance, probably due to antibiotic use for other purposes. Even when antibiotics are used, biofilms harbour so-called *persister* cells, nongrowing bacteria that are unaffected by antibiotics and can re-establish infection once the antibiotic treatment ceases.

Antibiotics are usually reserved for disease responding poorly to conventional treatment, usually with deep pockets, or for periodontal abscess. Overall, tetracyclines or a combination of metronidazole and amoxicillin seem to be the most effective and the incisor-molar pattern of periodontitis seems to be the most responsive pattern to antibiotic use.

Risks from antibiotic adverse effects and bacterial resistance must be weighed against their benefits and routine use for periodontitis cannot be justified.

Antibiotic use PMID: 26427574 and alternatives 36380339

Antibiotics after surgery PMID: 36472512

Complications of periodontitis

Complications can be local or systemic (Box 7.8). Locally, periodontitis causes tooth drifting and mobility, impaired masticatory function, halitosis and is a very common cause of tooth loss in adults.

Some systemic complications arise from the transient bacteraemia associated with mastication and tooth brushing. Bacteraemia is most severe when pockets are deep and inflamed, but it is still detectable in near heathy mouths. Infective endocarditis is the most significant complication and is discussed in Chapter 33 but sometimes abscesses in other organs, particularly the brain, are caused by periodontal bacterial species and are often assumed to originate in the gingival crevice.

Periodontitis has also been associated with a range of systemic conditions including cardiovascular disease, diabetes and obstetric complications (pre-term low birth weight, pre-eclampsia). There is a considerable challenge to establish whether any of these associations represent causal relationships or might reflect the presence of common risk factors. Intervention studies, demonstrating that periodontal treatment can reduce the associated complication are required but are very difficult to carry out.

Periodontitis is consistently associated with cardiovascular disease in many studies. It has been proposed that this might be mediated by either the overall bacterial burden or by specific bacterial species. However, it remains unclear whether this association might be caused by smoking or other risk factors that are common to both diseases. A number of systemic infections are thought to contribute to atheroma through lipopolysaccharide production and activation of systemic inflammatory mechanisms. Immune cross-reactivity between tissues and bacteria is often cited as a possible mechanism, as are inflammatory cell priming, lipid metabolism and nitric oxide. Whether periodontal treatment can reduce atheroma or its complications is unclear.

The suggestion that periodontitis affects diabetic control can now be considered proven, as discussed earlier.

Periodontitis and cardiovascular PMID: 36503487 and 35874771

SEVERE PERIODONTITIS

Distinctive patterns of severe periodontitis have been recognized and were previously called aggressive periodontitis. They no longer appear in the classification of periodontal disease because they appear to be the end of a spectrum of severity, rather than diseases in their own right. Such presentations include those where periodontitis seems out of proportion to the small amounts of plaque present, there is extensive destructive at a young age or an unusual incisor-molar or very localized distribution. Nevertheless, these patterns of disease can be distinctive.

The most characteristic is the localised pattern of deep pocketing previously called localised (juvenile) aggressive periodontitis, which has a number of distinctive features and is now classified as molar/incisor pattern periodontitis (Figs. 7.16 and 7.17). Typically, this has onset around puberty though it can be seen in adults, is much more frequent in individuals with an African heritage, may be familial, is often symmetrical and is associated with a particular bacterial species, *Aggregatibacter actinomycetemcomitans* leucotoxin-producing strains. It remains controversial whether this pattern of disease is a specific entity but it is

worth recognizing, since it is responsive to treatment including antibiotics, particularly tetracycline.

These severe types of periodontitis appear to be self-limiting. After a period of rapid attachment loss, the disease process often slows and becomes indistinguishable from periodontitis.

Early onset severe disease, affecting the deciduous dentition, is often associated with impaired neutrophil function, either of chemotaxis, phagocytosis or both, or hyperreactive macrophages that produce excessive cytokines. Causes are considered in the following sections.

Localised aggressive periodontitis PMID: 31668171

PERIODONTITIS AS A MANIFESTATION OF SYSTEMIC CONDITIONS

A diverse range of diseases can present with periodontal destruction, some simply predisposing to conventional periodontitis and others causing distinctive patterns of destruction. Predisposing conditions such as diabetes have been previously dealt with. All except Down's syndrome are uncommon or rare but are important to distinguish from severe periodontitis because the underlying disorder may threaten the patient's health or life. Recognised causes of premature periodontal destruction are summarised in Box 7.9 and some are discussed in more detail in separate sections. Many cause a widespread and rapidly destructive periodontitis in the deciduous dentition. Severe periodontitis in children is very unusual and always has an underlying systemic host defence defect, usually leucocyte adhesion deficiency.

Agranulocytosis and acute leukaemia may also be associated with necrotising periodontitis. Agranulocytosis is mainly a disease of adults, whereas the common childhood type of acute leukaemia (acute lymphocytic leukaemia) typically produces gingival enlargement rather than periodontal destruction. The importance of cyclic neutropenia has been greatly exaggerated and early-onset periodontitis is by no means always associated. All these immunodeficiency disorders are typically associated with abnormal susceptibility to non-oral infections.

Down's syndrome

In people with Down's syndrome (Ch. 40), gingivitis is exacerbated by excessive plaque formation and challenges establishing effective toothbrushing habits. In the past, progress to periodontitis between age 15 and 25 was usual

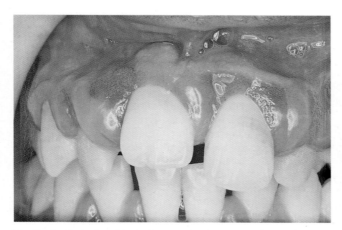

Fig. 7.16 Periodontitis, incisor-molar pattern. Drifting of upper central incisors due to gross loss of attachment. There is some marginal inflammation, but oral hygiene is good and the clinical appearance belies the periodontal destruction visible radiographically or on probing.

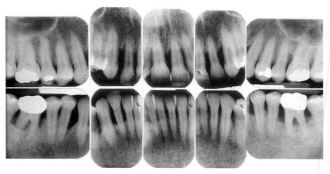

Fig. 7.17 Periodontitis, incisor-molar pattern. Young adult patient aged 20 years, showing severe bone destruction around three first permanent molars and upper and lower incisors. Probing depths exceeded 10 mm. *(Courtesy Dr R Saravanamuttu.)*

- Genetic disorders
  - Diseases associated with neutrophil disorders
    - Familial and cyclic neutropenia
    - Down's syndrome (Ch. 40)
    - Leukocyte adhesion deficiency
    - Papillon-Lefèvre syndrome
    - Haim-Munk syndrome
    - Chediak-Higashi syndrome
    - Glycogen storage diseases
    - Cohen syndrome
    - Infantile genetic agranulocytosis
    - Chronic granulomatous disease
  - Diseases affecting the connective tissues
    - Ehlers-Danlos syndrome type VIII (Ch. 14)
    - C-1 esterase inhibitor deficiency
  - Diseases affecting the periodontal tissues
    - Hypophosphatasia (Ch. 13)
    - Epidermolysis bullosa, Kindler syndrome type
- Acquired haematological disorders
  - Neutropenia (Ch. 28)
  - Haematological malignancy (Ch. 28)

and early tooth loss was a frequent consequence (see Fig. 40.4), but enhanced preventive regimes have proved effective and patients with Down's syndrome now retain more teeth into adulthood. Multiple immunodeficiencies and 'early ageing' of the immune system contribute, and there is early colonisation by periodontal pathogens. Small teeth with short roots predispose to tooth loss. Calculus used to be considered prevalent, but recent data suggests this is simply a reflection of oral hygiene and not a feature of the syndrome.

Papillon–Lefèvre syndrome

Papillon–Lefèvre syndrome is an exceedingly rare autosomal recessive disorder. The main features are, typically, hyperkeratosis of palms and soles starting in infancy and early-onset periodontal destruction caused by a loss-of-function mutation in the gene encoding cathepsin C. People with the disease are homozygous for the mutation and completely lack cathepsin C activity. Parents and carriers are heterozygous and have low cathepsin C activity but experience no ill-effects.

Cathepsin C is a lysosomal protease that plays an essential role in activating antibacterial compounds stored in an inactive form in neutrophils. Lack of activation impairs host responses to bacteria. Patients may also have learning disability, intracranial calcifications, hyperhidrosis and recurrent skin infections. Diagnosis is by genetic screening.

Leukocyte adhesion deficiency

Leukocyte adhesion deficiency results from lack of functional surface adhesion receptors on neutrophils, macrophages or both, preventing these inflammatory cells from emigrating into inflamed or infected tissues. This causes recurrent skin and fungal infections and delayed wound healing in addition to periodontitis. Periodontitis becomes evident soon after tooth eruption, and while the underlying deficiency persists,

treatment is ineffective. The only effective treatment is bone marrow transplantation.

Other causes of childhood periodontitis that might cause similar presentations include neutropenia, leukaemia, hypophosphatasia, Papillon–Lefèvre syndrome, HIV infection and acrodynia (heavy metal poisoning).

Periodontitis with neutrophil defects PMID: 30565245

PERIODONTAL (LATERAL) ABSCESS

A periodontal abscess results from acute infection of a periodontal pocket. It is less common than an apical abscess, but still a frequent dental emergency. The alternative name of lateral abscess indicates that the abscess lies at the side of the tooth rather than apically. The causes are uncertain but probably related to factors that tip the host-bacterial balance in favour of the bacteria. Thus, it sometimes follows treatment such as root debridement when trauma to the pocket lining may implant bacteria into the tissues or damage by a foreign body such as a fish bone or toothbrush bristle trapped in a pocket. Food packing down between the teeth with poor contact points may contribute. More often the cause is obscure. More generalised periodontitis is usually associated.

Spontaneous resolution by drainage through the pocket mouth is prevented by soft tissue swelling a constricting the pocket mouth.

Pericoronitis is a form of periodontal abscess beneath the operculum of a partially erupted molar.

Clinical features

The onset is rapid. Gingival tenderness progresses to throbbing pain. The tooth affected is vital and tender to percussion. The overlying gingiva is red and swollen. Pus may exude from the pocket, but a deeply sited periodontal abscess may point on the alveolar mucosa, forming a sinus. The vitality of the tooth and its less severe tenderness usually distinguish a lateral abscess from acute apical periodontitis. The great depth of the pocket helps make the diagnosis clear (Fig. 7.18).

Radiographic changes of infection are not visible until after approximately a week, after which the site shows a poorly demarcated radiolucency with loss of lamina dura of the bony pocket wall. However, an early radiograph may aid diagnosis of the pre-existing deep pocket.

Pathology

The bony wall of the pocket is actively resorbed by many osteoclasts. There is dense infiltration by neutrophils and pus formation (Figs 7.19) in the pocket and pocket wall. Alveolar bone in the floor of the original pocket is destroyed, and the pocket extends rapidly, destroying attachment and sometimes extending to the apex. Occasionally, pus tracks apically or from a deeply sited pocket so that a facial abscess or cellulitis results, though this is more likely to develop from a periapical abscess.

Treatment

A periodontal abscess should be drained, ideally through the pocket, by subgingival curettage and the root surface debrided. Incision through the overlying gingiva is best avoided unless drainage through the pocket fails, as a permanent soft tissue fenestration may result. However, if periodontal disease is severe and widespread, it may be more appropriate to extract the affected tooth. After treatment,

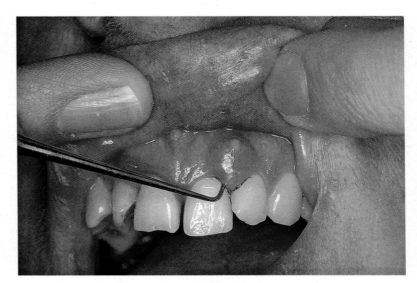

Fig. 7.18 Periodontal abscess. The abscess is pointing on the alveolar mucosa above the attached gingiva. The probe is inserted deeply in the pocket communicating with the abscess.

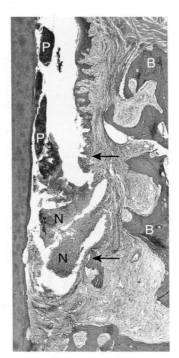

Fig. 7.19 **Acute periodontal abscess.** There is well-advanced periodontitis, with the tooth to the left, bone to the right (B) and the pocket wall with its epithelial lining centrally. The pocket contains plaque and calculus (P) towards the top of the image. Lower down, at the pocket base, a mass of neutrophils (N) form pus and inflammation extends up to a small island of residual lamina dura, which is being resorbed (lower arrow). The epithelial lining of the pocket stops at the abscess (upper arrow).

the site will have suffered significant acute attachment loss and bone loss.

Review PMID: 10883866 and 29926942

ACUTE PERICORONITIS

Incomplete eruption of a wisdom tooth produces a large stagnation area under the gum flap that anatomically mimics a pocket. It can easily become infected, causing pericoronitis.

Box 7.10   **Factors contributing to pericoronitis**
• Poor oral hygiene
• Impaction of food and plaque accumulation under the gum flap
• An upper tooth biting on the gum flap
• Periodontitis elsewhere in the mouth
• Necrotising (acute ulcerative) gingivitis (rarely)

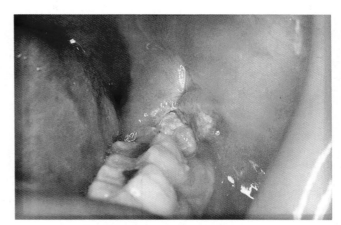

Fig. 7.20 **Pericoronitis.** A pocket has formed between the gingival operculum and the crown of a partially erupted third molar.

Pericoronitis is caused by a mixed infection by organisms typical of periodontitis and periodontal abscess, particularly anaerobes. Several factors (Box 7.10) may contribute.

Clinical features

Young adults are affected. The main symptoms are soreness and tenderness around the partially erupted tooth (Fig. 7.20). There is pain, swelling, difficulty in opening the mouth, lymphadenopathy, sometimes slight fever and, in severe cases, suppuration and abscess formation. Swelling and difficulty in opening the mouth may be severe enough to prevent examination of the area.

Management

Food debris should be removed from under the gum flap by irrigation. The position of the affected tooth, its relationship to the second molar and any complicating factors should be determined by radiography.

In mild cases, it may be enough for patients to keep the mouth clean and to use hot mouth rinses whenever symptoms develop, until the inflammation subsides. This may happen naturally by further eruption or by extraction of the tooth after the infection has been overcome.

If radiographs show that the third molar is badly misplaced, impacted or carious, it should be extracted after inflammation has subsided. Spread of infection (cellulitis or osteomyelitis) may follow extraction of the tooth while infection is still acute, but is rare.

When an upper tooth is biting on the flap, it is often preferable to extract it, especially if the both teeth are ultimately to be removed. If there are strong reasons for retaining the upper tooth, the cusps can be ground sufficiently to prevent it from traumatising the flap. In the past, caustic agents such as trichloroacetic acid were commonly used to reduce the operculum. This was very effective but carries a risk of accidental burns to adjacent mucosa or skin. Electrocautery may also be used. In severe cases, particularly when there is facial swelling, fever and lymphadenopathy, penicillin or penicillin and metronidazole should be given, but in most cases are unnecessary. Pericoronitis is a major cause of antibiotic overuse in dentistry.

Pus may track posteriorly from the operculum to cause serious fascial space infection as described in Chapter 9. In the pre-antibiotic era, acute infection from pericoronitis was a relatively common cause of death in young adults.

Both treated and untreated acute pericoronitis may become chronic if the operculum remains. In the absence of further acute episodes, there is extensive bone loss around the partially erupted tooth and its neighbours so that the second molar can be compromised.

Review and management PMID: 34202699

GINGIVAL RECESSION

Recession of the gingivae and exposure of the roots is common. It is sometimes progressive and worsens with age, but it is not a feature of ageing itself and susceptibility varies. The major predisposing factor is thinness of the gingival tissue, so recession is worst around lower incisors, upper canines buccally, and lingual to lower molars (Fig. 7.21). As recession progresses, the thickness of the gingiva increases so that recession may be self-limiting. Loss of attachment in areas of thick gingiva produces pockets whereas, in recession, the thin tissue is destroyed entirely (Figs 7.22 and 7.23).

The exact cause of recession is unclear, but the most common association is with plaque-induced inflammation. One hypothesis suggests that epithelial proliferation in inflamed junctional epithelium induces long rete processes that bridge across the narrow band of marginal connective tissue to fuse with rete processes of the external gingival epithelium. This is followed by remodelling of the gingival margin to preserve a normal epithelial thickness. Whether cervical abrasion caused by a stiff brush and abrasive toothpaste follows recession or causes it is impossible to ascertain, but the two are closely linked. Recession at the papilla, as opposed to in the thin buccal or lingual aspect of teeth is always associated with prior periodontitis.

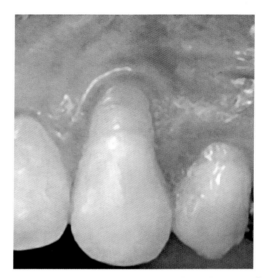

Fig. 7.21   Localised gingival recession. The buccal aspect of an upper canine is a typical site. Such localized recession is often blamed on trauma, but the very thin bone and soft tissue predispose to recession despite a mild degree of inflammation *(Courtesy Prof FJ Hughes)*

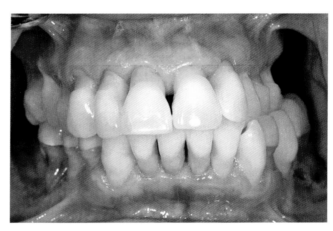

Fig. 7.22   Periodontitis with marked generalised recession *(Source: Block MS (2015). Implants for the maxillary edentulous patient. In: Color Atlas of Dental Implant Surgery, 4th ed, Philadelphia, Elsevier Inc.)*

Other hypothetical causes include acid regurgitation and minor tooth movements. The thin tissue is not very resistant to any insult and recession often follows direct trauma from factitial injury, trauma from oral piercings, and contact with topical tobacco or betel quid. Recession is also a complication of orthodontic treatment when tooth roots are inadvertently moved outside the alveolar bone.

Receded gingival margins often appear relatively uninflamed.

Treatment of gingival recession

Recession is primarily of cosmetic concern and often self-limiting. It can be managed by effective atraumatic cleaning to prevent additional inflammatory loss of attachment.

When recession extends past the mucogingival junction, a graft may be valuable to anchor the softer alveolar mucosa to bone and prevent rapid extension toward the apex. Free gingival grafting or advanced buccal flaps can be used for cosmetic reasons, just to cover the exposed root, but the graft lacks a

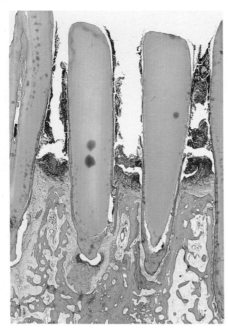

Fig. 7.23 Periodontitis with recession. In this case, gingival destruction is almost as great as the degree of bone resorption so that excessively long clinical crowns have been produced and there is only a thin layer of soft tissue over the interdental bone. Supragingival calculus and a dense inflammatory infiltrate in the gingiva can be seen. The tooth to the left of the midline appears non-vital. Although the pulp cannot be seen, there is a periapical granuloma and apical inflammatory hypercementosis.

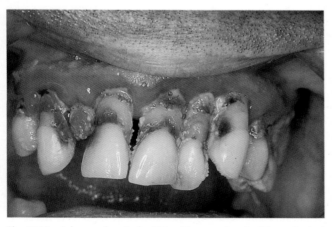

Fig. 7.24 Advanced periodontitis with recession. In this neglected mouth, deposits of plaque and supragingival calculus adhere to the exposed roots, which have active root caries. Probing depths are minimal despite the loss of attachment.

vascular tissue to support it, shrinks over time and success is unpredictable. Loss of interdental papillae can be restored using injected dermal filler, usually hyaluronic acid (Ch. 27).

Recession is often associated with dentine hypersensitivity from the exposed root. This results from additional demineralisation and can be tackled using dietary modification, fluoride or dentinal tubule blocking agents. The exposed root is also potentially at risk from later root caries (Fig. 7.24).

Recession review PMID: 21941318 and 34024328

> **Box 7.11   Typical features of necrotising ulcerative gingivitis and periodontitis**
>
> - In Western countries young adult healthy males mainly affected
> - Often cigarette smokers and/or with minor respiratory infection
> - In other parts of the world associated with malnutrition, immunosuppression, infectious disease and leukaemia
> - Cratered ulcers starting at the tips of the interdental papillae
> - Ulcers spread along gingival margins
> - Gingival soreness and bleeding
> - Foul breath
> - No significant lymphadenopathy
> - No fever or systemic upset
> - Smears from ulcers dominated by Gram-negative spirochaetes and fusiform bacteria
> - Responds to oral hygiene and metronidazole in immunocompetent patients
> - May develop into cancrum oris (noma) (Ch. 9)

NECROTISING PERIODONTAL DISEASES

Necrotising periodontitis is a distinct and specific disease that can cause significant periodontal tissue destruction.

Clinical features

The incidence of ulcerative or necrotising periodontal disease has declined sharply in the Western world in the last 60 years. It remains common where general health is often compromised and diseases such as malnutrition, measles or HIV infection act as predisposing factors. In the UK it typically affects apparently healthy young adults, usually with neglected mouths.

Typical features are summarised in Box 7.11.

Crater-shaped or punched-out ulcers form initially at the tips of the interdental papillae. Ulcers are sharply defined by erythema and oedema; their surface is covered by a greyish or yellowish tenacious slough. Removal of the slough causes free bleeding. The severe halitosis, likened to rotting hay, is characteristic.

Lesions remain restricted to the gingivae and supporting tissues. They mainly spread along the gingival margins and deeply, destroying interdental soft and hard tissues, but rarely spreading to alveolar mucosa (Fig. 7.25). Deep spread can cause rapid destruction of both soft tissues and bone, producing triangular spaces between the teeth.

If treatment is delayed, the end result is distortion of the normal gingival contour, promoting stagnation and predisposing to recurrences or later periodontal disease.

Aetiology

The bacteria responsible are said to be a complex of spirochaetes and fusiforms (Fig. 7.26). These organisms are present in small numbers in the healthy gingival flora and are also found in conventional periodontitis. With the onset of ulcerative gingivitis, both bacteria proliferate until they dominate the local bacterial flora. This, together with invasion of the tissues by spirochaetes and the sharp fall in their numbers with effective treatment indicate that they are the responsible agents. Nevertheless, it is still uncertain whether this 'fusospirochaetal complex' is the sole cause of

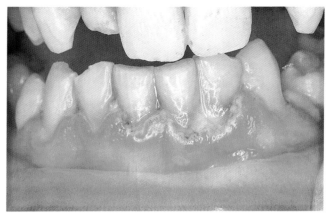

Fig. 7.25 Necrotising gingivitis (acute ulcerative gingivitis). Characteristic features, a crater-shaped ulcer starting at the tips of the interdental papillae and covered by an ulcer slough.

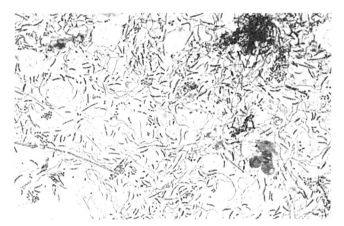

Fig. 7.26 Necrotising gingivitis (acute ulcerative gingivitis). A smear from an ulcer shows the dense proliferation of *Treponema vincentii* and *Fusobacterium nucleatum*.

> **Box 7.12   Bacteria implicated in acute ulcerative gingivitis**
>
> - *Treponema vincentii*
> - *Fusobacterium fusiformis*
> - *Prevotella intermedia*
> - *Porphyromonas gingivalis*
> - *Selenomonas sputigena*
> - *Leptotrichia buccalis*

ulcerative gingivitis and other bacteria have been implicated (Box 7.12).

Despite doubts about the precise identity of the bacterial cause of necrotizing periodontal disease, it is clearly primarily an anaerobic infection because it responds rapidly to metronidazole, as well as penicillins and improved oral hygiene.

Host factors. Ulcerative periodontal disease is a disease of otherwise healthy young adults associated with smoking, poor plaque control and stress. However, ulcerative gingivitis may also develop in children having immunosuppressive treatment and in patients with HIV infection (Ch. 30).

> **Box 7.13   Differential diagnosis of acute necrotising ulcerative gingivitis**
>
> - Primary herpetic gingivostomatitis (Ch. 15)
> - HIV-associated acute ulcerative gingivitis (Ch. 30)
> - Gingival ulceration in acute leukaemia or aplastic anaemia (Ch. 28)

Local factors appear to be important and ulcerative gingivitis does not appear to be transmissible. Ulcerative gingivitis ('trench mouth') was almost epidemic among soldiers in the 1914–1918 war and civilians subjected to bombing in the 1939–1945 war. Necrotising periodontitis is relatively rarely seen in the UK now, with the exception of patients presenting with untreated HIV infection (Box 7.13). Necrotising periodontitis is a precursor to cancrum oris (noma) discussed in Chapter 9.

PERIODONTITIS IN HIV INFECTION

HIV-associated periodontitis is associated with soft tissue necrosis and rapid destruction of the periodontal tissues. It is typically intensely painful. There is little deep pocketing because soft tissue and bone are destroyed virtually simultaneously. More than 90% of the attachment can be lost within 3–6 months, and the soft tissue necrosis can lead to exposure of bone and sequestration.

The pain of HIV-associated periodontitis is usually aching in character and felt within the jaw rather than in the gingivae. It may be felt before tissue destruction becomes obvious. HIV-associated gingivitis and periodontitis are usually generalised but are sometimes localised to one or more discrete areas.

Bacteriologically, HIV-associated periodontitis resembles classical periodontitis in HIV-negative persons, but poor resistance to viral infections may also contribute. It is typically associated with a low CD4 count and a poor prognosis unless the underlying HIV infection is treated effectively.

Management

Debridement and removal of any sequestra under local anaesthesia, chlorhexidine mouth rinses, systemic metronidazole and analgesics may be effective. Additional broad-spectrum antibiotics have been recommended by some but increase the risk of thrush to which these immunosuppressed patients are particularly susceptible. For persistent pain, oral analgesics are indicated.

People whose HIV infection is untreated are also at risk of acute ulcerative gingivitis.

Necrotising periodontitis PMID: 10863377, 10863376 and 29926942

GINGIVAL ENLARGEMENT

Gingival swelling is usually caused by inflammatory swelling, fibrous hyperplasia, medications or, less commonly, infiltration by neoplastic cells (Box 7.14).

Drug-induced gingival enlargement

Drug-induced gingival enlargement caused by the anticonvulsant drug phenytoin (Epanutin, Dilantin), has been recognized for over 70 years. More recently recognized causes

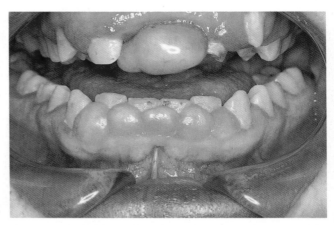

Fig. 7.27   Gingival hyperplasia due to phenytoin. Characteristically (and unlike Fig. 7.28), the fibrous overgrowth has originated in the interdental papillae, which become bulbous but remain firm and pale. Localised gross enlargement such as that around the upper central incisor may result and forms a plaque trap, exacerbating the overgrowth though inflammation.

include the immunosuppressive drugs ciclosporin and mycophenolate mofetil and the calcium-channel blocker drugs used for the management of hypertension and cardiac disease. Both the dihydropyridine calcium channel blockers, such as amlodipine and felodipine, and the non-dihydropyridines verapamil and diltiazem, have this effect.

These drugs are widely used. Calcium channel blocker drugs are the 4th most prescribed medication prescribed in the UK and the USA, taken by approximately 2 million people in the UK. Phenytoin is currently used relatively infrequently as a first line drug in epilepsy but is still taken by about 40,000 people in the UK, often long term. Ciclosporin is used particularly to prevent graft rejection following organ transplant, to control graft-versus-host disease after marrow transplant and, increasingly for autoimmune and inflammatory diseases such as rheumatoid arthritis and psoriasis. Thus, many individuals are potentially at risk of this adverse effect. Phenytoin and ciclosporin are the most potent stimulus with half of long-term users affected to some degree. Renal transplant patients often take both a calcium channel blocker and ciclosporin and are at particular risk.

Drug-induced enlargement affects primarily the papillae, whereas hereditary forms of gingival enlargement are diffuse. It is usually more prominent on the anterior teeth. The papillae become bulbous and in severe cases may reach the occlusal and incisal surfaces, partially or almost completely obscuring the crowns of the teeth (Fig. 7.27).

Classically, as seen with phenytoin, the gingivae are firm and pale, and the stippled texture is exaggerated, producing an orange-peel appearance. Histologically the tissue exhibits dense fibrous hyperplasia which may be uninflamed or show signs of secondary inflammation. Additionally, vascularity is increased in calcium channel blocker-induced enlargement and more markedly so in ciclosporin-induced enlargement, in which the gingiva appear redder and more inflamed.

The mechanisms are not fully understood, but there is assumed to be a genetic predisposition. All the causative drugs interfere with sodium or calcium transport, increasing cell proliferation, deplete folate and reduce degradation of collagen. Gingivitis contributes, and overgrowth of the gingivae can sometimes be prevented or kept under control by rigorous oral hygiene. Early changes can be seen after only 3 months of drug treatment, allowing intervention to prevent the condition.

If it is possible to stop the causative drug, slow resolution occurs over several months but is rarely complete. Frequently, gingivectomy is necessary to allow cleaning or for cosmetic reasons. The antibiotic azithromycin has recently been shown to reverse the fibrosis caused by ciclosporin.

Web URL 7.1 Review: http://emedicine.medscape.com/article/1076264

Drugs and gingival overgrowth PMID: 25680368 and 30198137

Management gingival overgrowth: PMID: 16677333

Hereditary gingival fibromatosis

Gingival fibromatosis is a feature of several heritable syndromes and is rare. As an isolated condition, hereditary gingival fibrosis is associated with mutation in the *SOS1* gene, which encodes a signalling pathway protein and other presentations are associated with multiple *GINGF* genes. When it develops as part of a syndrome, the most common association is hypertrichosis and learning disability. In other syndromes a range of features may coexist, including coarse and thickened facial features, simulating acromegaly, epilepsy, deafness, and cherubism.

Gingival enlargement may precede eruption of the teeth or may not develop until later in childhood. The gingivae may be so grossly enlarged as completely to bury the teeth or prevent eruption. The tissue is pale, firm and smooth or stippled in texture (Fig. 7.28).

Histologically, the gingival tissue consists of thick bundles of collagenous connective tissue with little or no inflammatory exudate (Fig. 7.29).

The excess gingival tissue can only be removed surgically but is likely to re-form. Gingivectomy should be delayed as long as possible, preferably until after puberty, when the rate of growth of the tissues is slower. Maintenance of oral hygiene is important to prevent infection becoming established in the deep false pockets. However, inflammation is frequently insignificant.

Other syndromes with generalised gingival enlargement due to other causes must be distinguished, such as hyaline fibromatosis, glycogen storage and other metabolic diseases, Cowden's syndrome and tuberous sclerosis.

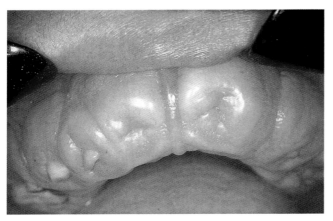

Fig. 7.28 **Hereditary gingival fibromatosis.** Fibrous overgrowth of the gingiva has covered the crowns of the teeth and almost buried them.

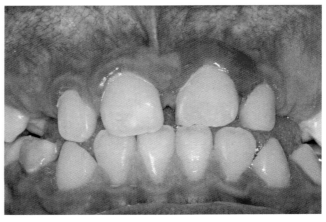

Fig. 7.30 **Localised juvenile spongiotic gingivitis.** Typical sharply demarcated spongy enlarged zone of gingiva extending away from the gingival margin. Note there is also some background conventional-appearing gingivitis.

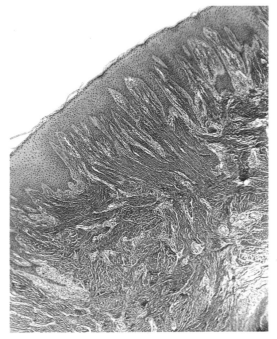

Fig. 7.29 **Gingival fibromatosis.** Both the genetic and drug-induced types share this histological picture of gross fibrous overgrowth. In this image the tissue has been stained with a Van Gieson stain that stains the collagen red. Note the absence of inflammation.

Review PMID: 34819125

Fibrous enlargement of the tuberosity

This rare condition is a poorly understood bilateral fibrous growth of the maxillary alveolus posterior to the premolar teeth. The bone is not enlarged. Some cases may have mild forms of hereditary gingival fibromatosis because bilateral fibrous tuberosity enlargement has been reported in family members of more typically affected individuals. However, it has also been reported as a reactive change when lower anterior teeth are opposed by complete dentures, in 'combination syndrome'.

Combination syndrome PMID: 30769080

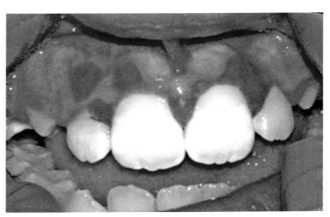

Fig. 7.31 **Localised juvenile spongiotic gingivitis.** In this more florid example there are several patches and some are sited away from the gingival margin. *(Fig. 18-13 from Law, C.S., Silva D.R., Duperon, D.F, et al., 2014. Gingival disease in Childhood. In: Newman, M.G., Takei, H.H., Klokkevold, P.R., et al. [Eds.], Carranza's clinical periodontology, twelfth ed. Saunders, Philadelphia, pp. 252-260.)*

LOCALISED JUVENILE SPONGIOTIC GINGIVITIS

This condition is rare, distinctive and does not respond to improvement in oral hygiene. The features are sessile rounded nodules of bright red, sharply demarcated and soft stippled or slightly papillary mucosa extending from the gingival margin to the mucogingival junction or beyond, a few millimetres in diameter (Figs 7.30 and 7.31). The buccal gingiva, usually maxillary, are most frequently involved, and most patients are female and between the ages of 6 and 18 years. The tissue bleeds easily. Most patients have a single focus.

The histological appearances are also distinctive, resembling inflammation of the junctional epithelium with a slightly papillary hyperplasia of the epithelium (Fig. 7.32).

The true nature of this condition remains to be determined. One suggestion is that it is a zone where junctional epithelium extends to the gingiva, and the epithelium shows altered keratinization, with loss of parakeratin and expression of keratin 19.

Lesions usually do not recur on excision, but whether they require any intervention or not is unclear as lesions may resolve spontaneously. It can occasionally be found in adults.

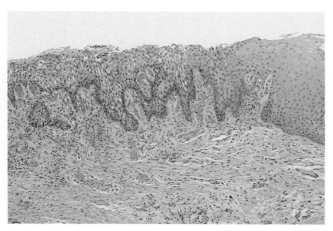

Fig. 7.32 **Localised juvenile spongiotic gingivitis.** The attached gingival epithelium is normal on the right, but there is a sharp demarcation to the affected epithelium on the left, which shows increased intercellular spaces and a loose poorly cohesive structure superficially. There are neutrophils in the epithelium but minimal inflammation in the underlying connective tissue.

Description PMID: 18602289

Multifocal adult disease PMID: 29512024

Conservative management 32918012

FOREIGN BODY GINGIVITIS

This condition is rare but probably underrecognised and can be puzzling to diagnose, even with a biopsy. The cause is implantation of foreign material into the gingiva, usually particles of prophylaxis paste, corundum, silica from air abrasion, crown cements, or zinc oxide pack as a complication of periodontal surgery. Prophylaxis paste probably enters the tissues following overenthusiastic use of cup or brush, abrading the marginal gingiva, crevice or pocket wall to implant the material. Gingiva with ulcers or atrophy, such as in lichen planus or pemphigoid, might be more susceptible to implantation.

Clinically, there is a red band of gingival inflammation, usually dusky red rather than brightly inflamed and sharply localised laterally. This is frequently mistaken for plaque-induced gingivitis, desquamative gingivitis or lichen planus (Fig. 7.33). Sometimes the changes are localised to a crown margin or other potential cause, but there may be a period of years before signs and symptoms develop and the history may not reveal a cause. The affected gingiva is characteristically symptomatic, usually sore or tender rather than painful, and slightly swollen.

On biopsy, the foreign material is often tiny fragments of crystalline or other opaque material that is difficult to see and may not be found without examination under polarised light. There is a classical granulomatous inflammatory response in only a quarter to a half of cases, the remainder having minimal changes, a light lymphocytic infiltrate or vascular changes that are easily mistaken for plaque-induced inflammation or, sometimes, lichen planus. Unfortunately, small particles of foreign material are quite a common chance finding in the gingiva and are often of no significance. Therefore, diagnosis requires clinical correlation, a number and distribution of the particles that matches the inflammation, and ideally a potential cause.

Treatment is difficult. Steroids are ineffective and surgical excision of the worst affected areas may be required if soreness

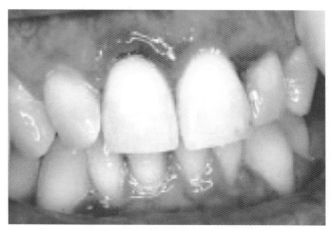

Fig 7.33 **Foreign body gingivitis.** Swelling and redness with soreness of affected areas. *(Source: Gravitis K, Daley TD, Lochhead MA. J Can Dent Assoc 2005; 71[2]:105–9)*

is severe or for cosmetic reasons. Eventually the inflammation may subside spontaneously, but over a long period. Prevention is key. Prophylaxis must be undertaken without physical trauma or heat trauma to the gingiva, and particularly carefully when desquamative gingivitis or other disease is present. Air abrasion is potentially particularly damaging, and the disease has also been reported to result from overpowerful domestic water jet oral cleaning devices.

Cases PMID: 9159816 and 30740500

Identification of materials PMID: 17305638

PLASMINOGEN DEFICIENCY GINGIVITIS

This rare inherited deficiency has a distinctive gingival presentation as described in Chapter 29.

OTHER INFLAMMATORY GINGIVAL SWELLING

Varying degrees of gingival swelling may accompany gingivitis and periodontitis. Typically, the swelling is mild or moderate, and is characterized by red, haemorrhagic gingival papillae. As discussed previously, pregnancy can frequently exacerbate inflammatory-mediated gingival swelling.

Granulomatosis with polyangiitis (Wegener's granulomatosis) is an uncommon, vasculitic disease described in Chapter 34. Occasionally, the first sign is a characteristic form of proliferative gingivitis, bright or dusky red in colour and with a granular surface, to which the term 'strawberry gums' has been applied. Early recognition may be life-saving.

Sarcoidosis and orofacial granulomatosis can give rise to generalised nodular gingival enlargement. These discussed in Chapters 31 and 35, respectively.

Acute leukaemia, particularly acute myelomonocytic leukaemia, causes gingival swellings. The abnormal white cells are unable to perform their normal defensive function and cannot control infection at the gingival margins. The abnormal leucocytes pack the area until the gingivae become swollen with proliferating leukaemic cells (Fig. 7.34). These cells are functionally defective, so that infection progresses leading to ulceration and breakdown of the tissues. Clinically, the gingivae are swollen, shiny, pale or purplish in colour and frequently ulcerated (Fig. 7.35). Other signs of leukaemia (pallor, purpura or lassitude) may also be seen. Topical antibiotics or

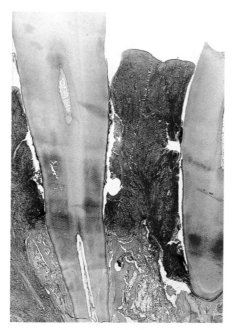

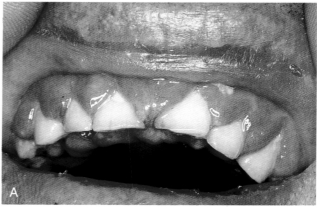

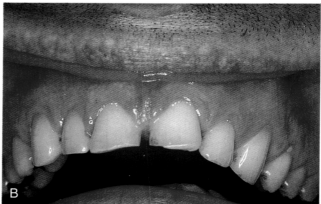

Fig. 7.34 Acute myelomonocytic leukaemia. The gingival swelling can be seen to be due to packing of the gingivae with leukaemic cells, immature and abnormal neutrophils or monocytes, stained dark blue. The periodontal tissues have broken down as a result of the poor resistance to infection.

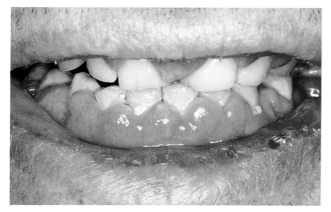

Fig. 7.35 Acute myelomonocytic leukaemia. The gingival margins are swollen and soft due to the leukaemic infiltrate.

Fig. 7.36 Acute leukaemia. (A) Gross leukaemic infiltration has caused the gingival margins to reach the incisal edges of the teeth. (B) The benefits of plaque control with chlorhexidine mouthwash and oral hygiene have restored the normal appearance, showing that these gingival manifestations are dependent on oral hygiene.

chlorhexidine and improved oral hygiene may lead to some improvement in the swelling (Fig. 7.36).

Other features of leukaemia are discussed in Chapter 28.

Scurvy causes grossly swollen and congested gingivae, and early tooth loss. Features are described in Chapter 36.

Glycogen storage diseases are rare inherited metabolic defects in which the gingiva are enlarged by accumulation of macrophages containing PAS positive glycogen. Type 1b is accompanied by neutrophil defects contributing to early onset periodontitis.

Osteomyelitis, osteitis and osteonecrosis of the jaws

8

Severe infections of bone are uncommon despite the numerous pathogenic bacteria in the mouth and the easy access to the medullary cavity through tooth roots and extraction sockets. Indeed, the bone of the jaws appears remarkably resistant to osteomyelitis. Oral and perioral soft tissue infections almost always originate in teeth or periodontium and in the past particularly, but occasionally today, they can be life-threatening or fatal by direct or haematogenous spread. Infection has been considered curable for decades, but the rise of antibiotic resistance poses a threat to the population, and dentists have important roles to play in antibiotic stewardship.

The processes of frustrated healing in a periapical granuloma are described in Chapter 5. Although the periapical granuloma is normally sterile, bacteria may enter the apical tissues sporadically to seed an infection. Dental extraction is often the precipitating factor in osteomyelitis, so understanding the normal healing processes is fundamental for prevention.

NORMAL HEALING OF AN EXTRACTION SOCKET

Stages in the normal healing of a single-rooted tooth extraction socket are shown in Fig. 8.1.

The first stage of healing is the formation of a clot. Normal clotting mechanisms produce a loose clot that fills the bony and soft tissue socket. Activated platelets trigger retraction of the clot, expressing fluid so that it becomes harder and shrinks below the level of the adjacent soft tissues, pulling any mobile soft tissue inward to reduce the area of the clot exposed. Clot retraction is usually complete in 4 hours, and the surface of the clot changes from shiny to matt. After retraction, the clot continues to stabilise by fibrin cross-linking, so avoiding rinsing is usually recommended for 24 hours until this process is complete. A socket containing early clot is shown at the top of Fig. 8.1 (A). Much of the clot (1) is bright red from trapped erythrocytes, and the periodontal ligament can still be seen around the socket periphery (2).

Lysis of the clot begins within 2 days, caused primarily by the fibrinolytic enzyme plasmin, generated by activation of plasminogen in the clot. A 2-day-old socket is shown in (B) and (C). In (B), the section is stained with haematoxylin and eosin and in (C) with a stain that shows fibrin in yellow, bone in red and the periodontal ligament in turquoise. The periodontal ligament is still sharply defined but, at higher power, the emigration of inflammatory cells into the clot would be seen. It is at this stage, when fibrinolysis has started but the clot is not well anchored to the wall, that the risk of dry socket from clot lysis or loss is highest. Note also how the thin buccal bone is being lost by resorption (B, C right). In normal socket healing, loss of bone around the socket is greater when the bone is thin and this leads to loss of alveolar bone height after healing is complete. When the buccal bone is very thin, as for instance in lower incisor

sockets, it is completely lost, allowing soft tissue to collapse into the socket and causing marked narrowing of the ridge.

At 4 days, capillaries and fibroblasts (granulation tissue) are growing into the blood clot from the periphery so that it is now firmly fixed to the socket wall. Macrophages migrate into the clot and start to demolish it ready for replacement by granulation tissue. The surface of the clot is white and porous clinically. Bacterial enzymes have lysed the surface fibrin, and there are bacteria in the superficial fibrin, which gradually disintegrates. Epithelium at the gingival margin undergoes hyperplasia and starts to grow over the intact clot, below the surface debris.

At 8 days (D), the socket is filled by granulation tissue (3) and the superficial layers contain inflammatory cells (4). The granulation tissue is soft or gelatinous and contains little collagen. It appears red if exposed ('socket granulations'). The periodontal ligament is no longer clearly identifiable. The lamina dura of the socket (5) is intact but, at higher power, osteoclasts would be seen on its surface. There is early surface resorption. Depending on the surface area of the socket mouth, epithelial migration is complete between 7 and 10 days; in this socket it is delayed and there is inflammation at the surface.

At 18 days (E), the socket is filled by granulation tissue and the fibroblasts within it have laid down a collagen network. The outline of the lamina dura is still visible (6) and woven bone is forming around the periphery of the socket. On the left, there is a thick layer of woven bone trabeculae (7) and a blue rim of cellular osteogenic tissue at the bone-forming front (8).

By 6 weeks (F), the woven bone has filled the socket and is in a phase of long-term remodelling to lamellar bone (9). The outline of the lamina dura (10) persists for a very variable length of time, depending on the bone turnover rate. By 3 months, it is usually not detectable radiographically, but socket outlines may persist for years in older people.

Wound healing general review PMID: 20139336

Socket healing PMID: 25867983

Socket grafting and ridge preservation PMID: 34176715 and 22405099

Extraction socket dressings

Materials may be put into fresh extraction sockets for three main purposes. To control bleeding (Ch. 29), for pain control in dry socket (Ch. 8) or in an attempt to induce bone formation for ridge preservation. Many pastes and dressings also contain antibacterial compounds, but their value is unclear. True infection of sockets, as opposed to a dry socket, is extremely rare and some patients may be allergic to iodine or other compounds used.

As a general principle, any material put into a socket will delay or impair healing. Non-resorbable materials should be regularly replaced, every one or two days, as the socket heals so as not to restrict granulation tissue formation and ultimate ridge height. Resorbable materials must be used in the

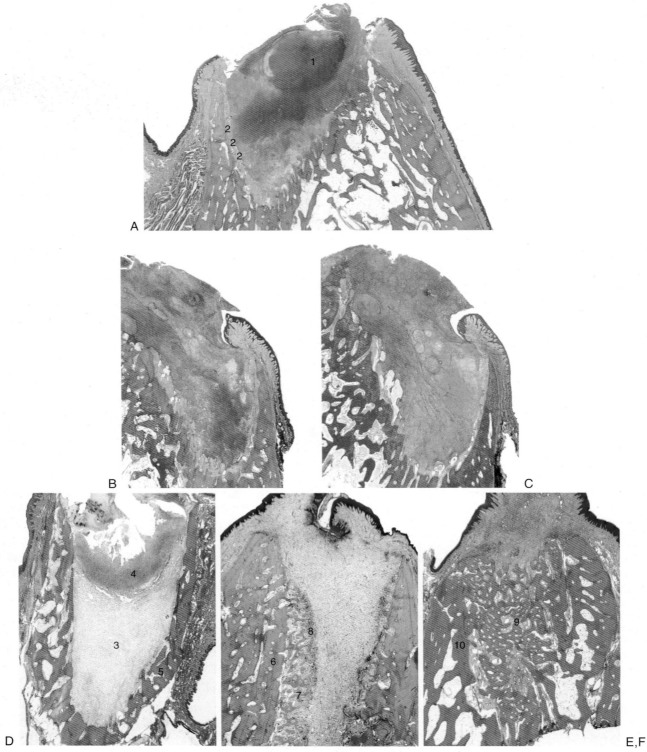

Fig. 8.1 Stages in the normal healing of a single-rooted tooth extraction socket. For explanation and annotations see text.

minimum required to be effective so that clot and granulation tissue can grow into the material and replace it. Excess or tightly packed material will not organize, forms a nidus for infection and may be treated as a foreign body leading to either extrusion of the material or persistent inflammation (Fig 8.2) and failure to heal. Adverse reactions to socket dressings are unpredictable. Apart from allergy to ingredients, they largely arise through local factors in the socket or misuse. Alternative socket sealing materials placed over rather than in the socket avoid some of these complications.

The loss of alveolar ridge dimension after extraction, noted above, is largely accounted for by resorption and loss of the

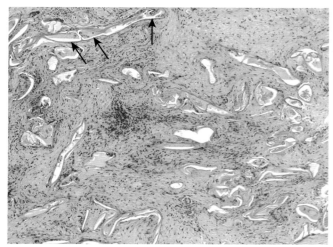

Fig 8.2   Haemostatic dressing found in a socket that failed to heal. The dressing comprises fibres that are iodinated, seen as the orange outline to the fibres (one arrowed). There is focal inflammation centrally and foreign body giant cells are seen adhering to fibres and inside their hollow centres (arrowed right).

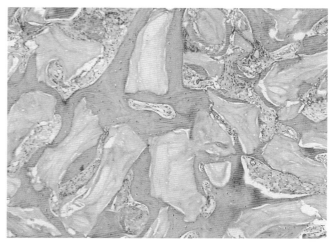

Fig 8.3   Bone inducing graft of anorganic bone removed from a socket at implant placement after 4 months healing. The graft material is pale pink and contains empty osteocyte lacunae. The irregular pieces of graft material have induced new bone formation over much of their surfaces, which stains a darker red colour and has osteocytes in the lacunae. The graft has successfully induced bone formation, but the graft has not yet been replaced by strong interconnected trabeculae of new bone after 4 months.

thinnest alveolar bone before bone formation has started in the socket. This may compromise the subsequent placement of implants and immediate implant placement or grafting materials may be used in an attempt to preserve ridge height and width. Many materials are used including hydroxyapatites, demineralized or deproteinized animal bone and platelet-derived agents. These are mostly intended to induce bone formation in the early phases and to be subsequently remodelled and replaced by normal bone, but often the graft material remains in the tissues for long periods. Although improvement can sometimes be demonstrated in individual patients, their use remains controversial and success unpredictable. Delayed healing or persistent inflammation caused by the material will increase bone loss (Fig 8.3). Use of these agents does not affect longer term bone remodelling and ridge resorption.

ALVEOLAR OSTEITIS

Alveolar osteitis ('dry' socket) is by far the most frequent painful complication of extractions. It is not really an infection but leads to superficial bacterial contamination of exposed bone and can progress to osteomyelitis, though extremely uncommonly. Osteitis simply means inflamed bone, not infection. Alveolar osteitis develops after 1%–2% of extractions, more frequently for lower-third molar extractions when, for difficult extractions, the incidence can reach 20%.

Aetiology

Alveolar osteitis is frequently unpredictable and without any obvious predisposing cause, but numerous possible aetiological factors exist (Box 8.1).

Alveolar osteitis is more likely to follow difficult disimpactions of third molars or traumatic extractions than uncomplicated extractions. However, the blood supply to the area often appears to be the critical factor. In healthy persons, alveolar osteitis virtually only affects the lower molar region, where the bone is more dense and less vascular than elsewhere. Alveolar osteitis is also an expected complication of extractions when the alveolar bone is sclerotic, as in Paget's disease, after radiotherapy and where vascular disease causes ischaemia of the bone. Alveolar

> **Box 8.1   Predisposing factors for alveolar osteitis**
>
> - Female patient
> - Excessive extraction trauma
> - Limited local blood supply
> - Gingival infection such as acute ulcerative gingivitis, pericoronitis or abscess
> - Local anaesthesia with vasoconstrictor
> - Smoking
> - Oral contraceptives
> - Osteosclerotic disease: Paget's disease, cemento-osseous dysplasia
> - Radiotherapy
> - History of previous dry socket

osteitis is also more frequent in susceptible patients when local anaesthesia is used, as a result of vasoconstriction.

The immediate cause is early loss of clot from the extraction socket due to excessive local fibrinolytic activity. The alveolar bone and gingiva have a high content of fibrinolysin activators (plasmin), that are released when the bone is traumatised, degrading the clot and leaving the socket empty. Once the clot has been destroyed, bacterial colonisation from the mouth is inevitable, and bacterial enzymes contribute to clot lysis.

The oestrogen component of oral contraceptives enhances serum fibrinolytic activity and interferes with clotting, and its use is associated with a higher incidence of alveolar osteitis. Similarly the higher oestrogen level of mid-menstrual cycle has been linked to increased risk.

Clinical features

Patients aged 20–40 years are most at risk, and women are more frequently affected. Pain usually starts a few days after the extraction, but sometimes may be delayed for a week or more. It is deep-seated, severe and aching or throbbing. The mucosa around the socket is red and tender. There is no clot in the socket, which contains, instead, saliva and often decomposing food debris (Fig. 8.4). When debris is washed away, whitish, dead bone may be seen or may be felt as a rough area with a probe and probing is painful. The appearance of an empty socket and exposed bone is diagnostic. Sometimes the socket becomes concealed by granulations growing in from the gingival margins, narrowing the opening and trapping food debris. Pain often continues for a week or two, or occasionally longer. Sequestration of parts of the socket wall may sometimes be seen radiographically (Fig. 8.5), but a radiograph performs no useful purpose except to exclude retention of a root fragment.

Pathology

Infected food and other debris accumulate in direct contact with the bone. Bone damaged during the extraction, particularly the dense bone of the lamina dura, dies. The necrotic bone and socket lodge bacteria which proliferate freely in the avascular spaces unhindered by host defences. In the surrounding tissue, inflammation prevents spread of infection beyond the socket walls. Dead bone is gradually separated by osteoclasts, and sequestra are usually shed in tiny fragments. Healing is slow. Granulation tissue cannot grow in from the socket walls and base until the necrotic bone is removed.

Although there is no infection within the tissues, the colonisation of the socket and sequestra by oral bacteria probably contributes to pain and slow healing. Anaerobes are thought to be significant and can produce fibrinolytic enzymes. However, antibiotics including metronidazole have not been shown to either prevent dry socket or speed healing reliably. Only chlorhexidine rinsing preoperatively has been shown to reduce incidence.

Prevention

Preventive measures are shown in Box 8.2. Because damage to bone is an important predisposing factor, extractions should be carried out with minimal trauma. Immediately after the extraction the socket edges should be squeezed firmly together and held for a few minutes until the clot has formed.

In the case of disimpactions of third molars, where alveolar osteitis is more common, prophylactic antibiotics are sometimes given. Their value is unproven, and there is no indication for using antibiotics for routine dental extractions. However, in patients who have had irradiation for oral cancer or have sclerotic bone disease, postoperative antibiotic cover should be given and the tooth removed surgically to cause as little damage as possible to surrounding bone. Antibiotics are given primarily to prevent osteomyelitis rather than dry socket.

There remain a few patients especially prone to alveolar osteitis, which follows every extraction under local anaesthesia including regional blocks. In such patients, dry socket may be preventable if general anaesthesia is used, although this is difficult to justify clinically.

Treatment

It is important to explain to patients that they may have a week or more of discomfort. It is also important to explain that the pain is not due, as patients usually think, to a broken root. Local conditions strongly favour persistence of infection, and the aim of treatment is to control symptoms until healing is complete, usually after approximately 10 days.

Treatment is to keep the open socket clean and to protect exposed bone from excessive bacterial contamination. The socket should be irrigated with mild warm antiseptic or

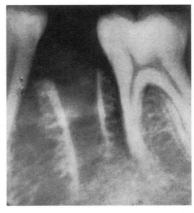

Fig. 8.5 Unusually severe sequestration in a dry socket. Almost the whole of the lamina dura and attached trabeculae have become necrotic, forming a sequestrum. Healing is delayed while the sequestrum remains in place. Most dry sockets are not associated with sequestration, or with only small sequestra.

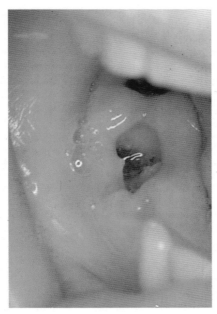

Fig. 8.4 Dry socket. Typical appearances of chronic alveolar osteitis; the socket is empty, and the bony lamina dura is visible.

Box 8.2   Prevention of dry socket

- Preoperative infection control
  - Scaling teeth before extraction
  - Chlorhexidine rinsing preoperatively and for 3 days postoperatively
- Atraumatic extraction
- Adherence to postoperative instructions
  - No rinsing or forceful spitting
  - No hot fluids
  - No smoking
- Postoperative antibiotics only for patients at particular risk

saline to remove all food debris. Chlorhexidine must not be used in the socket; allergy to chlorhexidine in this situation can be fatal. It is then traditional to place a dressing into the socket to deliver analgesia and close the opening so that further food debris cannot enter the socket. Many socket dressings have been formulated and should be antiseptic, obtundent, adhere to the socket wall, and be absorbable. Whatever is used, the minimum dressing to close the socket opening is used because dressing packed hard into the socket will delay healing. Non-absorbable dressings must be removed as soon as possible to allow the socket to heal. A dressing may only last 1–2 days, and the whole process needs repeating until pain subsides, normally after one or two dressings. Frequent hot saline mouthwashes also help keep the socket free from debris.

Key features of alveolar osteitis are summarised in Box 8.3.

Dry socket review PMID: 12190139 and 32348729

OSTEOMYELITIS OF THE JAWS

Unlike the long bones, osteomyelitis in the jaws is almost always of local origin and not caused by blood-borne infection. The classification of osteomyelitis is somewhat confusing, with a range of overlapping conditions. Their names are more descriptions of their clinical presentation based on the chronicity of the infection and effects on the bone. There are no strict definitions, and not all cases can be easily categorised.

Syphilitic, actinomycotic and tuberculous osteomyelitis of the jaws are distinct entities, but now seen only in resource-poor countries.

ACUTE OSTEOMYELITIS

→ Summary charts 5.1 and 13.1 pp. 81, 244

In acute osteomyelitis bacteria and inflammation spread through the medullary bone from a focus of infection.

By far the most common cause is spread of infection from a periapical infection, but there are other potential sources of infection (Box 8.4). The jaws are resistant to osteomyelitis, and most patients have a predisposing cause. These may be local factors, usually causing sclerosis and reducing the vascularity of the bone, or systemic predispositions to infection. The most important are summarised in Box 8.5.

The effect of immunodeficiency is variable, and acute osteomyelitis of the jaw is uncommon in HIV infection.

Clinical features

Most patients with acute osteomyelitis are adult males, who have more of the causative dental infections than females. Almost all cases affect the mandible, which is less vascular than the maxilla.

Early complaints are severe, throbbing, deep-seated pain and swelling with external swelling due to inflammatory oedema. Later, distension of the periosteum with pus and, finally, subperiosteal bone formation cause the swelling to become firm. The overlying gingiva and mucosa are red, swollen and tender.

Associated teeth are tender. They may become loose, and pus may exude from an open socket or gingival margins. Muscle oedema causes difficulty in opening the mouth and swallowing. Regional lymph nodes are enlarged and tender and anaesthesia or paraesthesia of the lower lip, caused by pressure on the inferior dental nerve, is characteristic.

Frequently, the patient remains surprisingly well but, in the acute phase, there may be fever and leucocytosis.

Radiographic changes do not appear until after at least 10 days, and radiographs can provide little useful information before this time except to identify any local cause. Later, there is loss of trabecular pattern and areas of radiolucency indicating bone destruction and sometimes widening of periodontal ligament. Affected areas have ill-defined margins and a moth-eaten appearance similar to a malignant neoplasm (Fig. 8.6). Areas of dead bone appear as relatively dense areas which become more sharply defined as they are progressively separated as sequestra. Later, in young persons particularly, subperiosteal new bone formation causes a buccal swelling

---

Box 8.4 Acute osteomyelitis of the jaws: potential sources of infection

- Periapical infection
- Pericoronitis
- Fracture through periodontal pocket or open to the mouth
- Acute necrotising gingivitis, cancrum oris and noma
- Penetrating, contaminated injuries (open fractures or gunshot wounds)

Box 8.5 Important predisposing conditions for osteomyelitis

Local damage to or disease of the jaws

- History of irradiation
- Causes of sclerosis of bone
  - Paget's disease
  - Fibro-osseous lesions, particularly cemento-osseous dysplasia
  - Osteopetrosis

Impaired immune defences

- Poorly controlled diabetes mellitus
- Sickle cell anaemia
- Chronic alcoholism or malnutrition
- Drug abuse
- Tobacco smoking
- Malignant neoplasms and their treatment

Box 8.3 Alveolar osteitis: key features

- The most common painful complication of dental extractions
- Onset usually 3–7 days after extraction
- Loss of clot normally filling extraction socket
- Loss of clot may be due to excessive local fibrinolytic action or bacterial enzymes or both
- Bare, whitish lamina dura exposed in socket
- Pain relieved by irrigation and repeated dressing of socket
- Dead bone usually shed as crumblike fragments
- Eventual healing of socket from its base by granulation

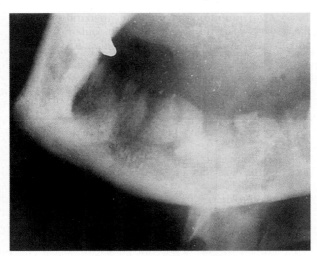

Fig. 8.6 Chronic osteomyelitis of the mandible following dental extractions. The outlines of the extraction sockets can be seen, together with dense sequestra of bone lying in a poorly circumscribed radiolucency. Oblique lateral view.

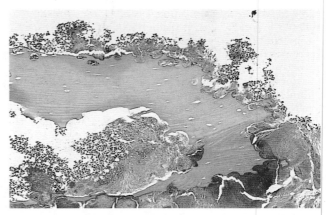

Fig. 8.7 High-power view of a sequestrum showing non-vital bone (the osteocyte lacunae are empty) and eroded outline with surface lacunae, produced by osteoclastic resorption, and a dense surface growth of bacteria.

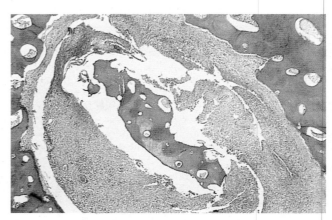

Fig. 8.8 Late-stage chronic osteomyelitis. A sequestrum trapped in a cavity within the bone. It is surrounded by fibrous tissue containing an infiltrate of inflammatory cells. Surgical intervention is needed to remove an infected sequestrum such as this.

and appears as a thin, curved strip of new bone below the lower border of the jaw in lateral or panoramic radiographs.

Osteomyelitis of the newborn is a very rare and distinctive variant affecting the maxilla shortly after birth, which is potentially fatal. The cause is either birth injuries or uncontrolled middle ear infection. Other than in children, the maxilla is very rarely affected.

Osteomyelitis of newborn PMID: 15125285

Pathology

Acute osteomyelitis is a suppurative infection with a mixed bacterial flora, much of which forms a biofilm on and within sequestra of bone. Oral bacteria, particularly anaerobes such as *Bacteroides*, *Porphyromonas* or *Prevotella* species, are important components of the flora. Staphylococci may be responsible when osteomyelitis follows an open fracture and the bacteria enter from the skin.

The mandible has a relatively limited blood supply and dense bone with thick cortical plates. Infection and acute inflammation cannot escape, and the pressure pushes infection through the marrow spaces. It also compresses blood vessels confined within the rigid boundaries of the vascular canals. Thrombosis and obstruction then lead to devascularization and further bone necrosis. Dead bone is recognisable microscopically by lacunae empty of osteocytes and medullary spaces filled with neutrophils and colonies of bacteria that proliferate in the dead tissue (Fig. 8.7).

Pus, formed by liquefaction of necrotic soft tissue and inflammatory cells, is forced along the medulla and eventually penetrates the cortex to reach the subperiosteal region by resorption of bone. Distension of the periosteum by pus stimulates subperiosteal bone formation, but perforation of the periosteum by pus and formation of sinuses on the skin or oral mucosa are rarely seen in developed countries and after effective treatment.

At the boundary between infected and healthy tissue, osteoclasts resorb the periphery of the dead bone, which eventually becomes separated as a sequestrum (Fig. 8.8). Once infection starts to localise, new bone forms around it, particularly subperiosteally.

Where bone has died and been removed or shed as sequestra, healing is by granulation tissue with formation of woven bone in the proliferating connective tissue. After resolution, woven bone is gradually replaced by compact bone and remodelled to restore normal morphology.

Osteomyelitis early diagnosis PMID: 21982609

Management

The key factor is to assess whether the infection is limited to the jaws or may be spreading systemically. A severely ill or very pale patient and a very high temperature suggest possible systemic spread and indicate a need to check for an underlying predisposing disease and consider blood culture to exclude septicaemia. The main requirements are summarised in Box 8.6.

Bacteriological diagnosis. A specimen of pus or a swab from the depths of the lesion must first be taken for culture and sensitivity testing, ideally by using an anaerobic sampling technique.

Antimicrobial treatment. Immediately after a specimen has been obtained, vigorous antibiotic treatment should be started. Initially, penicillin, 600–1200 mg daily can be given

> **Box 8.6 Summary of management of acute osteomyelitis**
>
> **Essential measures**
> - Remove source of infection, if possible
> - Bacterial sampling and culture
> - Vigorous (empirical) antibiotic treatment
> - Drainage
> - Analgesics
> - Give specific antibiotics once culture and sensitivities are available
> - Debridement
>
> **Adjunctive treatment**
> - Sequestrectomy
> - Decortication if necessary
> - Resection and reconstruction for extensive bone destruction

> **Box 8.7 Acute osteomyelitis of the jaws: key features**
>
> - Mandible mainly affected, usually in adult males
> - Infection of dental origin; mixed flora with anaerobes
> - Pain and swelling of jaw
> - Teeth in the area are tender: gingivae are red and swollen
> - Sometimes paraesthesia of the lip
> - Minimal systemic upset
> - After about 10 days, radiographs show moth-eaten pattern of bone destruction
> - Good response to prompt antibiotic treatment and debridement

by injection (if the patient is not allergic), with metronidazole 200–400 mg every 8 hours. Clindamycin penetrates avascular tissue better and is frequently effective. The regimen is adjusted later in the light of the bacteriological findings. Individual antibiotic resistant species are frequently found but this need not determine antibiotic choice in such a mixed flora.

Debridement. Removal of foreign or necrotic material and immobilisation of any fracture are necessary if there has been a gunshot wound or other contaminating injury.

Drainage. Pressure should be relieved by tooth extraction. Local analgesia is usually impossible in the presence of acute infection, but the earlier any causative tooth can be removed the better. Drainage may be achievable through the root canal as a temporary measure. If so, it may be possible to retain and restore the tooth at a later date. Alternatively bur holes through the cortex or decortication, as necessary, allow the exudate to drain out into the mouth or externally, reducing the pressure and preventing infection from being pushed further through the medullary bone. Such surgical drainage is rarely used now that high-dose and high-potency antibiotic regimes are available.

Removal of sequestra. Dead bone should not be forcibly separated, and vigorous curetting is inadvisable since non-vital bone may act as a useful scaffold for bone formation during healing. However, a loosened sequestrum may have to be removed. Teeth that are not the primary cause should be extracted only if severely loosened by bone destruction. With effective antibiotic treatment, areas of non-viable bone may not sequestrate and will be incorporated back into the healing bone. However, sequestra colonised by a bacterial biofilm will always eventually be shed.

Adjunctive treatment. Decortication or hyperbaric oxygen therapy, or both, may be attempted, particularly in radiation-associated osteomyelitis, although the effectiveness of hyperbaric oxygen is unproven. However, these are usually performed for chronic disease after other measures have failed.

Complications and resolution

Acute osteomyelitis usually resolves fully following aggressive treatment. Anaesthesia of the lower lip usually recovers with elimination of the infection. Rare complications include pathological fracture caused by extensive bone destruction, chronic osteomyelitis after inadequate treatment, cellulitis due to spread of exceptionally virulent bacteria or septicaemia in an immunodeficient patient.

Key features of acute osteomyelitis of the jaws are summarised in Box 8.7.

Review treatment PMID: 30509394

CHRONIC OSTEOMYELITIS

→ Summary charts 5.1 and 13.1 pp. 81, 244

Chronic osteomyelitis is much more common than acute osteomyelitis and arises from infection by weakly virulent bacteria or in avascular bone. Most cases develop without a prior acute phase, and only rarely does acute osteomyelitis lead to chronic osteomyelitis. When it does, it usually follows inadequate treatment.

Like the acute condition, there are usually predisposing factors such as those listed in Box 8.5. However, local bone sclerosis or irradiation are factors much more likely to predispose to chronic osteomyelitis than acute.

Clinical features

The picture is often dominated by persistent ache or pain, often relapsing, during a long period with a bad taste from pus draining to the mouth through sinuses. In more active phases there is swelling, increased pain and discharge, and increased tooth mobility. There may be exposed bone. Initially the tooth that was the original focus of infection can be identified, but chronic osteomyelitis may persist after its removal and the chronic infection becomes self-perpetuating in the bone.

Radiographic appearances are variable but sometimes distinctive (Fig. 8.9) with patchy and poorly defined radiolucency and sclerosis, sometimes resembling a malignant neoplasm. Sequestra may be identified, and there may be a periosteal new bone layer (see proliferative periostitis later in this chapter).

Pathology

Chronic osteomyelitis is a suppurative infection, but suppuration is generally limited and may cease in quiescent periods.

Persistent low-grade infection is associated with chronic inflammation, activation of osteoclastic bone destruction and granulation tissue formation. Healing is frustrated by inability of the inflammation and immune response to access

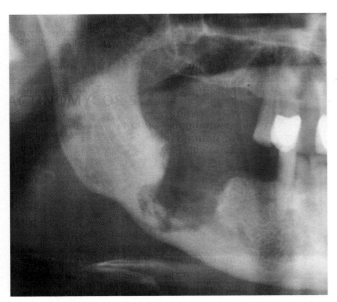

Fig. 8.9 Chronic osteomyelitis. The extent of destruction is much more readily apparent than in acute osteomyelitis. Note the sequestra lying close to the lower border and the peripheral sclerosis. A slight convexity of subperiosteal new bone formation is evident below the lower border.

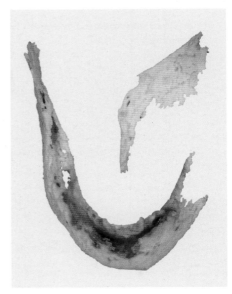

Fig. 8.10 Sequestration of the entire mandible following chronic osteomyelitis of odontogenic origin.

bacteria in dead avascular bone and by the slow separation of dead bone as sequestra. Sequestra will usually separate spontaneously during months or years and may be several centimetres in length. If antibiotic treatment is effective, sequestra may be sterilised and become reincorporated into healing bone. Conversely, infection may spread widely through abnormal bone or in a debilitated host but never develop the florid features of acute osteomyelitis (Fig. 8.10).

Chronic osteomyelitis is resistant to treatment and must be treated aggressively to overcome the factors noted previously that favour persistence of infection. The source of infection must be removed. Prolonged antibiotic treatment is the mainstay of treatment and must continue for at least 6 weeks and be tailored to the sensitivity of the micro-organisms. If sequestra are large, they must be removed surgically, and ideally all infected non-vital bone should be removed. Sometimes this requires corticectomy, which has the added advantage of opening the bone to healing from the periosteum. Thus, surgical intervention plays a much greater role in chronic than acute osteomyelitis. The response is slow, and antibiotics may be required for several months. If infection persists despite treatment, implantation of antibiotic-impregnated plastic beads provides a local slow release of antibiotic in high concentrations.

Key features of chronic osteomyelitis are shown in Box 8.8

DIFFUSE SCLEROSING OSTEOMYELITIS

This is an even lower intensity of infection, without formation of pus, in which low-virulence organisms or repeated inadequate antibiotic treatment may lead to longstanding widespread but very low-grade osteomyelitis. The presence of infection is not obvious, and chronic dull pain and swelling are often not severe enough to immediately suggest osteomyelitis. The main features are radiographic. There is extensive patchy sclerosis of the mandible, poorly localised and without a clear radiolucent focus of infection.

> **Box 8.8 Chronic osteomyelitis of the jaws: key features**
> - Mandible mainly affected
> - Infection of dental origin
> - Low-grade pain
> - Sclerosis or avascular bone often a predisposing factor
> - Resistant to treatment
> - Prolonged antibiotic treatment required
> - Role for surgery to remove sequestra and sclerotic bone

Diffuse sclerosing osteomyelitis is a controversial condition. In the past it has been confused with florid cemento-osseous dysplasia or fibrous dysplasia, and this confusion is understandable. The radiological features are similar, and the sclerosis of cemento-osseous dysplasia predisposes to infection. Diagnosis is difficult and should only be made when it is clear that there is infection present and not on the basis of radiological features alone. Biopsy may confirm inflammation in medullary spaces but is best avoided because of the risk of introducing further infection into the sclerotic bone. The distinction between diffuse sclerosing osteomyelitis and chronic non-bacterial osteomyelitis is difficult and there is considerable overlap in presentation; it remains possible that many patients thought to have infection actually have non-bacterial osteomyelitis

Treatment is to deal with any possible foci of infection with local measures and antibiotics. The key features of diffuse sclerosing osteomyelitis are shown in Box 8.9.

CHRONIC NON-BACTERIAL OSTEOMYELITIS

Many names have been applied to this controversial condition, including primary chronic osteomyelitis, acquired hyperostosis and chronic recurrent multifocal osteomyelitis, and it may overlap with diffuse sclerosing osteomyelitis. A key feature is

- No sex predilection
- Affects mandible almost exclusively
- Patchy diffuse sclerosis in the alveolar process
- Changes more marked around sites of periapical or
  periodontal chronic inflammation
- Persistent ache or pain but no swelling
- Radiographically resembles but is distinct from florid
  cemento-osseous dysplasia or fibrous dysplasia
- May be a presentation of the SAPHO (synovitis, acne,
  pustulosis, hyperostosis and osteitis) syndrome

Pathology

- Bone sclerosis and remodelling
- Scanty marrow spaces and little or no inflammatory
  infiltrate

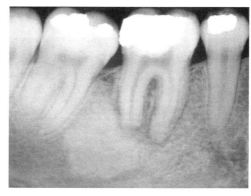

Fig. 8.11 Sclerosing osteitis. A focal zone of sclerosis associated with periapical inflammation from a non-vital lower first molar. *(Courtesy of Mr EJ Whaites.)*

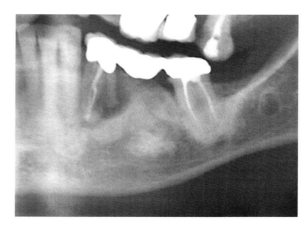

Fig. 8.12 Sclerosing osteitis. Multiple foci of sclerosis around the apices and roots of non-vital teeth, superficially resembling florid cemento-osseous dysplasia. *(Courtesy of Professor MP Foschini.)*

that more than jaw bones can be involved, often the sternum or spine or long bones in children. Some cases have a syndromic combination of synovitis, acne, pustulosis, hyperostosis and osteitis (SAPHO syndrome) or its childhood form of chronic recurrent multifocal osteomyelitis (CRMO). These cause zones of patchy radiolucency and sclerosis without clinical infection. These conditions are difficult to diagnose and require specialist investigation.

It is not always clear when confronted by a patient whether the presentation is infectious at all but antibiotic treatment must be tried initially. It has been suggested that the condition is due to tendon and periosteal inflammation rather than infection. Treatments have included antibiotics, non-steroidal and other anti-inflammatory drugs, steroids and bisphosphonates but none is reliably effective.

By definition, these types of osteomyelitis are inflammatory in nature, but there is also a range of genetic sclerosing bone dysplasias that are not caused by infection or inflammation and may look similar radiologically (Ch. 13).

Review PMID: 30456556

SAPHO syndrome PMID: 24237723

Tendoperiostitis PMID: 1437057

CHRONIC LOW-GRADE FOCAL OSTEOMYELITIS AND SCLEROSING OSTEITIS

➔ Summary charts 5.1, 13.1 and 12.2 pp. 81, 244, 229

In some cases, a focus of osteomyelitis is so small or caused by such low-virulence organisms that the clinical presentation is dominated by the local bone reaction to the infection rather than the infection itself. Focal sclerosing osteomyelitis is commoner in younger individuals because their bone is better vascularised and produces more reactive bone deposition around the infection. Suppuration and widespread infiltration of marrow spaces by inflammatory cells are absent, and bacteria are not readily cultivable. The key feature is a poorly defined zone of bony sclerosis. Centrally there is a nidus of infection, but it can be impossible to see it on plain radiographs, although it may be visualised on cone beam computed tomography (CT).

Sclerosing osteitis is a term given to a localised area of sclerosis without evidence of infection. These are probably a reaction to inflammation rather than infection and are frequently seen around the roots of non-vital teeth (Fig. 8.11). If multiple they resemble lesions of cemento-osseous dysplasia (Fig. 8.12). No treatment is required for the bone, but the causative tooth will usually prove to be non-vital and may be extracted or root-filled.

Key features of sclerosing osteomyelitis are listed in Box 8.10.

Sclerosing osteitis PMID: 23880262

OSTEORADIONECROSIS

When the predisposing cause for any type of osteomyelitis is radiotherapy, the condition is called *osteoradionecrosis*. Radiotherapy induces endarteritis of vessels causing a marked reduction in bone vascularity, inhibiting both an effective host response to infection and also the sclerotic response of the bone to infection. The risk of osteoradionecrosis rises with the radiation dose. At the normal doses of radical radiotherapy given for most oral carcinomas, approximately 60–65 Gy, approximately 3%–5% of patients may experience this distressing complication. Only directly irradiated bone is at risk, and it is almost always the mandible affected,

Box 8.10   Focal sclerosing osteomyelitis: key features

- Bony reaction to low-grade, usually periapical, infection
- Children and young adults affected
- Premolar or molar region of mandible affected
- Bone sclerosis associated with apex of a non-vital or pulpitic tooth
- Localised but uniform radiodensity related to tooth with widened periodontal ligament space or periapical area
- No expansion of the jaw

Pathology

- Dense sclerotic bone with scanty connective tissue or inflammatory cells

Treatment

- Elimination of the source of inflammation by extraction or endodontic treatment

Box 8.11   Prevention of osteoradionecrosis

- Following radiotherapy near salivary glands, xerostomia will worsen oral health
- Before radiotherapy around the jaws, all patients should have a dental examination
- Institute aggressive preventive regime of diet change and fluoride
- All potential foci of infection must be aggressively treated, usually by extraction
- Sockets must be epithelialised before radiotherapy starts
- Other treatment should be completed in a low risk 'window' of 10 weeks after radiotherapy
- Dentures and postoperative obturators must not traumatise mucosa
- Close monitoring for dental infection and to prevent trauma continues for life
- Extractions in irradiated bone must be atraumatic
- Antibiotics are required after any oral surgical procedure until healing is complete

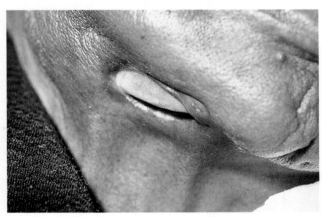

Fig. 8.13   Chronic osteomyelitis secondary to radiotherapy. Part of the necrotic portion of the mandible is visible, having ulcerated through the skin.

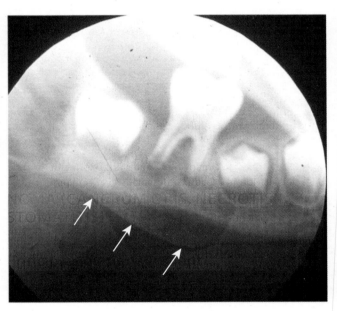

Fig 8.14   Proliferative periostitis. Oblique lateral radiograph of a 9-year-old girl showing bone destruction from infection around the first molar and onion-skin layer periosteal reaction below the lower border (arrowed). *(From Whaites, E. and Drage, N. 2021. Essentials of dental radiography and radiology, 6th ed, Edinburgh, Elsevier Ltd.)*

Treatment PMID: 23108891

Risk of development PMID: 22669065

Prevention after extraction PMID: 21115324

PROLIFERATIVE PERIOSTITIS

Proliferative periostitis is not an infection, but a response to it. Inflammation or infection cause the periosteum of the surrounding bone to become active and lay down layers of new bone around the cortex as a healing response. This new bone is rapidly formed and less well-mineralised than the normal cortex and may expand the bone by up to a centimetre or more in thickness. The process is intermittent, producing

following irradiation of oral, tonsil or major salivary gland cancers. Osteoradionecrosis is only a risk after radiotherapy is complete, and usually develops within a few years but radiotherapy patients have a risk for life.

The causative bacteria are oral flora and periodontal pathogens, which gain entry to the bone after minor trauma, dental infection, implant placement or tooth extraction. The mucosa is atrophic and heals poorly after radiotherapy so that teeth that require extraction must be removed a sufficient time before radiotherapy for the sockets to epithelialize and seal off the medullary cavity.

Infection spreads rapidly in irradiated bone and is difficult to treat. The clinical and radiographic features are those of chronic osteomyelitis (see Fig. 8.13) except that healing is impaired, sequestra separate much more slowly and there is no periosteal reaction. The course is often prolonged, and surgical intervention and aggressive antibiotic therapy are usually required. Pentoxifylline, a tumour necrosis factor antagonist, and hyperbaric oxygen are claimed to aid healing, but results are variable and the latter is very expensive and not widely available. Unfortunately, treatment is not always successful, and low-grade grumbling osteomyelitis may persist for the rest of a patient's life.

Prevention is key, and the dentist plays an important role by ensuring oral health (Box 8.11).

Box 8.12 Proliferative periostitis key features

- Children and adolescents mainly affected
- Usually associated with periapical but sometimes other inflammatory foci
- Periosteal reaction affecting lower border of mandible causing 'onion skin' thickening and swelling of bone
- Sometimes incorrectly called Garrè's osteomyelitis*

Pathology

- Parallel layers of highly cellular woven bone interspersed with scantily inflamed connective tissue
- Small sequestra sometimes present

Treatment

- Eliminate focus of infection
- Bone gradually remodels after 6–12 months

*Garrè's (note correct accent and spelling) osteomyelitis is a misnomer. In his original description he made no mention of proliferative changes in the lesion, X-rays had not been invented then, and he provided no histological back-up. This historic term has no place in current usage but persists in dentistry despite being long obsolete in medicine.
Reference PMID: 3041342

Box 8.13 Drugs associated with jaw osteonecrosis

- Antiresorptive
  - Bisphosphonates
    - Alendronate
    - Pamidronate
    - Risendronate
    - Zolendronate
    - And other high potency types
  - Denosumab (antibody RANKL inhibitor)
- Antiangiogenic
  - Tyrosine kinase inhibitors
    - Sorafenib
    - Sunitinib
  - Bevacizumab (vascular endothelial growth factor inhibitor)
  - Rapamycin (mTOR [mechanistic target of rapamycin] inhibitor)

Box 8.14 Risk factors for bisphosphonate-induced osteonecrosis

- Intravenous high-dose bisphosphonate treatment usually for bone metastases or hypercalcaemia of malignancy
- Immunosuppression from chemotherapy or steroids
- Anaemia
- Dental surgery or sepsis, ill-fitting dentures and poor oral hygiene
- Female patients
- Older patients
- Smoking

multiple parallel layers that can be seen radiographically as 'onion-skinning' (Fig. 8.14).

The ability to produce large amounts of periosteal new bone is more or less limited to children and adolescents. In older patients it forms more slowly and requires a long period to become evident. Chronic osteomyelitis in children and adolescents is often dominated by the periosteal reaction, which can be florid enough to cause facial asymmetry.

Proliferative periostitis develops over both malignant neoplasms and foci of chronic osteomyelitis, so the underlying cause must be identified. When it is osteomyelitis, vague pain is typical, and the focus of infection or a small sequestrum may only be detected on cone beam CT.

Key features are listed in Box 8.12.

Clinical description PMID: 289735 and 9768431

MEDICATION-RELATED OSTEONECROSIS OF THE JAWS (MRONJ)

Previously called *bisphosphonate-related osteonecrosis*, this condition is now known to be induced by a variety of drugs that inhibit either osteoclast activity or angiogenesis. It is also known as *antiresorptive-related osteonecrosis* (Box 8.13).

The majority of patients affected are elderly and have metastatic malignant disease because this is the main indication for the causative drugs (Box 8.14). Steroid use and smoking can also contribute.

Bisphosphonate drugs are concentrated in osteoclasts and bound into bone matrix by osteoblasts, where they remain active in bone for many years, being slowly released on bone turnover*. The osteoclast inhibition also delays bone healing.

---

* Bisphosphonate-induced osteonecrosis resembles the toxic necrosis of bone called *phossy jaw*, a scourge of match factory workers in Victorian times who ingested white phosphorus (P_4). They frequently died or lost a whole jaw from osteonecrosis. Public outrage and a famous strike in East London forced improvements in factory conditions and the introduction of the (slightly) safer red phosphorus match. Both white phosphorus and the two phosphonate groups in bisphosphonate drugs mimic pyrophosphate and act as inhibitors of enzymes that act on it.

Bisphosphonates inhibit osteoclasts and angiogenesis and are frequently used to treat metastases to bone, particularly from multiple myeloma, breast and prostate carcinoma. This is highly effective, constraining growth of metastases and inhibiting pathological fractures and their consequences, particularly nerve injury from spinal collapse. Risk is associated with high-potency bisphosphonates such as alendronate, pamidronate and zoledronate, especially when administered long term and in high doses intravenously. Osteonecrosis affects approximately 1% of patients on these regimes, although occasional cases have also been reported following oral administration for osteoporosis. The risk of developing MRONJ following a single extraction in a patient who has had intravenous high potency bisphosphonates is around 0.5%. Oral doses for osteoporosis carry a much lower risk

Exactly why bisphosphonates cause areas of bone to become non-vital is unclear. It has been thought that the drugs cause sterile necrosis, which then becomes infected. However, it is also possible that the effect is an osteomyelitis from the outset, modified by reduced healing capacity of the bone. The jaws are particularly at risk because of their poor blood supply in older people, potential foci of dental infection and covering of thin easily traumatised mucosa, but other bones have been affected.

In two-thirds of patients a dental extraction is the precipitating factor, and in most of the remainder there is no identifiable trigger. A striking presentation is painless

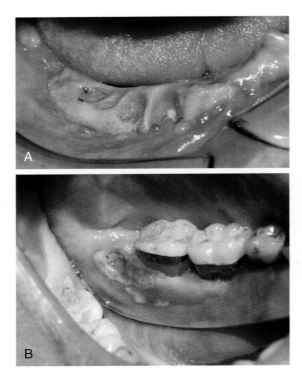

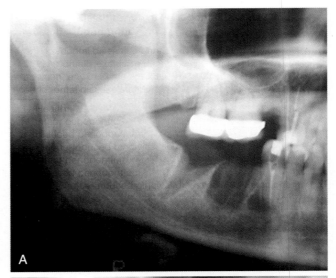

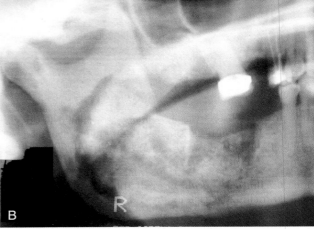

Fig. 8.15 Exposed necrotic bone in bisphosphonate-induced osteonecrosis, (A) following extraction and (B) apparently spontaneous. Despite exposure of large areas of necrotic bone, there is no overt infection in these early lesions. *(From Ruggiero, S.L., Fantasia, J., Carlson, E. 2006. Bisphosphonate-related osteonecrosis of the jaw: background and guidelines for diagnosis, staging and management. Oral surg oral med oral pathol oral radiol 102, pp. 433–441.)*

exposed bone without apparent infection (Figs 8.15 and 8.16); some patients may experience no acute symptoms or suppuration for prolonged periods. Once infection is introduced, the condition develops into acute or chronic osteomyelitis depending on the virulence of the organism and resistance of the patient. The drugs cause reduced bone turnover so that sequestra of necrotic bone separate very slowly and healing is inhibited. Later complications can include oroantral and cutaneous fistulas with suppuration.

The organisms colonising the dead bone are a mixed flora of oral bacteria in a biofilm, similar to conventional chronic osteomyelitis. Common species are *Actinomyces*, streptococci, *Serratia*, and enterococci, and facultative anaerobes predominate. As noted previously, it is unclear whether infection or necrosis is the primary disease process.

Review PMID: 16243172 and 20508948

Management

Prevention of infection is paramount. Potential problems should be eliminated before high dose bisphosphonate treatment, infective foci eliminated and teeth of dubious prognosis removed. Some authorities also suggest removal of tori and sharp ridges if prone to denture trauma.

After drug treatment, patients at risk are identified through their medical history. Additional predisposing factors will help gauge their risk (Box 8.5). Caries and periodontitis must be controlled. Ideally, all surgical dentistry should be avoided for as long as possible after drug administration. There is a role for attempting what might otherwise be considered heroic restorations and endodontics to avoid extractions. If

Fig. 8.16 **Bisphosphonate-induced osteonecrosis.** Non-healing extraction sockets in a breast cancer patient receiving bisphosphonate treatment. (A) There are minimal changes initially, but 12 months later, (B) there is a large sequestrum still incompletely separated extending from the premolar region, just above the lower border cortex and involving most of the ramus. *(From Ruggiero, S.L., Fantasia, J., Carlson, E. 2006. Bisphosphonate-related osteonecrosis of the jaw: background and guidelines for diagnosis, staging and management. Oral surg oral med oral pathol oral radiol 102, pp. 433–441.)*

extractions cannot be delayed, they are probably best followed by postoperative antibiotics and chlorhexidine rinses until the sockets are fully epithelialised. Unfortunately, these precautions are not always successful, and sometimes extraction of a tooth reveals an apparently already non-vital socket that does not bleed.

Discontinuation of the bisphosphonates either before extractions or long term does not appear to help because their effects last at least a year after administration and may be permanent, but a 2 month 'drug holiday' is sometimes recommended.

Management of established MRONJ is largely empirical. There is no reproducibly successful treatment, and the aim is to manage pain and favour the very slow healing that will take place if infection can be controlled. When bone is exposed but symptoms are minimal, long-term chlorhexidine mouth rinses reduce pain and the risk of infection. Attempts to remove necrotic bone surgically usually worsen the condition, and sequestra should only be removed when mobile. Uncomfortable sharp edges may be reduced with a bur. If there is infection or soft tissue swelling, aggressive and long-term antibiotic therapy based on the results of antibiotic culture and sensitivity is required to restore a stable chronic condition that can be controlled with topical treatments. If infection cannot be controlled, then more aggressive antibiotic regimes combined with surgery may be necessary. Severe complications including extraoral sinuses and pathological fractures may require surgical intervention. Many patients remain surprisingly asymptomatic, but managing pain may require potent analgesics in the short term.

Other treatments including hyperbaric oxygen, platelet derived growth factors and targeted sequestrectomy remain unproven.

Management PMID: 25234529 and 28983908

TRAUMATIC SEQUESTRUM

This is a rare but well-described oddity that often causes confusion in clinical diagnosis. It is also known as mylohyoid ridge sequestrum because the most common site is on the posterior part of a sharp mylohyoid ridge, inferior to the third molar (Fig. 8.17). Here the mucosa is thin and prone to trauma, and a traumatic ulcer can lead to devitalisation of a small area of the underlying cortical bone. This slows ulcer healing, but the dead bone eventually separates and the ulcer heals spontaneously. The sequestrum is usually only 1–2 mm in size. Mandibular tori may be similarly affected.

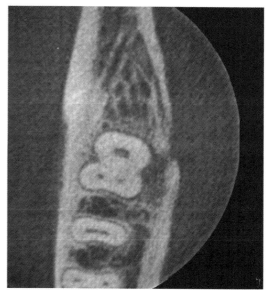

Fig. 8.17 Traumatic sequestration. Cone beam computed tomography axial view through lower molars showing loss of a small fragment of cortical bone lingual to the distal root of the last molar, caused by sequestration following trauma to the mucosa over the posterior edge of the mylohyoid ridge.

No treatment may be required. Once the sequestrum is loose, it may be removed to speed healing.

Case series PMID: 8515988

Major infections of the mouth and face

9

Although there are many types of facial infection, the vast majority of significant infections are odontogenic, that is, they arise by spread of infection from a tooth or the periodontium.

PERIAPICAL (DENTOALVEOLAR) ABSCESS

Usually, a non-vital pulp produces no more consequence than an asymptomatic and sterile periapical granuloma. Untreated, these may produce intermittent pain in periods of acute inflammation and persist as chronic inflammation for decades. However, infection may eventually develop into an acute periapical infection with abscess formation (Ch. 5).

In an abscess, bacteria cause localised tissue necrosis, and pus forms by the action of neutrophil proteolytic enzymes. The process is localised by granulation tissue forming the abscess wall. The surrounding soft tissues become oedematous with inflammatory exudate. Once an apical abscess is established, it is unlikely to resolve spontaneously.

It might be expected that the infection and oedema would spread through the path of least resistance into medullary bone and cause osteomyelitis, but this is unusual. For reasons that are not clear, the exudate usually tracks toward the adjacent cortex and perforates it, through the action of osteoclasts activated by the inflammation, and drains into the mouth.

The oedema in the periodontal ligament causes slight extrusion of the tooth, which comes into premature occlusion, is painful on biting and tender to percussion. There is throbbing intense pain, distinct from the sharp excruciating pain of any acute pulpitis that might have preceded pulp necrosis. Drainage of pus and exudate into the mouth, usually through the alveolar mucosa or gingiva, releases pressure, produces a bad taste, and the pain reduces to a dull ache.

The regional lymph nodes may be enlarged and tender, but systemic symptoms are usually slight or absent.

Apical abscesses are polymicrobial infections and frequent cultivable isolates include *Porphyromonas, Prevotella, Streptococcus, Fusobacterium* and *Actinomyces* species. However, culturing samples to test antibiotic sensitivity is not usually performed. Many uncultivable species, spirochaetes and obligate anaerobes are present, the flora is mixed and resides partly in the apical soft tissues and partly in the pulp canal of the causative tooth. Despite the mixed nature of the infection, penicillins remain the most effective antibiotics, with metronidazole reserved for patients allergic to penicillin. However, a localised apical abscess cannot be treated by antibiotics alone; the causative tooth or its pulp must be dealt with because bacteria in the pulp chamber are inaccessible to the drug. Local dental treatment, extraction or root canal treatment, is usually effective without the addition of antibiotics. Any localised collection of pus in the alveolar mucosa that has not yet drained spontaneously should be incised and drained surgically.

Radiographically, there may be minimal changes because bone loss takes time to develop, perhaps just some fuzziness around the apical periodontal ligament. In many cases the radiographic features of a pre-existing periapical granuloma may be visible, often with loss of the sharp definition of the peripheral bone margin.

Untreated, a localised periapical abscess causes a period of intense pain, which reduces once pus drains through a sinus. After this, the infection settles into a chronic state with minimal symptoms, resembling periapical periodontitis but with intermittent acute exacerbations and discharge of pus. This may persist indefinitely until the cause is treated.

Review and treatment PMID: 12013343

Review and sequelae PMID: 21602052

Microbiology PMID: 23554416

COLLATERAL OEDEMA

Even while the infection is limited to the bone, and continuing after it drains intraorally, there is oedema of the adjacent soft tissues (Fig. 9.1). Oedema is a purely inflammatory reaction, and the swollen tissues contain no bacteria. In children oedema is very prominent and gives the impression of cellulitis of the face, but the oedema is soft, unlike the firm brawny swelling of spreading infection, and there is no pyrexia. No specific treatment is required for a face enlarged by oedema. It resolves quickly when the causative tooth is dealt with.

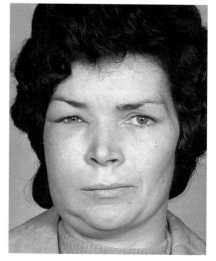

Fig. 9.1 Oedema due to acute apical periodontitis. An acute periapical infection of a canine has perforated the buccal plate of bone causing oedema of the face; this quickly subsided when the infection was treated.

'FASCIAL' OR TISSUE SPACE INFECTIONS

When pus from an apical abscess or pericoronitis breaks out into soft tissue, its path is guided by muscle attachments and fascia. These can divert the path of drainage away from the mouth into the tissues of the face, where pus and spreading infection can localise in the 'fascial spaces'. Anatomical descriptions of these spaces imply that fascia is a well-organised fibrous sheet dividing the face and neck into defined compartments and spaces. In reality, there are no spaces and the fascia is discontinuous and thin, but the inflammation and infection tend to localise reproducibly in tissue planes bounded by subcutaneous tissue, the masticatory muscles and muscles of the neck and the carotid sheath (Box 9.1). The fascial spaces are only potential spaces enlarged by accumulation of exudate or pus. Because the spaces have a large volume, pressure in the exudate is reduced, and it tends to accumulate rather than burrow onward to the surface. When the space is distended, its blood supply is disrupted, and the environment becomes avascular and anaerobic, favouring infection and inhibiting host defences.

The fascial spaces extend from the base of the skull to the mediastinum, and the inflammatory exudate acts as a vehicle to spread the infection into potentially life-threatening sites. The large volume of exudate and bacterial load produce pyrexia, toxaemia and symptoms of pain and trismus. There is an additional risk of spread to remote sites through lymphatics or blood vessels.

Once an infection penetrates into the tissue planes, it may spread or become localised depending on the causative bacteria and the resistance of the host.

Diabetes and immunosuppression are particular risk factors to develop fascial space infection. Infection from teeth tends to localise reproducibly in the spaces listed in Table 9.1, but it will be noted that these spaces intercommunicate, and infection may involve several of them (Figs 9.2 and 9.3). Infection spreads initially to the sublingual, submandibular, submental, buccal and canine spaces closest to the tooth apices, before extending to deeper spaces.

Nature of fascial spaces PMID: 23913739

Health services implications PMID: 22819453

FACIAL CELLULITIS

➜ Summary charts 5.1 and 35.1 pp. 81, 518

The great majority of fascial space infections are in the form of cellulitis in which, unlike a localised abscess, bacteria spread through the soft tissues (Fig. 9.4). Cellulitis causes gross inflammatory exudate and tissue oedema, associated with fever and toxaemia. Before the advent of antibiotics, the mortality was high. If treatment is delayed, the disease can still be life-threatening through airway compromise or erosion of the carotid sheath when the lateral pharyngeal space is involved. In Ludwig's angina particularly, airway obstruction can quickly result in asphyxia. In children particularly, spread from maxillary teeth may involve the orbit.

The characteristic features are diffuse swelling, pain, fever and malaise. The swelling is tense and tender, often described as 'brawny' meaning swollen and hard, with a characteristic board-like firmness. The overlying skin is taut and shiny. Pain and oedema limit opening the mouth and often cause

| Box 9.1 | The main structures directing spread of infection in the face and neck |

- Muscles
  - Buccinator
  - Mylohyoid
  - Masseter
  - Medial pterygoid
  - Superior constrictor of the pharynx
- Fascia
  - Investing layer of fascia
  - Prevertebral fascia
  - Pretracheal fascia
  - Parotid fascia
  - Carotid sheath

dysphagia (Fig 9.5). Systemic upset is severe with worsening fever, toxaemia, leucocytosis and raised serum C reactive protein. The regional lymph nodes are swollen and tender.

Pathology

The bacterial flora is similar to the dentoalveolar abscess from which it is derived. Anaerobic culture reveals streptococci, staphylococci and a dominance of anaerobes such as *Porphyromonas*, *Prevotella* and *Fusobacterium*. However, many uncultivable species are present. It is usual for at least one cultivable organism to show some antibiotic resistance.

Infection spreads most commonly from mandibular third molars, whose apices are closely related to several fascial spaces. In the early stages the infection does not localise, but after antibiotic treatment or time for a host response to develop, and depending on the organisms, small locules of pus develop scattered in the tissues.

Cellulitis, as opposed to abscess, is more frequent in patients with diabetes and immunocompromise.

Ludwig's angina

Ludwig's angina* is a severe form of cellulitis that usually arises from the lower second or third molars. It involves the sublingual and submandibular spaces bilaterally, almost simultaneously, and readily spreads into the lateral pharyngeal and pterygoid spaces and can extend into the mediastinum.

The main features are rapidly spreading sublingual and submandibular cellulitis with painful, brawny swelling of the upper part of the neck and the floor of the mouth on both sides (Fig. 9.6). With involvement of the parapharyngeal space, the swelling tracks down the neck and oedema can quickly spread to the glottis.

Swallowing and opening the mouth become difficult, and the tongue may be pushed up against the soft palate. Oral obstruction or oedema of the glottis causes worsening respiratory obstruction. The patient soon becomes desperately ill, with fever, respiratory distress, headache and malaise.

---

* Wilhelm Friedrich von Ludwig described the condition in 1836. He was physician to the royal family of King Wilhelm I, King of Prussia and the first German emperor. Although sometimes considered to have died of the condition that bears his name, this appears unlikely.

PMID: 16696873

Table 9.1   Tissue spaces commonly involved by dental infection*

Space	Anatomy	Usual sources of infection
Submental	Between mylohyoid and the skin, platysma and investing layer of fascia. Contains the submental lymph nodes	Lower incisors
Submandibular	Between mylohyoid, and the skin, platysma and investing layer of fascia and between the hyoglossus and body of mandible. It contains the submandibular gland and submandibular lymph nodes and communicates anteriorly with the submental and posteriorly and upward into the sublingual space	Lower canine, premolar and molar teeth, when their apices lie below the mylohyoid attachment
Sublingual	Between hyoglossus and the tongue muscles medially and mylohyoid and the body of mandible laterally. Contains the sublingual gland. Communicates posteriorly with the submandibular space around the posterior free edge of the mylohyoid, around the submandibular gland and duct	Lower incisor and canine teeth. Molars less frequently when apices are above the mylohyoid attachment
Buccal	Between buccinator muscle and the overlying skin, platysma and fascia. Posteriorly limited by ramus of mandible and masseter. Contains the buccal pad of fat. Communicates posteriorly with the pterygomandibular space	Usually upper molar and premolar teeth, sometimes lower molars when their apices lie below the buccinator attachment
Submasseteric	Between the lateral surface of the ramus of the mandible and the periosteum of masseter muscle	Rarely involved. Usually from pericoronitis around the lower third molar
Parotid	Contains the parotid gland, bounded by superficial fascia and base of skull	Only involved by spread from other spaces
Pterygomandibular	Between the medial surface of the ramus of the mandible and the medial pterygoid muscle with the lateral pterygoid forming its roof and the parotid gland posteriorly. Contains the lingual and inferior dental nerves and communicates upward with the infratemporal fossa	Pericoronitis around distally inclined lower third molars or upper third molars
Lateral pharyngeal	Between superior constrictor with the styloid muscles and medial pterygoid or submandibular gland. Limited posteriorly by the vertebral fascia. Contains the carotid sheath, along which infection can track to the mediastinum. Anteriorly there is communication along styloglossus with the sublingual and submandibular spaces	Pericoronitis around the lower third molar (and infections in the tonsil)
Canine fossa	In the canine fossa, bounded by the muscles of lips and face	Upper lateral incisors, canines or first premolars, including periodontal abscesses
Palate	Between the mucosa and periosteum and palatal bone	Upper molars

*The canine fossa and palate are not classed as tissue spaces, but pus frequently collects at these sites.

Management

The principles of treatment for cellulitis are to provide immediate aggressive antibiotic treatment to prevent further spread of infection and to remove the causative tooth or deal with pericoronitis as soon as possible. Teeth with apical infection are usually removed, draining any pus localised in the bone. Teeth can sometimes be preserved by obtaining drainage through the pulp chamber, but teeth cannot be left open for more than 48 hours because this will compromise the success of subsequent root treatment, making retention pointless. For this reason, many teeth are extracted, and emphasis must be on effective drainage. Impacted teeth with pericoronitis must be dealt with after the infection has resolved because surgery cannot be performed in an infected field without risking further spread. General anaesthesia may be required for extractions as local anaesthetic may not be effective in the inflamed tissues.

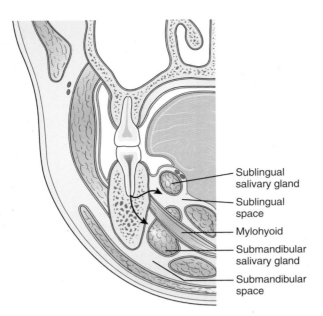

Fig. 9.2 Paths of infection spread from lower molars. By penetrating the lingual plate of the jaw below the attachment of mylohyoid, infection immediately enters the submandibular space. Below the mylohyoid is the main body of the submandibular salivary gland with its deep process curving around the posterior border of the muscle; infection from the third molar can follow the spaces around the gland to enter the sublingual space.

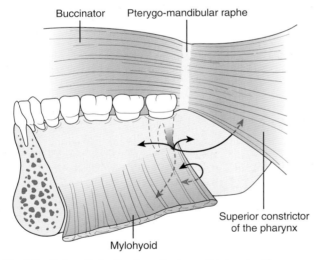

Fig. 9.3 Paths of infection from the lower third molar. The diagram shows the lingual aspect of the jaw and indicates how infection penetrating from the lingual plate of bone can enter the sublingual space above, or the submandibular space below, the mylohyoid muscle, which forms the major structure of the floor of the mouth. Moreover, because this point is at the junction of the oral cavity and pharynx, infection can also spread backward to reach the lateral surface of superior constrictor, the lateral pharyngeal space.

Antibiotic treatment is empirical initially with high-dose penicillins or other broad-spectrum antibiotics, but a sample for culture and sensitivity must be obtained before commencing treatment in case a change of antibiotic is required subsequently. Only occasionally is the flora unresponsive to first-line antibiotics, even if some species show antibiotic resistance on testing.

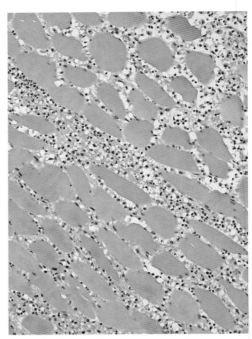

Fig. 9.4 Cellulitis. Infection spreading through the tissues is accompanied by a dense infiltrate of neutrophils, macrophages and fibrin exudate, here separating muscle fibres and bundles (stained red) in a facial muscle. The muscle bundles are normally closely packed with minimal space between them.

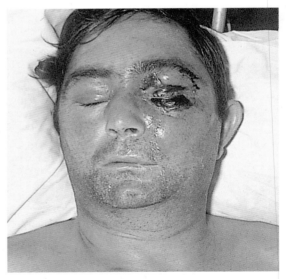

Fig. 9.5 Facial cellulitis arising from an infected upper tooth. The tissues are red, tense and shiny, and the patient is incapacitated by the systemic effects of infection. *(Courtesy Professor JD Langdon)*

Drainage plays little role in treatment of pure cellulitis because there is no collection of pus. However, when there is potential compromise of the airway or a suggestion that pus may be localising (see later in this chapter), then drains may be placed to allow oedema fluid to escape to relieve tissue tension (Fig 9.7). A microbiological sample can be obtained at the same time.

In Ludwig's angina, or when the airway is compromised by any infection, the main requirements are immediate admission to hospital, securing the airway by intubation

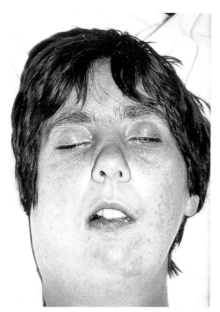

Fig. 9.6 Ludwig's angina. There is cellulitis and gross oedema of the right submandibular and sublingual spaces extending on to the left side and into the neck and parapharyngeal space. *(Courtesy Professor JD Langdon.)*

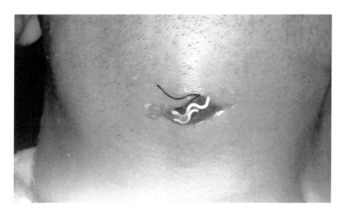

Fig. 9.7 Ludwig's angina. Incision and drainage of the front of the neck to relieve the pressure of exudate which compromises the airway. The neck is grossly swollen, shiny and dusky in hue; the edges of the wound have pulled apart, indicating the distension of these normally lax tissues.

or tracheostomy if necessary, procurement of a sample for culture and sensitivity testing, aggressive antibiotic treatment and drainage of the swelling to reduce pressure.

Key features of fascial space infections are summarised in Box 9.2.

Ludwig's in children PMID: 19286617

Fatal outcome PMID: 17828174

Airway compromise PMID: 10326823

Antibiotic choice PMID: 30836194

FACIAL ABSCESS

Depending on the micro-organisms and effectiveness of host defences, pus from an apical abscess or pericoronitis may localise in the tissues to form a discrete abscess rather than spreading. Systemic signs are less marked and inflammation

> **Box 9.2   Fascial space cellulitis: key features**
> * Commonest cause is odontogenic infection
> * Potentially life-threatening infections due to spread of bacteria into tissue planes
> * Infection usually arises from lower second or third molars
> * Ludwig's angina comprises bilateral involvement of sublingual and submandibular spaces and readily spreads into lateral pharyngeal and pterygoid spaces
> * Affected tissues swollen and of board-like hardness
> * Severe systemic upset
> * Glottic oedema, carotid sheath erosion or spread into the mediastinum may be fatal

and swelling less extensive in abscess than in cellulitis. The collection of pus is surrounded by compressed fibrous and granulation tissue, which prevent spread but also natural drainage. Eventually an abscess will point to a surface and drain spontaneously, but this is best prevented by early intervention because formation of a sinus to the skin is usually followed by disfiguring scarring.

When pus starts to collect in the tissues after cellulitis, the brawny diffuse swelling of oedema and cellulitis can still be present, but a localised zone of softening develops over the pus, with a darker red zone of inflammation. Pyrexia increases. If left too long before drainage, the overlying skin becomes fluctuant just before the abscess drains spontaneously.

The principles of management of abscess are the same as for cellulitis, except that early surgical drainage of pus is essential. Small abscesses may resolve with high-dose antibiotics alone, but better and more rapid resolution will follow surgical drainage in most cases.

ANTIBIOTIC ABSCESS

The antibiotic abscess or 'antibioma' is an abscess that has been controlled but not eliminated by antibiotic treatment. This may arise after inadequate, often prolonged intermittent antibiotic treatment, particularly at insufficient dose. It may also arise from effective antibiotic treatment provided without ensuring that a collection of pus has been drained. The pus can be rendered sterile or nearly so, and the surrounding granulation tissue matures to dense scar tissue, producing a thick zone of fibrosis around the pus.

The patient has a hard mass, with puckering of the overlying skin if superficially located, and either mild symptoms of intermittent pain and swelling or no symptoms at all. Treatment may be conservative, but resolution takes many months, and it is usually better to excise the whole mass. Drainage alone removes any residual infection, but the main signs arise from the surrounding fibrosis. Antibioma is commoner in countries where antibiotics are available without prescription and self-medication is common.

Microbiology antibiotic choice PMID: 16916672 and 30836194

NECROTISING FASCIITIS

➔ Summary chart 5.1 p. 81

Necrotising fasciitis is an uncommon, rapidly spreading, potentially lethal infection causing necrosis and rapid dissolution of

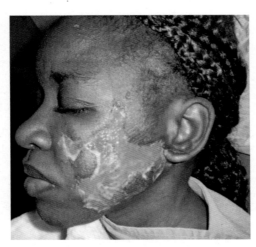

Fig. 9.8 Necrotising fasciitis. Necrosis and loss of skin and subcutaneous tissue exposing underlying muscle *(Source: Balaji SM, Balaji PM (2017). Head and Neck Space Infections, Part -III. In: Textbook of oral and maxillofacial surgery, 3rd ed. New Delhi: Elsevier.)*

subcutaneous tissues and fascia with loss of attachment of the overlying skin. Muscles are relatively spared (Fig. 9.8). Rarely, the infection can have a dental source and may threaten the airway. Most patients are of middle age or older, and the majority have some predisposing factor such as immunosuppression, steroid use, chronic disease or smoking.

The virulence factors of the causative organisms seem to be the key factor. Many types of bacteria, both aerobic and anaerobic, can be responsible. Samples usually reveal mixed infections; a quarter of cases are caused by single organisms, usually Group A streptococci or staphylococci, particularly methicillin-resistant *Staphylococcus aureus*. The remainder have a mixed flora including anaerobic pathogens such as *Porphyromonas* and *Prevotella* species.

Clinically, there is initially a rapidly spreading area of erythema of the skin. The margins soon become ill-defined. Thrombosis and necrosis in small vessels cause the skin to become painful and oedematous, dusky red then purplish and black. Undermining of the skin causes separation from the underlying connective tissue and accumulation of subcutaneous gas, which may be visible on radiographs. Early infection deeper in the tissue is difficult to differentiate from simple cellulitis but unusually raised C-reactive protein and white cell counts give a clue.

The airway may need protection by tracheostomy, and immediate admission to hospital is required. Unusually in an infection, aggressive surgery is undertaken as soon as the condition is recognised as spread is so rapid. The extent of undermining of the skin should be explored and widely opened to drainage, debridement and for removal of necrotic tissue. Penicillin and metronidazole or clindamycin should be given empirically until bacteriological findings dictate alternatives. Hyperbaric oxygen provides additional benefit, if available.

Untreated or ineffectively treated, necrotising fasciitis proceeds to systemic spread of infection with toxic shock and death.

Case report PMID: 23821623

Microbiology and management PMID: 10760723

CAVERNOUS SINUS THROMBOSIS

→ Summary chart 5.1 p. 81

Cavernous sinus thrombosis is an uncommon life-threatening complication of infection that can sometimes originate from infection from an upper anterior tooth, the sinuses or nose. The path of infection from the anterior teeth is to the canine space, and then by retrograde flow through the low-pressure venous system around the eye to the cavernous sinus. Infection may also spread to the cavernous sinus from its posterior aspect following infection in the infratemporal fossa, again via the venous system. Skin abscesses on the face are another source of infection.

Clinically, gross oedema of the eyelid is associated with pulsatile exophthalmos due to venous obstruction. Cyanosis, proptosis, a fixed dilated pupil and limited eye movement develop rapidly. There is pain around the eye, over the maxilla, and headache with vomiting in late stages. The patient is seriously ill with rigors, a high swinging fever and deteriorating sight.

Early recognition and treatment of cavernous sinus thrombosis are essential. Magnetic resonance imaging with contrast is the imaging modality of choice. The main treatment measures are use of prolonged intravenous antibiotics, drainage of pus and removal of any causative tooth. Anticoagulation, usually with heparin, is sometimes used but has risks and equivocal benefit. In developed countries, aggressive antibiotic treatment has reduced the mortality to 20%, but spread to the contralateral sinus followed by meningitis or clotting in the cerebral sinuses are potentially fatal complications. Without antibiotics, almost all cases are fatal. As many as half of survivors may lose the sight of one or both eyes, even when correctly treated. Progression is often very rapid, with death in less than 24 hours if untreated.

Case report PMID: 2685213

Treatment PMID: 22326173

NOMA (CANCRUM ORIS, NECROTISING STOMATITIS)

Noma** is a severe oral infection, starting in the gingiva as acute necrotising ulcerative gingivitis and extending onto and destroying part of the jaw or face. It progresses rapidly and may be fatal if inadequately treated.

Noma is widespread in sub-Saharan Africa and also found in South America and the Far East. The World Health Organization has estimated the worldwide incidence to be nearly 140,000 cases a year.

The main bacteria isolated are anaerobes including *Fusobacterium necrophorum*, *Prevotella intermedia* and spirochaetes. *F. necrophorum* is a commensal in the gut of herbivores and also a cause of necrotising infections in animals. It may play an important role in noma in Africa as a result of patients living in close proximity to, and often sharing drinking water with, cattle. The flora is often referred to as a 'fusospirochaetal complex' because no particular species alone appears to account for the disease, which is a true polymicrobial infection.

** Noma was first described in 1595 in Holland where, as in other parts of Europe, severe malnutrition and debilitating diseases were widespread. The term 'noma' was coined in 1680. Since then, noma has virtually disappeared from Europe, reappearing only briefly in concentration camps during World War 2.

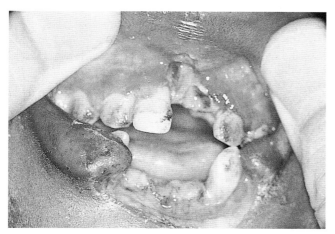

Fig. 9.9 Noma. In the maxilla there is extension of necrotising gingivitis into the alveolar process and in the lower arch anteriorly, resulting in destruction of much of the lower lip.

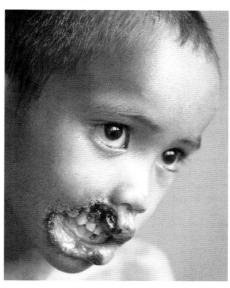

Fig. 9.11 Noma. A six-year-old child with noma extending onto the lips and cheek. *(Source: Srour, M.L., Wong, V., Wyllie, S. 2014. Noma, actinomycosis and nocardia. In: Farrar, J., White, N.J., Hotez, P.J., et al. eds. Manson's tropical diseases. St. Louis: Elsevier, pp. 379-384.e1.)*

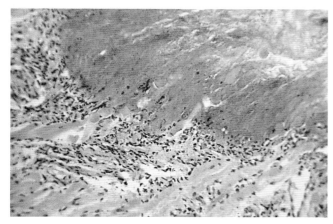

Fig. 9.10 Noma. Muscle has been invaded by spirochaetes and fusiforms. There is rapid necrosis, seen top right, and only a light inflammatory response of neutrophils.

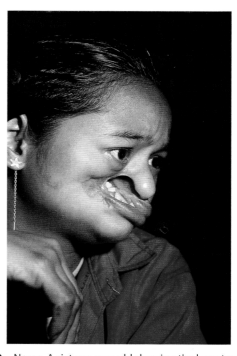

Fig. 9.12 Noma. A sixteen-year-old showing the long-term effects of facial tissue loss following noma at age 4 years. *(Source: Srour, M.L., Wong, V., Wyllie, S. 2014. Noma, actinomycosis and nocardia. In: Farrar, J., White, N.J., Hotez, P.J., et al. eds. Manson's tropical diseases. St. Louis: Elsevier, pp. 379-384.e1.)*

Malnutrition due to poverty and climatic disasters is the major factor in the aetiology. Other factors are poor oral hygiene and other infections, particularly measles and herpesviral diseases. Noma affects children younger than 10 years. The few cases in adults are likely to be secondary to HIV infection, but it remains a rare complication despite the immune deficiency.

Noma starts in the oral cavity from an acute necrotising ulcerative gingivitis (Ch. 7) or a painful, small, reddish-purple spot or indurated papule that ulcerates. There is extensive oedema. The infection and necrosis extend outward, rapidly destroying soft tissues and bone (Fig. 9.9). Diffuse oedema of the face, foetor and profuse salivation are associated. While the overlying tissues become ischaemic, the skin turns blue-black.

The gangrenous area becomes increasingly sharply demarcated and ultimately sloughs away. Muscle, invaded by the micro-organisms, undergoes rapid necrosis associated with only a weak inflammatory response (Fig. 9.10). The slough is cone-shaped, with its apex superficially so that the underlying destruction of hard and soft tissues is more extensive than external appearances suggest. The slough separates, the bone dies; sequestration and exfoliation of teeth follow. A gaping facial defect is left (Fig. 9.11) that heals poorly with scarring and distortion of tissues (Fig. 9.12).

Management

Malnutrition and underlying infections must be treated. A combination of penicillin or an aminoglycoside and metronidazole will usually control the local infection, but light surgical debridement of necrotic soft tissue is also needed. After control of the infection and recovery of health, reconstructive surgery is usually required to prevent permanent disfigurement. However, there is a significant mortality, almost all cases if untreated and 5%–10% if treated.

Noma review PMID: 16829299 and 34905547

ACTINOMYCOSIS

Actinomycosis is a chronic, suppurative infection caused by *Actinomyces sp.* Although common in the past, it has become rare in the UK. Half of all cases of actinomycosis affect the face and neck.

Clinically, men are predominantly affected, typically between the ages of 30 and 60 years. A chronic soft tissue swelling near the angle of the jaw in the upper neck is the usual complaint. In the past this would progress to a dusky-red or purplish, firm and slightly tender swelling with multiple discharging sinuses (Fig. 9.13). Pain is minimal. In the absence of treatment, a large fibrotic mass can form, covered by scarred and pigmented skin, on which several sinuses open.

However, such a florid picture is rarely seen now. Currently, the usual clinical features are a persistent subcutaneous collection of pus or a sinus, unresponsive to conventional, short courses of antibiotics.

Pathology

The key microbiological signature is the presence of *Actinomyces israelii* or *Actinomyces gerencseriae* in a mixed infection with aerobic and anaerobic organisms. These are slow-growing aerobic organisms, and simple conventional cultures may only grow the accompanying organisms, usually coagulase-negative staphylococci, *S. aureus* and both α- and β-haemolytic streptococci. This may lead to a false-negative diagnosis, and pus samples for culture must be sent to the laboratory with a form indicating a suspicion of actinomycosis; otherwise the true nature of the infection may be missed.

A. israelii is a long filamentous Gram-positive bacterium, not a fungus as its name suggests. The classification of this genus of bacteria is complex, and many so-called oral Actinomyces species are now reclassified and not thought pathogenic. However, pathogenic species can still be isolated from the mouth and are the likely source for actinomycosis of the head and neck. Injuries, especially dental extractions or fractures of the jaw can provide a pathway and sometimes

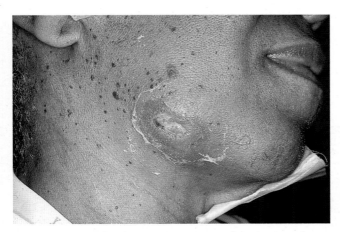

Fig. 9.13 Cervicofacial actinomycosis. Sinus draining centrally over a firm persistent swelling *(Source: Pfaller MA, Murray PR, Rosenthal KS (2021). Non–spore-forming anaerobic bacteria. In: Medical microbiology, 9th ed. Philadelphia: Elsevier Inc.)*

precede infection but rarely do so. Most patients will have been previously healthy.

Actinomycosis spreads by direct extension through the tissues and does not follow tissue planes or spread to lymph nodes like other odontogenic infections. The infection is chronic and suppurative. In the tissues, colonies of *Actinomyces* form rounded colonies of filaments with peripheral, radially arranged club-shaped thickenings seen at higher power (Fig. 9.14).

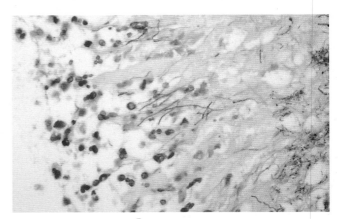

Fig. 9.14 Actinomycosis. Individual branching filaments of *Actinomyces* seen at high power as blue threads in the edge of this sulphur granule stained with Gram stain. The red objects on the left are inflammatory cells on the surface of the colony.

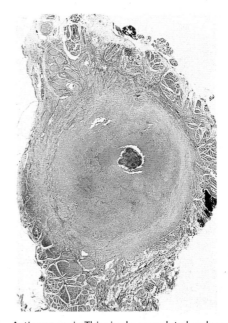

Fig. 9.15 Actinomycosis. This single, complete loculus was from an early case of actinomycosis that followed dental extraction. The colony of actinomyces with its paler staining periphery (a 'sulphur' granule) is in the centre; around it is a dense collection of inflammatory cells, surrounded in turn by proliferating fibrous tissue, stained pinkish red. It will be apparent that an antibiotic cannot readily penetrate such a fibrous mass and must be given in large doses to be effective.

Neutrophils mass round the colonies, pus forms, chronic inflammatory cells surround the pus and an abscess wall of fibrous tissue forms (Fig. 9.15).

The abscess eventually points on the skin, discharging pus in which so-called *sulphur granules* (colonies of *Actinomyces sp.*) may be visible with the naked eye as yellow flecks. The abscess continues to discharge, infection spreads laterally to cause further abscesses and surrounding tissues become fibrotic. Untreated, the area can become honeycombed with abscesses and sinuses, in widespread fibrosis.

Microbiology PMID: 25045274

Management

Actinomycosis should be suspected if a skin sinus fails to heal after a possible focus of infection has been found and eliminated. A fresh specimen of pus is needed. A positive diagnosis can rarely be made without 'sulphur granules', which may be found by rinsing the pus with sterile saline. The laboratory should be warned that actinomycosis is suspected to enable appropriate media to be used and the culture maintained long enough for these slow-growing organisms to be detected.

Frequently, penicillins will have been given but in doses insufficient to control the infection. This makes subsequent bacteriological diagnosis difficult. In the correct clinical setting, empirical treatment as actinomycosis is logical even if bacteriological confirmation is not forthcoming.

The mainstay of treatment is penicillin, which should be continued for a minimum of 4–6 weeks, renewed as necessary, because pockets of surviving organisms may persist in the depths of the lesion to cause relapse. Abscesses should be drained surgically as they form and sinuses excised. Combined surgical and antibiotic treatment is most effective. For patients allergic to penicillin, erythromycin can be given.

Healing leads to scarring and puckering of the skin at the sites of sinuses, and these often have to be excised for cosmetic reasons.

The key features of actinomycosis are given in Box 9.3.

Complication of extraction PMID: 32820354

Treatment PMID: 25045274

Biopsy diagnosis PMID: 24870370

Other 'actinomycoses'

Infections with other non-pathogenic filamentous Gram-positive bacteria can be misclassified as actinomycosis. Examples are extraradicular infection in periapical granulomas,

in which a colony of bacteria very occasionally grows beyond the root apex. The colony is like a sulphur granule, but isolated in the cavity where it may remain localised for a long period to cause failure of root canal treatment. Similar colonies may be found in tonsil crypts and growing around sequestra as they exfoliate into the mouth. However, none are spreading infections, none require intensive antibiotic treatment and none are true actinomycosis.

Extraradicular 'actinomycosis' PMID: 12738954

THE SYSTEMIC MYCOSES

Deep tissue oral mycoses are rare in Britain but may be seen in immunocompromised patients or in people from endemic areas such as South America and other tropical regions (Box 9.4). Cryptococcosis is a common mycosis in HIV infection. Clinically, most of the systemic mycoses can cause oral lesions at some stage, and often then give rise to a nodular and ulcerated mass, which can be tumour-like in appearance (Fig. 9.16).

The most characteristic oral infection is the nodular mulberry-like gingival hyperplasia and ulceration of paracoccidioidomycosis, or South American blastomycosis, a fungal infection of lungs, lymph nodes, bone and mucosa that is endemic in Brazil (Fig. 9.17). Clinically, this has a superficial resemblance to gingival lesions of Wegener's granulomatosis (Ch. 34).

Microscopically, most deep mycoses give rise to granulomas similar to those of tuberculosis, but there may also be abscess formation. Characteristic yeast forms or hyphae may sometimes be seen with special stains such as periodic

---

> **Box 9.4   Some systemic mycoses that can affect the mouth**
>
> - Histoplasmosis
> - Rhinocerebral mucormycosis
> - Rhinocerebral aspergillosis
> - Cryptococcosis
> - Paracoccidioidomycosis (South American blastomycosis)

> **Box 9.3   Actinomycosis: key features**
>
> - Rare chronic infection by filamentous Gram-positive bacterium, usually *Actinomyces israelii*
> - Infection spreads direct through the tissues, not along fascial planes
> - Multiple abscesses and sinuses, in severe cases
> - More usually now, there is only a localised subcutaneous collection of pus
> - Microscopy shows large radially arranged colonies of actinomyces
> - Pus forms surrounded by a fibrotic abscess wall
> - Sulphur granules (colonies of *Actinomyces sp.*) from the pus are best for culture
> - Responds to prolonged treatment with penicillin
> - Surgical drainage of locules of pus may be needed

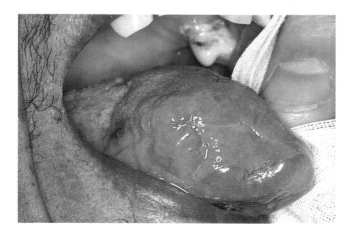

Fig. 9.16   Histoplasmosis. The gross nodular swelling of the tongue and ulceration are typical of many of the systemic mycoses.

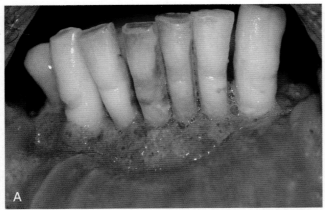

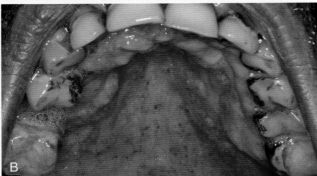

Fig. 9.17 South American blastomycosis. Characteristic nodular enlargement of gingiva seen in the upper image (A); note extension to labial mucosa. The lower figure (B) shows nodular lesions and erythema extending onto the palate. *(Courtesy of Prof. RS Gomez and Dr BC Durso)*

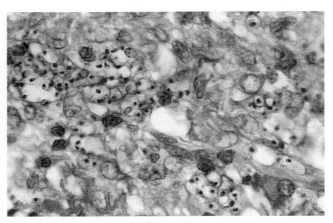

Fig. 9.18 Histoplasmosis. Part of an oral biopsy under high power, showing numerous typical round yeast forms with their clear haloes (periodic acid–Schiff stain).

acid–Schiff (PAS) (Fig. 9.18). However, microscopy may not be diagnostic, and culture of unfixed material may be necessary. Treatment requires systemic antifungal drugs, which have significant adverse effects.

Systemic mycoses in HIV PMID: 1549312

Histoplasmosis case reports PMID: 23633697 and 23219033

Paracoccidioidomycosis PMID: 8464610

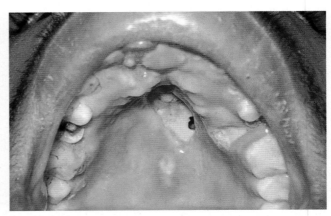

Fig. 9.19 Mucormycosis. There is necrotic ulceration in several areas reflecting more widespread necrosis of the underlying maxilla. In this case the infection started in the maxillary sinus. *(Source: Bansal S, Sardana K (2014). Palatal ulceration. CID. 32(6): 827-838.)*

Mucormycosis

This rare disease is the most significant deep mycosis of the head and neck because of its rapid progression and frequently fatal outcome. The causative fungi are environmental, often soil saprophytes that can only infect a debilitated or immunocompromised host. Many unrelated genera and species, including *Mucor sp.* and *Rhizopus sp.*, can cause the infection, and the name of the condition is difficult to align with the organisms; mucormycosis and zygomycosis are considered synonymous.

Most patients have poorly controlled diabetes, iron overload or a cause for immunosuppression. Recently, like other fungal diseases, mucormycosis became common in patients suffering severe COVID-19, usually those with concomitant diabetes or steroid treatment and particularly in India. The infection often starts in the sinuses or nose from inhaled spores but may occasionally follow tooth extraction, even in immunocompetent patients. The fungi invade blood vessels and so cause rapidly spreading tissue necrosis and large tissue defects (Figs. 9.19 and 9.20). Treatment requires surgical clearance and aggressive antifungal treatment, but a third of patients have a fatal outcome.

Review PMID: 8464609 and 18248590

In COVID-19 PMID: 34829397 and 34507870

SYSTEMIC INFECTIONS BY ORAL BACTERIA

The mouth harbours a great variety of microbes and virulent pathogens, particularly in periodontal pockets, but high levels of immunity and the fact that many of these organisms can only thrive in a mixed bacterial ecosystem keep them localised. It is almost always in the immunocompromised that oral commensals can spread and cause septicaemia or remote infections.

Infective endocarditis

A special example of a systemic infection of dental origin is infective endocarditis, which can occasionally follow dental operations, particularly extractions, and cause irreparable damage to heart valves (Ch. 33).

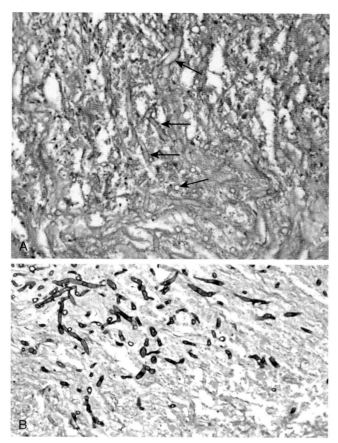

Fig. 9.20 Mucormycosis. The tissue is necrotic and infiltrated by the very pale, broad, knobbly branching hyphae of *Mucor* spp., seen as broad ribbons or circles in cross-section (*arrowed*). These are difficult to see in routine stains (A) but revealed by Grocott staining, which stains their cell walls black (B).

Lung and brain abscesses

Some abscesses at these sites are due to oral anaerobic bacteria that are probably aspirated during sleep to cause a lung abscess and then a secondary brain abscess. Isolated brain abscesses caused by oral bacteria are recognised but difficult to explain otherwise, though organisms previously considered limited to the oral cavity or periodontal pocket are increasingly recognised in infections at other body sites.

Cysts in and around the jaw 10

Cysts are the most common cause of chronic swelling of the jaw. A cyst comprises a wall of fibrous tissue and a central lumen, or space, lined by epithelium. Cysts are more common in the jaw than in any other bone because only the jaw contains epithelium during and remaining after tooth formation.

Definition Cysts are pathological fluid-filled cavities lined by epithelium.

CLASSIFICATION OF CYSTS

There are many types of cysts, and those in the head and neck are difficult to classify neatly and comprehensively. There is not currently a complete classification that is accepted internationally. A classification based on the current WHO classification is given in Box 10.1.

Cysts can be classified into two groups based on the origin of the epithelium that lines the central cavity. **Odontogenic cysts** are lined by odontogenic epithelium derived from the dental lamina and its derivatives. The epithelial lining originates by the proliferation of rests of Serres, reduced enamel epithelium or rests of Malassez. Odontogenic cysts therefore can only affect the tooth-bearing regions of the jaw. Odontogenic cysts account for most cysts of the jaw. By far, the most common is the radicular cyst, and this and the dentigerous cyst are common enough to present regularly in general dental practice (Box 10.2).

Odontogenic cysts can be further divided into inflammatory and developmental types depending on their cause. In reality, most of the developmental cysts are of unknown cause, and the developmental aetiology is assumed, though some are caused by specific gene mutations.

Non-odontogenic cysts are lined by other types of epithelia, and they are usually developmental in origin. The sources of non-odontogenic epithelium in the jaw include developmental residues in the incisive canal, glands and ducts and maxillary sinus lining epithelium.

Some of the odontogenic tumours, notably ameloblastoma, also contain cysts lined by epithelium, and these mimics need to be considered in differential diagnosis (Ch. 11).

Although the classification of cysts provides a logical way to list and understand them, it has little bearing on diagnosis and treatment, which are determined by the individual cyst type. It is not possible to identify odontogenic epithelium under the microscope unless it has basal cells resembling ameloblasts or fortuitously forms Rushton bodies (hyaline bodies), an enamel matrix-like secretory product that can only be formed by odontogenic epithelium (Fig. 10.11).

There are many other causes of circumscribed areas of radiolucency in the jaw that mimic cysts (Box 10.3).

General reference work ISBN-13: 978-1-119-35499-4

Incidence of cysts PMID: 23766099

Box 10.1   Cysts of the jaw, face and neck
ODONTOGENIC CYSTS
Cysts of inflammatory origin

Radicular cyst
  Residual radicular cyst
Inflammatory collateral cysts

Cysts of developmental or unknown origin

Dentigerous cyst
  Eruption cyst
Odontogenic keratocyst
Orthokeratinised odontogenic cyst
Lateral periodontal cyst
  Botryoid odontogenic cyst
Glandular odontogenic cyst
Calcifying odontogenic cyst
Gingival cysts
  Gingival cyst of infants
  Gingival cyst of adults

NON-ODONTOGENIC CYSTS

Nasopalatine duct cyst
Surgical ciliated cyst
Nasolabial cyst
Sublingual dermoid cyst
Thyroglossal duct cyst
Branchial cyst
Foregut cysts

Box 10.2   Relative frequency of different types of jaw cysts

Radicular*	45%
Residual radicular	7%
Dentigerous	16%
Odontogenic keratocyst	10%
Incisive canal	10%
Collateral	3%
Lateral periodontal	<1%

*The relative proportion of each cyst type in different countries is considerably affected by the incidence of non-vital teeth in the population, as this determines the incidence of radicular cysts. These are estimates from the United Kingdom, and radicular cysts are less common than in previous decades. Incidence in published studies is also affected if some cysts are classified as odontogenic tumours instead.

COMMON FEATURES OF JAW CYSTS

Many features are shared by all types of cysts. All cysts enlarge slowly, and there are two main mechanisms of enlargement: expansion under internal hydrostatic pressure and growth of the epithelial lining.

Hydrostatic pressure is the mechanism of cyst growth in almost all cysts. The luminal contents are under pressure for a variety of reasons. There is poor lymphatic drainage from the cavity, the wall and lining have partial properties of a semipermeable membrane, and the lumen contains many degraded inflammatory proteins and dead lining cells. These and other factors produce an osmotic pressure that expands the cyst. The pressure is probably intermittent and of the order of 70 cm of water and therefore higher than the capillary blood pressure, able to compress veins and lymphatics in the wall so that fluid cannot escape. Expansion is slow. It takes five years for a cyst in the mandible to enlarge to a few centimetres in diameter in an adult (Fig. 10.1), but growth is faster in children because bone turnover is more rapid and the bones less dense, providing less resistance to enlargement.

Enlargement resorbs bone around the periphery and once the cortex is perforated, pushes the periosteum outward.

Growth of the wall is a less common mechanism, seen primarily in odontogenic keratocysts. In this cyst, the epithelial lining has a high mitotic rate, and the lumen is filled with keratin, which is resistant to degradation, insoluble and thus exerts little osmotic pressure. Instead, the wall enlarges by growing, budding and insinuating finger-like processes or developing outpouchings that extend into adjacent bone. Glandular odontogenic cysts grow in a similar way.

Growth pattern and effects on adjacent structures differ with the mechanism of enlargement. Hydrostatic pressure acts equally in all directions, and all cysts that grow this way enlarge equally in all directions until the surrounding structures restrict them. Initially, they will enlarge like a balloon, forming a hollow sphere by resorbing medullary bone. Later, enlargement is restricted by cortical bone, tooth roots or the cortical layer around the inferior dental canal. The pressure will then push out the cyst in other directions with less resistance, but pressure is exerted on the resisting structures, and eventually, the cyst will move teeth orthodontically, resorb the cortex and push the inferior dental canal out of the way. Over a longer period, tooth roots may be resorbed. Conversely, the odontogenic keratocyst, without any internal pressure, burrows along the path of least resistance in the medullary bone around the teeth without displacing them and partly constrained by the cortex to produce a long thin shape.

Expansion of the jaw results from resorption of the cortex and pushing out of the periosteum. The periosteum is a tough resistant elastic layer that the cyst cannot penetrate. As it expands, it forms a new cortical bone layer around the cyst. There is not time to form a well-organised lamellar bone layer, and the 'periosteal new bone layer' is mostly soft

> **Box 10.3 Radiographic mimics of cysts**
> - Anatomical structures (maxillary antrum and foramina)
> - Large periapical granulomas
> - Odontogenic tumours, particularly ameloblastoma (Ch. 11)
> - Simple bone cyst and aneurysmal bone cyst (Ch. 12)
> - Giant cell lesions (Ch. 12)
> - Cherubism (Ch. 12)

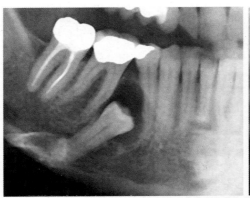
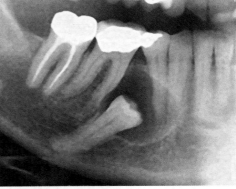
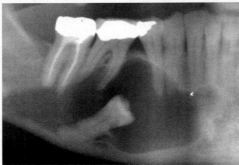

Fig. 10.1 Growth of an untreated cyst. This dentigerous cyst was identified at the size shown *upper left*. After 15 months, it had grown to the size shown *upper right*. It took a further five years and four months to grow to the size in the lower radiograph. Generally cysts enlarge slowly, but enlarge more quickly when inflammation is present. *(Courtesy Mr O Obisesan.)*

woven bone. Palpation of the new bone layer can cause it to crack, and the fragments rubbing together give rise to the clinical sign of 'eggshell crackling'. Cysts expand the cortex closest to their site of origin first. Cysts arising in the alveolus expand buccally first, except in the lower molar region, where the lingual cortex is closer and thinner. The periosteal new bone layer can be seen in radiographs.

Expansion is rarely seen in odontogenic keratocysts until a late stage because their lack of internal hydrostatic pressure renders them unable to resorb the cortex, or at least resorb it only with difficulty. Expansion is seen, but it is a late sign in cysts that have reached a comparatively large size. It is more marked in children where the bone is less dense and turning over more rapidly or when a cyst becomes inflamed and develops increased internal pressure.

Tooth vitality is not affected by cysts. The radicular cyst is caused by a non-vital tooth, but all cysts can tip and resorb the adjacent teeth without causing a loss of vitality. The neurovascular bundles to their apices are either displaced to the periphery of the cyst or run across the lumen, where they are prone to damage on surgical removal of the cyst.

A bluish colour is characteristic of cysts that have expanded beyond the cortex and results from their fluid content (Fig. 10.2). It may be possible to transilluminate cysts or demonstrate fluctuance if they expand through the cortex in two places.

Radiological features are common to most cysts. All produce sharply defined evenly radiolucent lesions with a smooth rounded outline. The surrounding bone forms a reactive thin cortical or sclerotic layer around any cyst that grows slowly enough, and this is seen as cortication, a distinct white line around the edge of the lesion. Cysts may be unilocular (one cavity) or multilocular (many cavities). Multilocular cysts have a scalloped outline, and septa may be visible, dividing the locules from one another. The radiological appearances provide an opportunity to assess the growth pattern and effects on the cortex, teeth and other structures that give clues to diagnose individual types of cysts.

Signs and symptoms. Cysts in bone may enlarge without signs or symptoms for a long period, and approximately one-third of cysts are chance radiographic findings. A further third present with painless jaw expansion or displacement of teeth. The remaining third becomes infected, either through communication with a non-vital tooth or pocket or by rupturing into the soft tissues. Cysts may therefore present as abscesses, and their cystic nature may not be immediately evident. A 'cyst abscess' has a fuzzy rather than a corticated outline radiographically. Very large cysts may precipitate a pathological fracture.

Fluid content. Aspiration of cyst fluids for diagnosis is obsolete as an investigation, but any thick white paste found in a cyst is probably keratin and indicates a likely diagnosis of odontogenic keratocyst. Most cyst fluids are watery and opalescent but sometimes more viscid and yellowish, and they sometimes shimmer with cholesterol crystals (see later in this chapter). A smear of this fluid may show typical notched cholesterol crystals microscopically (Fig. 10.8). In infected cysts, an aspirate of pus should be taken for bacterial culture and sensitivity.

Key features of jaw cysts are shown in Box 10.4.

TREATMENT OF JAW CYSTS

Most types of cysts are treated in the same way, the exceptions being odontogenic keratocyst and a few other rare types that have a risk of recurrence. Their special treatment is discussed later in this chapter with each entity. The remaining types of cysts have limited treatment options.

It may seem odd to be discussing treatment before a definitive diagnosis, but in clinical practice, treatment is often performed before a definitive diagnosis, based on clinical and radiological features. The dentist therefore needs sufficient knowledge to make an accurate differential diagnosis on these findings and be alert for features of cysts that might recur, as these would require a biopsy and definitive diagnosis to plan treatment. Otherwise, if a confident differential diagnosis is made, and if the cyst is small, it may be treated and the final diagnosis confirmed by histopathology subsequently.

Enucleation and primary closure is the usual method of treatment and is usually entirely effective (Box 10.5). A mucoperiosteal flap over the cyst is raised, and a window is opened in the bone large enough to give adequate access. The soft tissue of the cyst wall is then separated from the bony wall. In thick-walled cysts, it separates cleanly with a

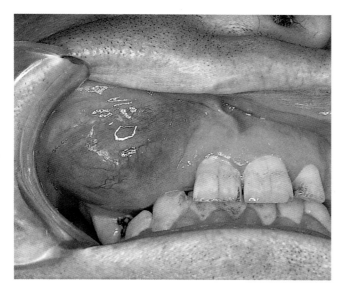

Fig. 10.2 Typical clinical appearance of a large cyst. This radicular cyst in the right maxillary alveolar process forms a rounded swelling with a bluish colour.

> **Box 10.4 Key features of jaw cysts**
>
> - Form sharply defined radiolucencies with corticated smooth borders
> - Cysts close to the mucosal surface may be transilluminated and appear bluish
> - Grow slowly, displacing rather than resorbing teeth
> - Symptomless unless infected and frequently chance radiographic findings
> - Rarely large enough to cause pathological fracture
> - Form compressible and fluctuant swellings if extending into soft tissues
> - Aspiration can confirm fluid contents, excluding a solid lesion
> - Not all types have diagnostic biopsy features, and clinical and radiological information is required for diagnosis
> - Often treated prior to histological confirmation of diagnosis

blunt instrument and scoops out easily; in thinner-walled cysts, more care is needed. The entire cyst is removed intact and should be sent for histological examination. If there is a non-vital tooth associated, as in a radicular cyst, this is treated as described later in this chapter. If there are apices of other teeth extending into the cavity, these teeth are usually either root treated preoperatively or on cyst removal by a retrograde approach. Alternatively, they may be extracted.

The edges of the bone cavity are smoothed off, free bleeding is controlled, and the cavity is irrigated to remove debris. The mucoperiosteal flap is replaced and sutured in place on sound bone around the margin of the bony window. The cavity fills with blood and organises. The sutures should be left for at least ten days.

Any disadvantages are largely theoretical, and in competent hands even very large cysts can be enucleated safely. Recurrence is remarkably rare unless the cyst has been misdiagnosed. There are few contraindications, and they are relative rather than absolute.

Marsupialisation. Marsupialisation, or decompression, was a largely outmoded treatment but has regained popularity for very large odontogenic keratocysts. The cyst is opened essentially as for enucleation, but the lining is left in place and sutured to the oral mucous membrane at the margins of the opening to produce a wide communication into the mouth. The aim is to decompress the cavity, eliminating any internal pressure, and make it into a pouch continuous with the oral mucosa. The cavity gradually closes by the ingrowth of bone from the periphery and the replacement of the lining epithelium by the ingrowth of the oral epithelium.

However considerable aftercare is needed to keep the cavity clean. The cavity is initially packed with ribbon gauze, and after the margins have healed, a plug or extension to a denture is made to close the opening loosely. Food debris has to be regularly washed out, and the opening shrinks with healing, making this difficult. A further disadvantage is that the complete lining is not available for histological examination.

Decompression is a partial marsupialisation in which the cavity is opened and a permanent narrow drain inserted rather than leaving a pouch with a deliberately large oral communication, reducing some of the disadvantages of marsupialisation but achieving the same outcome.

The main application of decompression and marsupialisation is for large odontogenic keratocysts to avoid more aggressive surgery or for temporary decompression of exceptionally large cysts where fracture of the jaw is a risk. When the cyst has shrunk and enough new bone has formed, the remaining lining can be enucleated. Occasionally, retention of the tooth in a dentigerous cyst is needed, and marsupialisation may allow it to erupt.

Advantages and limitations are given in Box 10.6.

Case series marsupialisation PMID: 25631867

Systematic review marsupialisation PMID: 34749963

Curettage. Curettage is the scraping of the bony cavity after enucleation or piecemeal removal of a lesion. It is not necessary in most cysts because the soft tissue separates easily from the smooth bony wall of the cavity. When the lining is friable, as in odontogenic keratocyst, a light curettage may help dislodge any remaining small fragments that could seed recurrence, but it is only a precautionary measure after attempting removal of the entire lining.

Infection is a secondary change and must be treated first by antibiotics and drainage to avoid performing surgery in an infected field. Once the infection is controlled, the cyst is treated as normal.

TREATMENT OF SOFT TISSUE CYSTS

Soft tissue cysts are almost always benign. Unlike cysts in bone, they need to be removed with a small amount of surrounding normal tissue to avoid bursting them or leaving small fragments in the tissues to seed a recurrence. Soft tissue cysts are therefore excised (removed by cutting around them) with a small margin of normal tissue shaped to facilitate wound closure.

ODONTOGENIC CYSTS

RADICULAR CYST → Summary chart 10.1 p. 163

Radicular cysts, or periapical cysts, are the most common type of cyst in the jaw and also the most common cause of major, chronic jaw swellings. They are odontogenic and inflammatory in type. The radicular cyst is defined by its location at the apex of a non-vital tooth.

> **Definition** A radicular cyst is a cyst on the apex of a non-vital tooth.

Clinical features

The age at presentation is wide, ranging from 20–60 years. Radicular cysts are more common in males than females, roughly in the proportion of 3:2. The maxilla is affected more than three times as frequently as the mandible. These features reflect the frequency and location of non-vital teeth. Although deciduous teeth are often devitalised by caries, radicular cysts are rarely seen before the age of ten years, probably because of the time required for them to form.

There is a slowly enlarging painless swelling, with no symptoms until the cyst becomes large enough to be noticed (Fig. 10.2). The swelling is rounded and at first hard. Later, when the bone has been reduced to eggshell thickness, a crackling sensation may be felt on pressure. Finally, part of the cortex of the bone is resorbed entirely, leaving a soft fluctuant swelling, bluish in colour, beneath the mucous membrane. The dead tooth from which the cyst has originated is (by definition) present, and its relationship to the cyst will be apparent in a radiograph (Fig. 10.3). Infection may develop in the cyst cavity because of communication with the pulp cavity of the associated non-vital tooth, and the swelling becomes painful and may expand rapidly, partly due to inflammatory oedema.

Key features of radicular cysts are summarised in Box 10.7.

Radiography

A radicular cyst appears as a rounded, radiolucent area with a sharply defined outline. A condensed radiopaque corticated periphery is present only if growth is slow and is usually more prominent in longstanding cysts. The dead tooth from which the cyst has arisen can be seen and often has a large carious cavity or other cause for loss of vitality evident. Adjacent teeth may be tilted or displaced and can become slightly mobile as their bony support is reduced.

Pathogenesis

Epithelial proliferation. A non-vital tooth is present by definition. Most non-vital teeth persist in a symptomless state for many years, causing no more than a periapical granuloma. However inflammation in the granuloma is sufficient to induce proliferation in the epithelial rests of Malassez, the network of strands of epithelium that remain after breakdown of the root sheath of Hertwig. Rests of Malassez are more frequent around the apical third of the root and vary in number between individuals, perhaps explaining why some individuals develop multiple radicular cysts.

Cavitation. When the epithelial rests proliferate, they grow into larger islands of epithelium that break down to form a cavity in the centre. This is because the proliferating

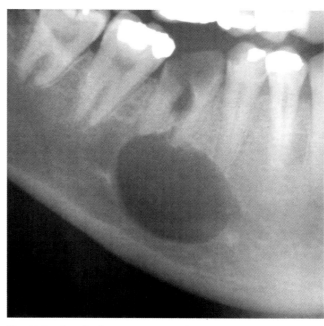

Fig. 10.3   A radicular cyst on a grossly carious and non-vital first permanent molar.   A rounded and sharply defined area of radiolucency is associated with the apices of the roots.

Box 10.7   Radicular cyst: key features

- Form in bone in relation to the root of a non-vital tooth
- Arise by epithelial proliferation in an apical granuloma
- Are usually asymptomatic unless infected or large
- Diagnosis is by the combination of radiographic appearances, a non-vital tooth and appropriate histological appearances
- Clinical and radiographic features are usually adequate for planning treatment
- Do not recur after enucleation
- Residual radicular cysts are radicular cysts that remain after the causative tooth has been extracted
- Cholesterol crystals often seen in the cyst fluid but only indicate inflammation and are not specific to radicular cysts

---

cells lie peripherally in the basal cell layer and move toward the centre of the island as they mature. Eventually they die and autolyse, producing a central cavity.

Fluid accumulation. As soon as a cavity forms, tissue fluid collects, and debris from dead epithelial cells and inflammatory exudate produce the hydrostatic pressure that causes cyst expansion. Radicular cysts enlarge in a balloon-like fashion producing the signs noted earlier, expansion and pressure effects on bone and teeth.

Secondary inflammation. This develops because of the non-vital tooth. Lymphocytes, plasma cells and macrophages collect in foci in the fibrous wall. There is always inflammation somewhere in the wall of a radicular cyst. Leakage from inflamed blood vessels allows erythrocytes to pass into the wall and cyst cavity. Unlike most other cell types, red cells have free cholesterol in their membranes. When the red cells in the cyst lumen or wall degenerate, their membranes release their cholesterol, which crystallises and

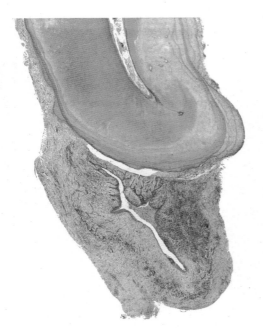

Fig. 10.4   The earliest stages of the formation of a radicular cyst. Tooth root, above, and a periapical granuloma, below, containing darkly-stained proliferating strands of odontogenic epithelium. The epithelium has broken down centrally to form a small epithelium-lined space.

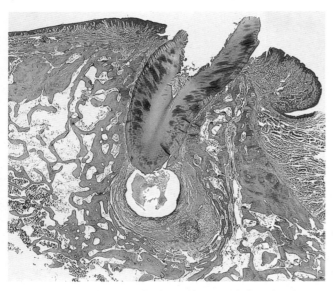

Fig. 10.5   A developing radicular cyst. An epithelium-lined cavity has formed in this large periapical granuloma. There is a thick fibrous capsule infiltrated by chronic inflammatory cells. The alveolar bone has been resorbed and remodelled to accommodate the slowly expanding swelling. The lumen contains debris and may or may not communicate directly with the pulp cavity.

induces a foreign body inflammatory reaction with giant cells and macrophages. The other lipid from the erythrocytes' membrane is taken up by macrophages that develop a foamy cytoplasm of engulfed fat droplets. Clusters of crystals and inflammatory cells form nodules in the wall ('mural nodules') that hang into the cyst cavity. Inflammation induces the cyst lining epithelium to become hyperplastic.

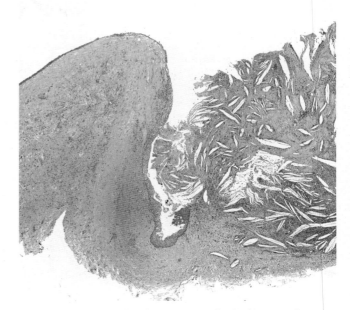

Fig. 10.6   Cholesterol clefts in a cyst wall. The lumen is above, and the darkly-stained epithelial lining is visible on the left. A large collection of cholesterol crystals has formed in the fibrous wall. The epithelium overlying this focus has broken down, and the cholesterol can leak into the cyst lumen.

Bone-resorbing factors. Experimentally, cyst tissues in culture release bone-resorbing factors. These are predominantly prostaglandins E2 and E3. Different types of cysts and tumours may produce different quantities of prostaglandins, but it is unclear whether this aids growth of the cyst *in vivo*.

Histopathology

The smallest and earliest cysts are no more than a periapical granuloma containing a few strands of proliferating epithelium (Figs 10.4 and 10.5). Later, a well-organised thick cyst wall with epithelial lining and dense inflammatory infiltrate develops.

The fibrous wall consists of collagenous connective tissue with variable inflammation, usually plasma cells and macrophages. Mural nodules of cholesterol clefts (Figs 10.6 and 10.7) and cholesterol crystals are found in the wall and lumen (Fig. 10.8). Peripherally, osteoclasts resorb the inner aspect of the bony cavity to allow expansion. Beyond that, in the adjacent medullary cavity, osteoblasts react to the inflammation by increasing bone deposition, producing the line of cortication seen radiographically.

The lumen is lined by a non-keratinising epithelium of variable thickness. More inflamed cysts have a more hyperplastic epithelium that appears net-like (Fig. 10.9), forming rings and arcades (Fig. 10.10). Hyaline bodies may be seen in the epithelium, confirming that it is odontogenic in origin (Fig. 10.11), and mucous cells may be present as a result of metaplasia (Fig. 10.12).

Longstanding cysts, or those in which the non-vital tooth has been root treated, typically have a thin flattened epithelial lining, a thick fibrous wall and less inflammatory infiltrate.

Differential diagnosis

Radicular cysts are usually readily recognised by their clinical and radiographic features, so a confident preoperative

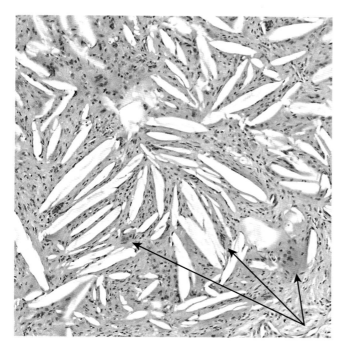

Fig. 10.7　Cholesterol clefts at a higher magnification.
Cholesterol has been dissolved out during the preparation of the
section, leaving empty clefts. The spaces between crystals are
filled by macrophages removing erythrocyte debris following
haemorrhage. The crystals are treated as foreign bodies, and
flattened multinucleate foreign body giant cells are seen along the
edges of several clefts (arrowed).

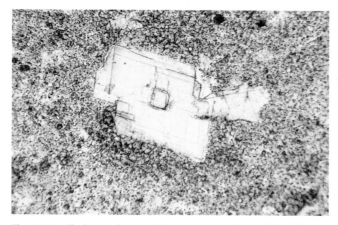

Fig. 10.8　Cholesterol crystals from a cyst aspirate. This indicates
the presence of inflammation. The rectangular shape with a
notched corner is characteristic.

diagnosis makes biopsy unnecessary unless there are unusual features such as root resorption or a poorly defined
margin.

Histological examination is essential after removal to
confirm the diagnosis, even though the histological features
are not entirely specific; it is really undertaken to exclude
unsuspected diagnoses.

Treatment

Radicular cysts are almost always treated by enucleation
and primary closure (mentioned previously). The associated
non-vital tooth is usually extracted because radicular cysts

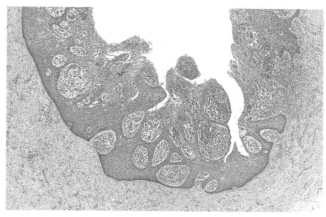

Fig. 10.9　Radicular cyst. The epithelial lining often assumes this
arcading pattern with numerous inflammatory cells beneath its
surface.

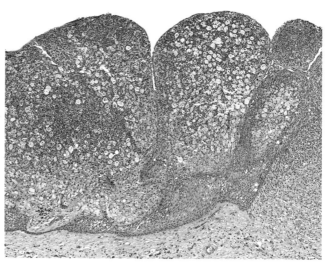

Fig. 10.10　Higher power of the lining of a radicular cyst. The
arcading epithelium contains numerous neutrophils emigrating
into the lumen, and there are pale-staining areas of foamy
macrophages in the inner wall.

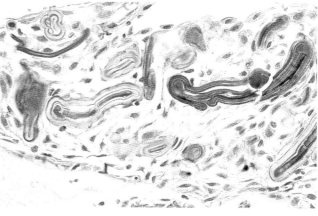

Fig. 10.11　Hyaline or Rushton bodies. These translucent or pink-
staining lamellar bodies are secreted by the cyst lining epithelium
and indicate the odontogenic origin of a cyst.

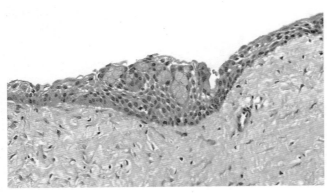

Fig. 10.12 Mucous metaplasia in a radicular cyst. Some epithelial cells in the slight thickening of the lining have become goblet cells and contain pale blue-stained mucin. This change is of no clinical significance and happens in a proportion of all cyst types but is most typical of dentigerous cysts and those arising in the maxilla.

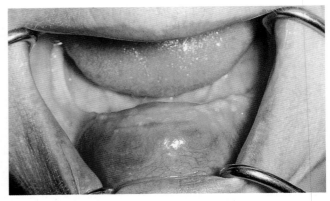

Fig. 10.13 Residual cyst. The causative tooth was extracted, leaving a small unsuspected cyst in the alveolar process, enlarging over many years to reach this size. See also Fig. 10.14.

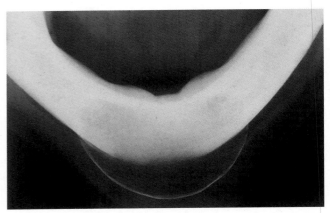

Fig. 10.14 Radiographic appearance of the residual cyst shown in Fig. 10.13. Note the thin bulging periosteal new bone layer, which can give rise to the clinical sign of eggshell crackling. *(Figs 10.13 and 10.14 Courtesy Mr P Robinson)*

tend to develop in irregular dental attenders, and the tooth is often unrestorable. However it can be preserved in most cases by placing an orthograde root filling before surgery and performing an apicectomy and retrograde filling, usually with mineral trioxide aggregate, when the cyst is enucleated. Healing may take several months before bone fills the cavity, and any cortical expansion slowly reduces with remodelling.

The treatment of suspected radicular cysts by root filling alone is somewhat contentious. Animal studies suggest that small cysts may resolve if the causative tooth is effectively root treated. Unfortunately, this is difficult to prove in humans as the presence of a cyst can only be confirmed histologically after removal. Because periapical granulomas can also attain a significant size (several centimetres), it is never certain exactly what has been treated. Although the size of a periapical radiolucency does affect the chances of it being a cyst rather than a granuloma, there is no definite threshold size that accurately indicates a cyst. Sometimes even a lesion a few millimetres in diameter can be a well-organised radicular cyst. Sharp definition of the lesion radiographically is also a poor indicator because definition is partly a function of size; larger periapical granulomas always appear better defined radiographically.

However it is clear that what *appear* to be cysts as large as approximately 20 mm in diameter can often resolve after endodontic treatment. It is therefore worth trying conservative treatment for small suspected radicular cysts, provided the patient accepts the risk of failure and will wait to assess the response. This may avoid surgery but carries some risks: infection in the periapical granuloma or cyst and failing to diagnose a completely different unsuspected lesion that just happens to be at the apex of a non-vital tooth.

General reference ISBN 978-1-119-35499-4

Size cyst v granuloma PMID: 18634946 and 20171356

Lateral radicular cyst

➜ Summary chart 10.1 p. 163

A so-called *lateral radicular cyst* is a radicular cyst that forms at the side of a non-vital tooth root at the opening of a lateral branch of the root canal rather than at the apex. They are rare and need to be distinguished from lateral periodontal cysts, a different type of cyst (later in this chapter) that forms beside tooth roots.

Residual radicular cyst

➜ Summary chart 10.1 p. 163

A residual radicular cyst is a radicular cyst that has persisted after extraction of the causative tooth. The features are identical to other radicular cysts, except that the key diagnostic feature has been removed; this may complicate differential diagnosis. Residual cysts are more frequent in older persons (Figs 10.13 and 10.14) and present with expansion of the jaw, often many years after the extraction. Once the causative tooth has been removed, inflammation subsides (Fig. 10.15) so that residual cysts grow very slowly.

INFLAMMATORY COLLATERAL CYSTS

These are cysts adjacent to the cervical area or furcation of molars buccally or distobuccally, particularly on mandibular molars, often those partially or recently erupted (Fig. 10.16). One presentation is buccal to erupting first or second permanent molars in children (often called 'mandibular buccal infected cyst'). Another is a cyst adjacent to the furcation in the molars of young adults expanding the alveolus (paradental or bifurcation cyst). They can reach several centimetres in diameter and then tip the tooth roots lingually and the crown buccally. In both types, the affected tooth is vital but typically shows pericoronitis or gingival inflammation.

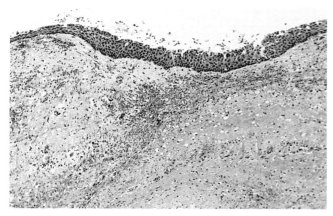

Fig. 10.15   Lining of a residual cyst. There is only a minor degree of inflammation, and the epithelium forms a thin regular layer.

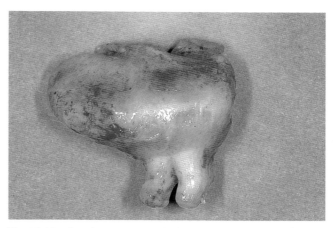

Fig. 10.17   Dentigerous cyst. This cyst has been removed intact together with its associated lower molar tooth. The cyst surrounds the crown and is attached at the cementoenamel junction, leaving the roots projecting through the wall.

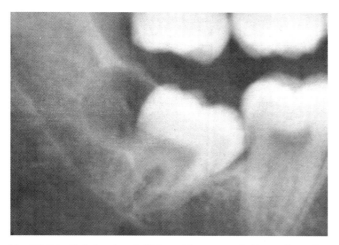

Fig. 10.16   Collateral cyst. This cyst has expanded buccally and distobuccally from the furcation area of the third molar. Although the cyst seems to originate at the cementoenamel junction, the periodontal ligament posteriorly and follicle anteriorly are not expanded, showing that the cyst lies outside the follicle, and so cannot be a dentigerous cyst.

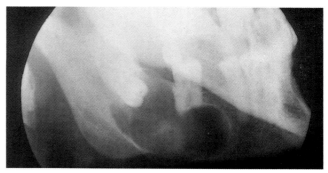

Fig. 10.18   Dentigerous cyst. Oblique lateral view showing a cyst that has developed around the crown of the buried third molar (*left*) but has extended forward around the root of a vital second molar. The vitality of the second molar is a key feature in differentiating whether this is a dentigerous cyst associated with the third molar or radicular cyst associated with the second molar.

These cysts are poorly understood but are probably inflammatory in origin. A proportion are bilateral, and a few are associated with enamel spurs or pearls in the buccal bifurcation (Ch. 2). Many are 'pocket cysts' communicating with a periodontal pocket and lined by junctional epithelium. They expand by internal pressure similarly to a radicular cyst, which they resemble histologically. Enucleation is effective, and the tooth can be conserved. Mandibular buccal infected cysts communicating with a pocket may resolve spontaneously.

Review PMID: 15128056

Paradental type PMID: 1065342

DENTIGEROUS CYSTS

➜ Summary chart 10.1 p. 163

This common cyst surrounds the crown of an unerupted tooth and is an expansion of the follicle caused by the separation of the reduced enamel epithelium from the enamel (Figs 10.17 and 10.18). The cyst is therefore odontogenic and is considered developmental in type. The cyst wall is attached to the neck of the tooth and the lining epithelium to the cervical enamel ('dentigerous relationship').

Definition The dentigerous cyst is a cyst around the crown of an unerupted tooth, with the epithelial lining attached around the cemento-enamel junction.

Clinical features

Dentigerous cysts are the most common developmental odontogenic cysts. They are more than twice as common in males as females, and two-thirds develop on lower third molars. Upper canines and lower premolars are also affected, reflecting the most frequently impacted teeth. These cysts present mostly between the ages of 10 and 30 years. They grow by internal pressure and cause the same clinical features as other cysts that expand the jaw, expansion with displacement of adjacent structures. They are often a chance radiographic finding when the cause is sought for an unerupted tooth.

Radiography

The cavity is circumscribed, rounded and always unilocular and contains the crown of the tooth (Fig. 10.18). Dentigerous cysts grow slowly and have a corticated outline. Cysts may attain a very large size, larger than 10 cm, and large

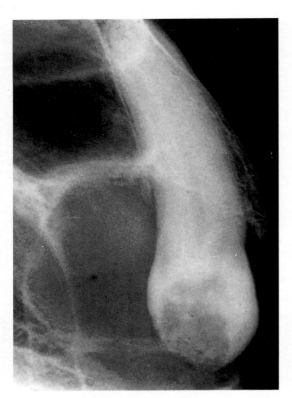

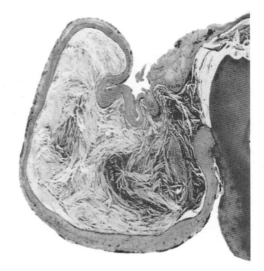

Fig. 10.20   Dentigerous cyst. The cyst surrounds the crown of this lower molar, the cusp tip visible top right and the wall is attached to its cementoenamel junction. There is a uniform, thin epithelial lining with minimal inflammatory infiltrate. Cholesterol clefts are numerous in the lumen, a result of haemorrhage in the wall.

Fig. 10.19   Resorption of tooth associated with a dentigerous cyst. The crown of this buried canine within the cyst shows resorption. This is seen only in longstanding cysts, as in this otherwise edentulous patient.

cysts may appear to be multilocular on radiographs (pseudoloculation) because ridges on the inside of the bony cavity are superimposed on the image. The affected tooth is often displaced a considerable distance, lower third molars to the lower border of the mandible or high in the ramus. In longstanding cysts, the enclosed tooth may become resorbed (Fig. 10.19). Because dentigerous cysts are often treated on the basis of a radiological differential diagnosis, it is critical to confirm that the cyst wall joins the tooth at its cementoenamel junction.

Pathogenesis

Dentigerous cysts are considered to be developmental, but inflammation from pericoronitis or an adjacent non-vital tooth may initiate some. Multiple dentigerous cysts are seen in people with cleidocranial dysplasia (Ch. 13) who have many unerupted teeth.

The earliest event is separation of the reduced enamel epithelium from the crown to form the cyst space. The epithelium is tightly bound to the enamel during formation but more loosely attached after the normal time of eruption, but the reason for separation is unclear. As the reduced enamel epithelium stops at the cementoenamel junction, the lining epithelium is attached there, and the fibrous wall is continuous with the periodontal ligament (Figs 10.20 and 10.21).

The cyst enlarges by internal pressure, expanding the dental follicle, displacing adjacent structures and the associated tooth and eventually expanding the jaw.

Histopathology

The wall of a dentigerous cyst in its early stages comprises an uninflamed fibrous wall lined by a thin, sometimes

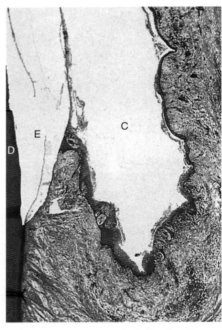

Fig. 10.21   Dentigerous cyst. To the left is the dentine (D). E is the enamel space left after decalcification and is separated from the cyst cavity (C) by a thin layer left by the inner enamel epithelium. The cyst itself appears to have formed as a result of the accumulation of fluid between the inner and outer enamel epithelium and by the continued proliferation of the latter to form the cyst lining, which joins the tooth at the epithelial attachment to the enamel.

bilaminar, epithelium that resembles reduced enamel epithelium (Figs 10.22 and 10.23). While the cyst enlarges, a degree of inflammation usually develops, and inflammatory or metaplastic changes can develop to differing degrees in different cysts. There may be frequent mucous cells or focal keratinisation. Once significant inflammation supervenes,

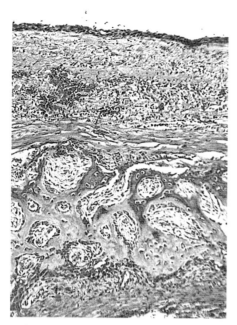

Fig. 10.22 The wall of a dentigerous cyst. There is minimal inflammation, and the darkly-stained epithelium is only two or three cells thick (at the top, lumen above). Beyond the fibrous tissue, the outermost layer of the wall is formed by woven bone induced by expansion through the cortex, a feature common to most types of intraosseous cyst.

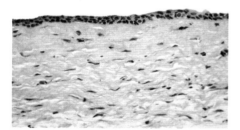

Fig. 10.23 Dentigerous cyst. In this uncomplicated cyst, there is no inflammation, and the wall comprises a layer of fibrous tissue lined by a thin layer of darkly-stained stratified squamous epithelium two cells thick (at the top, lumen above).

they can come to resemble a radicular cyst, and the diagnosis can no longer be made on biopsy alone.

Differential diagnosis

The key diagnostic feature is the dentigerous relationship to the tooth. It is normally possible to make a confident diagnosis radiographically and proceed to treatment without biopsy, confirming the diagnosis after enucleation. However care must be taken not to be caught out by other lesions simulating a dentigerous relationship. An odontogenic keratocyst, ameloblastoma or other radiolucent lesion may occasionally grow around the crown of an unerupted tooth to create a similar radiographic appearance (Fig. 10.33). Identifying a clear attachment at the cementoenamel junction will reduce the likelihood of this error. Because of this risk, the diagnosis should always be confirmed by histological examination, primarily to exclude other unexpected lesions.

It is also sometimes necessary to differentiate an enlarged follicle from a dentigerous cyst. The width of a normal follicle

---

> **Box 10.8   Dentigerous cyst: key features**
>
> - Arise in bone and contain the crown of an unerupted tooth, which is usually displaced
> - Cyst wall is attached to the tooth around the cemento-enamel junction
> - Are most frequently associated with unerupted third molars and canines
> - Clinical and radiographic features usually provide an accurate preoperative diagnosis, but confirmation is histological
> - May be mistaken radiographically for other cysts or tumours that grow around the crown of an unerupted tooth
> - Respond to enucleation or marsupialisation and do not recur after treatment

radiographically can be 2–3 mm. If there is uncertainty about whether a cyst space has developed, radiographic follow-up rather than intervention is appropriate.

Treatment

Dentigerous cysts are usually treated by enucleation with removal of the unerupted tooth, there usually being no reason to conserve the impacted lower third molar. However for other teeth, such as maxillary canines that are in a favourable position, it may be possible to marsupialise, decompress or surgically remove a dentigerous cyst to allow the tooth to erupt, providing space and traction orthodontically if necessary. Alternatively, the tooth can be removed and transplanted but with a risk of resorption in the long-term.

It remains unresolved whether leaving disease-free unerupted third molars *in situ*, according to current guidelines, risks the development of dentigerous cysts in later life. This would appear to be so, but the risk must be very low.

Key features of dentigerous cysts are summarised in Box 10.8.

Review PMID: 20605411

General reference ISBN 978-1-119-35499-4

ERUPTION CYST

An eruption cyst is a superficial dentigerous cyst arising on a tooth during eruption. They are therefore seen in children, forming a soft, rounded swelling on the alveolus. Trauma to the cyst causes internal bleeding and a dark blue colour (Figs 10.24 and 10.25).

Most eruption cysts burst spontaneously, and the tooth erupts normally, but if very large, the cyst roof may be incised or removed. Haemorrhage around an erupting tooth is much more likely to be traumatic than indicate an eruption cyst.

Case series PMID: 28160586

ODONTOGENIC KERATOCYST

→ Summary charts 10.1 and 10.2 pp. 163, 164

The odontogenic keratocyst has a characteristic clinical, radiological and histological appearance. It is important to recognise because it may recur after treatment, can grow

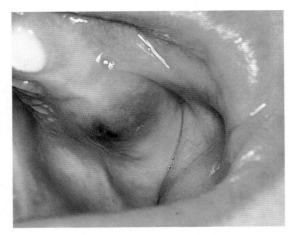

Fig. 10.24 An eruption cyst over an erupting upper molar. There has been bleeding into the cyst cavity as a result of trauma.

Feature	Odontogenic keratocyst	Orthokeratinised odontogenic cyst
Type of keratinisation	Parakeratin	Orthokeratin
Relative frequency (%)	90	10
Male: female ratio	1.5:1	2:1
Association with impacted tooth (%)	35	70
Location near the midline (%)	6	16
Radiographic appearance	Usually multilocular unless small	Almost always monolocular
Recurrence rate (%)	3–20	2

Table 10.1 The two types of odontogenic cysts that keratinise

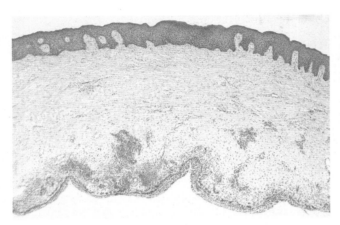

Fig. 10.25 Roof of an eruption cyst. At the upper surface is the keratinised epithelium of the alveolar ridge and, below, separated by a thin layer of relatively uninflamed fibrous tissue, the lining of an eruption cyst. The red patches in the inner wall are erythrocytes from haemorrhage.

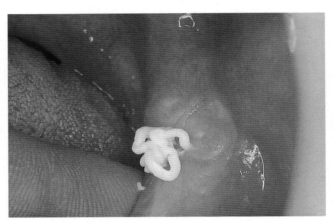

Fig. 10.26 An odontogenic keratocyst. Perforation of and pressure on the cyst roof has caused keratin, which fills the lumen, to extrude, and the characteristic appearance helps confirm the diagnosis.

to a very large size without symptoms, and is sometimes associated with a syndromic presentation.

The name of this cyst indicates that its epithelial lining keratinises, but this alone is not specific. Another less common cyst, the ortho-keratinising odontogenic cyst, also has this feature, and minor focal keratinisation can be seen in other odontogenic cysts. The differences between the two keratinising cysts are summarised in Table 10.1. Sublingual dermoid cysts are also heavily keratinised, but these are soft tissue cysts and readily differentiated.

> **Definition** The odontogenic keratocyst is a developmental odontogenic cyst with a tendency to recur, characterised by a histological appearance of parakeratinised lining epithelium with palisaded ameloblast-like basal cells.

Keratin filling the cyst lumen is bright white and, when seen during surgery, is a useful diagnostic feature indicating

these cyst types. It may be appreciated on opening a cyst for biopsy or if the cyst is punctured (Fig. 10.26), and its nature may be confirmed by histology. It should not be mistaken for pus, which is fluid rather than paste and has a characteristic smell.

Clinical features

Peak incidence is between ages 10 and 30 years, but the age range is very broad. The mandible is usually affected. At least 50% of odontogenic keratocysts form in the posterior body and lower ramus. Odontogenic keratocysts, like other jaw cysts, are symptomless until the bone is expanded or they become infected, both unusual features in this cyst type.

Radiography

Odontogenic keratocysts produce well-defined radiolucent areas with a more or less rounded or scalloped margin. Some are unilocular, but the majority are multilocular (Fig. 10.27). The margin is sharply demarcated and corticated radiographically.

The characteristic growth pattern is evident radiologically and is almost diagnostic. There is extensive spread forward and backward along the medullary cavity with minimal

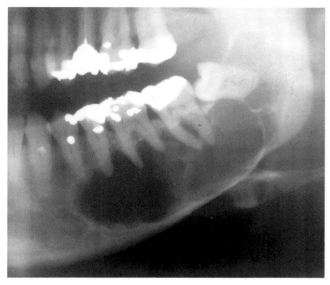

Fig. 10.27 Odontogenic keratocyst. Part of a panoramic tomograph showing typical appearances. The cyst is multilocular and has extended a considerable distance along the medullary cavity without appreciable expansion or displacement of the teeth.

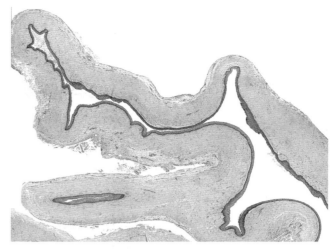

Fig. 10.29 Odontogenic keratocyst. Typical folded cyst outline with darkly-stained epithelium lining the lumen and a satellite cyst lying in the wall on the lower left. The fibrous tissue is uninflamed and thin.

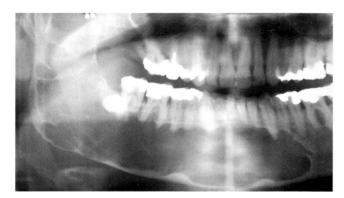

Fig. 10.28 Odontogenic keratocyst. Huge cyst extending from coronoid to the opposite molar region with minimal tooth displacement or expansion of bone.

expansion until the whole of the medulla is replaced. There is minimal displacement and no resorption of teeth or the inferior dental canal (Fig. 10.28). In a minority of cases, the cyst may arise at the site of a tooth that has failed to develop.

The lack of expansion results in many odontogenic keratocysts being large at the time of discovery.

Pathogenesis

Odontogenic keratocysts arise from the various rests of odontogenic epithelium that remain in the alveolus after tooth development, usually the rests of Serres.

Most odontogenic keratocysts are caused by mutation, deletion or other inactivation of the patched 1 (*PTCH1*) gene on chromosome 9q, a tumour suppressor gene. This gene is discussed in more detail in the following section. Loss of *PTCH* gene activity releases a brake on the cell cycle, mediated through the sonic hedgehog pathway. Mutation of the gene is found in 80% of odontogenic keratocysts, and the remainder may have other genetic faults in this signalling pathway, such as in the *PTCH2* gene. Mutation results in permanent activation of the sonic hedgehog pathway,

causing a relatively high proliferative activity in the cyst lining epithelium. This has two consequences. First, the cysts appear to enlarge by growth of the wall rather than internal pressure. Second, epithelial proliferation probably favours recurrence if small pieces of epithelium are left after incomplete removal.

The lining becomes folded because growth of the wall exceeds that of the cavity containing the cyst (Fig. 10.29). Extensions of the lining penetrate the wall to form small daughter cysts that enlarge to produce a multilocular lesion. The cyst wall produces bone-resorbing factors that resorb the surrounding medullary bone, allowing the cyst to enlarge slowly but relentlessly along the medullary cavity.

The possible neoplastic nature of odontogenic keratocysts

There has always been a tendency to regard these cysts as 'aggressive' on grounds of recurrence and the fact that they may grow to a very large size before detection. This, together with the fact that odontogenic keratocysts are caused by the inactivation of a tumour suppressor gene, has led some to classify them as benign neoplasms. The term *keratocystic odontogenic tumour* was proposed in 2005 to signify its neoplastic status. However this never gained wide acceptance, and the name *odontogenic keratocyst*, which has a long history, is again the official name.

Although the arguments for a neoplasm are more numerous and, in some ways, convincing, neoplasms are defined by their relentless growth and not by their molecular genetics. The odontogenic keratocyst responds well to marsupialisation, provided all of the locules are opened to the surface. This is the best evidence that the cyst is not a neoplasm. It is notable that some odontogenic tumours also harbour apparently neoplastic genetic alterations but are not considered neoplasms either (see Ch. 11).

The evidence for and against a neoplastic nature is listed in Table 10.2.

Cyst or neoplasm PMID: 21270459

Histopathology

Unlike the common cysts, odontogenic keratocyst has a diagnostic histological appearance (Box 10.9), so that biopsy

Table 10.2 Evidence for and against odontogenic keratocyst being a neoplasm

In favour of neoplasm	Against neoplasm
Recurrence	Other factors favour recurrence, thin friable lining and satellite cysts. Recurrence is thought to follow incomplete removal
Infiltrative ('aggressive') growth pattern	Growth is relentless but not aggressive or destructive
High proliferative activity of epithelial lining	Responds to marsupialisation
Caused by mutation or deletion of PTCH tumour suppressor gene	Similar molecular changes are present in non-neoplastic lesions of other tissues
May contain defects of *p16*, *p53* and other tumour suppressor genes	Similar molecular changes are present in non-neoplastic lesions of other tissues
Associated with other neoplasms in the basal cell naevus syndrome	Many other features of the syndrome are developmental and non-neoplastic
Squamous cell carcinoma may rarely develop within an odontogenic keratocyst	Squamous cell carcinoma may also develop in radicular and dentigerous cysts

Box 10.9   Typical histological features of odontogenic keratocyst

- Diagnosis may be made on histological features alone
- Epithelial lining of uniform thickness with flat basal layer
- Thin eosinophilic layer of parakeratin with corrugated surface
- Clearly defined basal layer of tall cells, at least focally with reversed polarity (Fig. 10.30)
- Epithelial lining weakly attached to the fibrous wall
- Thin fibrous wall
- Lumen filled by keratin
- Satellite cysts in the wall (Fig. 10.29)
- Inflammatory cells typically absent or scanty

is the definitive diagnostic investigation (Fig. 10.30). In a typical cyst, the fibrous wall is very thin and uninflamed. The lining epithelium has a corrugated, thinly parakeratinised surface and a palisaded basal layer of columnar cells that show reverse polarity, at least focally. The basal cells resemble pre-ameloblasts and indicate the cyst's odontogenic origin. The epithelium often separates from the wall on removal. In the fibrous tissue of the wall, there are usually scattered islands of odontogenic epithelium. These can form small 'satellite' or 'daughter' cysts, each of which will enlarge to become a separate locule in a multilocular cyst.

However if inflammation develops, the epithelial lining undergoes hyperplasia, loses its characteristic features and resembles that of a radicular cyst (Figs 10.31 and 10.32), making histological diagnosis more difficult. Because there is often focal inflammation in cysts, as large a biopsy sample as possible should be obtained for diagnosis.

The typical features are also lost after treatment by marsupialisation because the oral epithelium grows in to replace the cyst lining epithelium.

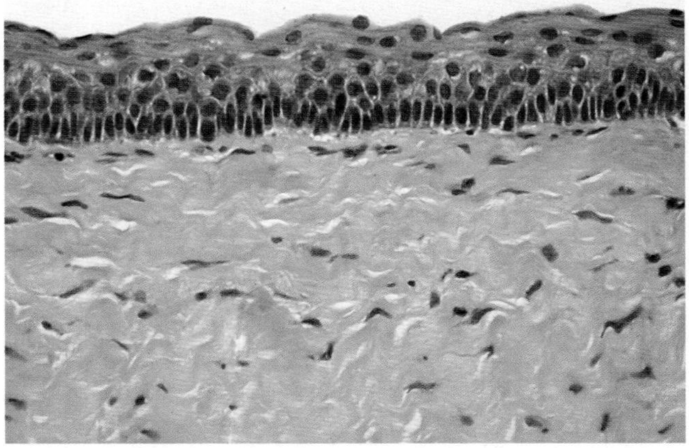

Fig. 10.30   Odontogenic keratocyst. High power, showing the diagnostic features of the epithelial lining: a flat basement membrane; elongated palisaded basal cells with focal reverse polarity; 10–20 cells in thickness and with a corrugated parakeratinised surface.

Differential diagnosis

The odontogenic keratocyst is usually correctly identified radiologically unless small and unilocular, in which case it may resemble any other cyst or well-defined radiolucent lesion. If the diagnosis is suspected, or if there is doubt, a biopsy is required to confirm the diagnosis. Correct preoperative diagnosis is necessary to select the special treatment given to this cyst type.

Occasionally, an odontogenic keratocyst may envelop an unerupted tooth or entrap a tooth and prevent its eruption, superficially producing a radiographic resemblance to a dentigerous cyst (Fig. 10.33). Odontogenic keratocysts with many locules may simulate an ameloblastoma radiographically (Fig. 10.34), but the relative lack of expansion aids identification of the cyst.

General reference ISBN 978-1-119-35499-4

Treatment and recurrence

If the diagnosis is not suspected preoperatively and the cyst is treated by simple enucleation, recurrence is likely. Recurrence has several contributing causes (Box 10.10). Historically, recurrence rates of more than 50% were reported, but with the current techniques described later in this chapter, recurrence rates of 2%–3% can be achieved.

Probably the major factor leading to recurrence is the difficulty in removing every trace of the epithelial lining, which is thin, friable and has a complex outline. Any fragments missed may survive and grow because of their proliferative activity. Larger cysts have a higher risk of recurrence because complete removal is more difficult. When the cyst extends around multirooted teeth, these usually have to be sacrificed to ensure complete removal.

Even if effectively removed, it is possible for a completely new cyst to form from residual dental lamina rests, explaining apparent recurrence as long as 40 years after removal. Otherwise, recurrence is often within the first five years after treatment. Vigorous treatment is likely to reduce the risk of recurrence, but there is no absolute certainty of a cure in one operation, and patients need long-term radiographic follow-up.

Ideally therefore diagnosis should be confirmed by biopsy preoperatively to allow appropriate treatment.

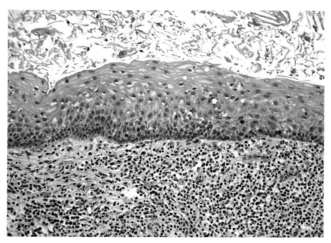

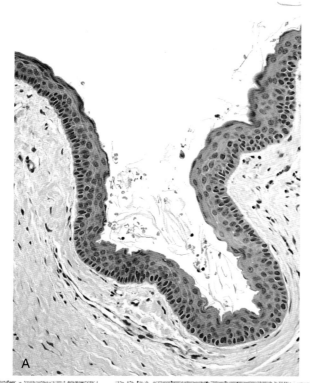

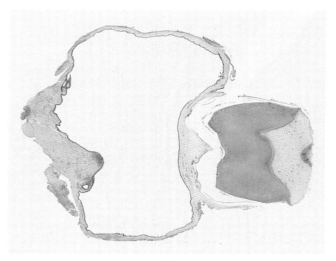

Fig. 10.32 Inflamed odontogenic keratocyst. Higher power of a more inflamed cyst with complete loss of diagnostic histological features. The epithelial lining resembles that of a radicular or inflamed dentigerous cyst, with only a hint of keratin on the left to give a clue to the correct diagnosis.

Fig. 10.33 A cyst arising in the follicle of an unerupted developing tooth. Radiographically, the cyst might have appeared to be in a true dentigerous relationship with the crown. However this is not a dentigerous cyst; its lining does not join the tooth at the amelocemental junction (as in Figs 10.19 and 10.20). A higher power view would reveal the characteristic lining of an odontogenic keratocyst.

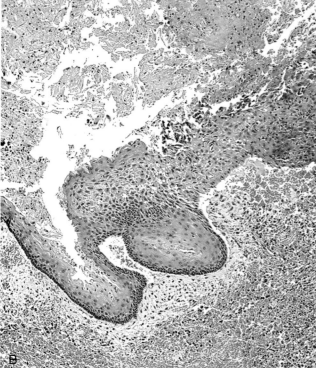

Fig. 10.31 Inflamed odontogenic keratocyst. Some areas of the lining show typical features (A), but in (B), inflammation has induced epithelial thickening and loss of the basal palisading and keratin.

Treatment depends largely on the extent of the cyst and the degree of multilocularity. Unilocular and small multilocular cysts can be treated conservatively and are usually enucleated and the bony cavity curetted vigorously to remove every fragment of cyst lining.

A useful additional precaution is the treatment of the cavity wall with an agent to kill any residual lining. Traditionally this was a fixative (Carnoy's solution) applied on gauze to the cyst cavity for a few minutes. This had the advantage of also toughening the lining for removal. It kills and denatures tissue to a depth of approximately 1–2 mm, far enough to kill the full thickness of the wall. However it is a caustic mixture of ferric chloride in alcohol, chloroform and highly concentrated acetic acid and must be used with care near vital structures such as the inferior dental neurovascular bundle. The inclusion of chloroform makes Carnoy's solution controversial, and a modified formula without it appears to be equally effective. Some authorities claim no added benefit versus careful mechanical removal and curettage of the cavity, but most consider that adding Carnoy's solution reduces recurrence by about half. A recent alternative to Carnoy's solution

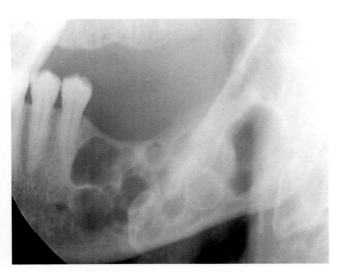

Fig. 10.34 **Odontogenic keratocyst with multiple locules.** Note the cortication around each cavity. The appearances resemble ameloblastoma, though the lack of expansion gives a clue to the correct diagnosis. *(Courtesy Mr EJ Whaites.)*

Box 10.11 **Odontogenic keratocyst: key features**

- Caused by mutations in *PTCH1* or *PTCH2* genes that activate the hedgehog signalling pathway in the cyst lining epithelium
- 5%–11% of jaw cysts
- Incidence peaks in the second and third decades, mean age of 38 years
- Form most frequently in the posterior alveolar ridge, body or lower ramus of the mandible
- 75% are in the mandibular premolar and molar region
- Grow around teeth without displacing them
- Often multilocular and this is usually seen radiographically
- Spread extensively along marrow spaces before expanding the jaw
- May recur after enucleation
- Radiographic features often characteristic
- Definitive diagnosis only by histopathology
- May be confused with ameloblastoma or with dentigerous cysts radiographically
- Multiple or childhood cysts are a sign of basal cell naevus (Gorlin's) syndrome

---

Box 10.10 **Possible reasons for the recurrence of odontogenic keratocysts**

- Thin, fragile linings, difficult to enucleate intact
- Finger-like cyst extensions into cancellous bone
- Multilocularity - small locules and satellite cysts may be left *in situ*
- More rapid proliferation of keratocyst epithelium
- Experience of surgeon
- Late formation of new cysts from other dental lamina remnants

---

is 5% 5-fluorouracil (5FU), an antimetabolite drug applied as a cream to gauze packed into the cavity for 24 h after cyst removal. This appears very effective and may carry less risk of inferior dental nerve damage.

Recently, a more conservative approach has been proposed. It has been recognised that a low risk of recurrence is better than a mandibular resection and consequent morbidity. Although recurrences are seen as a failure of treatment, if detected early, they may be easily managed by minor surgery, and a second curettage will often be effective.

Perhaps surprisingly, given the so-called *aggressive* nature of this cyst and its lack of internal pressure, marsupialisation has been found to be effective. Marsupialisation is followed by slow shrinkage of the cyst, allowing enucleation of a much smaller cyst with less morbidity and preservation of teeth. Reduction in size is associated with ingrowth of oral epithelium into the cavity, replacing the typical keratinised epithelium with non-keratinising stratified squamous epithelium. This makes surgical separation of the remaining cyst much easier, and recurrence after marsupialisation followed by enucleation is less frequent than after enucleation alone. Teeth displaced by the cyst often regain an upright position.

Complete resolution after marsupialisation is possible but takes a long time, as long as 20 months, and it requires cooperative patients who will irrigate the cavity and keep it open and clean until it resolves. However use as a primary treatment is increasing because the morbidity is considerably less than radical surgery, and the procedure is simpler than trying to enucleate the lining from a large cavity with a complex shape.

For the most extensive cysts, resection and reconstruction with a bone graft may be required. This controls recurrence and has the advantage of cure in one operation but carries significant morbidity. Posterior maxillary cysts may be treated more aggressively as they can be difficult to eradicate if they escape the confines of the bone, and occasionally these extend to the skull base.

If an unsuspected odontogenic keratocyst is accidentally enucleated, radiographic follow-up is appropriate, and any recurrence can be treated appropriately.

Key features of odontogenic keratocysts are summarised in Box 10.11.

Marsupialisation PMID: 8863300

Recurrence and treatment PMID: 15883937

Treatment with 5FU PMID: 33795069 and 32866486

Basal cell naevus syndrome

This syndrome, often called Gorlin's or Gorlin-Goltz syndrome, is inherited as an autosomal dominant trait. It is defined by the triad of multiple basal cell carcinomas, odontogenic keratocysts and various skeletal anomalies.

The syndrome is caused by any one of many germline mutations in, or occasionally deletions in, the patched genes (*PTCH1 or PTCH2*) on chromosome 9q. These changes inactivate the patched receptor and constitutively activate the sonic hedgehog pathway that is important in developmental patterning. Families with the syndrome have inactivation of one allele, causing skeletal anomalies. The genes are also tumour suppressor genes and modulate the cell cycle via the same signalling pathway. Inactivation or mutation of the second copy or of a related pathway gene is associated with development of multiple basal cell carcinomas and odontogenic keratocysts. Mutations in *PTCH1* and *2* are also be found in almost all odontogenic keratocysts in patients without the syndrome.

- Caused by a germline mutation in *PTCH1, PTCH2,* or other genes that activate the hedgehog signalling pathway
- Characteristic facies with frontal and parietal bossing and broad nasal root (Fig. 10.35)
- Multiple odontogenic keratocysts of the jaw (Fig. 10.37)
- Multiple naevoid (early onset) basal cell carcinomas of the skin
- Skeletal anomalies (usually of a minor nature) such as bifid ribs and abnormalities of the vertebrae
- Intracranial anomalies may include calcification of the falx cerebri and abnormally shaped sella turcica
- Cleft lip and palate in approximately 5%

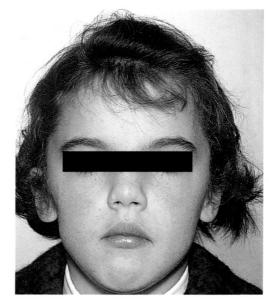

Fig. 10.35   Basal cell naevus syndrome. The typical facies with a broad nasal root and mild frontal bossing.

The main features of the syndrome are listed in Box 10.12, and the facial appearance is shown in Fig. 10.35, although a great many other abnormalities may be present. Although the genetic changes are highly penetrant, they show considerable variation in expressivity, so the effects vary between families and individuals. There is no clear correlation between the features seen and the particular gene mutation. One of the most consistent features, and one useful in confirming the diagnosis, is the presence of palmar pits, small round pinpoint depressions on the palms and soles of feet 1–2 mm in diameter. These are caused by focal lack of keratin and may appear red or a dark colour as they fill with dirt. Although these may be seen in other diseases, three or more pits is a diagnostic feature for the syndrome.

In view of the great variety of abnormalities that may be present, the effects on the patient depend on the predominant manifestation.

The number of basal cell carcinomas is very variable, but in some cases, they number hundreds or thousands over the lifetime of a patient. The face is a common site. The carcinomas are sometimes termed 'naevoid' because a linear cluster of them in their early stages looks like a birthmark and because they often present in children, but they behave as conventional basal cell carcinomas (Fig 10.36).

Almost all patients have odontogenic keratocysts, necessitating repeated operations. The presence of an odontogenic keratocyst in a child or multiple cysts should raise suspicion of the syndrome (Fig. 10.37). The cysts are identical to the non-syndromic equivalents and have the same tendency to recur. Cleft lip or palate or both is seen in a small proportion of these patients.

Case series PMID: 8042673

Diagnostic criteria management PMID: 21834049

Multiple basal cell carcinomas PMID: 33957740

Web URL 10.2 Genetics: http://omim.org/entry/109400

ORTHOKERATINISED ODONTOGENIC CYST

The second type of keratinising jaw cyst is the orthokeratinised odontogenic cyst (Fig. 10.38). It is less common than the parakeratinised type and used to be thought of as a variant.

This cyst differs in several respects from the true odontogenic keratocyst, having a lower proliferative activity, no

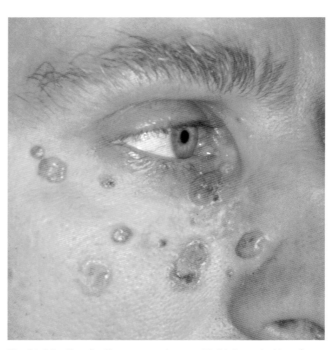

Fig. 10.36   Basal cell nevus syndrome. Multiple typical basal cell carcinomas presenting as pearly to flesh-coloured papules and nodules with rolled border and telangiectasia and some crusting and ulceration *(Source: Miller J. J., Marks J. G. (2019). Epidermal growths. In: Lookingbill and Marks' principles of dermatology, 6th ed, Philadelphia, Elsevier Inc)*

association with basal cell naevus syndrome and no *PTCH* gene changes. Differences are summarised in Table 10.1, and the most important difference is that orthokeratinised cysts are less likely to recur than parakeratinised cysts. The cyst has no particular clinical or radiological features that would allow preoperative diagnosis. Most are misdiagnosed as dentigerous cysts radiographically because they often arise in a dentigerous relationship to a lower third molar. Enucleation is curative.

Case series PMID: 20121617 and 34511349

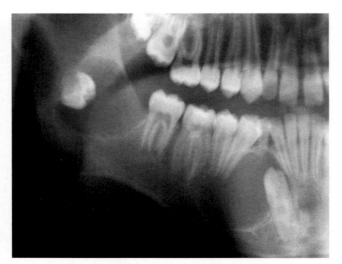

Fig. 10.37 Basal cell naevus syndrome. These two odontogenic keratocysts appear to be dentigerous but are not convincingly attached to the amelocemental junction of the teeth. Biopsy revealed odontogenic keratocysts and the presence of two in one patient, or in a child, indicates the syndrome.

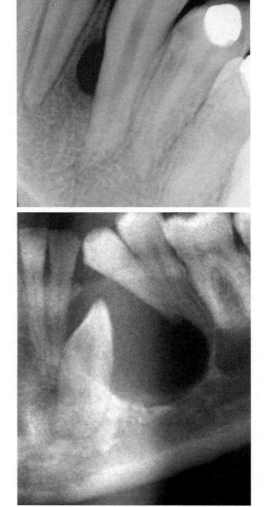

Fig. 10.39 Lateral periodontal cyst. Two typical examples of lateral periodontal cysts in the usual site adjacent to the roots of lower canines and premolars.

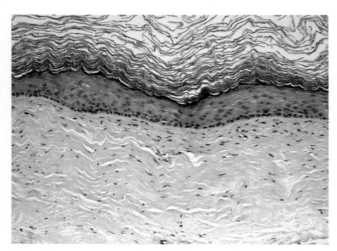

Fig. 10.38 Orthokeratinised odontogenic cyst. Uninflamed wall with a thickly orthokeratinised epithelium. Keratin fills the lumen, but the other characteristic features of odontogenic keratocyst are not present; for example there are no palisaded basal cells.

LATERAL PERIODONTAL AND BOTRYOID ODONTOGENIC CYSTS

These uncommon developmental odontogenic cysts form in the periodontal ligament beside the mid portion of the root of a vital tooth, presumably arising from a rest of Malassez. The botryoid odontogenic cyst is less common and is a lateral periodontal cyst that is multilocular.

Both types affect adults who are middle-aged and elderly and are usually chance radiographic findings when small. More than three-quarters of the unilocular lateral periodontal cysts arise in the lower canine and premolar region, and their location is characteristic and almost diagnostic (Fig. 10.39). Multilocular botryoid odontogenic cysts have a slightly broader distribution (Fig 10.40) but are still most common in the anterior mandible. If multilocularity is noted radiographically, the cyst is usually mistaken for an odontogenic keratocyst preoperatively. Occasional examples of both unilocular and multilocular variants reach several centimetres in diameter and expand the jaw and displace teeth.

Both the unilocular and multilocular variants have a diagnostic histological appearance. The lining is squamous or cuboidal epithelium that is mostly only one or two cells thick but has focal rounded thickenings or plaques (Fig. 10.41). In the plaques, the cells are arranged with a swirling appearance, sometimes with clear cytoplasm resembling the dental lamina.

Lateral periodontal cysts should be enucleated and do not recur. If the cyst is small, the related tooth, which is vital, can be retained. However the multilocular botryoid variant has a tendency to recur.

The features are summarised in Box 10.13.

Case series PMID: 29156092

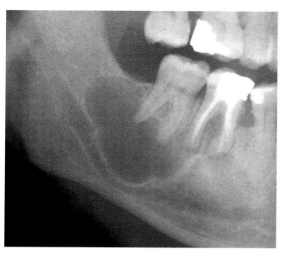

Fig. 10.40 Botryoid odontogenic cyst. There is a corticated and well-defined radiolucency with a scalloped outline as evidence of possible multilocularity but no other clue as to the cyst type.

> **Box 10.13 Key features of lateral periodontal and botryoid odontogenic cysts**
>
> **Lateral periodontal cysts**
> - Developmental cysts that form beside a vital tooth
> - Affect the mandibular premolar to canine region
> - Usually seen by chance in radiographs
> - Resemble other odontogenic cysts radiographically
> - Diagnostic histological appearance
> - Respond to enucleation
>
> **Botryoid odontogenic cysts**
> - Rare variant of lateral periodontal cyst
> - Microscopically, as lateral periodontal cyst but multilocular*
> - Tend to recur after enucleation
>
> *Multilocularity not necessarily visible in radiographs

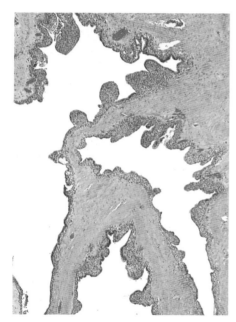

Fig. 10.41 Botryoid odontogenic cyst. A cyst with several locules and the characteristic lobular thickenings or plaques of the lining epithelium. A lateral periodontal cyst has the same appearance but a single cyst cavity.

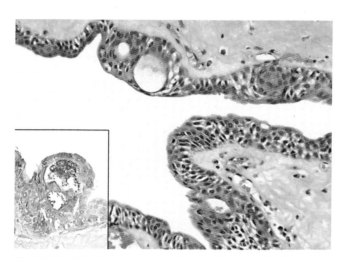

Fig. 10.42 Glandular odontogenic cyst. The epithelial lining has an occasional plaque similar to those in lateral periodontal cysts, but these contain small glands or duct-like spaces. *Inset*, glands contain mucin revealed by staining with Alcian blue and periodic acid–Schiff producing a bright blue reaction.

> **Box 10.14 Glandular odontogenic cyst**
> - Rare developmental odontogenic cyst
> - Frequently multilocular*
> - Diagnostic histological appearance
> - Has a strong tendency to recur
> - Small lesions may be enucleated with curettage
> - Large multilocular lesions are excised conservatively
>
> *Multilocularity not necessarily visible in radiographs

GLANDULAR ODONTOGENIC CYST

The glandular odontogenic cyst is a rare odontogenic cyst previously known as the *sialo-odontogenic cyst*. Glandular odontogenic cysts are diagnosed in middle-aged patients and usually in the mandible, anterior to molars. The cysts are unilocular or multilocular and expand the jaw and displace and resorb teeth.

The cyst has a diagnostic histological appearance with small glands that are lined by mucous cells and secrete mucin and lie in the thickenings of the epithelial lining (Fig. 10.42).

Approximately a third of cases recur after enucleation and additional curettage and sacrifice of teeth or conservative excision may be necessary. Clinical and radiographic misdiagnosis of multilocular examples as odontogenic keratocyst will fortuitously result in more aggressive treatment, and this is usually sufficient to prevent recurrence. The features are summarised in Box 10.14.

Systematic review PMID: 28744957

Diagnosis and recurrence PMID: 21915706

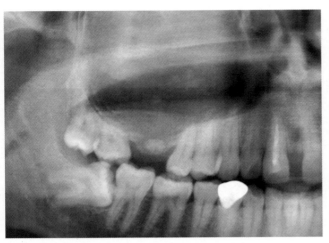

Fig. 10.43 Calcifying odontogenic cyst. This typical large corticated maxillary example is mostly radiolucent but contains some patchy mineralisation, both centrally and around the periphery, especially around the inferior margin in the first molar region.

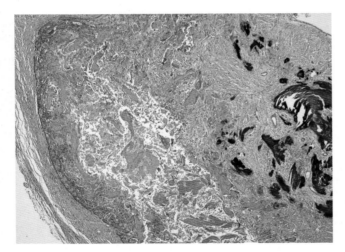

Fig. 10.44 Calcifying odontogenic cyst. The fibrous wall and dark blue-stained epithelium run vertically along the left, with the lumen filled by ghost cells (stained orange-red). Some ghost cells have become incorporated into the fibrous wall (*right*) and are calcifying (seen as very dark blue). The lumen (*centre*) is filled by ghost cells shed into the cyst cavity.

CALCIFYING ODONTOGENIC CYST

The calcifying odontogenic cyst is rare. Clinically, almost any age and either jaw can be affected. The site is most often in the bone anterior to the first molar, but occasionally, it can develop extraosseously as a small nodule on the gingiva that indents the underlying bone.

On radiographs, the appearance is usually unilocular but may be multilocular and contain flecks or, more rarely, dense masses of calcification (Fig. 10.43). Occasionally, roots of adjacent teeth are resorbed. Unless mineralisation is present, the radiographic appearances are not diagnostic.

The lining of the cyst looks like ameloblastoma (see Ch. 11) with an epithelium with cuboidal or ameloblast-like basal cells (Figs 10.44 and 10.45) and often a thick layer of stellate reticulum. The diagnostic feature is a peculiar form of abnormal keratinisation producing clusters of pale, swollen, eosinophilic cells with a hole centrally. The hole is

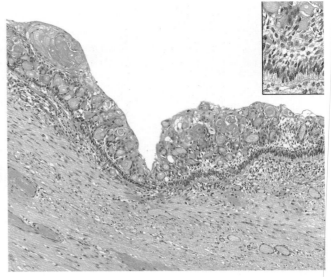

Fig. 10.45 Calcifying odontogenic cyst. The lumen (above) has a thin lining of epithelium with a basal layer of palisaded ameloblast-like columnar cells with stellate reticulum-like suprabasal cells and numerous pale-pink round ghost cells singly and in clusters. At high power (*inset*) the columnar cells show reversed polarity.

produced by degeneration and loss of the nucleus, leaving a pale 'ghost' of the cell (Fig. 10.46). The ghost cells often stack up in layers and may calcify in a patchy fashion, giving the cyst its name and producing the spotty radiopacities that give a clue to the diagnosis. Where this keratin-like material comes into contact with connective tissue, it induces a dentine-like matrix or mineralised tissue called dentinoid.

The cyst has mutations in the *CTNN1* gene, a proto-oncogene that encodes beta-catenin, an adhesion and gene transcription factor. Mutations are associated with several tumour types, and other benign and malignant odontogenic tumours that contain ghost cells.

Approximately 10% of calcifying odontogenic cysts arise in continuity with an odontome or other odontogenic tumour.

The behaviour of a calcifying odontogenic cyst is benign, and enucleation is usually effective. However very similar histological features may be found in a solid odontogenic tumour from which the calcifying odontogenic cyst must be differentiated. These solid dentinogenic ghost cell tumours (Ch. 11) have a risk of recurrence on removal, whereas the cysts usually do not.

Key features are summarised in Box 10.15.

Case series PMID: 1716354

Ghost cell lesions PMID: 18221328

CARCINOMA ARISING IN ODONTOGENIC CYSTS

Extremely rarely, a carcinoma arises from the epithelium of a cyst lining. In such cases, the cyst has usually been untreated for a long period of time. Radicular, dentigerous and odontogenic keratocysts can all undergo malignant change, and the carcinomas are usually squamous in type (Fig. 11.48). Such cases are often diagnosed only after removal but if allowed to progress, will present with the typical features of carcinoma in the jaw, patchy bone destruction, nerve signs, tooth root resorption and mobility.

Review PMID: 21689161

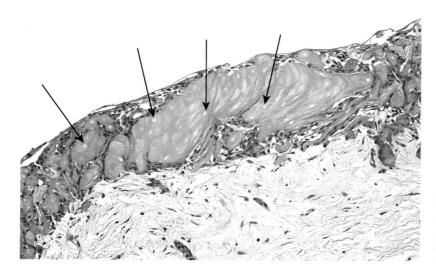

Fig. 10.46   Calcifying odontogenic cyst, the fibrous wall below, lumen above. The epithelial cells in this area are inconspicuous, the epithelium being almost replaced by numerous ghost cells. *Arrows* indicate the nuclear holes that give these cells their name.

Box 10.15   Calcifying odontogenic cyst: key features

- Rare odontogenic cyst
- Wide age range
- Radiographically unilocular often indistinguishable from other jaw cysts
- Calcifications in the cyst wall may suggest the diagnosis
- Forms at any site in the alveolar ridge, usually posteriorly
- Occasionally forms in the soft tissue of the gingiva
- Diagnosed by finding the ghost and ameloblast-like cells histologically
- Usually responds to enucleation
- Intraosseous solid lesions are distinct and more aggressive (Ch. 11)

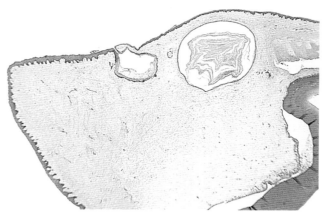

Fig. 10.47   Gingival cyst of the newborn (Bohn's nodules). This section from an embryo shows cyst formation in the rests of Serres superficial to the developing teeth. The cysts are lined by keratinising epithelium.

GINGIVAL CYST OF THE NEWBORN

Also known as Bohn's nodules, these small cysts of the dental lamina can be found in as many as 80% of newborn infants. They form small nodules on the alveolar ridge, each up to 2 mm diameter. Their whitish colour is caused by their content of keratin. They are considered to be due to the proliferation of the epithelial rests of Serres (Fig. 10.47) and can arise on the lateral aspects of the ridge and the crest. They resolve spontaneously by rupture over a few days and are of no significance but may be mistaken for natal teeth.

Incidence PMID: 21995277

Epstein's pearls

Epstein's pearls are similar to small cysts along the midpalatine raphe in the newborn. They may enlarge sufficiently to appear as creamy-coloured swellings a few millimetres in diameter but also resolve spontaneously in a matter of weeks or months.

GINGIVAL CYST OF ADULTS

Gingival cysts in adults are rare and present after the age of approximately 40 years, most often in the lower canine and premolar region. Clinically, they form dome-shaped swellings less than 1 cm in diameter and sometimes erode the underlying bone by pressure (Fig. 10.48). They are lined by very thin, flat, stratified squamous epithelium and may contain fluid or layers of keratin, and sometimes the epithelium forms plaques similar to those in lateral periodontal cysts. They do not recur on excision.

Case series PMID: 26233969 and 29156092

NON-ODONTOGENIC CYSTS

NASOPALATINE DUCT CYST

The formation of a cyst in the incisive canal is surprisingly common in some studies, accounting for around 5% of jaw cysts and making this the most common non-odontogenic cyst of the jaw. They are also known as *incisive canal cysts*.

Clinical features

These cysts arise in the incisive canal, and the presentation depends on where in the canal they form. They may form

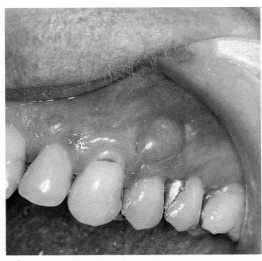

Fig. 10.48   Gingival cyst in an adult. Typical presentation as a superficial cyst in the attached gingiva of a premolar tooth.

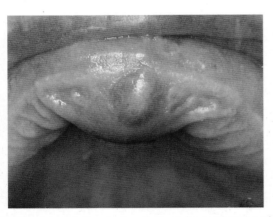

Fig. 10.49   Nasopalatine duct cyst. Typical presentation with a dome-shaped bluish enlargement overlying the incisive canal, extending forward under the incisive papilla.

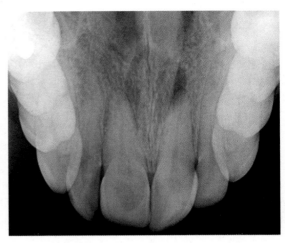

Fig. 10.50   Nasopalatine duct cyst. The usual appearance is a rounded or ovoid radiolucency at the site of the incisive canal.

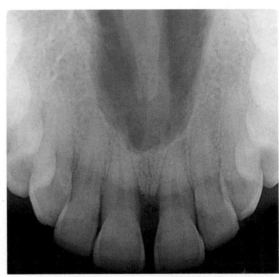

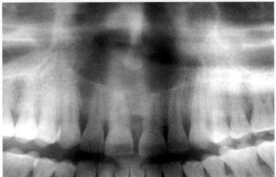

Fig. 10.51   Nasopalatine duct cyst. This example is so large that it is visible on a panoramic radiograph and extends beyond the posterior limits of an occlusal view.

a superficial soft tissue cyst in the incisive papilla if at the oral end (Fig. 10.49), grow primarily into the nose if at the superior end or grow slowly in the bone of the anterior palate if they arise in the middle. Often, they burst into the mouth or nose, producing intermittent salty discharge. Cysts from the middle of the canal expand the bone of the palate downward and upward while they grow forward, over or between the central incisor apices to expand the anterior alveolus in the midline.

Radiography shows a rounded radiolucent area with a corticated outline at the site of the incisive canal (Figs 10.50 and 10.51). In anterior occlusal or periapical films, they may appear heart-shaped because of the superimposition of the anterior nasal spine. They are usually symmetrical but become asymmetrical when large (Fig. 10.52). The root apices of the central incisors are often pushed apart.

The normal incisive canal appears as large as 10 mm in diameter radiographically because of magnification and distortion. In deciding from a radiograph whether or not an unusually large incisive canal is a cyst or not, a cut-off value of 6–8 mm is usually taken, but there is no need for immediate surgical exploration as radiographic follow-up will detect enlargement when a cyst is present.

Key features of nasopalatine duct cysts are summarised in Box 10.16.

Case series PMID: 1995816

Patent nasopalatine duct PMID: 2185448

Pathogenesis and pathology

The nasopalatine duct is an air passage between the mouth and the organ of Jacobson, a sense organ for pheromones in

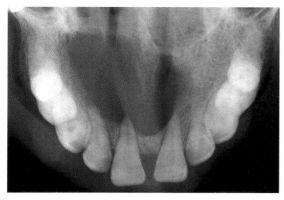

Fig 10.52 Nasopalatine duct cyst. This cyst has become asymmetrical and involves the apices of the incisors, which may suggest incorrectly that the cyst is a radicular cyst associated with a non-vital tooth.

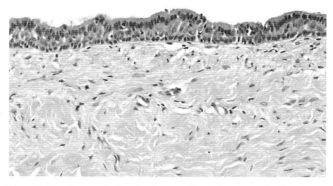

Fig. 10.53 Nasopalatine duct cyst. The lining, in part at least, may consist of respiratory (ciliated columnar) epithelium, as here.

> **Box 10.16   Nasopalatine duct cyst: key features**
> - Often asymptomatic, chance radiographic findings
> - Form in the incisive canal
> - Arise from vestiges of the embryological nasopalatine duct
> - Lined by squamous or columnar respiratory epithelium
> - The long sphenopalatine nerve and vessels in the canal may be removed with the cyst
> - Can usually be recognised radiographically
> - Do not recur after enucleation

the nasal septum of many animals, including cats and cattle. Humans have no Jacobson's organ, though the duct forms in embryos and then involutes. Remnants of the vestigial duct sometimes persist. Very occasionally a complete duct exists, dividing into two at its upper end with a canaliculus opening each side of the nasal septum. More often the duct is blind ending, or just a few islands of cells may remain in the bony canal to occasionally give rise to nasopalatine duct cysts.

The epithelial lining is usually either stratified squamous epithelium or ciliated columnar (respiratory) epithelium with mucous glands (resembling either oral or nasal mucosa, respectively; Fig. 10.53).

The long sphenopalatine nerve and vessels that pass through the incisive canal are often removed with the cyst and seen histologically (Fig. 10.54), but no noticeable deficit results.

Nasopalatine duct cysts can be enucleated without recurrence.

SURGICAL CILIATED CYST

This benign cyst, sometimes called the postoperative cyst of the maxilla, is a complication of surgery or trauma. The usual triggering events are surgery around the sinus, including the Caldwell-Luc procedure, LeFort 1 osteotomy or fracture, sinus or pre-implant surgery or surgical tooth extraction. During all these events, sinus lining epithelium can be implanted into the jaw, where it may develop into a cyst, often two or three decades later. Surgical ciliated cysts are usually diagnosed in older adults and present as an asymptomatic radiolucency or with expansion and tooth displacement.

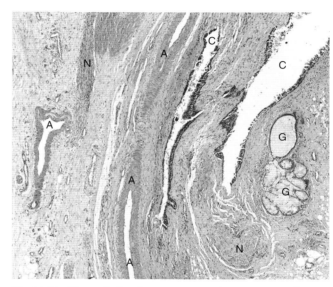

Fig. 10.54 Nasopalatine duct cyst. Surgical treatment usually removes the adjacent neurovascular bundle, which can be seen in the wall. C cyst, G glands associated with the cyst lining, A artery, N nerve.

Enucleation is curative and the cyst is lined by epithelium resembling that lining the maxillary antrum, pseudostratified with cilia and mucus-secreting goblet cells (Fig. 10.55).

Review PMID: 22310457 and 25109584

NASOLABIAL CYST

This very uncommon cyst forms outside the bone in the soft tissues, deep to the nasolabial fold. It probably arises from the lower end of the nasolacrimal duct and is occasionally bilateral. It presents over a wide age range, mostly in middle-aged adults and much more commonly in females. The cysts form soft tissue swellings in the upper lip, distort the nostril (Fig. 10.56) and cause pressure resorption of the anterior maxilla if large (Fig. 10.57).

The lining is pseudostratified columnar respiratory epithelium, like the nasolacrimal duct. The cyst is excised, usually from an intraoral approach through the labial sulcus.

Review and treatment PMID: 26153269

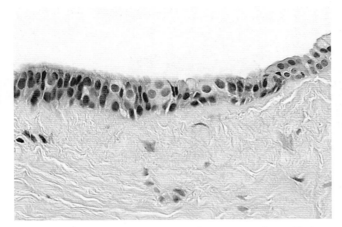

Fig 10.55 Surgical ciliated cyst. The lining is pseudostratified columnar epithelium of respiratory type.

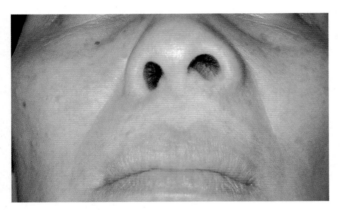

Fig. 10.56 Nasolabial cyst. Typical fullness of the nasolabial fold and in the lateral wall and floor of the nasal cavity caused by this cyst on the patient's left. *(Adapted from Yuen HW, et al. 2006. Nasolabial cysts: Clinical features, diagnosis, and treatment, Fig. 1 British Journal of Oral and Maxillofacial Surgery, 45[4], 293-297)*

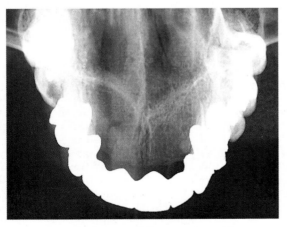

Fig. 10.57 Nasolabial cyst. A different patient with a cyst on their right, showing pressure resorption of the anterior lip of the nasal cavity, seen as asymmetry and a scooped-out concavity to the patient's right of the anterior nasal spine.

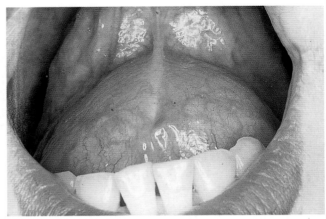

Fig. 10.58 Sublingual dermoid cyst. This is an unusually large specimen but appears even larger because the patient is raising and protruding her tongue. This cyst, unlike a ranula, can be seen to have a thick wall because it has arisen in the deeper tissues of the floor of the mouth.

SUBLINGUAL DERMOID CYST

These are cysts above the hyoid and mylohyoid, immediately beneath the tongue (Fig. 10.58), usually in the midline, occasionally to one side (Fig. 10.59). They are lined by a keratinising stratified squamous epithelium like skin, complete with associated sebaceous glands, sweat glands and sometimes hair follicles. Those without skin adnexae are called *epidermoid cysts*.

A sublingual dermoid is more deeply placed than a ranula (Ch. 22), lacks the bluish appearance and is firmer. They are asymptomatic when small, enlarge to interfere with speech or eating and can attain a large size over many years, completely concealed by the tongue in its normal resting position. Most present in the second or third decade.

These cysts are removed by excision.

Review PMID: 20392029

Case series PMID: 15018452

THYROGLOSSAL DUCT CYST

Thyroglossal or thyroglossal duct cysts develop from embryological epithelial remnants of the thyroglossal duct, anywhere along its rather convoluted path of migration from the dorsum of the tongue to the site of the thyroid gland (Fig. 10.60). The duct forms at week four *in utero* and by week eight has reached the site of the normal thyroid gland. By week ten it has involuted, leaving only occasional small nests of epithelium in approximately 10% of individuals.

Thyroglossal cysts are the commonest neck cysts, and almost all present in the area of the body of the hyoid bone, very rarely in the floor of the mouth or at the foramen caecum. Those around the hyoid bone form swellings in the midline neck skin in adolescents and young adults (Fig. 10.61). Classically the cyst rises on swallowing while the tongue moves upward.

Histologically, the cysts are lined by stratified squamous epithelium or respiratory epithelium, and there are often clusters of ectopic thyroid tissue in the wall.

These cysts are removed surgically with the body of the hyoid bone and tissue along the line of the tract down to the gland to ensure that all remnants and any ectopic gland are removed. This prevents recurrence, development of new

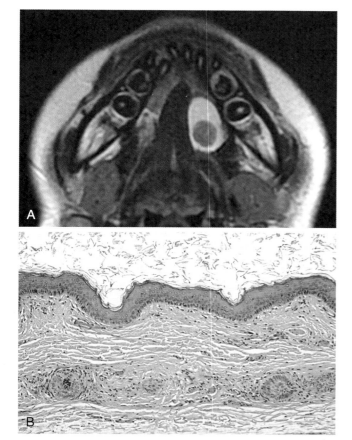

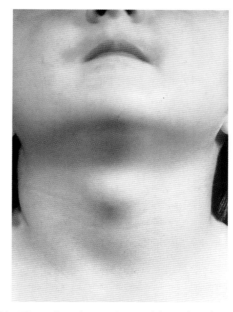

Fig. 10.61 **Thyroglossal cyst.** A typical thyroglossal cyst in the midline close to the body of the hyoid bone and just below the skin. *(From Chummy, S.S., 2011. Last's Anatomy: Regional and Applied, 12th edition. Churchill Livingstone, Edinburgh)*

Fig. 10.59 **Sublingual dermoid cyst.** In the magnetic resonance imaging scan of a different example, the fluid contents produce a bright signal showing a circumscribed cyst on one side of the floor of the mouth (A). On biopsy (B), the cyst is lined by a thin ortho-keratinising epithelium like that of the skin, and a few islands of glandular epithelium lie in the wall. The lumen is filled by keratin flakes.

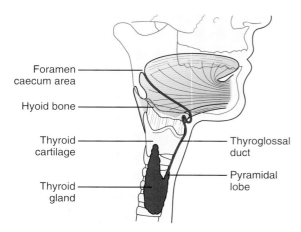

Fig. 10.60 **Path of the thyroglossal duct.** Ectopic thyroid, cysts, and occasionally thyroid carcinomas can be found anywhere along the line of the tract but are the most common where it loops below and behind the body of the hyoid. The path of the tract is convoluted in adults, but in early embryos, it is a short straight line.

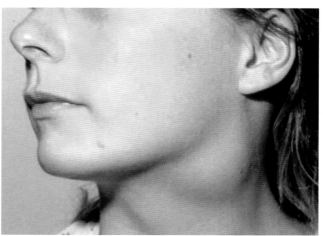

Fig. 10.62 **Branchial cyst.** A typical branchial cyst at the junction of level 2 and level 3 in the neck, and just anterior to the sternomastoid muscle. *(From Myers, E.N., 2008. Operative Otolaryngology: Head and Neck Surgery, 2nd Edition. Elsevier, Edinburgh.)*

BRANCHIAL CYST

The five pharyngeal arches develop between weeks two to six *in utero* and give rise to many structures in the head and neck. Failure of fusion of the arches can leave embryological remnants in the neck that can give rise to branchial cysts. These occur at reproducible sites. By far the most common is the second branchial arch cyst, which is visible externally at the anterior border of the sternomastoid muscle (Fig. 10.62), just below the angle of the mandible. Genuine branchial cysts, as opposed to lymphoepithelial cysts arising in lymph nodes at a similar site, extend deeply, sometimes between the branches of the carotid or even as far as the pharynx, the embryological path of the second arch cleft. Sometimes the cysts open to the skin and are then known as *branchial clefts*.

cysts and ensures the removal of all ectopic microscopic thyroid tissue, which can rarely be the site of the development of thyroid cancer.

See also lingual thyroid in Chapter 37.

Review: PMID: 25439547

Branchial cysts can attain a large size and present in adolescents or adults up to 40 years of age. They are lined by non-keratinising squamous epithelium and often have lymphoid tissue in their wall.

A branchial cyst in an adult older than 45 years would be extremely unlikely, but an identical presentation may develop when tonsil or base of tongue carcinomas metastasise to a cervical lymph node. These metastases are often cystic and can be difficult to tell from a benign cyst clinically and histologically. This is discussed further in Chapter 21.

Origin and imaging PMID: 26661849

FOREGUT CYST

These very rare cysts are developmental anomalies in children and adolescents, usually in the midline ventral tongue or floor of the mouth. The cyst is lined by gastric or other intestinal mucosa and is treated by excision. Several other hamartomas and partly cystic developmental anomalies occur in the tongue (Ch. 17).

OTHER CYSTS IN OTHER CHAPTERS

Ameloblastoma is an odontogenic tumour that can be solid or contain cysts and appear unilocular or multilocular. It may be clinically and radiologically indistinguishable from other types of cysts (Ch. 11).

Mucous retention and extravasation cysts are considered in Chapter 22.

Malignant neoplasms can arise in radicular, dentigerous and odontogenic keratocysts, though exceedingly rarely, and this topic is covered in Chapter 11.

A further group of cysts common in the head and neck are skin cysts, epidermoid and dermoid cysts ('sebaceous' cysts) arising from inflammation or trauma to the skin.

There are two bone cysts that are cystic in their radiographic appearances but lack an epithelial lining, the simple bone cyst and aneurysmal bone cyst, covered in Chapter 12.

A number of other cysts are historical concepts and are now abandoned. It is now considered that there is no such entity as a globulomaxillary cyst, median mandibular cyst or median palatal cyst.

Summary chart 10.1 Differential diagnosis of the common and important causes of a well-defined monolocular radiolucency in the jaw.

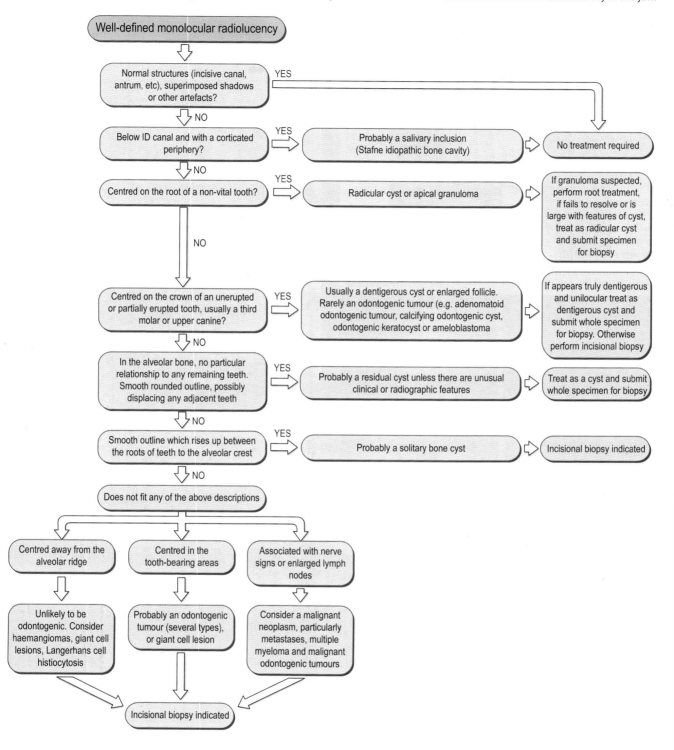

Summary chart 10.2   Differential diagnosis of a multilocular radiolucency at the angle of the mandible.

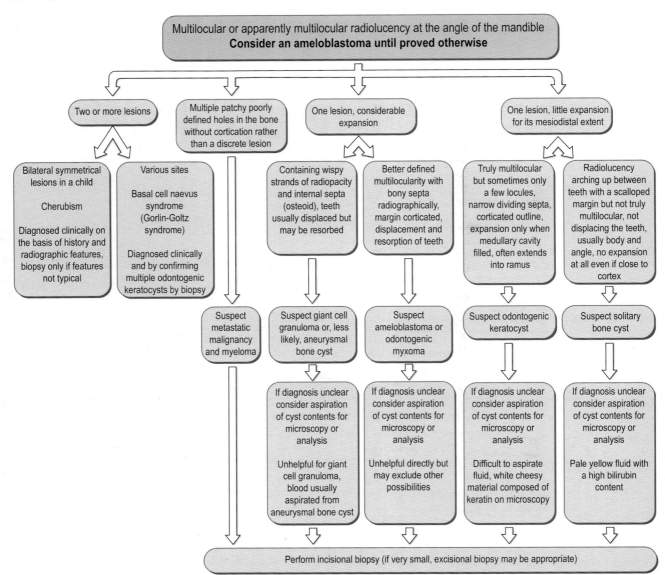

Odontogenic tumours and related jaw lesions

11

Neoplasms and other tumours affecting the jaws can be odontogenic, derived from odontogenic tissues, or non-odontogenic (Box 11.1). It is not usually obvious whether a swelling is odontogenic or not clinically. Radiology provides important clues but, in many instances, the origin and nature of a particular lesion may not be clear until biopsy.

Odontogenic tumours are the most common neoplasms of the jaws but all are considered rare. Odontogenic cysts are much more common than odontogenic tumours. There are many types of odontogenic tumour but only the odontomes and ameloblastoma are seen fairly frequently. Odontogenic tumours are derived from either odontogenic epithelium (dental lamina, reduced enamel epithelium, rests of Serres, rests of Malassez), products of odontogenic mesenchyme (dental follicle, dental papilla, pulp, periodontal ligament) or both in varying proportions. The dental follicle gives rise to the inner half of the lamina dura of the socket, so odontogenic lesions may produce tissue that resembles bone.

The accepted standard classification of odontogenic tumours is that of the World Health Organization (WHO). A simplified version of the current classification is shown in Box 11.2, and the whole classification is given in Appendix 11.1 together with brief details of the rarer lesions. It should be noted that this is a classification of *tumours* (swellings), not only of neoplasms, and it therefore includes lesions of differing types and behaviour. It is also important to realise that the nature and classification of some diseases is unclear. Therefore, the classification includes important conditions that resemble odontogenic tumours but are included in subsequent chapters. To aid understanding, the tumours are classified and listed in a simplified order here.

PATHOGENESIS OF ODONTOGENIC TUMOURS

Odontogenic tumours result from excess proliferation and abnormal development of the dental lamina and odontogenic mesenchyme. The mechanisms are early somatic (post-zygotic) genetic changes, either mutations or deletions of individual genes or chromosomal translocations that deregulate specific genes. Several genes are implicated in different odontogenic cysts and tumours as shown in Table 11.1. Though the genetics are complex, it is striking that the genetic changes tend to affect a limited number of signalling pathways that are known to be involved in tooth development.

The primary causes of these genetic changes are unknown but they are probably random spontaneous events.

The mere presence of molecular changes does not indicate whether any odontogenic cyst or tumour is either neoplastic or malignant. Some of the genetic changes found in cysts or hamartomatous odontogenic tumours are also found in neoplasms, sometimes malignant neoplasms. This apparently anomalous finding is explained by context in which the genetic changes act. A genetic change may produce different results in adult or developing tissues or when present in only some cells (mosaicism). It has already been noted in Chapter 10 that odontogenic keratocyst is caused by mutation in the *PTCH1* tumour suppressor gene, but that in odontogenic keratocyst this mutation may act via a developmental function. Similarly, the adenomatoid odontogenic tumour, which has a completely benign hamartomatous growth pattern, harbours *KRAS* mutations that are frequently found in cancers.

Molecular analysis of odontogenic tumours is still in its infancy. Although some single gene changes are associated with specific cysts or tumours but it is not yet known what additional important or modifying genetic changes might be present elsewhere in their genomes.

The genetic causes of odontogenic tumours are not esoteric science but are of considerable significance to clinicians. They are already used in diagnosis and some can be targeted with specific and highly effective drugs.

Box 11.1   Important causes of tumours (swellings) of the jaws

- Cysts, predominantly odontogenic cysts
- Odontogenic tumours
- Giant cell lesions
- Fibro-osseous lesions
- Primary (non-odontogenic) neoplasms of bone
- Metastatic neoplasms

Box 11.2   Simplified classification of commoner and more important odontogenic and jaw tumours*

Benign epithelial tumours
- Ameloblastomas
  - Ameloblastoma, conventional
  - Ameloblastoma, unicystic
  - Ameloblastoma peripheral/extraosseous
- Calcifying epithelial odontogenic tumour
- Adenomatoid odontogenic tumour

Benign mixed epithelial and mesenchymal tumours
- Ameloblastic fibroma
- Odontome (developing/compound and complex)

Benign mesenchymal tumours
- Odontogenic fibroma
- Cementoblastoma
- Cemento-ossifying fibroma
- Odontogenic myxoma / myxofibroma

Malignant neoplasms
- Ameloblastic carcinoma
- Primary intraosseous carcinoma NOS
- Odontogenic sarcomas

* For the full classification, see Appendix 11.1

Table 11.1   Genetic changes associated with odontogenic cysts and tumours

Cyst / Tumour	Molecular changes	Pathway
Calcifying odontogenic cyst*	*CTNNB1* mutation	Wnt
Odontogenic keratocyst*	*PTCH1 (or PTCH2)* mutations	SHH
Adenomatoid odontogenic tumour	*KRAS* mutations	MAPK/ERK
Squamous odontogenic tumour	? *AMBN* mutation	? Notch
Calcifying epithelial odont. tumour	?? *PTEN, CDKN2A, JAK3, MET, AMBN, PTCH1* mutation	Unclear
Ameloblastoma, conventional and unicystic	*BRAF* mutation, mostly p.V600E but also sometimes with *KRAS / NRAS / HRAS + FGFR2* mutation. Some cases in maxilla have *SMO* mutation instead	MAPK/ERK and/or SHH
Ameloblastic fibroma (Ameloblastic fibro-dentinoma and -odontoma)	*BRAF* mutation in half of cases *BRAF* mutation in two thirds and one third of cases respectively	
Odontomes	Lack *BRAF* mutation	Wnt
Cementoblastoma	*FOS* rearrangement, c-FOS overexpression	
Cemento-ossifying fibroma	Various genes in syndromes *HRPT2, GDD1.* varies in sporadic cases, but differ from other types of ossifying fibroma in other bones	Wnt
Odontogenic myxoma	Unknown	MAPK/ERK
Ameloblastic carcinoma	*BRAF* mutation, usually p.V600E	MAPK/ERK
Clear cell odontogenic carcinoma	*EWSR1:: ATF* rearrangement, less frequently *EWSR1::CREB1* or *EWSR1::CREM*	
Ghost cell odontogenic carcinoma	*CTNNB1* mutation, rarely *APC, SHH* and loss of *RB1, FHIT, PTEN, ATM* and *CHEK2*	Wnt, possibly SHH
Odontogenic sarcomas	*BRAF* p.V600E mutation in the mesenchymal component	MAPK/ERK

*see chapter 10

Mutations in odontogenic tumours need not signify neoplasia PMID: 27059373

Review molecular changes PMID: 25409852 and 35048058

WHO Classification of Tumours Editorial Board. Head and neck tumours, published by International Agency for Research on Cancer; 2022 Vol. (WHO classification of tumours series, 5th ed.; vol. 9, 978-92-832-4514-8)

BENIGN EPITHELIAL TUMOURS

AMELOBLASTOMAS → Summary chart 10.2 p. 176

Several types of ameloblastoma are recognised. All are benign epithelial neoplasms in which the epithelium contains ameloblast-like cells and stellate reticulum-like cells, indicating its odontogenic nature.

Conventional ameloblastoma

This is the most common type and the most common neoplasm in the jaws. It is also known as the solid/multicystic type. Ameloblastomas are usually first recognised between the ages of 30 and 50 years and are rare in children and old people, overall accounting for about 1% of head and neck neoplasms. There is a higher incidence in individuals of African heritage. Eighty percent form in the mandible; of these 75% develop in the posterior molar region and often involve the ramus. They are symptomless until the swelling is noticed (Fig. 11.1). Ameloblastomas can grow to enormous size and cause major disfigurement.

Practical Point Ameloblastoma should be included in the differential diagnosis for any radiolucency in the posterior alveolus and lower ramus of the mandible.

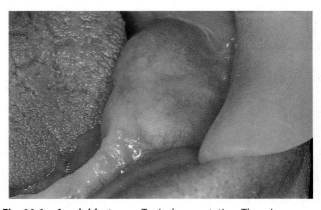

Fig. 11.1   Ameloblastoma. Typical presentation. There is a rounded, bony swelling of the posterior alveolar bone, body and angle of the mandible without ulceration.

Radiographically, ameloblastomas typically form rounded, cyst-like, radiolucent areas with well-defined margins. The smallest appear unilocular, larger ameloblastomas may comprise a few large, clustered cysts ('soap-bubble' multilocularity) or numerous small cysts a few millimetres across ('honeycomb' multilocular pattern) or a mixture of patterns (Fig. 11.2). Multilocularity is evident radiographically in about three quarters of cases and seen best in CT imaging. Expansion may be both lingual and buccal. Other multilocular lesions that may mimic ameloblastoma radiologically include odontogenic keratocyst, giant-cell granuloma and odontogenic myxoma. Ameloblastomas with a single bony cavity simulate many of the much more common types of cysts and tumours radiographically, but tooth root resorption and cortical perforation suggest ameloblastoma.

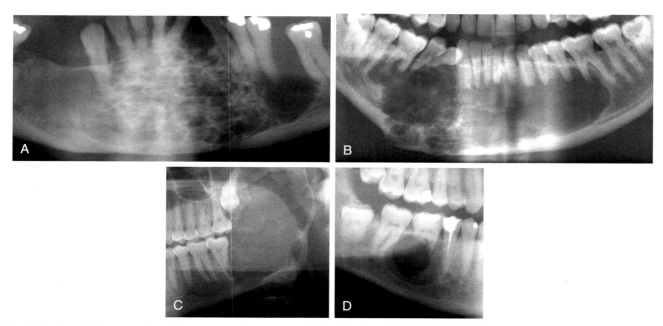

Fig. 11.2 Ameloblastoma. Four different ameloblastomas (A-D) showing the range of radiographic features, including honeycomb, multilocular, and apparently unicystic. All were typical solid/multicystic ameloblastoma on biopsy.

Pathology

The origin of conventional ameloblastoma differs with site. The majority in the mandible are caused by the *BRAF* p.V600E mutation in the Braf signalling protein gene in odontogenic epithelium, less frequently mutation in *RAS* genes or *FGFR2*. Maxillary ameloblastomas usually lack this mutation and most have mutations in the *SMO* gene, a protein in the hedgehog signalling pathway. The effect of all these mutations is to promote cell division and dysregulate differentiation. A minority of ameloblastomas have multiple genetic changes and these are more likely to recur after treatment. Perhaps counterintuitively, ameloblastomas with the *BRAF* p.V600E mutation are less likely to recur after conventional surgery than those without, and also tend to arise in younger patients.

Conventional ameloblastomas are a mixture of solid neoplasm and cysts (Fig. 11.3), and either component may predominate.

The solid areas comprise fibrous tissue containing islands or interconnected strands and sheets of epithelium with a peripheral layer of palisaded preameloblast-like cells that, at least focally, have nuclei at the opposite pole from the basement membrane (reversed polarity, a feature seen in ameloblasts just before secretion of enamel matrix). There are two histological patterns.

In the *follicular* pattern, the most common and most readily recognisable type (Fig. 11.4), there are islands with an outer layer of tall, columnar, ameloblast-like cells with reversed polarity surrounding a core of loosely arranged polyhedral or angular cells, resembling stellate reticulum (Fig. 11.5). In the *plexiform* pattern the epithelium forms strands and interconnected sheets and the ameloblast cells are often less prominent (Fig. 11.6). These two histological patterns are generally considered to be of no significance and many ameloblastomas show both, and other, patterns. The follicular type may have a slightly higher risk of recurrence after surgery.

Cyst formation is common, and there are usually several cysts as large as a few centimetres in diameter. Even apparently solid ameloblastomas contain numerous microscopic cysts. In the follicular pattern, the cysts develop in the stellate reticulum inside the epithelial islands, whereas in the

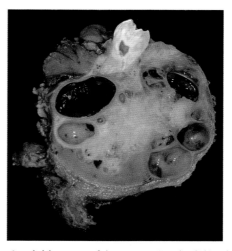

Fig. 11.3 Ameloblastoma of the conventional solid/multicystic type in a resection specimen showing multiple cysts.

plexiform pattern the cysts are caused by degeneration of the connective tissue stroma (Fig. 11.4 and 11.7).

Other less common histological variants include the *acanthomatous* type, in which prickle cells replace the stellate reticulum and sometimes form keratin (Fig. 11.8). The rare *basal cell* variant and consists of more darkly staining basal cells with little evidence of ameloblasts. In the *granular cell pattern* the epithelium in the central areas of the tumour islands degenerates into sheets of large eosinophilic granular cells (Fig. 11.9).

The most important histological feature is that islands of ameloblastoma can extend into the medullary spaces of surrounding bone. This behaviour is not expected in a benign neoplasm because it resembles infiltration by a malignant neoplasm. Only a minority of ameloblastomas have this feature, but it determines the necessary treatment. The islands of ameloblastoma may extend into bone marrow spaces for several millimetres beyond the edge of the main bony cavity. If left behind after surgery, they will seed recurrence (Fig. 11.10).

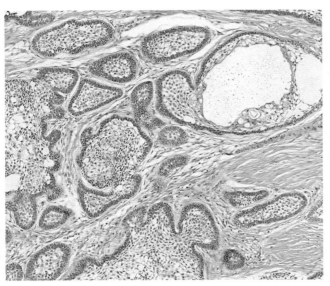

Fig. 11.4   Ameloblastoma. Islands of follicular ameloblastoma comprising 'stellate reticulum' and a peripheral layer of elongate ameloblast-like cells. The island top right shows early cyst formation in the epithelium.

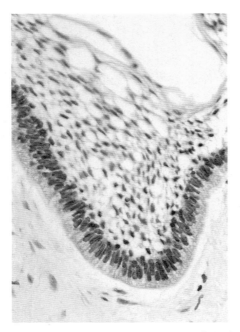

Fig. 11.5   Ameloblastoma. At high power in this follicular ameloblastoma, the palisaded, elongate peripheral cells with reversed polarity are seen to be very similar in appearance to ameloblasts.

Additional types of ameloblastoma are listed in Appendix 11.1.

Key features are shown in Box 11.3.

Extensive review PMID: 7633291

Genetic changes in ameloblastoma PMID: 24374844 and 24859340

Behaviour and treatment

Ameloblastomas enlarge the jaw slowly, displacing and often resorbing tooth roots, perforating the cortical bone and, if

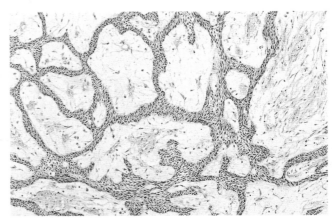

Fig. 11.6   Ameloblastoma, plexiform type. There are thin, interlacing strands of epithelium, but typical ameloblasts are often not obvious or widespread in this pattern.

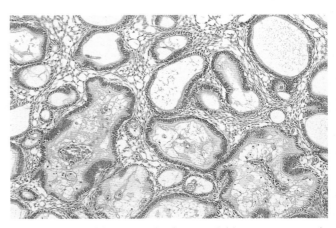

Fig. 11.7   Ameloblastoma. Plexiform ameloblastoma composed of interconnecting strands of epithelium surrounding islands of connective tissue. Several of the stromal islands have degenerated to form small cysts.

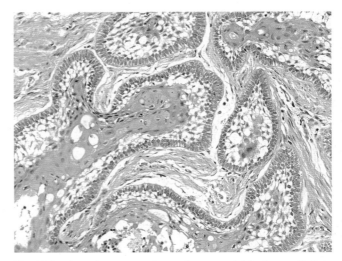

Fig. 11.8   Acanthomatous change in an ameloblastoma. Stellate reticulum-like cells have undergone squamous metaplasia to form keratin and appear red in H&E stain. This is called *acanthomatous* because it looks like prickle cells in keratinising epithelium.

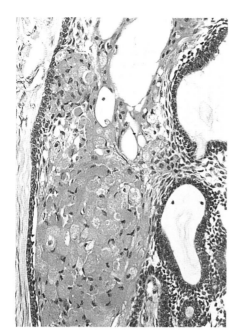

Fig. 11.9   Ameloblastoma with granular cell change. Ameloblastoma and stellate reticulum-like cells have undergone degenerative change to form large pink granular cells. In some tumours this change is extensive, and the term 'granular cell ameloblastoma' is applied.

Box 11.3   Conventional ameloblastoma: key features
- Benign neoplasm of odontogenic epithelium
- Caused by somatic mutation activating MAP kinase pathway, often in *BRAF*
- The most common odontogenic neoplasm
- Usually presents between ages 30 and 50 years
- Permeates into surrounding medullary bone
- Typically asymptomatic
- Radiographically, most present as a multilocular cyst
- Most commonly forms in posterior mandible
- Conventional definitive treatment by excision with a margin of normal bone
- Conservative removal possible for small well-circumscribed mandibular lesions
- Anti-Braf drugs shrink V660E mutation positive ameloblastomas allowing conservative surgery
- Maxillary ameloblastomas can invade the cranial base and be lethal

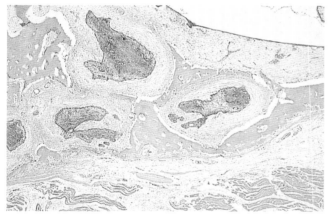

Fig. 11.10   Ameloblastoma. Islands of ameloblastoma penetrating surrounding bone at the periphery of the lesion. Such bony infiltration demands that ameloblastoma is excised with a margin rather than curetted.

large, expanding into soft tissue constrained only by the periosteum. Although benign, recurrence can make them difficult to eradicate.

The diagnosis must be confirmed by biopsy. The permeation of adjacent medullary bone previously discussed cannot usually be detected preoperatively, but if seen in a biopsy indicates a need for more aggressive surgical treatment.

Maxillary ameloblastomas are particularly dangerous, partly because the bones are considerably thinner than those of the mandible and present weak barriers to spread. Maxillary ameloblastomas tend to form in the posterior region and to grow backwards and upwards to invade the sinonasal passages, pterygomaxillary fossa, orbit and eventually the

cranium and brain. They are thus occasionally lethal despite being benign.

These occasional adverse outcomes and recurrence caused by extension of ameloblastoma into medullary bone determine treatment. The standard of care for ameloblastoma is currently wide surgical excision, preferably removing 10 mm of apparently normal bone around the margin to ensure that any medullary bone containing ameloblastoma is removed. Complete excision of a large ameloblastoma may therefore require partial resection of the jaw, often with the condyle and bone grafting. Smaller lesions may be excised, leaving the lower border of the jaw intact and extending the resection subperiosteally. Bony repair then causes much of the jaw to re-form. These extensive operations normally guarantee cure and have the advantage of completing treatment in one episode.

In recent years there has been a tendency to try to treat ameloblastoma more conservatively to avoid the morbidity of large surgical excisions, especially in adolescents. Case selection for conservative treatment is paramount. Small mandibular lesions can sometimes be enucleated, the cavity curetted and the lower border and much of the cortex preserved. Such treatment must be undertaken in the expectation that there may be recurrence. Advocates of conservative surgery point out that subsequent resection will be required only for a few recurrences and that the majority of patients will benefit. Conversely, recurrence carries risks if ameloblastoma escapes into soft tissue or extends posteriorly into the infratemporal fossa as these are potentially fatal complications. Conservative management remains somewhat controversial and requires long follow-up. Marsupialisation is ineffective, since it does not affect the solid component and because enlargement depends on tissue growth rather than hydrostatic pressure in the cysts.

A more recent and dramatic change in treatment results from discovery of the *BRAF* p.V600E mutation in some ameloblastomas because the mutation can be targeted by specific drugs. Tumour DNA is first sequenced to confirm the presence of the *BRAF* p.V600E mutation. Ameloblastomas with other *BRAF* mutations can be treated but the usual drug, Dabrafenib, is most effective on the V600E mutation. This means that mandibular ameloblastomas and those in patients at the younger end of the age spectrum are most likely to respond. Anti-Braf therapy can be applied to unicystic and conventional ameloblastoma with the appropriate mutation.

Anti-Braf treatment is still in the experimental phase but appears highly effective and is likely to become the standard of care. Currently, best evidence suggests using anti-Braf treatment in younger patients and anti-Braf with anti-MEK combination treatment in adults. Only a few months to a year of treatment will often reduce the size of an ameloblastoma significantly, up to 90% of its diameter. The bone around the ameloblastoma remodels as the tumour shrinks. Once drug treatment has produced a localised residual ameloblastoma surrounded by bone, conservative surgical enucleation is possible with minimal morbidity. Following this, recurrence seems not to occur though the follow-up period achieved so far is relatively short.

Resistance to anti-Braf drugs occurs and adverse effects, while generally mild and limited, can require cessation of the drug, but some shrinkage is usually achieved.

Whatever method is used to treat ameloblastoma, long-term regular radiographic follow-up is essential because recurrence may not appear for many years.

Key features of ameloblastomas are summarised in Box 11.3.

Literature review PMID: 7633291

Surgical treatment PMID: 16487813

Anti-Braf treatment PMID: 30208863 and 37966914

Benign but sometimes fatal PMID: 7718524

Desmoplastic ameloblastoma

The desmoplastic ameloblastoma is a distinctive histological pattern of conventional ameloblastoma, though it is not classified separately. These ameloblastomas arise with equal frequency in both jaws and often present in the anterior regions as a fine honeycomb radiolucency resembling a fibro-osseous lesion. The islands of epithelium are sparse, do not show obvious ameloblasts and the lesion is dominated by densely collagenous ('desmoplastic') tissue (Fig. 11.11) in which fine bone trabeculae can form to produce the honeycomb radiographic appearance (Fig. 11.12). Behaviour and treatment are the same as for the conventional ameloblastoma and its main significance is in radiological misdiagnosis as a fibro-osseous lesion.

Systematic review PMID: 31810564

Adenoid ameloblastoma

Adenoid ameloblastoma is a rare and recently characterised tumour with an uncertain relationship to conventional ameloblastoma. It appears to be a distinct tumour type because it is associated with *CTNNB1* rather than *BRAF* mutations and is probably related to dentinogenic ghost cell tumour and not an ameloblastoma at all. Histologically it is characterised by epithelium forming a lace-like plexiform pattern of thin strands and sheets containing whorled cellular condensations and ducts (Fig. 11.13). Clear cells and ghost cells may be minor features and ameloblasts are inconspicuous. The epithelium induces dentinoid in the connective tissue, a poorly organized mineralised tissue that may be a very dysplastic attempt to form dentine. It has been suggested that adenoid ameloblastoma behaves in a more aggressive fashion than conventional ameloblastoma, with more frequent recurrence, but this remains unproven. The name

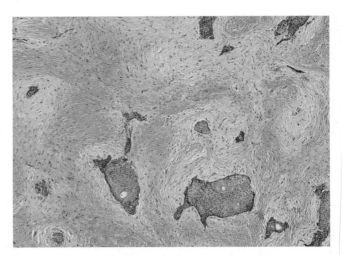

Fig. 11.11 Desmoplastic ameloblastoma. Most of the lesion is densely collagenous stroma, containing dispersed strands and spiky irregular islands of epithelium without the typical peripheral ameloblasts. Ameloblasts may be found focally, but they, and stellate reticulum, are sparse.

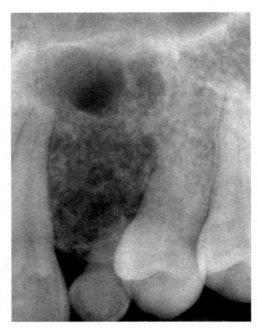

Fig. 11.12 Desmoplastic ameloblastoma. The radiographic appearance is not as radiolucent as typical conventional ameloblastoma with a fine honeycomb pattern and an indistinct margin, strongly resembling fibro-osseous lesions such as fibrous dysplasia.

and histological appearances must not be confused with adenomatoid odontogenic tumour.

Case series PMID: 26297394

Biology and behaviour PMID: 34282559 and 34549835

Metastasising ameloblastoma

This is a very rare curiosity, a histologically typical ameloblastoma which, although apparently benign, gives rise to distant metastases. The metastases are usually in the lung. Some cases appear to have resulted from aspiration and others follow surgical disruption at the primary site or repeated incomplete removal, suggesting that they result from surgical implantation into the circulation and are not truly malignant.

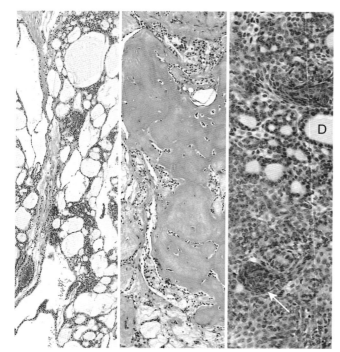

Fig. 11.13 Adenoid ameloblastoma. Left, the typical fine lace-like pattern of epithelium, centre, dentinoid and right at higher power, solid epithelium containing ducts (D) and whorled condensations (arrowed).

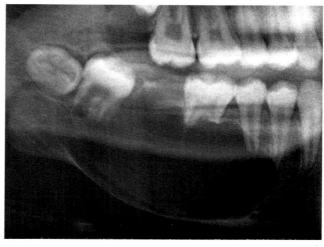

Fig. 11.14 Unicystic ameloblastoma. This ameloblastoma forms a monolocular radiolucency in a young adult, with expansion and root resorption. Its unicystic nature was confirmed after removal, but cannot be determined radiographically.

Both the primary tumour and the 'metastases' look histologically identical to conventional benign ameloblastomas, and metastasis cannot be predicted from an incisional biopsy. Because the 'metastases' are really benign, local excision of the secondary deposit(s) can be curative and patients can survive decades with disseminated disease.

Case series PMID: 20970910

Anti-Braf treatment PMID: 37966914

> **Box 11.4 Unicystic ameloblastoma: key features**
>
> - Benign neoplasm of odontogenic epithelium
> - Caused by the same genetic changes as conventional ameloblastoma
> - Single cyst cavity radiologically AND histologically
> - No solid component and no extension into surrounding bone
> - Present at a slightly younger age than conventional ameloblastoma
> - Amenable to enucleation but do sometimes recur
> - Respond to anti-Braf treatment if appropriate mutation present
> - Difficult to diagnose confidently until the entire cyst is removed

---

Unicystic ameloblastoma

➜ Summary chart 10.1 p. 175

The unicystic ameloblastoma is an ameloblastoma that has a single cyst cavity and no solid component. Such ameloblastomas present at a younger age than conventional ameloblastoma, in the second and third decades and may account for 10% of all ameloblastomas. Many present in a true dentigerous relationship to an unerupted third molar. The remainder may simulate any odontogenic cyst type depending on location but, often, suggestive features of root resorption, cortical perforation or large size may give clues to the diagnosis (Fig. 11.14).

Key features are shown in Box 11.4

In theory, the single cyst structure should mean that these ameloblastomas could be treated by simple enucleation with a low risk of recurrence. Unfortunately, making a preoperative diagnosis of unicystic ameloblastoma is difficult, and there remains controversy about exactly what constitutes a unicystic structure.

An ameloblastoma with only one bony cavity radiographically can be a conventional solid or multicystic ameloblastoma. This will not become apparent until the lesion has been opened surgically or examined histologically and the multiple cysts seen. It is therefore important to bear in mind the various configurations of an ameloblastoma that could present radiologically as a single cyst. These are shown in Fig. 11.15.

An ameloblastoma where the epithelium is limited to a single layer lining the lumen is termed a *luminal type* of unicystic ameloblastoma. If there are papillary projections into the cyst lumen, but no islands within the wall, this is termed an *intraluminal unicystic* or *plexiform unicystic ameloblastoma*. In these types, ameloblastoma epithelium is limited to the lumen or inner cyst wall and they are truly unicystic.

The danger of making this diagnosis on radiological grounds alone is shown by the third diagram in Fig. 11.15. Here a conventional ameloblastoma has developed one very large dominant cyst. However, there is a focus of solid/multicystic ameloblastoma in one area of the wall that might penetrate its full thickness or even into surrounding bone. This has been called the *mural type* of unicystic ameloblastoma, but in reality it is a conventional ameloblastoma that could easily be misdiagnosed as a unicystic one.

The histological appearances of the true unicystic ameloblastomas are similar and are shown in Fig. 11.16. The tumour cells forming the cyst wall are often flattened and easily mistaken for those of a non-neoplastic cyst.

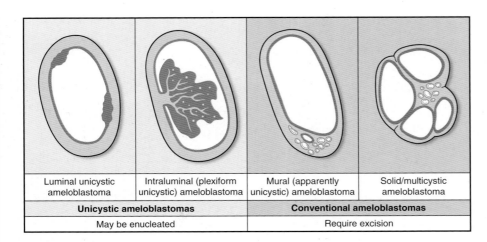

Fig. 11.15 Explanations for a radiological presentation of apparently unicystic ameloblastoma. The two patterns on the left are true unicystic ameloblastomas, whereas those on the right are conventional ameloblastomas with one or more large cysts. See the text for a further explanation of the significance.

Luminal unicystic ameloblastoma	Intraluminal (plexiform unicystic) ameloblastoma	Mural (apparently unicystic) ameloblastoma	Solid/multicystic ameloblastoma
Unicystic ameloblastomas		**Conventional ameloblastomas**	
May be enucleated		Require excision	

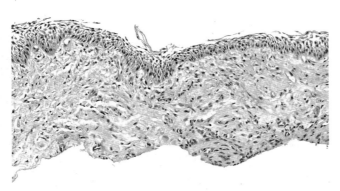

Fig. 11.16 Unicystic ameloblastoma. Part of the lining of a large unicystic ameloblastoma. The epithelium is often stretched and loses its typical features, with only a few ameloblast-like basal cells.

It has often been assumed that unicystic ameloblastomas may be enucleated without recurrence. This is sometimes true, but there are two factors that indicate that this is oversimplistic. The first factor is the difficulty in making the diagnosis preoperatively. The diagnosis can only be made confidently after removal because it requires detailed histological examination of the whole wall. A single biopsy of a stretched cyst lining is insufficient for diagnosis. In many cases unicystic ameloblastomas are not recognised before surgery and are enucleated on the assumption that they are dentigerous or other types of cysts. After diagnosis, it is usually sufficient to monitor radiographically, and most will heal without problems. Any recurrence should be treated as conventional ameloblastoma.

The second factor to consider is that unicystic ameloblastoma is biologically very similar to conventional ameloblastoma. Most carry the same activating *BRAF* p.V600E mutation and a minority *SMO* mutation. Unicystic ameloblastoma also has a recurrence rate, lower than for conventional ameloblastoma but still significant, up to 30% after simple enucleation.

The presence of *BRAF* p.V600E mutation opens the possibility of drug treatment as discussed above, and early evidence suggests that unicystic ameloblastoma responds well.

Review PMID: 9861335

Genetic changes PMID: 30216733

Surgical treatment and recurrence PMID: 16782308

Anti-Braf treatment PMID: 34599642

SQUAMOUS ODONTOGENIC TUMOUR

This rare tumour mainly affects young adults and involves the alveolar process of either jaw, close to the roots of teeth.

Radiographically, the squamous odontogenic tumour can mimic severe bone loss from periodontitis if it develops near the alveolar crest or produce a unilocular or multilocular cyst-like cavity if more deeply placed.

Histologically, it is composed of rounded islands of squamous epithelium with flattened peripheral cells (there are no elongate ameloblasts) in a fibrous stroma (Fig. 11.17). No keratin should be present in the epithelium, which may contain laminated calcifications or globular eosinophilic structures. Unfortunately, the histology is not very specific, and squamous odontogenic tumour is prone to overdiagnosis because there are histological mimics found next to cysts and in inflammatory lesions.

This tumour is benign and removed by curettage and extraction of any teeth involved.

Case and review PMID: 27632187

Review PMID: 8915020 and 29311021

CALCIFYING EPITHELIAL ODONTOGENIC TUMOUR → Summary chart 11.1 p. 185

This rare tumour, also known as a *Pindborg tumour* after its discoverer, is important because it can be mistaken for a carcinoma microscopically.

It arises over a wide age range, most frequently in middle age, usually in the posterior body of the mandible, which is twice as frequently involved as the maxilla. Presentation is either with swelling or as an asymptomatic chance radiographic finding. There is a well-defined radiolucent area initially, sometimes corticated, that may develop increasing internal radiopacity when it mineralises. Most present as a mixed radiolucency (Fig. 11.18).

Pathology

This unusual tumour sometimes resembles a carcinoma but is benign. It comprises sheets or strands of epithelial cells in fibrous tissue. The epithelial cells have a prickle cell morphology with intercellular bridges and appear very eosinophilic. In a proportion of cases, their nuclei show gross variation in nuclear size, including giant nuclei, and hyperchromatism, mimicking malignancy (Fig. 11.19). At

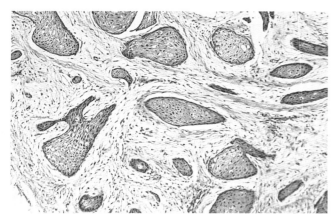

Fig. 11.17   Squamous odontogenic tumour. Islands of squamous epithelium without peripheral palisaded cells or stellate reticulum.

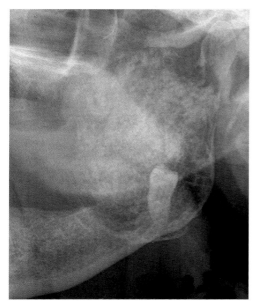

Fig. 11.18   Calcifying epithelial odontogenic tumour (Pindborg tumour). This posterior mandibular example is a mixed radiolucency.

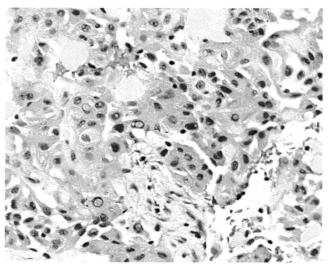

Fig. 11.19   Calcifying epithelial odontogenic tumour. At higher power the epithelial cells are eosinophilic and resemble prickle cells and sometimes have hyperchromatic and irregularly sized nuclei, often with nuclear vacuoles, as seen here. A few rounded deposits of pale pink amyloid are present.

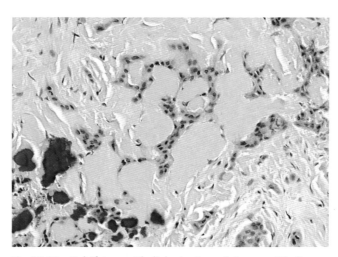

Fig. 11.20   Calcifying epithelial odontogenic tumour (Pindborg tumour). The tumour is composed of strands and sheets of polyhedral epithelial cells, in the centre with rounded deposits of secreted pale pink-staining amyloid. Toward the lower left, some of this material has mineralised, stains a darker-blue colour and gives rise to radiopacities within the lesion.

the periphery these cells can extend into adjacent medullary spaces, in a similar manner to conventional ameloblastoma, appearing to be infiltrative. Despite these alarming features, mitoses are very rare.

The diagnosis is aided by areas of amyloid deposited in the connective tissue. This amyloid material is pink, homogeneous and often mineralises, producing rounded densely mineralised masses with concentric 'Liesegang' rings (Fig 11.20). The amyloid may be sparse or a dominant feature and can be identified with Congo Red staining. It is a precipitated secretory product of the epithelial cells, a defective truncated protein called *odontogenic ameloblast-associated protein* (ODAM) that is normally found in tooth germs in small quantities, confirming the odontogenic nature of this tumour. It is the mineralisation of the amyloid that produces the dense radiopacities seen on radiographs. Because the mineralisation is dystrophic and not actively caused by the tumour cells, the amount of mineralisation is very variable. Some tumours remain completely radiolucent, most are mixed radiolucencies and some become densely radiopaque.

Calcifying epithelial odontogenic tumours extend into adjacent bone medullary spaces like ameloblastomas, and complete excision of the tumour with a border of normal bone should be curative, but recurrence will follow incomplete excision or curettage.

Key features of calcifying epithelial odontogenic tumour are summarised in Box 11.5.

Review PMID: 10889914 and 28601296

Box 11.5   Calcifying epithelial odontogenic tumour: key features

- Rare neoplasm of odontogenic epithelium
- Usually presents between ages 40 and 70 years
- Most commonly forms in posterior mandible
- Solid tumour, radiolucent, becoming a mixed radiolucency with time
- Histopathologically can resemble carcinoma
- Contains amyloid that may mineralise
- Locally infiltrative like ameloblastoma but rarely recurs
- Treated by excision with a small margin

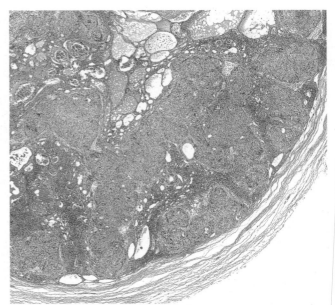

Fig. 11.22   Adenomatoid odontogenic tumour. Low magnification shows an encapsulated tumour with microcysts and convoluted ring structures of epithelium. The supporting connective tissue stroma is scanty.

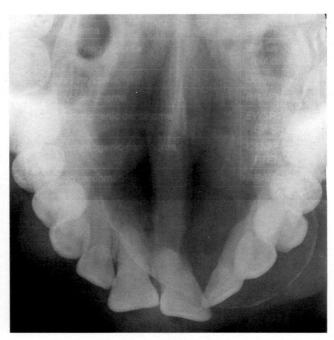

Fig. 11.21   Adenomatoid odontogenic tumour. A typical cyst-like presentation in the anterior maxilla. No mineralisation is evident in this example.

ADENOMATOID ODONTOGENIC TUMOUR

→ Summary charts 10.1 and 11.1 pp. 175 and 194

Adenomatoid odontogenic tumour is uncommon, completely benign and a hamartoma not a neoplasm. Its name comes from its histological resemblance to a gland because it contains duct-like structures.

Adenomatoid odontogenic tumours present in late adolescence or young adulthood and are more common in females than males. Most develop in the anterior maxilla and form a very slow-growing swelling resembling a dentigerous or radicular cyst (Fig. 11.21) or are chance findings in the follicle of an extracted unerupted tooth. When in the wall of a cyst, a subtle radiographic clue is fine speckled mineralisation around the wall.

Multiple tumours can occur in the very rare Schimmelpenning syndrome, with sebaceous naevi of the skin and neurological, ocular and cranial anomalies.

Pathology

Adenomatoid odontogenic tumours have mutations that activate the MAPK/ERK pathway, mostly *KRAS* p.G12V and

KRAS p.G12R. These mutations are common in malignant neoplasms but their role in this benign hamartoma remains undefined.

A well-defined capsule encloses sheets, whorls and arcading strands of epithelium, among which are microcysts, resembling ducts cut in cross-section and lined by columnar cells similar to ameloblasts (Figs 11.22 and 11.23). These microcysts may contain homogeneous eosinophilic material. Fragments of amorphous or crystalline calcification may also be seen among the sheets of epithelial cells.

Adenomatoid odontogenic tumours shell out readily, enucleation is curative and recurrence is almost unknown.

Key features of adenomatoid odontogenic tumour are summarised in Box 11.6.

Reviews PMID 22869356 and 32680811

Genetic changes PMID: 30643167

BENIGN EPITHELIAL AND MESENCHYMAL TUMOURS

The odontogenic tumours discussed so far are epithelial in origin. Those in the following section contain both odontogenic epithelium and mesenchyme and so are sometimes called 'mixed' odontogenic tumours. This allows the possibility of inductive interaction between the tissues to form matrix, enamel and dentine, though in practice this happens only in two of the four described below.

Ameloblastic fibroma

→ Summary chart 10.1 p. 175

Although rare, this tumour is important as one that is much more common in children and can be very destructive in the growing facial bones.

Ameloblastic fibromas affect young persons, usually aged 7–25 years, and usually develop in the posterior mandible. They form multi- or unilocular radiolucencies that expand

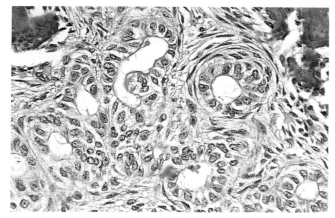

Fig. 11.23 Adenomatoid odontogenic tumour. At higher power the duct-like spaces, which give the tumour its name, are seen.

the jaw slowly and displace teeth or prevent their eruption, later perforating the cortex and resorbing tooth roots.

Pathology

Unusually, it is considered that both epithelium and connective tissue components are neoplastic. Both components may harbour the *BRAF* p.V600E mutation also found in ameloblastomas, but it is much more frequent in the epithelium than the mesenchymal component. Histologically, ameloblastic fibroma comprises interconnected strands and small islands of odontogenic epithelium in a cellular mesenchymal tissue resembling dental papilla. The epithelial strands and islands are composed of cuboidal cells where the strands are thin, but they broaden out and may have peripheral buds resembling cap stage tooth germs, though there are always only small amounts of central stellate reticulum and few peripheral elongate ameloblast-like cells and no formation of dentine or enamel (Figs 11.24).

Ameloblastic fibroma is benign and separates readily from the surrounding bone. Conservative resection is effective but, if incomplete, recurrence follows. In the maxilla, an excision margin of bone is often taken because the bones are thin and confident excision is more difficult than in the mandible. Large lesions are best treated by resection with a margin.

There is a potential for malignant change following repeated incomplete removal (see odontogenic sarcomas).

Key features are summarised in Box 11.7.

Systematic review PMID: 28776760

Genetics PMID: 32966885

AMELOBLASTIC FIBRODENTINOMA AND FIBRO-ODONTOME

When a tumour resembling an ameloblastic fibroma forms enamel and dentine, the lesion has been described as an *ameloblastic fibro-odontome*. If one forms only dentine, the term *ameloblastic fibrodentinoma* has been used.

Whether these represent distinct entities or not is highly controversial. However, it is clear that when dental hard tissue is found in this context, the most likely explanation is that the tumour is the very early stage of a developing odontome (below) and that, given time, this would become obvious as more enamel and dentine mineralized and the soft tissue components involuted, mimicking normal tooth

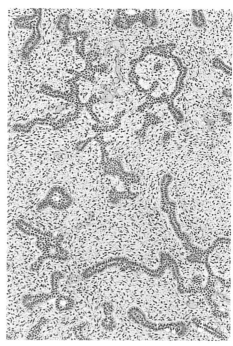

Fig. 11.24 Ameloblastic fibroma. The appearance is somewhat similar to that of ameloblastoma, but the pattern of budding strands is distinctive, and the hypercellular connective tissue resembles the undifferentiated mesenchyme of the dental papilla.

Box 11.6 Adenomatoid odontogenic tumour: key features

- Rare
- Hamartoma of odontogenic epithelium
- Usually presents between ages 15 and 30 years
- Most common in the anterior maxilla
- Often appears radiographically as a dentigerous cyst
- Encapsulated – treated by enucleation

Box 11.7 Ameloblastic fibroma: key features

- Rare
- Neoplasm of both odontogenic epithelium and mesenchyme
- Usually seen in children or young adults
- Solid lesion but appears as unilocular or multilocular radiolucency
- Treated by excision with a small margin
- Can undergo malignant change to ameloblastic sarcoma

---

development. Since the earliest stages of a developing odontome appear almost identical to ameloblastic fibroma and because odontomes are so common, this is almost always the correct explanation.

This does not mean that occasional lesions resembling ameloblastic fibroma with dental hard tissue do not exist or never behave in a neoplastic fashion, but they must be extremely rare. In order to prevent misdiagnosis and

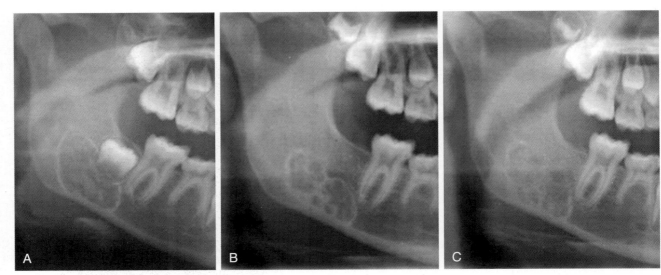

Fig. 11.25 **A developing complex odontome.** These three panoramic radiographs (A–C) were taken 2 years between each and show the progressive development and mineralisation of an odontome, which has been left in situ because of its size and close relationship to the inferior dental nerve canal. *(Courtesy Mr D Falconer.)*

overtreatment of the commoner and less significant developing odontome, these variants are now classified as developing odontomes.

Molecular analysis has revealed considerable heterogeneity in these lesions, which often contain a *BRAF* mutation, resembling ameloblastic fibroma rather than odontomes. It seems likely that reclassification will be required as a better understanding develops.

Are developing odontomes PMID: 6938886 and 24055148

Genetic analysis PMID: 32966885

PRIMORDIAL ODONTOGENIC TUMOUR

This very rare and recently described odontogenic tumour of children and adolescents produces a large expanding radiolucency in the posterior mandible and ramus. It is often associated with an unerupted tooth and then appears radiographically as a dentigerous cyst.

Histologically, the tumour resembles a giant solid mass of dental papilla with a thin layer of ameloblasts around the periphery but no odontoblasts, dentine or enamel matrix, or only very small amounts. This outer epithelial layer often folds inwards to produce a lobulated surface. The few cases reported have been treated by enucleation or conservative surgery without recurrence.

Original description and review PMID: 24807692 and 32040459

ODONTOMES (ODONTOMAS*)

➜ Summary charts 11.1 and 12.1 pp. 185, 202

Odontomes are developmental malformations (hamartomas) of dental tissues and not neoplasms. They are

---

*In the UK, the term *odontome* is traditionally used, but the international terminology is *odontoma*. Odontoma incorrectly suggests a benign neoplasm. These lesions are hamartomatous and show no progressive growth.

the most common odontogenic tumours and are chance radiographic findings or present having prevented tooth eruption in children and adolescents. In their early stages they are radiolucent, developing opaque flecks and then dense opaque masses as enamel and dentine form internally (Fig. 11.25). Occasionally they may erupt and then often become infected because of their convoluted shape and because no organised epithelial attachment can form. Most odontomes are small, a centimetre or two in diameter, but very large examples can expand the jaw and resorb tooth roots. Microscopic examples sometimes form in the follicle or normal molars, often over the crown.

Genetic analysis of odontomes in humans is hampered by their dense mineralization. Animal models and the development of multiple odontomes in patients with Gardner's syndrome (Ch. 12) implicate overactivation of Wnt signalling, known to be important in tooth development.

Case series PMID: 21840103

Review PMID: 1067549

Genetics PMID: 26411543

The two common types of odontome are compound and complex odontomes. Both are easily enucleated and do not recur. If odontomes are left untreated in the jaw, cysts of dentigerous type may form by separation of reduced enamel epithelium from enamel.

There is an ill-defined borderland between odontomes and some malformed teeth. *Dens in dente*, invaginated odontomes, tuberculate mesiodens, dilated odontomes and connate teeth are distinctive minor tooth malformations discussed in Chapter 2.

Key features of compound and complex odontomes are summarised in Box 11.8.

Compound odontome

These are clusters of many separate, small, tooth-like structures (denticles) within one crypt, the whole lesion usually no larger than 20 mm in diameter (Figs 11.26 and 11.27). This type is usually found in the anterior maxilla and causes minimal swelling.

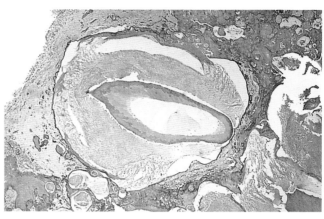

Fig. 11.28 Compound odontome. A denticle of dentine surrounded by enamel matrix is lying within more irregular calcified tissues.

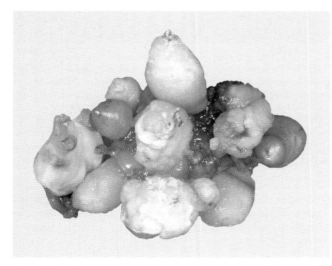

Fig. 11.26 Compound odontome. A cluster of small deformed teeth or denticles.

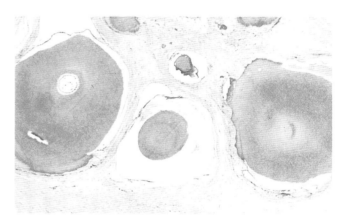

Fig. 11.29 Compound odontome. Sections from the odontome, seen in the radiograph shown in Fig. 11.27, show denticles of dentine and enamel cut in various planes, a denticle root on the left has a central pulp chamber with a rim of odontoblasts just visible.

Histologically, the denticles are embedded in fibrous connective tissue and have a fibrous capsule around the entire lesion (Figs 11.28 and 11.29). Each denticle has an organised structure with pulp centrally and an enamel cap over the abnormally shaped dentine. The denticles develop like normal teeth, mineralise fully and, once mature, stop growing.

Complex odontome

Complex odontomes consist of a single irregular mass of hard and soft dental tissues, having no morphological resemblance to a tooth and frequently forming a cauliflower-shaped disorganised nodule of enamel and dentine. These may reach several centimetres in size and often expand the jaw.

Radiographically, when calcification is complete, an irregular radiopaque mass is seen containing areas of densely radiopaque enamel (Fig. 11.30).

Histologically, the mass consists of all the dental tissues in a disordered arrangement, but frequently with a radiating structure. The pulp is usually finely branched so that the mass is perforated, like a sponge, by small branches of pulp (Fig. 11.31).

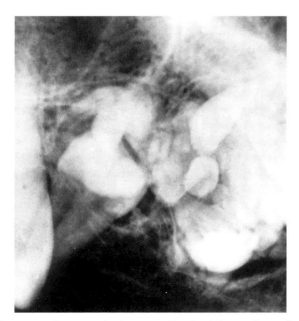

Fig. 11.27 Compound odontome. The denticles overlap each other in the radiograph but are, nevertheless, just visible as individual tooth-like structures.

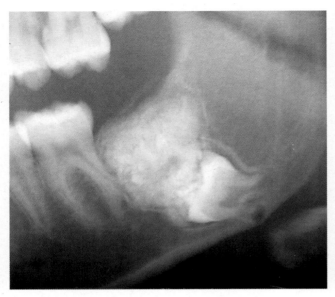

Fig. 11.30   Complex odontome. In this radiograph, the odontome overlies the crown of a buried molar and shows the typical dense amorphous area of radiopacity. Note the radiolucent rim of follicle and lamina dura of a 'crypt' extending around the lesion.

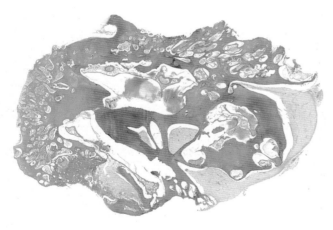

Fig. 11.31   Complex odontome. A disorganised mass of dentine, enamel and cementum penetrated by fine divisions of pulp. The apparently empty spaces were filled with enamel before decalcification to produce the section and the other spaces contain pulp with odontoblasts.

Other types of odontome

Ameloblastic fibrodentinoma and *ameloblastic fibro-odontome* were discussed with ameloblastic fibroma. As noted, they resemble the early stages of development of a complex odontome (Fig. 11.32) and have a major component of soft tissue resembling ameloblastic fibroma. Genetic analysis suggests these lesions have more in common with ameloblastic fibroma than odontomes but many eventually mature like odontomes with increasing mineralization and cessation of growth. The explanation for this apparent inconsistency is that the great majority of such lesions are probably developing odontomes while a few are true neoplasms, but classification and nature remain contentious.

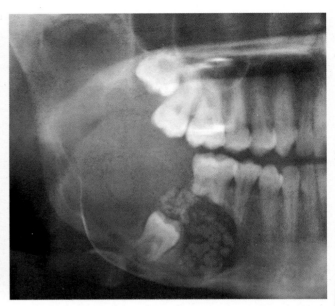

Fig. 11.32   Developing complex odontome. This large lesion has both a mineralising odontome component above and anterior to the unerupted tooth and a significant radiolucent soft tissue portion distally. The soft tissue element has the histological appearance of ameloblastic fibroma, and such lesions were previously called *ameloblastic fibro-odontome.*

CALCIFYING ODONTOGENIC CYST

→ Summary chart 11.1 p. 185

The calcifying odontogenic cyst is rare and has been considered both an odontogenic tumour and an odontogenic cyst, but it is currently classified with cysts (Ch. 10) as it rarely recurs on removal. However, it is easily confused with odontogenic tumours radiographically and histologically (Box 11.9).

DENTINOGENIC GHOST CELL TUMOUR

→ Summary charts 11.1 and 13.1 pp. 185, 222

This very rare odontogenic tumour is technically a benign neoplasm but, like ameloblastoma, infiltrates adjacent tissues and has an aggressive growth pattern. It arises most frequently posteriorly in either jaw with swelling and a mixed radiolucency with a variably well-demarcated border and often with tooth root resorption. Incidence is higher in people of Asian heritage, particularly males and individuals in middle age.

Histologically, dentinogenic ghost cell tumour appears like ameloblastoma but with additional ghost cells (see calcifying odontogenic cyst [Ch. 10]) and formation of dentinoid, or dysplastic dentine. Dentinoid is an osteoid-like material formed by the connective tissue but induced by the epithelium in a similar way to dentine (Fig. 11.33). Ghost cells are found in a spectrum of lesions from the benign calcifying odontogenic cyst, the benign but aggressive dentinogenic ghost cell tumour and the extremely rare malignant ghost cell odontogenic carcinoma. Distinction between the three is based on size, cystic or solid destructive growth, mitotic activity and cytological atypia.

Surgical excision with a margin of normal tissue is recommended because of a marked tendency to recur, even after resection and often after many years.

Box 11.9 Calcifying odontogenic cyst and dentinogenic ghost cell tumour compared

Calcifying odontogenic cyst

- Classified as a cyst not a neoplasm
- Radiographically and histologically unilocular
- Calcified ghost cells can be seen radiographically, the internal mineralisation suggesting an odontogenic tumour
- Rarely recurs after enucleation

Dentinogenic ghost cell tumour

- Benign odontogenic neoplasm but permeates medullary bone like ameloblastoma
- Solid structure
- Poorly defined border radiologically, at least focally
- Resorbs adjacent tooth roots
- Recurs frequently unless resected with a margin of surrounding bone

Features in common

- Arise in either jaw, usually posteriorly
- Ameloblastoma-like areas with ghost cells present histologically
- May induce dentinoid
- Mutations in the *CTNNB1* gene

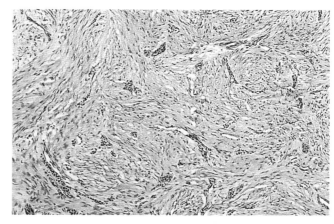

Fig. 11.34 Odontogenic fibroma. This rare mesenchymal odontogenic tumour consists of fibrous tissue containing rests and strands of odontogenic epithelium resembling those found in the periodontal ligament.

BENIGN MESENCHYMAL TUMOURS

These tumours do not contain any true mesenchyme, that is an embryonic tissue, but rather are tumours of its derivatives: the fibroblasts and osteoblasts of dental follicle, pulp, periodontal ligament and cementum.

ODONTOGENIC FIBROMA

➔ Summary chart 10.1 p. 175

The odontogenic fibroma is a benign neoplasm of fibrous tissue.

Clinically, odontogenic fibroma arises across a wide age range, more frequently affects females and the mandible and forms a slow-growing asymptomatic mass that may eventually expand the jaw. It appears as a sharply defined, rounded radiolucent area in a tooth-bearing region, displacing and later resorbing tooth roots.

Pathology

Odontogenic fibromas consist of spindle-shaped fibroblasts and bundles of whorled collagen fibres (Fig. 11.34). Some contain rests of odontogenic epithelium. These epithelial islands are not required for diagnosis; they just reflect the odontogenic origin. Occasionally epithelial islands are a prominent feature and the explanation for this is unclear. It is possible that the fibrous tissue promotes epithelial growth, but the epithelium has minimal proliferative activity. The epithelial component is important because islands may be seen in adjacent medullary bone and closely associated with, sometimes even within, adjacent nerves leading to misdiagnosis of malignancy, particularly as sclerosing odontogenic carcinoma.

A number of unusual variants have been described, including one containing prominent amyloid, a mineralising variant, one with giant cells and one with numerous Langerhans cells in the epithelium. Whether these are variants or separate tumour types remains to be determined.

Odontogenic fibromas are benign, enucleate easily from surrounding bone and do not recur.

Case series PMID: 32988809

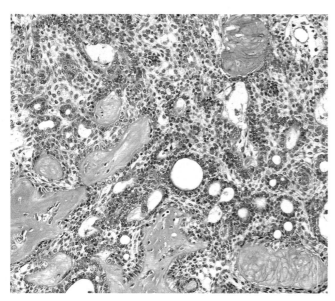

Fig. 11.33 Dentinogenic ghost cell tumour. Solid sheets of ameloblastoma-like epithelium, with stellate reticulum, two islands of ghost cells (*top and bottom right*) and irregular islands of dentinoid (*left*).

A histologically similar solid nodule on the gingiva is sometimes referred to as a peripheral variant. These have an indolent behaviour and can be simply excised without recurrence.

Key features are summarised in Box 11.9.

Ghost cell lesion spectrum PMID: 18221328

Review PMID: 26341683

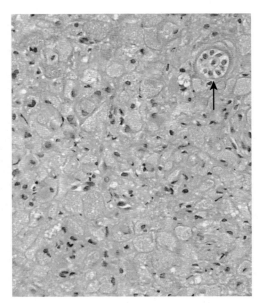

Fig. 11.35 Granular cell odontogenic tumour. There are sheets of pale, slightly grey cells with granular cytoplasm dispersed in collagen. An occasional rest of odontogenic epithelium may be found (*arrowed*), but as is the case for odontogenic fibroma, these are not required for diagnosis.

Granular cell odontogenic tumour

This odd and very rare tumour shares many features with odontogenic fibroma, but the fibroblasts become rounded and enlarged with prominent granular cytoplasm (Fig. 11.35). It is not known whether this is a degenerative change in an odontogenic fibroma or a distinct tumour type. Treatment is as for odontogenic fibroma.

Case series PMID: 12424457

ODONTOGENIC MYXOMA

→ Summary chart 10.2 p. 176

The odontogenic myxoma is a benign neoplasm, the third most common odontogenic tumour after odontomes and ameloblastoma. Most arise between the ages of 10–30 years and produce asymptomatic swellings of the jaws, usually posteriorly in the mandible.

Myxomas cause radiolucent areas with scalloped indistinct margins or a soap-bubble or honeycomb appearance (Figs 11.36 and 11.37). They displace teeth after destroying their supporting bone and are more extensive than is appreciated radiographically. Magnetic resonance imaging gives a more accurate estimation of extent because of its high water content. Expansion is usually prominent.

Pathology

This is the odontogenic tumour that most deserves the name of a mesenchymal tumour because its appearance is exactly that of the mesenchyme of the developing dental follicle and papilla. The bulk of the myxoma is loose myxoid (mucous) ground substance, containing dispersed spindle-shaped or angular fibroblasts with long, fine, anastomosing processes (Figs 11.38 and 11.39). The ground substance is hyaluronic acid and chondroitin sulphate, as in normal tissue, but excessive in amount. A few collagen fibres may also form, and more collagenous examples are sometimes called fibromyxomas. There are often small, scattered islands of

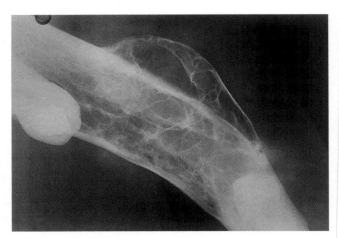

Fig. 11.36 Odontogenic myxoma. An occlusal view showing the finely trabeculated, honeycomb appearance and expansion of the mandible. Evidence of residual tumour was still present after 35 years in spite of vigorous treatment, both surgery and radiotherapy, in its earlier stages.

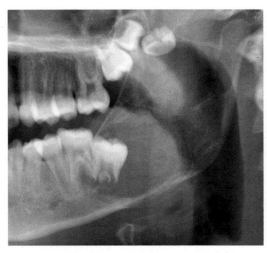

Fig. 11.37 Odontogenic myxoma. Another example from a panoramic view, this has a less honeycomb appearance, but characteristic straight septa are seen within it towards its superior margin.

odontogenic epithelium. The margins of the tumour are ill-defined, and peripheral bone is progressively resorbed.

Myxomas are benign but grow by secretion of the ground substance by the fibroblasts rather than cell proliferation. The gelatinous consistency allows the tumour tissue to permeate widely between medullary bone trabeculae without a clear margin, making removal very difficult. Excision with a margin of normal bone and removal of associated teeth is required but, despite vigorous treatment, some myxomas recur.

Key features are summarised in Box 11.10.

Radiology PMID: 9482003

Review PMID: 32506377 and 29683236

Treatment and recurrence PMID: 31551163

Normal dental follicle

The normal dental follicle resembles odontogenic myxoma histologically and sometimes shows enlargement, often on

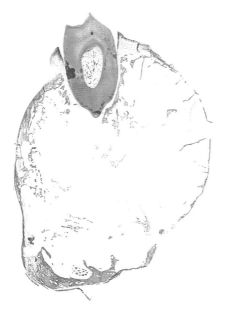

Fig. 11.38 Odontogenic myxoma. This cross-section of the mandible through a myxoma shows extensive bony resorption and gross expansion. The pale-staining myxoid lesion gives the tumour an empty appearance.

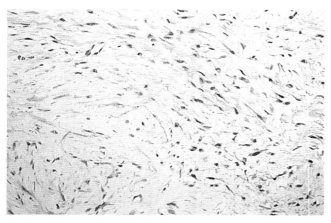

Fig. 11.39 Odontogenic myxoma. High-power view showing the typical appearance of sparse fibroblasts lying in a bluish staining myxoid ground substance-rich matrix.

> **Box 11.10 Odontogenic myxoma: key features**
> - Benign neoplasm of odontogenic myxoid fibrous tissue
> - Usually seen in young adults
> - Forms a multilocular, or honeycomb or soap-bubble radiolucency
> - Most common site is posterior mandible
> - Resembles normal dental follicle histologically
> - Treated by excision but prone to recurrence

impacted unerupted teeth ('hyperplastic follicle'). If removed on suspicion of a dentigerous cyst or other odontogenic tumour, it can be mistaken for myxoma if the pathologist is not aware of the clinical presentation. The shape, size and location are diagnostic and should prevent misdiagnosis and overtreatment.

Misdiagnosis risk PMID: 10587272

CEMENTOBLASTOMA

➔ Summary charts 11.1 and 12.1 pp. 185, 202

Cementoblastoma is a benign neoplasm of cementoblasts that forms a mass of cementum on a tooth root.

Clinically, cementoblastomas mainly affect young adults, particularly males, typically younger than 25 years of age. They are slow growing, sometimes painful and expand the jaw or are chance radiographic findings. The lower first permanent molar is the tooth that is almost always affected.

Radiographically, there is a radiopaque mass, with a thin radiolucent margin, fused to the root of a tooth (Fig. 11.40). The mass may be rounded or irregular in shape and mottled in texture. Resorption of the associated tooth root is almost always seen, but the tooth remains vital.

Pathology

Cementoblasts, though odontogenic in origin, are functionally osteoblasts and cementoblastoma has close similarity to osteoblastoma, a neoplasm of osteoblasts found in long bones and the vertebral column. Cementoblastoma and osteoblastoma both have *FOS* oncogene rearrangements and overexpress c-FOS, a transcription factor that causes osteoblast proliferation. Cementoblastoma seems to have less growth potential than osteoblastoma, even though the histopathology and genetic causes seem almost identical.

Histologically, the mass consists of cementum fused to a resorbed tooth root. The cementum often has many reversal lines, resembling Paget's disease centrally, and a radiating structure of unmineralised matrix at the periphery. The cementoblasts are larger and more darkly stained than normal osteoblasts, and often several cell layers lie on the surface of the matrix. Outside the actively growing rim is a thin fibrous capsule (Figs 11.41 and 11.42).

Cementoblastomas are benign and treated by extraction of the tooth and enucleation and curettage of the bony cavity. Recurrence is unusual, but incomplete removal leads to regrowth.

Key features are summarised in Box 11.11.

Review PMID: 28869132

Genetics PMID: 33653978

'Cementomas'

Some sources refer to a group of lesions called *cementomas*. This historic designation used to be applied to all localised cementum lesions, but it is no longer used because the causes have become better characterised and require different treatments. Current terms for 'cementomas' are shown in Box 11.12.

CEMENTO-OSSIFYING FIBROMA

➔ Summary charts 11.1 and 12.1 pp. 185, 202

The name *cemento*-osseous fibroma has recently been reinstated for this lesion to emphasise its odontogenic nature. In the past is has been classified with the ossifying fibromas of bone that arise in both the jaws and facial skeleton (Ch. 12), but the genetics and presentation and restriction to the tooth bearing parts of the jaws suggest an odontogenic origin. These lesions are presumed to originate from periodontal ligament or lamina dura bone of the socket, part of which

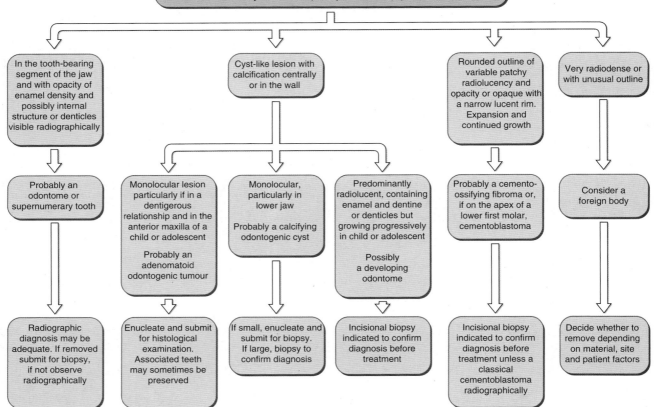

Mixed radiolucency and radiopacity with *sharply defined* periphery

In the tooth-bearing segment of the jaw and with opacity of enamel density and possibly internal structure or denticles visible radiographically

Cyst-like lesion with calcification centrally or in the wall

Rounded outline of variable patchy radiolucency and opacity or opaque with a narrow lucent rim. Expansion and continued growth

Very radiodense or with unusual outline

Probably an odontome or supernumerary tooth

Monolocular lesion particularly if in a dentigerous relationship and in the anterior maxilla of a child or adolescent

Probably an adenomatoid odontogenic tumour

Monolocular, particularly in lower jaw

Probably a calcifying odontogenic cyst

Predominantly radiolucent, containing enamel and dentine or denticles but growing progressively in child or adolescent

Possibly a developing odontome

Probably a cemento-ossifying fibroma or, if on the apex of a lower first molar, cementoblastoma

Consider a foreign body

Radiographic diagnosis may be adequate. If removed submit for biopsy, if not observe radiographically

Enucleate and submit for histological examination. Associated teeth may sometimes be preserved

If small, enucleate and submit for biopsy. If large, biopsy to confirm diagnosis

Incisional biopsy indicated to confirm diagnosis before treatment

Incisional biopsy indicated to confirm diagnosis before treatment unless a classical cementoblastoma radiographically

Decide whether to remove depending on material, site and patient factors

Summary chart 11.1   Differential diagnosis and management of sharply defined mixed radiolucencies in the jaws.

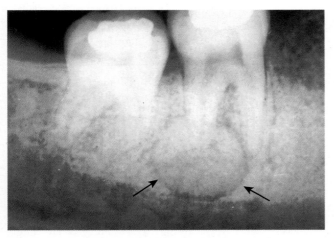

Fig. 11.40   Periapical radiograph showing the typical appearances of a cementoblastoma. A radiopaque mass with a radiolucent rim is attached to the root apex. *(Courtesy Mr E Whaites.)*

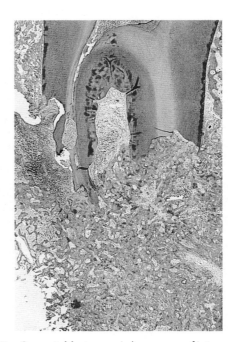

Fig. 11.41   Cementoblastoma. A dense mass of interconnected trabeculae of osteoid is fused to the resorbed roots of the first permanent molar.

is odontogenic in origin. The cemento-ossifying fibroma is one of several neoplasms and dysplasias that have a fibro-osseous appearance histologically and these other lesions (Ch. 12) need to be considered in the differential diagnosis. It is a common feature of all such lesions that clinical, radiological and histological information is required for accurate diagnosis.

Cemento-ossifying fibromas are uncommon benign neoplasms that typically cause a painless swelling in the mandibular premolar or molar region. Patients are usually between 20 and 40 years of age on diagnosis, but the range is wide. Females are affected several times more frequently than males.

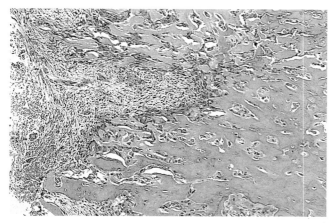

Fig. 11.42   Cementoblastoma. At high power at the periphery of the lesion there are seams of osteoid radiating from the centre of the lesion (to the right) with a thick layer of atypical cementoblasts on their surface. The capsule of the lesion is to the left.

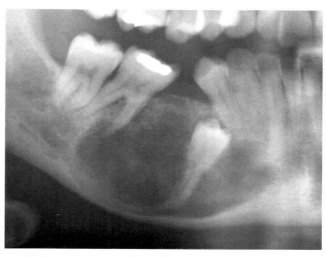

Fig. 11.43   Cemento-ossifying fibroma. The tumour forms a characteristic rounded well-circumscribed lesion radiographically. This less heavily mineralized example is cloudily radiolucent and has displaced erupted and unerupted teeth.

Box 11.11   Cementoblastoma: key features

- Benign neoplasm of cementoblasts
- Related to the long bone neoplasm osteoblastoma but less destructive
- Caused by overexpression of the c-FOS transcription factor
- Usually seen in young adults
- Most commonly at the apex of a vital lower first molar
- Fused to the resorbed root
- Radiopaque with a narrow lucent rim
- Treated by enucleation without recurrence

Box 11.12   Localised lesions of cementum

- Cementoblastoma
- Cemento-osseous dysplasia
  - Periapical form
  - Focal form
  - Florid form
  - Familial florid form
- Hypercementosis
  - Paget's disease
  - Inflammatory hypercementosis

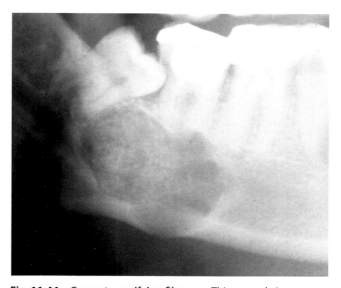

Fig. 11.44   Cemento-ossifying fibroma. This example is more densely mineralised, and the peripheral corticated margin is readily apparent.

Pathology

Being a fibro-osseous lesion, it has histological similarity to fibrous dysplasia and cemento-osseous dysplasias, and it cannot always be differentiated from them on the basis of its microscopic appearances alone. One key distinguishing feature is the well-demarcated periphery, sometimes with a fibrous capsule between the lesion and surrounding bone. Clinical and radiographic findings are required for definitive diagnosis.

The histological appearances vary widely and range from hypercellular but predominantly fibrous tumours to densely calcified masses depending on size and duration of growth. Cemento-ossifying fibromas grow slowly and mitoses are not usually seen.

Both trabeculae of woven bone with a peripheral osteoblast layer and dense rounded islands of acellular bone are seen,

Like other fibro-osseous lesions, the cemento-ossifying fibroma starts as a small radiolucency containing fibrous tissue and expands slowly. Calcification develops centrally while the lesion enlarges, initially as woven bone but eventually becoming bone that is densely calcified and radiopaque. At all stages, the lesion has a sharply defined margin, often with a thin radiolucent rim surrounded by a narrow zone of cortication. This circumscription is a key diagnostic feature and can be detected both radiographically (Figs 11.43 and 11.44) and histologically (Figs 11.45 and 11.46). Roots of related teeth can be fused to the lesion or displaced and there is localized jaw expansion, occasionally gross.

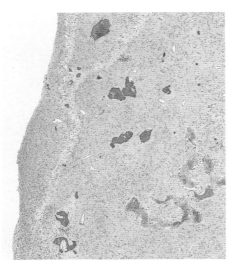

Fig. 11.45 Cemento-ossifying fibroma. This example is mostly fibrous with developing trabeculae of woven bone forming centrally, towards the bottom right. Scattered elsewhere are small densely mineralised and darkly staining islands of dense cementum-like bone. The lesion has shelled out easily and the smooth well-defined periphery is seen on the left.

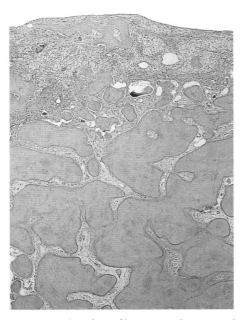

Fig. 11.46 Cemento-ossifying fibroma. In this mature lesion, there are large coalescing islands of dense bone and little fibrous tissue. Note the well-demarcated periphery of fibrous tissue which has shelled away from the adjacent bone during removal.

usually a mixture of both (see Fig. 11.45). Foci of bone grow gradually, fuse and, ultimately, form a dense mass (Fig. 11.46).

Occasional lesions develop cystic degeneration following haemorrhage, enlarge more rapidly and parts resemble aneurysmal bone cyst histologically (Ch. 12).

Management

Cemento-ossifying fibromas can usually be readily enucleated, separating from surrounding bone in the plane of their capsule. Occasionally, large tumours that have distorted the jaw require local resection and bone grafting. Recurrence is rare. Densely mineralised lesions are relatively avascular and can become a focus for chronic osteomyelitis following extraction of teeth with roots in or close to the mass.

Review PMID: 3864113 and 34184157

Treatment PMID: 27311848

Multiple and syndromic cemento-ossifying fibromas

Cemento-ossifying fibromas are found in several syndromes and these should be suspected when there is presentation in childhood, multiple cemento-osseous fibromas, or a family history of similar lesions or other bone disease. These syndromes are caused by mutations in several different genes including the *HRPT2* parafibromin gene and the same genetic alterations can also cause a minority of non-syndromic cemento-ossifying fibromas.

Causes and associated features are shown in Table 11.2. Malignant neoplasms of parathyroid gland and the possibility of renal disease are the main significant risks in the hyperparathyroidism jaw tumour syndrome. Jaw lesions in hyperparathyroidism might be expected to be brown tumours as a result of high parathormone levels (Ch. 13), but in this syndrome the jaw lesions are fibro-osseous, not giant cell lesions. The cemento-ossifying fibromas and hyperparathyroidism can arise in different relatives.

Gnathodiaphyseal dysplasia is easily misdiagnosed as osteogenesis imperfecta. Treatment of these cemento-ossifying fibromas is as for the non-syndromic type.

CDC73/HRPT2 OMIM #145001 and case report PMID: 16448924

CDC73/HRPT2 as cause PMID: 12434154

Gnathodiaphyseal dysplasia OMIM #166260 and PMID: 28176803

Table 11.2 Syndromes with cemento-ossifying fibromas

Syndrome	Cause and inheritance	Additional features
Hyperparathyroidism jaw tumour syndrome OMIM #145001	Inactivating mutation in the *CDC73*(*HRPT2*) encoding parafibromin, a tumour suppressor gene in the Wnt signalling pathway. Inherited as an autosomal dominant but with very variable phenotype and expressivity	Hyperparathyroidism caused by parathyroid adenomas or carcinomas, renal cysts, renal tumours and uterine tumours. Cemento-ossifying fibromas in both mandible and maxilla, often multiple, sometimes in childhood
Gnathodiaphyseal dysplasia OMIM #166260	Mutation in the *GDD1* (*ANO5*) gene, which encodes a transmembrane ion channel, inherited as an autosomal dominant	Presents in infants or children. Frequent bone fractures with normal healing, bowing and cortical thickening of the long bones
Familial ossifying fibroma	Unknown, possibly associated with Wnt signalling pathway	Jaw lesions only. It is possible some of these cases are mildly affected patients with the two other syndromes in this table.

MALIGNANT ODONTOGENIC TUMOURS

Malignant odontogenic tumours are very rare, and there are several histological types. A malignant equivalent exists of most of the odontogenic tumours except adenomatoid odontogenic tumour and odontome.

The malignant tumours, either carcinomas or sarcomas, can present with typical signs of malignancy, such as progressive growth of a swelling of the jaw, pain, ulceration, loosening of teeth, nerve signs and invasion beyond bone into soft tissues. However, some are low-grade, not clinically evident as malignant, and sometimes the diagnosis is not suspected until a biopsy is examined. The main significance is to be aware of their existence and be alert for minor features of malignancy in the clinical and radiographic appearance of jaw tumours: nerve signs, an indistinct moth-eaten outline and tooth root resorption.

Key learning point: Malignant neoplasms in the jaws are usually metastatic

Most arise in the posterior jaws, more frequently in the mandible. All are more common in older people.

Treatment is primarily by surgery, with radiotherapy added for incomplete excision, but recurrence and metastatic spread are relatively common.

Malignant neoplasms in the jaws are much more likely to be metastatic than odontogenic (Ch. 12). Metastases tend to develop in the bone marrow below the inferior dental canal in the mandible. The malignant odontogenic tumours usually develop above the canal in the alveolar bone or in the retromolar region.

Ameloblastic carcinoma is a carcinoma that resembles an ameloblastoma histologically, with palisaded basal cells (Fig. 11.47) and often expresses the *BRAF* p.V600E mutation seen in the benign ameloblastoma.

Primary intraosseous carcinoma is a carcinoma arising in the jaws with no resemblance to a specific odontogenic tumour. Almost all are squamous carcinomas, and approximately 40% appear to arise in odontogenic cysts, radicular, dentigerous or odontogenic keratocysts (Fig. 11.48).

Sclerosing odontogenic carcinoma is an extremely rare primary intraosseous carcinoma that induces a dense collagenous stroma and shows prominent spread along nerves. Despite this, the carcinoma is relatively indolent and has a good prognosis, with only very rare cases recurring or metastasizing. Some doubt its existence and great care is required for diagnosis, many cases appearing to be misdiagnoses, particularly of odontogenic fibroma.

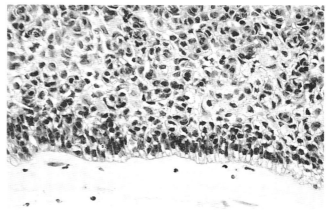

Fig. 11.47 Ameloblastic carcinoma. Very rarely a malignant variant of the ameloblastoma is encountered. Histologically, they may be indistinguishable from other carcinomas but, in some cases, as here, a peripheral layer of palisaded ameloblast-like cells remains, indicating the tumour's odontogenic nature.

Clear cell odontogenic carcinoma is a carcinoma comprising sheets and islands of cells with clear cytoplasm (Figs 11.49 and 11.50).

Ghost cell odontogenic carcinoma is a carcinoma containing scattered islands of ghost cells. It is the malignant counterpart of dentinogenic ghost cell tumour.

Ameloblastic fibrosarcoma is the rare malignant counterpart of ameloblastic fibroma. It is invasive and destructive but has little tendency to metastasise. As many as half of cases seem to develop in ameloblastic fibromas that have been repeatedly inadequately treated. In these sarcomas the epithelial component remains benign, but the dental-papilla like component becomes very cellular and atypical (Fig. 11.51). Those that contain mineralisation are known as *ameloblastic fibro-dentinosarcoma* or *odontosarcoma*, but behave similarly.

Odontogenic carcinosarcoma is extremely rare, with both epithelium and mesenchymal components being malignant. Most cases arise from pre-existing benign odontogenic tumours and are probably the result of higher grade transformation rather than genuine carcinosarcomas.

Review all types PMID: 10587275

Primary intraosseous carcinoma PMID: 33044723

Ameloblastic carcinoma PMID: 17448710 and 31444935

Clear cell carcinoma cases PMID: 26232924 and 31227275

Clear cell carcinoma translocation PMID: 23715163

Arising in cysts PMID: 21689161

Odontogenic sarcomas PMID: 10587276

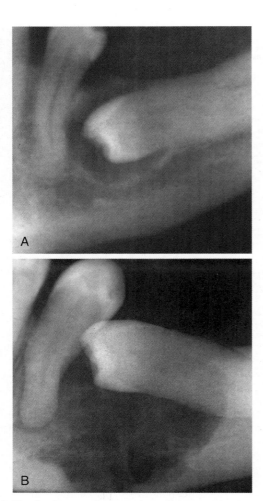

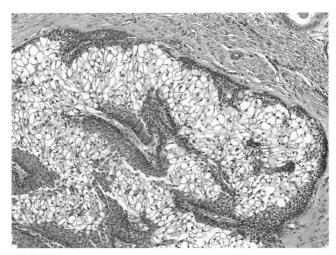

Fig. 11.50 **Clear cell odontogenic carcinoma.** This rare epithelial odontogenic tumour contains cells with vacuolated clear cytoplasm either in sheets, as here, or narrow strands.

Fig. 11.48 **A primary odontogenic carcinoma** arising in a cyst or enlarged follicle. A. initially the radiological appearance is almost benign, but with subtle erosion of the cortication around the cyst. B. Two years later the carcinoma has enlarged to destroy surrounding bone and caused a pathological fracture.

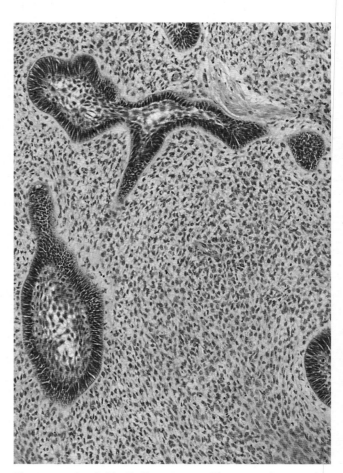

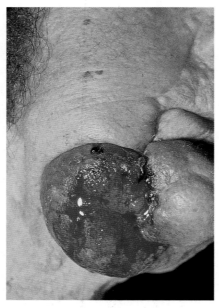

Fig. 11.49 **Clear cell odontogenic carcinoma.** This neglected tumour has fungated through the cheek.

Fig. 11.51 **Ameloblastic fibrosarcoma.** The tumour has strands and islands of epithelium with ameloblasts and stellate reticulum, as seen in ameloblastic fibroma, but the dental papilla-like mesenchymal tissue in the background is malignant, showing hypercellularity, enlarged cells and, seen only at higher power, frequent mitoses.

Appendix 11.1

World Health Organization classification of odontogenic and maxillofacial bone tumours 2022*

Name	Growth pattern†	Relative incidence‡	Notes
Odontogenic Cysts			See Ch. 10
Benign epithelial odontogenic tumours			
Adenomatoid odontogenic tumour	H	Common	
Squamous odontogenic tumour	BN	Rare	
Calcifying epithelial odontogenic tumour	BN	Rare	
Ameloblastoma, unicystic type	BN	Common	No longer includes the 'mural' type
Ameloblastoma peripheral/extraosseous type	BN	Rare	
Ameloblastoma, conventional	BN	Common	Previously called solid/multicystic type
Adenoid ameloblastoma	BN	Not yet clear	New entity in 2022 classification
Metastasizing ameloblastoma	BN	Very rare	Classification contentious (see text)
Benign mixed epithelial and mesenchymal odontogenic tumours			
Odontome (developing/compound and complex)	H	Common	Includes ameloblastic fibrodentinoma and fibro-odontome, removed from classification in 2017
Primordial odontogenic tumour	?BN or H	Very rare	New entity in 2017 classification
Ameloblastic fibroma	BN	Rare	
Dentinogenic ghost cell tumour	BN	Very rare	
Benign mesenchymal odontogenic tumours			
Odontogenic fibroma	BN	Rare	
Cementoblastoma	BN	Rare	
Cemento-ossifying fibroma	BN	Common	Reinstated as an odontogenic tumour
Odontogenic myxoma	BN	Common	
Malignant Odontogenic tumours			
Sclerosing odontogenic carcinoma	MN	Very rare	New entity in 2017 classification
Ameloblastic carcinoma	MN	Very rare	
Clear cell odontogenic carcinoma	MN	Very rare	
Ghost cell odontogenic carcinoma	MN	Very rare	
Primary intraosseous carcinoma NOS	MN	Very rare	Includes those arising in cysts
Odontogenic carcinosarcoma	MN	Very rare	
Odontogenic sarcomas	MN	Very rare	

The classification of some odontogenic tumours is contentious and will only be resolved by their genetic analysis. In the current version of the classification, tumours with more aggressive behaviour are towards the end of each section of the classification, though accurate ordering is not possible for all. In 2005 the odontogenic keratocyst was renamed keratocystic odontogenic tumour, but lack of evidence of neoplastic nature has led to reinstatement of its original name of odontogenic keratocyst and reclassification with odontogenic cysts. Similarly, the calcifying odontogenic cyst was previously called calcifying cystic odontogenic tumour.

The equivalent table for non-odontogenic tumours of the jaws and facial skeleton is at the end of Chapter 12.

* WHO Classification of Tumours Editorial Board. Head and neck tumours (ISBN 978-92-832-4514-8)
Publisher: International Agency for Research on Cancer; 2022 Vol. (WHO classification of tumours series, 5th ed.; vol. 9)
† MN malignant neoplasm; BN benign neoplasm; H hamartoma; D Dysplasia. B Borderline – benign but can infiltrate locally, R reactive, U unknown
‡ Refers to incidence in jaws and is relative. Overall, all these tumours are rare.

Non-odontogenic tumours of the jaws and facial skeleton

12

Tumours of the jaws and facial bones are conventionally divided into odontogenic, as in the previous chapter, and non-odontogenic types. This is helpful in diagnosis since odontogenic tumours only arise in the tooth-bearing parts of the jaws. However, it artificially separates clinically, radiologically or histologically similar lesions, as is seen with cemento-ossifying fibroma and other ossifying fibromas.

The exact nature of some of the diseases in this chapter remains unclear and there is no good overall classification. Some are grouped based on their histological similarities and others on radiological presentation or behaviour. In some cases, the exact diagnosis may only be determined after biopsy gives a clue as to which group a particular lesion belongs, so a histological-based grouping is logical in terms of differential diagnosis.

Some conditions that follow are exclusive to the jaws or arise there much more commonly than in other bones. Only the more important examples are considered here, classified as shown in (Box 12.1). The classification of the WHO is given in Appendix 12.1.

As noted in the previous chapter, malignant neoplasms in the jaws are much more likely to be metastatic than primary.

BENIGN MAXILLOFACIAL BONE AND CARTILAGE TUMOURS

EXOSTOSES AND TORI

These localised developmental swellings of bone are very common. They are extensions of the normal bone structure, with a surface cortical compact bone layer and, if large, a core of normal medullary bone. No clear genetic inheritance has been shown, although there is some genetic contribution to developing a torus palatinus.

A *torus mandibularis* develops on the lingual aspect of the mandible above the mylohyoid muscle and floor of mouth mucosa, usually lingual to the canine and premolars (Fig. 12.1). When small, they are smooth, but larger examples have a lobular shape and can also form a row of nodules extending back to the third molars. Mandibular tori are almost always symmetrical.

Torus palatinus commonly forms toward the posterior of the midline of the hard palate (Fig. 12.2). The swelling is rounded and symmetrical, sometimes with a midline groove or lobular surface if large. It is not usually noticed until middle age. Palatal tori tend to arise in people with larger bones and are associated with some rare sclerosing bone dysplasias, disorders of enhanced bone growth (Ch. 13).

Other small exostoses are occasionally seen, usually on the surface of the alveolar processes of the maxilla buccally (Fig. 12.3). Sometimes these are multiple and symmetrical, forming a row of nodules.

Some exostoses are acquired and probably triggered by inflammation inducing proliferation of the periosteum. Gingival exostoses may very rarely develop at the site of free gingival graft placement or on the crest of the alveolar ridge below the pontic of a bridge.

Until recently, tori have been considered insignificant, but their thin mucosal covering is prone to damage. Their prophylactic removal has been suggested to prevent medication-related osteonecrosis (Ch. 8), which develops more commonly in areas of mucosal trauma. This would only seem justified for the largest and most trauma-prone examples.

Complication free grafts: PMID: 16192951

Below bridges: PMID: 31283810

Box 12.1   Non-odontogenic tumours of jaw and facial bones.

Benign maxillofacial bone and cartilage tumours
- Exostoses and tori*
- Osteoma and dense bone island*
- Osteochondroma

Giant cell lesions of bone
- Central giant cell granuloma*
- Brown tumour of hyperparathyroidism (Ch. 13)
- Cherubism*

Bone cysts
- Simple bone cyst
- Aneurysmal bone cyst
- Cystic haemorrhagic degeneration in other tumours

Fibro-osseous neoplasms and dysplasias
- Cemento-osseous dysplasia*
- Fibrous dysplasia
- Juvenile trabecular ossifying fibroma*
- Psammomatoid ossifying fibroma*
- Familial gigantiform cementoma*

Soft tissue tumours in the jaws
- Haemangioma
- Melanotic neuroectodermal tumour of infancy*
- Ewing's sarcoma

Haematological tumours in the jaws
- Langerhans cell histiocytosis
- Myeloma
- Solitary plasmacytoma
- Lymphoma

Primary malignant maxillofacial bone and cartilage tumours
- Osteosarcoma
- Chondrosarcoma
- Intraosseous rhabdomyosarcoma*
- Metastases to the jaws

Those marked * are more common in the jaws than in other bones.

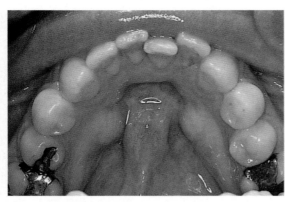

Fig. 12.1 **Mandibular tori.** The typical appearance of bilateral tori lingual to the lower premolars.

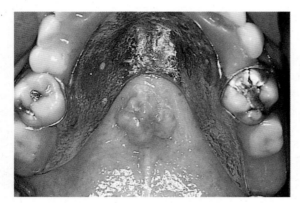

Fig. 12.2 **Torus palatinus.** Palatal tori range from small smooth elevations to lobular swellings such as this. The bone is covered by only a thin mucosa that is prone to trauma.

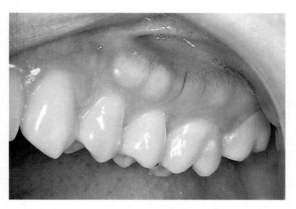

Fig. 12.3 **Exostoses.** Bony exostoses, aside from tori, are found most frequently buccally on the alveolar bone and are often symmetrically arranged.

DENSE BONE ISLANDS

These areas of sclerosis, also known as bone islands, enostoses or idiopathic osteosclerosis, are found mostly in long bones and occasionally in the jaws. They are commoner in males and often chance findings in routine, particularly panoramic, radiographs (Fig. 12.4). Though often considered normal anatomical variants they are currently thought

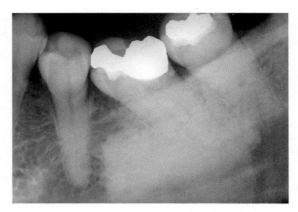

Fig. 12.4 Sclerotic bone island in the posterior mandible, a relatively dense example. The periphery may be sharply or less well-defined. *(Courtesy Mr EJ Whaites)*

to be intramedullary osteomas, benign neoplasms that show slow but progressive enlargement.

Histologically, they comprise an island of normal but dense cortical bone within the medullary cavity.

Their main clinical significance is that similar sclerotic areas of bone in the jaws are a feature of the Gardner variant of familial adenomatous polyposis, and this may need to be excluded. Dense bone islands resemble sclerosing osteitis but are not associated with a focus of infection or inflammation and should not be mistaken for a low-grade bone infection (particularly if first noticed after a surgical procedure). Otherwise, they may be mistaken for cemento-osseous dysplasia (Ch. 11). Their density slows orthodontic tooth movement.

Operative interference should be avoided. Repeat radiographic follow up will confirm the diagnosis.

Large case series PMID: 21912499

In children PMID: 33423206

OSTEOMAS

→ Summary chart 12.1 p. 202

Osteomas are benign bone neoplasms that arise on the surface of bones but, unlike tori and exostoses, grow progressively. Osteomas almost always arise in skull or facial bones and less frequently in the jaws (Fig. 12.5). The sinuses are a site of predilection. The bone in osteomas is histologically normal, but often dense.

Compact osteomas are a nodule of histologically normal bone, sometimes in parallel layers like bone cortex rather than in Haversian systems. This dense bone contains only occasional vascular spaces and grows very slowly. **Cancellous osteomas** have a peripheral cortical layer and central zone of medullary bone with marrow spaces (Figs. 12.6 and 12.7). Osteomas can be excised if they become large enough to cause symptoms or interfere with the fitting of a denture or for diagnosis.

Differential diagnosis in jaw PMID: 18602294

Review PMID: 21820784

Gardner's syndrome

Gardner's syndrome is a variant of familial adenomatous polyposis (FAP) caused by mutation in the *APC* gene and inherited as an autosomal dominant trait. The mutation carries a high risk of colon carcinoma. Only a small

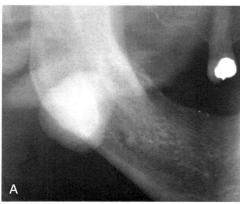

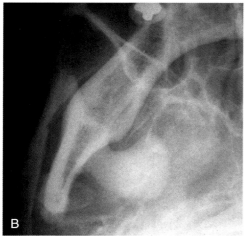

Fig. 12.5   Compact osteoma. A large mass seen on a panoramic film (A) is seen to be pedunculated from the medial aspect of the mandible in an axial computed tomography scan (B).

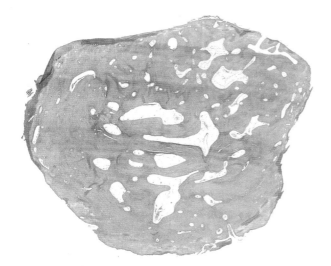

Fig. 12.6   Cancellous osteoma. A thick cortex of bone with few medullary spaces centrally, the broad dense trabeculae of bone around them contributing to an overall very dense bone nodule.

proportion of individuals with FAP have the Gardner variant with the additional signs of multiple osteomas of the jaw, fibromas and epidermal cysts, together with a range of other less frequent signs. These extra features are associated with

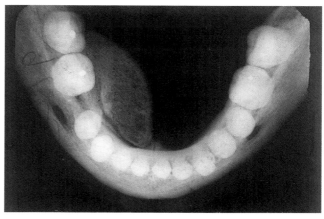

Fig. 12.7   Cancellous osteoma of the mandible. The tumour has arisen from a relatively narrow base lingually to the molars but has been moulded forward during growth by pressure of the tongue. The trabecular pattern of cancellous bone can be seen. A torus mandibularis would arise further forward on the jaw, have a broad base and does not enlarge.

mutations at specific codons in the gene. Dental features include odontomes, supernumerary teeth and sclerotic zones of bone in the jaws, in addition to the typical osteomas.

Osteomas and dental features are visible radiographically (Fig 12.8) before the colonic polyposis becomes evident in the second decade of life. Early recognition may save the life of a patient, particularly in the 30% of patients who have a spontaneous mutation and thus no family history. The dental changes, when present, are easily identified; the jaws, facial bones and skull are the most common site for osteomas. Superficial osteomas cause visible deformity, and the multiple skin cysts and nodules also often affect the face.

Genetic carriers may also have jaw osteomas.

The risk of colonic adenocarcinoma is approximately 10% by age 21 years and 95% by age 50 years, and prophylactic colectomy is indicated.

Review oral features PMID: 17577321

Treatment PMID: 20594634

Genetics supernumerary teeth PMID: 24124058

Web URL 12.1 Syndrome and genetics http://omim.org/ and enter 175100 into search box

OSTEOCHONDROMA

These are small protruding columns of bone with a core of medullary bone and a cartilaginous cap at the outer growing end. They only form at sites of endochondral ossification and so are much commoner in long bones than in the jaws, where they only arise around the mandibular condyle. Those at the anteromedial aspect of the condyle limit mouth opening or cause displacement. If located laterally, they cause a swelling over the joint. They can be detected at almost any age and are considered benign neoplasms.

Osteochondroma is characteristic radiologically and may be diagnosed with reasonable certainty on cone beam computed tomography, even though the radiolucent cartilage cap is not visible.

Diagnosis is confirmed after surgical removal. The lesion is subperiosteal and has a cap of hyaline cartilage or fibrocartilage similar to the condyle, showing normal endochondral

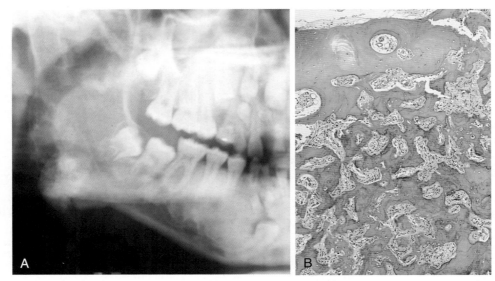

Fig. 12.8 Gardner's syndrome. A, Panoramic radiograph showing multiple unerupted supernumerary teeth and sclerotic bone areas in the jaws, the same patient as shown in Fig. 2.40. B, Patch of sclerotic bone from the maxilla covered by normal cortex.

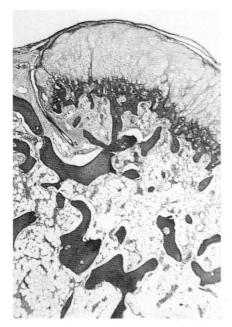

Fig. 12.9 Osteochondroma. There is a superficial cap of pale, blue-stained hyaline cartilage which undergoes endochondral ossification to form normal trabeculae of lamellar bone. The marrow spaces contain normal marrow continuous with those in the underlying bone.

ossification with vertical rows of aligned cartilage cells (Fig. 12.9). With time the mass progressively ossifies.

In the jaw, these benign bony growths grow more slowly after skeletal maturation. Removal is curative.

Cases PMID: 20346630 and 3159417

GIANT CELL LESIONS OF BONE

The giant cell lesions of bone are defined by their histological appearance, with numerous osteoclast-type multinucleate giant cells lying in a haemorrhagic stroma of mononuclear

> **Box 12.2 Differential diagnosis of the giant cell lesions of the jaws***
>
> **Giant cell lesions likely to be found in the jaws**
>
> - *Central giant cell granuloma.* Almost only develops in the jaws, usually solitary. No serological or radiographic features of hyperparathyroidism
> - *Cystic haemorrhagic degeneration* developing as a complication of fibro-osseous lesions and other vascular bone tumours
> - *Cherubism.* Lesions are multiple, symmetrical, near the angles of the mandible, family history usually present, patients have mutations in the *SH3BP2* gene
> - *Brown tumour of hyperparathyroidism.* Serum calcium levels and parathormone levels are raised (Ch. 13)
>
> **Giant cell lesions of bone that are rare in the jaws**
>
> - *Aneurysmal bone cysts* may contain many giant cells but consist predominantly of multiple blood-filled spaces, most lesions have a characteristic t(16;17) translocation
> - *Giant cell tumour of bone.* A rare benign bone tumour affecting long bones and almost never the jaws or head and neck, caused by mutation in the *H3F3A* gene
>
> **Giant cell lesions in soft tissues**
>
> - *Giant cell epulis,* a reactive hyperplastic lesion of the gingiva (Chap. 24)
> - Some soft tissue tumours elsewhere in the body such as *tenosynovial giant cell tumour,* a tumour of tendons

* Conditions in which giant cells may be found as a minor feature, such as sarcoidosis, tuberculosis and foreign body reactions, are not considered giant cell lesions. True giant cell lesions are really lesions of the mononuclear stromal cells that promote osteoclast formation through aberrant cell signalling.

cells, some of which are precursor cells that fuse to form the giant cells. The histological pattern of a giant cell lesion is seen in all the lesions shown in Box 12.2. All giant cell lesions have a dusky maroon or purplish colour clinically caused by haemorrhage within them.

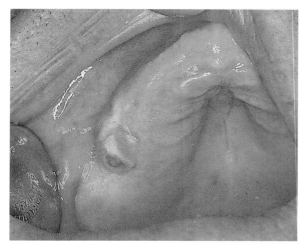

Fig. 12.10   Giant cell granuloma. This maxillary lesion has perforated the cortex and formed an ulcerated bluish soft tissue mass on the alveolar ridge. The underlying alveolar bone is considerably expanded.

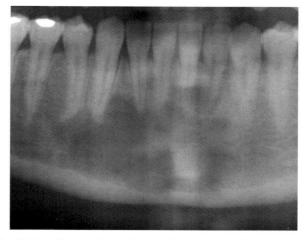

Fig. 12.11   Giant cell granuloma. Characteristic radiographic appearance of a radiolucency with scalloped margins and apparently multilocular.

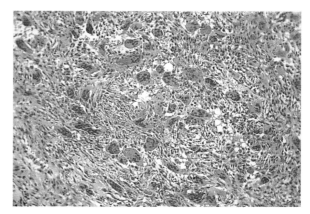

Fig. 12.12   Giant cell granuloma. This tissue is vascular and contains much extravasated blood, around which giant cells are clustered.

In small biopsy samples it may be impossible to differentiate these giant cell–rich lesions, and radiological features, blood chemistry, and sometimes genetics are necessary to make a definitive diagnosis.

CENTRAL GIANT CELL GRANULOMA

→ Summary chart 10.2 p. 176

The central giant cell granuloma is a localised benign tumour of fibrous tissue containing numerous osteoclasts that arises almost exclusively in the jaws.

Giant cell granuloma is seen in females twice as frequently as males and usually in people younger than 30 years, although there is a broad age range. Two-thirds of lesions develop in the mandible, anterior to the first molars, where the teeth have had deciduous predecessors. There is frequently only a painless swelling, but growth is sometimes rapid, and the mass can, rarely, erode through the bone, particularly of the alveolar ridge, to produce a purplish soft tissue swelling (Fig. 12.10). Lesions are typically several centimetres across.

Radiographs show a rounded cyst-like radiolucent area, often faintly loculated or with a soap-bubble or honeycomb appearance and usually at least partly corticated (Fig. 12.11). Roots of teeth can be displaced but are only occasionally resorbed.

Pathology

A giant cell granuloma is a lobulated mass of proliferating vascular connective tissue packed with osteoclast giant cells (Figs 12.12 and 12.13). The giant cells are arranged in clusters around areas of haemorrhage and deposits of haemosiderin from breakdown of erythrocytes. The lobules are separated by fibrous tissue septa, sometimes containing a thin layer of osteoid or bone, giving the lesion its characteristic faint honeycomb or multilocular appearance radiographically. Although the histological appearances are very similar to the brown tumour of hyperparathyroidism, there is no association with hyperparathyroidism.

Giant cell granuloma is caused by activation of the MAPK-pathway, caused by somatic mutations in one of the genes

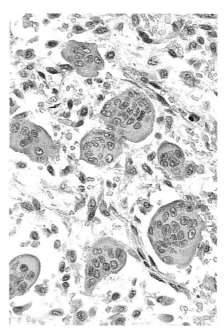

Fig. 12.13   Giant cell granuloma. High power showing the osteoclast-like giant cells with numerous, evenly dispersed nuclei.

KRAS, *FGFR1* or *TRPV4*. These induce osteoclast precursors and increase bone resorption through the parathormone pathway.

Management

Many giant cell granulomas grow slowly, and some have even been shown to resolve spontaneously. However, the majority enlarge and require removal by curettage. Approximately 15% of lesions recur, but a second curettage is usually curative.

Some granulomas enlarge rapidly, perforate the cortex, and resorb tooth roots. Such behaviour indicates a higher risk of recurrence, and the surgeon may elect to excise the lesion with surrounding bone, particularly in the maxilla and facial bones where effective curettage in thin bones is difficult to achieve. Very large lesions may require en bloc resection. In the majority of cases, complete removal is not necessary for effective treatment.

A variety of medical treatments are available that have been shown to partially control growth, and these may be used for particularly rapidly enlarging examples, when patient factors prevent immediate surgery or in children where facial growth might be affected by surgery. Injection of corticosteroids converts the lesions to fibrous tissue, usually in about three doses during several months, and calcitonin, interferon alpha and bisphosphonates all slow growth. However, residual lesion may still require surgery.

Key features are summarised in Box 12.3.

Review PMID: 29751369

Genetic basis PMID: 31705763

Noonan and other syndromes

Multiple giant cell granulomas occur in Noonan syndrome, the genetic cause of which is known to be mutation of the *PTPN11* gene or others in the RAS pathway, inherited in an autosomal dominant pattern. Patients have cardiac anomalies, short stature and learning disability and a characteristic facial appearance. Patients with the giant cell granulomas are a minority of patients who have a variant of the syndrome.

Further syndromes associated with giant cell granulomas include neurofibromatosis type 1, LEOPARD, cardiofaciocutaneous and Jaffe–Campanacci, which are also caused by mutations activating the MAPK-pathway.

Multiple histologically similar giant cell lesions in the jaws are seen in cherubism, but with a different cause and outcome.

Noonan's syndrome case and review PMID: 22848035

OMIM # 163950

PERIPHERAL GIANT CELL GRANULOMA

The peripheral giant cell granuloma is an epulis, a nodule on the gingiva, comprising a focus of tissue histologically identical to giant cell granuloma covered by normal epithelium. Despite the histological similarity, these lesions have not been previously thought to be an extraosseous type of giant cell granuloma as they often arise in inflammatory foci, do not recur on simple excision and may resolve spontaneously. This lesion has been thought to be an unrelated gingival hyperplastic lesion and better called *giant cell epulis* to avoid confusion. However, the giant cell epulis has identical *KRAS* mutations as the intraosseous giant cell granuloma, though it lacks some of the other genetic changes seen in the central type. This suggests that there is a relationship between the two types of lesions. Giant cell epulis is discussed in Chapter 24.

CHERUBISM

→ Summary chart 10.2 p. 176

Cherubism causes multiple multilocular bone lesions in the mandible and maxilla that develop in early childhood, enlarge and then regress over many years. Cherubism is caused by one of several mutations in the *SH3BP2* gene that encodes a signalling protein involved in bone turnover. It is inherited as an autosomal dominant trait.

Although a dominant condition, there may be no family history because of variable expressivity and penetrance. As a result of weaker penetrance of the trait in females, the disease is approximately twice as frequently clinically evident in males. Non-familial cases may also be new mutations. Usually, only isolated cases are encountered, but a family with 20 affected members has been reported.

Clinical features

The onset is typically between the ages of 6 months and 7 years, but rarely is delayed until late teenage or after puberty. Typically, symmetrical swellings are noticed at the age of 2–4 years in the region of the angles of the mandibles and, in severe cases, in the maxilla bilaterally. The symmetrical mandibular swellings give the face an excessively chubby appearance (Fig. 12.14). The alveolar ridges are expanded, and the mandibular swellings may sometimes be so gross lingually as to interfere with speech, swallowing or even breathing, but the rapidity and extent of growth is very variable. Erupted teeth are frequently displaced and loosened and teeth fail to develop in the affected areas of the jaws.

Maxillary involvement is uncommon and is usually associated with more severe mandibular disease. Extensive maxillary lesions cause the eyes to appear to be turned heavenward; this, together with the plumpness of the face, is the reason for these patients having been likened to cherubs. The appearance of the eyes is due to the maxillary masses pushing the floors of the orbits and eyeballs upward, exposing the sclera below the pupils. Expansion of the maxillae may also cause stretching of the skin and some retraction of the lower lids.

There is frequently cervical lymphadenopathy. This is typically seen in the early stages and may completely subside by puberty.

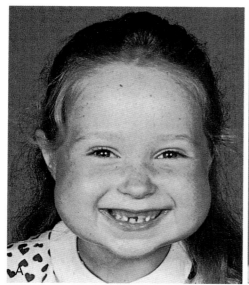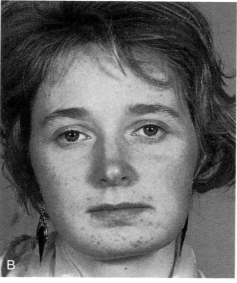

Fig. 12.14 Cherubism. The typical expansion of the mandibular rami in a child have regressed 10 years later. *(From Cawson, R.A., Binnie, W.H., Barrett, A.W., et al., 2001. Oral disease. Third ed. Mosby, St. Louis.)*

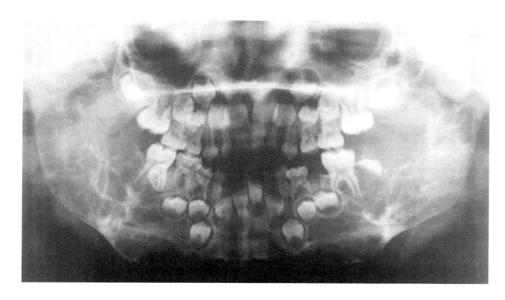

Fig. 12.15 Cherubism. Both rami, much of the body of the mandible and the posterior maxillae are expanded by multilocular radiolucent lesions that have displaced and destroyed developing teeth.

Radiology

Radiographic changes may be seen considerably earlier than clinical signs and are usually more extensive than the clinical swelling would suggest. The body and ramus of the mandible are particularly involved by large radiolucent lesions with fine bony septa producing a multilocular appearance (Fig. 12.15). Lesions often destroy the involved tooth germs, leading to missing teeth. Maxillary involvement is shown by diffuse rarefaction of the bone and extension to obliterate the sinuses. Extent is most clearly visualised by computed tomography scanning.

Pathology

The jaw lesions consist of loose fibrous tissue containing clusters of multinucleate giant cells (Fig. 12.16), overall resembling giant cell granulomas or hyperparathyroidism. With the passage of time, giant cells become fewer and there is bony repair of the defect (Fig. 12.17).

Management

Growth is rapid for a few years and then slows down until puberty is reached. There is then slow regression until, by

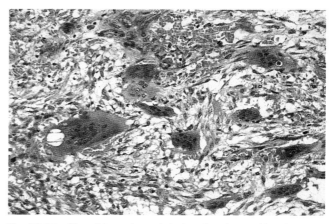

Fig. 12.16 Cherubism. An early lesion showing multinucleate giant cells lying in haemorrhagic oedematous fibrous tissue. The appearances are indistinguishable histologically from giant cell granuloma.

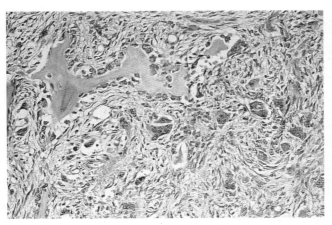

Fig. 12.17 Cherubism. In a late lesion, there is formation of woven bone by the fibrous tissue and giant cells are less numerous. Eventually bone remodelling will restore the contour and quality of the bone.

> **Box 12.4 Cherubism: key features**
> - Inherited as autosomal dominant trait caused by *SH3BP2* mutation
> - Jaw swellings appear in infancy
> - Angle regions of mandible affected symmetrically giving typical chubby face
> - Symmetrical involvement of maxillae in more severe cases
> - Radiographically, lesions appear as multilocular cysts
> - Histologically, lesions consist of giant cells in vascular connective tissue
> - Lesions regress with skeletal maturation
> - Normal facial contour recovers unless severely affected

adulthood, a typical facial contour is typically completely restored, although bone defects may persist radiographically. Severely affected patients may develop permanent facial alteration, particularly if bony support for the eye has been destroyed.

Because of natural regression of the disease, treatment can usually be avoided. If disfigurement is severe, the lesions respond to curettage or to paring down of excessive tissue. Treatment in the early stages is likely to lead to recurrence.

Key features are summarised in Box 12.4.

General review PMID: 22640403 and 32620450

Natural history PMID: 11113824

BONE CYSTS

The bone cysts produce well-defined radiolucencies in the jaws and other bones that appear cyst-like, but they lack an epithelial lining. When these lesions are detected radiologically, they are often thought to be other types of cysts and are not recognised until opened for biopsy. Whether the lack of an epithelial lining makes these lesions pseudocysts as opposed to cysts is a common but futile discussion because it depends on which definition of cyst is accepted.

SIMPLE BONE CYST

➔ Summary charts 10.1 and 10.2 pp. 175, 176

Simple bone cysts, also known as solitary bone cysts, are cavities in bones, either filled with fluid or apparently empty.

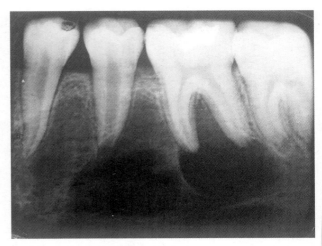

Fig. 12.18 Simple bone cyst. Typical appearance showing a moderately well-defined but non-corticated radiolucency extending up between the roots of the teeth.

Simple bone cysts are almost always single lesions and are found mostly in teenagers and individuals younger than 25 years. They are most common in long bones, usually the femur or humerus. When the jaws are affected, cavities are found almost exclusively in the mandible and in the alveolus and body rather than the ramus. Males and females are equally affected by jaw lesions and bilateral or multiple cysts are occasionally found.

Most jaw simple bone cysts are asymptomatic and are often chance radiographic findings. Approximately one-quarter of patients have a painless swelling. The vitality of adjacent teeth is not affected despite their apices extending into the cavity. The apices are sometimes superficially resorbed.

Radiographically, the cavities form rounded, radiolucent areas that tend to be less sharply defined than odontogenic cysts and have two unusual features. First, the area of radiolucency is typically much larger than the size of any swelling suggests. Second, the cavity often arches up between the roots of the teeth and may as a consequence be seen first on a bitewing radiograph (Figs 12.18 and 12.19). Cavities usually appear unilocular but larger examples, which can be as large as 10 centimetres across, may appear multilocular because of bony ridges in their walls.

Pathology

Simple bone cysts are of unknown cause but long bone, and probably jaw, simple cysts contain a chromosomal translocation involving the *NFATC2* gene. This is surprising because the same translocations are also found in some high-grade malignant sarcomas and there is no evidence from its behaviour that the simple bone cyst might even be a benign neoplasm. However, it appears that simple bone cysts in the jaws lack this specific translocation and may have other genetic changes with similar effects. There is no evidence to support the old theory that they result from injury, haemorrhage and defective repair in bone.

The cavity has a smooth bony wall with a thin connective tissue lining containing a few red cells, blood pigment or giant cells detached from the bone surface (Fig. 12.20). There are often no cyst contents, but there may sometimes be a little fluid and some fibres of collagen and fibrin. There is no epithelial lining.

Key features of simple bone cysts are summarised in Box 12.5.

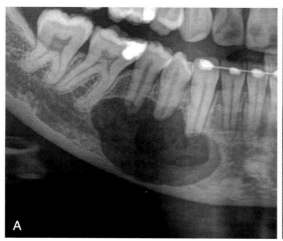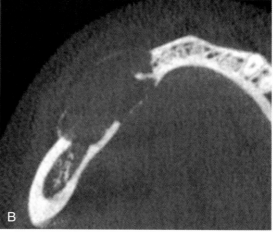

Fig. 12.19 Simple bone cyst. Panoramic radiograph (A) showing a rounded expansile radiolucent lesion with a tendency to dip up between the roots of the teeth. This example shows minor root resorption; most cause none. In axial computed tomography (B), the minimal lingual expansion and limited buccal expansion can be seen, outlined by a thin periosteal new bone layer. *(Courtesy Prof. D Baumhoer)*

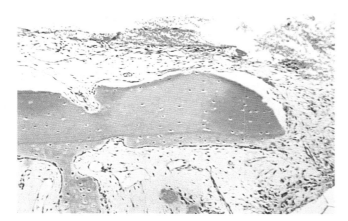

Fig. 12.20 Simple bone cyst. The scanty cyst lining comprises bone and a thin layer of fibrous tissue. Epithelium is not present, and in some cases even the fibrous lining is lacking.

Review genetic causes PMID: 34081036

Jaw lesion radiology PMID: 9503460

General Review PMID: 30792085

Management

When radiological features are typical, there may be no need for intervention, and some lesions resolve spontaneously. Biopsy plays no role in diagnosis because there is minimal tissue to sample but opening the cyst will reveal the characteristic empty cavity, and the usual treatment is light curettage to remove a sample for histological examination and to trigger bleeding and subsequent healing. Recurrence is minimal.

A radiographic change simulating simple bone cyst is seen in the osteoporotic bone marrow defect (Ch 13).

Cysts similar to simple bone cysts may develop in florid cemento-osseous dysplasia (see below).

ANEURYSMAL BONE CYST

→ Summary chart 10.2 pp. 176

Aneurysmal bone cyst is a benign neoplasm in which bone is replaced by an expansile mass of highly vascular tissue

Box 12.5 Simple bone cysts: key features

- Often chance radiographic findings
- Rarely expand the jaw
- Are of unknown aetiology but associated with genetic changes
- Have no epithelial lining. Appear empty at operation or contain pale fluid
- Arch up between tooth roots
- Histology confirms the lack of epithelial lining
- Resolve after surgical opening and closure, or occasionally spontaneously

containing clusters of giant cells. The cause is a chromosomal translocation involving the *USP6* gene, which becomes up-regulated and activates multiple signalling pathways.

Aneurysmal bone cysts are much more common in long bones; jaw lesions account for only 1%–2% of the total. The usual site is posterior body and ramus of mandible, sparing the condyle.

Most patients are between 10 and 20 years of age, and there appears to be no strong predilection for either sex. The main manifestation is usually a rapidly growing painless swelling. The name aneurysmal is given to indicate the ballooning expansion that is characteristic in long bones, similar to the shape of a dilated vascular aneurysm.

Radiographically, the radiolucent cavity may appear multilocular or be divided by faint septa (Fig. 12.21). Adjacent teeth are displaced, occasionally resorbed but vital. Extensive 'blow out' periosteal expansion with a thin cortex is usual, rather than cortical perforation. The large fluid filled vascular spaces in the lesion can be visualized on computed tomography (CT) or magnetic resonance imaging (MRI).

Key features of aneurysmal bone cysts are summarised in Box 12.6.

Pathology

How USP6 upregulation produces the lesion is unclear, possibly by triggering fibroblast proliferation, bone resorption and inflammation.

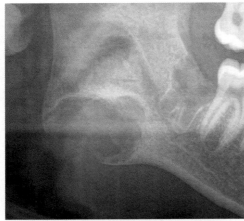

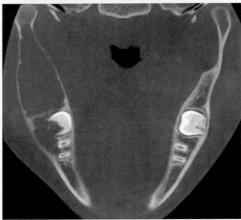

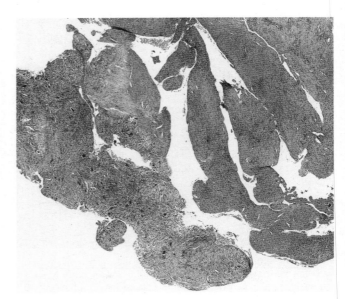

Fig. 12.22 Aneurysmal bone cyst. Strips of fibrous tissue collapsed together after loss of blood from the intervening spaces, with giant cells seen as small dark dots in the tissue lower left.

Fig 12.21 Aneurysmal bone cyst. Two different examples, both of which contained the diagnostic *USP6* translocation, showing the range of radiological appearances. The panoramic radiograph shows a localized but very expansile osteolytic lesion with a scalloped outline, cortical perforation and peripheral bone sclerosis. The lesion in the axial CT has filled and expanded the posterior body and ramus of the mandible in a more diffuse fashion. *(Courtesy Prof. D Baumhoer)*

Box 12.6 Aneurysmal bone cyst: key features

- Benign neoplasm caused by upregulation of *USP6* gene
- Rare in the jaws
- Jaw lesions are usually in the mandibular ramus and angle
- Affects patients usually between 10 and 20 years of age
- Form very expansile soap-bubble radiolucencies
- Histologically, consist of a mass of blood-filled spaces with scattered giant cells
- Are treated by curettage but sometimes recur
- Radiologically and histologically similar lesions associated with fibro-osseous and other lesions are thought to arise from cystic haemorrhagic degeneration and are not true aneurysmal bone cysts

---

Histologically, there is a highly cellular mass of cavernous blood-filled spaces without an endothelial lining. When seen at operation, the appearance has been likened to a blood-filled sponge (Fig. 12.22). The spaces are separated by fibrous septa formed by the causative fibroblasts. However,

the histology is dominated by other cell types without the genetic changes: osteoclast-type giant cells and osteoblasts that form osteoid and woven bone. These other cells cluster in the fibrous tissue and are presumably attracted by cytokines, haemorrhage or inflammation.

Biopsy is necessary for diagnosis. Detecting the genetic changes is not usually necessary for diagnosis but may be helpful in difficult cases or to differentiate aneurysmal bone cyst from giant cell granuloma or cystic haemorrhagic degeneration in other tumours.

Treatment consists of thorough curettage, which may need to be repeated because the lesion recurs in approximately 20% of cases. Very large examples may require resection.

Case series PMID: 24931106 and 19233862

CYSTIC HAEMORRHAGIC DEGENERATION IN OTHER TUMOURS

Some jaw lesions, notably fibro-osseous lesions and giant cell lesions and osteoblastomas may develop expansile vascular cystic changes that closely resemble aneurysmal bone cyst. Fibrous dysplasia, ossifying fibromas and giant cell granulomas are particularly prone. Cystic haemorrhagic degeneration may be just as expansile as true aneurysmal bone cyst and reach a very large size but is more easily treated without recurrence (Fig. 12.23).

These cysts lack the genetic translocations of aneurysmal bone cyst but have almost identical radiographic and histological features. Prior to the discovery of the aneurysmal bone cyst genetic translocation, such cysts were called 'secondary' aneurysmal bone cysts. Lacking the genetic changes, this secondary change is now ascribed to haemorrhage (most of the associated lesions are very vascular) but evidence of their true cause and nature is lacking. These apparently secondary lesions are far commoner than true aneurysmal bone cysts in the jaws, accounting for almost all cases. The histopathological features are very similar to the true aneurysmal bone cyst and the thin fibrous septa may contain foci of the associated fibro-osseous or giant cell lesion (Fig 12.24).

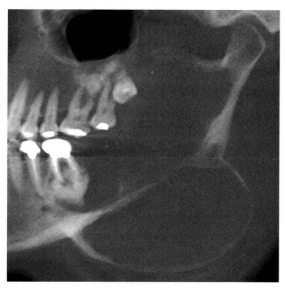

Fig. 12.23   Secondary cystic haemorrhagic degeneration resembling aneurysmal bone cyst. Part of a panoramic radiograph showing an expansile radiolucency with faint internal septa. The sclerotic bone masses associated with the molar tooth apices show that the cysts have arisen as an element of florid cemento-osseous dysplasia.

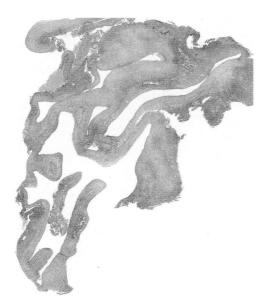

Fig 12.24   Secondary cystic haemorrhagic degeneration. The features are indistinguishable from aneurysmal bone cyst, a sponge-like cluster of large spaces, in life filled with blood, separated by fibrous septa that contain occasional giant cells or fibro-osseous tissue. See also Fig. 12.22.

Florid cemento-osseous dysplasia is prone to develop another different type of secondary cystic change that resembles simple bone cyst (see below).

Different cause PMID: 15509545

Box 12.7   Fibro-osseous lesions of the head and neck

Fibrous dysplasia
- Monostotic, polyostotic and Albright's syndrome

Cemento-osseous dysplasias
- Periapical, focal, florid and familial florid cemento-osseous dysplasia

Fibro-osseous neoplasms
- Cemento-ossifying fibroma, solitary and syndromic (Ch. 11)
- Ossifying fibroma, juvenile trabecular and psammomatoid types

Proliferative periostitis (Ch. 8)

FIBRO-OSSEOUS NEOPLASMS AND DYSPLASIAS

A fibro-osseous lesion is one in which bone is replaced by a mass of cellular fibrous tissue that grows and then gradually matures back to bone. The degree of maturation varies between diseases and takes many months or years. Sometimes the maturation never proceeds beyond woven bone, or the woven bone may mature further to disorganised lamellar bone or very dense sclerotic amorphous mineralisation. Fibro-osseous lesions are therefore defined by their histological appearance and can be reactive proliferations, neoplasms or dysplasias.

Defining fibro-osseous lesions histologically is not very helpful in clinical differential diagnosis since it requires biopsy. However, the characteristic clinical and radiological features and behaviour of these diseases allows fairly confident diagnosis. Fibro-osseous lesions are listed in Box 12.7.

Review all types PMID: 30887390

CEMENTO-OSSEOUS DYSPLASIAS

These poorly understood diseases are non-neoplastic disturbances of growth and remodelling of bone and cementum. They are, by far, the most common fibro-osseous diseases of the jaws and are common enough to be seen from time to time in general dental practice. They have similar histological and radiological features and differ mainly in their extent and radiographic appearances. The cause is alterations in one of several related genes, varying between subtypes. The florid form is associated with *HRAS* and *KRAS* mutation and the focal form with *NRAS*, *FGFR3* and *BRAF* mutation, while the periapical form is not yet characterized.

All types affect the bone around tooth root apices and have a strong predilection for females, accounting for more than 90% of cases, particularly people of African descent. Patients tend to present between 30 and 50 years of age, but probably after many years of asymptomatic disease. Although classified as though diseases of cementum, all types are really diseases of the lamina dura and periapical bone and an intact periodontal ligament separating the lesions from the tooth root is seen radiologically, though it may be absent in the earliest stages.

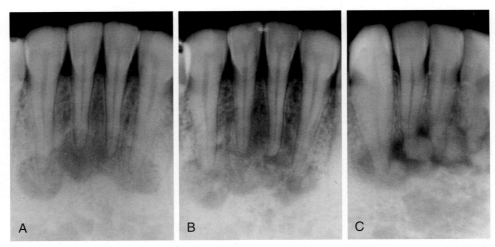

Fig. 12.25 **Periapical cemento-osseous dysplasia.** Three films taken over a period of years showing, (A) the early radiolucent stage resembling periapical granulomas, (B) intermediate stage with patchy mineralisation and (C) the late stage with well-defined masses of cementum in the centre of lesions. *(Courtesy Mr EJ Whaites)*

Periapical cemento-osseous dysplasia

→ Summary chart 13.1 p. 244

In the periapical form, several adjacent teeth are affected, usually lower incisors.

The condition is asymptomatic and often a chance radiographic finding of rounded radiolucent areas related to the apices of the teeth. These simulate periapical granulomas but the related teeth are vital. The separate lesions enlarge, may fuse and develop internal calcification over a period of years or decades. Mineralisation starts centrally and gives each lesion a target-like appearance radiographically. Eventually the lesions cease to enlarge, rarely exceeding 8–10 mm, and become densely radiopaque (Fig. 12.25). All stages of development may be seen at the same time in different lesions in the same patient. The teeth remain vital throughout.

Natural history PMID: 25425097

Florid cemento-osseous dysplasia

→ Summary chart 13.1 p. 244

In the florid form, multiple teeth are affected in more than one quadrant. The affected areas are frequently symmetrically distributed and may involve all teeth in all four quadrants, although the mandibular teeth are more commonly and more severely affected in most cases.

Individual lesions develop around the root apices exactly as in the periapical form but become larger and occasionally expand the jaw. The target-like appearance with central sclerosis resembling cementum on the root apex, surrounded by a radiolucent trim with a further outer zone of sclerosis in the surrounding bone is characteristic. Eventually, dense radiopaque, somewhat irregular masses of sclerotic bone without a radiolucent border develop, producing a radiographic appearance similar to chronic osteomyelitis (Fig. 12.26). As in the periapical form, tooth vitality is not affected.

The florid form becomes the most sclerotic and is particularly liable to become infected after extraction of involved teeth (Ch. 8).

Some patients also develop cysts that resemble simple bone cysts in association with the lesions and these may cause expansion and can recur after treatment unlike conventional simple bone cysts.

Radiology PMID: 9927089 and 29284472

Review PMID: 9377196 and 27422424

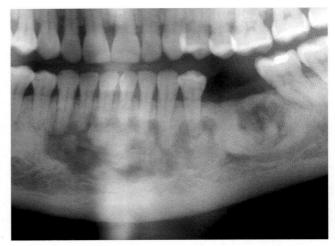

Fig. 12.26 **Florid cemento-osseous dysplasia.** Section of a panoramic tomogram showing the typical appearances of multiple irregular radiopaque masses centred on the roots of the teeth. The periphery of each is radiolucent, and the surrounding bone shows some sclerosis. Similar lesions were present in the contralateral molar region and on some maxillary teeth.

With cyst formation PMID: 16182928

With jaw expansion PMID: 21237426

Familial florid cemento-osseous dysplasia

A familial background is recognized in this form of the disease and mutation of the *ANO5* gene, which encodes a membrane ion channel, has been found in a few cases. The familial florid form resembles the florid form but is more extensive, has earlier onset, often causes marked jaw expansion and may have a less restricted ethnic distribution than the florid form.

Review PMID: 32315206

Cause PMID: 30996299

Focal cemento-osseous dysplasia

→ Summary chart 13.1 p. 244

This term is given to changes similar to florid osseous dysplasia but forming a single lesion on one or a few adjacent teeth. The lesion resembles a cemento-osseous fibroma

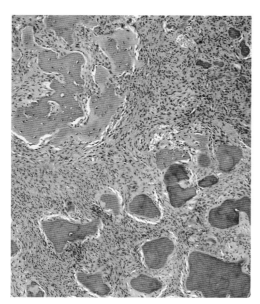

Fig. 12.27 Cemento-osseous dysplasia. All three types have the same histological appearances, a very cellular fibrous tissue containing trabeculae of woven and sclerotic bone and islands of dense basophilic cementum-like bone. In early lesions the fibrous component predominates; late lesions become densely mineralised and sclerotic.

radiographically but shows the maturation sequence typical of this group of lesions. Lesions are usually in the posterior mandible.

Review PMID: 7838469

Microscopy

It must be emphasised that biopsy should **not** be performed for diagnosis. The diagnosis should be made radiographically, and biopsy avoided because it risks introducing infection into the sclerotic bone (Ch. 8). It must also be remembered that the histological features of all fibro-osseous lesions are very similar and so diagnosis is not possible on the biopsy appearances alone.

If a biopsy is required, it shows multiple small curettings of very cellular fibrous tissue containing woven bone trabeculae and islands of dense cementum-like bone like other fibro-osseous lesions. Progressive calcification leads to the formation of a solid, bony mass with prominent resting and reversal lines (Fig. 12.27).

Management of cemento-osseous dysplasias

No treatment is usually required. Osteomyelitis starting in these lesions following tooth extraction or implant placement must be avoided because the widespread sclerosis in the late stages makes infection to eradicate and surgery causes significant morbidity. Wide excision may then be required to allow resolution. Treatment is indicated rarely for cosmetic reasons, if there is marked expansion or if cystic change develops.

Infection as a complication PMID: 31011984

FIBROUS DYSPLASIA AND ALBRIGHT'S SYNDROME → Summary chart 12.2 p. 229

Fibrous dysplasia is a growth disturbance of bone caused by mutation in the *GNAS1* gene. This gene encodes a G protein

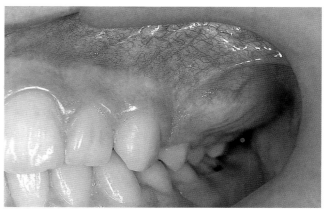

Fig. 12.28 Fibrous dysplasia. Typical presentation with a poorly defined, rounded expansion of the maxilla with no displacement of teeth and intact overlying mucosa.

signalling molecule, and the mutation inactivates the G protein, allowing cyclic AMP to levels to rise, activating the affected cell.

The mutation is not inherited but occurs in a stem cell in the very early embryo, as early as a week or two after fertilisation, before placenta and embryonic tissues have started to form. The clone of cells carrying the mutation develops normally, and its daughter cells become distributed and incorporated into different tissues so that any patient is a mosaic for the mutation. Mutation can occur at such an early stage of development that it can be transmitted on to mesodermal, endodermal or ectodermal cells and affect almost any tissue. If the mutation arises later in development, after tissues have started to differentiate, then the affected daughter cells will be limited to one germ cell layer or, if later still, one tissue at one body site. The extent of the mosaicism, that is, the number of cells affected by the mutation, defines the clinical presentation.

There is no family history for any of the following presentations because this is a somatic or post-zygotic mutation.

Fibrous dysplasia review PMID: 17982387

Mosaicism general review PMID: 34637327 and 32916079

Monostotic fibrous dysplasia

Monostotic fibrous dysplasia causes enlargement of one bone or part of one bone. This typically starts in childhood but usually stops growing in early adulthood. The jaws are the most frequent sites in the head and neck region and a common site overall, followed by skull bones, ribs and femur. Males and females are almost equally frequently affected. It is the commonest presentation of fibrous dysplasia, six times commoner than the polyostotic form.

In monostotic disease the *GNAS1* mutation arises late in development, so that the clone of affected cells is present in only one bone, forming both the osteoblasts and the fibrous tissue in the marrow spaces. In the affected region, the activated fibroblasts and osteoblasts grow excessively, but they remain under some degree of growth control, and the increased growth usually develops at a time when the bone would normally be growing and ceases at around the time the bone would normally be mature.

When the jaws are involved, a painless, smoothly rounded swelling, usually of the maxilla, is typical (Fig. 12.28). This is often centred around the zygomatic region or more posteriorly. Initially, the teeth are aligned but, if the mass becomes very large, it will displace teeth. Patients with fibrous dysplasia may have missing teeth and enamel hypoplasia, but the dental defects are mild and poorly described. Lesions affecting the maxilla may spread to involve contiguous skull bones causing deformity of the orbit, base of skull and cranial nerve lesions (craniofacial fibrous dysplasia). The swelling usually grows very slowly, but with occasional rapid growth spurts.

Radiographically, the features reflect the structure of the abnormal bone described later in this chapter, and this varies depending on the stage of the process. Early lesions are patchy radiolucencies but develop into weak radiopacities, with a ground glass or fine orange-peel texture while the lesion mineralises. The degree of radiopacity increases, and late lesions are sclerotic and lack the trabecular pattern of normal bone. A fingerprint pattern of coarse trabeculae may be seen in very old lesions. The cortex and lamina dura are affected by the process, and their definition is lost radiographically. The cortex is expanded but thin and barely discernible during growth (Fig. 12.29). Two key diagnostic features are that the margins merge imperceptibly with the surrounding normal bone and that there is always expansion of the bone (Fig. 12.30).

Pathology

The microscopic appearances vary with stage. In the early radiolucent phase there is loose cellular fibrous tissue that forms slender trabeculae of osteoid and woven bone. These link together in complex and variable shapes. At the margin there is a gradual imperceptible merging into surrounding normal bone (Figs 12.31 and 12.32). During this phase the bone enlarges and radiographically has a featureless ground glass appearance with no cortex or lamina dura.

After several years, while skeletal growth slows, the bone gradually starts to mature, though abnormally. The woven bone trabeculae are larger and more heavily mineralised but only develop a minimal peripheral osteoblast layer and a little thin lamellar bone. Radiographically, the bone is visible as the coarse trabecular pattern of the orange peel appearance. In addition, there may be islands of very dense heavily mineralised bone, but these are not cementum as sometimes claimed. Occasional loose foci of giant cells can also be seen, but these are not a major feature as they are in giant cell lesions. Gradually a partial cortex reforms and growth ceases.

The bone remains mostly woven in type for many years but eventually develops into lamellar bone and slowly remodels. By middle age, only subtle radiographic features remain.

Biopsy is required to confirm a fibro-osseous lesion, but cannot distinguish fibrous dysplasia from other fibro-osseous lesions with certainty. However, biopsy provides tissue for identification of the *GNAS1* mutation by DNA sequencing or PCR, which is diagnostic. The combination of a fibro-osseous lesion on biopsy, radiological features and the clinical presentation are usually conclusive. The vascular soft bone may bleed significantly on biopsy.

Very occasionally lesions can reactivate and grow in later life, but the reasons are unknown. Fibrous dysplasia can also be complicated by the development of haemorrhagic cystic degeneration that produces very expansile vascular lesions resembling aneurysmal bone cysts, though this is unusual in the jaws.

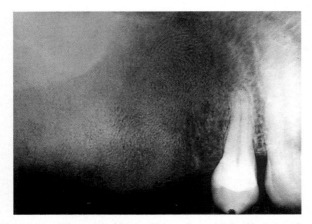

Fig. 12.29 Fibrous dysplasia. This well-established lesion with a rounded swelling merges imperceptibly with normal bone surrounding the canine. There is loss of lamina dura and cortex in the affected area, and the fine trabecular pattern produces an orange-peel or thumb-print appearance.

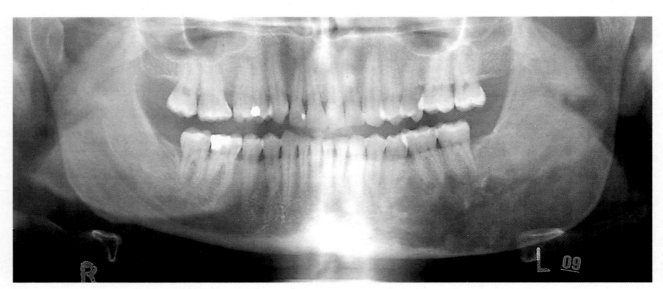

Fig. 12.30 Fibrous dysplasia affecting the left mandible with a patchy radiolucency. No lesion border can be identified.

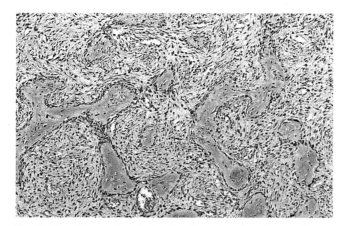

Fig. 12.31 Fibrous dysplasia. Slender trabeculae of woven bone, said to resemble Chinese characters or be C-, S- and Y-shaped, lying in a very cellular fibrous tissue. With maturation there is progressively more bone formation.

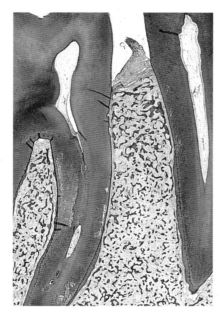

Fig. 12.32 Fibrous dysplasia. There is loss of lamina dura around the teeth and its replacement by affected bone. These numerous small trabeculae give rise to the ground-glass and orange-peel appearances radiographically.

Jaw lesions PMID: 25409854 and 27493082

Craniofacial involvement PMID: 22771278

Treatment

The disease is self-limiting, but lesions become quiescent rather than resolve. The lesion is not well demarcated and cannot be excised. Disfiguring lesions may be pared down to a more cosmetic contour, but this should be delayed until the process has become inactive, usually just after the end of the second decade, slightly earlier in females. Surgery to active or recently active lesions risks reactivation and rapid growth. However, extraction of teeth from affected bone does not increase bone growth, fractures heal normally and implants can be placed.

The late sclerotic bone is prone to osteomyelitis, and the long-term success of implants is unclear, in part because they lack the support of a well-organised cortical bone layer.

During growth the bone may be painful. In rapidly enlarging lesions treatment with bisphosphonates reduces pain and may be used to limit growth but is rarely used for jaw lesions.

There is a small risk of sarcomatous change in later life. This complication is more frequent in craniofacial bones but not the jaws and affects less than 1% of patients. Osteosarcoma is the usual type of sarcoma to develop.

Key features are summarised in Box 12.8

Treatment and dental treatment PMID: 22640797

Polyostotic fibrous dysplasia

Polyostotic fibrous dysplasia is rare and, unlike the monostotic form, females are affected three times more frequently than males and onset is at a slightly younger age.

Polyostotic fibrous dysplasia involves the head and neck region in over 50% of cases. A jaw lesion may then be the most conspicuous feature and polyostotic disease may not be suspected initially. Thus, all patients with an apparently solitary jaw lesion should be screened for involvement of other bones and for the features of Albright's syndrome.

Long bone involvement causes most problems, with bowing of weight bearing bones, bone pain and pathological fractures.

Histologically and radiographically, the individual lesions are indistinguishable from the monostotic form.

Albright's syndrome

Albright's syndrome (also known as *McCune-Albright syndrome*) comprises polyostotic fibrous dysplasia, skin pigmentation and endocrine disturbances. Most patients are girls aged less than 10 years at onset.

The bone lesions are more numerous than in non-syndromic polyostotic fibrous dysplasia, and more than three-quarters of cases have one or both jaws involved and nearly all have skull involvement. Skin pigmentation consists of brownish macules with irregular outlines that frequently overlie affected bones and appear especially on the back of the neck, trunk, buttocks or thighs, and only very occasionally on the oral mucosa (Fig. 12.33). These are caused by melanocytes carrying the *GNAS1* mutation, which activates melanin synthesis.

Endocrine dysfunction is usually manifest as precocious puberty, but other thyroid, pituitary and adrenal anomalies may develop. Hypothyroidism, Cushing's syndrome and acromegaly can all be found. Malignant neoplasms in the

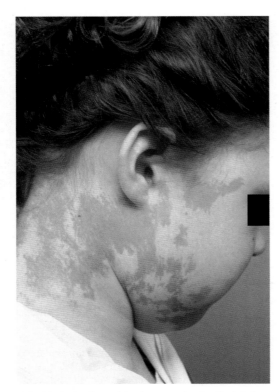

Fig. 12.33 Typical cafe-au lait pigmentation in Albright's syndrome, the patches characteristically have irregular margins. *(Courtesy of the Institute of Dermatology, London, UK).*

Table 12.1 Types of ossifying fibromas

Type	Origin	Sites
Conventional cemento-ossifying fibroma	Odontogenic	Alveolus and adjacent bone of jaw
Juvenile trabecular cemento-ossifying fibroma	Unclear, possibly odontogenic	Alveolus and adjacent bone of jaw including ramus of mandible
Psammomatoid ossifying fibroma	Non-odontogenic	Facial bones, sinuses, skull and jaws

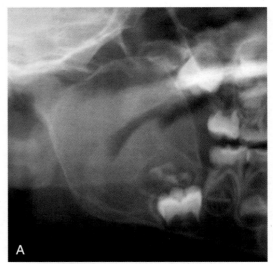

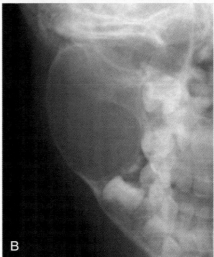

affected organs are very rare; only the bone lesions have a significant risk. The risk is higher in Albright's syndrome than in the monostotic form but is still very low.

Histologically and radiographically, the individual bone lesions are indistinguishable from the monostotic form.

Review PMID: 22640971

OSSIFYING FIBROMAS

→ Summary charts 11.1 and 12.1 pp. 194, 228

The group of ossifying fibromas is somewhat confusing because, despite similarities and a common name, some types develop only in the jaw and are considered odontogenic tumours (cemento-ossifying fibromas, see Ch. 11), whereas others develop in facial or long bones and must therefore be non-odontogenic (ossifying fibromas; Table 12.1). All types are also classified as fibro-osseous lesions because of their histological appearances.

Juvenile trabecular ossifying fibroma

It is controversial whether this is just a histological variant of cemento-ossifying fibroma, reflecting diagnosis at a younger age, but it is currently considered a rare but distinct entity without the genetic changes of other ossifying fibromas. It arises in children aged 8–15 years and causes a rapidly expanding jaw swelling in either jaw. Radiologically there is a well-defined and usually partly corticated radiolucency with tooth displacement and, if large, cortical perforation (Fig. 12.34).

The histological appearance can be worrying, resembling osteosarcoma (Fig 12.35). This misdiagnosis can be avoided by noting the radiological circumscription. The loose, fibroblastic stroma contains very fine, lace-like trabeculae of

Fig 12.34 Juvenile trabecular ossifying fibroma. This example in the mandible shows a typically very large expansile lesion (A). In this young child the lesion is in an early phase and no internal mineralisation is evident radiographically. The postero-anterior jaws projection shows marked expansion of the ramus lingually and buccally (B)..

immature osteoid entrapping plump osteoblasts. Mitoses may be seen, and focal collections of giant cells are common.

The juvenile type grows rapidly, but it responds to enucleation and curettage despite the worrying presentation.

Juvenile trabecular type PMID: 11925539 and 23052375

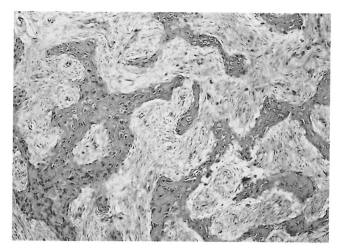

Fig 12.35   Juvenile trabecular ossifying fibroma. The tumour consists of trabeculae of woven bone in fibrous tissue, usually with minimal mineralization, and resembles osteosarcoma.

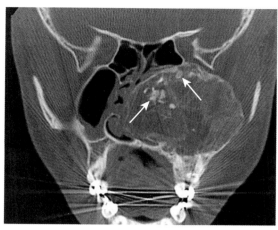

Fig. 12.37   Psammomatoid ossifying fibroma. Computed tomography showing a lesion in the typical site involving maxilla, maxillary and ethmoid sinuses and nasal cavity, and expanding the maxilla toward the coronoid process. This example has internal mineralisation visible (arrowed). *(From Wenig, B.M., Mafee, M.F., Ghosh, L., 1998. Fibro-osseous, osseous, and cartilaginous lesions of the orbit and paraorbital region. Correlative clinicopathologic and radiographic features, including the diagnostic role of CT and MR imaging. Radiol. Clin. North Am. 36, 1241-1259, xii.)*

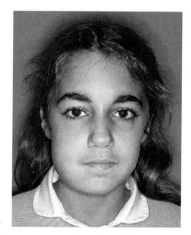

Fig. 12.36   Psammomatoid ossifying fibroma. A lesion in the mandible of a 12-year-old girl producing asymmetry by expansion of the mandibular ramus. *(Fig. 8 from Papadaki, M., Troulis, M.J., and Kaban, L.B. 2005. Advances in diagnosis and management of fibro-osseous lesions. Oral Maxillofac Surg Clin North Am 17(4):415-434.)*

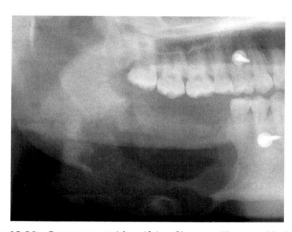

Fig. 12.38   Psammomatoid ossifying fibroma. This mandibular lesion extends from the premolars to the ramus with considerable buccal and lingual expansion and perforation of the cortex. There is only thin cortication reflecting rapid growth and it appears relatively radiolucent. *(Courtesy Dr L Collins).*

Psammomatoid ossifying fibroma

This ossifying fibroma has also been called juvenile (active) ossifying fibroma but is now known to develop at all ages, though most present between 15 and 35 years of age. It affects the maxilla, facial bones and base of skull, particularly the ethmoid region, more frequently than the mandible. The cause is unclear, but likely to be rearrangements of the *SATB2* gene, an unusual cause since alterations in this gene are generally considered to cause developmental problems rather than neoplasms.

Lesions cause asymptomatic, often rapid, expansion of bone, displacing adjacent structures such as teeth, sinuses or orbit (Fig. 12.36). Radiological appearance depends on the degree of mineralisation, but most are radiolucent or of even mixed density (Figs 12.37 and 12.38).

Histologically, the lesion has a very distinctive pattern with a highly cellular fibroblastic tissue containing compact, rounded dense calcifications, larger than, but reminiscent of, the so-called *psammoma bodies* in thyroid carcinomas (Fig. 12.39). These small, mineralised balls often have an

eosinophilic rim of matrix collagen and do not usually fuse together as the lesion matures.

The treatment is enucleation and curettage. There is a risk of recurrence, perhaps because these lesions often arise in thin facial bones that make treatment difficult. However, any recurrence is usually eradicated by a second or third curettage, so that conservative surgery is all that is required.

Review PMID: 31285096

Detailed description PMID: 1843064

Familial gigantiform cementoma

This extremely rare disease is probably inherited as an autosomal dominant condition and causes very large and disfiguring lesions, usually in multiple quadrants and presenting in early childhood. The term *gigantiform cementoma* has often been used incorrectly for florid cemento-osseous dysplasia with expansion or for its familial form. In familial gigantiform cementoma the multiple tumours reach 10

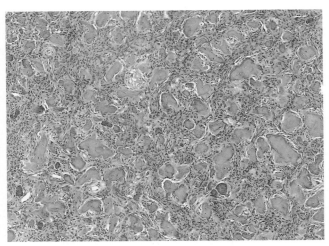

Fig. 12.39 Psammomatoid ossifying fibroma, comprising small darkly stained mineralised nodules of bone in a cellular fibrous tissue. Whether mineralisation is psammomatoid or not can be detected histologically but not radiographically.

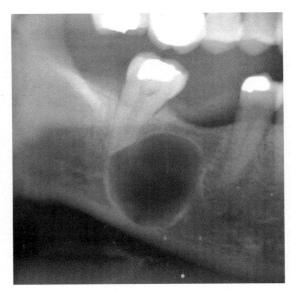

Fig. 12.40 **Haemangioma of bone.** This very well corticated and rounded radiolucency was thought to be an odontogenic cyst and opened for biopsy. Luckily it was a low-pressure type of haemangioma.

or 20 cm in diameter and affect multiple quadrants. The few genuine cases appear to affect mostly children of Asian heritage.

In at least some cases, the origin appears to start at the tooth roots but lesions grow progressively and recur after incomplete removal, so that the condition is similar to multiple cemento-ossifying fibromas rather than a type of cemento-osseous dysplasia and is probably a distinct, but extremely rare, disease.

Cases and review PMID: 11312460

URL: internet image search: novemthree tzuchi

SOFT TISSUE TUMOURS IN THE JAWS

HAEMANGIOMA OF BONE

Intraosseous haemangiomas are rare, and it is unclear whether they are hamartomas or benign neoplasms, but they tend to present in patients younger than 30 years of age, and more frequently in females. They are common in the craniofacial skeleton and three-quarters of head and neck lesions arise in the mandible.

Clinically, haemangiomas in bone are usually asymptomatic and are often chance radiographic findings. However, some cause progressive painless swellings which, when the overlying cortex is resorbed by pressure from the lesion, may form a pulsatile bluish soft tissue swelling. Teeth may be loosened, and there may be bleeding, particularly from any involved gingival margins. Extensive multiple haemangiomas can cause complete resorption of their bone ('vanishing bone disease').

Radiographically, the features of haemangioma are extremely varied. They range from a sharply defined cyst-like appearance (Fig. 12.40) to poorly defined lobulated radiolucencies or even a soap-bubble appearance (Fig. 12.41). A serpiginous shape is particularly suggestive.

Pathology

Haemangiomas of bone are essentially the same as those in soft tissues (Ch. 25). They are usually cavernous, with low flow and pressure (Fig. 12.42), but there is also an arteriovenous type (fast-flow angioma) which has large feeder

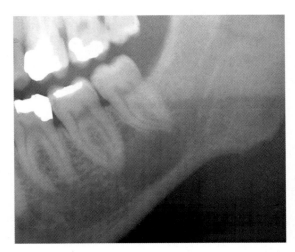

Fig. 12.41 **Haemangioma of bone.** This haemangioma below the second and third molars was thought to be a simple bone cyst. Clues as to its real nature are few. It is not as radiolucent as a cyst, and it communicates with the inferior dental canal, where its feeder vessels originate. Biopsy was associated with considerable bleeding.

arteries, tends to expand rapidly and is likely to bleed severely if opened.

Intrabony vascular malformations PMID: 25703595

Management

A haemangioma may not be suspected if its vascularity is not obvious. Opening it or extracting a related tooth may therefore release torrents of blood, occasionally with fatal results.

If there are identifiable feeder vessels, selective arterial embolisation can be performed either as a treatment or to reduce size and blood flow before surgery. However, the complexity of the arterial tree in the head and neck makes this a skilled procedure and often only partial embolisation can be achieved. Surgery after embolisation is considerably

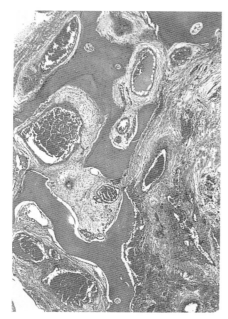

Fig. 12.42   Haemangioma of bone. The marrow spaces contain very large blood-filled sinuses with thin walls; the lesion is poorly localised and permeates between the bony trabeculae.

safer. For the largest haemangiomas, a wide en bloc resection may be the only practical treatment.

Treatment PMID: 12729771

MELANOTIC NEUROECTODERMAL TUMOUR OF INFANCY

➔ Summary chart 26.1 p. 435

This rare benign but destructive neoplasm develops almost exclusively in the jaws and craniofacial bones and affects children in the first few months of life. Two-thirds of lesions arise in the maxilla, usually anteriorly, with occasional examples in the mandible, skull or brain. It is usually painless and expands quickly forming a bluish-black pigmented mass (Fig. 12.43) that interferes with feeding. Its causes and origin are unknown but it shows a range of neural crest differentiation patterns.

Radiographically, there is an area of bone destruction, frequently with ragged margins, and displacement of the developing teeth (Fig. 12.44) that can simulate a malignant neoplasm.

Pathology

Microscopy reveals that the tumour has two components and a very striking appearance. The first is melanin-containing epithelium, comprising cuboidal epithelial cells forming islands and lining slit-like spaces (Figs 12.45 and 12.46). The second is a population of small darkly stained cells with round nuclei and little cytoplasm. These grow either in the centre of the small epithelial lined cysts or in clusters in the fibrous tissue that supports both components. Some degree of atypia and infrequent mitotic figures are often seen. The round cells resemble neuroblasts and secrete vanillylmandelic acid (VMA), which can be detected in the urine and aids diagnosis. This is a metabolic degradation

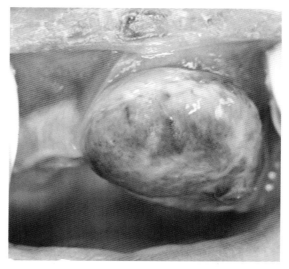

Fig. 12.43   Melanotic neuroectodermal tumour of infancy. This example has become ulcerated, and the dark pigment can be seen as speckles in the tissue. *(Fig. 9.36 from Woo, S.B., 2012. Oral pathology: a comprehensive atlas and text. Saunders, Philadelphia, p. 215.)*

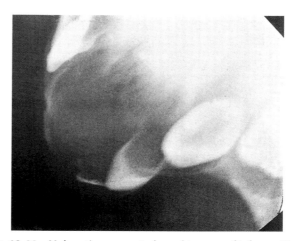

Fig. 12.44   Melanotic neuroectodermal tumour of infancy. The anterior maxilla of this neonate contains an expansile radiolucency that has displaced tooth germs and eroded the alveolar bone.

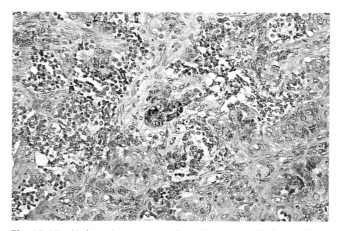

Fig. 12.45   Melanotic neuroectodermal tumour of infancy. Pale pink-staining epithelial cells, some of which are pigmented (centrally), arranged in clusters and surrounded by small, round, darkly staining tumour cells.

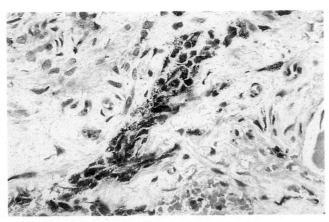

Fig. 12.46 Melanotic neuroectodermal tumour of infancy. Higher power showing the melanin pigment granules within a strand of epithelium.

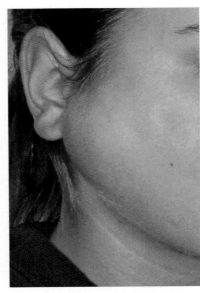

Fig. 12.47 Rapidly enlarging swelling of the ramus caused by Ewing's sarcoma in a patient aged 12 years.

> **Box 12.9 Melanotic neuroectodermal tumour of infancy: key features**
>
> - Very rare
> - Congenital or appears in first few months of life
> - Presents as expansion of anterior maxilla, typically bluish in colour
> - Benign but destroys bone
> - Treated by conservative excision or curettage initially
> - May recur

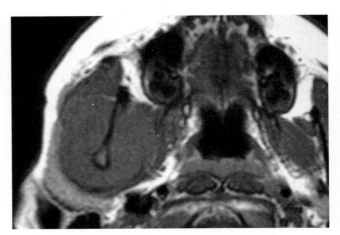

Fig. 12.48 Axial magnetic resonance imaging scan of Ewing's sarcoma in the mandibular ramus. The features are not specific but indicate a rapidly growing lesion because the cortex of the ramus is still visible in the centre of the large round tumour mass.

product of the epinephrine pathway produced by many neuroendocrine tumours.

Frequent mitotic figures and loss of differentiation of the melanocyte-like cells suggest more aggressive behaviour.

Case series PMID: 12142876

Management

After confirmation of diagnosis by biopsy, surgery is the treatment of choice. The extent of the resection is controversial and can range from local excision and curettage to total maxillectomy because the behaviour of the tumour is unpredictable. Though unencapsulated, it usually separates easily from the bone at operation and conservative surgery can be curative for small tumours. Incomplete excision is not always followed by recurrence, but a third will recur. Occasional tumours act as though malignant and may be fatal, but this cannot be reliably predicted in advance so that initial treatment is conservative.

Serum levels of epinephrine, norepinephrine and urinary VMA return to normal after treatment and may be monitored for evidence of recurrence.

Key features are summarised in Box 12.9

Review PMID: 30170777

Surgical management PMID: 19070747 and 30871849

EWING'S SARCOMA

Ewing's sarcoma of bone and its near relative, the primitive neuroectodermal tumour of soft tissue, are members of a group of malignant neoplasms that are essentially undifferentiated but show some neural features and are defined by their genetic causes.

Ewing's sarcoma is rare overall, and only 1% or so of these already rare lesions arise in the jaws with a further 3%–4% in craniofacial bones. It tends to arise in the body of the mandible in children or young adults, aged 10–30 years. Typical symptoms are bone swelling and often pain, progressing over a period of months to perforate the cortex and form a soft tissue mass (Fig. 12.47). Teeth may loosen, and the overlying mucosa ulcerate. Fever, leukocytosis, a raised erythrocyte sedimentation rate (ESR) and anaemia may be associated and indicate a poor prognosis.

Radiographically there is a very poorly defined radiolucency that can be difficult to see in its early stages on plain radiographs or panoramic views but later may produce a prominent 'onion-skin' periosteal reactive bone visible on CT or cone beam CT (Fig. 12.48).

Table 12.2   Presentations of Langerhans cell histiocytosis

Classification	Presentation	Features
Chronic unifocal form	Solitary eosinophilic granuloma	Adults, usually bones (80%), lymph nodes or lungs affected
Chronic multifocal form	Multifocal eosinophilic granuloma (including Hand–Schuller–Christian disease)	Young adults and adolescents. Single system involvement but multiple lesions, usually in skull, skin, nodes, brain, liver, pituitary
Acute disseminated form	Letterer–Siwe disease, multisystem disease with diffuse tissue involvement	Young children and infants. Multiple organ involvement, particularly liver, spleen and bone marrow and, to a lesser extent, bone

Genetics

Ewing's sarcoma is caused by one of several similar characteristic reciprocal translocations. In 85% this is a t(11,22) translocation that fuses two genes (Ewing's sarcoma gene *EWSR1* and *Fli1*) that then produce an abnormal transcription factor responsible for transforming the cells. Many other causative translocations are recognised between related genes in the same gene families and genetic diagnostic tests are performed routinely on biopsy samples.

Pathology

Ewing's sarcoma cells resemble lymphocytes but are approximately twice their size. They have a darkly staining nucleus and a rim of cytoplasm, which is typically vacuolated and contains glycogen. The cells form diffuse sheets or loose lobules, separated by septa, and are occasionally organized into rosettes. A rare 'adamantinoma-like' variant is more frequent in the head and neck, has more varied features, the same translocation but is probably a distinct tumour type.

The initial treatment is chemotherapy followed by wide excision and radiotherapy. Chemotherapy improves the survival but, unfortunately, increases the risk of lymphoid tumours in later life. If the disease is localised, 70% of patients will survive 5 years, but the survival in patients with disseminated disease is less than 20%. Jaw lesions have a better prognosis than long bone lesions, probably because they are diagnosed at a smaller size; this is the main prognostic indicator. Distant spread is usually to the lungs and other bones rather than lymph nodes.

Case series PMID: 21107767

HAEMATOLOGICAL TUMOURS IN THE JAWS

LANGERHANS CELL HISTIOCYTOSIS

Langerhans cells are dendritic antigen-presenting cells that function within epithelia. They derive from monocyte precursors in the tissues and can also differentiate from the bone marrow when additional cells are required after injury. In this group of conditions they proliferate excessively and localise in bone, organs and skin. Three main forms are recognised, and their features are shown in Table 12.2 but, in practice, this is a continuous spectrum of disease severity and no single classification has yet proved satisfactory.

Key features of oral lesions are summarised in Box 12.10.

The cause is unknown, but in about a third of cases with the systemic forms the disease is neoplastic because the cells are clonal and approximately half of cases carry mutations in the *BRAF* oncogene. It seems that mutation in the bone

Box 12.10   Langerhans cell histiocytosis: oral lesions

- Eosinophilic granulomas form isolated or multifocal tumours of Langerhans cells, eosinophils and other inflammatory cells
- Sharply demarcated radiolucencies
- Alveolar bone around teeth may be destroyed (teeth floating in air appearance)
- May also mimic the periodontal destruction pattern of localised juvenile periodontitis radiographically
- Diagnosis is by biopsy
- Solitary lesions respond to curettage or resection

marrow precursors leads to neoplastic disseminated disease in bone and soft tissue, whereas mutation in the mature or maturing dendritic cell in the tissues causes localised forms that are mostly in bone and of much lower risk. Localised lesions may occasionally resolve spontaneously.

Oral involvement is present in approximately 10% of both child and adult patients, and the mandible is affected in nearly 75%, either alone or in polyostotic disease. Langerhans cell histiocytosis restricted to the oral mucosa, as opposed to bone, is extremely rare and causes ulcers.

Pathology

Biopsy is required for diagnosis. There are varying proportions of Langerhans cells and eosinophils, sometimes with other types of granulocytes. The Langerhans cells have pale, vesicular and often lobulated nuclei and weakly eosinophilic cytoplasm (Fig. 12.49). Langerhans cells in all types of the disease can be identified in a biopsy by immunocytochemistry for the CD1a surface marker or the CD207 receptor langerin found in the cell membrane and cytoplasmic granules. Diagnostic electron microscopy for the characteristic cytoplasmic Birbeck granules has been superseded by these stains. There may also be necrosis.

Langerhans cells are a minority of cells in the lesion; most cells are inflammatory cells including many activated T cells. The lesion and adjacent tissue destruction is therefore caused by immune dysregulation directed by the abnormal Langerhans cells as well as their proliferation.

Solitary or unifocal eosinophilic granuloma

An eosinophilic granuloma of the jaw causes localised bone destruction with swelling and often pain (Fig. 12.50). Lesions are often centred in the alveolar bone and destroy the bone and soft tissue of the periodontium to expose the roots of the teeth. A rounded area of radiolucency with indistinct margins (Figs 12.51 and 12.52) and an appearance of teeth 'floating

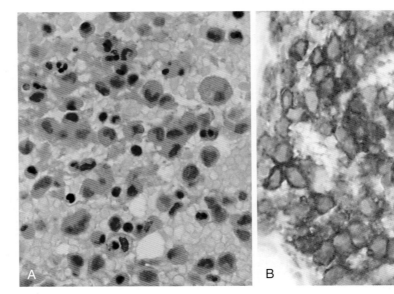

Fig. 12.49   Langerhans cell histiocytosis. High power showing the large round paler-staining Langerhans cells with their characteristic folded, bilobed (coffee bean) nuclei and some eosinophils, smaller and brighter red (A). The Langerhans cells are more easily identified by positive brown immunohistochemical staining for their membrane protein CD1a (B).

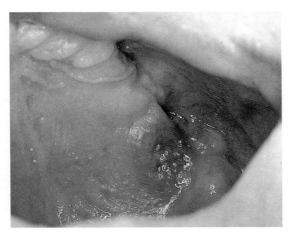

Fig. 12.50   Langerhans cell histiocytosis. This localised lesion (eosinophilic granuloma) has produced an ulcerated mass on the maxillary alveolar ridge. The clinical appearances are non-specific.

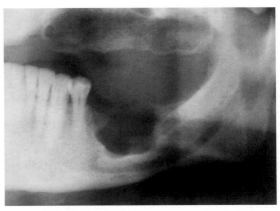

Fig. 12.52   Langerhans cell histiocytosis. This localised lesion (eosinophilic granuloma) shows the characteristic appearance of a well-defined radiolucency scooped out of the alveolar bone. The margin is corticated in places, but less well-defined elsewhere.

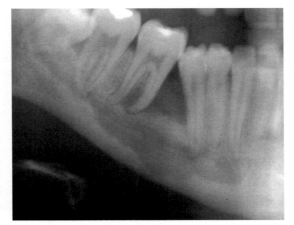

Fig. 12.51   Langerhans cell histiocytosis. Destruction of interdental bone and extension down to a scalloped margin at the lower border of the mandible.

in air' are typical. Young and middle-aged adults are mainly affected, and the lesion is most frequently in the mandible. When one lesion is found, a search for others should be made.

Chronic multifocal Langerhans cell histiocytosis

In this form, the skull, axial skeleton, femora, and also sometimes the viscera (liver and spleen) or the skin may be involved. When the skull is affected, there are multiple lesions in the jaws and base of skull and a minority of patients are seen with the Hand–Schuller–Christian triad of exophthalmos, diabetes insipidus and lytic skull lesions. Exophthalmos and diabetes result from involvement of orbital tissues and base of skull extending to the pituitary gland. The histological features are the same as eosinophilic granuloma.

Acute disseminated Langerhans cell histiocytosis

This aggressive form of histiocytosis, previously called *Letterer–Siwe syndrome*, affects infants or young children and behaves as a lymphoma of Langerhans cells. Progression to widespread disease, with involvement of skin, viscera and bones, can be rapidly fatal, despite treatment by irradiation and/or chemotherapy. Depending on extent, survival may be as low as 50% at 5 years.

Treatment

Overall, the behaviour of Langerhans cell histiocytosis is unpredictable, but the younger the patient and the greater the number of organ systems affected, the worse the prognosis. All affected patients should be investigated for multifocal disease with a skeletal survey or bone scan.

For eosinophilic granulomas in the jaw, the traditional treatment has been curettage or steroid injection, and the response is usually good. However, spontaneous regression during months or years is also reported, and currently conservative medical treatment with azathioprine or methotrexate, with or without a chemotherapeutic such as mercaptopurine, is under evaluation. These treatments seem to work well for skin lesions and some jaw lesions and should be first-line treatment. Whether destructive lesions threatening many teeth may require surgical intervention is unclear. Intralesional injection of corticosteroids may be given as adjunctive treatment and may be safe and effective for monostotic disease. Multifocal bone disease may require vinblastine with systemic steroids. Irradiation may be given if other measures fail or for inaccessible lesions of the skull base. Prolonged follow-up is desirable because of the risk of recurrence and because the apparently single lesion may have been an early manifestation of multifocal disease.

For multisystem disease, a combination of cytotoxic chemotherapy, corticosteroids and irradiation of active bone lesions is required. The poor survival and rapid progression in infants with acute disseminated disease was noted previously. Patients surviving long enough may benefit from marrow transplantation.

General review PMID: 30157397

Oral lesions PMID: 19758405 and 33751219

Treatment PMID: 20188480

MYELOMA

Multiple myeloma is a malignant neoplasm of plasma cells. The malignant plasma cells localise in the bone marrow, multiply to displace the normal marrow and cause multiple foci of bone destruction. Myeloma is a systemic disease from the outset. It is rare for a jaw lesion to cause the initial symptoms, but the skull is a common site of involvement in later disease and a third of patients may have a focus in the jaws. Myeloma is usually diagnosed in patients older than 60 years of age.

Clinically, myeloma lesions may be asymptomatic or cause bone pain and tenderness, weakening of bones and pathological fracture. The malignant plasma cells secrete immunoglobulin in great quantities causing a markedly raised ESR. The excess immunoglobulin is detectable by serum electrophoresis for diagnosis.

Radiologically myeloma lesions are radiolucencies, traditionally multiple 'punched out' radiolucencies in the vault of the skull. Presentation with jaw lesions is uncommon, but multiple small foci of bone destruction is a common presentation after treatment or in relapse (Fig. 12.53).

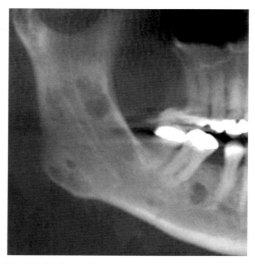

Fig. 12.53 Multiple myeloma. There are multiple small relatively well-defined radiolucencies in the ramus, alveolus, body and near the angle. *(Courtesy Mrs J Brown.)*

Genetics

Myeloma arises by one of several mechanisms involving chromosomal translocations. These bring together one of a variety of oncogenes, often CCND1 encoding the cell cycle regulator cyclin D1, with genes for immunoglobulins, both transforming the cell and inducing the excessive immunoglobulin synthesis. Myeloma arises from a single cell, and so all the malignant plasma cells are monoclonal; they all secrete antibody of the same immunoglobulin (Ig) class and antigen specificity.

Pathology

Myeloma lesions are masses of neoplastic plasma cells that may be well or poorly differentiated. Because the cells are monoclonal and secrete only one type of immunoglobulin light chain, either kappa or lambda, this is helpful in diagnosis (Fig. 12.54). Diagnosis can also be aided by serum electrophoresis showing a monoclonal band. Light chain overproduction is usual and leads to Bence-Jones proteinuria and often amyloidosis. Biopsy of a lesion or an aspirate of bone marrow is required to characterise the myeloma for treatment selection.

General review PMID: 23803862

Treatment

Myeloma is considered incurable, but treatment has developed to the stage that life can be extended for many years. Initially, most patients will be treated with combination chemotherapy including steroids and a thalidomide analogue and the proteasome inhibitor bortezomib, and there is frequently a good initial response. Remission is maintained and prolonged with a progression of drug regimens selected to match disease progression and avoid adverse effects.

If patients are fit enough, autologous stem cell transplants provide the best survival. During remission, the patient's own stem cells are harvested, either from blood or bone marrow, and reintroduced after high-dose chemotherapy. Localised lesions may be treated with radiotherapy or occasionally surgery if they threaten adjacent important structures or fracture. When bone deposits are

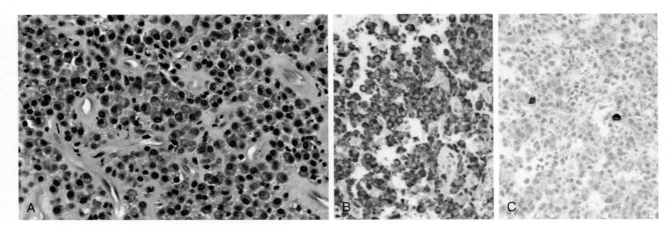

Fig. 12.54 Multiple myeloma. A. the tissues are infiltrated by a uniform population of plasma cells, slightly larger than normal cells. Myeloma is confirmed by immunohistochemistry for immunoglobulin light chains in the right panels. **B.** staining for kappa light chain and, **(C),** lambda light chain; brown stain is positive (see also Fig. 1.8 for method). It can be seen that almost all the plasma cells are secreting kappa light chain containing antibody, whereas only an occasional cell (probably inflammatory plasma cells not part of the myeloma) contains lambda light chain. The plasma cell population is therefore clonal and neoplastic.

> **Box 12.11   Multiple myeloma: key features**
>
> - Myeloma is a disseminated malignant neoplasm of plasma cells
> - Radiographically, punched-out lesions develop, particularly in the skull
> - Similar lesions may appear in the jaws
> - Monoclonal immunoglobulin (usually immunoglobulin G) produced
> - Anaemia, purpura or immunodeficiency may develop as bone marrow is gradually replaced by myeloma
> - Excess immunoglobulin light chain production can lead to amyloidosis
> - Many implications for dental treatment

widespread or symptomatic, they may be treated with bisphosphonates to reduce bone resorption, reduce bone pain and hypercalcaemia, and prevent fractures and collapse of vertebrae. Median survival for patients recently diagnosed is 8 years, and 20 years is currently the likely maximum.

Dental aspects

A myeloma deposit in the jaws or amyloid deposition in the oral soft tissues can be the first manifestation of the disease.

Complications of disease and its treatment affect delivery of dental treatment. Bone marrow replacement by myeloma plasma cells causes thrombocytopenia, anaemia, bleeding and purpura. Immunosuppression from steroids and loss of normal lymphocytes predispose to opportunistic infections. Antibiotic prophylaxis may be required for surgery depending on stage of disease. High-potency bisphosphonates given intravenously include pamidronate and zoledronic acid, and this treatment carries a risk of medication-induced osteonecrosis (see Ch. 8).

Key features are summarised in Box 12.11.

Oral presentations PMID: 24048519

Amyloidosis

Amyloidosis is most frequently a complication of myeloma resulting from deposition of excess secreted Ig light chains in the tissues; this is discussed in Chapter 17.

SOLITARY PLASMACYTOMA

A plasmacytoma is a solitary neoplasm of plasma cells that can be thought of as a localised form of myeloma. Approximately 80% of these rare tumours form in the soft tissues of the head and neck region, often in the nose and sinuses. Circulating immunoglobulin light chains are less frequently found than in myeloma. Patients are usually in their 50s or 60s.

Multiple myeloma develops in as many as 50% of patients with jaw plasmacytoma within 2 years but only 5%–10% of soft tissue and sinus plasmacytoma. This progression demonstrates the link between these conditions and suggests that intraosseous plasmacytoma is often the initial and presenting lesion of myeloma.

Solitary plasmacytoma occasionally affects the jaws and nasal cavity, and the signs and symptoms are as for a deposit of multiple myeloma. Treatment is by combinations of surgery and radiotherapy depending on site. More than 65% of patients survive for 10 or more years, but multiple myeloma develops in the majority eventually, sometimes many years later.

Histologically, the appearances of plasmacytoma and multiple myeloma are the same (Fig. 12.54).

Jaw plasmacytoma PMID: 34503289

Soft tissue plasmacytoma PMID: 24339430

LYMPHOMA

As discussed later, lymphomas of the oral soft tissues are uncommon except in association with HIV infection and are more likely to present as enlarged cervical lymph nodes (Ch. 28) or parotid gland swelling, the latter in Sjögren's syndrome (Ch. 22).

PRIMARY MALIGNANT NEOPLASMS OF BONE

OSTEOSARCOMA

➔ Summary chart 13.1 p. 244

Osteosarcoma is defined as a malignant neoplasm that forms bone or osteoid. Most osteosarcomas arise in long

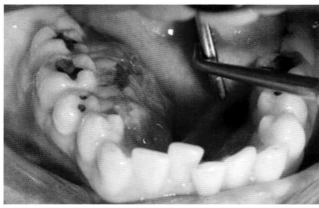

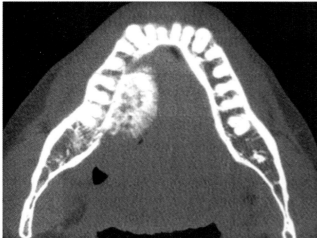

Fig. 12.55   Osteosarcoma of the jaw. Upper panel, a bony hard expansion of the alveolus. Lower image, computed tomography showing the original outline of the mandible to be intact, but the expanded tissue contains bone and has a radiating 'sun ray' appearance. *(Figure from Fernandes, R., et al., 2007. Osteogenic sarcoma of the jaw: a 10-year experience. J. Oral Maxillofac. Surg. 65 (7), 1286-1291.)*

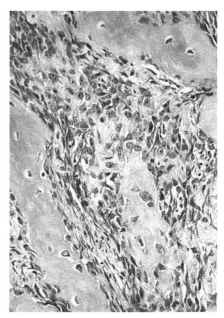

Fig. 12.56   Osteosarcoma. Trabeculae of abnormal woven bone surrounded by atypical cells in which mitoses are frequent and pleomorphism is conspicuous.

the periodontal ligament may cause widening radiologically as an early feature.

Pathology

The cause is unknown, but the tumour cells have marked chromosomal instability with numerous genetic changes.

The sarcoma comprises disorganised neoplastic osteoblasts that vary in size and shape, from spindle cells to angular or large and hyperchromatic (Fig. 12.56). Bone formation is not necessarily prominent, and a search must be made for the diagnostic zones of osteoid and disorganised woven bone. Mitoses may be seen, particularly in the more highly cellular areas. Cartilage and clusters of osteoclasts may also be found. The variable appearance and sparse osteoid in some lesions make diagnosis difficult in a small biopsy. Several histological variants are recognized.

Longstanding Paget's disease predisposes to osteosarcoma, but because the jaws are rarely affected by Paget's disease, this is not a significant risk factor. However, osteosarcoma may develop in skull and facial bones affected by Paget's disease, and also occasionally many years after head and neck irradiation for another cancer.

Key features are summarised in Box 12.12

Case series PMID: 10982954

Management

Treatment is by radical surgery, a wide en bloc resection including any soft tissue extension, usually a minimum of a hemimandibulectomy or a total maxillectomy. In recent years, it has been common to add radiotherapy and/or chemotherapy as would be provided for long bone sarcoma. However, distant metastasis from jaw lesions is much less frequent than from long bone sarcomas and the additional benefit is marginal, being beneficial only in cases with incomplete excision or in the few high-grade sarcomas. The prognosis depends mainly on the extent

bones of children and adolescents, are highly malignant, metastasise early to lung and are frequently fatal. In contrast, osteosarcomas of the jaws tend to arise between 30–50 years of age, seem to grow more slowly, rarely metastasize and have a much better prognosis. Osteosarcoma of other craniofacial bones has the same prognosis as in long bones.

Only about 5% of osteosarcomas arise in the jaws; males are slightly more frequently affected, and the body of the mandible is a common site.

There is typically a firm swelling that grows noticeably in a few months and becomes painful (Fig. 12.55). Teeth may be loosened, and there may be paraesthesia or loss of sensation in the mental nerve area.

Radiographically, appearances are variable but irregular bone destruction with a poorly defined moth-eaten margin is usual. Bone formation within osteosarcomas varies in extent, but when the sarcoma extends beyond bone into soft tissue, even small amounts of bone can be seen clearly and aid diagnosis (see Fig. 12.55). Rapid enlargement pushes the periosteum away from the bone and triggers formation of a periosteal new bone layer over the tumour, giving rise to a sun-ray appearance and Codman's triangles at the margin. Although characteristic, this reflects rapid growth and is not specific to osteosarcoma. Spread along

- Rare
- Patient mean age is approximately 35 years
- Usually affects the mandible
- Radiographically, bone formation is seen in a soft tissue mass
- Treated by radical surgery, sometimes with additional chemotherapy
- Most are low grade and very rarely metastasize
- Better prognosis than osteosarcoma of the long bones
- Occasionally develops as a post-irradiation tumour

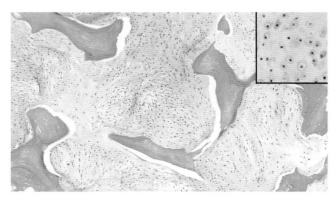

Fig. 12.57   Chondrosarcoma. The residual trabeculae of medullary bone, stained red, are surrounded by bluish cartilage-like tissue that has replaced all the marrow. At higher power, inset, the resemblance of the tumour cells to chondrocytes in lacunae is seen.

of the tumour and deteriorates with spread to the soft tissues, to lymph nodes (in about 10% of cases) or to the base of the skull. In approximately 50%, there is local recurrence within a year of treatment. The 5-year survival rate may range from 70% for tumours less than 5 cm in diameter to zero for tumours greater than 15 cm, and death usually follows local recurrence rather than distant metastasis.

Treatment PMID: 24246156 and 12237918

CHONDROSARCOMA

→ Summary chart 13.1 p. 244

The chondrosarcoma family of malignant neoplasms includes several quite diverse types, with the common feature of forming cartilage. Those that form both cartilage and osteoid or bone are considered osteosarcomas and because most jaw osteosarcomas produce both mineralised tissues, distinction can be difficult. Chondrosarcomas of the jaws behave in a similar fashion to those in the commoner sites in the vertebrae, ribs and skull.

Chondrosarcomas of the jaws are even rarer than osteosarcomas and affect adults at an average age of approximately 45 years. Only about 3% of chrondrosarcomas arise in the head and neck and the anterior maxilla is the site of 60% of them. A painless swelling or loosening of teeth associated with a radiolucent area are typical. The radiolucency can be well or poorly circumscribed or may appear multilocular. Calcifications are frequently present and may be widespread and dense, aiding radiological diagnosis.

Pathology

The commoner types are all associated with mutations in the genes *IDH1* or *IDH2* which are normally involved in citrate metabolism and generate NADPH. Mutated enzymes lose normal activity and generate substances that interfere with chromosome structure and gene regulation. Chondrosarcomas are graded based on how well the cartilage is differentiated and how pleomorphic and mitotically active the cells are. Jaw chondrosarcomas are usually at the low-grade end of the spectrum. The cartilage is lobular and comparatively well formed, with mild atypia in chondrocytes and only an occasional mitosis (Figs 12.57).

Chondrosarcomas must be widely excised as early as possible as radiotherapy and chemotherapy have no effect on low-grade tumours. Greater margins are required with increasing grade, from 1–3 cm. Survival is good, and the 75% 5-year survival is better than for the higher-grade

chondrosarcomas that arise elsewhere in the skeleton. Death usually follows repeated recurrence and extension to the skull. Metastasis is unusual.

Mesenchymal chondrosarcoma is a rare but highly malignant variant. It is a highly cellular tumour in which there are only small foci of tissue recognisable as poorly formed cartilage. The jaws are common sites, and patients are usually younger than for other chondrosarcomas, in their second or third decade.

Case series PMID: 8635057 and 24213203

All cartilaginous lesions PMID: 20614285

Mesenchymal chondrosarcoma PMID: 17681487

INTRAOSSEOUS RHABDOMYOSARCOMA

This recently described malignant neoplasm of striated muscle arises within bone, particularly in the jaws and, to a lesser extent, other craniofacial bones. It is caused by a translocation of the *TFCP2* gene that encodes a transcription factor.

Mainly adolescents and young adults are affected with a rapidly growing destructive jaw mass with features of malignancy. The histological features are very variable but obviously those of a high-grade malignant neoplasm with uniform cytological atypia, abnormal nuclei and frequent mitoses. These features being relatively non-specific, diagnosis depends on immunohistochemistry and often on genetic analysis.

The prognosis is very poor. Most patients have metastases at presentation and response to all treatments tested to date has been limited.

Cases PMID: 33382123

METASTASES TO THE JAWS

→ Summary chart 13.1 p. 244

Blood-borne metastasis to bone is almost always from a carcinoma, usually an adenocarcinoma. Cancer types that metastasize to the jaws (Box 12.13) do so because of specific biological properties, they are not simply the commonest malignant neoplasms. Metastasis to bone affects those bones with the greatest medullary volume – the spine, pelvis, ribs

- Breast
- Bronchus
- Prostate
- Thyroid
- Kidney

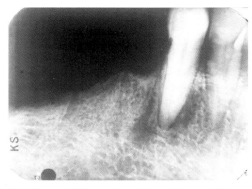

Fig. 12.59 Metastatic bronchogenic carcinoma. This small metastasis in the alveolar bone has produced a poorly demarcated, patchy radiolucency and destroyed the lamina dura around a root apex. Such small lesions could easily be mistaken for periapical granulomas radiographically, but have ragged margins.

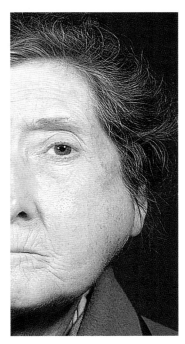

Fig. 12.58 Metastatic carcinoma of the mandible. Swelling developed in the ramus quite suddenly in this apparently fit patient. Investigations showed a deposit of poorly differentiated carcinoma in the jaw and signs of a bronchial carcinoma.

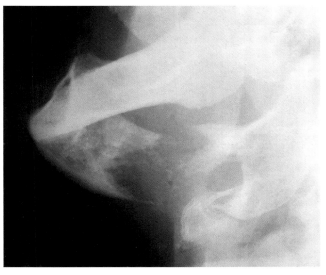

Fig. 12.60 Metastatic carcinoma in the mandible. A large and poorly defined radiolucent metastasis has destroyed most of the posterior body of the mandible, resulting in a pathological fracture. Oblique lateral view.

and femur. Jaw metastases are, therefore, relatively unusual and almost always signify late-stage disease and widespread metastases in other bones. It is rare that a metastasis to the jaw is the first sign leading to diagnosis of the primary malignancy.

Jaw metastases are much more common than primary malignant neoplasms of bone.

Patients are usually middle-aged or elderly, reflecting the age distribution of carcinoma at the primary sites. The vast majority of metastases are in the mandible. Common symptoms are pain or swelling of the jaw (Fig. 12.58), trismus and paraesthesia or anaesthesia of the lip. A non-healing tooth socket is an important presentation for dentists.

There is typically an area of radiolucency with a hazy outline (Figs 12.59 and 12.60). This sometimes simulates an infected cyst or may be quite irregular and simulate osteomyelitis. One key feature is that metastases seed in the marrow spaces and, in the mandible, most of the marrow lies below the inferior dental canal. This localisation helps distinguish potential metastases from lesions associated

with the teeth. However, it is important to be alert for metastases mimicking infection or dental disease if the radiographic features are unusual or treatment is ineffective. Sometimes the entire mandible may have a moth-eaten appearance from complete replacement of the medulla, usually by lymphoma.

While most jaw metastases are destructive and radiolucent, some types induce bone sclerosis, notably prostatic carcinoma and less frequently breast or bladder metastases.

Pathology

Diagnosis requires biopsy unless a primary cancer with extensive bony metastases is already known. In such circumstances a biopsy is confirmatory but will not alter the treatment. In new lesions, biopsy is required and the histological appearances will be those of the primary carcinomas. The malignant tissue infiltrates adjacent marrow spaces and induces osteoclastic bone resorption (Fig. 12.61).

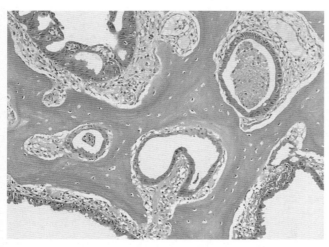

Fig. 12.61 Metastatic carcinoma in the jaw. All the medullary spaces contain adenocarcinoma, forming glands and duct-like spaces.

When a new metastasis is found, others are probably present elsewhere and a skeletal survey, bone scan, positron emission tomography scan or other survey technique will show the extent of the disease. Few patients survive more than a few months after diagnosis of a jaw metastasis and patients are treated palliatively unless they have one of the few carcinomas that respond to hormonal or other targeted treatment, such as prostate or breast. This may induce a relatively long remission. Palliative radiotherapy may sometimes make the lesion in the jaw regress for a time and lessen pain.

Case series PMID: 17138711 and 25409855

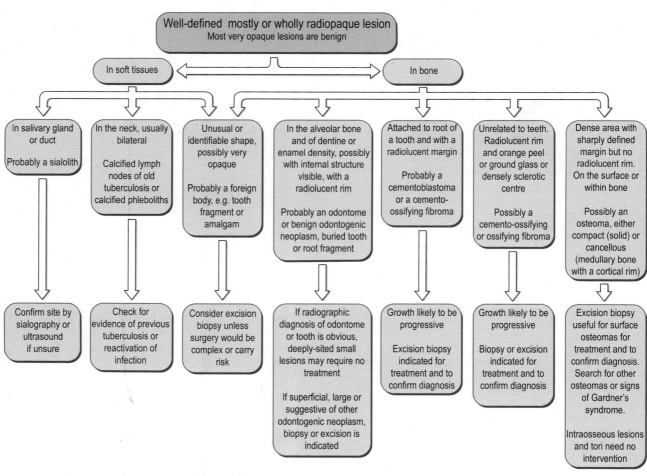

Summary Chart 12.1 Differential diagnosis of a well-defined radiopaque lesion in the jaws or soft tissues.

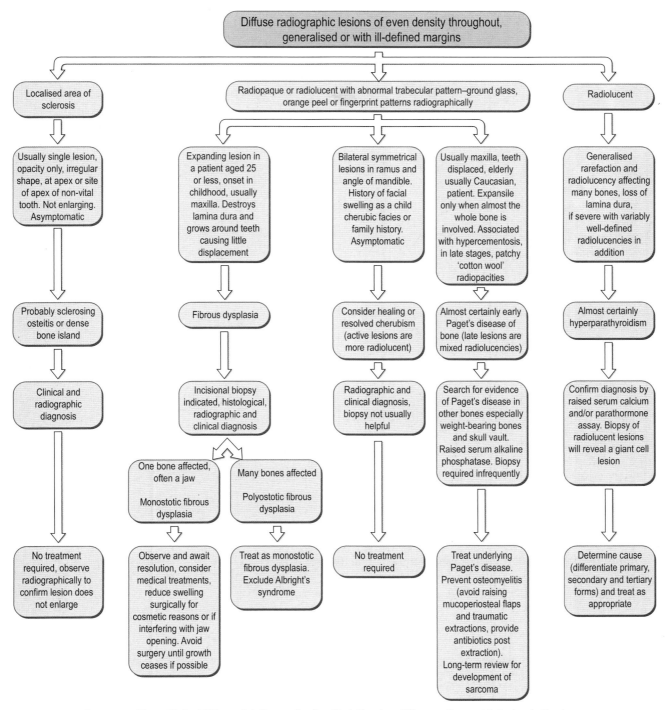

Summary Chart 12.2 Differential diagnosis of an ill-defined or diffuse radiographic lesion in the jaws.

Appendix 12.1

World Health Organization classification of non-odontogenic maxillofacial bone tumours 2022*

Name	Growth pattern[†]	Relative incidence[‡]
Giant cell lesions and bone cysts (all non-odontogenic)		
Central giant cell granuloma	U	Common
Peripheral giant cell granuloma	R	Common
Cherubism	D	Rare
Aneurysmal bone cyst	BN	Rare
Simple bone cyst	U	Rare
Fibro-osseous tumours and dysplasias (all non-odontogenic)**		
Cemento-osseous dysplasia	D	Very common
Segmental odontomaxillary dysplasia (Ch. 2)	D	Very rare
Fibrous dysplasia	D	Rare
Juvenile trabecular ossifying fibroma	BN	Rare
Psammomatoid ossifying fibroma	BN	Rare
Familial gigantiform cementoma	BN	Extremely rare
Benign maxillofacial bone and cartilage tumours		
Osteoma	BN	Rare
Osteochondroma	BN	Rare
Osteoblastoma	BN	Rare
Chondroblastoma	BN	Rare
Chondromyxoid fibroma	BN	Rare
Desmoplastic fibroma of bone	BN	Rare
Malignant maxillofacial bone and cartilage tumours		
Osteosarcoma of the jaw	MN	Rare
Chondrosarcoma family	MN	Rare
Mesenchymal chondrosarcoma	MN	Rare
Rhabdomyosarcoma with TFCP2 rearrangement	MN	Very rare
Tumours of uncertain histogenesis		
Melanotic neuroectodermal tumour of infancy	BN	Very rare
Vascular soft tissue tumours		
Haemangioma	BN	Rare in bone
Undifferentiated small round cell sarcomas of bone and soft tissue		
Ewing's sarcoma	MN	Very rare
Haematolymphoid: Histocytic and dendritic cell tumours		
Langerhans cell histiocytosis	U (some MN)	

*WHO Classification of Tumours Editorial Board. Head and neck tumours. Publisher: International Agency for Research on Cancer; 2022 Vol. (WHO classification of tumours series, 5th ed.; vol. 9, 978-92-832-4514-8)

[†]MN malignant neoplasm; BN benign neoplasm; H hamartoma; D Dysplasia. B Borderline – benign but can infiltrate locally, R reactive, U unknown

[‡]Refers to incidence in jaws and facial bones and is relative. Overall, all these tumours are rare.

**an odontogenic origin for cemento-osseous dysplasia and familial gigantiform cementoma is possible.

Inherited, metabolic and other non-neoplastic bone diseases

13

Some inherited conditions are not included in this chapter. Gardner's, Albright's and Noonan syndromes, cherubism and the familial forms of cemento-osseous dysplasia and ossifying fibroma are dealt with in Chapter 12. These diseases either have similar non-inherited forms or clinical, radiological or histological similarities with other groups of diseases. From the point of view of differential diagnosis, they are better described elsewhere. Bone diseases of dental significance are summarised in Box 13.1.

INHERITED DISEASES OF BONE

Osteogenesis imperfecta

Osteogenesis imperfecta is a group of genetic conditions in which the bones have reduced bone density and fracture easily. The term *brittle bone disease* is usually taken to mean this genetic condition but has also been applied to osteoporosis.

Pathology

Most types are inherited as an autosomal dominant trait, and the more common causal genes are the *COL1A1* and *COL1A2* procollagen genes. Procollagen in the bone matrix fails to form a normal alpha helix, polymerise into normal type 1 collagen and the collagen cannot mineralise. Without appropriate matrix, osteoblasts are unable to form normal amounts of bone, leading to fractures. However, there is remarkable molecular and clinical diversity, and the classification now extends to over 20 types in six clinically defined groups, based on inheritance pattern, genes affected and severity of the clinical phenotype. Even within one type there is variability of the effects. No gene is known for some types (Table 13.1). Mutations in genes for collagen processing, post-translational modification, cytoskeletal function and osteoblast differentiation account for additional types. Many of the more recently described gene defects produce additional effects reflecting their fundamental roles in other cellular processes. All types together affect approximately 1 in every 20,000 live births.

The bones are thin and lack the usual cortex of compact bone (Fig. 13.1), but development of epiphyseal cartilages is unimpaired so that bones in most types can grow to their normal length. Nevertheless, they may become grossly distorted by multiple fractures and result in restricted growth. The most severe cases (type II) usually die at birth or soon after; mild cases (type V) may have little disability. In the more common form (type I), the many fractures can cause severe deformity (Figs 13.2 and 13.3). The sclera of the eyes may also appear blue because their thinness allows the pigment layer to show through (Fig. 13.4). Deafness also develops.

The majority of individuals with milder disease have relatively good health. Apart from occasional fractures, approximately 60% have joint hypermobility and many tend to experience back and joint pain due to osteoarthritis.

Natural history and types PMID: 24754836

Types and genetics PMID: 34169326

Dental effects

Because collagen type 1 is a major matrix protein of dentine too, some patients have affected teeth. It is difficult to be certain about the exact relationship between the two conditions because some types are described in few families, and often there has only been clinical examination and no examination of extracted teeth. Mild cases may have radiographic features of affected teeth but appearance is normal. Types III and IV account for most cases with affected teeth. The effects on teeth are described in Chapter 2 and appear identical to those in dentinogenesis imperfecta, though they result from mutations in different genes. The dental changes in osteogenesis imperfecta are currently called 'osteogenesis imperfecta with hereditary opalescent teeth', whereas those affecting the teeth alone caused by other mutations are called 'dentinogenesis imperfecta'. Some forms are also associated with missing teeth and deciduous teeth are shed at a younger age, because of their smaller roots and less densely mineralized dentine.

Dental effects PMID: 7285471 and 24700690

Management

Treatment with a bisphosphonate may be given to prevent resorption of what bone does form. The benefits vary between different mutations and use carries a long-term risk of osteonecrosis. Denosumab, another antiresorptive drug acting on osteoclasts, and teriparatide, recombinant parathormone that stimulates osteoblasts, are occasionally used. The TGF-β-targeted treatment fresolimumab is available for patients with mutation in the *COL1A2* or *CRTAP* genes, but effectiveness is not yet defined. No other treatment is effective, except to protect the child from even minor injuries and to minimise deformity by attending to fractures. Care

---

Box 13.1   Bone diseases of dental significance

- Osteogenesis imperfecta – associated dentinogenesis imperfecta
- Osteopetrosis – anaemia and risk of osteomyelitis
- Cleidocranial dysplasia – multiple unerupted teeth
- Cherubism – cyst-like giant cell lesions
- Rickets – hypocalcification of teeth in severe cases
- Scurvy – purpura, swollen, bleeding gingivae
- Hyperparathyroidism – 'cyst-like' giant cell lesions
- Paget's disease – overgrowth of maxilla
- Fibrous dysplasia – typically, hard swelling of maxilla
- Gardner's syndrome – risk of colon carcinoma
- Osteoporosis – treatment with bisphosphonates

Table 13.1   Types of osteogenesis imperfecta

Type	Inheritance	Phenotype	Mechanism	Gene	Hereditary opalescent teeth
I	AD	Mild	Defective collagen synthesis	COL1A1	rare
II	AD	Severe, perinatal onset, ultimately lethal	Defective collagen synthesis	COL1A1 or COL1A2	no
	Various, AR or unknown	Severe, perinatal onset, ultimately lethal	Collagen post-translational modification, gene regulation	CRTAP, LEPRE1; PPIB; OASIS	Unclear and variable, DI some animal models, some patients missing teeth
III	AD	Progressive deformity	Defective collagen synthesis	COL1A1 or COL1A2	frequent
	AR	Progressive deformity	Extracellular collagen processing	BMP1	Present
	AR	Progressive deformity	MAPK signalling	CCDC134	unclear
	unknown	Progressive deformity	Collagen post-translational modification	CRTAP, FKBP10, LEPRE1, PLOD2, PPIB, SERPINH1, TMEM38B and others	Variable, Frequent (SERPINH1); mild (FKBP10), or unknown, some animal models suggest tooth ankylosis in addition (CRTAP)
	unknown	Progressive deformity	Osteoblast differentiation	WNT1	unclear
IV	AD	Moderate	Defective collagen synthesis	COL1A1 or COL1A2	frequent
	X linked	Moderate	Actin cytoskeleton formation	PLS3	no
V	AD	Moderate, hypertrophic callus and ossification of the interosseous membrane	Matrix mineralisation	IFITM5	no*
Atypical	AD	Additional systems involved, optic atrophy, immunodeficiency	Endoplasmic reticulum function	NBAS	unclear

*Type V has no opalescent teeth but does show hypodontia and short roots in some families.
AD, autosomal dominant; *AR*, autosomal recessive.
Additional rare types are known

must be taken during dental extractions, but fractures of the jaws are uncommon. Implants appear to osseointegrate in the few cases reported, enabling treatment of late dental effects.

Key features are summarised in Box 13.2.

Dental implants PMID: 35162583

Gnathodiaphyseal dysplasia

This very rare autosomal dominant condition was previously thought to be a variant of osteogenesis imperfecta with frequent fractures but normal healing. Its other features include bowing and cortical thickening of the long bones and multiple ossifying fibromas of the jaws. The teeth are normal (Ch. 11).

Case series PMID: 4014312

Osteopetrosis

Osteopetrosis, or marble bone disease, is a rare genetic disease in which the bones become solid and dense (Fig. 13.5) but brittle, because of increased bone deposition. The condition is caused by a variety of mutations in proteins that inactivate osteoclasts, preventing normal bone resorption and remodelling. There are several types of variable severity and inheritance pattern, and the disease can present in children or adults.

Medullary spaces are compressed by progressive deposition of bone on the trabeculae, reducing the marrow spaces until they are minute (Fig. 13.6), and the epiphyseal ends of the bones are club shaped. Loss of marrow space causes the liver and spleen to take on blood-cell formation, but anaemia is common, and defective white cells can lead to abnormal susceptibility to infection.

Curative treatment is limited to bone marrow transplant, which must be undertaken at a very young age and can only be countenanced in potentially fatal forms of the disease.

General review PMID: 23877423

Dental aspects

There may be compression of cranial nerve canals so that trigeminal or facial nerve neuropathies result. Despite its density, the bone can be brittle so that the jaw may fracture

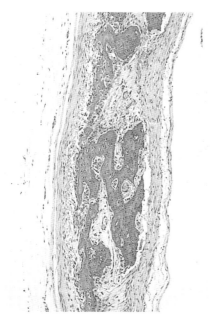

Fig. 13.1 Osteogenesis imperfecta. A section from the vault of the skull of a stillborn infant with type II disease. In this most severe form of osteogenesis imperfecta the bone is small in amount, woven in type and shows no differentiation into the normal structure with cortical plates and medullary space.

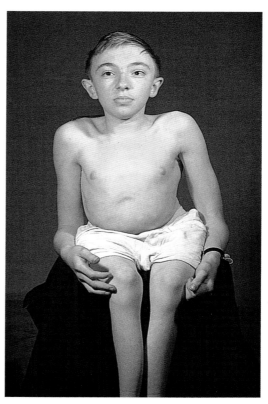

Fig. 13.3 Clinical appearance of a severely affected child with osteogenesis imperfecta type III in which there is progressive deformity.

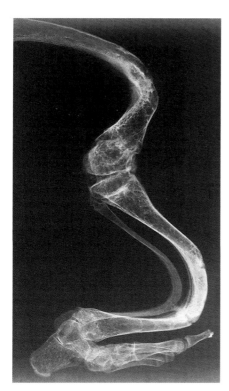

Fig. 13.2 Osteogenesis imperfecta. Leg of an infant with a severe type of osteogenesis imperfecta showing severe bending as a result of multiple fractures under body weight.

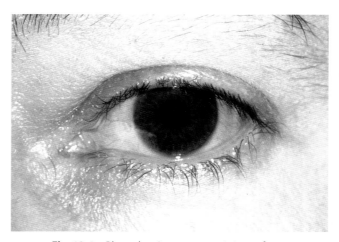

Fig. 13.4 Blue sclera in osteogenesis imperfecta.

treat so that prevention of dental infections is important and implants carry a high risk.

Tooth eruption is delayed and may fail, tooth shape may become distorted and there may be enamel hypoplasia depending on causative gene.

Key features are summarised in Box 13.3.

Dental changes PMID: 27858309

Sclerosing bone dysplasias

Many other genetic conditions are recognized that are associated with bone sclerosis and generalized increased bone mass (Box 13.4), but all are rare. They may be inherited as autosomal recessive or dominant conditions and are often

during extractions. Osteomyelitis of the jaws is surprisingly rare despite the almost complete sclerosis and reduced vascularity, but affects approximately 10% of patients. It usually develops in the mandible and is very difficult to

caused by mutations in genes of the Wnt signalling pathway. The best characterised are sclerostosis and van Buchem disease, caused by mutations or dysregulation of the *SOST* gene that encodes sclerostin, a signalling protein that normally inhibits bone formation. Patients often have a Dutch or Afrikaaner heritage.

Both these diseases are associated with a large skeleton but particularly enlargement of the mandible and cranial bones and development of tori. Mandibular enlargement may be the presenting feature in early adulthood. The large mandible has increased angle producing a long mandible with prognathism and a very thick and patchily sclerotic cortex (Fig. 13.7). In later life, skull bone growth causes cranial nerve palsies, deafness and headaches from compression of the brain. Other sclerosing bone dysplasias can be associated with more disparate developmental alterations.

When only the mandibular involvement is noted in a young patient, the radiographic appearances resemble chronic non-bacterial osteomyelitis and SAPHO (Ch. 12).

Autosomal dominant endosteal hyperostosis PMID: 30028190

SOST-related sclerosing bone dysplasias PMID: 36508511

LRP5 high bone mass PMID: 37659026

Box 13.2   Osteogenesis imperfecta: key features

- Thin fragile bones
- Usually an autosomal dominant trait, but many inheritance patterns
- Multiple fractures lead to gross deformity in severe types
- Mild types may be unrecognized until adulthood
- Teeth affected, especially in types III and IV
- Affected teeth resemble those in dentinogenesis imperfecta
- Jaw fractures are uncommon
- Some patients treated with bisphosphonates or other antiresorptive drugs

---

Achondroplasia

Achondroplasia is the most common type of genetic skeletal disorder and causes reduced long bone growth, so that affected individuals have short-limbs while the

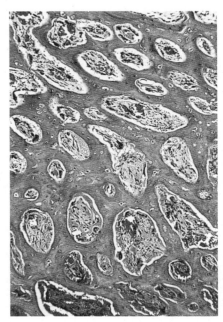

Fig. 13.6   Osteopetrosis. Almost solid bone with only small medullary spaces.

Box 13.3   Osteopetrosis: key features

- Rare genetic defect of osteoclastic activity
- Bones lack medullary cavities, are very dense but brittle
- Anaemia is common
- Osteomyelitis a recognised complication
- Delayed tooth eruption

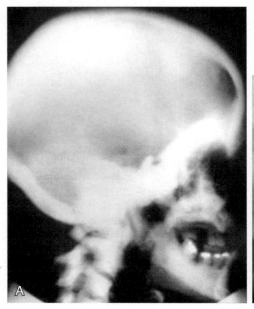

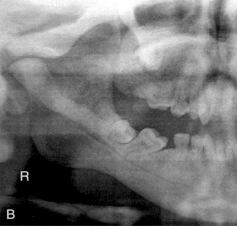

Fig. 13.5   Osteopetrosis. (A) True lateral skull showing the cranial features of radiopaque, dense vault and thickened base. (B) Right side of a panoramic radiograph showing loss of the normal trabecular pattern and replacement with dense thickened bone. *(From Whaites E, Drage N, 2021. Essentials of dental radiography and radiology, 6th ed. Oxford: Elsevier Ltd)*

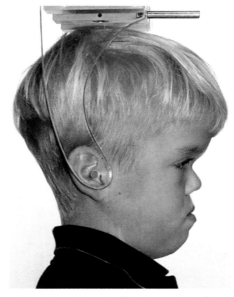

Fig. 13.8 Achondroplasia. Maxillary hypoplasia, the retruded maxilla and nose do not grow forwards because of reduced cartilaginous growth in the skull base. *(From Cohen MM, Jr, MacClean RE, 2000. Craniosynostosis: diagnosis, evaluation, and management. New York: Oxford University Press)*

Box 13.5 Achondroplasia: key features
- A common genetically determined growth restriction
- Failure of proliferation of cartilage in epiphyses and base of skull
- Short limbs but skull and trunk unaffected
- Middle third of face retrusive due to reduced growth of skull base
- Relative prognathism
- Malocclusion often severe

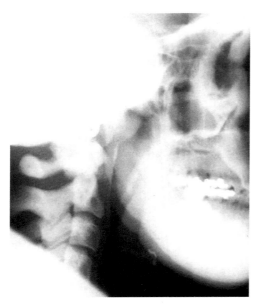

Fig. 13.7 Sclerostosis. Lateral view showing enlarged and very dense mandible and involvement of cranial bones.

size of the trunk and head is unaffected. The cause is a homozygous mutation in the gene encoding fibroblast growth factor receptor 3, that prevents bone forming from cartilage at the epiphyses and in the base of the skull. Inheritance is autosomal dominant, but homozygous mutation is lethal.

Dental aspects

The head size is unaffected but with a high forehead, and reduced growth at the base of the skull causes the middle third of the face to be retrusive (Fig 13.8). The mandible is often protrusive, and there is usually severe malocclusion and sometimes posterior open bite. Associated macroglossia has been described. All these features predispose to a high incidence of sleep apnoea, affecting a third of individuals.

Key features are summarised in Box 13.5.

Case and review: PMID: 24151409

Cleidocranial dysplasia

In this rare familial disorder, there is a mutation or deletion in the *RUNX2* gene that encodes a transcription factor that controls osteoblast and chondroblast proliferation and differentiation. Development of the clavicles is attenuated and there is delayed closure of fontanelles, sometimes retrusion of the maxilla and a range of other features, many affecting the skull. Partial or complete absence of clavicles allows the

patient to bring the shoulders together in front of the chest (Fig. 13.9).

Dental aspects

Cleidocranial dysplasia is one of the few identifiable causes of delayed eruption of the permanent dentition. Many permanent teeth may remain embedded in the jaw (Fig. 13.10) and frequently give rise to dentigerous cysts (see Ch. 10). The deciduous teeth are retained. The *RUNX2* gene that is mutated in this condition normally controls alveolar bone remodelling, tooth and periodontal ligament development, all required for tooth eruption. Orthodontic traction to induce eruption is very slow because the mutation affects bone remodelling.

Key features are summarised in Box 13.6.

Case series and review PMID: 22023169

Hypophosphatasia

Hypophosphatasia is an uncommon recessive genetic disorder caused by one of many mutations in the *TNAP* gene that encodes the enzyme non-specific alkaline phosphatase required to liberate inorganic phosphate for mineralisation. Inheritance is autosomal and either dominant or recessive. There are several types of variable severity, milder forms presenting at an older age. While the severe forms are rare, the milder forms are relatively common with an incidence of 1:500–3000. The early-onset type causes rickets-like skeletal disease with defective mineralization causing multiple fractures that heal slowly and muscle weakness. Teeth lack cementum and therefore periodontal attachment to bone, causing premature loss. This is sometimes the only sign of the disease (see Fig. 2.38). Diagnosis is made by the low levels of plasma alkaline phosphatase. Late-onset hypophosphatasia presents with bone fractures. See also Chapter 2.

General review PMID: 34884378

Dental effects PMID: 19232125

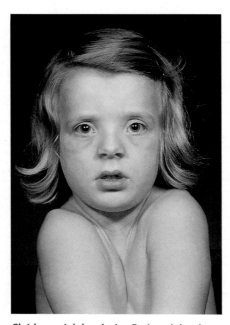

Fig. 13.9 Cleidocranial dysplasia. Reduced development of the clavicles allows this excess mobility of the shoulders. Other members of the family were also affected.

Sickle cell anaemia and thalassaemia major

Both these haemoglobinopathies can cause bone changes, but only in the most severely affected. Thalassaemia is the more likely to do so but the classical changes are now rarely seen. In thalassaemia, the bone marrow becomes hyperplastic, responding to chronic hypoxia, expanding the marrow spaces in all bones. Trabecular bone becomes less dense, and in untreated cases there is painless expansion of bones, with eventual obliteration of the maxillary sinuses. Bones are thus larger but osteoporotic. Skull radiographs may show a 'hair-on-end' appearance (Fig 13.11) caused by periosteal growth expanding the bone, large maxilla and a thin cortex in all bones. In severe cases frontal bossing develops (Fig 13.12). The teeth may be displaced, causing malocclusion. Treatment with bisphosphonates or recombinant parathormone reduce bone loss, preventing long bone fractures. Bisphosphonate use carries a long-term risk of jaw osteonecrosis.

In sickle cell anaemia, the changes are less marked but, in addition, the abnormal erythrocytes sludge in vessels under low oxygen tension, block them and cause painful infarcts in the bones. Symptomatically and radiographically, infarcts can mimic osteomyelitis. Bone infarcts may appear relatively radiolucent at first but become sclerotic.

Box 13.6   Cleidocranial dysplasia: key features

- Caused by mutation or deletion in *RUNX2* gene
- Absent clavicles, delayed closure of fontanelles
- Many or most permanent teeth typically fail to erupt
- Delayed eruption then prolonged retention of deciduous teeth
- Many supernumerary unerupted teeth also present
- Long-term risk of developing dentigerous cysts
- Sinuses reduced in size
- High arched palate and sometimes cleft palate
- Large skull with frontal bossing
- Ocular hypertelorism
- Short stature

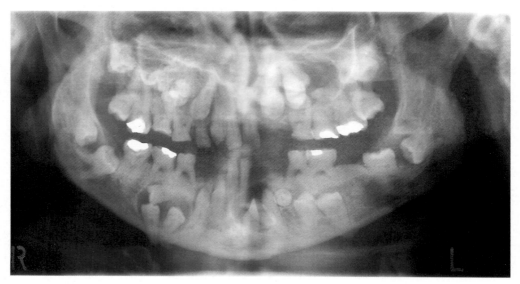

Fig. 13.10   Cleidocranial dysplasia. There are many additional teeth but widespread failure of eruption and possibly development of dentigerous cysts.

Gigantism and acromegaly

Overproduction of pituitary growth hormone, usually by an adenoma, before the epiphyses fuse, gives rise to gigantism with overgrowth of the whole skeleton. After fusion of the epiphyses, overproduction of growth hormone gives rise to acromegaly. The main features are continued growth at the mandibular condyle, causing marked prognathism, macroglossia, thickening of the facial soft tissues and overgrowth of the hands and feet (see Ch. 37).

METABOLIC BONE DISEASE

Rickets

Rickets in resource-poor countries is usually due to deficiency of dietary calcium, whereas in developed countries it is rare and caused by deficiency of vitamin D, either in the diet or through lack of exposure to sunlight (Ch. 36). Rickets causes defective calcification and development of the skeleton. Similar changes may also result from excess mineral excretion in chronic renal diseases (renal rickets) including renal tubular acidosis, hypophosphatemic rickets and defects in vitamin D metabolism in the kidney.

The onset of rickets is usually in infancy. The main effects are broadening of the growing ends of bones and prominent costochondral junctions due to the epiphyseal changes (Figs 13.13 and 13.14). The weakened bones bend readily. Typical changes in the skull are wide fontanelles, bossing of the frontal and parietal eminences and thinning of the back of the skull.

Treatment of rickets is with vitamin D and calcium supplements.

Dental aspects

Teeth have priority over the skeleton for minerals, and the teeth are rarely affected by rickets except in the most severe cases. Hypocalcification of dentine, with a wide band of

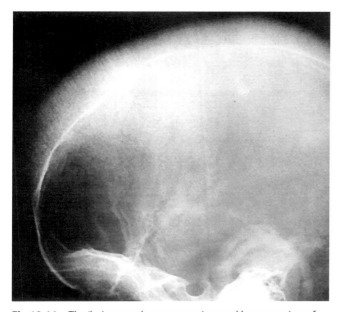

Fig 13.11   The 'hair on end appearance' caused by expansion of the marrow space in the skull and rapid periosteal bone growth to accommodate it, in this case in a patient with sickle cell disease. *(Courtesy H. G. Poyton, DDS, Toronto, Ontario, Canada).*

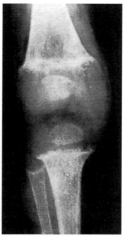

Fig. 13.13   **Rickets.** Overgrowth of cartilage causes the epiphyseal plate to be broad, thick and irregular, and the ends of the bone become splayed. The growing end of the bone is ill-defined and calcification defective.

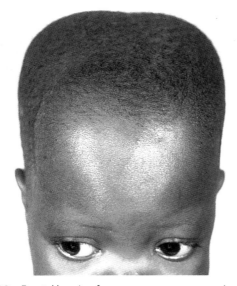

Fig 13.12   Frontal bossing from marrow space expansion, in this case in sickle cell anaemia. *(Courtesy Professor R. Hendrickse).*

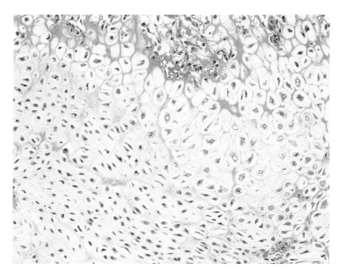

Fig. 13.14   **Rickets.** Microscopically, the epiphyseal plate has become disorganised with loss of the normal alignment of the chondrocytes. There is proliferation, but no calcification.

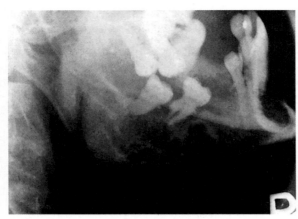

Fig. 13.15 Hyperparathyroidism. A patient of 51 years with hyperparathyroidism as a result of a parathyroid adenoma. There is an area of bone destruction simulating a multilocular cyst. The radiograph quality is low because of the loss of bone mineral.

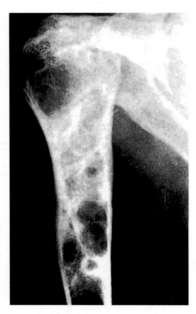

Fig. 13.16 Hyperparathyroidism. Generalised bone radiolucency and *osteitis fibrosa cystica*, multiple brown tumours, in the humerus of the same patient with a parathyroid adenoma.

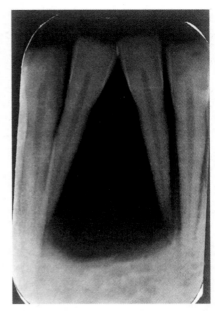

Fig. 13.17 Hyperparathyroidism. In this patient with hyperparathyroidism as a result of rejection of a kidney graft, there is a well-defined area of bone loss caused by a brown tumour.

predentine and extensive interglobular spaces, may be seen in unusually severe rickets. Eruption of teeth may also be delayed in such cases. Teeth with changes of rickets are not predisposed to dental caries.

Dental effects PMID: 23939820

Vitamin D–resistant rickets

This condition caused by genetic failure of reabsorption of phosphate in the kidney is associated with characteristic dental effects and is discussed in Chapter 2.

Hyperparathyroidism

➜ Summary charts 10.2 and 12.2 pp. 176, 229

Overproduction of parathormone (PTH) mobilises calcium from the skeleton and raises the plasma calcium level. In primary hyperparathyroidism the cause is usually an adenoma of the parathyroid glands, uncommonly hyperplasia of

the gland and rarely a parathyroid carcinoma. Mostly elderly women are affected. This is less common than secondary hyperparathyroidism, in which PTH secretion is maintained by the normal homeostatic response to low calcium levels, usually caused by vitamin D deficiency or chronic renal failure (because the kidney enzymatically activates vitamin D). The major symptoms of all types result from renal damage which leads to hypertension or cardiovascular disease.

Bone disease is identical in primary and secondary disease but is rarely seen now because of early treatment. Radiographically there is diffuse bone loss: thinning of bone trabeculae, subperiosteal resorption of the bone of the fingers and resorption of the terminal phalangeal tufts. Dental radiographs may reveal reduced bone density, loss of trabecular pattern and definition of the lamina dura around the teeth. In severe disease these changes are more marked, and in addition the patient may develop one or more brown tumours. These cyst-like radiolucencies may appear unilocular or multilocular (Figs 13.15–13.17) and are now more likely to be seen in secondary disease because of its long-term course. Bony changes can cause pathological fractures but reverse with treatment (Figs 13.18 and 13.19). A second effect seen in hyperparathyroidism secondary to renal disease is localized or diffuse mandibular enlargement, sometimes dramatic (see Ch. 38).

Hyperparathyroidism is also present in 95% of patients with multiple endocrine neoplasia type 1 (MEN 1) syndrome (Ch. 37) and is a feature of the hyperparathyroidism jaw tumour syndrome with multiple cemento-ossifying fibromas (Ch. 12).

Teeth primary hyperparathyroidism PMID: 13912943

Diffuse and localized mandibular enlargement PMID: 22676829 and 9127383

Pathology

Histologically, the altered bone architecture can be seen, with thin trabeculae and cortex and frequent osteoclasts resorbing the bone surfaces.

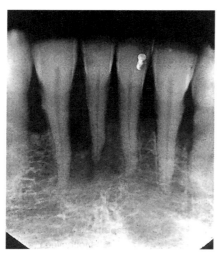

Fig. 13.18 Hyperparathyroidism. A periapical view reveals the relative radiolucency of the bone. There is loss of lamina dura around the roots, loss of trabeculae centrally and coarsening of the trabecular pattern elsewhere.

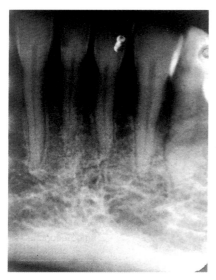

Fig. 13.19 Hyperparathyroidism. The same patient after treatment shows improved bone density and reformation of the lamina dura and cortex.

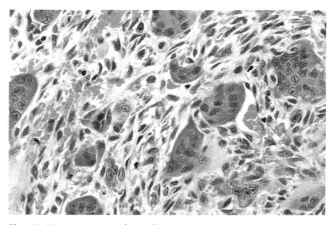

Fig. 13.20 Hyperparathyroidism. Multinucleate osteoclast-like giant cells are lying in a haemorrhagic fibrous tissue. The appearances are indistinguishable histologically from giant cell granuloma.

Box 13.7 Biochemical findings in primary hyperparathyroidism

- Raised plasma calcium, usually above 10 mg/dl
- Low serum phosphorus
- Raised plasma parathyroid hormone levels
- Raised serum alkaline phosphatase

Box 13.8 Hyperparathyroidism: key features

- Overproduction of parathyroid hormone due to hyperplasia or adenoma of parathyroid glands
- Calcium mobilised from bone to serum, then lost in urine
- Common effects are malaise, hypertension or peptic ulcer and kidney stones
- Significant bone disease now uncommon with early diagnosis
- Generalised rarefaction of bone, loss of density and lamina dura
- In severe disease, brown tumours in the jaw appear radiographically as multilocular cyst-like areas
- Histologically, brown tumours are indistinguishable from giant cell granulomas
- Diagnosis confirmed by raised parathyroid hormone and serum calcium levels

---

The brown tumour comprises foci with complete bone loss filled by soft tissue containing numerous osteoclasts in a highly vascular stroma (Fig. 13.20). There is extensive internal haemorrhage. Breakdown of erythrocytes produces haemosiderin pigment and colours the lesion brown, hence its name. The histological appearances are indistinguishable from a giant cell granuloma of the jaws (see Ch. 12)

Diagnosis cannot, therefore, depend on histology alone, and radiographs and blood chemistry are essential whenever histology reveals a giant cell lesion (Box 13.7), with a search for involvement of other bones if test results suggest hyperparathyroidism.

The increased excretion of calcium leads ultimately to renal stone formation and renal damage. Other clinical features also result from the hypercalcaemia. The severe complications make early diagnosis of this disease particularly important.

Features in jaws PMID: 35181256

Brown tumours in jaws PMID: 16798410

Management

In primary hyperparathyroidism, surgical removal of the causative adenoma is curative. A sestamibi scan (a form of technetium 99 scan) can often identify the hyperactive gland to target it for surgery. For secondary hyperparathyroidism, treatment depends on the success of management of the renal failure. Bone lesions may respond to oral administration of vitamin D, whose metabolism is abnormal as a result of the renal disease. Surgery may also become necessary in late-stage renal failure to remove parathyroid glands that enlarge and secrete excessively and autonomously in response to the low serum calcium, so-called *tertiary hyperparathyroidism*.

Key features are summarised in Box 13.8.

OTHER BONE DISEASES

Paget's disease of bone*

→ Summary chart 13.1 p. 222

Paget's disease of bone (osteitis deformans) is a disturbance of bone turnover that causes irregular resorption and softening followed by sclerosis of bone. Paget's disease affects older people, with onset after the age of 45 years. Anglo-Saxon races and their migrated descendants have the highest incidence. In Britain, as many as 2% of people older than 50 years may have radiographic signs and incidence doubles with each decade of age. Men are more frequently affected than women. Pagets's disease in young people develops only as part of rare syndromes.

The possibility that Paget's disease is caused by a virus, possibly measles or a canine virus, is now considered less likely than genetic causes. However, there must be environmental factors because the incidence and severity have decreased dramatically in the UK during the last 50 years. This, together with effective treatment, has made clinically evident disease uncommon.

Cases often show familial clustering and about 15% of cases in Britain probably have an inherited genetic cause or predisposition and this rises to half of cases in some emigrant Anglo-Saxon populations. Familial cases tend to be affected more severely. Several genes are thought to account for familial cases and the main candidates are the *SQSTM1* and *RANK* genes that regulate osteoclast differentiation and function through the NFκB signalling pathway. Non-familial cases are associated with somatic mutations in these and other functionally related genes.

The bones most frequently affected are the sacrum, spine, skull, femora and pelvis, the skull being involved in almost half of cases. The disease may be widespread and is usually symmetrical, but sometimes a single bone is affected. In a severely affected patient, the main features are an enlarged head, thickening of long bones, which bend under stress, and tenderness or aching bone pain which can be severe. However, over half people affected are asymptomatic.

Paget's disease is now largely effectively treated by bisphosphonates, either orally or given as intravenous infusion during active disease. Calcitonin can also be used to inactivate osteoclasts but is no longer used for long-term treatment because there is a risk for cancer of various types, although the risk is low. It is reserved for disease not responding to bisphosphonates or for rapid pain relief and limited to 3 months of treatment. Calcium and vitamin D supplementation are also required.

General review PMID: 25585180 and 28339664

Pathological process and genetics PMID: 33768371

Pathology

Resorption, softening and then sclerosis of bones develop in sequence. A focus of diseased bone gradually enlarges, spreading along a bone like a wave, leaving an enlarging central zone of the bone sclerotic and distorted. Bone resorption and replacement becomes rapid, irregular, exaggerated and purposeless, and the ultimate result is diffuse thickening of

---

* Sir James Paget (1814–1899), pioneer surgical pathologist, described several diseases that bear his name: Paget's disease of the nipple (intraductal breast carcinoma involving the nipple), extramammary Paget's disease, Paget's abscess and Paget's disease of bone. In general usage, the additional 'of bone' is understood when Paget's disease is referred to, but may need to be specified to avoid confusion.

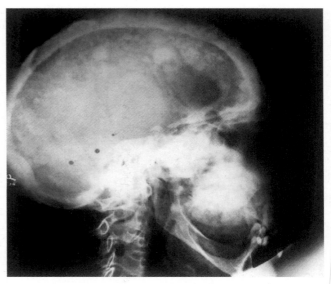

Fig. 13.21   Paget's disease of the skull and maxilla. The thickening of the bone and the irregular areas of sclerosis and resorption, which give it a fluffy appearance, are in striking contrast to the unaffected mandible.

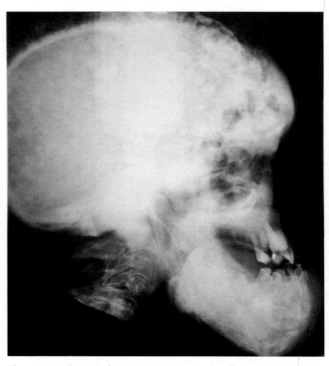

Fig. 13.22   Paget's disease. A very severely affected individual with extensive sclerosis and enlargement of all skull bones and jaws including, unusually, the mandible.

affected bones. Closely adjacent parts of the bone may show different stages of the disease; a common result is therefore patchy areas of osteoporosis and of sclerosis (Figs 13.21 and 13.22).

Repeated bone resorption and deposition is marked histologically by blue-staining resting and reversal lines. Their irregular pattern characteristically produces a jigsaw puzzle ('mosaic') appearance in the bone (Fig 13.23). Both osteoclasts and osteoblasts are more prominent than in normal bone, and the osteoclasts are abnormally large and with more nuclei than normal. In the late stages, affected

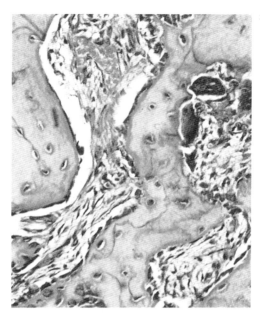

Fig. 13.23   Paget's disease. There is a well-marked irregular ('mosaic') pattern of reversal lines due to repeated alternation of resorption and apposition. The marrow has been replaced by fibrous tissue; many osteoblasts and osteoclasts line the surface of the bone.

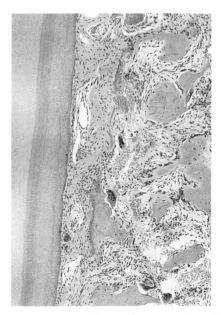

Fig. 13.24 Paget's disease affecting the jaw results in destruction of the cortex including the lamina dura surrounding the teeth and, at a later stage, causes hypercementosis (see Fig. 6.17) and sometimes ankylosis.

bones are thick, the cortex (Fig 13.24) and medulla are not distinguishable and the whole bone is spongy in texture. There is also fibrosis of the marrow spaces and increased vascularity with large vessels. These shunt the majority of the blood flow direct from the arterial to venous circulation, reducing the perfusion of bone and lowering peripheral resistance. This places a strain on the heart and may lead to eventual high-output cardiac failure.

Serum calcium and phosphorus levels are usually normal, but the alkaline phosphatase level is particularly high and

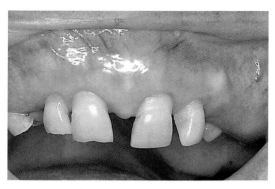

Fig. 13.25   Paget's disease. Characteristic features of the involved maxilla are the broadening and deepening of the alveolar process, generalised bone enlargement and spacing of the teeth.

may reach 700 IU/L. This is the primary diagnostic test for Paget's disease, and with typical radiological appearances, no biopsy is necessary.

The development of osteosarcoma is a recognised but rare complication of Paget's disease, affecting about 0.25% of cases. This is the commonest cause of osteosarcoma in older people, in whom osteosarcoma is otherwise very rare, and it carries a very poor prognosis. Osteosarcoma developing in the jaws is extremely rare in comparison with other bones but it does arise there occasionally.

Many patients live to an advanced age in spite of their disabilities.

Pathology review PMID: 24043712

Dental aspects

The skull is the most frequently affected bone in the head and neck. The softened skull vault deforms under the weight of the brain and sags down around the sides to produce the radiological sign of *Tam O'Shanter* skull, said to resemble the Scottish hat of the same name. Involvement of the skull base narrows foramina and in severe cases leads to cranial nerve deficits, commonly deafness.

Approximately 20% of patients used to have jaw involvement but reducing severity during the last decades seems to have reduced the incidence in the jaws. When they are affected, the maxilla is considerably more frequently and severely affected than the mandible (see Fig. 13.21). The jaw and alveolar process becomes symmetrically and grossly enlarged (Figs 13.25-13.26). The sinuses are obliterated in severe cases, and the nasal airway can be reduced in size. Outward expansion of the alveolus carries the teeth with it so that spacing develops and old dentures no longer fit. When the maxilla and base of skull are greatly enlarged, the orbits are pushed laterally. Hypertelorism and the additional facial height contribute to the appearance known as 'leontiasis ossea', a deformity somewhat incongruously likened to the appearance of a lion's face and a degree of severity that is now of only historical interest.

There may also be gross and irregular hypercementosis of teeth. The increased turnover in cementum extends to resorption and replacement of the tooth root and cementum can extend through the widened apex into the pulp. The lamina dura around the teeth is lost, and teeth may become ankylosed if the hypercementosis becomes fused to sclerotic areas of surrounding bone. Attempts to extract affected teeth may succeed only by fracturing away a large mass of bone. Severe bleeding from the vascular bone may follow. In

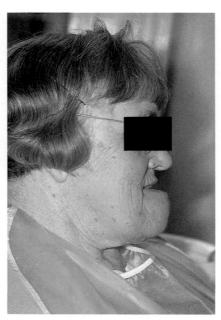

Fig. 13.26 Paget's disease. A rare example of severe mandibular involvement.

the longer term the dense cemental and bone sclerosis are prone to osteomyelitis and heal slowly. Antibiotic cover is necessary for extractions if the alveolus is sclerotic. Biopsy of involved jaws is not necessary for diagnosis and should be avoided for the same reason.

The main radiographic features are lower density of the bone in the early stages and sclerosis in the later stages. Changes are unevenly distributed, and loss of normal trabeculation and patchy sclerosis cause the characteristic 'cotton-wool' appearance.

Prolonged bisphosphonate treatment gives patients with Paget's disease a risk of medication-induced osteonecrosis (Ch. 8).

In the diagnosis of Paget's disease in the jaws, alternatives to consider are fibro-osseous lesions, particularly florid cemento-osseous dysplasia (see Ch. 12). The patchy radiolucent and sclerotic appearances are very similar, but cemento-osseous dysplasia always starts in the alveolar processes of the jaws and is much more common in the mandible. Paget's disease in the jaws is now so rare that alternative causes of sclerosis are much more likely, but initial presentation to a dentist is still possible.

Key features are summarised in Box 13.9.

Dental relevance PMID: 6459433

Osteoporosis

Osteoporosis (meaning porous bones) is an extremely common and initially asymptomatic condition in which bone mineral density is reduced. The cause is a result of imbalance between deposition and resorption, usually caused by one or more of multiple factors including aging, low initial bone mass, post-menopausal oestrogen loss, smoking, alcohol use, malnutrition, vitamin D deficiency and physical inactivity. Spongy bones deform and are at increased risk of fracture. Up to 40% of females and 15% of males have osteoporosis in developed countries.

The jaws are affected more than weight bearing bones and the diagnosis can be made on panoramic radiography that shows thinning of the cortex, reduced trabeculation

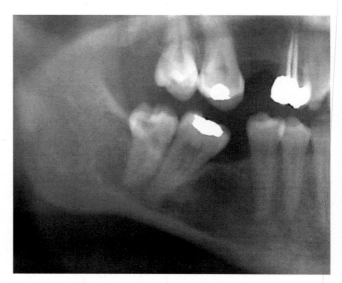

Fig. 13.27 Osteoporotic bone marrow defect affecting a typical site. Large lesions with well-defined borders such as this are often subjected to biopsy for diagnosis.

and overall bone density. In severe cases a uniform ground glass pattern results that resembles that seen in hyperparathyroidism but, unlike hyperparathyroidism, the bone loss in osteoporosis is diffuse and discrete radiolucent lesions do not form.

This reduced bone density does not appear to be a significant predisposing factor for chronic periodontitis.

The main significance for dentistry is treatment with oral low potency oral bisphosphonate and other antiresorptive drugs. Although the dose appears to carry almost no risk for medication-related osteonecrosis, it is prudent to take it into account in planning treatment if there has been very long-term exposure. Osteoporosis does not significantly reduce the success of implant placement but osseointegration is slower. The presence of osteoporosis in the rest of the skeleton does not contraindicate implant placement.

Dental significance PMID: 33048242 and 37043030

Osteoporotic bone marrow defect

This is an anatomical variant rather than a lesion and is included here because it may be misdiagnosed radiographically for simple bone cyst (Fig. 13.27).

The defect is simply a very large marrow space without bony trabeculae and filled with haemopoietic or fatty marrow. The common site is the posterior body of mandible, and there are no symptoms. There is no association with generalized osteoporosis. No treatment is required, but large and radiographically well-defined examples are often submitted to biopsy assuming the changes to be pathological.

Cases and review PMID: 4528570

Summary chart 13.1   Mixed patchy radiolucent and radiopaque lesion with poorly defined margin.

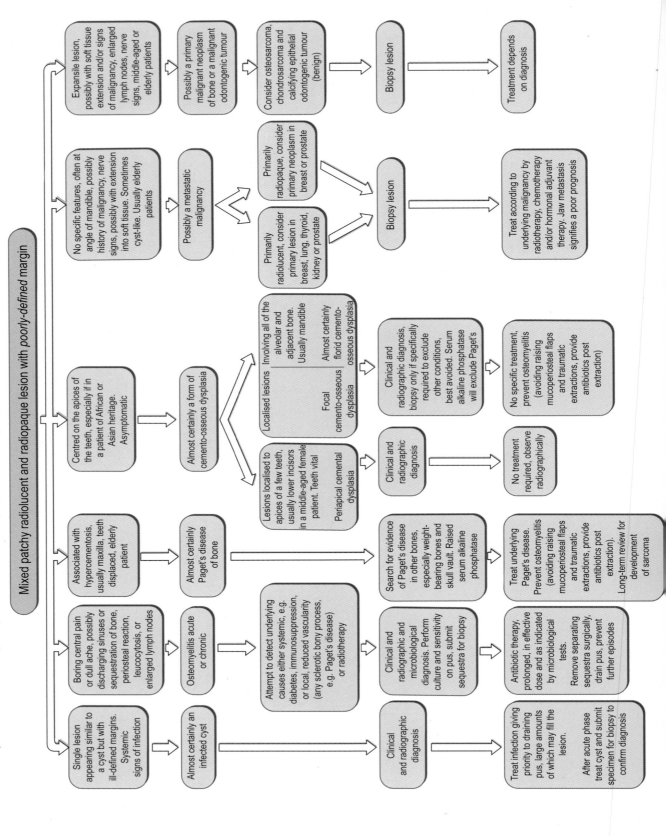

Disorders of the temporomandibular joints and trismus

14

Temporomandibular joint (TMJ) disorders can cause various combinations of limitation of movement of the jaw, pain, locking or clicking sounds. Pain, in particular, is a frequent cause of limitation of movement. These complaints are rarely due to organic disease of the joint, but diagnosis requires organic disease to be excluded. Important causes of limitation of mandibular movement are summarised in Boxes 14.1 and 14.2.

Trismus is correctly defined as inability to open the mouth due to muscle spasm, but the term is often used for limited movement of the jaw from any cause and usually refers to temporary limitation of movement. The term *ankylosis* means fusion between condyle and fossa within the joint, usually bony or fibrous union as a result of infection or trauma, and results in complete or near complete trismus (see Box 14.2). Inability to open the mouth fully is usually temporary, and causes are summarised in the following sections. Pain dysfunction syndrome is by far the most common cause of temporary limitation of movement of the temporomandibular joint.

TEMPORARY LIMITATION OF MOVEMENT

Infection and inflammation in or near the joint

Any infection or inflammation involving the muscles of mastication will lead to trismus, either by making opening painful or because oedema or swelling prevent movement. The main causes are surgical extraction of third molars, acute pericoronitis and infections of dental origin in fascial spaces (Ch. 9).

Submasseteric abscess results in profound trismus. Mumps makes eating painful and limits movement because the parotid gland is compressed by the mandibular ramus on opening. Rare causes include suppurative arthritis, osteomyelitis, cellulitis and suppurative parotitis.

Mandibular block injections may cause inflammation and oedema in medial pterygoid muscle, usually through bleeding. Needle-track infections are now only of historic interest since single-use sterile needles have been used.

Box 14.1   Causes of limitation of mandibular movement

Pericapsular and remote causes

- Infection and inflammation in adjacent tissues
- Injury, condylar neck or zygoma fracture
- Irradiation and other causes of fibrosis
- Fibrous ankylosis in the periarticular tissues
- Oral submucous fibrosis
- Systemic sclerosis

Intracapsular causes

- Traumatic arthritis and disk damage
- Infective arthritis
- Rheumatoid and osteoarthritis
- Intracapsular condylar fracture
- Neoplasms of the joint
- Loose bodies in joint
- Intracapsular fibrous ankylosis, caused by any of the above

Muscular

- Temporomandibular joint pain-dysfunction syndrome
- Myalgia caused by bruxism
- Cranial arteritis
- Tetanus and tetany
- Haematoma from ID block

Other

- Drugs
- Dislocation
- Craniofacial anomalies involving the joint

Box 14.2   Extracapsular causes of limitation of temporomandibular joint movement ('false ankylosis')

Mechanical interference with jaw movement

- Trauma: depressed fracture of the zygomatic bone or arch
- Hyperplasia: developmental overgrowth of the coronoid process
- Neoplasms: osteochondroma, osteoma of the coronoid process
- Irradiation fibrosis
- Miscellaneous:
  - myositis ossificans in masticatory muscles
  - taut skin in systemic sclerosis
  - taut mucosa in oral submucous fibrosis
  - congenital anomalies of the jaw or face

Capsular causes

- Trauma: periarticular fibrosis from wounds or burns
  - Posterior or superior dislocation
  - Longstanding anterior dislocation
- Infection: fibrosis from chronic periarticular suppuration
- Joint capsule fibrosis
  - Irradiation
  - Post-surgical scarring

Injuries

The common causes of mandibular condyle fracture are cycle accidents and assault. Unilateral condylar neck fracture usually produces only a mild limitation of opening with deviation of the jaw to the affected side but closing into intercuspal occlusion may be difficult. Bilateral displaced condylar fractures cause an anterior open bite with limited movement. A major 'guardsman's fracture' (bilateral condylar and symphysis fracture) with damage to the fossa causes severe restriction of all movements. Less severe injuries frequently result in an effusion into the temporomandibular joint; both wide opening and complete closure are then prevented during the acute phase.

Bleeding into the joint space after a condylar fracture fills the joint with blood clot and organisation can lead to bone formation in the clot, either in one compartment of the joint or both, the latter resulting in bony ankylosis. Early mobilisation of condylar fractures prevents this complication. Treatment of condylar fractures is controversial, with little evidence to support either open or closed reduction. Treatment in children is conservative to avoid later growth disturbance

Any unstable mandibular fracture causes protective muscle spasm and limitation of movement. Patients with displaced Le Fort II or III fractures often complain of limited opening. In reality, they are half open at rest with the jaws wedged apart by the posteriorly and inferiorly displaced maxillary fragment. Reduction of the fracture allows closure.

Condylar fractures PMID: 34809889

Drugs

Tardive dyskinesia is an adverse effect of long-term treatment with drugs, causing uncontrollable repetitive involuntary movements. These often affect the face and muscles of mastication and produce trismus. The antiemetic metoclopromide and antipsychotics including butyrophenones and phenothiazines are causes. These effects may reverse on drug withdrawal, if that is possible, but may also persist long after cessation of treatment.

Tardive dyskinesia PMID: 25556809

PERSISTENT LIMITATION OF MOVEMENT: EXTRACAPSULAR CAUSES

Extracapsular causes of persistent limitation of opening are caused by some degree of mechanical interference to mandibular movement (see Box 14.2).

Irradiation

Radiation-induced trismus is a common effect of head and neck radiotherapy and results primarily from damage to the muscles of mastication, particularly the pterygoid muscles. The severity is proportional to the dose, and the cause is inflammation followed by fibrosis. The effect is long term, developing during months and years, and is slowly progressive. Irradiation of the joint itself does not appear to be as significant.

Modern intensity modulated radiotherapy allows accurate delivery of radiotherapy dose, and this effect is likely to be less common in future. However, it is impossible to deliver curative doses to tumours of the posterior oral cavity, maxilla, tonsil, pharynx and salivary glands without irradiating the masticatory muscles, and as many as half of patients suffer this adverse effect.

Jaw exercises and stretching are ineffective once the process is established but are prescribed prophylactically. Stretching is painful, and dedication is required to achieve a good result. Stretching devices (Fig. 14.1) or a trismus screw may aid the process. Otherwise, surgical treatment is difficult and may involve division of muscle attachments from the jaw or section of the angle or body of the mandible to produce a false joint. Bone surgery is complicated by the risk of osteoradionecrosis and infection (see Ch. 8).

Treatment in cancer patients PMID: 26876238 and 32435968

Oral submucous fibrosis

Oral submucous fibrosis, caused by betel nut habits, causes limitation of opening and predisposes to oral carcinoma. Fibrosis of the buccal mucosa, soft palate and the pillars of the fauces render the mucosa firm and hard and prevents opening. Fibrosis extends deeply into muscles of mastication and is progressive. Ultimately, opening the mouth may be completely impossible, and tube feeding may become necessary. There is no effective treatment. This condition is considered in detail in Chapter 19.

Systemic sclerosis (scleroderma)

Systemic sclerosis is an uncommon connective tissue disease characterised by immunologically mediated vascular damage and widespread fibrosis, particularly of subcutaneous and submucous tissues. Although the most obvious feature is the progressive stiffening of the skin, the gastrointestinal tract, lungs, heart and kidneys can also be affected.

Clinically, women between the ages of 30 and 50 years are predominantly affected. Raynaud's phenomenon is the most common early manifestation, often associated with arthralgia.

Systemic sclerosis has autoimmune and environmental causes, and probably a genetic predisposition. Autoantibodies are found against centromeres, topoisomerase (anti Scl70) and RNA polymerase, but the cause of the fibrosis appears to be a dysregulated wound healing process involving persistent inflammation. T lymphocytes secrete excessive transforming growth factor beta, to which the patient's

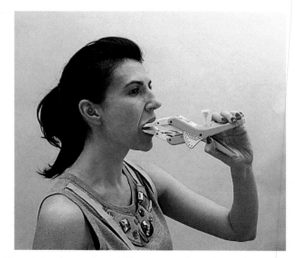

Fig. 14.1 A muscle and fibrosis stretching device for trismus.

fibroblasts are particularly sensitive. Endothelial cell function is disturbed and blood vessel formation is reduced and adhesion molecules upregulated, enhancing inflammatory cell emigration into the tissues. The initial cause remains unknown, but occasionally anti-cancer drugs, including taxanes, trigger onset.

The skin becomes thinned, stiff, smooth, tethered, pigmented and marked by telangiectases (Fig. 1.3). A hallmark of the disease is involvement of the hands causing such changes as atrophy of, or ischaemic damage to, the tips of the fingers. Contractures prevent straightening of the fingers.

The head and neck are involved in more than three-quarters of patients and, in a minority, symptoms start there. Narrowing of the eyes and taut, mask-like limitation of movement can give rise to a characteristic appearance ('Mona Lisa face'). The lips may be constricted ('fish mouth') or become pursed with radiating furrows. Occasionally, involvement of the periarticular tissues of the temporomandibular joint together with the microstomia may greatly limit opening of the mouth (Fig. 14.2). Involvement of the oral submucosa may cause the tongue to become stiff and narrowed ('chicken tongue'). Oesophageal stiffness causes dysphagia and allows gastric reflux.

Widening of the periodontal ligament space is another change characteristic of systemic sclerosis but is seen in fewer than 10% of cases. The mandibular angle and ramus are resorbed in an unusual pattern in 15% of patients, and more rarely, there is gross extensive resorption of the jaw with a risk of pathological fracture. Tooth root resorption is also reported but appears rare. Sjögren's syndrome develops in a significant minority.

Histologically, there is great thickening of the subepithelial connective tissue, degeneration of muscle fibres and atrophy of minor glands. The collagen fibres are swollen and eosinophilic. There are scattered infiltrates of chronic inflammatory cells around vessels, and arterioles typically show thickening of their walls.

Features of systemic sclerosis relevant to dentistry are shown in Box 14.3.

General review PMID: 23806160

Oral features PMID: 27659631 and 33448431

Jaw radiology PMID: 9084272

Complications and prognosis

Skin disease alone, although debilitating, is rarely fatal. The main disabilities are dysphagia or result from pulmonary, cardiac or renal involvement. Pulmonary involvement leads to impaired respiratory exchange and, eventually, dyspnoea and pulmonary hypertension. Cardiac disease can result from the latter or myocardial fibrosis. Renal disease secondary to vascular disease is typically a late effect; it leads to hypertension and is an important cause of death. The overall 10-year survival rate is 70%, but much reduced if there is visceral involvement.

No specific treatment has been available and conventional treatments are provided specific to the complications suffered. Immunosuppressive drugs are frequently used including mofetil mycophenylate, methotrexate or cyclophosphamide for musculoskeletal involvement but general immunosuppression does not affect the underlying disease process. Penicillamine has previously been given to depress fibrosis but can cause loss of taste, oral ulceration, lichenoid reactions and other complications and immunosuppressants are now preferred. Multiple novel drugs are in trial, including cytokine antagonists and inflammatory receptor blockers and fibroblast inhibitors, with some proving effective. Tyrosine kinase inhibitors are the most commonly prescribed in the UK but have significant adverse effects including stomatitis.

Clinical review PMID: 28413064

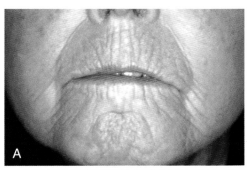

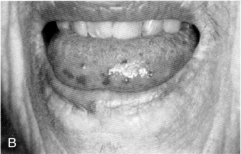

Fig. 14.2   Systemic sclerosis. Fibrosis of perioral skin with furrowing (A), telangiectases of lips and tongue and (B) limitation of opening. *(From Varga, J., 2015. Systemic sclerosis (scleroderma). In: Goldman, L., Schafer, A.I. Goldman-Cecil medicine, 25ᵗʰ ed. Elsevier Saunders, New York, pp. 1777–1785.e2.)*

Box 14.3   Dental relevance of systemic sclerosis

- Limitation of opening
- Limited oral access from microstomia
- Prominent gingival recession in a minority
- Coup de sabre linear scars of face and tongue
- Firm whitish-yellow fibrotic mucosal plaques, very rarely
- Widening of periodontal ligament radiographically in 7% cases
- Dental erosion from gastric reflux
- Mandibular resorption at angle and ramus
- Dry mouth
- Risk of Sjögren's syndrome (Ch. 22)
- Dentally relevant effects of drug treatment may include
  - Nifedipine given for Raynaud's phenomenon
  - Immunosuppression from ciclosporin, methotrexate or steroids
  - Lichenoid reactions to angiotensin-converting enzyme inhibitors for hypertension or penicillamine
  - And others depending on specific presentation

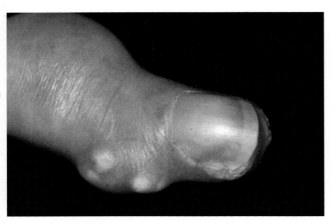

Fig. 14.3 **Calcinosis cutis,** a feature of CREST syndrome. The nodules are usually small, a millimetre or so across, but may fuse and form larger masses that can ulcerate the skin. *(From Gravallese EM, Hochberg MC, Smolen JS et al, 2019. Rheumatology, 7th ed. Philadelphia: Elsevier Inc.)*

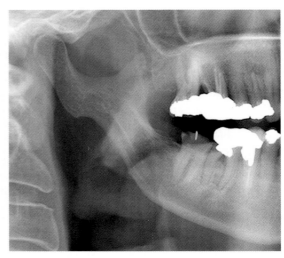

Fig. 14.5 **Scleroderma.** Resorption of the posterolateral ramus is characteristic but seen only in severe cases. *(Courtesy Dr M Payne.)*

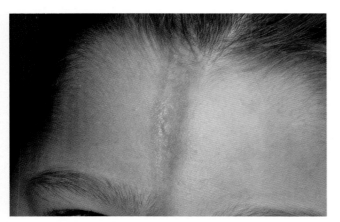

Fig. 14.4 **Scleroderma en coup de sabre.** Linear atrophy and fibrosis across the forehead. *(From Paller, A.S., Mancini, A.J., 2016. Collagen vascular disorders. In: Paller, A.S., Mancini, A.J. 2016. Hurwitz clinical pediatric dermatology, 5th ed. Elsevier, Philadelphia, pp. 509–539.e8.)*

CREST syndrome

CREST syndrome is the combination of **C**alcinosis, **R**aynaud's phenomenon **E**sophageal dysfunction, **S**clerodactyly and **T**elangiectasia and can be thought of as a limited cutaneous form of scleroderma with a better prognosis. It affects elderly females. Calcinosis is seen as calcified skin nodules a few millimetres to a centimetre in diameter (Fig 14.3); telangiectasia can result in prolonged bleeding. The remaining features are as seen in systemic sclerosis.

Oral features PMID: 8217427

Morphoea

Morphoea, or localised scleroderma, is considered a very limited skin form of systemic sclerosis producing scar-like fibrosis, as oval patches or sometimes linear deep scars with a characteristic *scleroderma en coup de sabre* ('sabre cut') morphology (see Fig. 14.4). This latter type often affects the forehead or scalp, with hair loss, deep contraction and resorption of underlying bone (Fig. 14.5), and it occasionally affects the tongue. Childhood morphoea is a possible cause of facial hemiatrophy.

> **Box 14.4** **Important causes of ankylosis ('true' or intracapsular ankylosis)**
>
> **Trauma**
> - Intracapsular fracture of the condyle
> - Penetrating wounds
> - Trauma from forceps delivery at birth
>
> **Infection**
> - Otitis media/mastoiditis
> - Osteomyelitis of the ramus/condyle
> - Haematogenous – pyogenic arthritis
>
> **Arthritides**
> - Systemic juvenile arthritis
> - Psoriatic arthropathy
> - Osteoarthritis (rarely)
> - Rheumatoid arthritis (rarely)
>
> **Neoplasms of the joint**
> - Osteochondroma
> - Osteoma
>
> **Miscellaneous**
> - Synovial chondromatosis

Morphoea review PMID: 24048434

Oral features PMID: 27776552

PERSISTENT LIMITATION OF MOVEMENT: INTRACAPSULAR CAUSES

Almost all intracapsular causes of limited opening are caused by ankylosis, due to fibrous or bony union of the condyle and temporal bone. Causes of ankylosis are shown in Box 14.4. A few, such as neoplasms of the joint itself or synovial chondromatosis, produce mechanical interference without ankylosis.

Box 14.5 Rheumatoid arthritis: systemic and joint features

- Onset in middle age. Sometimes acute
- Morning stiffness
- Symmetrical involvement of several joints
- Involvement of hand joints with eventual ulnar deviation
- Joint inflammation and rheumatoid nodules
- Rheumatoid factor and anti-citrullinated protein antibodies frequently positive
- Muscle wasting and osteoporosis
- Frequently malaise, fatigue, fever and anaemia
- Pain and disability usually severe, but *not* in the TMJ
- Sjögren's syndrome in about 15%

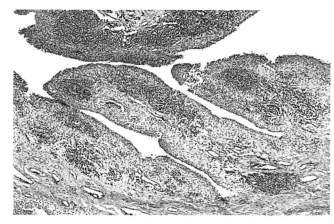

Fig. 14.6 Rheumatoid arthritis. Inflamed villi of pannus growing across the surface of a temporomandibular joint severely affected by rheumatoid arthritis.

Treatment of ankylosis

Ankylosis is treated in a similar fashion regardless of which of the following causes is responsible, and relatively aggressive surgical intervention is necessary. All the fibrous or bony tissue causing ankylosis is removed, and interposition of a temporalis muscle flap or other implant material prevents healing across the joint space. In the growing patient, joint reconstruction using a free costochondral bone graft gives better results because, in many cases, the graft will grow with the patient, reducing subsequent facial deformity. Early mobilisation with aggressive physiotherapy is required to prevent the ankylosis reforming.

Arthritis

The main causes are:

Traumatic arthritis. Follows dislocation or fracture. Surprisingly, undisplaced fractures of the neck of the condyle can remain unnoticed for many weeks until pain of arthritis develops.

Infection and inflammation. Acute pyogenic arthritis is exceedingly rare but exceedingly painful.

Rheumatoid and other arthritides. These are discussed below.

Rheumatoid arthritis

Rheumatoid arthritis is an autoimmune disease of unknown cause that affects approximately 2% of the population. It has a strong genetic background and environmental risk factors include smoking. The disease target is the synovial membrane, which is infiltrated by inflammatory cells, enlarges and grows across the joint surface causing resorption and joint destruction.

The initial inflammation appears non-specific. Deposition of immune complexes of immunoglobulin M complement-activating autoantibody against immunoglobulin receptor (rheumatoid factor) may be an initiating factor, but the disease is self-perpetuating as a result of systemic immune activation. Persistent inflammation causes the synovial fibroblasts to contribute to the inflammation, secrete damaging proteases and recruit osteoclasts that resorb the joint surface.

The main features (Box 14.5) are chronic inflammation of many joints, pain and progressive limitation of movement of small joints. Rheumatoid arthritis is the only important inflammatory disease of the temporomandibular joints, but is rarely symptomatic in this joint.

General review PMID: 22150039

Clinical features

Women are affected, particularly in the third and fourth decades. The smaller joints are mainly affected (particularly those of the hands), and the distribution tends to be symmetrical. Extra-articular manifestations include vasculitis and involvement of almost any organ system. Loss of weight, malaise and depression are common as secondary effects.

The temporomandibular joints are never involved alone, and temporomandibular joint involvement is usually a late sign. Although three-quarters of patients have clinical or radiological abnormalities of the temporomandibular joints, pain and swelling are not features. When there are symptoms of temporomandibular joint involvement, they are crepitus and limitation of movement with pain on clenching or chewing, rather than opening and closing. The shape of the condyle is flattened at first. In severely involved joints, the shape of both condyle and glenoid fossa can be lost, predisposing to dislocation.

Radiography shows flattening of the condyles with loss of contour and irregularity of the articular surface as typical findings. The joint space may be widened by exudate during phases of acute exacerbation but later narrowed. The underlying bone is often osteoporotic, and the margins of the condyles become irregular.

Biopsy is not used for diagnosis because joint involvement is always seen in established cases. If examined histologically, there is proliferation of the synovial lining cells and infiltration of the synovium by dense collections of lymphocytes and plasma cells (Fig. 14.6). The synovial fluid contains neutrophils and fibrinous exudate from the hyperaemic vessels in the synovial membrane. A vascular, inflamed mass of granulation tissue (pannus) spreads over the surfaces of the articular fibrocartilages from their margins and is followed by death of chondrocytes and loss of intercellular matrix. Fibrous adhesions form between the joint surfaces and the meniscus. The meniscus may eventually be destroyed, and inflammatory changes in the ligaments and tendons can then lead to fibrous or bony ankylosis, though this very rare. Collapse of the joint is a more likely outcome in severe disease, with development of an anterior open bite as a consequence.

TMJ radiology PMID: 8734713 and 11426029

Management

Diagnosis is based on the clinical, radiographic and auto-antibody findings, notably rheumatoid factor and anti-citrullinated protein antibodies. Systemic treatment previously relied on various drugs selected on the basis of individual response and disease severity. These included non-steroidal anti-inflammatory drugs, penicillamine, antimalarial drugs and colloidal gold injections. Many of these drugs had severe oral adverse effects (Box 14.6). More recently, treatment has emphasized early diagnosis with intensive rapid intervention to induce remission by modifying lifestyle factors (smoking and obesity) and using 'disease-modifying' antirheumatic drugs. Methotrexate is now the primary drug, with glucocorticoids if necessary and if remission is not achieved in a few months, many other biological agents may be used, including interleukin 6 pathway antagonists, golimumab (anti-tumour necrosis factor α monoclonal antibodies) and janus kinase-inhibitors such as facitinib and rituzimab to deplete B cells. Low-dose methotrexate is a popular maintenance treatment for severe disease in remission. These disease modifying drugs may have diverse and sometimes severe adverse effects, but aside from oral lichenoid drug reactions appear to have no major oral effects. Low dose methotrexate maintenance does not cause immunosuppression clinically, but disease modifying drugs can cause sufficient immunosuppression to reactivate or predispose to tuberculosis.

If joint symptoms are severe, a corticosteroid injection into the joint space may reduce pain and swelling but cannot be repeated frequently without inducing bone resorption. There is no effect of steroids on disease progression and no evidence that they can allow normal condylar growth in juvenile rheumatoid arthritis.

Joint surgery is rarely performed, but if required, a functional joint may be restored with various implant materials or a custom-made artificial joint. Replacement joints tend to be reserved for patients with mandibular growth disturbance as a result of juvenile rheumatoid arthritis, as part of an orthognathic treatment plan to advance the hypoplastic mandible.

Box 14.6 Rheumatoid arthritis: dental implications

- Difficulty with oral hygiene, reduced manual dexterity and limited range of movement
- Oral access reduced by limited opening
- Difficulty lying in dental chair
- Anaemia
- Sjögren's syndrome in about 15%
- Mild bleeding risk from thrombocytopenia
- Cervical lymph nodes may be enlarged during active disease
- Risk of atlantoaxial subluxation if cervical spine involved
- Adverse effects of drug treatment
  - Lichenoid reactions from older medications: gold, antimalarials and penicillamine
  - Immunosuppression from ciclosporin, methotrexate and infliximab
  - Candidosis from immunosuppression and anaemia
  - Oral ulceration from methotrexate
  - Anaemia from non-steroidal anti-inflammatory drugs
  - Interactions with drugs prescribed for dentistry

Dental aspects

The nature of any link between rheumatoid arthritis and chronic periodontitis remains controversial but the enhanced systemic inflammatory reaction is seen to be active at both sites.

Generally speaking, although rheumatoid arthritis is a common disease, specific treatment of TMJ symptoms is unlikely to be necessary but any gross abnormalities of occlusion, such as overclosure, should be corrected to reduce abnormal movement at the temporomandibular joints.

Sjögren's syndrome is associated in approximately 15%. Involvement of small joints of the hand makes oral hygiene a challenge. Important features of rheumatoid arthritis are summarised in Box 14.6.

Medical review PMID: 27156434

Dental care PMID: 27857093

Osteoarthritis

Osteoarthritis is a disorder of cartilaginous repair. Joints are more susceptible than normal to daily wear, so that large weight-bearing joints are the most frequently affected. The temporomandibular joint is occasionally affected after trauma. Alterations in cartilage matrix appear to be the cause and are linked to several gene defects. Erosion of cartilage causes resorption of the underlying bone, which distorts, collapses and becomes sclerotic in response. New bone grows at the edge of the joint (osteophytes), limiting movement, and the capsule and ligaments are thickened. Inflammation is mild.

In diseases in which joint movement is abnormal or a joint is malformed, osteoarthritis may develop as a secondary complication, for instance in congenital hip disease or Ehlers-Danlos syndrome. Trauma and diabetes also predispose.

Osteoarthritis is very common. Severe disease affects 2% of the population, but by the age of 70 years, three-quarters of individuals have some radiographic features. Presentation is usually in middle age or older people because it takes many years of cumulative damage for the effects to become significant. Stress, particularly on weight-bearing joints, is the main cause of pain, but frequently joints with radiographic signs of osteoarthritis are painless. A characteristic feature is the presence of Heberden's nodes (bony swellings) of the terminal interphalangeal joints. Affected joints are swollen and warm when the disease is active and produce crepitus on movement.

Osteoarthritis of the temporomandibular joint is occasionally seen by chance in radiographs but is not a cause of significant symptoms. The unusual structure of the joint, with a fibrocartilage disk rather than hyaline cartilage, and the lack of weight bearing seem to protect it. The disk suffers the worst damage (Fig. 14.7). Any significant limitation of movement is likely to be from osteophytes around the joint or fragments of osteophytes that have fractured and become loose bodies in the joint.

In the rare event that a patient has severe pain and joint deformity associated with osteoarthritis of the temporomandibular joint, any factor contributing to stress on the joint should be relieved. Treatment is symptomatic, and topical agents and anti-inflammatory analgesics are the main line of treatment. Corticosteroid or hyaluronate injections have been tried but, in general, the more conservative the approach the better.

Important features of osteoarthritis are summarised in Box 14.7.

Natural history joint damage PMID: 7621016

Dental aspects

Although the temporomandibular joint rarely causes problems, the disease has significant dental implications as shown in Box 14.8.

Dental care PMID: 18511715

Other types of arthritis

Many other types of arthritis can affect the temporomandibular joints but rarely do so. They include psoriatic arthritis, the juvenile arthritides, gout, ankylosing spondylitis, Lyme disease and reactive arthropathy. Psoriatic arthropathy can cause ankylosis of the temporomandibular joint. Juvenile arthritis can be severe and disabling, and destruction of the condylar head leads to severely limited opening and secondary micrognathia.

Condylar hyperplasia

Condylar hyperplasia is a rare, usually unilateral, overgrowth of the mandibular condyle (Fig 14.8). Hyperplasia may be evident as overgrowth during the normal growth period or seen later if growth fails to stop at the appropriate time. It causes facial asymmetry, deviation of the jaw to the unaffected side on opening and a crossbite (Fig. 14.9). The condition usually manifests itself after puberty and is slowly progressive. Pain in the affected joint is variable. If the condition is still active at the time of diagnosis, an intracapsular condylectomy should be performed to remove the active growth cartilage of the condylar surface. If the disease has stabilised – usually at the end of puberty or shortly afterward – corrective

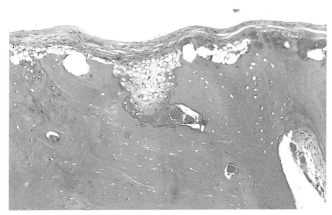

Fig. 14.7 Osteoarthritis. The fibrocartilage layer is thin and split, and the underlying bone shows resorption centrally.

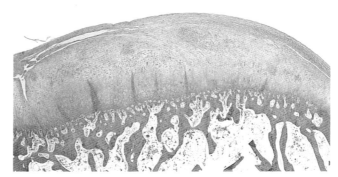

Fig. 14.8 Condylar hyperplasia. The condyle retains an immature structure with a thick cartilage layer, calcification and new bone formation, reflecting the continued growth. The thick cortical bone layer found below the cartilage in adults is not present.

Box 14.7 Important features of osteoarthritis

- Onset mainly older than 60 years
- Slow development of pain and wear of weight-bearing joints
- Usually, one or a few joints involved
- Heberden's nodes
- Palpable coarse crepitus of affected joints
- Bony swelling and deformity
- Secondary muscle weakness and wasting
- Little or no inflammation and no systemic effects

Box 14.8 Dental implications of osteoarthritis

- Pain on movement restricts access to care
- Difficulty with oral hygiene, reduced manual dexterity and limited range of movement
- Difficulty lying in dental chair
- Joint replacements do not require antibiotic prophylaxis unless there are specific patient indications. Prophylaxis may be *considered* in diabetics, individuals who are immunosuppressed or had previous joint infection
- Adverse effects of drug treatment
  - Anaemia from non-steroidal anti-inflammatory drugs
  - Bleeding tendency in people on aspirin

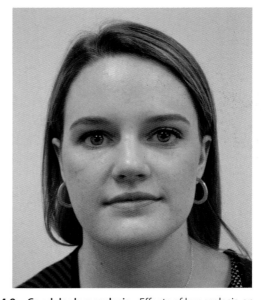

Fig. 14.9 Condylar hyperplasia. Effects of hyperplasia on the right side, note the increased facial height on the affected side, midline shift of the mandible to the left and tilted maxillary occlusal plane. *(From Baker SB, Weinzweig J, Patel PK, 2022. Aesthetic surgery of the facial skeleton. Philadelphia: Elsevier Inc.)*

osteotomies may be needed to restore the occlusion and facial symmetry. This may be difficult. The mandible grows down, forward and laterally, tilting the occlusal plane and allowing the maxillary alveolus and teeth to grow down into the space producing a complex asymmetry.

Coronoid hyperplasia can also occur but is rarer and usually bilateral.

Review and treatment PMID: 25483450

Tissue changes PMID: 3461098

Neoplasms

Osteochondroma (Fig. 14.10) is probably the most common tumour of the condyle or coronoid process, but even that is very rare. Osteoma and chondroma and their malignant counterparts may develop and are treated in the same way as elsewhere in the skeleton (see Ch. 12).

Synovial chondromatosis and loose bodies

Loose bodies (or 'joint mice') are fragments of bone or cartilage floating free in the joint space. Compared with other joints, they are rare in the temporomandibular joints where the main causes are synovial chondromatosis and osteochondritis dissecans.

In **synovial chondromatosis** multiple nodules of cartilage develop in the synovial membrane, each up to 1–2 mm in diameter (Fig.14.11). The nodules become separated and fall into the joint space to cause locking, deviation to the affected side on opening, and crepitus, followed eventually by pain and swelling when the joint is damaged. Synovial chondromatosis is rare and probably a benign neoplasm because it harbours gene rearrangements, but pressure resorption from the nodules is destructive and can erode into the cranial cavity from the joint.

The nodules are seen best on magnetic resonance image scanning because they may not be mineralised. More than 100 may be present in the joint capsule.

Histologically, the nodules of cartilage are well organized, cytologically benign (Fig. 14.12) and may calcify. Diagnosis is by imaging, and the diagnosis is confirmed after surgical removal of the loose bodies and the whole of the affected synovium. Endoscopic removal is sometimes possible, but incomplete excision can be followed by recurrence.

Osteochondritis dissecans is primarily a disease of weight-bearing joints and extremely rare in the temporomandibular joint. It results from trauma or loss of blood supply to the bone below the articular surface, always in the condyle. The bone becomes necrotic, and pieces of the overlying fibrocartilage layer separate to form loose bodies. Diagnosis is by imaging, and the patient has discomfort and episodes of locking. Conservative management may be successful in the young, but surgical removal of the loose body may be required.

Synovial chondromatosis series PMID: 16003619

Osteochondritis dissecans PMID: 16997094

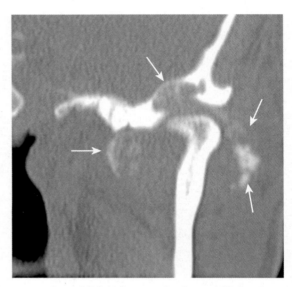

Fig. 14.11 Synovial chondromatosis. Coronal CT showing the joint capsule expanded by numerous small nodules, some mineralized and others less dense. Superiorly, the glenoid fossa has been eroded. *(From Hatcher D, Tamimi D, 2017. Specialty imaging: Temporomandibular joint. Oxford, Elsevier Ltd.)*

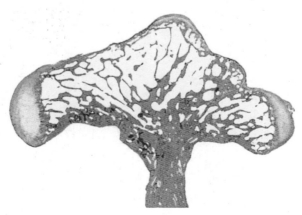

Fig. 14.10 Osteochondroma of the condyle. Two cartilage-capped exostoses arising near the condyle have grown progressively sideways to form a distorted condylar head several centimetres across.

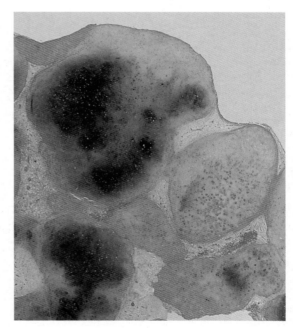

Fig. 14.12 Synovial chondromatosis of the temporomandibular joint. Multiple rounded nodules of benign cartilage growing in the joint capsule.

LIMITATION OF MOVEMENT: MUSCLE CAUSES

Temporomandibular pain dysfunction

This is one of the most controversial areas in dentistry and cause and optimum treatment are unclear. Many interventions appear effective and the condition is very common, making this the most common cause of trismus and limited jaw movement.

The differing views of this condition are reflected in its many names. In the UK the terms *temporomandibular pain dysfunction syndrome*, *facial arthromyalgia* or *myofascial pain* are used. In the United States, the more generic *temporomandibular disorders* indicates that this is a group of related presentations, but this term includes organic joint disease excluded in other definitions. None of the names is satisfactory; many emphasise the joint when it is not the primary cause of the condition.

Presentation

Pain dysfunction syndrome comprises a collection of symptoms of pain and tenderness in the muscles of mastication and in or around the joint, limitation of movement and clicking or other sounds from the joint. Onset is occasionally ascribed to violent yawning, laughing or trauma but is usually insidious.

It is estimated that 25% of the population may experience at least some of the symptoms at some time in their life and half may show signs, although this is perhaps a reflection of the poor specificity of the diagnostic criteria. Although the symptoms are common, treatment is much more likely to be sought by young or early adult women. The condition is often considered of low significance and difficult to treat, but it can cause significant discomfort, stress and depression and have a major impact on quality of life. It also consumes significant healthcare resources. The symptoms and signs wax and wane, sometimes peaking with almost acute severity. They are:

Muscle and joint tenderness felt during jaw movement or mastication, and on palpation. The joint pain may be referred from the muscles or associated with their tendons rather than originating in the joint. The pain is not severe, more an ache or tenderness and often poorly localised by the patient. Muscle symptoms are usually worse on one side or completely unilateral. Pain is classically preauricular.

Limitation of mandibular movement characterised by reduced opening and lateral excursion, associated with pain, making mastication difficult. The mandible deviates to the side of the pain, reflecting muscle spasm. Trismus may be complete in severe phases.

Joint noises are usually clicks or crepitus on movement. The noises can be impressive and surprise the patient but are not painful. They indicate poor coordination of movement of the disk and mandible. Clicks are very common and do not alone indicate pain dysfunction syndrome.

A series of secondary symptoms have an unclear relationship to the central disorder:

Bruxism is most closely associated and is an understandable cause of muscle spasm (see Ch. 6). Patients who brux at night wake with worse limitation of movement and pain that slowly reduces during the day. Other parafunctional activity or jaw posturing is also sometimes associated.

Headache may be misinterpreted temporalis pain, referred pain or relate to stress, possibly causing, or possibly a result

of, the disorder. Migraine is also associated in an ill-defined way (Ch. 39).

Locking of the joint. This does not necessarily indicate organic disease in the joint, but rather uncoordinated movements of the condyle, disk and muscles. Most locking is in an open position. Closed lock is rarer and more likely to indicate internal joint derangement.

Ear pain is probably referred pain from the joint and does not indicate damage to the ear itself. Tinnitus can also be associated.

Symptoms are recurrent in two-thirds of patients and only 15% recover completely after a single episode.

Features are summarised in Box 14.9.

Aetiology

The aetiology is unknown and probably multifactorial. Psychosocial factors seem to play a significant role. Some authorities consider the problem to be within the spectrum of chronic facial pain, sharing psychological aetiological factors with burning mouth and atypical facial pain, but this only partly explains the condition and probably not in all patients. Stress and anxiety are well-recognised causes of clenching and bruxing, with constant contraction of facial and masticatory muscles. More than half of patients recognise a stressful life event preceding their symptoms, and many have other stress-associated disorders such as stress headache, irritable bowel, insomnia, depression or chronic fatigue. The predisposing factors most strongly associated relate to joint stretching and include excessive yawning, prolonged dental treatment or mandibular trauma, or holding an abnormal mandibular posture to avoid pain from pericoronitis or a tooth.

The joint is almost always normal, and it is unclear whether any derangements of the meniscus are primary or secondary changes in the small proportion of patients who have them. If the joint is abnormal, it should be treated as joint disease and not temporomandibular pain dysfunction.

Previous suggestions that the occlusion is a primary cause have not been validated in studies. However, there is clearly some poorly understood relationship between the patterns of movement of the jaw, muscle tenderness and the effect the occlusion exerts on them, as demonstrated by the diagnostic value of splints. Abnormal neuromuscular coordination, causing areas of spasm of the masticatory muscles, appears to be a likely main cause.

Investigation

In view of the absence of objective signs, diagnosis is largely by exclusion. The pain character and distribution are typical

---

Box 14.9   Typical features of pain dysfunction syndrome

- Female to male preponderance of nearly 4 to 1
- Most patients are between 16 and 40 years
- Onset is usually gradual
- Pain usually one-sided, rarely severe
- Typically, a dull ache is made worse by mastication
- Pain typically felt in front of the ear and in the temporal region
- Frequently also limitation of opening
- Clicking or crepitus in the joint
- Ultimately self-limiting
- Causes no long-term damage to joint

and the main function of the history and examination are to exclude organic disease. As in all cases of pain in the region of the jaws, referred pain from the teeth should be carefully excluded. Structured questionnaires are useful for pain diagnosis and monitoring.

The muscles should be palpated to identify tender areas that can be confirmed by the patient as the correct source when the pain is poorly localised. Check the movements of the mandible to identify postural positions, limitation of movement and asymmetry.

The temporomandibular joint should be palpated for tenderness or swelling which, if present, suggest organic disease. Crepitus may be felt but is not specific and is not necessarily a sign of significant joint disease.

Radiographs of the joints may be taken to make sure that movements are not excessive in either direction and are equal on both sides. However, the main value of radiographs is to exclude such changes as fluid accumulation (widening of the joint space) or damage or deformity of the joint surfaces, indicating organic disease.

Palpation of the temporal artery will aid exclusion of giant cell arteritis.

Management

Temporomandibular pain dysfunction is ultimately self-limiting and does not progress to permanent damage or degenerative arthritis later in life. No irreversible treatment should be undertaken. Surgery, orthodontics and occlusal adjustment in particular are to be avoided.

There is a strong placebo effect in any form of treatment and reversible treatments, usually in combination, will usually reduce trismus and pain. Possible interventions include exercises and stretching, massage, physiotherapy, soft diet, application of heat to muscles, ultrasound therapy, cognitive behavioural therapy, hypnosis, relaxation and many more. Dividing patients into those who have primarily muscle or joint symptoms for different types of treatment seems logical but is not always easy to do. Botulinum toxin injection into masticatory muscles reduces spasm but requires many injections and, while helpful in some patients, has limited effect in metanalysis (Ch. 27).

The provision of various types of splints has long been a popular dental intervention. There are many types, but specific indications for particular types remain largely without an evidence base. Splints perform two roles, diagnostic and therapeutic. They are perhaps most useful for diagnosis, interfering with the neuromuscular control of jaw movement and breaking learned habits so that a short period of wear may quickly change the pain and joint symptoms to confirm the diagnosis (whether improving or occasionally worsening them). Soft vacuum-formed splints are easily provided for night wear to reduce bruxism, but only last a short time between the teeth of a dedicated bruxist. Hard splints are more complex to make and may either permit movement in all directions – removing the occlusal guidance of jaw movement – or attempt to guide the jaw to some artificial 'correct' posture. Partial coverage splints and flat anterior bite planes risk allowing overeruption of the uncovered teeth in only a few weeks, and full coverage splints are generally preferred, but all types are of limited value.

A broad range of analgesics including non-steroidal anti-inflammatory drugs are used but have no proven benefit. Medication targeting stress, anxiety or depression, such as benzodiazepines or tricyclic antidepressants, also provide minimal or no benefit.

| Box 14.10 | Principles of management of pain dysfunction syndrome |

- Exclude referred pain and infection of dental origin
- Exclude joint disease
- Exclude giant cell arteritis (in older people)
- Reassurance and education
- Conservative management – reversible treatments only
- Soft diet and jaw exercises
- Consider need for a splint
- Analgesics or anxiolytics in selected cases

Unless joint disease is identified by imaging, arthroscopy should be avoided.

In practice, a combination of education and reassurance, a soft diet and a soft splint worn at night for 3 months, with some simple jaw exercises, is sufficient intervention to allow the patient to manage the condition until it wanes in severity. More severely affected patients may merit a trial of non-steroidal anti-inflammatory drugs or a brief course of a benzodiazepine if anxiety is severe. Most cases are amenable to management in primary care, but patients with clear psychological factors, widespread pain or locking of the joint are best treated in a specialised centre.

Explaining that the condition may recur and relapse during many years is important for patient acceptance of mild symptoms in the long term.

The main principles of management of pain dysfunction syndrome are summarised in Box 14.10.

Update review PMID: 34853604

Review UK perspective PMID: 27024901

Symptoms PMID: 8995904 and 9973710

Association with pain sensitivity PMID: 26928952

Management advice PMID: 24386767 and 34674093

Meta-analysis splint therapy PMID: 32065109

Occlusal adjustment ineffective PMID: 9656902

Psychosocial model PMID: 9610309

Web URL 14.1 UK clinical guideline: https://www.rcseng.ac.uk/dental-faculties/fds and use search box for 'Temporomandibular disorders' and select the clinical guideline

Web URL 14.2 NICE guidance: http://cks.nice.org.uk/ and enter TMJ in search box

Web URL 14.3 US Guidance for younger patients: https://www.aapd.org/globalassets/media/policies_guidelines/bp_tempdisorders.pdf

Web URL 14.4 Multilingual evidence-based diagnosis: http://www.rdc-tmdinternational.org/ and follow menus to TMD assessment/Diagnosis and select 'translations'

Botulinum toxin PMID: 34743162 and 35775414

Acute temporomandibular pain dysfunction

In patients with an acute onset there is often a clear cause such as trauma or a prolonged period of forced mouth opening, usually for dental surgery. In such cases analgesics, soft diet and reassurance with instructions to avoid yawning or forced opening for 2 months are usually sufficient.

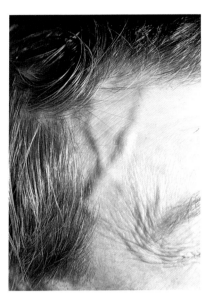

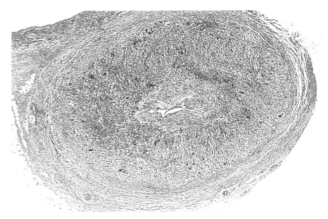

Fig. 14.14 Giant cell (temporal) arteritis. The structure of the artery is disrupted by inflammatory cells, and the lumen is much reduced in size.

Fig 14.13 Giant cell arteritis. Firm, tortuous and nodular temporal artery. *(From Klippel JH, Dieppe PA, 1997. Rheumatology, 2ⁿᵈ ed. Maryland Heights, MO: Mosby.)*

Giant cell arteritis (temporal arteritis)

Giant cell arteritis is an autoimmune inflammatory disease of large arteries, particularly the cranial arteries causing swelling and narrowing of the lumen.

Clinically, women older than 55 years are predominantly affected and the incidence is 1:10,000. The disease may start with malaise, weakness, low-grade fever and loss of weight. Severe throbbing headache is the most common symptom. The temporal artery is the most frequently affected artery of relevance to dentists and becomes red, tender, firm, swollen, and tortuous on palpation (Fig 14.13).

In 20% of patients, there is ischaemic pain in the masticatory muscles, that worsens on mastication, sometimes called 'jaw claudication'.* This characteristic combination of headache and pain on mastication can be misdiagnosed as temporomandibular joint dysfunction. Ophthalmic artery involvement is found in as many as half of patients and can cause disturbance of vision or sudden blindness. Reduced blood flow can cause pale ischaemic patches and complete obstruction causes infarcts and ulceration, both sometimes seen in the tongue.

Histologically, the arterial media and intima are oedematous and inflamed and contain macrophages and multinucleate giant cells. Intimal damage leads to formation of thrombi, and the internal elastic lamina becomes disrupted and eventually destroyed for short lengths of the artery (Figs 14.14–14.16). Healing is by fibrosis and partial recanalisation of the thrombus.

General review PMID: 24461386

Intraoral involvement PMID: 21176820 and 34880035

Management

Biopsy is not required for diagnosis in a typical presentation. The diagnosis should be made from the clinical features, raised erythrocyte sedimentation rate (seen in 90%) and

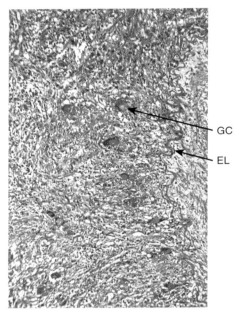

Fig. 14.15 Giant cell (temporal) arteritis. At higher power the internal elastic lamina of the artery may be seen together with giant cells, lymphocytes and neutrophils in the media. GC, giant cell; EL, elastic lamina.

Doppler flow ultrasound, which reveals lumen narrowing and wall thickening of the temporal arteries. If a biopsy is required, it must be at least 1 cm and ideally 3 cm long to ensure that it includes the short lengths of affected wall necessary for diagnosis, but still has low sensitivity.

Treatment should not be delayed because blindness, which develops in as many as 50% of untreated patients, stroke and cardiac complications make it essential to start treatment immediately. Giant cell arteritis should be treated with urgency.

Systemic corticosteroids are given on the basis of inflamed scalp vessels and a high (>70 mm/hour) erythrocyte sedimentation rate (ESR). Corticosteroids are usually quickly effective and are continued until the ESR falls to normal but adverse effects of the high doses are common. Interleukin 6 receptor antibodies may be used in patients susceptible to steroid adverse effects.

Review PMID: 32168069

---

* The term is based on the intermittent claudication in the calves on arterial insufficiency, but is something of a misnomer because claudication means limping.

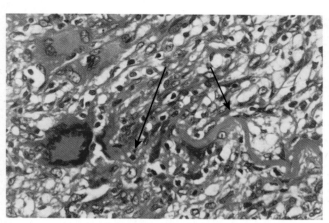

Fig. 14.16   Giant cell (temporal) arteritis. At high power, multinucleate giant cells, lymphocytes and neutrophils may be seen among the remnants of the artery's internal elastic lamina (wavy red line, arrowed).

Polymyalgia rheumatica

Half of patients with temporal arteritis have this more extensive condition with weakness, stiffness and pain of the shoulder or pelvic girdles associated with malaise and low fever. The ESR is usually greatly raised.

General review PMID: 23579169

Tetanus and tetany

These are rare causes of masticatory muscle spasm. Lockjaw (trismus) is a classical early sign of tetanus which, although rare, must be excluded because of its high mortality. In 2020, two of the reported seven cases in the UK died. The trismus is associated with extreme muscle contraction and typically causes spasms of a few minutes at a time. This possibility should be considered whenever a patient develops acute severe limitation of movement of the jaw without local cause, but has had a penetrating wound, particularly a contaminated one, in the previous 4 weeks (Box 14.11).

Immunisation has almost eradicated the disease in most countries but neonatal tetanus is still a significant cause of infant mortality worldwide Following a full course of five toxoid doses, booster vaccination is not required. However, patients with contaminated facial, or other, injury whose vaccination status is not known should be offered anti-tetanus immunoglobulin to provide passive immunity. Immunised or partially immune subjects may develop localized tetanus, with spasm of muscles only around the injury and 'cephalic' tetanus may follow facial or neck injury.

Tetany is most likely to be seen as a result of anxiety and hyperventilation. Tetany is usually associated with typical carpal spasm, and tapping on the facial nerve may trigger spasm of facial muscles (Chvostek's sign).

Tetanus with trismus, case PMID: 26869628

PAIN REFERRED TO THE JOINT

Salivary gland disease, otitis externa, otitis media and mastoiditis are potent causes of pain referred to the temporomandibular joint. Temporomandibular pain dysfunction illustrates referred pain from muscles of mastication, and any disease in these muscles may produce joint pain; indeed joint and ear pain may be referred from almost anywhere in the sensory distribution of the trigeminal nerve. Excluding

---

Box 14.11   Wounds at risk of *Clostridium tetani* infection

- Compound fractures
- Puncture wounds
- Wounds with foreign bodies, such as splinters
- Wounds with systemic sepsis
- Wounds contaminated by soil
- Animal bites from agricultural animals
- Wounds with extensive tissue necrosis

dental causes for any ear or joint pain is therefore an essential step in diagnosis.

DISLOCATION

The temporomandibular joint may become fixed in the open position by anterior dislocation, when the condyle slides over the anterior articular eminence. Causes include forcible opening of the mouth by a blow on the jaw or during dental extractions under general anaesthesia or sedation. People with epilepsy sometimes dislocate during seizures. A minority of patients have a small articular eminence or lax joint capsule and dislocate relatively easily, for instance on yawning or taking a large bite. This may be frequent in conditions with generalised hypermobile joints, such as Ehlers–Danlos and Marfan's syndromes, but recurrent dislocation does not necessarily indicate any underlying condition.

Dislocation is usually readily diagnosed clinically, but radiography will confirm the condyle position if unclear (Fig. 14.17).

Dislocation is very painful, and the dislocation should be reduced immediately if possible, but muscle spasm and guarding by the patient tend to maintain the dislocation.

The traditional method to reduce the dislocation is to press downward and backward on or behind the lower posterior teeth with the thumbs while standing behind the patient. This is difficult and sedation may be required. Sudden reflex closing in a conscious patient risks a major bite injury to the thumbs, which must be protected with padding.

Occasionally, the dislocation remains unnoticed and, surprisingly, a patient may tolerate the disability and discomfort for weeks or even months (Figs 14.18–14.19). In these cases, effusion into the joint, following injury, becomes organised to form fibrous adhesions. When this happens, manual reduction may be impossible and open surgical reduction, with division of adhesions, must be carried out.

For recurrent dislocation, augmentation of the eminence by bone graft or down-fracture of the zygomatic arch to enlarge the eminence are overall the most successful procedures. If recurrent dislocation is associated with abnormal muscle activity, botulinum toxin may be used to induce atrophy of the causative muscle fibre group (Ch. 27).

Review PMID: 25483448

Treatment recurrent dislocation PMID: 34768586

Ehlers–Danlos syndrome

Ehlers–Danlos syndrome (see also Ch. 2) is a heritable disease of collagen formation causing, among other features, hyper-extensibility of the skin, lax joint capsules and ligaments, impaired healing and scar formation. Almost all cases are caused by mutation in the gene for type 5

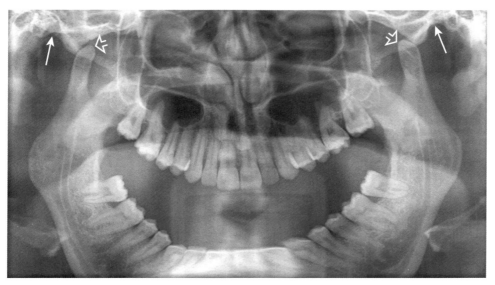

Fig. 14.17 **Bilateral dislocation of jaw** seen in a panoramic radiograph, the condyles (open arrows) are anteriorly displaced from the glenoid fossae (solid arrows) and the mouth is widely propped open. *(From Whaites E, Drage N, 2013. Essentials of dental radiography and radiology, 5th ed. Oxford, Churchill Livingstone.)*

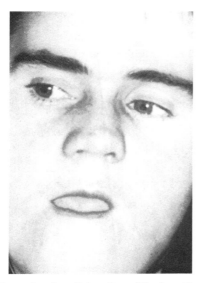

Fig. 14.18 **Longstanding dislocation of the jaw.** The teeth had been extracted about a month previously; in spite of the patient's inability to close her mouth and the distorted appearance, the dislocation remained unrecognised.

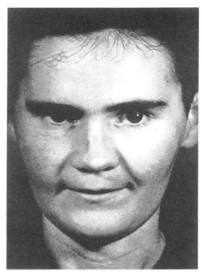

Fig. 14.19 Reduction of the dislocation (performed by open operation because of development of fibrous adhesions) restores the patient's normal appearance and movements of the jaw.

collagen but numerous rarer types are recognised, all with slightly different combinations of features (see Table 14.1). Not all patients have typical lax skin and joints. Pulp stones seem to affect only some families and are not closely associated with any one type. Short roots and small teeth are also reported, as are enamel hypoplasia, dentine dysplasia and early onset severe periodontitis (Fig 14.20). Wrist mobility may impair toothbrushing, leading to poor oral health.

Review oral features PMID: 17052632

Oral and TMJ effects PMID: 15817074

Case, multiple dental defects PMID: 16937863

Periodontal type PMID: 34324282 and 28836281

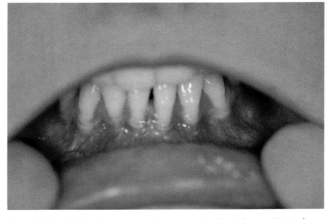

Fig. 14.20 **Ehlers Danlos syndrome,** periodontal type. Note the thin or absent attached gingiva. *(From Paller A, Mancini A, 2021. Paller and Mancini - Hurwitz Clinical Pediatric Dermatology, 6th ed. St. Louis, Elsevier Inc.)*

Table 14.1   Types and features of Ehlers-Danlos syndrome

Type	Inheritance and gene	Features	Dental significance
Classical	Autosomal dominant Mutations in collagen 5, rarely in collagen 1	Skin and joint hypermobility, bruising	Poor healing Temporomandibular joint (TMJ) dislocation frequent Pulp stones
Classical-like	Autosomal recessive Mutation in tenascin XB	Skin and joint hypermobility, bruising	Dislocations rare
Cardiac-valvular	Autosomal recessive Mutations in collagen 1	Progressive aortic and mitral valve failure, skin and joint hypermobility,	Mitral valve prolapse predisposes to endocarditis Poor healing TMJ dislocations rare
Vascular	Autosomal dominant Mutation in collagen 3, rarely in collagen 1	Thin skin, arterial and bowel rupture, bruising, joints mostly unaffected	Bleeding risk Marked gingival bleeding on toothbrushing Occasional rapidly progressing periodontitis Poor healing TMJ dislocation, bruising without trauma often on cheek
Hypermobility	Autosomal dominant, Mutation unclear, possibly in collagen 3	Skin and severe joint hypermobility Weak scars	TMJ dislocation frequent Early-onset arthritis High narrow palate
Arthrochalasia	Autosomal dominant Mutations in collagen 1	Severe joint hypermobility and skin extensibility	TMJ dislocation frequent Poor healing, weak scars
Dermatosparaxis	Autosomal recessive Mutations in collagen 1 processing enzyme gene ADAMTS2	Severe skin fragility and sagging skin, severe bruising Exophthalmos with periorbital excess skin and oedema, blue sclera, large fontanelles, delayed closure cranial sutures	Haematoma formation Anterior open bite, small mandible Abnormal teeth similar to dentinogenesis imperfecta
Kyphoscoliosis	Autosomal recessive Mutation in PLOD1 collagen processing enzyme gene	Joint hypermobility, muscle hypotonia, progressive scoliosis from birth	Poor healing Some cases facial dysmorphology
Brittle cornea syndrome	Autosomal recessive Mutation in transcriptional regulator ZNF469	Cornea thin with scarring, blue sclera	
Spondylodysplastic	Autosomal recessive Mutation in galactose transferase enzyme genes	Reduced growth, muscle hypotonia and bowing of limbs, exopthalmos, delayed closure fontanelles, blue sclera	Some genetic types enamel hypoplasia
Musculocontractual	Autosomal recessive Mutation in protein processing genes	Congenital multiple contraction of muscles, bruising, weak scars	Small oral opening and retruded small mandible, high palate
Myopathic	Autosomal dominant or recessive Mutation collagen 1	Muscle hypotonia, contractures and joint hypermobility, weak scars	
Periodontal	Autosomal dominant Gain of function mutations in Complement C1 genes	As classical with rapidly progressive periodontitis, Marfanoid facial features	Premature loss of permanent teeth and marked alveolar bone resorption. Only a thin band of attached gingiva

Diseases of the oral mucosa: mucosal infections

15

Few diseases are specific to the oral mucosa. Mucosal changes can be part of an underlying systemic disease, a marker of internal malignancy, specific to the mouth or of almost no significance. Occasionally mucosal signs indicate potentially life-threatening disease.

The oral mucosa has a limited range of responses to injury. The epithelium may thicken (acanthosis), thin (atrophy), proliferate (hyperplasia), keratinise, detach or break down to form an ulcer. This restricted range of changes means that many oral diseases appear similar. The end result of damage caused by many diseases is ulceration.

ULCERS → Summary charts 15.2, 16.2 and 16.3

Many oral diseases are characterised by ulcers. An ulcer is a break in the continuity of the epithelium, exposing the connective tissue to the oral environment. Ulcers may have sharp well-defined borders or ragged margins, but all are covered by a fibrin slough. The slough has a characteristic grey-yellow appearance, which with experience is readily distinguished from the brighter white colour of keratinisation. Ulcers have a superficial bacterial contamination by oral flora, but the tissue below very rarely becomes infected. The rapid turnover of oral epithelium allows uncomplicated ulcers to heal rapidly, but ulceration may be chronic or persistent if the cause persists.

Important causes are summarised in Table 15.1.

General review diagnosis ulcers PMID: 26650694 and 30701449

HERPESVIRUS DISEASES

The herpesvirus group can cause many oral and head and neck diseases, listed in Table 15.2. All herpesvirus infections are more common in immunosuppression, particularly HIV infection. Infection can then be more severe, persistent or recurrent and carry higher risks of significant complications.

Oral hairy leukoplakia, which may occur with or without immunosuppression, is discussed with white lesions in Chapter 18.

PRIMARY HERPETIC STOMATITIS

→ Summary chart 15.2

Primary infection (systemic infection in a non-immune individual) of the mouth is usually caused by *Herpes simplex* virus type 1. Herpesviruses have been considered almost ubiquitous and globally almost all individuals are infected with either type 1 or type 2 virus. Free virus is transmitted by close living conditions, usually through saliva in early childhood. In resource-poor communities, 90% of individuals have been exposed to the virus by adolescence, as demonstrated by antibody levels. In the UK, the proportion of the population who are exposed to the virus before the age of 20 years, and are therefore immune, has reduced to 60%. The consequence is that though the incidence of herpetic stomatitis has declined, lack of immunity developed in childhood allows the disease to present in adolescents or adults, rather than in children only.

Table 15.1   Important causes of oral mucosal ulcers

	Ulceration preceded by vesicles or bullae	Ulceration without preceding vesiculation
Infectious	Primary herpetic stomatitis	Measles
	Herpes labialis	Glandular fever
	Herpes zoster and chickenpox	Tuberculosis
	Hand-foot-and-mouth disease	Syphilis
	Herpangina	
Non-infectious	Pemphigus vulgaris	Traumatic
	Mucous membrane pemphigoid	Aphthous stomatitis
	Linear IgA disease	Behçet's disease
	Dermatitis herpetiformis	HIV-associated mucosal ulcers
	Bullous erythema multiforme	Lichen planus
		Lupus erythematosus
		Eosinophilic ulceration
		Wegener's granulomatosis
		Some mucosal drug reactions
		Necrotising sialometaplasia (Ch. 22)
		Carcinoma (Ch. 20)

Table 15.2   Herpesvirus diseases relevant to dentistry

Human Herpesvirus type	Common name	Diseases	
1	Herpes simplex	Primary herpetic stomatitis Herpes labialis Herpetic whitlow	This chapter
2	Herpes simplex	A rarer cause of oral diseases as type 1, more commonly genital infections of similar type	This chapter
3	Varicella zoster	Chicken pox Shingles (zoster)	This chapter
4	Epstein–Barr virus	Infectious mononucleosis (glandular fever) Hairy leukoplakia Lymphoma, of several types including nasal type Nasopharyngeal carcinoma Hodgkin's disease Lymphoepithelial carcinoma of salivary glands Mucosal ulcers	Infectious mononucleosis Ch. 32 Hairy leukoplakia Ch. 18
5	Cytomegalovirus	Salivary infection in neonates Infectious mononucleosis-like disease	This chapter
8	Kaposi sarcoma virus	Kaposi sarcoma Multicentric Castleman's disease	Kaposi sarcoma Ch. 25 Castleman's disease Ch. 32

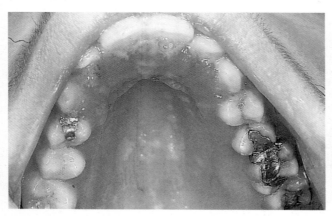

Fig. 15.1   Primary herpetic gingivostomatitis. Pale vesicles and ulcers are visible on the palate and gingivae, especially anteriorly, and the gingivae are erythematous and swollen.

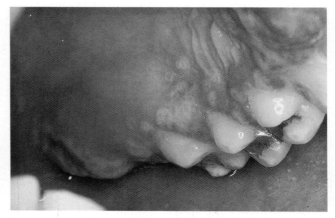

Fig. 15.2   Primary herpetic gingivostomatitis. A group of recently ruptured vesicles on the hard palate, a characteristic site. These early individual lesions are of uniform size, but several have coalesced to form larger irregular ulcers.

Herpes simplex virus type 2 is more commonly found in, and causes similar disease in, the genital tract, but the viruses are not strictly site specific and both types may cause infection at any other site, though less frequently. The virus type is not of clinical significance.

Clinical features

The great majority of primary infections are subclinical or completely asymptomatic. Only 1% of people infected develop any symptoms, and these are often minimal. Most patients with clinical infection are children aged younger than 6 years.

In clinical disease, vesicles develop on the oral mucosa approximately 7–10 days after transmission. The hard palate, gingiva and dorsum of the tongue are favoured sites (Figs 15.1–15.3). The vesicles are dome-shaped, tense and filled with clear fluid and increase from 1 mm in diameter to 2–3 mm. There are usually tens or more than 100 tiny vesicles. Rupture of vesicles after a day or two leaves circular, sharply defined, shallow ulcers with yellowish or greyish floors and red margins. Initially round, the ulcers enlarge and coalesce to produce more irregular but shallow ulcers. The gingival margins are swollen and red, with or without ulcers.

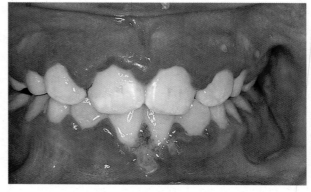

Fig. 15.3   Primary herpetic gingivostomatitis. There is diffuse reddening of the attached gingiva with ulceration in the lower incisor region extending beyond the attached gingiva.

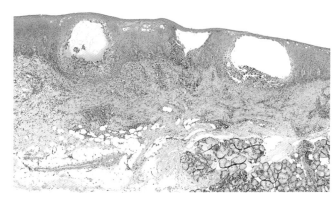

Fig. 15.4 Herpetic vesicles. A strip of mucosa with underlying normal salivary gland. This is an early infection and three vesicles about half a millimetre across are seen within the epithelium. The vesicle is formed by accumulation of fluid within the prickle cell layer. Virus infected cells and debris from lysed epithelial cells are floating freely in the vesicle fluid.

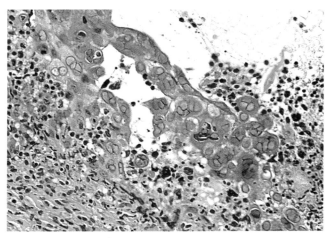

Fig. 15.5 Herpetic vesicle at higher power. Running from top left to bottom right is epithelium lining the vesicle. The epithelial cell nuclei are ballooned and pale stained ('mulberry nuclei').

Symptoms depend on extent of ulceration, but the ulcers are painful and often interfere with eating. There is usually a degree of fever and systemic upset with enlarged cervical lymph nodes and sometimes a non-specific macular rash. Systemic features can be severe, particularly in adults.

Oral lesions usually resolve within a week to 10 days, but malaise can persist so long that an adult may not recover fully for several weeks.

Clinicopathological features PMID: 18197856

Pathology

The DNA virus targets epithelial cells, and replication leads to cell lysis. Clusters of infected cells break down to form the vesicles within the epithelium (Fig. 15.4). Virus-damaged epithelial cells with swollen nuclei and marginated chromatin (ballooning degeneration) are seen in the floor of the vesicle and in direct smears from early lesions (Figs. 15.5 and 15.6). Infected cells fuse with normal adjacent cells, spreading the infection and forming multinucleate cells. Later, the full thickness of the epithelium is destroyed to produce a sharply-defined ulcer associated with an in-flammatory infiltrate.

Diagnosis

The clinical picture is usually distinctive (Box 15.1). A smear showing virus-damaged cells provides additional diagnostic evidence. A rising titre of antibodies reaching a peak after 2–3 weeks provides absolute, but retrospective, confirmation of the diagnosis, as does viral culture of vesicle fluid.

In cases of severe disease, when the patient is immuno-suppressed or complications such as spread to the eye are suspected, rapid definitive diagnosis can be obtained by PCR DNA amplification, ELISA assays or electron microscopy. These virus-specific tests have the additional ability to reveal that approximately 15% of cases are caused by the type 2 virus that normally causes genital infection, but the symptoms, signs and treatment are identical.

Obtaining a definite diagnosis may not be essential. Hand, foot and mouth disease and herpangina (later in this chapter) produce similar features and, if mild, all are treated only by supportive measures.

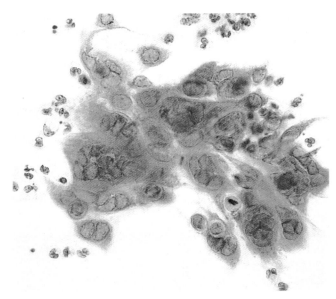

Fig. 15.6 A smear from a herpetic vesicle. The distended degenerating nuclei of the epithelial cells cluster together to give the typical mulberry appearance.

Treatment

Patients feel very unwell, and children fail to eat or maintain fluid intake, sleep poorly and are fractious. Addressing these concerns is important for children and stressed parents. Because the disease is ultimately self-limiting, supportive treatment may be all that is required. Bed rest, soft bland diet, drinking through a straw and paracetamol elixir are effective. A non-prescription sedative antihistamine will aid sleeping. Chlorhexidine mouthwash is sometimes used in an attempt to reduce pain by controlling secondary infection of ulcers. It also helps maintain gingival health while tooth brushing is impossible. The saliva is infectious, and transfer to the eye must be avoided because ocular herpes infections may develop into encephalitis by direct spread along the optic nerves.

Treatment with antiviral drugs is highly effective, but only if administered during the first 48 hours or so after vesicles appear, a maximum of 5 days after prodromal symptoms appear or if new vesicles are developing. Aciclovir is a nucleoside analogue that is only phosphorylated by viral DNA-encoded enzymes in infected cells. The activated drug blocks viral DNA synthesis, preventing viral replication. Aciclovir suspension can be used as a rinse and then swallowed for systemic effect or given in tablet form at 400 mg, three times per day for 5 days in adults and children older than 2 years. Routine use of antiviral drugs in children is not recommended and cases should be selected on the basis of severity accepting that the evidence base is weak and suggests only limited reduction in healing time.

Older topical antiviral drugs are no longer recommended.

Aggressive treatment is essential in people who are immunosuppressed to prevent infection spreading onto the skin or eye and other systemic complications. Valaciclovir is then the preferred drug for its higher blood level and longer half-life.

Unusually prolonged or severe infections or failure to respond to aciclovir suggest immunodeficiency, and herpetic ulceration persisting for more than a month is an AIDS-defining illness.

Aciclovir for child patients PMID: 27255621

US treatment guidance PMID: 27181443

Web URL 15.1 UK NICE treatment guidance: http://cks.nice.org.uk/herpes-simplex-oral

Latency

Herpes simplex and zoster are neurotropic as well as epitheliotropic viruses. After the immune response develops and mucosal infection subsides, the virus can remain hidden from the immune response in the sensory nerves that supply the site of the primary infection. Virus is transported back along the nerves from the mucosa to the neurone cell bodies in the ganglia where it establishes a lifelong latent infection. During latency there are no symptoms, no virus replication occurs and the patient is not infectious.

Reactivation of the latent infection depends on the host cell, not the virus, and triggers (discussed later in this chapter) switch the virus back into replicative infection, after which it travels back down the neurones to reinfect the skin or mucosa. Only a small proportion of the latently infected neurones are able to reactivate, so that recurrent lesions develop only in small foci within the area involved by the primary infection. They are almost always on the lip (herpes labialis) but occasionally in the mouth or on the skin. Rare intraoral recurrence is most frequently on the palate.

Many in the population shed virus intermittently into saliva indicating reactivation of latent infection. They suffer no symptoms but can transmit the infection.

Persistent infection and infectivity PMID: 17703961 and 24167660

HERPES LABIALIS → Summary chart 15.2 p. 280

Herpes labialis is a secondary infection, that is an infection in an immune individual following reactivation of latent virus. The neutralising antibodies and T-cell responses produced in response to the primary infection are not protective because the virus travels along the nerves inside neurones from the trigeminal ganglion to infect the lip epithelial cells directly.

Reactivation of latent virus to produce a herpes labialis lesion ('cold sore') happens in up to 30% of the population, many more than have ever had a clinically evident primary infection. Recurrent lesions must therefore usually follow a subclinical infection. Triggering factors include the common cold, other febrile infections, exposure to ultraviolet light, menstruation, emotional stress, local trauma, hypothermia, dental treatment and immunosuppression, but often none is identified.

Clinically, changes follow a consistent course with prodromal paraesthesia or burning sensations, then erythema at the site of the infection. Vesicles form after an hour or two, usually in clusters along the mucocutaneous junction of the lips and extending a short distance onto the adjacent skin (Fig. 15.7).

The vesicles enlarge, coalesce and weep exudate. After 2 or 3 days they rupture and crust over, but new vesicles frequently appear for a day or two only to scab over and finally heal, usually without scarring. The whole cycle may take as long as 12 days. In patients who are immunocompromised, lesions are larger, more painful and last longer.

Secondary bacterial infection may induce scarring. Infectious virus is shed from the lesion until it is completely healed, so a dentist with a cold sore should not work.

Recurrent infection can trigger erythema multiforme (Ch. 16).

Treatment

The need for treatment depends on extent. Many stoical patients manage cold sores with over-the-counter preparations of minimal value. Docosanol is a fatty alcohol with a mild effect. In the UK aciclovir, 5% cream, is available without prescription and may be effective if applied before vesicles appear, when premonitory sensations are felt. Penciclovir, on prescription, applied every 2 hours is more effective. These agents must be dabbed and not rubbed onto the lesions to avoid spreading the infectious exudate more widely.

Sunscreen on the lips prevents lesions in people susceptible to ultraviolet light reactivation.

Patients who experience frequent, multiple or large cold sores may benefit from more aggressive treatment with antiviral drugs. Repeated early high-dose treatment both treats the lesion and reduces the risk of future attacks.

Vaccines are in trial and have greatest potential benefit in the developing world where herpes simplex infections are a common cause of blindness and are common sexually transmitted diseases, but none is yet approved.

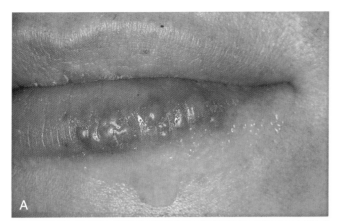

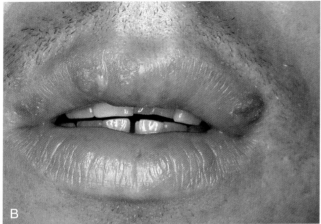

Fig. 15.7   Herpes labialis. (A) Typical vesicles. (B) Crusted ulcers affecting the vermilion borders of the lips.

Web URL 15.1 NICE treatment guidance: http://cks.nice.org.uk/herpes-simplex-oral

US treatment guidance PMID: 27181443

Herpetic whitlow

Both primary and secondary herpetic infections are contagious. *Herpetic whitlow* (Fig. 15.8) is a skin infection in a non-immune host after inoculation from another infected site, either another individual or by autoinoculation. Children with a primary infection may transfer the infection by finger sucking. Routine glove wear has made this a much less common occupational hazard for dental surgeons and their teams.

Antiviral drugs should be prescribed as for a primary infection.

Case and image PMID: 22546886

HERPES ZOSTER OF THE TRIGEMINAL NERVE → Summary chart 15.2 p. 280

The varicella zoster virus causes chickenpox in the non-immune, mainly children (later in this chapter), while reactivation of the latent virus in the nerves of immune individuals causes zoster (shingles), mainly in older people. The mechanism of latency is as described above for herpes simplex, but unlike simplex virus, reactivation is a relatively rare phenomenon, and most patients only ever experience a single attack of zoster. Although zoster affects as many

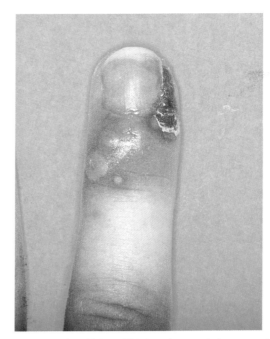

Fig. 15.8   Herpetic whitlow. This is a characteristic non-oral site for primary infection in a non-immune individual as a result of contact with infected vesicle fluid or saliva. The vesiculation and crusting are identical to those seen in herpes labialis.

as one in three adults, the face and mouth are relatively unusual sites.

Clinical features

Zoster usually affects adults of middle age or older. The first signs are pain and irritation or tenderness in the dermatome supplied by the nerve in which the virus has reactivated after latent infection. Unlike simplex infection there is severe neuralgic, often burning, pain initially while the virus replicates in the nerve and travels to the skin or mucosa. After 2–3 days the pain is felt in the skin and a vesicular rash develops, sharply limited to the dermatome. Facial rash or stomatitis is therefore sharply defined along, and limited by, the midline.

Vesicles are usually numerous and can become confluent and pass through the same sequence of rupture, ulceration, crusting and healing as described for herpes simplex infections over 7–10 days (Figs 15.9 and 15.10). The regional lymph nodes are enlarged and tender. Pain continues until the lesions crust over and start to heal, but secondary infection may cause suppuration and scarring of the skin. Malaise and fever are usually associated.

In its prodromal phase the acute neuralgic pain of trigeminal nerve zoster is a classic mimic of pulpitis, and patients may well present for dental treatment. If no dental cause is evident, this possibility should be considered. This has given rise to the myth that dental extractions can precipitate facial zoster.

Pathology

The varicella zoster virus produces epithelial lesions similar to those of herpes simplex.

A national programme of vaccination against varicella zoster started in the UK in 2013 for people aged between 70 and 80 years and has been recommended in the US since 2017 for those aged over 50 years. Vaccination reduces

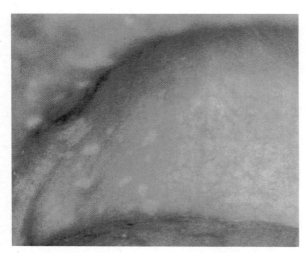

Fig. 15.9 Herpes zoster. Erythema and ulcers on the hard and soft palate on the right side and stopping abruptly at the midline.

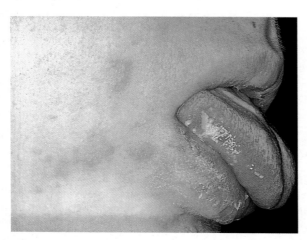

Fig. 15.10 Herpes zoster of the trigeminal nerve. There are vesicles and ulcers on one side of the tongue and facial skin supplied by the first and second divisions. The patient complained only of toothache.

attacks by approximately half and reduces severity in the remaining patients.

Management

Herpes zoster is an uncommon cause of stomatitis, but readily recognisable without laboratory investigation (Box 15.2), although viral culture and other more rapid tests such as polymerase chain reaction (PCR) are available if required.

Mild attacks may require only analgesia and topical soothing cream. Facial infections are usually treated because of the risk of scarring and higher risk of complications. Oral aciclovir, 800 mg, 5 times a day for 7 days is effective. In patients who are immunocompromised the drug is continued until 2 days after healing and famciclovir or valaciclovir may be preferred. The drug must be given at the earliest opportunity for maximum effect, ideally within 72 hours, and complemented with analgesics. Addition of prednisolone speeds recovery and reduces the incidence of post-herpetic neuralgia (Ch. 39) but is not usually recommended because the evidence is weak. Use should be limited to older people who are most at risk of post-herpetic neuralgia. Any patient who is immunosuppressed, develops complications, has eye involvement or bacterial infection of

---

| **Box 15.2** | **Herpes zoster of the trigeminal area: key features** |

- A recurrent latent *Varicella zoster* infection
- Prophylactic vaccination available
- Typically in older people
- Pain precedes the rash
- Facial rash accompanies the stomatitis
- Lesions localised to one side, within the distribution of any of the divisions of the trigeminal nerve
- Malaise can be severe
- Can be life-threatening in immunosuppression
- Treat with systemic aciclovir
- Antibiotics required if the rash becomes secondarily infected
- Sometimes followed by post-herpetic neuralgia, particularly in older people

---

skin lesions or is very old or infirm should be managed in a specialist centre. Intravenous aciclovir may be required.

Treatment PMID: 19691461

Use of corticosteroids PMID: 29431387

Web URL 15.2 NICE guidance: http://cks.nice.org.uk/shingles#!scenario:1

Complications

Zoster of the trigeminal nerve will occasionally cause tooth devitalisation and even bone necrosis in the affected area, during or after the clinical infection, particularly when the prodromal symptoms included toothache.

Involvement of the tip and lateral tip of the nose indicates involvement of the external nasal branch of the nasociliary nerve, a branch of the ophthalmic division of the trigeminal that also supplies the cornea. This is Hutchinson's sign*, and it indicates a high risk of ocular involvement and need for specialist treatment from the outset (Fig. 15.11).

Zoster in immunosuppression can be a lethal infection if encephalitis develops. Thus, zoster in very old people, organ transplant patients, patients treated for malignant disease or in HIV infection require aggressive treatment and follow up. Vaccination for people with immunosuppression must use newer recombinant vaccine rather than the live virus vaccine used routinely.

Post-herpetic neuralgia mainly affects older people and is difficult to relieve (Ch. 39).

Case devitalisation teeth PMID: 16054735

Rare oral complications PMID: 20692192

Ramsay Hunt syndrome

Ramsay Hunt** syndrome is zoster infection reactivated in the facial nerve. Virus is latent in the geniculate ganglion, which houses both sensory and motor fibres. On reactivation, patients develop unilateral facial paralysis, loss of taste on one side of the anterior tongue and vesicles on the

---

*This is named after the same Sir Jonathan Hutchinson (1828–1913) who described the characteristic incisors of syphilis and who has over a dozen eponymous signs, disease and syndromes named after him.
**There is no hyphen in the name of this disease because it is named after James Ramsay Hunt (1872–1937), not after two people.

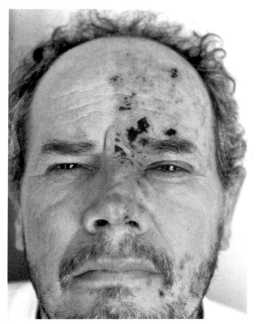

Fig. 15.11   Typical unilateral zoster rash, sharply defined at the midline, and affecting all three divisions of the trigeminal nerve and the tip of the nose (Hutchinson's sign). *(From Mannis MJ, Holland EJ, 2022. Cornea, 5ᵗʰ ed. Oxford: Elsevier Inc)*

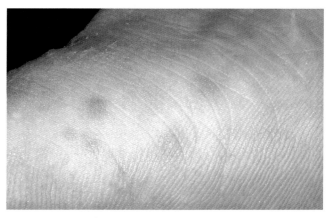

Fig 15.12   Hand-foot-and-mouth disease. The rash consists of vesicles or bullae on the extremities; often they are relatively inconspicuous erythematous patches as here.

tongue, hard palate and in the external auditory canal, all on the same side. It must be differentiated from Bell's palsy. Pain is severe.

Treatment is as for zoster of the trigeminal nerve, but the chances of full recovery are lower than for Bell's palsy.

CYTOMEGALOVIRUS ULCERS

Cytomegalovirus, or herpesvirus type 5, is another almost ubiquitous virus that causes an acute primary disease, usually in the newborn, and can remain latent to cause recurrent infection. Almost all infections are asymptomatic. In the few with clinical disease, primary infection resembles infectious mononucleosis, sometimes with painful swelling and infection of salivary glands.

The main interest is cytomegalovirus ulceration of the oral mucosa in immunodeficiency, particularly in HIV infection. These ulcers show no specific clinical features but are usually large and shallow and solitary. In people who are immunosuppressed they heal slowly, and biopsy is usually undertaken to identify a cause. The virally infected cells have typical inclusions in their nuclei and can be identified on immunohistochemistry (see Fig. 1.8).

Cytomegalovirus infection in immunosuppression is treated with the aciclovir analogue ganciclovir or related drugs. No treatment is required in immunocompetent adults.

Review oral signs PMID: 8385303

In immunosuppression PMID: 8705589

HAND-FOOT-AND-MOUTH DISEASE

→ Summary chart 15.2 p. 280

Hand-foot-and-mouth disease is a common viral infection caused by several related strains of enteric viruses, notably coxsackie A16 and enterovirus 71. These are RNA viruses

spread by faecal-oral contact and, distantly, related to poliovirus.

The disease is highly infectious and often causes minor epidemics among school children and an occasional parent or teacher, often in the autumn. Spread is by droplet, contact and faecal-oral transmission with an incubation period probably between 3 and 10 days. Patients remain infectious for several weeks. The disease is unrelated to foot-and-mouth disease of cattle.

Clinical features

This is a mild viral infection characterised by ulceration of the mouth and a vesicular rash on the extremities. Regional lymph nodes are not usually enlarged, and systemic upset is typically mild or absent, but there may be diarrhoea and vomiting. The main features are small, scattered oral ulcers in all areas of the mouth, usually with little pain and an erythematous background. Unlike herpetic stomatitis, intact vesicles are rarely seen and gingivitis is not a feature.

The rash develops after the oral ulcers and consists of vesicles, sometimes deep-seated, or occasionally bullae, mainly seen on palms and soles and around the base of fingers or toes, but any part of the limbs may be affected (Fig. 15.12). The rash is often the main feature, and such patients are unlikely to be seen by dentists. In some outbreaks, either the mouth or the extremities alone may be affected.

The disease typically resolves within a week. No specific treatment is available or needed, but myocarditis and encephalitis are rare complications. In India and South-East Asia disease caused by the less common Coxsackie A6 and A10 is associated with neurological complications and is occasionally fatal.

Key features are summarised in Box 15.3.

Clinical review PMID: 26087425

Oral features PMID: 1061921

More severe variant PMID: 24932735 and 27406374

HERPANGINA

This can be considered related to hand-foot-and-mouth disease, and the features described above also apply. It is slightly less common than hand-foot-and-mouth disease and is caused by enteroviruses, of often the same types, but most often by coxsackie A strains.

Box 15.3 Hand-foot-and-mouth disease: key features
- Caused mainly by enteric viruses
- Highly infectious
- School children predominantly affected
- Typically mild vesiculating stomatitis
- Vesicles and erythema on palms and soles of feet
- Rarely severe enough for dental opinion to be sought
- No specific treatment available or needed
- Herpangina is similar but with no rash and fewer ulcers

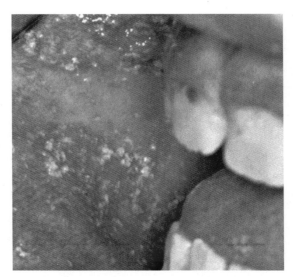

Fig. 15.14 Koplik's spots in measles. White pinpoint spots on an erythematous background, likened to the appearance of grains of salt. *(Fig. 16.7 From Paller, A.S., and Mancini, A.J. 2011. Hurwitz clinical pediatric dermatology: a textbook of skin disorders of childhood and adolescence. Philadelphia: Saunders.)*

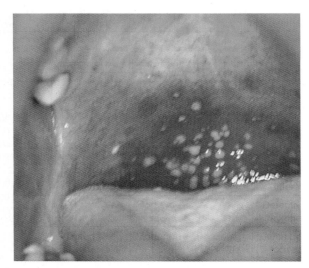

Fig 15.13 Herpangina. Typical cluster of ulcers on an erythematous background on the soft palate. *(From Cohen J, Powderly WG, 2004. Infectious diseases. 2nd ed. St Louis: Mosby)*

The presentation is a similar mild viral disease with a cluster of a few larger ulcers usually limited to the soft palate, tonsils or posterior mouth but no rash (Fig. 15.13). As after hand, foot and mouth disease, occasional complications can occur.

Herpangina review PMID: 20118685

MEASLES

Measles, once a common childhood illness, is now rare following introduction of vaccination schemes in many countries, but there are still approximately 2000 cases each year due to poor uptake in the UK. Occasional epidemics still occur, but death from measles is now limited to adults, people who are immunocompromised or experience late complications. Worldwide, despite a global vaccination campaign, measles is still the leading cause of vaccine-preventable death.

In the prodromal stage of measles, toward the end of a 14-day incubation period, there is fever lasting about 4 days during which Koplik's spots form on the buccal mucosa and soft palate. These are characteristic pinpoint foci of epithelial necrosis on a red background (Fig. 15.14). Classically, while these break down into ulcers, the patient develops the typical fever and rash starting on the face. However, the spots are very variable, have been reported to be absent in vaccinated children and also to occur late in the disease. Recognising Koplik's spots is therefore very helpful,

but the oral lesions require no treatment. The main effects are the fever, extensive maculopapular rash and cough. Measles resolves in about 3 weeks.

Measles is highly infectious and has many severe complications and in the UK is a notifiable disease. In the developing world and in people who are immunosuppressed it is potentially fatal and predisposes to cancrum oris (noma, Ch. 9).

Case and image PMID: 25754702

Case series, images PMID: 22236551

CHICKEN POX

Chicken pox is caused by infection with varicella zoster virus in a non-immune host, usually a child younger than 12 years. The UK does not have a universal chicken pox vaccination scheme, and the disease remains endemic whereas childhood vaccination is recommended routinely in the US. An effective vaccine is available but use in the UK is limited to protecting those at particular risk of complications, primarily people who are immunosuppressed, women who are pregnant and non-immune healthcare workers. The formulation of chicken pox vaccine is different from the shingles vaccine because the target populations are different. It is not expected to protect against shingles and may even increase risk of shingles in later life.

After a 2-week incubation period, there is malaise, nausea, fever, sore throat and the rash appears on the face and trunk producing intensely itchy blisters that break down into ulcers. The oral lesions usually appear before the rash and appear like herpes simplex vesicles and ulcers except that they tend to occur on the buccal mucosa and palate. There are normally only a few, and numerous ulcers signify a more severe systemic infection.

Treatment is mostly supportive, with aciclovir or related drugs if the diagnosis is made early enough or the patient is at risk of complications.

Review and cases PMID: 1068230, 6931841 and 11314207

MPOX

Mpox, previously called monkeypox, is a disease of rodents and primates caused by the mpox virus and previously found only in some African countries around the Congo basin. Smallpox vaccination produces a cross-reactive immunity, as the viruses are closely related, and when vaccination ceased following smallpox eradication in 1980, the disease appeared and has gradually become more widespread in central and West Africa. It only occasionally spread to distant countries until 2020 when mpox appeared in several countries and spread in epidemics, often in men who have sex with men. It is now found in almost all countries but remains rare.

Key features are shown in Box 15.4.

Shortly after infection there are fever, lymphadenopathy (unlike chickenpox), myalgia, backache and fatigue. Then a rash resembling that of chickenpox appears, particularly on the face and limbs. On the skin the lesions are initially flat, becoming raised to form painful papules that often have an umbilicated central depression after 1–2 days. These develop into fluid filled blisters in 5–7 days that burst to form an ulcer and crust over. The number ranges from a few to hundreds and they may be small, as in chickenpox, or over 10 mm in diameter. In severe disease they coalesce, ulcerating large areas of skin. Healing takes 2–4 weeks and is usually uneventful with supportive care. In patients with severe disease, children and people who are immunosuppressed the untreated disease can be fatal, though anti-smallpox and specific antivirals are available. People vaccinated against smallpox have less severe disease.

About half to three quarters of patients develop oral lesions and these usually appear before those on the skin. They are less typical than the skin lesions and quickly break down to form ulcers on any part of the mouth, often the lips. Oral lesions often seem to show ulceration spreading from the centre like the umbilication seen in skin lesions (Fig. 15.15). As skin lesions are frequent, presentation in a dental setting would be limited to people who have a few lesions on the lips or intraorally or are recently infected. Cases have been reported with a single skin lesion.

Oral lesions PMID: 36096397 and 37232783

Infection control dentistry PMID: 35934521

TUBERCULOSIS

Mucosal infection is described here; tuberculous lymphadenopathy is dealt with in Chapter 32.

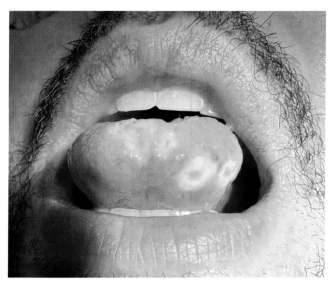

Fig. 15.15   Mpox. Target or umbilicated lesions with early breakdown to ulcers seen 2 days after onset of symptoms *(From Benslama L, Foy J-P, Bertolus C, 2022. Journal of stomatology, oral and maxillofacial surgery. 123(6): 596)*

The recrudescence of tuberculosis is partly a consequence of the HIV epidemic, partly explained by multiple drug-resistant mycobacteria and partly due to the variable and reduced effectiveness of the BCG (bacillus Calmette-Guérin) vaccination. Vaccination is only routine in countries with a high incidence and, when indicated, must be given immediately or soon after birth.

Though tuberculosis is common, with over 10 million new cases each year worldwide, oral tuberculosis is rare and only seen as a complication of active pulmonary disease in which the mucosa is infected from the sputum. Trauma is probably required to allow the organisms to access the underlying tissue. Open active tuberculosis itself is now rare in developed countries and tends to be seen in older men with pulmonary infection and a chronic cough that has progressed unrecognised, people who have neglected treatment or are immunosuppressed. They are likely to show typical signs of pulmonary infection: chest pain, malaise, weight loss and haemoptysis.

The typical lesion is an ulcer on the mid-dorsum of the tongue; the lip or other parts of the mouth are infrequently affected. The ulcer is typically angular or stellate, with overhanging edges and a pale indurated floor, but can be ragged and irregular (Fig. 15.16). It is painless in its early stages, and regional lymph nodes are usually unaffected. A second typical presentation is a non-healing extraction socket. In both cases the presentation may resemble a malignant neoplasm. Irregular nodular gingival enlargement, with or without ulceration, is seen more rarely (Fig. 15.17).

Primary oral tuberculosis is extremely rare, seen essentially only in high incidence countries, and affects non-immune children and young adults. The presentation is variable with ulcers, and gingival swelling.

The diagnosis is rarely suspected before biopsy.

Case series PMID: 22014940 and 31879619

Review PMID: 20486998

Primary oral tuberculosis PMID: 33456244 and 33110314

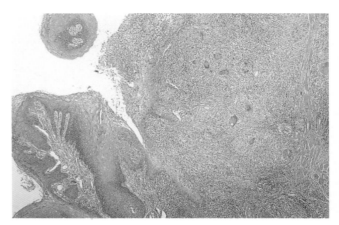

Fig. 15.18 Tuberculous ulcer. At the margin, numerous pale staining granulomas are present in the ulcer bed, which fills the right half of the image. The darkly stained multinucleate Langhans giant cells are visible even at this low power.

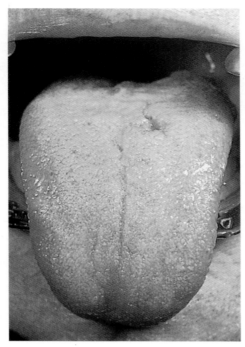

Fig. 15.16 A tuberculous ulcer of the tongue. The rather angular shape and overhanging edges of the ulcer are typical. The patient was a man aged 56 years with advanced but unrecognised pulmonary tuberculosis.

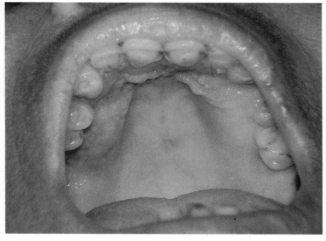

Fig 15.17 Diffuse gingival enlargement caused by infection from pulmonary tuberculosis *(From Pai K, Pai KM, Manu MK et al, 2018. The lancet infectious disease. 18(11): 1288)*

Pathology

Typical non-caseating tuberculous granulomas containing occasional Langhans-type giant cells are seen in the floor of the ulcers (Fig. 15.18). Mycobacteria are sometimes identifiable in the oral lesion by using special stains but can be demonstrated more easily in the sputum. Chest radiographs usually show advanced infection. In tropical countries and in immunosuppression, similar histological features arise from fungal or atypical mycobacterial infections.

Management

Diagnosis is confirmed by biopsy, chest imaging and a specimen of sputum. Mycobacterial infection is confirmed by culture or PCR. Interferon gamma release assays used in latent infection are not used to diagnose active infection.

Oral lesions clear up rapidly if vigorous multidrug chemotherapy is given for the pulmonary infection. No local treatment is needed.

SYPHILIS

As a result of contact tracing and early treatment, fewer than 150 cases a year of primary or secondary syphilis were seen in England and Wales in the 1980s. However, since the mid-1990s, the prevalence has risen steadily in developed countries. There are currently approximately 8000 new cases of syphilis a year in the UK, the highest levels since the 1950s with incidence tripling since 2010. There are 10,000 a year in the United States, but there is no accurate estimate for Africa where the incidence is highest. This increase is a worldwide trend, and the disease has, for example, become widespread in Eastern Europe.

Most of these increases parallel rates of HIV infection and, in developed countries, two-thirds to three-quarters of cases are in men who have sex with men. HIV infection predisposes to a fulminant form of the disease and also renders some diagnostic tests based on antibody levels inaccurate.

Oral lesions in each stage of syphilis are clinically quite different from each other. Oral lesions in the UK probably often pass unrecognised outside specialist clinics.

Congenital syphilis

Congenital syphilis arises when an infected mother transmits the infection to her child in utero or during birth. After almost vanishing in the developed world, congenital infection is now seen again, even in developed countries, and worldwide it causes the death of half a million infants each year. Survivors usually develop either latent or tertiary syphilis. The widespread infection produces many signs and developmental disturbances, classically diffuse rash, lymphadenopathy, rhinitis, radial scarring around the mouth and periostitis of many bones producing a saddle nose and frontal bossing. The classical triad of interstitial keratitis of the cornea, sensorineural hearing loss and dental anomalies is diagnostic.

Dental anomalies are discussed in Chapter 2.

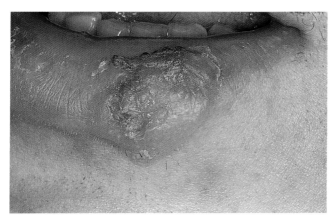

Fig. 15.19 Primary chancre. The lower lip is a typical site for extragenital chancres, but they are rarely seen.

UK incidence PMID: 26931054

US incidence PMID: 26562206

Primary syphilis

Oral chancres are found in 5%–10% of all cases of primary syphilis. They appear 2–10 weeks after infection and may form on the lip, tip of the tongue or, rarely, other oral sites. A chancre consists initially of a firm nodule about a centimetre across (Fig. 15.19). The surface breaks down after a few days, leaving a rounded ulcer with raised indurated edges. Chancres are usually solitary, and multiple lesions suggest immunosuppression. A chancre is typically painless. Regional lymph nodes are enlarged, rubbery and discrete.

A biopsy may only show non-specific inflammation, but sometimes there is conspicuous perivascular infiltration by plasma cells. If infection is suspected, immunohistochemical staining can reveal the treponemal organisms in the epithelium, but the diagnosis is easily missed if not suspected clinically. Diagnosis is best made by serological tests or polymerase chain reaction. Biopsy can be diagnostic, though rarely performed, but direct examination of smears from oral lesions is not recommended because *Treponema pallidum* cannot be confidently distinguished from other oral commensal spirochaetes.

After 8 or 9 weeks the chancre heals, often without scarring, but while present is highly infectious. Unfortunately, the diagnosis of syphilis is rarely made at the primary stage.

Secondary syphilis

The secondary stage develops 1–4 months after infection as the causative spirochaetes spread to other tissues. It typically causes mild fever with malaise, headache, sore throat and generalised lymphadenopathy, soon followed by a rash and stomatitis.

The rash is variable but typically consists of asymptomatic pinkish ('coppery') macules, symmetrically distributed and starting on the trunk. It may last from a few hours to several weeks, and its presence or history is a useful aid to diagnosis. Oral lesions, which rarely appear without the rash, mainly affect the tonsils, lateral borders of the tongue and lips. They are usually flat ulcers covered by greyish membrane and may be irregularly linear (snail's track ulcers) or, most commonly, coalesce to form well-defined rounded areas (mucous patches) (Fig 15.20). *Condyloma lata* are raised mucous patches

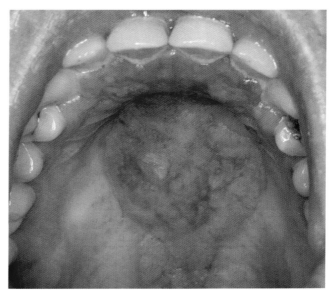

Fig. 15.20 Secondary syphilis. A large mucous patch on the palate.

(Fig 15.21) that resemble large flat papillomas. Oral lesions may mimic pemphigoid, pemphigus, lichen planus, erythema multiforme and other causes of widespread ulcers and inflammation.

Discharge from the ulcers contains many spirochaetes, and saliva is highly infectious. Serological reactions (see later in this chapter) are positive and diagnostic at this stage, and biopsy is diagnostic using *T. pallidum*-specific immunohistochemical stains (Fig 15.22).

Untreated secondary syphilis becomes latent, non-infectious and asymptomatic but carries the risk of developing tertiary disease.

Tertiary syphilis

Late-stage syphilis develops in patients approximately 3 or more years after infection in as many as a third of untreated patients but not in those treated effectively. The onset is insidious, and during the latent period the patient may appear well. The late tertiary stage is now very rare in developed countries but remains common worldwide. Leukoplakia of the tongue may develop during this late stage (Ch. 19) and other effects of syphilis such as aortitis, tabes or general paralysis of the insane may be associated.

The characteristic oral lesion is the gumma, usually of the palate, tongue or tonsils. This starts as a swelling a few to several centimetres in diameter sometimes with a yellowish centre that undergoes necrosis, leaving a painless indolent deep ulcer. The ulcer is rounded, with soft, punched-out edges. The floor is depressed and pale ('wash-leather') in appearance. It eventually heals with severe scarring that may distort the soft palate or tongue, perforate the hard palate (Fig. 15.23) or destroy the uvula.

Microscopically, there is non-specific inflammation with endarteritis and sparse granulomas. However, the appearances can be completely non-specific, and diagnosis depends on laboratory tests. Biopsy is often not diagnostic because the number of *T. pallidum* is very small, a gumma being primarily an immunologically driven hypersensitivity reaction rather than an infected focus.

Review oral lesions PMID: 15953910 and 33459991

Case series PMID: 24045192 and 34263964

Tertiary syphilis cases PMID: 24891485 and 33911527

Management

Management of syphilis in the dental setting is limited to maintaining suspicion to identify cases and screening diagnosis in secondary care. Definitive diagnosis and treatment must be provided by specialists. Clinical diagnosis and biopsy diagnosis with confirmation of *Treponema* by immunohistochemistry is the likely pathway in most cases presenting to dentists as the diagnosis is not usually suspected and a biopsy may well be taken.

When the diagnosis is suspected, specialist testing must be sought as interpretation of the results is complex. Positive test results may indicate past rather than active disease and other sexually transmitted diseases or HIV infection may also be present. The organism cannot be cultured, and serological tests are used. Until recently the specific fluorescent antibody tests and *T. pallidum* haemagglutination or particle agglutination assays were the most specific. Although widely used, the VDRL test is a screening test of low positive predictive value and multiple tests had to be used. Gradually these tests are being replaced by PCR-based rapid molecular assays of very high sensitivity and specificity. Tests indicate the infection, but not the stage.

Benzathine penicillin is the drug of choice, an intramuscular preparation with slow absorption. Syphilis in HIV infection requires more aggressive treatment.

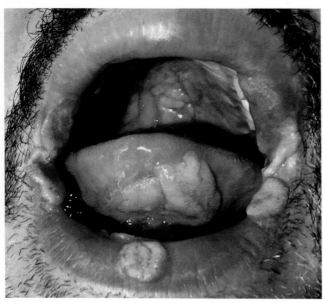

Fig. 15.21   Secondary syphilis. Multiple raised flat mucous patches or condyloma lata *(Courtesy Dr J Setterfield)*

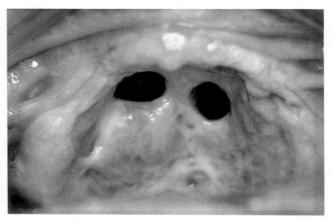

Fig. 15.23   Tertiary syphilis. Gummas of the palate. Necrosis in the centre of the palate has caused perforation of the bone and two typical round punched-out holes.

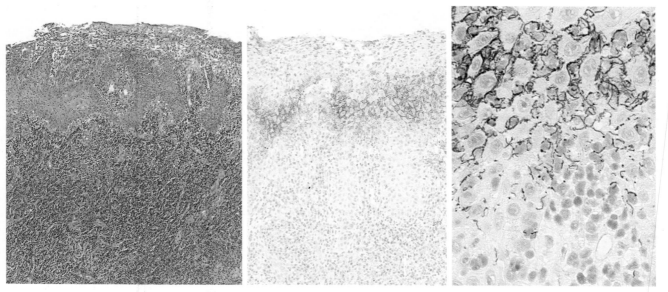

Fig. 15.22   Secondary syphilis. On the left in routine H&E stain the features are non-specific, with numerous neutrophils in the epithelium and a dense plasma cell infiltrate below. Immunohistochemistry for *T. pallidum*, in the centre, reveals very abundant spirochaetes in the epithelium seen as yellow-brown staining. Right, at high power, the shape of individual spirochaetes can be seen around the epithelial cells.

CANDIDOSIS

Candidosis* can be caused by several species of candida but in 80% of infections the organism is *Candida albicans*. All are normal commensals in the mouths of a third or more of the healthy population, and many more among denture wearers, individuals with dry mouth and older people. This candida 'carriage' is not associated with symptoms or disease and the number of organisms existing as commensals is relatively small.

Candida sp. is dimorphic. Carriage is associated with the yeast ('blastospore') form but only the invasive hyphal form causes disease. The reasons for the organism switching to a pathogenic form ('phenotype switching') are unclear, but disease seems to follow some change to the oral environment. Thus, host factors are probably more important than fungal factors. After switching, Candida becomes more adhesive, secretes pathogenic enzymes and is more resistant to killing by neutrophils.

The most common pathogenic species is *Candida albicans*. *Candida glabrata, tropicalis* and *krusei* and other less frequent species account for some 20% of disease between them. Some of the less frequent isolates are reported to be more likely to develop resistance to antifungal drugs, but this remains a relatively rare problem clinically.

The concept that candidosis is a 'disease of the diseased' dates from 1868, and many medical factors are recognised to predispose to infection (Box 15.5). These are likely to influence adhesion of the yeast form to the epithelial cells, which seems to trigger development of invasive hyphae. When the yeasts adhere, they trigger host cell receptors to activate an innate host response and attract neutrophils into the epithelium. Hyphae are only able to invade a limited distance into the epithelium, only within keratin and the upper prickle cell layer. Oral candidosis is a very superficial infection, explaining its mild symptoms. However, weakened innate and adaptive immunity carry a risk of invasive deep infection and hematogenous spread.

Microbiology candida biofilms PMID: 21134239

Controversies in candidosis PMID: 22998462

There are various classifications of oral candidosis, but in reality these diseases merge into one another and can coexist. Thus, infection causes a spectrum of distinctive presentations, rather than separate diseases (Box 15.6). The commonest forms are thrush, chronic hyperplastic candidosis and denture stomatitis. Chronic mucocutaneous candidosis is discussed later in this chapter and in Chapter 37.

Thrush ➜ Summary chart 15.1 and 19.1 pp. 279, 347

Thrush**, a disease recognised by Hippocrates, is also sometimes called the acute pseudomembranous type of candidosis because of the thick white layer of candidal hyphae, dead and dying epithelial and inflammatory cells and debris that covers the mucosa like a membrane.

Thrush is common in neonates, caused by lack of an immune response and infection acquired during passage through the birth canal. It is also common in people who are

---

*Candidosis not 'candidiasis' because it is a mycosis. Named fungal infections usually end in –osis, for instance histoplasmosis and cryptococcosis. The '-iases' are in general parasitic infections such as trypanosomiasis.
**Thrush is not a mere nickname or household term but is a medical term of respectable antiquity though its origin is uncertain.

> ### Box 15.5 Oral candidosis: important predisposing factors
>
> - Develops often at the extremes of age
> - Immunodeficiency (diabetes mellitus, HIV infection, chemotherapy)
> - Immunosuppression (including steroid inhalers)
> - Anaemia, of any type
> - Suppression of the normal oral flora by antibacterial drugs
> - Xerostomia
> - Denture wearing, orthodontic appliance wearing, poor oral hygiene
> - Smoking
> - High carbohydrate diet
> - Epithelium with increased keratin, for instance in lichen planus and dysplasia
> - Almost any severely debilitating illness
> - Treatment for malignant disease

> ### Box 15.6 Spectrum of oral candidosis
> **Acute candidosis**
> - Thrush
> - Acute antibiotic stomatitis
>
> **Chronic candidosis**
> - Denture-induced stomatitis
> - Chronic hyperplastic candidosis
> - Erythematous candidosis
> - Chronic mucocutaneous candidosis
>
> **Angular stomatitis**

very old or very debilitated and on the soft palate of asthmatic steroid inhaler users who spray their palate rather than inhale the drug. It may also follow antibiotic treatment.

Rarely, persistent thrush is an early sign of chronic mucocutaneous candidosis or candida-endocrinopathy syndrome (Ch. 37).

Clinical features

Although classified as acute, thrush may have a rapid onset or develop insidiously from a chronic infection and in people who are immunosuppressed it may become chronic. Thrush forms soft, friable and creamy coloured plaques on the mucosa (Fig. 15.24), and the pseudomembrane can be scraped or wiped off exposing the erythematous mucosa below. This differentiates thrush from chronic forms of candidosis in which the white surface layer is keratin. The extent of pseudomembrane varies from isolated small flecks to widespread confluent plaques and the buccal mucosa, palate and dorsal tongue are the most commonly affected sites. Angular stomatitis is frequently associated, as it is with any form of intraoral candidosis.

The condition is not painful; rather it is uncomfortable, sometimes with a bad taste or burning sensation.

Pathology

A Gram- or periodic acid-Schiff (PAS)-stained scraping from the pseudomembrane shows large masses of tangled hyphae,

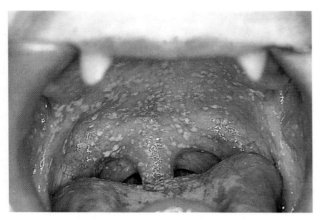

Fig. 15.24 Thrush. The lesions consist of soft, creamy patches or flecks lying superficially on an erythematous mucosa. This soft palate distribution is particularly frequent in patients using steroid inhalers.

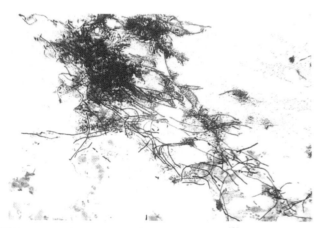

Fig. 15.25 Direct scraping from thrush. The tangled mass of Gram-positive hyphae of *Candida albicans* is diagnostic. A few yeast cells may be present as well, but it is the presence of hyphae that is diagnostic.

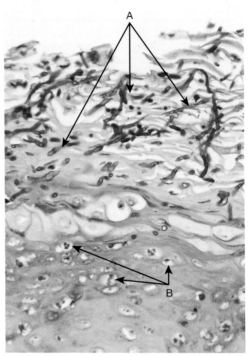

Fig. 15.26 Thrush. At high power the surface layers of the epithelium are separated by inflammatory oedema and are colonised by fungal hyphae *(A)* and infiltrated by neutrophils *(B)*. The infection is always very superficial; the lower edge of the image is at the level of the epithelial prickle cells.

detached epithelial cells, fibrin exudate and neutrophils (Fig. 15.25), and finding hyphae is diagnostic. Biopsy is not necessary but would show hyperplastic oedematous epithelium infiltrated by neutrophils. Staining with PAS shows many candidal hyphae growing down through the epithelial cells to the upper prickle cell layer (Fig. 15.26). More deeply, the epithelium is hyperplastic, with long slender rete processes extending down into the corium and a lymphoplasmacytic infiltrate below.

Key features are summarised in Box 15.7.

Management

The diagnosis is made on clinical features supported by microscopy of a scraping.

The infection itself is managed by dealing with any identifiable predisposing factors, and this alone may allow thrush to resolve. However, usually a course of topical antifungal is first line treatment. The treatments for candida infection, and their indications are given in Appendix 15.1.

A search must also be made for predisposing condition(s) in the medical history and oral examination, and they must be treated or ameliorated if possible. Denture wearers will benefit from the denture hygiene regime outlined below for denture-induced stomatitis.

Box 15.7 Thrush: key features

- Acute onset candidosis
- Sore rather than painful
- Secondary to various predisposing factors (Box 15.4)
- Common in HIV infection and indicates weak immunity
- Creamy soft patches, readily wiped off the mucosa
- Smear shows many Gram-positive hyphae
- Histology shows hyphae invading superficial epithelium
- Responds to topical antifungals though systemic often used

Anaemia or some cause of immunosuppression, usually HIV infection, should be suspected when thrush is seen in an adult in whom there is no detectable predisposition. These are also suggested by failure to respond to treatment or recurrent disease. In immunosuppression, specialised advice must be sought as recurrent thrush indicates marked suppression and extension to the oesophagus is a significant complication.

Web URL 15.3 NICE treatment guidance UK: http://cks.nice.org.uk/candida-oral

US guideline PMID: 26679628, see section XVI inside

Angular cheilitis → Summary chart 15.1

Angular cheilitis or angular stomatitis is an infection at the commissure of the lips, typically caused by leakage of candida-infected saliva at the angles of the mouth. It can be

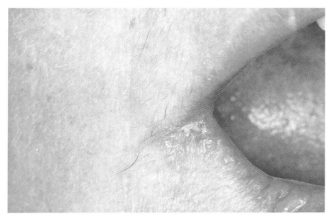

Fig. 15.27   Angular stomatitis. Cracking and erythema at the commissure is due to leakage of saliva containing *Candida albicans*, constantly reinfecting the saturated skin.

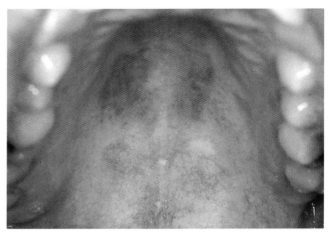

Fig. 15.28   Erythematous candidosis. Irregular patches of erythema on the palate of a patient using a steroid inhaler.

seen with thrush in infants, in denture wearers, in association with chronic hyperplastic candidosis or alone. It is a characteristic sign of candidal infection though a minority of cases are caused by bacteria.

Clinically, there is mild inflammation at the angles of the mouth with painful fissuring or cracking and sometimes a soft crust. Severe lesions may bleed.

The morphology of the lips, commissure and skin contribute to the condition. The commissure is normally dry and lightly keratinised, but in patients with angular cheilitis it is usually wet, either from saliva leakage or from deliberate licking or application of moisturisers or similar materials. Saturation of the keratin allows candida to infect the epithelium. In older people the commissure communicates with folds of skin caused by loss of elasticity and sagging of the facial tissues with age and inflammation and infection may then extend onto the skin (Fig. 15.27).

Management

Angular cheilitis is a mixed infection. Candida is found in as many as 90% of cases, but the proportion varies in different populations, being higher in denture wearers. Staphylococci, streptococci or other pathogens are frequently present and exactly which organisms are causative is unclear.

Treatment is targeted at the intraoral reservoir of candidal infection using local measures and antifungal drugs as appropriate. In mild cases this alone causes angular stomatitis to resolve. Miconazole gel is the ideal first-line treatment for the commissures as it has additional activity against several Gram-positive bacterial species including staphylococci and can be expected to successfully treat almost all cases. Failure is more likely due to incomplete treatment of the intraoral infection, but if this appears controlled, changing to 2% fusidic acid cream for the angles on assumption of staphylococcal or streptococcal infection is logical.

There is a particularly high proportion of patients with anaemia as a predisposing cause in angular cheilitis and iron, folate and vitamin B_{12} levels should be checked.

In people who are edentulous, have lost lip support or have prominent skin folds, attempts to correct vertical dimension or thicken the labial flange cannot usually remove these susceptible areas. Dermal fillers haven been tried, produce good cosmetic results but so far remain without a good evidence base for preventing infection.

Box 15.8   Types of erythematous candidosis

- Acute antibiotic stomatitis
- Median rhomboid glossitis
- Denture stomatitis
- Erythematous candidosis

Erythematous candidosis

→ Summary charts 15.1 and 19.3 pp. 279, 349

This term is now applied to any candidal infection that produces red mucosa. Originally the name was used to describe the chronic red form of candidosis seen on the palate and gingiva of HIV-positive patients (see Fig. 30.6). However, the name was not very specific, and similar changes can arise in the immunocompetent, sometimes caused by a mixed infection with a bacterial and candida component.

The term is now taken to include a number of presentations with a primarily red mucosa, either localised or generalised. There may be occasional white flecks on the red background, but no 'pseudomembrane' (Fig. 15.28).

If a candidal infection produces a red area but does not fit the descriptions of the specific conditions listed in Box 15.8, it can simply be described as erythematous candidosis. Such lesions are usually on the hard palate, dorsum of the tongue and soft palate and are usually associated with immunosuppression or steroid inhalers as an underlying factor.

Web URL 15.3 NICE treatment guidance UK: http://cks.nice.org.uk/candida-oral

US guideline PMID: 26679628, see section XVI inside

Acute antibiotic stomatitis

→ Summary chart 15.1 p. 279

This condition is also known as antibiotic sore mouth and acute atrophic candidosis. It follows overuse or topical oral use of antibiotics, especially broad-spectrum drugs such as tetracycline. These suppress the normal oral flora that competes with *Candida* in the mouth, allowing its overgrowth.

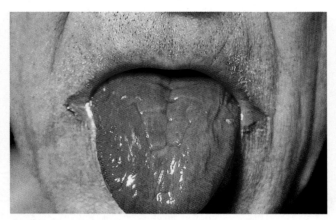

Fig. 15.29 **Glossitis in antibiotic-induced candidosis.** The tongue is red, smooth and sore as in anaemia, but the appearance results from inflammation and oedema. Similar changes affect other parts of the mouth, and there is angular cheilitis.

Clinically, the whole mucosa is red and sore, but the tongue is typically worst affected and appears smooth, having lost its filiform papillae (Fig. 15.29). A few flecks of thrush may be present. Resolution may follow withdrawal of the antibiotic but is accelerated by topical antifungal treatment. A similar but chronic generalised candidal erythema can also be a consequence of xerostomia and is a typical complication of Sjögren's syndrome.

Web URL 15.3 NICE treatment guidance UK: http://cks.nice.org.uk/candida-oral

US guideline PMID: 26679628 see section XVI inside

Median rhomboid glossitis

➔ Summary charts 15.1 and 19.3 pp. 279, 349

Median rhomboid glossitis produces a red patch in the midline of the dorsum of the tongue at the junction of the anterior two-thirds with the posterior third, classically in a diamond shape. It has historically been proposed to be a developmental condition, but it is not seen in children and has nothing to do with persistence of the tuberculum impar or development of the thyroid. However, not all lesions can be shown to be infected with candida. It seems that this presentation has a very low level of infection. Infection is probably intermittent and permanently damages the mucosa so that it loses its ability to form papillae and appears red even when infection is absent or inactive. Median rhomboid glossitis is relatively common and is found in 1%–2% of the population.

Clinically, median rhomboid glossitis is seen in adults and is typically symptomless. Its colour ranges from pink to red, and the affected area has lost its filiform papillae (Fig. 15.30). Usually the patch is smooth, flat or appears slightly depressed, but in longstanding lesions it may develop nodules. In the few cases with more intense infection, white flecks may be seen (Fig. 15.31). A florid lesion may appear worrying and be mistaken for a carcinoma, particularly when nodular, but squamous carcinoma virtually never develops at this site.

One factor that may predispose to infection at this site is that, in many individuals, this part of the tongue rests against the soft palate, trapping saliva, and so is not as self-cleansing as the rest of the tongue. Sometimes a matching patch of candidosis is present on the soft palate at the site of contact.

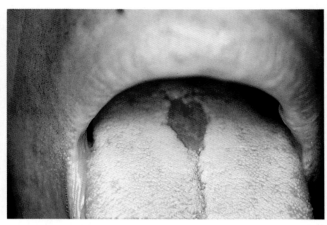

Fig. 15.30 **Median rhomboid glossitis.** The typical lozenge-shaped area of depapillation in the midline of the tongue, made more prominent in this patient because of the prominent tongue furring.

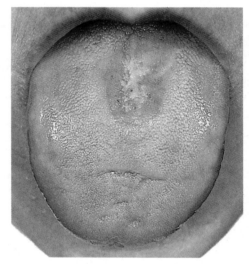

Fig. 15.31 **Median rhomboid glossitis.** There is a whitish patch centrally in the depapillation, overall with sharply demarcated borders in the midline of the tongue at the typical site.

Histologically, the appearances are variable. The primary change is epithelial atrophy with loss of filiform papillae and often broad parallel-sided rete process hyperplasia. Fungal hyphae should be sought but are often not found or are very sparse. Below the epithelium in longstanding cases there is a broad band of dense scarred fibrous tissue (Fig. 15.32) that makes the lesion feel indurated. Nodules arise by inflammation-induced fibroepithelial hyperplasia.

Case series and images PMID: 21912494

Case series PMID: 366496

Management

Diagnosis is based on clinical appearance, and reassurance is usually the main requirement. Antifungal treatment does not usually resolve the lesion and should not be considered unless a scraping is positive for hyphae on microscopy. Nodular or lobulated lesions do not resolve on antifungal treatment and filiform papillae may be lost permanently. A biopsy should not be required.

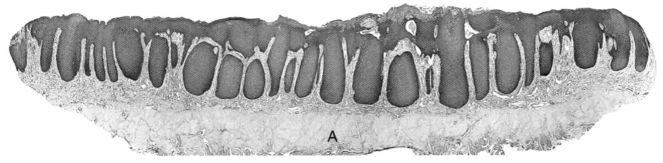

Fig. 15.32 Median rhomboid glossitis with epithelial rete process hyperplasia, light inflammation below and a band of scar tissue (A).

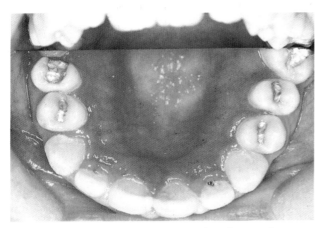

Fig. 15.33 Typical denture stomatitis. Clear demarcation between the erythema of the mucosa covered, in this instance, by an orthodontic appliance and the palate behind the posterior margin is clearly seen.

Denture-induced stomatitis

➔ Summary charts 15.1 and 19.3 pp. 279, 349

A well-fitting upper denture cuts off the underlying mucosa from the protective action of saliva and provides a space in which the oral flora, including candida, can proliferate freely. In susceptible patients, particularly smokers, this can promote candidosis, seen as a symptomless area of erythema. The erythema is sharply limited to the area of mucosa occluded by the upper denture or orthodontic appliance (Fig. 15.33). Similar inflammation is not seen under the more mobile lower denture, which allows a relatively free flow of saliva beneath it.

The exact relationship between the denture, candidal infection and denture-induced stomatitis remains somewhat contentious. In the past, the denture has been seen as the cause, either through poor fit, 'allergy' or irritation. *Candida* infection is definitely present, but hyphal forms are sparse and the inflamed mucosa may be reacting to either candida or bacteria in the biofilm adherent to the denture rather than being invaded. Biopsy shows inflammation in the tissues and occasional fungal hyphae at the surface. Evidence for the importance of candida comes from the fact that angular stomatitis is frequently associated.

Management

The clinical picture is distinctive, but the diagnosis can be confirmed by finding candidal hyphae in a smear from the inflamed mucosa or the fitting surface of the denture. Quantification of candida in saliva is of little value as candidal

carriage is common and counts are higher in denture wearers.

The infection responds to antifungal drugs but recurs unless the denture factors are addressed. Topical agents such as nystatin can only gain access to the palate if the patient leaves out the denture while the medication is in the mouth. Systemic fluconazole is often used (Appendix 15.1).

Porosity voids in methylmethacrylate denture bases also harbour *C. albicans* and dentures may therefore form a reservoir that can reinfect the mucosa. Elimination of *C. albicans* and bacterial biofilm from the denture base is important and can be achieved by brushing and soaking the denture in dilute chlorhexidine mouthwash overnight. A key predisposing factor is night wear of dentures. Ceasing this alone may allow resolution.

A simpler alternative is to coat the fitting surface of the denture with miconazole gel while it is being worn. The denture should be removed and scrubbed clean at intervals and miconazole re-applied three times a day. This treatment should be continued until the inflammation has cleared and *C. albicans* has been eliminated. This is likely to take 1–2 weeks, but patients should be warned not to continue this treatment indefinitely. Resistance to miconazole is growing and the oral gel can be absorbed. Using miconazole gel on a denture in this way is contraindicated in patients taking warfarin or phenytoin because sufficient miconazole is absorbed to enhance their effects.

Lack of response may be due to poor patient compliance or to an underlying disorder, particularly iron deficiency. Systemic antifungal drugs without local measures are ineffective. Key features are summarised in Box 15.9.

Web URL 15.3 NICE treatment guidance UK: http://cks.nice.org.uk/candida-oral

US guideline PMID: 26679628, see section XVI

Treatment PMID: 24971864

Papillary hyperplasia of the palate

Extensive nodular fibroepithelial hyperplasia of the palate has often been considered a complication of candidosis, but candida alone is not the cause. This condition is discussed in Chapter 24.

Chronic hyperplastic candidosis

➔ Summary charts 15.1, 19.1 and 19.2 pp. 279, 347, 348

The alternative name of *candidal leukoplakia* reveals the controversial nature of this condition, in which chronic low level candidosis induces a localised zone of epithelial keratosis. Unfortunately, candida will also readily infect the keratotic lesions of true leukoplakia (Ch. 19) to produce the

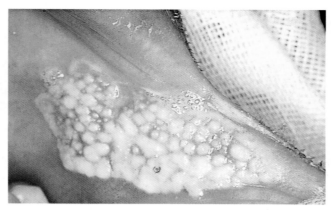

Fig. 15.35   Chronic hyperplastic candidosis. This more florid infection is white and nodular with erythema, suggesting fungal infection clinically but also raising concern about potential malignancy. Candidal hyphae would be frequent in a biopsy.

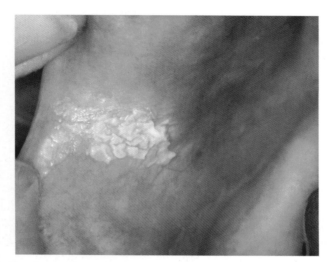

Fig 15.34   Chronic hyperplastic candidosis. Typical appearance and site just behind the commissure. The surface is usually flat or may be tessellated as here. In longstanding infection the surface may become slightly nodular. No erythema is present and candida hyphae would be sparse on biopsy.

same clinical appearance. As many leukoplakias have no specific features, it may not be possible to tell these two situations apart. However, a white patch caused entirely by candidal infection carries a minimal or no risk of developing squamous carcinoma.

Clinical features

Adults, typically males of middle age or older, are affected, and most are smokers. The usual sites are the post-commissural buccal mucosa and the dorsum of the tongue. The plaque is variable in thickness, often rough or irregular in texture and tightly adherent (Fig. 15.34). It will not rub off. Angular stomatitis may be confluent with plaques on the post-commissural mucosa.

When the candida infection is more florid, lesions develop an erythematous background or speckling and resemble speckled leukoplakia, strongly resembling a high-risk lesion for developing carcinoma (Fig. 15.35).

Pathology

The surface epithelium is parakeratotic and contains candidal hyphae. They are often sparse and elicit little or no inflammatory response, just a few neutrophils focally. PAS stain shows the hyphae growing (as in thrush) directly through the epithelial cells of the keratin layer (Figs 15.36 and 15.37) to the prickle cell layer, but no further. Candida induces mild epithelial hyperplasia, and often there long parallel-sided rete processes. Inflammation in the connective tissue is mild.

If dysplasia is present on biopsy, the lesion is a leukoplakia with superimposed candidal infection and not chronic hyperplastic candidosis.

Management

After confirmation of the diagnosis by histology or a scraping for hyphae, antifungal treatment is provided, but eradication of infection is difficult in this chronic infection. Usually, miconazole gel is effective but may need supplementing with a systemic antifungal drug such as fluconazole for two weeks. Accompanying angular cheilitis needs concurrent treatment, and denture hygiene and efforts to reduce the oral load of candida are required as described for denture stomatitis. Underlying anaemia may contribute and should be treated first, and ideally smoking should cease. These interventions not targeted to the lesion itself are often the key to success.

Long-term intermittent antifungal therapy may be required. Excision of the candidal plaque alone is of little value, as the infection can recur in the same site even after skin grafting.

If, after all these interventions, the plaque remains, consideration must be given to the fact that it may be a leukoplakia with superimposed candida infection and require follow up as a potentially malignant lesion. Although a potential for malignant change is generally thought to exist, this is contentious and the risk is very low and probably absent.

Review PMID: 12907694

Chronic mucocutaneous candidosis syndromes → Summary chart 15.1 p. 279

These syndromes are all rare, but difficult to manage. Classification is complex now that many types can be classified by their causative genes.

The significance of these conditions is to recognise them when **chronic** *Candida* infection presents with very florid

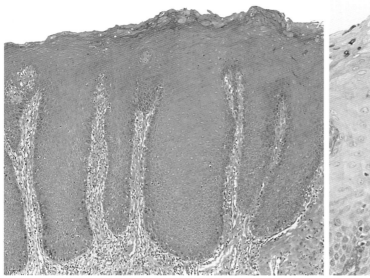
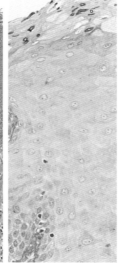

Fig. 15.36 Chronic hyperplastic candidosis. Thin parakeratin at the surface, long parallel-sided rete processes and a few inflammatory cells immediately below the epithelium (left). At higher power (right), a few Candida hyphae are in the keratin, appearing as magenta-coloured tubes in cross section in periodic acid Schiff (PAS) stain.

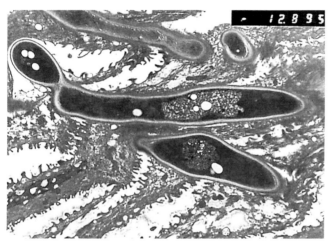

Fig. 15.37 Electron micrograph showing two Candida hyphae (very dark) growing through superficial keratinocytes of the oral mucosa. Note how they penetrate through the cells and do not grow around them.

Box 15.10   Features of autoimmune polyendocrine syndrome I

- Genetic: usually autosomal recessive
- Hypoparathyroidism
- Adrenocortical insufficiency
- Chronic mucocutaneous candidosis
- Type 1 diabetes
- Autoimmune keratitis of the eye
- Malabsorption and diarrhoea
- Autoimmune hepatitis

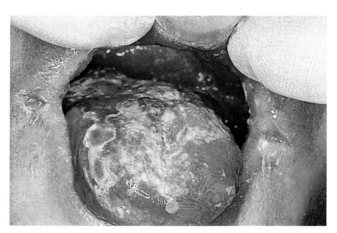

Fig. 15.38 Chronic mucocutaneous candidosis. Extensive red and white patches throughout the oral mucosa and angular cheilitis.

involvement, particularly of skin, nails and mucosa, proves resistant to treatment, or presents in childhood or adolescence.

All seem to be caused by immunodeficiency that is relatively selective for fungi or candida in particular, and one type is autoimmune. Family history is variable.

General review PMID: 20859203

Autoimmune polyendocrine syndrome I or endocrine candidosis syndrome is defined by hypoparathyroidism, adrenocortical insufficiency and chronic mucocutaneous candidosis, though many other features can present before the classical features are evident (Box 15.10). Inheritance can be autosomal recessive or dominant, and onset is in the first two decades of life. Failure of an immune regulator gene allows autoreactive T cells to escape deletion in the thymus during development. There are multiple autoantibodies to endocrine glands and against interferons, which are diagnostic. Candidosis is usually the presenting feature with thick plaques and red areas at any or all sites in the mouth (Fig. 15.38), spreading to the pharynx and oesophagus.

This form of candidosis is potentially malignant, and 20% of patients develop oral or oesophageal carcinoma.

Treatment of the candida infection must be aggressive and involves multiple agents. In children care must be taken to avoid finger sucking as infection will spread to wet skin and may then be intractable (Fig 15.39). Hypoplastic dental defects are frequently also present.

General review PMID: 15141045 and 30510552

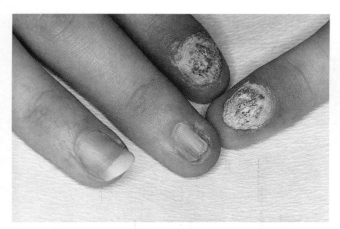

Fig. 15.39 **Chronic mucocutaneous candidosis.** Damage to fingernails through chronic infection in one of the more severe types.

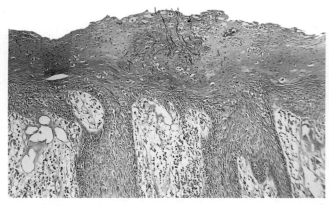

Fig. 15.40 **Chronic mucocutaneous candidosis.** At high power the thick parakeratin layer at the surface of this lesion is seen to be invaded by numerous fungal hyphae, as seen in simple chronic hyperplastic candidosis.

Pathogenesis PMID: 34455138

Other types of mucocutaneous candidosis are recognised, with variable inheritance, severity and specific gene defects. Some arise from autoimmune failure as a result of major histocompatibility complex gene mutations, and others are associated with autoantibodies to interleukin 17, STAT1 mutations reducing levels of interleukin (IL)-17 or other cytokines, or defects that compromise killing of candida by neutrophils. Mild forms are indistinguishable from sporadic cases of chronic hyperplastic candidosis histologically (Fig. 15.40). More severe forms may have susceptibility to bacterial infection or a range of other diseases. Thymoma and myasthenia gravis are associated with those types with autoantibodies against IL-17.

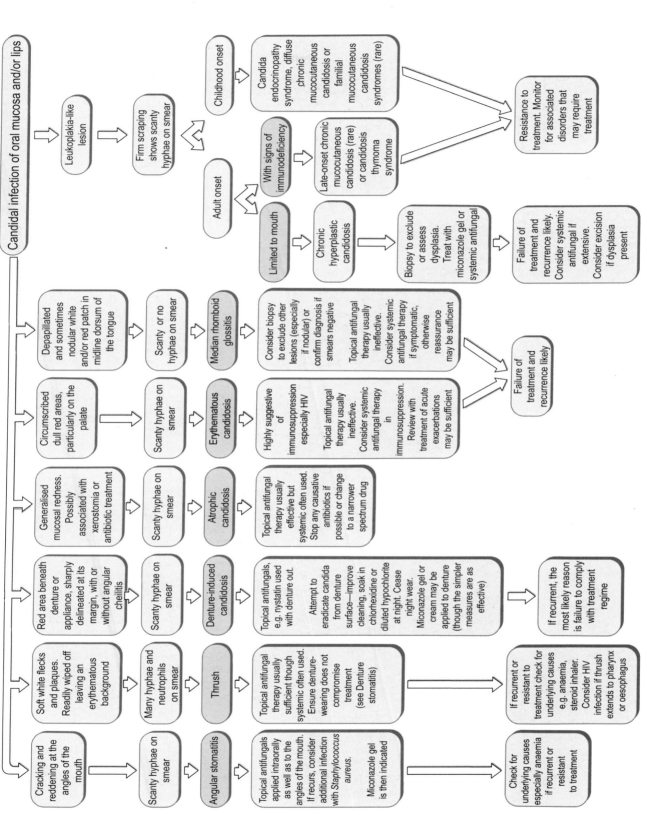

Summary chart 15.1   Summary of the types of oral Candida infection and their management.

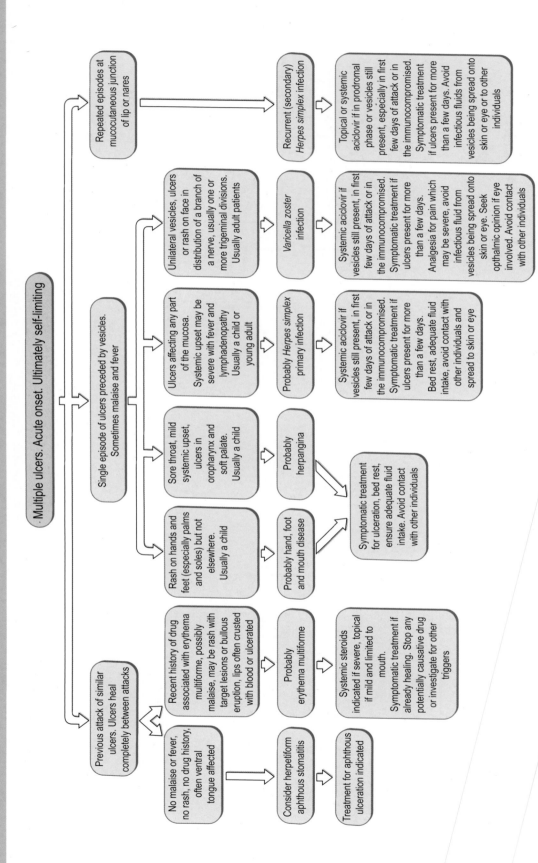

Multiple ulcers. Acute onset. Ultimately self-limiting

Repeated episodes at mucocutaneous junction of lip or nares

Recurrent (secondary) *Herpes simplex* infection

Topical or systemic aciclovir if in prodromal phase or vesicles still present, especially in first few days of attack or in the immunocompromised. Symptomatic treatment if ulcers present for more than a few days. Avoid infectious fluids from vesicles being spread onto skin or eye or to other individuals

Single episode of ulcers preceded by vesicles. Sometimes malaise and fever

Unilateral vesicles, ulcers or rash on face in distribution of a branch of a nerve, usually one or more trigeminal divisions. Usually adult patients

Varicella zoster infection

Systemic aciclovir if vesicles still present, in first few days of attack or in the immunocompromised. Symptomatic treatment if ulcers present for more than a few days. Analgesia for pain which may be severe, avoid infectious fluid from vesicles being spread onto skin or eye. Seek opthalmic opinion if eye involved. Avoid contact with other individuals

Ulcers affecting any part of the mucosa. Systemic upset may be severe with fever and lymphadenopathy Usually a child or young adult

Probably *Herpes simplex* primary infection

Systemic aciclovir if vesicles still present, in first few days of attack or in the immunocompromised. Symptomatic treatment if ulcers present for more than a few days. Bed rest, adequate fluid intake, avoid contact with other individuals and spread to skin or eye

Sore throat, mild systemic upset, ulcers in oropharynx and soft palate. Usually a child

Probably herpangina

Symptomatic treatment for ulceration, bed rest, ensure adequate fluid intake. Avoid contact with other individuals

Rash on hands and feet (especially palms and soles) but not elsewhere. Usually a child

Probably hand, foot and mouth disease

Previous attack of similar ulcers. Ulcers heal completely between attacks

Recent history of drug associated with erythema multiforme, possibly malaise, may be rash with target lesions or bullous eruption, lips often crusted with blood or ulcerated

Probably erythema multiforme

Systemic steroids indicated if severe, topical if mild and limited to mouth. Symptomatic treatment if already healing. Stop any potentially causative drug or investigate for other triggers

No malaise or fever, no rash, no drug history, often ventral tongue affected

Consider herpetiform aphthous stomatitis

Treatment for aphthous ulceration indicated

Summary chart 15.2 Differential diagnosis and management of the common and important causes of multiple oral ulcers with acute onset.

Appendix 15.1

Recommendations for treatment of oral candidosis.

Confirm diagnosis with smear (most types) or biopsy (chronic hyperplastic candidosis) unless presentation is typical

Check history for predisposing causes which may require treatment

If candidosis is recurrent or not responsive to treatment, test for anaemia, folate and vitamin B_{12} deficiency and perform a urine test for diabetes

If a denture is worn:
- Stop night-time wear
- Check denture hygiene and advise
- Soak denture overnight in antifungal (dilute hypochlorite or chlorhexidine mouthwash) or, less effective, apply miconazole gel to denture fit surface while worn

If a steroid inhaler is used, check it is being used correctly, preferably with a spacer. Advise to rinse mouth out after use.

If immunosuppression is known, ensure no evidence of systemic illness that might be due to candidaemia, breathlessness or difficulty swallowing and refer for immediate hospital care if so.

This table illustrates principles of treatment but cannot include all detail. Always check the prescribing guidance for your institution or country.

	Drug treatments			
Presentation	Generalised or severe	Localised or mild infection including chronic hyperplastic form	Angular stomatitis	Immunosuppression or otherwise resistant to treatment*
Drug of choice and regime	Fluconazole 50 mg/day for 7 days, repeated if necessary. *or* Nystatin suspension 100,000 units/mL (less effective) *or* miconazole oral gel in children aged over 4 years	Miconazole gel 24 mg/mL Apply QDS** if lesion localised *or* Nystatin suspension 100,000 units/mL (less effective)	Apply miconazole gel 24 mg/mL QDS to the angles of the mouth 10 days or fusidic acid cream	Start with miconazole or nystatin, consider fluconazole 50–100 mg/day for 7–14 days
Notes	Amphotericin is no longer recommended as first-line treatment in primary care due to poor evidence base and is no longer available in the UK Fluconazole is reserved for severe infections because of the risk of resistance	Most effective if lesion accessible for application For recurrent infection in white patches fluconazole may be required simultaneously	Must treat intraoral infection simultaneously. This is always present even if not evident	Itraconazole has a higher risk of adverse effects and is not recommended for use in primary care
Cautions	Avoid in liver dysfunction and in patients taking drugs metabolised by the liver including warfarin, statins and some immunosuppressants. Avoid in pregnancy	Miconazole oral gel is absorbed, particularly if applied to denture fit surface. Avoid in liver dysfunction and patients taking drugs metabolised by the liver including warfarin, statins and some immunosuppressants. Avoid in pregnancy	No adverse effects if only small amounts are applied as described above	Seek advice before prescribing for patients on immunosuppressive drugs, especially ciclosporin and with known immunosuppression of any cause

If there is conspicuous papillary hyperplasia of the palate, consider treatment (cryosurgery or excision) after treatment when inflammation has subsided. The irregular surface predisposes to recurrence of candidosis.

Recommendations are aligned with UK NICE guidance http://cks.nice.org.uk/candida-oral

* Candidal resistance to azole drugs is possible, but failure of treatment is more likely to result from non-compliance with local measures such as denture wear and cleaning or an untreated underlying condition.

** *Quater in die sumendus*, meaning take four times a day.

Diseases of the oral mucosa: non-infective stomatitis

16

ULCERS

→ Summary charts 16.2 and 16.3 pp. 311, 312

Ulcers are full-thickness breaks in the continuity of the epithelial covering of the mucosa, exposing connective tissue to the mouth, and their general features are discussed at the start of Chapter 15.

Clinically, dividing ulcers into those that are persistent and those that are recurrent is a useful first step in differential diagnosis. Most oral ulcers heal after a few days to 2 weeks depending on their size, more rapidly on the floor of mouth or buccal mucosa than on the palate or gingiva. Recurrent oral ulcers are those that recur singly or in crops at the same or different sites. Recurrent ulcers have few common causes.

It is important to distinguish recurrent oral ulceration, a presentation of several diseases, from recurrent aphthous ulceration (recurrent aphthous stomatitis), which is a specific condition.

General review diagnosis ulcers PMID: 26650694

TRAUMATIC ULCERS

→ Summary charts 16.2 and 16.3 pp. 311, 312

Traumatic ulcers are usually caused by biting, denture trauma or chemical trauma and arise at trauma-prone sites such as lip, buccal mucosa or adjacent to a denture flange. They are tender, have a yellowish-grey floor of fibrin slough and red margins (Fig. 16.1). Inflammation, swelling and erythema are variable, depending on the cause and time since trauma. There is no induration unless the site is scarred from repeated episodes of trauma. Occasionally, a large ulcer is caused by biting after a dental local anaesthetic (see Fig. 40.1). Biting trauma may produce two small adjacent ulcers matching cusps of upper and lower opposing teeth (Fig 17.17).

Chemical trauma is usually accidentally self-inflicted or iatrogenic. Very corrosive agents such as silver nitrate and trichloroacetic acid are now rarely used in dentistry but etchant, hypochlorite and some tooth whitening agents are just a few of the caustic agents that can cause mucosal ulcers after sometimes quite short contact time (Fig 16.2). Some patients continue to believe that aspirin is effective for toothache if held against the alveolus to dissolve. The result is local whitening caused by epithelial necrosis, followed by ulceration.

Traumatic ulcers heal in days after elimination of the cause. If they persist for more than 10 days without reduction in size and symptoms, or there is any other cause for suspicion as to the cause, biopsy should be carried out to exclude other diseases. Biopsy is not otherwise helpful because the histological features of traumatic ulcers are of non-specific inflammation and repair only.

Eosinophilic ulcers and traumatic ulcerative granuloma

This is a related series of presentations with confusing names. When presenting as a flat or deeper punched out ulcer the name eosinophilic ulcer is used. When an ulcerated mass forms, the names traumatic ulcerative granuloma or traumatic ulcerative granuloma with (stromal) eosinophilia (TUGSE) may be used. However, these conditions have nothing to do with eosinophilic granuloma of bone and do not contain granulomas histologically. The cause is unknown, but an unusual response to trauma is suspected though a history of trauma is not always obtained.

Eosinophilic ulcers have a worrying presentation, often resembling carcinoma and exceeding 10 mm in diameter and enlarging rapidly before stabilising. The ulcers are usually on the tongue but also develop on the gingivae and, occasionally, other sites. Most are in adults of middle age or older, but a

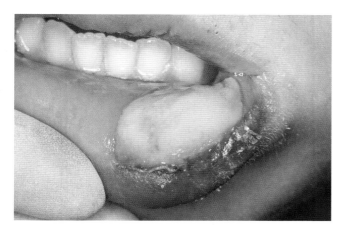

Fig. 16.1 A large traumatic ulcer on the lower lip. Note the colour of the fibrin slough, distinct from the keratin of a white patch, and the well-defined epithelial margin with minimal inflammation.

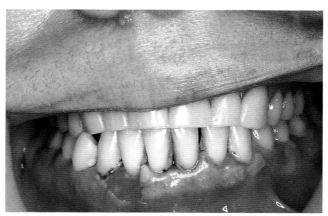

Fig. 16.2 Chemical burn. The gingivae are white and necrotic around the central incisors, left lateral incisor and canine following injudicious use of a caustic agent. On the patient's right side an ulcer is present around the lateral incisor and canine.

characteristic presentation is in infants in the first year of life where erupting lower incisors repeatedly traumatise the ventral tongue or lower lip on feeding (Riga-Fede disease, Fig. 16.3). A concerning feature is failure to heal, and eosinophilic ulcers may persist for many months, during which the cellular inflammatory infiltrate in the deeper tissues proliferates, raising the mucosa to produce an ulcerated nodule. It is these nodular ulcerated lesions that are sometimes called *traumatic ulcerative granulomas* (with stromal eosinophilia or TUGSE). The dense inflammatory infiltrate produces firmness in the underlying tissues, which may be misinterpreted as induration and the clinical appearance strongly suggests carcinoma or other malignant disease (Fig. 16.4).

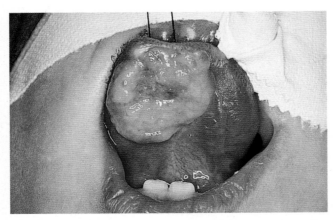

Fig 16.3 Traumatic ulcerative granuloma of the tongue caused by the lower incisors ('Riga-Fede disease'). *(From Eichenfield LF, Frieden IJ, Esterly NB, 2008. Neonatal Dermatology, 2nd ed. Edinburgh: Saunders)*

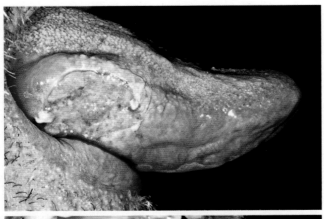

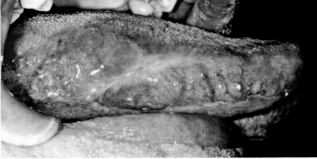

Fig. 16.4 **Traumatic ulcerative granuloma** on the lateral border of tongue (above) strongly resembling squamous carcinoma. Despite the mass and ulcer enlarging further, it resolved completely in 6 weeks (below).

In practice, lesions usually heal spontaneously within 3–10 weeks, but biopsy will often trigger more rapid resolution.

Pathology

Biopsy is usually undertaken to exclude carcinoma or malignant disease because of size, induration and failure to heal. It is therefore unfortunate that the histological appearances can also be worrying and somewhat resemble some types of lymphoma. A mixed inflammatory infiltrate of eosinophils and pale macrophages and endothelial cells extends deeply, disrupting underlying tissues, and there may be suspicion of cytological atypia and mitotic activity. The presence of CD30+ activated lymphocytes and clonal T cell receptor populations in some cases are suggestive of lymphoma but probably reflect an abnormal inflammatory or immunological response causing persistence of inflammation and recruiting the numerous eosinophils into the tissues. It is the prominent eosinophils histologically that give the condition its name.

Eosinophilic ulcer case series PMID: 8515985 and 24269143

Traumatic ulcerative granuloma PMID: 19846813 and 31672390

Factitious ulceration (self-inflicted oral ulcers)

Factitious ulcers in the mouth are rare and usually associated with psychosocial disorders in which the patient gains 'benefit' from producing their lesions in some way or another. The dentist must be aware that this presentation may signal a significant mental health condition with a risk of other types of self-harm including suicide.

The usual presentation is a non-healing ulcer in the anterior mouth, often easily visible, caused by repeated physical trauma, but presentation and methods of inducing the injury are diverse (Box 16.1). Even self-extraction of teeth has been reported.

Biopsy may be performed to exclude organic disease or when persistent trauma causes fibrosis that is mistaken for induration of malignant disease. Underlying mental health conditions are typically concealed, and definitive diagnosis is often difficult. Once suspected, multidisciplinary management with medical specialties should be initiated without delay.

Self-harm is also a recognised manifestation of a variety of medical conditions: autism spectrum disorders, familial dysautonomia, Lesch-Nyhan and Tourette syndromes and other causes of learning disability and is common in people living in institutions.

Unintended factitious injury can also follow repetitive habits such as picking at the gingival margin with a fingernail, but the degree of trauma is then minor and ulcers rarely develop, though considerable damage to the periodontium may result, even causing tooth exfoliation. Mouth guards,

---

Box 16.1 Features suggestive of factitious oral lesions
- Lack of correspondence with any recognisable disease
- Bizarre configuration with sharp outlines
- Usually in an otherwise healthy mouth
- Clinical features inconsistent with the history
- In areas accessible to the patient
- Lack of response to any or all conventional treatments

barrier appliances and cognitive behaviour therapy may be required.

Case series PMID: 7776171

RECURRENT APHTHOUS STOMATITIS

→ Summary charts 15.2 and 16.2 pp. 280, 311

Recurrent aphthous stomatitis is the most common oral mucosal disease and affects as much as 25% of the population at some time in their life. Many cases are mild, and no treatment is sought.

There are three presentations of recurrent aphthous stomatitis (often called *recurrent aphthous ulceration* or just *recurrent aphthae*), each of which is defined by its clinical presentation.

Ulcers similar and sometimes identical to aphthous stomatitis can be a feature of other diseases or syndromes. Whether these are truly aphthous stomatitis or mimics is unclear (Table 16.1).

PFAPA case series PMID: 24237762 and 19889105

MAGIC case series PMID: 4014306 and 34972595

Clinical features

Ulcers frequently start in childhood. Recurrences increase in frequency until early adult life or a little later, then gradually wane. Recurrent aphthae are rare in older people, particularly the edentulous, unless affected by a haematological deficiency. The great majority of patients are of high or middle socioeconomic status and are non-smokers.

Many patients have prodromal symptoms of pricking or sensitivity at the site for a few hours or a day before the ulcer forms. There is a brief period of erythema before the ulcer appears. The ulcers have a smooth sharply defined margin with an erythematous rim in the enlarging phase. The erythematous rim reduces once the ulcer reaches its full size, and while it heals, the margin becomes irregular or less well defined. Typical features common to all types of recurrent aphthae are summarised in Box 16.2.

Table 16.1 Diseases in which the ulcers have the features of recurrent aphthous stomatitis (not including those associated through deficiency states)

Disease	Features
Behçet's disease	See text
MAGIC syndrome	**M**outh **A**nd **G**enital ulcers with **I**nflamed **C**artilage, a variant of Behçet's disease with relapsing polychondritis
PFAPA syndrome (Ch. 31)	**P**eriodic **F**ever, **A**phthous stomatitis, **P**haryngitis, and cervical **A**denitis, a disease of young children of unknown cause, usually treated with steroids, ultimately self-limiting. Probably a genetic auto-inflammatory disease mediated by an abnormal interleukin 1β response. Monthly fever rising as high as 41°C for 3–5 days with mucosal inflammation and enlarged nodes. Completely asymptomatic between attacks
HIV infection (Ch. 30)	Often associated with ulcers of major aphthous type

Minor aphthous stomatitis is the most common type, and the usual history is a single, or crops of several, painful ulcers recurring at intervals of a few weeks. Minor aphthae affect almost exclusively the non-keratinised mucosa, usually the labial and buccal mucosa, sulcuses, or lateral borders of the tongue (Fig. 16.5). Individual minor aphthae persist for 7–10 days, then heal without scarring. Often all ulcers in a crop develop and heal more or less synchronously. Unpredictable remissions of several months may be noted. In severe cases, ulcers are more numerous, and new crops may develop and heal continuously at different sites, without remission.

Major aphthous stomatitis is rare and causes single large ulcers or occasionally two or three at a time. These are much larger than in the minor form, 20 mm diameter is not unusual, and persist for many weeks. The pain of major aphthae can interfere with eating. They usually affect the soft palate, fauces, buccal mucosa and lateral tongue (Figs 16.6 and 16.7). This type may occasionally develop on keratinised mucosa and often heal with scarring. Ulcers can be designated as major form on the basis of size, duration or both. A cut-off diameter of 10 mm is often taken as the upper limit of the minor form, but size should not be an absolute criterion.

Herpetiform aphthous stomatitis is also rare and causes crops of many tiny ulcers, as many as 100 at a time, usually in the floor of mouth and ventral tongue (Fig. 16.8). The background mucosa is red, giving a resemblance to herpetic ulceration, but viral infection is not the cause.

The three types are summarised in Box 16.3.

Box 16.2 Typical features of recurrent aphthae

- Onset frequently in childhood but peak in adolescence or early adult life
- Attacks at variable but sometimes relatively regular intervals
- Most patients are otherwise healthy
- A few have haematological deficiency
- Most patients are non-smokers
- Usually self-limiting eventually
- Ulcers often preceded by prodromal symptoms
- Ulcers almost never occur on keratinised mucosa

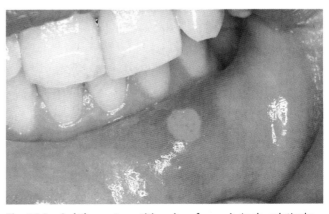

Fig. 16.5 Aphthous stomatitis, minor form. A single, relatively large shallow ulcer in a typical site. There is a narrow band of periulcer erythema. These features are non-specific, and the diagnosis must be made primarily on the basis of the history.

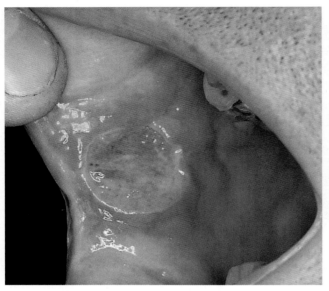

Fig. 16.6   Aphthous stomatitis, major type. This large, deep ulcer with considerable surrounding erythema has been present for several weeks.

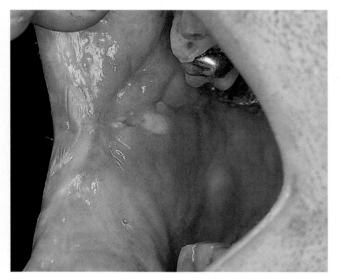

Fig. 16.7   Recurrent aphthous stomatitis, major type. The same ulcer shown in Fig. 16.6, but healing. The ulcer is much smaller, but there is puckering of the surrounding mucosa from scarring.

Aetiology

The main factors thought to contribute are shown in Box 16.4. None completely explain the disease, but different factors may apply to different individuals or subgroups of patients.

   Genetic factors. There is good evidence for a genetic predisposition. The family history is often positive, and the disease affects identical more frequently than non-identical twins. No genetic marker has been found though polymorphisms in inflammatory signalling genes have been proposed and some patients have abnormal interleukin 1β and interleukin 6 levels. A number of genetic autoinflammatory diseases are known to be caused by loss of function in genes controlling inflammation (Ch. 31), and several include aphthous stomatitis-like ulcers, but with additional

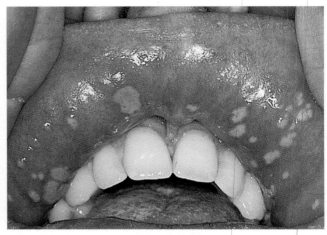

Fig. 16.8   Recurrent aphthous stomatitis, herpetiform type. There are numerous small, rounded and pinpoint ulcers, some of which are coalescing. The surrounding mucosa is lightly erythematous and the overall picture is highly suggestive of viral infection, but the attacks are recurrent and no virus can be isolated.

Box 16.3   Types of recurrent aphthae

Minor aphthae

- The most common type
- Non-keratinised mucosa affected
- Ulcers are shallow, rounded, 3–7 mm across, with an erythematous margin and yellowish floor
- One or several ulcers may be present

Major aphthae

- Uncommon
- Ulcers frequently several centimetres across
- Sometimes mimic a malignant ulcer
- Ulcers persist for several months
- Masticatory mucosa, such as the dorsum of the tongue or occasionally the gingivae, may be involved
- Scarring may follow healing

Herpetiform aphthae

- Uncommon
- Non-keratinised mucosa affected
- Ulcers are 1–2 mm across
- Dozens or hundreds may be present
- May coalesce to form irregular ulcers
- Widespread erythema round the ulcers

Box 16.4   Possible aetiological factors for recurrent aphthae

- Genetic autoinflammatory predisposition
- Exaggerated response to trauma
- Infections
- Immunological abnormalities
- Gastrointestinal disorders
- Haematological deficiencies
- Hormonal disturbances
- Stress

systemic features. The concept that aphthous stomatitis is a genetically mediated autoinflammatory disease is appealing, but, as yet, unproven. In the possibly related Behçet's disease (see later in this chapter), the evidence for a genetic predisposition is much stronger.

Trauma is often blamed by patients. There is some evidence that minor trauma is more likely to develop into an ulcer in a susceptible individual, and most ulcers are on the less trauma-resistant lining mucosa. The evidence for this is stronger in Behçet's disease.

Infections. There is no evidence that aphthae are directly due to any microbes either causing infection or triggering immune reactions. An extensive range of oral commensals, pathogens, bacteria, viruses and unusual organisms such as mycoplasmas and L-forms have been investigated fruitlessly.

Immunological abnormalities. The formation and healing of an ulcer involves inflammatory and immune mechanisms, but there is no evidence any are causal, and the disease is not autoimmune. There is no association with atopy or other known allergens despite many patients linking ulcers to dietary components. Aphthae lack virtually all features of typical autoimmune diseases. They also fail to respond reliably to immunosuppressive drugs and become more severe in the immune deficiency state induced by HIV infection.

Food allergy is often claimed by patients but not supported by direct evidence. It is possible that gastrointestinal effects of food allergy could cause mild deficiency states and that these could predispose or worsen pre-existing aphthous stomatitis. Dietary elimination of individual suspected allergens has not been shown to affect severity or incidence, but response has been shown with strict general exclusion diets.

Gastrointestinal disease. Aphthae are only rarely associated with gastrointestinal disease such as coeliac disease, and then as a result of a deficiency secondary to malabsorption, particularly of vitamin B_{12} or folate.

Haematological deficiencies. Deficiencies of vitamin B_{12}, folate or iron have been reported in as many as 20% of patients with aphthae (though they can also be common in the healthy population). Such deficiencies are more frequent in patients whose aphthae start or worsen in middle age or later, have more than three ulcers at a time or very frequent or unremitting attacks. In many such patients, the deficiency is latent, the haemoglobin is within normal limits, and the main sign is micro- or macrocytosis of the red cells. In patients who thus prove to be iron, vitamin B_{12} or folate deficient, remedying the deficiency may bring rapid resolution of the ulcers.

Zinc deficiency. Zinc deficiency has been found to be more common in aphthous stomatitis patients but the significance is unclear.

Hormonal factors. In a few women, aphthae are associated with the luteal phase of the menstrual cycle, but there is no strong evidence that hormone treatment is reliably effective. Pregnancy is often associated with remission.

'Stress' is often related to exacerbations according to patients, and some studies have reported a correlation. However, stress is notoriously difficult to quantify, and some studies have found no association.

HIV infection. Aphthous stomatitis is a recognised feature of HIV infection. Its frequency and severity are related to the degree of immune deficiency, as discussed later.

Not smoking. It has long been established that recurrent aphthae is a disease, almost exclusively, of non-smokers, and this is one of the few consistent findings. Recurrent aphthae may also start when smoking is abandoned (but restarting does not induce remission), and quitting using nicotine supplements seems to prevent this. The reasons are unclear.

In summary deficiencies of iron, folate or vitamin B_{12} are the most significant predisposing factors because these may be secondary to another more significant condition and because addressing them may cure or ameliorate the condition.

Pathology

Biopsy plays no role in the diagnosis except to exclude carcinoma in the case of clinically worrying major aphthae or to exclude viral infection in herpetiform aphthae.

If performed, biopsy in the prodromal phase reveals an initial lymphocytic infiltration of the epithelium, followed by destruction of the epithelium and non-specific acute and chronic inflammation (Fig. 16.9). Aphthae are not preceded by vesicles.

Diagnosis

Diagnosis is almost exclusively by history, primarily recurrences of self-healing intraoral ulcers at fairly regular intervals. Almost the only other condition with this history is Behçet's disease. Usually occasional ulcers are tolerated, and it is an increase in frequency of ulcers that brings the patient to seek treatment. A detailed history of the ulcer number, shape, size, site, duration, frequency of attacks is required.

Most patients appear well, but haematological investigation is particularly important in older patients and those with recent exacerbations in frequency of crops, ulcer size or pain. Routine blood indices are informative, and usually the most important finding is an abnormal mean corpuscular volume (MCV). If macro- or microcytosis is present, further investigation is necessary to find and remedy the cause. Treatment of vitamin B_{12} deficiency or folate deficiency is sometimes sufficient to control or abolish aphthae. Applying the most sensitive tests for iron, folate and B_{12} deficiency identifies more patients who can benefit from treatment, and they will often respond to supplementation despite apparently having very mild or early deficiency.

Key features for diagnosis are shown in Table 16.2.

Medical conditions associated PMID: 9421219

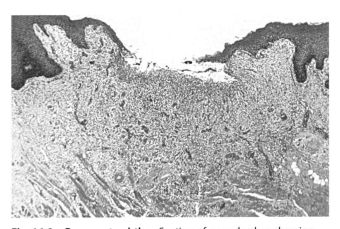

Fig. 16.9   Recurrent aphtha. Section of an early ulcer showing the break in the epithelium, the inflammatory cells in the floor and the inflammatory changes more deeply where numerous dilated vessels can be seen.

Table 16.2   Checklist for diagnosis of recurrent aphthous stomatitis

	Check for	Comments
History	• Recurrences • Pattern? Minor, major or herpetiform type? • Onset as child or teenager • Family history • Distribution only on non-keratinised mucosa • Signs or symptoms of Behçet's disease (ocular, genital, skin, joint lesions) (Table 16.3)	The history is all-important
Examination	• Discrete well-defined ulcers • Scarring or soft palate involvement suggesting major aphthae	Exclude other diseases with specific, appearances, e.g., lichen planus or vesiculobullous disease
Investigations	• Anaemia, iron, red cell folate and vitamin B_{12} status • History of diarrhoea, constipation or blood in stools suggesting gastrointestinal disease, e.g., coeliac disease or malabsorption	Used to exclude underlying conditions, especially in patients with onset in later life or exacerbation of pre-existing disease

Management

Apart from the minority with underlying systemic disease, treatment is empirical and palliative only. Despite numerous clinical trials, no medication gives completely reliable relief. Low-potency and topical agents should be tried first. Some patients report that changing toothpastes is helpful.

Reassurance and education. Patients need to understand that the ulcers may not be curable but can be made bearable with symptomatic treatment. Reducing the number of attacks is more difficult to address, but some treatments are successful, particularly if attacks are frequent. The condition usually wanes eventually of its own accord, although after many years.

Corticosteroids. Some patients get relief from hydrocortisone, 2.5 mg, oromucosal tablets allowed to dissolve next to the ulcer three times per day. These low-potency corticosteroids adhere to the mucosa to provide a high local concentration of drug and are suitable for use in dental practice. They probably reduce the painful inflammation but do not speed healing much or reduce frequency of attacks. They are best applied in the very early, asymptomatic stages.

Triamcinolone dental paste. Triamcinolone dental paste (Adcortyl in Orabase) acts similarly but is no longer available in the UK and is superseded by the previously mentioned mucosal adhesive tablets.

Tetracycline mouth rinses. Trials in both Britain and the United States showed that tetracycline rinses significantly reduced both the frequency and severity of aphthae. However, the reasons are unclear and this is best reserved for herpetiform aphthae as these respond reliably. The contents of a tetracycline capsule can be stirred in a little water and held in the mouth for 2–3 minutes, three or four times daily. However, there are few easily soluble tetracycline preparations, and repeated use carries a risk of superinfection by *Candida albicans*. Doxycycline, 100 mg, dispersible tablets are a suitable preparation. The solution should not be swallowed.

Chlorhexidine. A 0.2% solution has also been used as a mouth rinse for aphthae. Used three times daily after meals and held in the mouth for at least 1 minute, it has been claimed to reduce the duration and discomfort of aphthous stomatitis.

Topical salicylate preparations. Salicylates have an anti-inflammatory action and also have other local effects. Preparations of choline salicylate in a gel can be applied to aphthae. These preparations, which are available over the counter, appear to help some patients.

Local analgesics. These provide only symptomatic relief, but benzydamine mouthwash or spray helps some patients. Topical lidocaine or benzocaine sprays and gels are more effective but can only be used in limited doses and for a short time. They do not require prescription in the UK.

Treatment of major aphthae. Major aphthae, whether or not there is underlying disease such as HIV infection, may sometimes be so painful, persistent and resistant to conventional treatment as to be disabling. Reportedly effective treatments include azathioprine, ciclosporin, colchicine and dapsone, but thalidomide is probably most reliably effective. Their use may be justified for major aphthae even in otherwise healthy persons if they are disabled by the pain and difficulty of eating. However, such drugs can only be given under specialist supervision.

Complementary and experimental treatments. Common, relatively inconsequential diseases that are difficult to treat will always be used to promote treatments without a good evidence base. While the disease remits spontaneously and unpredictably, and measurement of symptoms is imprecise, it is difficult to prove whether such treatments are effective or not.

Possible treatments for recurrent aphthae are summarised in Appendix 16.1.

RAS review PMID: 21812866 and 17850936

Disease associations PMID: 22233487

Cochrane review treatment PMID: 22972085

BEHÇET'S DISEASE → Summary chart 16.2 p. 311

Behçet's disease was originally defined as a triad of oral aphthous stomatitis, genital ulceration and uveitis. However, it is a systemic vasculitis of small blood vessels and affects many more organ systems than suggested by this limited definition.

The importance of making the diagnosis is indicated by the life-threatening risk of thrombosis, of blindness or brain damage in a small number of patients.

Clinical

Behçet's disease is particularly common in Turkey*, central Asia, the Middle East and Japan but is less common in

---

* Hulusi Behçet (1889-1948) was a Turkish dermatologist.

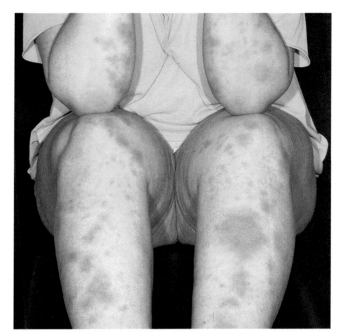

Fig. 16.10 Erythema nodosum. This is the commonest skin manifestation of Behçet's disease. *(From Habib, F., 2004. Clinical Dermatology: A colour guide to diagnosis and therapy, fourth ed. Mosby, Philadelphia.)*

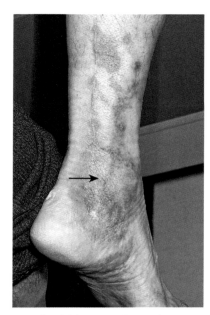

Fig. 16.11 Thrombophlebitis in Behçet's disease. Inflammation and pigmentation highlight the sites of veins (arrow) and their valves.

emigrants from these areas and is rare in people from Europe, the Americas and Africa. This matches the geographic incidence of the human leukocyte antigen (HLA)-B51 allele (see later in this chapter).

Patients are usually young adult males between 20 and 40 years old and they can develop one or more of four patterns of disease.

Mucocutaneous. Oral aphthae are the most consistent feature, are not distinguishable from common aphthous stomatitis and may be of any of the three types. There is often genital ulceration and a variety of rashes including erythema nodosum (Fig. 16.10) and vasculitis (Fig. 16.11).

Arthritic. Joint involvement with or without mucocutaneous involvement. The large weight-bearing joints are most affected. There is pain, but no destructive arthritis and only a few joints are involved. The pain may be relapsing or constant.

Neurological. This type may occur with or without other features and is usually a late stage. Vasculitis within the brain causes a variety of neurological symptoms including sensory and motor disturbances, confusion and seizures. Thrombosis of vessels causes raised intracranial pressure, blurred vision and headache.

Ocular. This type may also be solitary or accompany other types. There may be uveal inflammation or vasculitis and thrombosis of the retinal arteries, either of which can lead rapidly to blindness if not treated.

Behçet's review PMID: 34524077 (updated annually) and 34531393

Aetiology

The aetiology is unknown, but the disease has features including circulating immune complexes, high levels of cytokine secretion and activation of lymphocytes and macrophages in the circulation. These suggest an immune-mediated reaction, and it is presumed that this may be a response to an unknown infectious agent, possibly through immune cross reaction between pathogen and host heat shock proteins.

The ethnic distribution suggests a strong genetic component and HLA tissue types are linked, most strongly to HLA-B51. This is a common allele in the healthy population and so is not of use in diagnosis but can predict ocular lesions in those who do have the disease.

Diagnosis and management

Oral aphthae are frequently the first manifestation. Behçet's disease should therefore be considered in the differential diagnosis of aphthous stomatitis, particularly in patients in an ethnic group at risk, and the medical history should be checked for the features shown in Table 16.3. The frequency of other manifestations is highly variable.

As a result, there are no absolute criteria or reliable tests for the diagnosis, but in a dental setting, aphthous stomatitis in combination with any two of the other major features can be regarded as likely indicators meriting referral of the patient.

Tests are not helpful in diagnosis, apart from the pathergy test. The test is positive if there is an exaggerated response to a sterile needle puncture of the skin. However, the test must be interpreted by an experienced clinician and tends to be positive only in patients from the Mediterranean region. Moreover, a positive pathergy test does not correlate with the presence of oral lesions or with the overall severity of the disease and is rarely positive in patients from the UK. It is also not entirely specific for Behçet's disease but has a specificity over 90% in susceptible populations.

The International Criteria for Behçet's Disease System is shown in Table 16.3.

Diagnostic criteria PMID: 23441863

Treatment PMID: 34321904

Treatment

Treatment is difficult and requires a multidisciplinary approach. Ciclosporin and tacrolimus are the main treatments, with steroids for acute exacerbations. Thalidomide or topical

Table 16.3 The International Criteria for Behçet's Disease 2014 together with their overall incidence in all patients*

Sign group	Criteria	Points	Incidence
Oral aphthous stomatitis	Three attacks or more in one year	2	80%[†]
Genital ulceration	Recurrent ulcers or scarring	2	80%
Ocular lesions	Uveitis or retinal vasculitis	2	50%
Skin lesions	Follicular pustular rash or erythema nodosum	1	75%
Central nervous system involvement	Any involvement	1	10%
Vascular manifestations	Superficial phlebitis, deep vein thrombosis, large vein thrombosis, arterial thrombosis, and aneurysm	1	30%
Positive pathergy test (optional to include)		1	5%–60%[‡]

*A score of 4 or more points predicts Behçet's disease with 95% certainty, 98% if the pathergy test is performed. Incidence of features varies between populations.
[†]100% using older criteria, previously a requirement for diagnosis.
[‡]The higher figure is for patients from the middle East and central Asia.

tacrolimus are most effective for oral ulcers. Anti-tumour necrosis factor α drugs such as infliximab are a promising recent option, but a wide range of treatments are used for specific conditions.

Complications include blindness, rupture of large-vessel aneurysms, thrombosis and embolism, but in the absence of these and other significant complications, relapses become less frequent, and the disease may eventually burn out.

HIV-ASSOCIATED ORAL ULCERS

People with HIV infection (Ch. 30) are susceptible to severe recurrent aphthae that are not otherwise distinguishable from common aphthae. They may be of any of the three types, but most are either major or herpetiform aphthae. With declining immune function, the ulcers become more frequent and severe but improve on effective anti-retroviral treatment. Aphthae are no more frequent in HIV infection than in the healthy population and are classified with group 3 lesions (Ch. 30). Ulcers whose presentation does not match the three patterns of aphthae are classified just as 'HIV ulceration' (previously 'atypical' ulceration).

Biopsies should be taken from non-healing ulcers to exclude opportunistic infections and other HIV-associated conditions including lymphoma, Epstein-Barr virus or cytomegalovirus ulcers and deep fungal infections.

Treatment with potent topical steroids is frequently effective. In severe cases ulcers require the higher potency drugs listed for aphthous ulcers, often systemically (Appendix 16.1).

Description PMID: 1545960

Treatment PMID: 9154767 and 14507229

HIV-associated lesions PMID: 24034072

NICORANDIL-INDUCED ULCERS

The potassium channel activator Nicorandil, used to dilate arterioles in angina, causes ulcers of skin and oral mucosa. Ulcers have been reported to affect 5% of patients on the drug, but this is likely an overestimate. Ulcers usually appear within 24 months of starting the drug, often after a few weeks, and are usually solitary and on the lateral tongue, buccal mucosa, gingivae or fauces. Perianal or vulval skin are the usual skin sites. Ulcers can arise at relatively low doses, although they are commoner at higher dose.

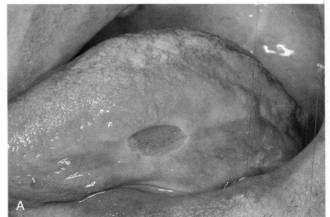

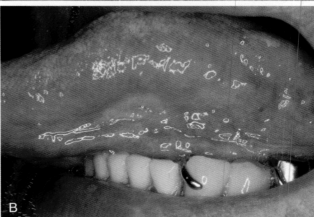

Fig. 16.12 Nicorandil-induced ulcer. The ulcer appears sharply demarcated and has no well-organised slough or granulation tissue in the base (A). Healing took 9 weeks after drug withdrawal and a scar remains (B). *(From Yamamoto, K., Matsusue, Y., Horita, S., et al., 2011. Nicorandil-induced oral ulceration: report of 3 cases and review of the Japanese literature. Oral Surg. Oral Med. Oral Pathol. Oral Radiol. Endod. 112, 754–759.)*

The oral ulcers have a characteristic clinical appearance and are strikingly painful (Fig. 16.12). They are deep, with a punched-out or overhanging margin, and range from 1–3 cm in diameter. They may be mistaken for major aphthae or carcinoma. Ulcers do not usually respond to local medications and persist for several months unless the drug is withdrawn, when they heal within a few weeks depending on their size.

Nicorandil is known to delay wound healing, and biopsy shows reduced formation of granulation tissue in the ulcer base. However, the features are non-specific, and biopsy does not aid diagnosis other than to exclude other causes.

Case series PMID: 15920586 and 29767853

MISCELLANEOUS MUCOSAL ULCERS

Wegener's granulomatosis

Mucosal ulceration is occasionally a feature of this disease but mainly in its established stage (Ch. 34). Clinically, ulceration may be widespread but is otherwise non-specific. Biopsy is diagnostic.

LICHEN PLANUS AND SIMILAR CONDITIONS

Lichen planus is a common chronic inflammatory disease of skin and mucous membranes. Although in most patients the features are characteristic, they are varied and not very specific. A number of other diseases appear similar or identical. This is confusing both clinically and terminologically. Pathologists often group these conditions under the umbrella term of 'lichenoid processes' based on their histopathology, but in clinical parlance 'lichenoid' is usually reserved for conditions that mimic lichen planus clinically. The terms used here are shown in Table 16.4, but it has to be accepted that is it is sometimes impossible to differentiate a number of lichen planus-like conditions when only oral lesions are present.

'DESQUAMATIVE GINGIVITIS'

→ Summary chart 19.3 p. 349

Desquamative gingivitis is a clinical description, not a diagnosis. Its meaning is erythematous gingiva with peeling or blistering of the surface epithelium, and the most common causes are lichen planus, mucous membrane pemphigoid or pemphigus. In clinical practice, peeling and blistering are usually only detected in pemphigoid, which is therefore the commonest cause if these are accepted as a defining characteristic. In practical use, the term tends to be used for any gingivae that appear red or raw across the full width of gingiva, whether or not peeling can be seen or revealed in the history. Using this definition, lichen planus is the commonest cause. Gingiva around varying numbers of teeth can be affected (see Figs 16.13, 16.29 and 16.33).

The gingivae appear smooth, from matt dull red to shiny bright red and translucent due to the thinness of the atrophic epithelium. When lichen planus is the cause, there may be white flecks or faint striae on the red background. Peeling or blistering may be seen as bullae or small tags of epithelium at the margins of zones of epithelial separation. The appearances are strikingly different from simple marginal gingivitis.

Desquamative gingivitis almost always indicates a mucocutaneous disease, but the appearance is not specific, and occasionally topical lichenoid reactions to restorations, foreign body gingivitis and toothpaste reactions appear similar. The correct underlying diagnosis should be confirmed by biopsy.

Review causes PMID: 18166088 and 26225114

Delay in diagnosis 32651518

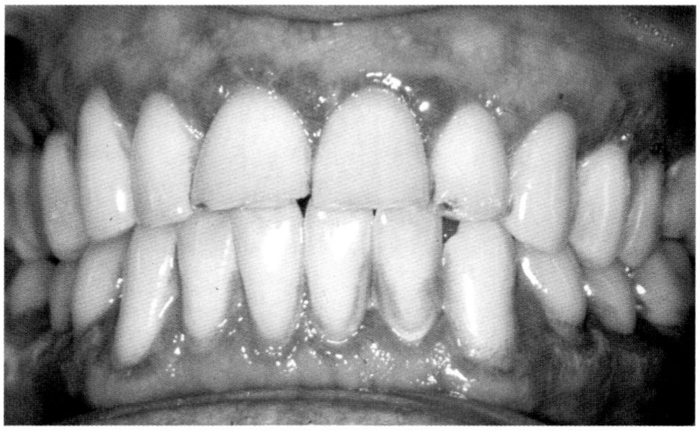

Table 16.4 Lichen planus and lichenoid processes

Lichen planus	The prototypical disease pattern with no cause found
Lichenoid reaction	A disease that appears as lichen planus clinically and histologically but has a defined cause, usually a drug or a topical agent
Lupus erythematosus	A distinct disease, but one that shares clinical and histological features with lichen planus. When these features are incomplete, it may not be possible to distinguish it from either lichen planus or a lichenoid reaction
Graft versus host disease	A distinct disease following bone marrow transplant. Its clinical and histological features mimic lichen planus
Lichen sclerosus et atrophicus	A rare and distinct disease. Its clinical and histological features mimic lichen planus but skin lesions are usually characteristic
Lichenoid lesion	A controversial term describing disease with incomplete or unusual features, resembling lichen planus clinically but possibly indicating a risk of malignant transformation and presence of dysplasia. There are no well-defined diagnostic criteria
Epithelial dysplasia	Lesions of leukoplakia and erythroplakia are occasionally indistinguishable clinically from lichen planus or lichenoid reactions when features of dysplasia are mild or subtle. The relationship between lichen planus and oral carcinoma is discussed in this chapter and Chapter 19

Fig. 16.13 Desquamative gingivitis caused by lichen planus. A well-defined band of patchy erythema extends around several teeth, in places affecting the full width of the attached gingiva and limited at the mucogingival junction. This change may be localised or widespread. Within the red areas faint white flecks and striae are sometimes visible to suggest lichen planus as the cause, as seen around the lower left premolars.

LICHEN PLANUS → Summary charts 16.1, 16.3, 19.1, 19.2 pp. 296, 312, 347, 348

Lichen planus is a very common chronic inflammatory disease of skin and mucous membranes found in 1%–2% of the population. It affects mainly patients of middle age or older and is slightly more common in females.

Aetiology and pathogenesis

The aetiology of lichen planus remains unknown. This may well be because there are many different causes producing the same clinical and histological outcome. Lichen planus has been associated with polymorphisms in genes for many cytokines, HLA-B and -DR antigens suggesting that immune or inflammatory dysregulation is an underlying factor.

In contrast, the pathogenesis is relatively well understood. Basal cells in epidermis and mucosal epithelium are destroyed by an immunologically mediated process in which cytotoxic T cells (CD8[+]), and smaller numbers of helper T cells, migrate into the basal layers and destroy the basal cells. It is unclear whether this process is driven by an antigen-specific mechanism or not, or whether it is autoimmune or a reaction to an extrinsic antigen in the tissues.

The T cells destroy the basal cells either by direct cytotoxicity using perforin and enzymes released directly onto the cell, or through secretion of tumour necrosis factor α or other cytokines. The basal epithelial cells die by apoptosis. This leaves the epithelium with fewer proliferating cells to renew itself, and it becomes thinner. It also destroys the cells best adapted to adhere to the connective tissue. Prickle cells take the place of the basal cells, but production of the basement membrane is compromised. The basement membrane is important in maintaining the basal epithelial cells and signalling between connective tissue and epithelium. Loss of this interaction inhibits repair and weakens the attachment of epithelium, sometimes causing it to separate.

The thin epithelium becomes keratinized and the keratinization is "premature", that is it starts lower in the epithelium than normal and eosinophilic cytoplasm of partial keratinization is seen throughout the prickle cell layer and even down to the basement membrane when the basal cells are lost.

Epithelial damage induces cytokine production to attract lymphocytes to form a dense band-like infiltrate below the epithelium. Here CD4[+] helper cells predominate, with smaller numbers of cytotoxic CD8[+] T cells and a few macrophages, but the infiltrate is characteristically almost exclusively lymphocytic.

The process is in a state of balance. When destruction of basal cells dominates, the epithelium becomes atrophic or ulcerates, non-specific inflammation supervenes and symptoms increase. When the immunological reaction wanes, the remaining basal cells proliferate and recover, the epithelium thickens and becomes more heavily keratinised and symptoms may vanish. What causes this cyclical course is unclear, but patients often identify stress and trauma, including dental treatment, as factors causing the condition to flare up.

There is a poorly understood link between hepatitis C and lichen planus. This association is only found in countries with a high incidence of hepatitis C such as Southern Europe and Japan. The cause may be either an immunological cross reaction or a T cell immune response against hepatitis C virus replicating in oral epithelium. There is a suggestion that anti-HCV treatment may cause this type of lichen planus to resolve. This supports the concept that lichen planus may be the consequence of immune reactions to a variety of systemic, topical or epithelial antigens, and not a single disease.

Another disease associated with lichen planus is hypothyroidism, but again the significance is unclear.

General review PMID: 25216164 and 27349424

Detailed pathogenesis PMID: 12191961

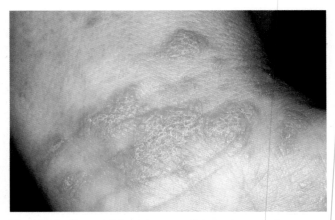

Fig. 16.14 Dermal lichen planus on lightly pigmented skin. This, the flexor surface of the wrists, is a characteristic site. The lesions consist of confluent papules with a pattern of minute white striae on their surface and background erythema.

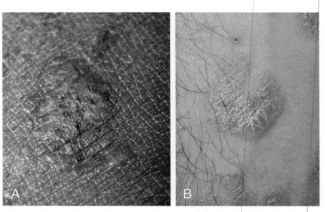

Fig. 16.15 Lichen planus on pigmented skin (left) has a much darker appearance than on lightly pigmented skin (right). Erythema and striae are less obvious. The lesion and surrounding skin become more heavily melanin-pigmented because of the chronic inflammation, producing a very different appearance. *(From Bolognia J, Schaffer J, Cerroni L, 2018. Dermatology, 4th ed. London: Elsevier Ltd)*

Skin lesions

During the course of the disease, about one-third of patients have skin lesions only, one-third have oral lesions only and the remaining third have both. Skin lesions on lightly-pigmented skin are typically purplish papules, 2–3 mm across with a glistening surface marked by minute fine 'Wickham's striae'* and are usually itchy (Fig. 16.14). Striae are fine white randomly orientated lines caused by keratinisation. On pigmented skin, the inflammation often induces increased pigmentation so that lesions appear dark and the erythema and striae are less easily seen (Fig 16.15). Typical sites are the flexor surface of the forearms and especially the wrists , shins and small of back.

Skin lesions help in diagnosis if present but can be identical in drug-induced lichenoid reactions. Skin lesions are relatively easy to treat with steroids, and many patients only suffer them for a few years. It is therefore important to ask about previous rashes when taking a history.

Review skin lichen planus PMID: 34790675

---

* Louis Wickham (1861–1913) was a French dermatologist and pathologist. The name applies to the striae on skin and oral mucosa.

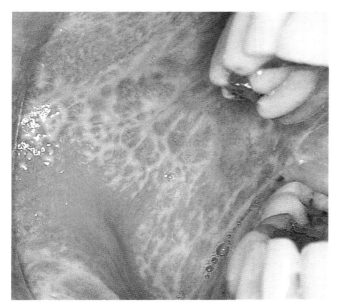

Fig. 16.16 Lichen planus, striated pattern. This is the most common site and type of lesion, a lacy network of white striae on the buccal mucosa. The lesions are usually symmetrically distributed. This is a florid example, often there are only a few striae posteriorly.

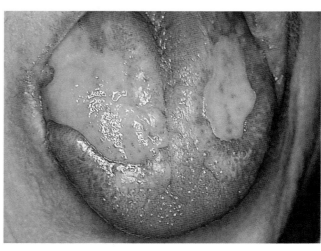

Fig. 16.18 Ulcerated lichen planus of the tongue. Two extensive areas of shallow ulceration have formed symmetrically on the tongue. Lingual involvement is seen usually in severe cases where the buccal mucosa and other sites are also affected.

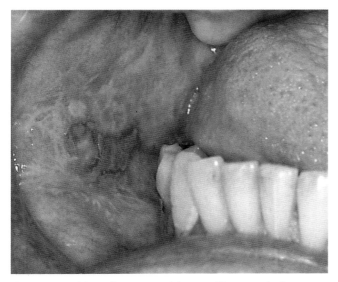

Fig. 16.17 Lichen planus, atrophic type. There are shallow irregular zones of ulcer and erythema surrounded by poorly defined striae.

Oral lesions

The oral lesions have a characteristic but not entirely specific appearance and distribution (Figs 16.16–19).

Lesions are usually bilateral and very often symmetrical, sometimes strikingly so. The buccal mucous membranes, particularly posteriorly, are by far the most frequently affected site, but lesions may spread forward almost to the commissures. The next most common site is the tongue, either the lateral margins or, less frequently, the dorsum. The gingivae are often affected, at least focally, by desquamative gingivitis (discussed previously in this chapter), and this is fairly frequently the only oral site involved. Only gingiva

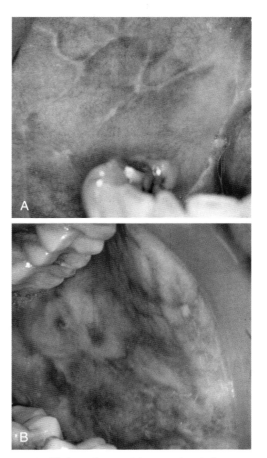

Fig. 16.19 Oral lichen planus with secondary inflammatory pigmentation in patients with dark skin colour. In the upper panel it can be seen how melanin pigmentation follows the distribution of the striae. In the lower panel pigmentation dominates the appearance, lichen planus is less obvious and the condition could be mistaken for a pigmented lesion.

around teeth is affected; lichen planus resolves on extraction of teeth and rarely affects edentulous ridges. The floor of the mouth and palate are usually uninvolved and apparent extension to floor of mouth should raise suspicion of either misdiagnosis (of a potentially malignant dysplastic process) or a drug reaction.

Depending on the balance between destruction and resolution, the disease presents with a range of appearances. These are not different types of lichen planus, only presentations or phases of disease. Any one patient may have several presentations at the same time that change from one pattern to another over time. The patterns help determine treatment need but have no other significance.

Unlike skin lesions, oral lesions are difficult to treat, and most patients will experience oral lesions for life, although severity may wane with age.

Patients with darker skin tones often develop pigmentation, which can be a very marked feature in all the presentations noted below. The appearance is not as markedly different as it is on the skin because the oral mucosa is mostly non-pigmented. However, inflammation triggers melanin pigmentation in the melanocytes normally present in the epithelium and the more heavily inflamed atrophic and ulcerated presentations and desquamative gingivitis may become very dark (Fig. 16.19).

Reticular lichen planus comprises a meshwork pattern of *striae*, fine white lines caused by keratinisation, between 0.1–2 mm wide that criss-cross randomly. They are sharply defined snowy white and form lacy, radiating or annular patterns (Figs 16.16 and 16.19 upper panel). They may occasionally be interspersed with minute, white papules. If the keratinisation is thick, striae may be felt as slightly raised and patients feel them as roughening or a 'dry' area.

Atrophic or erythematous lichen planus produces red areas of epithelial thinning (Fig. 16.17), often combined with striae. The inflamed submucosa is visible through the thin epithelium, appearing red. Atrophic (and ulcerated) lichen planus is often incorrectly called *erosive* lichen planus. Erosions are partial loss of epithelial thickness from the surface, as in pemphigus, whereas the red areas in lichen planus are due to epithelial thinning, with the surface layers intact.

Ulcerated lichen planus results from severe basal cell destruction to the extent that the epithelium cannot renew itself and ulcers develop. The ulcers are shallow and irregular and covered by a smooth, slightly raised yellowish layer of fibrin (Fig. 16.18). Ulcers are usually surrounded by atrophic areas, and striae may be seen around the margins.

Plaques are continuous areas of keratinisation that appear white and often affect the dorsum of the tongue or the buccal mucosa. Whether plaque-type lichen planus exists or is a misdiagnosis of leukoplakia caused by clinical and histological similarity is contentious. The plaques themselves are clinically indistinguishable from other leukoplakias, so that the diagnosis should only be accepted if other typical presentations of lichen planus are present elsewhere in the mouth.

Desquamative gingivitis is most commonly caused by lichen planus. The gingivae appear shiny, inflamed and smooth across the full width of the attached gingiva (see Fig. 16.13). The gingivae are occasionally the only site involved by lichen planus.

Bullous lichen planus results from detachment of the epithelium because of loss of basal cells and the weakened basement membrane. Gingiva is the site most likely to produce blisters, but they quickly break down into ulcers

---

Box 16.5   Oral lichen planus: typical features

- Females account for at least 65% of patients
- Patients usually older than 40 years
- Untreated disease can persist for 10 or more years
- Lesions in combination or isolation, comprise:
  - Striae
  - Atrophic areas
  - Ulcers
  - Plaques
- Common sites are:
  - Buccal mucosae
  - Dorsum of tongue
  - Gingivae
- Lesions usually bilateral and often symmetrical
- May be cutaneous lesions or history of rash
- Asymptomatic lesions require no treatment
- Usually, good symptomatic response to corticosteroids
- No curative treatment

---

leaving small tags of epithelium at the ulcer margin. This is not a special type of lichen planus, it reflects severity, but it does require differentiation from the other immunobullous diseases (discussed later in this chapter).

Typical features of lichen planus are summarised in Box 16.5.

Clinical features and management PMID: 16269024 and 27349424

Pathology

Histologically, a series of common features are seen in varying proportions matching the clinical presentations. There is usually a dense sharply defined band-like infiltrate of lymphocytes running along beneath the epithelium. Smaller numbers of lymphocytes infiltrate the basal cell layers and are seen adhering to basal cells undergoing apoptosis. Apoptotic bodies are seen along the basal cell and immediately superficial layers, and where they cluster there are 'holes' in the epithelium from loss of cells (*liquefaction degeneration* is a historical term for this: there is no liquefaction).

Where basal cells are completely destroyed, prickle cells form the basal layer, and the basement membrane is thickened. The epithelium may be thin if basal cell destruction dominates. If the process is mild and there is minimal basal cell destruction, the epithelium may thicken, develop rete processes as part of a healing response and show prominent keratosis. Zones of affected mucosa are sharply defined laterally. A cross cut stria shows a short zone of keratinisation overlying a matching zone of basal cell loss and underlying infiltrate with normal mucosa on each side. Complete loss of epithelium and non-specific inflammation are seen in ulcers.

Typical histological features of keratotic and atrophic lesions are summarised in Box 16.6 and shown in Figs 16.20–16.23.

Diagnosis

The diagnosis can usually be made on the history, the appearance of the lesions and their distribution, ideally confirmed by biopsy. A biopsy is usually considered mandatory

Box 16.6   Lichen planus: typical histological features

White lesions (striae and plaques)

- Hyperkeratosis or parakeratosis
- Apoptotic degeneration of the basal cell layer
- Compact, band-like lymphocytic (predominantly T cell) infiltrate cells hugging the epithelial-connective tissue interface
- CD8 + lymphocytes predominate in the epithelium

Atrophic lesions

- Severe thinning and flattening of the epithelium
- Minimal or no keratin
- Marked destruction of basal cells
- Compact band-like, subepithelial inflammatory infiltrate hugging the epithelial-connective tissue interface

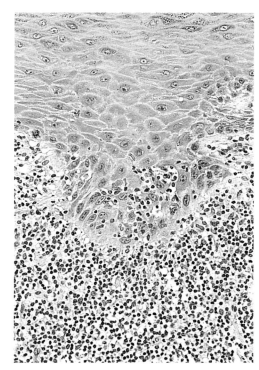

Fig. 16.21   Lichen planus. The basement membrane is thickened, and lymphocytes from the dense infiltrate below emigrate into the basal cells of the epithelium where they are associated with focal basal cell destruction.

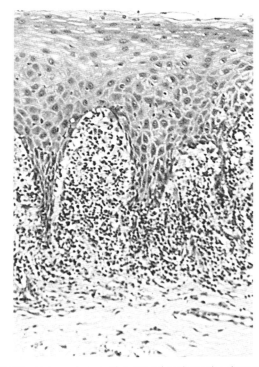

Fig. 16.20   Lichen planus. The rete ridges have the characteristic pointed (sawtooth) outline which is frequent in the skin but uncommon in mucosal lichen planus.

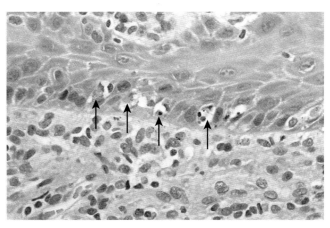

Fig. 16.22   Lichen planus. Lymphocytes infiltrating the basal cells are associated with basal cell apoptosis, loss of a prominent basal cell layer and prickle cells abutting the basement membrane. A cluster of apoptotic bodies is visible (arrows), each consisting of a shrunken bright pink cell with a condensed and fragmented nucleus.

Management

There is no treatment for the underlying disease process; treatment is symptomatic to manage any flare up in symptoms and complications. Asymptomatic striae and keratotic lesions usually require no treatment. Atrophic and ulcerated lesions are painful, are sensitive to acid, spicy or irritant foods and can make eating difficult.

There are several treatment options. It is usual to start with low-potency topical treatments. Medium-potency steroids should be provided in a specialist centre, not only because of the adverse effects of the drugs but because the

for any oral white lesion to exclude dysplasia but is often avoided in completely typical lichen planus. This is acceptable provided follow-up is to be provided, and the problem of malignant transformation is understood (discussed later in this chapter). Biopsy is required in plaque-type lesions or when lesions are in any other way unusual. Differential diagnosis is from other lesions described in this section and is summarised in Summary chart 16.1. Even with biopsy, foreign body gingivitis can be difficult to distinguish from desquamative gingivitis caused by lichen planus (Ch. 7).

***Diagnosis and management** PMID: 23399399*

***Controversies** PMID: 22788669*

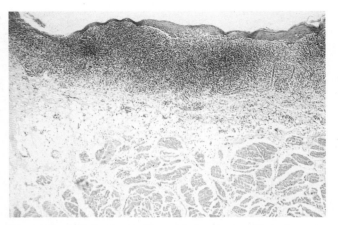

Fig. 16.23 Lichen planus. The epithelium is atrophic and greatly thinned. A well-demarcated, dense, broad band of lymphocytes extends along the superficial corium immediately below the epithelium.

more severe disease may benefit from a broader range of treatments.

No best treatment PMID: 22242640

Reassurance and education. Patients need to understand that lesions will persist for many years, but that symptoms can be managed. They can be reassured that lichen planus is not infectious. Education about the risks of malignant transformation is difficult given the uncertainties surrounding this, but the risk is extremely low. Patients need to be told to return if the pattern changes or symptoms worsen.

Oral hygiene. Gingival lichen planus is difficult to treat. Sensitivity prevents toothbrushing, but accumulation of plaque worsens inflammation and symptoms. Chlorhexidine mouthwash may be useful to get the condition under control, and non-astringent toothpaste will produce less sensitivity. However, such toothpastes may not contain fluoride and need to be chosen with care or fluoride supplemented in another way. Buccal mucosal lesions can also be worsened

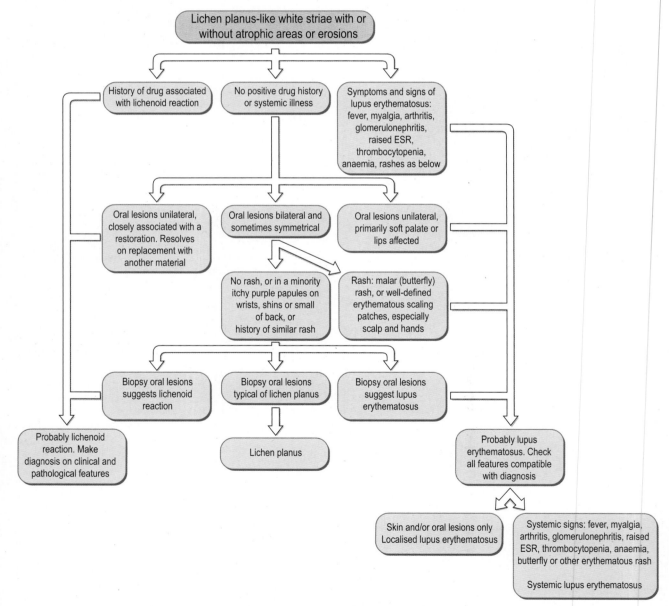

Summary chart 16.1 Differential diagnosis of oral lichen planus and conditions which mimic it clinically.

by plaque if the affected mucosa rests against the teeth. Improving oral hygiene should be an important element of treatment.

Topical low-potency steroids. A few patients gain benefit from hydrocortisone, 2.5 mg oromucosal adhesive tablets, used as described for aphthous stomatitis, but these are only suitable for mild localised and intermittently atrophic disease.

Chlorhexidine mouthwash. Because at least some symptoms are the result of bacterial surface colonisation of atrophic mucosa or ulcers, some patients benefit from chlorhexidine.

Topical medium-potency steroids. These are the mainstay of treatment for most lesions with atrophy or ulcers and are used short-term to control disease exacerbations in mild disease. Localised lesions are best managed with a topical agent. Triamcinolone is no longer available in orabase (Adcortyl), but a similar gel to apply to the lesions is available without prescription in some countries. However, this is not very effective because it does not stick well.

A better alternative is beclomethasone sprayed onto the lesions, using the same types of inhalers as are used for asthma. Approximately six puffs each day from an inhaler can be used to deliver enough of the corticosteroid to an ulcer. For gingival lesions, application of steroid gels in a vacuum formed tray increases effectiveness by keeping high doses in contact with affected mucosa for longer periods. For most patients with moderate disease, 0.5 mg betamethasone dissolved in 5–10 mL water and used as a mouthwash for 1–2 minutes four times daily before spitting out, is effective.

Topical high-potency steroids. For more severe or generalised disease, a mouthwash preparation is required to reach a wide area of mucosa. Because mouthwashes are only in contact with the mucosa for a limited time, high-potency steroids are required. Patients should not rinse but hold the preparation in the mouth for a minute over the affected mucosa and then spit it out to avoid systemic effects. Fluocinonide or clobetasol are often used. Clobetasol cream can be mixed 1:1 with plain orabase to make a topical preparation, but it is difficult to apply, messy and the orabase formulation can be considered uncomfortable in the mouth.

Systemic steroids. Systemic prednisolone is used for severe disease. Patients can also use topical preparations but swallow the dose for an initial period of 1–2 weeks to get severe disease under control and then continue with topical application.

Disease-modifying agents. These are potent and partly experimental treatments often not supported by a good evidence base, but they can be dramatically effective in some cases. Ciclosporine and tacrolimus or pimecrolimus are available as topical and systemic agents. Mycophenolate immunosuppression is also used. These may be used alone or as 'steroid sparing' additional medication.

Unproven and ineffective remedies. Unproven and ineffective remedies abound because the disease remits unpredictably, and benefit is difficult to measure. There is a strong placebo effect to any treatment in mild disease.

Monitoring for complications is critical. Candidal infection is frequent because of increased keratinisation and steroid treatment. A sudden exacerbation of symptoms or a switch from keratotic to atrophic or ulcerated form may well indicate superimposed candidosis. A scraping for hyphae is diagnostic, and antifungal treatment alone is likely

> **Box 16.7 Checklist for management of lichen planus**
> * Reassure patients that the condition is not usually of great consequence despite the fact that it can cause constant irritating soreness. Tell patients that the severity waxes and wanes unpredictably and the condition may persist for many years
> * Always check for drugs which might cause a lichenoid reaction. This is indistinguishable clinically but may respond to a change of medication
> * When inflammation worsens or symptoms become more severe, consider the possibility of superinfection with *Candida*
> * Biopsy lesions that appear unusual, form homogeneous plaques or are in unusual sites
> * Check for skin lesions that may aid diagnosis
> * Be aware that squamous carcinoma may develop in lesions closely resembling lichen planus, although very rarely
> * Follow-up lesions associated with reddening, or with unusual site, appearance or severity

to allow the lichen planus to return to its less symptomatic state.

A checklist for the management of lichen planus is given in Box 16.7.

Vulvovaginal-gingival syndrome

This is a very severe but uncommon pattern of lichen planus defined by atrophic and ulcerative involvement of genital mucosa and gingiva. Buccal mucosa and tongue are also frequently affected, and unusual sites such as scalp, oesophagus or eye are involved in 20% of patients. This form leads to scarring and significant complications outside the mouth. It is also resistant to treatment, often requiring higher-potency steroids or topical tacrolimus on non-oral sites.

Cases and treatment PMID: 16781300 and 7979437

Malignant change in lichen planus

The risk of, and possible frequency of, squamous cell carcinoma developing in lichen planus has long been controversial. It is currently generally accepted that patients with oral lichen planus have a risk of developing oral squamous carcinoma, but the risk is extremely low. It is certainly well below the 1% figure commonly reported and probably 10–100 times lower than this — otherwise the rate of malignant change would greatly exceed the actual incidence of oral cancer.

Difficulty arises in assessing this risk for several reasons. First, lichen planus, as noted previously, has characteristic but not specific features, both clinically and histologically. Some dysplastic lesions have a streaky or 'pumice' appearance that can be mistaken for striae. Many cases of lichen planus are not subjected to biopsy, so the presence or absence of dysplasia from the outset cannot be confirmed. Plaque-type lichen planus is difficult to distinguish from a leukoplakia. It is the author's experience that most cases of carcinoma apparently arising in lichen planus are accounted for by misdiagnosis of mild degrees of dysplasia in lesions that clinically mimic lichen planus, particularly the early stages of proliferative verrucous leukoplakia.

It is important to remember that biopsy alone cannot make a definitive diagnosis of lichen planus. Biopsy is required primarily to exclude other conditions and there is no such thing as 'biopsy proven lichen planus' though this term is often used in the context of evidence to support malignant transformation.

It is clear that a number of patients develop carcinoma in a background of keratosis and atrophy that either is lichen planus, is indistinguishable from it, or is misdiagnosed as it. Specific risk factors have not been identified, and both keratotic and atrophic lesions resembling lichen planus have preceded carcinoma. Patients with lesions in sites that are unusual for lichen planus but high-risk sites for squamous carcinoma, such as ventral tongue or floor of mouth or in smokers, should be kept under review, the diagnosis of lichen planus treated with scepticism and changes in appearance regarded with suspicion. Since lichen planus usually has onset between the ages of 30 and 60 years, new lichen planus-like lesions in older people should be considered potentially malignant and investigated as such by biopsy. The diagnosis of lichen planus affecting the ventral tongue or floor of mouth should never be accepted unless there are typical changes elsewhere, even if the biopsy appears to indicate lichen planus.

Two large studies PMID: 17112770 and 19362039

Prediction PMID: 27084261

Risk of transformation is overestimated PMID: 35858493

LICHENOID LESION

This term has been proposed to describe oral changes resembling lichen planus but without definite diagnostic features, in an attempt to define disease that might carry a risk of malignant transformation. Unfortunately, the same term is used for other purposes clinically and histologically and clear defining diagnostic criteria are lacking.

LICHENOID REACTIONS → Summary charts
16.1, 16.3, 19.1, 19.2 pp. 296, 312, 347, 348

This term is given to lichen planus-like lesions caused by a known trigger, usually a drug. Lichenoid reactions cannot always be confidently distinguished from lichen planus either clinically or histologically. However, lichenoid reactions are often more severe and *may* possess one or more suggestive features (Box 16.8), though these apply mostly to severe reactions.

In practice, trying to draw a distinct dividing line between lichen planus and lichenoid reactions is somewhat artificial. The diagnostic criterion would be resolution on removal of the stimulus, followed by relapse on re-challenge. However, whether the cause is a drug or an amalgam restoration, this may not be possible. Many patients with lichen planus are on potentially causative drugs, but their relevance is never determined and may not influence treatment.

Lichenoid reactions may produce any of the patterns of lichen planus described previously.

Lichenoid drug reactions

A very wide range of drugs can cause lichenoid reactions of the skin, mucous membranes or both (Box 16.9), and a complete drug history is mandatory in all patients thought to have lichen planus. Often a causative drug is not even

---

Box 16.8   Features suggesting a lichenoid reaction

- Onset closely associated with potential cause
- Unilateral lesions or unusual distributions
- Unusual severity
- Widespread skin lesions
- Localised lesion in contact with potential cause

Box 16.9   Some drugs capable of causing lichenoid reactions

These are only the more common causes:
- Colloidal gold (now rarely used)
- Beta-blockers
- Oral hypoglycaemics
- Allopurinol
- Non-steroidal anti-inflammatory drugs
- Antimalarials
- Methyldopa
- Penicillamine
- Some tricyclic and serotonin uptake inhibitor antidepressants
- Thiazide diuretics
- Captopril
- Many new targeted anti-inflammatory, immunosuppressant and chemotherapy drugs including TNF blocking antibodies, interleukin antagonists and tyrosine kinase inhibitors

---

suspected because it has been taken without prescription and over-the-counter medication must also be sought in the history. Reactions may not develop for months after a drug is first taken. They often also persist months or years after administration, especially after colloidal gold injection, so drugs taken in the preceding years should also be identified.

The list in Box 16.9 is by no means exhaustive, but those listed are commonly implicated.

Proof of causation requires withdrawal and re-challenge after healing, but the medical risk is hardly ever justified. Changing to another drug may be helpful, but alternatives from the same class of drug may also cause the same reaction.

The cause of drug reactions is unclear. It is possible that the drug itself becomes bound to the epithelial cells and elicits an antigen-specific response. It is also possible that the drug is metabolised idiosyncratically in the epithelium of susceptible patients, triggering the immune reaction.

Biopsy can sometimes distinguish lichenoid reactions from lichen planus, but the distinction is relatively subtle and not completely specific. The role of biopsy is to exclude other conditions, rather than distinguish lichen planus from a lichenoid reaction.

Lichenoid reactions are treated in exactly the same way as lichen planus with withdrawal of drug(s) if possible. Thus, the absolute distinction between lichen planus and a lichenoid reaction is not always necessary for treatment. Drug cessation will sometimes lead to resolution, but it may take many months.

Review PMID: 12494560 and 31241804

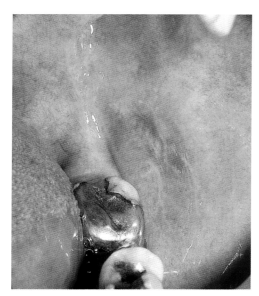

Fig. 16.24 Lichenoid reaction to amalgam. A patch of atrophy and striae in close association with a large amalgam. *(From Allen, C.M., Camisa, C., 2012. Oral Disease. In: Bolognia, J.L., Jorizzo, J.L., Schaffer, J.V. (Eds.), Dermatology, third ed. Elsevier, Saunders, Philadelphia.)*

Topical lichenoid reactions

The commonest topical cause of lichen planus-like clinical lesions is dental restorations, particularly amalgam, but mouthwashes, toothpastes, lipstick and other agents have been implicated.

Restoration reactions

Topical lichenoid reactions to restorative materials are usually triggered by amalgam but may be to polymeric materials, gold alloys or nickel. The clinical appearances are similar or identical to lichen planus or lupus erythematosus, but lesions are localised to the mucosa in contact with, not just close to, restorations (Fig. 16.24). For this reason, most develop on the posterior buccal mucosa or posterior ventral tongue.

Lesions may comprise only striae or a plaque, but more severe reactions have ulceration or atrophy centrally, surrounded by a zone of erythema and then striae. The more sharply defined a lesion is, the more atrophic or ulcerated, and the more closely related to a restoration, the more likely it is that the restoration is the cause and that its removal will be curative.

Corroded amalgam restorations are those most likely to trigger reactions, but which components of restorative materials are responsible remains unclear. Several metals in amalgams are haptens, and patients with amalgam reactions are more likely to show hypersensitivity to metals on skin testing. It is assumed that tiny amounts of these metals pass into the mucosa and bind to the epithelium to trigger the cell-mediated immune reaction.

Biopsy often shows large sharply defined rounded perivascular infiltrates deep in the tissues and the epithelium is often very atrophic, but the features are not always distinguishable from lichen planus (Fig. 16.25). Patch testing for metal hypersensitivity is not completely specific as the skin can react to a substance that causes no reaction in the mouth. A majority of patients with amalgam-induced lesions will react to mercury, but a negative test does not rule out the diagnosis.

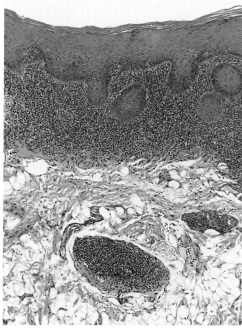

Fig. 16.25 Lichenoid reaction to amalgam. The features are similar or identical to lichen planus. Amalgam reactions often have dense perivascular infiltrates of inflammatory cells deeper in the tissue, two of which are seen here.

Lichenoid reactions to restorations are confirmed when healing follows removal of the restoration. The decision whether to remove a restoration or not has to be made almost completely on clinical grounds.

Amalgam reactions cases PMID: 2371051

Amalgam reactions review PMID: 2002442

Amalgam reactions treatment PMID: 12627099

Cinnamon stomatitis and plasma cell gingivitis

Cinnamon is a common cause of topical lichenoid reactions in the United States where strong cinnamon flavours are popular and used extensively, including in toothpastes, chewing gums and confectionery.

Although the histological features are lichen planus-like, the clinical appearance is more likely to be patchy irregular keratosis without significant erythema.

Gingiva affected by cinnamon toothpaste or chewing gum reactions are bright red across the full width of the gingiva and onto adjacent alveolar mucosa, and a biopsy shows plasma cell dominated gingivitis. Plasma cells are common in simple gingivitis, but this condition has an unusually florid and extensive infiltrate. The diagnosis is based on clinical resolution after withdrawal of the allergen or irritant, not on the histopathological appearance. This condition is rare and can be also associated with a variety of other toothpastes and foods.

Clinical and histology PMID: 1437042

Case series PMID: 3164031

GRAFT-VERSUS-HOST DISEASE

In graft-versus-host disease, lymphocytes transplanted in a bone marrow transplant proliferate and circulate to attack the recipient's tissues. Bone marrow transplant

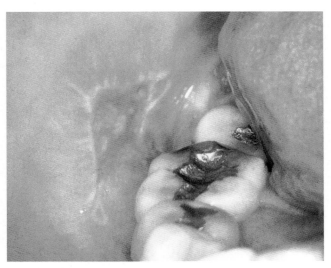

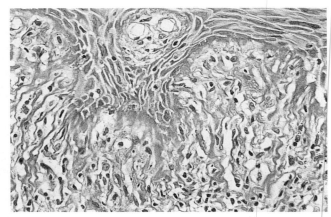

Fig. 16.27 Lupus erythematosus stained with periodic acid–Schiff to show the thickened basement membrane, which is magenta coloured with a fibrillar consistency.

Fig. 16.26 Lupus erythematosus. The clinical presentation is often very similar to lichen planus, with ulceration, atrophy and striae. Lesions on the soft palate or with radiating striae, as here, should be investigated for lupus erythematosus.

(hematopoietic stem cell transplantation) is increasingly used for diseases including leukaemias, myeloma and non-malignant diseases including sickle cell and Fanconi anaemia and thalassaemia. Graft versus host disease may therefore be seen in children as well as adults.

Acute graft versus host disease is only seen in specialized centres. The mouth is extensively ulcerated and erythematous.

Chronic graft versus host disease develops weeks or months after grafting in over half of transplant recipients and is less florid. The clinical and histological appearances are identical to lichen planus and the treatment is the same. Diagnosis is made primarily on the basis of history and any effects in other organs.

Occasional cases of malignant transformation have been reported and marrow-transplanted patients are also at risk of lip and oral carcinoma regardless of the development of oral graft versus host lesions. Further complications include dry mouth and salivary gland destruction similar to Sjogren's syndrome from graft lymphocytes attacking salivary tissue, and viral infections as a result of immunosuppression.

Review oral lesions PMID: 9167093 and 31425593

Treatment PMID: 20859645

Risk of oral carcinoma PMID: 35565303

LUPUS ERYTHEMATOSUS

➜ Summary charts 16.1, 16.3 pp. 296, 311

Lupus erythematosus is an autoimmune connective tissue disease with two main forms, systemic and cutaneous. Either can give rise to oral lesions that resemble oral lichen planus.

Systemic lupus erythematosus has varied systemic effects discussed in Chapter 31; oral lesions are discussed here. Discoid lupus is essentially a skin disease with rare oral lesions.

Clinically, oral lesions appear in approximately 20% of cases of systemic lupus and can, rarely, be the presenting sign (Fig. 16.26). Patients are usually female and the disease is more common in people of African heritage.

Oral changes are variable patterns of white and red areas. They may be identical to lichen planus, with ulcers, erythema and striae, although the striae are typically less well-defined than in lichen planus. Features suggestive of lupus erythematosus are lesions forming a discrete patch, unilateral lesions, symmetrical ulcers with surrounding erythema and radiating striae. The most indicative presentation is patches of atrophy and keratosis on each side of the hard/soft palate or a single midline palatal patch. Palate is a site that lichen planus typically spares so this distribution aids diagnosis. Lesions often involve primarily the gingiva but extend from it to adjacent mucosa. As with lichen planus, lesions may show increased melanin pigmentation in individuals with dark skin.

Pathology

Histologically, the features are as lichen planus, with some subtle differences. If the lesion is associated with the systemic form of lupus erythematosus, there may be marked thickening of the basement membrane zone (Fig. 16.27) and around blood vessels due to fibrosis and inflammation triggered by deposition of antigen/antibody complexes. The inflammatory infiltrate is highly variable in density, may not be closely applied to the epithelium and typically extends deeply into the connective tissue and may have a perivascular distribution (Fig. 16.28). There may be oedema below the epithelium. In the epithelium, the surface keratin layer may dip down into the central area of rete processes and irregular rete hyperplasia with deep clusters of keratinising cells is characteristic. In florid cases, these changes can mimic dysplasia or carcinoma, but are seen in only a minority of cases; in most the histopathological features are indistinguishable from lichen planus.

The lupus band test is immunofluorescent detection of a band of immunoglobulins and complement C3 with a granular texture deposited along the basement membrane. It works well in sun-exposed skin but is usually negative in oral lesions where it does not aid diagnosis.

Diagnosis depends on clinical features and biopsy. Autoantibodies are helpful in systemic disease, particularly antibodies to double-stranded (native) DNA, antinuclear antibodies of other types and the anti-Smith (Sm) autoantibody. There may also be a raised erythrocyte sedimentation rate (ESR), anaemia and, often, leukopenia or thrombocytopenia. If only oral lesions are present, these tests are likely to be negative. However, they should be performed to ensure that a case of systemic

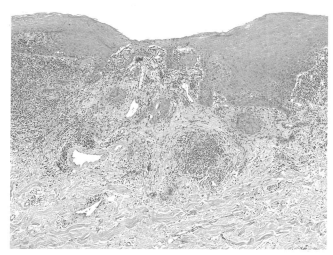

Fig. 16.28 Lupus erythematosus. The histological picture is similar to that seen in lichen planus, with a subepithelial band of lymphocytes, basal cell degeneration and epithelial atrophy. Features sometimes seen, and shown here, are dense perivascular infiltrates of lymphocytes in the deeper tissues and epithelial proliferation with irregular rete processes with keratinizing cells at their ends, overall resembling dysplasia or carcinoma.

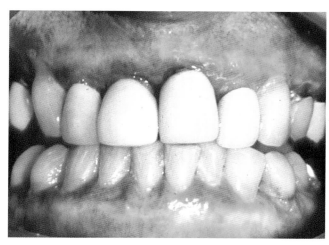

Fig. 16.29 Chronic ulcerative stomatitis. The appearance of desquamative gingivitis is identical to that caused by lichen planus, and only detection of the specific autoantibody by immunofluorescence can establish the diagnosis. *(From Newman, M.G., Takei, H., Klokkevold, P.R., et al. 2012. Carranza's Clinical Periodontology. Philadelphia:Saunders. Courtesy Dr Douglas Damm, University of Kentucky, Lexington)*

lupus presenting with oral lesions is not missed, as systemic disease has significant complications.

Oral lesions may respond to topical corticosteroids as used for lichen planus, but those in systemic disease tend to be resistant.

General review PMID: 17307106

Oral lesions review PMID: 15567365 and 17576335

Histological diagnosis PMID: 6584819

CHRONIC ULCERATIVE STOMATITIS

This rare mucosal disease mimics lichen planus and is probably underdiagnosed. It is an immunobullous disease like those in the next section but is considered here because of its clinical similarity to lichen planus.

The cause is an autoimmune reaction with immunoglobulin (Ig) G antibodies to a protein called CUSP, an isoform of the p63 cell cycle control protein normally expressed in the nuclei of the mucosal epithelium. This protein plays many roles in cell cycle control, preventing apoptosis and controlling differentiation. Binding of the antibody could have many effects, but it seems that the main pathogenic effect is to cause the epithelium to detach from the connective tissue.

Clinically, females older than 40 years are mainly affected. Lesions are usually shallow ulcers, erosions or erythema affecting the tongue. Buccal mucosa and gingiva are the next most frequently affected (Fig. 16.29). The lesions resemble lichen planus both clinically and histologically, even with striae in some cases. Skin involvement is uncommon.

There are no features to differentiate chronic ulcerative stomatitis from lichen planus in routine biopsy. However, immunofluorescence reveals the causative autoantibody, either bound in the tissues using direct, or in serum using indirect, immunofluorescence. The autoantibody is bound to the nuclei of the basal and immediately suprabasal cells.

Box 16.10 Chronic ulcerative stomatitis: key features
- Females older than 40 years mainly affected
- Lesions resemble lichen planus
- Direct immunofluorescence shows autoantibodies to squamous epithelial nuclear protein
- Chloroquine or hydroxychloroquine moderately effective

Diagnosis starts by suspecting the condition in a patient with apparent severe lichen planus that does not respond to steroids. Immunofluorescence, or detection of circulating antibody by ELISA, completes the diagnosis.

Steroids are relatively ineffective. Hydroxychloroquine, originally an antimalarial drug but now used in rheumatoid arthritis and autoimmune disease, is considered the most effective treatment. However, resolution may be followed by relapses and combination therapy with tacrolimus is sometimes used. Adverse effects of these drugs require treatment to be in a specialist centre.

Key features of chronic ulcerative stomatitis are summarised in Box 16.10.

Review PMID: 18593454 and 35092104

Immunodiagnosis PMID: 19682320

IMMUNOBULLOUS DISEASES

Immunobullous diseases are autoimmune diseases in which autoantibodies directed against components of the skin or oral epithelium cause epithelial separation to produce blisters. These diseases were previously called *vesiculo-bullous diseases* (a vesicle is a small blister, and a bulla is one more than 10 mm diameter). The two main diseases are pemphigus and pemphigoid, each of which has several variants (Box 16.11). Chronic ulcerative stomatitis is related and discussed in the previous section. Other diseases of different types producing vesicles and bullae include viral infections (Ch. 15), erythema multiforme and epidermolysis bullosa.

Box 16.11 The immunobullous diseases

- Pemphigus
  - Pemphigus vulgaris
  - Pemphigus foliaceous
  - IgA pemphigus
  - Drug-induced pemphigus
  - Paraneoplastic pemphigus
- Pemphigoid
  - Bullous pemphigoid
  - Mucous membrane pemphigoid
  - Linear IgA disease
  - Drug-induced pemphigoid
  - Anti-P200 pemphigoid
- Epidermolysis bullosa acquisita
- Dermatitis herpetiformis

PEMPHIGUS VULGARIS

→ Summary charts 16.2, 16.3 pp. 311, 312

Pemphigus vulgaris is an uncommon autoimmune disease causing vesicles or bullae on skin and mucous membranes. Almost all cases of oral pemphigus are of the pemphigus vulgaris type.

Aetiology

Pemphigus vulgaris is a classical autoimmune disease. Autoantibodies are directed against desmoglein 1 or 3, two proteins of the desmosomes that hold epithelial cells together. Skin epithelial integrity depends on both proteins, but mucosa has only desmoglein 3. The relative abundance of the autoantibodies against the two antigens determines the relative effects on skin and mucosa. Antibody from the circulation passes into tissue fluid and can permeate into the epithelium where it binds to desmosomes and causes detachment of the cells from one another. Exactly how this occurs is unclear, but the antibody binding may interfere with structure or affect turnover of desmosomes. The epithelium loses its cohesion and disintegrates.

The process starts in the suprabasal and prickle cells, forming a vesicle in which fluid accumulates. Gradually vesicles enlarge to become bullae and eventually burst. Epithelial cells that have lost their attachment collapse into a round shape and fall into the bullae and can be seen in a smear of the fluid, in which they are known as acantholytic or Tzanck cells.

When the bulla bursts, a layer of basal cells remains stuck to the basement membrane because they are attached by hemidesmosomes, which do not contain desmogleins. However, these cells quickly become abraded, and an ulcer develops.

Loss of the epithelium occurs almost without inflammation and without damage to the connective tissue so that there is only a limited wound healing response and tissue fluid exudes continuously from the burst bulla. Protein, fluid and electrolytes can be lost in great quantities from affected skin, and the raw areas readily become secondarily infected. Untreated, the condition can be fatal when skin involvement is extensive.

Clinical

Females aged 50–60 years are predominantly affected, and people of Indian and Jewish heritage are predisposed. Blisters first appear in the mouth in two-thirds of patients and then

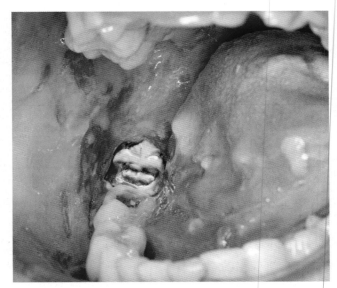

Fig. 16.30 Pemphigus vulgaris. Typical oral presentation with erythema, erosions and persistent ulcers. The surrounding epithelium is friable and disintegrates on gentle stroking.

Box 16.12 Pemphigus vulgaris: key clinical features

- Females predominantly affected, usually aged 40–60 years
- Commoner in people from Mediterranean, Middle Eastern countries and Indian subcontinent and their descendants
- Lesions often first in the mouth but spread widely on the skin
- Lesions consist of fragile vesicles and bullae
- Ruptured vesicles form irregular erosions on the mucosa
- Nikolsky's sign may be positive
- Widespread skin involvement is fatal if untreated
- Good response to prolonged immunosuppressive treatment

develop widely on the skin. Blisters on the skin have a tough layer of keratin as their roof and often persist for some time, filled with clear fluid, before bursting. Blisters in the mouth are less frequently seen because they usually develop on the non-keratinised lining mucosa, and their roofs disintegrate quickly, leaving very painful erosions or superficial ulcers with ragged edges (Fig. 16.30). On the keratinized gingiva, the appearances are those of desquamative gingivitis. The ulcers heal very slowly, over weeks or even months, but rarely scar as they are so superficial.

Progress of the disease is very variable. At its most rapid it progresses from widespread oral ulceration to involve the eyes and then skin in a few days, but some patients have oral blisters only for many months. A few patients with antibodies only to desmoglein 3 may have minimal or no skin involvement.

Key clinical features are summarised in Box 16.12.

Management

The diagnosis must be confirmed as early as possible. When skin blisters are present, the picture is distinctive. When

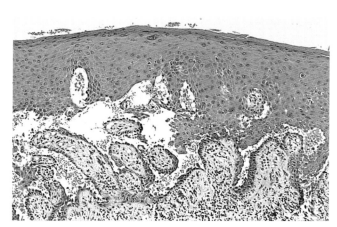

Fig. 16.31 Pemphigus vulgaris. The edge of a bulla formed by separation of the epithelium just above the basal cells. There is acantholysis centrally, and a layer of basal cells remains, covering the dermal papillae.

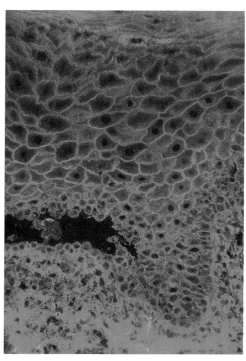

Fig. 16.32 Pemphigus vulgaris. Fresh frozen biopsy tissue stained with fluorescent antibody to immunoglobulin G shows green fluorescence along the lines of the intraepithelial attachments of the keratinocytes typical of pemphigus. (See Fig. 1.6.)

oral ulcers suggest the disease but no blisters have been noticed, gently stroking the weakened epithelium of mucosa or skin can sometimes cause a vesicle or bulla to develop (Nikolsky's sign).

Diagnosis requires biopsy and immunofluorescence findings. Trauma on biopsy will cause disintegration of the affected epithelium so that the specimen must be taken from more normal perilesional mucosa. Though clinically normal, histologically this will show splits and acantholysis (disintegration of the prickle cell layer) above the basal cells (Fig. 16.31). Immunofluorescence (Ch. 1) confirms the diagnosis and distinguishes the different variants (Fig. 16.32). In pemphigus vulgaris the autoantibody is seen to bind around the edges of prickle cells at the site of the desmosomes. A separate unfixed biopsy for immunofluorescence is required and is best taken from apparently normal buccal mucosa.

Histological findings are summarised in Box 16.13.

Once the diagnosis has been confirmed, initial treatment is with systemic steroids, usually prednisolone starting at around 80–100 mg/day, plus azathioprine as a steroid-sparing drug. Treatment must continue, reducing the dose after initial response, until all blisters are healed. Withdrawal too soon causes relapse, and a maintenance dose must be titrated against the patient's response or, better, the level of circulating autoantibody measured by ELISA on serum. Oral lesions respond more slowly than skin lesions. Almost all immunosuppressive drugs can be effective. The anti-CD20 drug rituximab depletes B lymphocytes, reducing autoantibody titres, and is effective in treatment-resistant cases. Eventually severity wanes, and patients may be maintained on low doses of steroid or immunosuppressants, either systemic or topical oral preparations.

Pemphigus vulgaris review PMID: 15888101

Controversies PMID: 22335787

Treatment PMID: 25934414 and skin 29192996

Pemphigus variants

These resemble pemphigus vulgaris clinically, but differ in their histological features, target antigens and response to treatment. Pemphigus vegetans is a benign localised form of pemphigus vulgaris that causes thickened papilloma-like

---

Box 16.13 Pemphigus vulgaris: pathology

- Loss of intercellular adherence of suprabasal prickle cells (acantholysis)
- Formation of clefts immediately superficial to the basal cells
- Extension of clefts to form intraepithelial vesicles
- Rupture of vesicles and bullae to form ulcers
- High titre of circulating antibodies to desmogleins
- Binding of antibodies to desmosomes detectable by immunofluorescence staining

---

lesions on the lips and only occasionally intraorally. IgA pemphigus has autoantibodies of IgA class instead of the usual IgG4, and mucosal involvement is rare. Pemphigus foliaceous has no mucosal involvement because the target antigen is only desmoglein 1.

Occasionally drugs trigger pemphigus; many can, but penicillamine is the usual cause.

Paraneoplastic pemphigus

Paraneoplastic pemphigus is a rare type of pemphigus seen in patients with malignant neoplasms, particularly lymphomas, leukaemias or Castleman's disease. There is severe mucosal involvement, often including nasal or oesophageal mucosa or the eye but very variable skin severity. The pathogenesis is the same as pemphigus vulgaris except that, in addition to the desmoglein autoantibodies, there are antibodies against other desmosome components such as periplakins, envoplakins, desmoplakins and also antibasement membrane antibodies, producing a confusing clinical picture with features of pemphigus, pemphigoid and erythema multiforme and graft versus host disease. Lichen planus-like presentations may also develop.

Histologically, the biopsy shows correspondingly mixed features with both suprabasal acantholysis and splitting along the basement membrane. Immunofluorescence is required for diagnosis. Indirect immunofluorescence using rat bladder as a substrate is the most specific test because it detects autoantibodies against the desmoplakin proteins, but is only positive in 75% of cases. The presence of antibodies against multiple target proteins is the most helpful feature.

The malignant neoplasm is usually known, but a third of cases present with pemphigus and a search for an underlying malignancy must be made. This type of pemphigus is very difficult to treat, may be intractable and often fatal because aggressive immunosuppression is required.

Review PMID: 15063382 and 18940624

MUCOUS MEMBRANE PEMPHIGOID

→ Summary charts 16.2, 16.3 pp. 311, 312

Diseases of the pemphigoid group are uncommon chronic autoimmune diseases causing bullae and painful erosions as a result of separation of epithelium from the connective tissue (Box 16.14). An obsolete name for mucous membrane pemphigoid is *cicatricial pemphigoid*, meaning scarring pemphigoid, but scarring is not a prominent feature in the mouth, though it is frequent in the eye.

Aetiology

In mucous membrane pemphigoid, the autoantibodies are directed against several basement membrane components, mostly against the BP180 antigen or less frequently integrins, laminin or type VII collagen. The antibodies are of IgG class and fix complement. Binding to the basement membrane causes complement activation, attracting and activating neutrophils to degrade the basement membrane. The result is that the epithelium falls off the connective tissue on the slightest trauma.

Clinical

Mucous membrane pemphigoid affects mostly women and has onset between the ages of 50 and 80 years. Blisters develop on the oral mucosa and in the eye, and less frequently in the vagina, pharynx, nose, pharynx and oesophagus. Signs and symptoms often develop slowly over months or years with cyclical exacerbations and remissions.

Intraorally the common sites are gingivae, buccal mucosa, palate and tongue. Desquamative gingivitis (this chapter) is the commonest oral manifestation (Fig. 16.33) and occasionally the only intraoral sign in mild disease. Vesicles and blisters are rarely seen on the gingiva, but form on other

affected sites. They may be seen for a short while before they burst (Fig. 16.34) because the roof of the blister is formed by an intact relatively resilient full thickness layer of epithelium, unlike the blisters in pemphigus. However, the blisters soon break down to leave shallow ulcers with ragged margins (Fig. 16.35), sometimes with small flaps or tags of separated epithelium at their edges. Bleeding into bullae can cause them to appear as blood blisters.

The severity is very variable. Individual erosions are very painful and heal slowly over several weeks, but new blisters and erosions develop continuously.

The eye is involved less frequently than the mouth, producing conjunctivitis, erythema and erosions. Blisters inside the eyelids and over the sclera heal with scarring, distorting the lids and causing adhesions between the lids and the sclera. Approximately one-quarter of patients will develop eye lesions in the first 5 years of disease. Severity of eye involvement determines treatment because ultimately

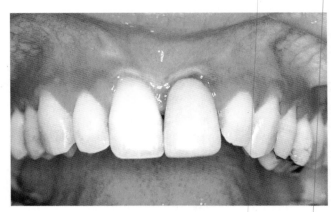

Fig. 16.33 Desquamative gingivitis as a result of mucous membrane pemphigoid. There is patchy reddening involving the attached gingivae around several teeth and in places the erythema extends to the alveolar mucosa. Unlike desquamative gingivitis caused by lichen planus, no white flecks or striae are present. Occasionally, tags of separating epithelium may be found.

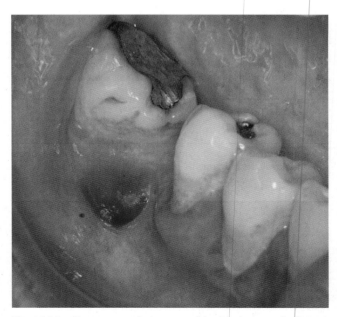

Fig. 16.34 **Mucous membrane pemphigoid.** An intact bulla at the junction of the attached gingiva and alveolar mucosa. The bulla fluid is lightly blood stained and visible through the intact pale yellow epithelial roof.

Box 16.14   Mucous membrane pemphigoid: typical features

- Females mainly affected and usually aged over 50 years
- Oral mucosa often the first site
- Involvement of the eyes, may cause scarring and blindness
- Skin involvement absent or minimal
- Indolent, non-fatal disease
- Oral bullae are subepithelial and sometimes seen intact

scarring and secondary keratinization of the cornea can lead to blindness.

The skin is very rarely involved.

Clinical features are summarised in Box 16.14.

Diagnosis and management

In addition to the typical presentation, Nikolsky's sign (see pemphigus section) is typically positive.

The diagnosis is confirmed by biopsy and immunofluorescence microscopy and requires either an intact vesicle or a sample from the margin of a blister. Unfortunately, biopsy of such involved tissue is difficult because the epithelium may separate from the underlying tissue during biopsy, rendering it useless for diagnosis. Great care must be taken to obtain an intact specimen. A normal buccal mucosa biopsy is best for immunofluorescence, though a skin biopsy is usually preferable if skin lesions are present.

Histologically, there is loss of attachment and separation of the full thickness of the epithelium from the connective tissue at basement membrane level. The roof of a bulla is formed by intact epithelium (Fig. 16.36). The floor is formed by connective tissue alone, infiltrated by inflammatory cells.

Direct immunofluorescence reveals the site of autoantibody binding, its immunoglobulin class and any complement activation. In almost all cases immunoglobulin IgG and/or complement component 3 can be found along the basement membrane (Fig. 16.37). When autoantibodies of both IgA and IgG antibody classes are present, the clinical course is usually more severe and resistant to treatment.

Indirect immunofluorescence is less useful than in pemphigus as the autoantibodies circulate only at very low concentration. It is positive in just more than half of cases. Indirect immunofluorescence can be used to differentiate the target antigen by using a substrate of normal skin split along its basement membrane zone by incubation in concentrated salt solution. Whether the autoantibodies bind to the floor or roof of the split gives information on the localisation of the target antigen. Binding to the floor indicates the variant called *epidermolysis bullosa acquisita* (discussed later).

Treatment should be multidisciplinary. Mild disease or disease in remission can often be effectively controlled with topical corticosteroids. Doses are low and without systemic effects, and application in a vacuum-formed tray enhances effectiveness for gingival lesions. Moderate disease requires a high-potency steroid topically or dapsone if this is ineffective. If there is severe oral disease or involvement of other sites, systemic steroids with azathioprine as a steroid-sparing agent are used to induce remission before moving to less potent drugs. Non-responsive disease requires immunosuppressants such as mycophenolate.

Because of the possible risk to sight, ocular examination is necessary if early changes in the eyes are suspected. Minor eye involvement also responds to dapsone, but severe eye disease requires potent immunosuppression with steroids and azathioprine, cyclophosphamide, mycophenolate mofetil or infliximab to induce remission.

General review PMID: 15984952

Treatment PMID: 25953640

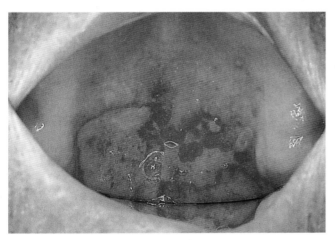

Fig. 16.35 **Mucous membrane pemphigoid.** Typical but more severe oral presentation with persistent erythema and ulceration of the palate.

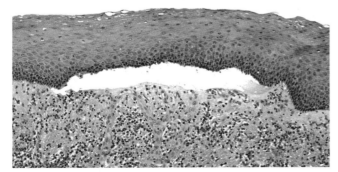

Fig. 16.36 **Mucous membrane pemphigoid.** Biopsy from clinically normal mucosa. The full thickness of the epithelium has separated cleanly from the underlying connective tissue to form a microscopic fluid-filled bulla. The weakened attachment of epithelium to connective tissue has separated with the slight trauma involved in biopsy.

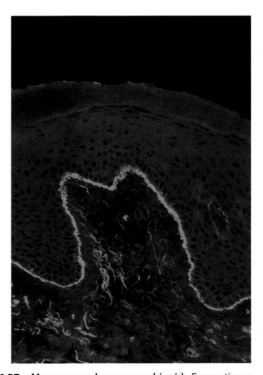

Fig. 16.37 **Mucous membrane pemphigoid.** Frozen tissue stained with fluorescent anti-C3 shows a line of fluorescence along the basement membrane indicating complement activation there. Intact mucosa is required for immunofluorescence, and biopsy is best performed in apparently normal mucosa, not in a lesion. (See Fig. 1.6.).

Bullous pemphigoid

Bullous pemphigoid is the commonest blistering disease of skin. It affects a similar population to mucous membrane pemphigoid, and the signs are similar. However, it affects the mouth in less than 10% of patients, producing similar but transient superficial erosions to mucous membrane pemphigoid, and is treated in the same way. The eye is involved only very rarely.

Other pemphigoid variants

Linear IgA disease or linear IgA bullous dermatosis is a form of pemphigoid in which the autoantibodies binding to the basement membrane are of IgA class. Half of patients have intraoral blistering, and the eye may be involved. It can also arise in children.

Lichen planus pemphigoides is a hybrid condition resembling both lichen planus and pemphigoid, usually affecting the skin and very occasionally the mouth.

Epidermolysis bullosa acquisita is unrelated to the developmental condition epidermolysis bullosa and presents in the same way as bullous pemphigoid. The autoantibodies are directed against the collagen type VII anchoring fibrils below the basement membrane. Both skin and mouth are often involved, and there is a mucosa-predominant form. Oral lesions affect any part of the mouth and resemble the bullae and ulcers in other immunobullous diseases. Desquamative gingivitis is unusual.

Drug-induced pemphigoid may be caused by many drugs, notably vancomycin and other antibiotics, amiodarone, captopril and other anti-hypertensive drugs and non-steroidal anti-inflammatory drugs. Linear IgA disease is particularly frequently drug-associated.

TOOTHPASTE AND MOUTHWASH-INDUCED EPITHELIAL PEELING

Superficial epithelial peeling or desquamation can be mistaken for blistering by patients. It is probably far commoner than is recognized and may be caused by detergents in toothpastes, particularly sodium lauryl sulphate, and is best managed by patient education and acceptance, or changing brand. However, the sloughing is often unnoticed or blamed on astringent or sharp foods. This condition appears to be of no significance, and it is not established whether it is an irritant or allergic phenomenon. The common sites are the lingual alveolar mucosa and buccal mucosa. The main importance is not to overdiagnose this condition as a more significant immunobullous disease. When florid, as for example caused by a mouthwash, it may resemble diffuse keratosis like leukoedema (Ch. 18).

Review PMID: 31246938 and experimental series 8811477

ERYTHEMA MULTIFORME

→ Summary charts 15.2 and 16.2 pp. 280, 311

This mucocutaneous hypersensitivity reaction affects the mouth in many cases and, in patients presenting to dentists, oral lesions may be the only sign. Erythema multiforme is one of the few causes of *recurrent* oral ulceration and also produces blisters.

Aetiology

Though the mechanism is unclear, erythema multiforme appears to be a cell-mediated hypersensitivity reaction. It is

Box 16.15   Triggers for erythema multiforme

- *Herpes simplex* infection, usually a cold sore
- Genital recurrent herpes
- Mycoplasmal pneumonia
- *Varicella zoster* infections
- Rarely drugs; penicillins, barbiturates, sulphonamides, allopurinol and others

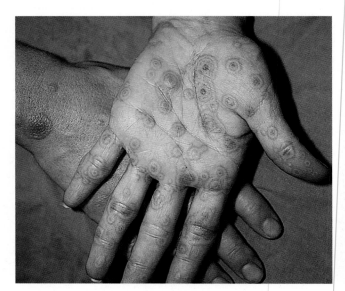

Fig. 16.38   Typical target lesions on the skin in erythema multiforme. *(From Swartz M, 2014. Textbook of Physical Diagnosis, 7th ed. Philadelphia: Saunders)*

more likely in immunosuppression, HIV infection, systemic lupus erythematosus and during radiotherapy and chemotherapy.

Erythema multiforme may be triggered by many agents (Box 16.15), but 90% of attacks are precipitated by an infection, usually *Herpes simplex* infection. Patients with herpes infections as the trigger have a genetic predisposition, the HLA-DQw3 allele. The triggering agent is not present in lesions, they result from a cross reacting immunological response.

When patients have a triggering stimulus, it is usually present 9–14 days before onset of erythema multiforme.

Clinical

Most patients are aged between 20 and 40 years, with a slight male predominance. Two forms are recognised. In the *minor form*, only skin is involved and this is a relatively mild self-limiting condition. In the *major form* there are florid lesions on skin and oral, nasal and genital mucosae.

There is acute onset, sometimes preceded by vague arthralgia or slight fever for a day in the major form. Then the characteristic 'target' lesions may appear (Fig. 16.38), initially on arms and legs and spreading to the trunk. Each is a well-defined red macule a centimetre or more in diameter. During a period of a few hours to days, the centre becomes raised, with a bluish cyanotic centre. In severe cases, skin lesions blister and ulcerate centrally. New crops of lesions develop during a period of approximately 10 days. However, classical target lesions are often absent and the rash is very variable (Fig 16.39). Oral and lip lesions appear a few days

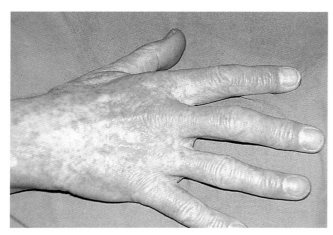

Fig. 16.39   Erythema multiforme. As the name suggests, the rash is variable and here shows only patchy erythema.

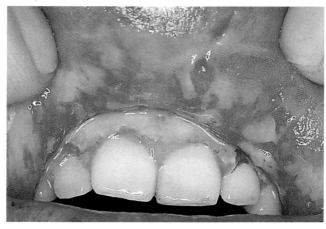

Fig. 16.41   Erythema multiforme. There is ulceration, erythema, sloughing of epithelium and a small vesicle centrally. The anterior part of the mouth and the lips are typically affected.

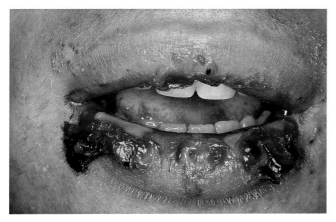

Fig. 16.40   Erythema multiforme. Ulceration of the vermilion of the lip with bleeding, swelling and crusting is characteristic.

> **Box 16.16   Erythema multiforme: typical clinical features**
>
> - Adolescents or young adults, particularly males, mainly affected
> - Lips frequently grossly swollen, split, crusted and bleeding
> - Widespread irregular fibrin-covered erosions and erythema in the mouth
> - Conjunctivitis may be associated
> - Cutaneous target lesions or erythematous patches
> - Attacks may recur at intervals of several months
> - Recurrent but usually ultimately self-limiting

into the attack, most commonly anteriorly in the mouth on the buccal and labial mucosa and tongue. Target lesions are not seen intraorally; the oral lesions are inflamed patches with irregular blistering and broad, shallow irregular ulcers (Figs 16.40 and 16.41). On the lips, fibrin oozes continually from the inflamed tissues and forms haemorrhagic crusts. There is severe pain.

Features are summarised in Box 16.16 .

General review PMID: 22788803

Oral review PMID: 17767983 and 24034067

Difference from Stevens Johnson PMID: 7741539 and 15567361

Diagnosis and management

Diagnosis relies on the typical presentation, history of previous recurrent episodes and a trigger, if present. When only the mouth is involved, a biopsy may be required, but the appearances are very variable and this aids most by excluding alternative causes, particularly pemphigus.

The histological appearances are variable. There are lymphocytes below the epithelium and basal cell degeneration with apoptosis similar to that in lichen planus, but with additional acute inflammation and accumulation of oedema fluid in and below the epithelium, producing intraepithelial vesicles or bullae (Figs 16.42 and 16.43).

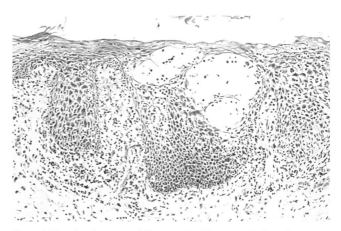

Fig. 16.42   Erythema multiforme. In this example there is necrosis of prickle cells, producing intraepithelial vesicles, much oedema but few inflammatory cells.

The attack usually lasts for 3 or 4 weeks and is self-limiting without treatment in the minor form. Oral lesions are painful, interfere with eating and fluid intake must be maintained. Unless already resolving, lesions seem to benefit from treatment with corticosteroids. A short reducing dose of prednisolone starting at around 60 mg/day for 3 days, tapering off over a week, is frequently given but has no good evidence base. Chlorhexidine will prevent

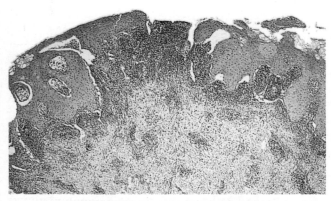

Fig. 16.43   Erythema multiforme. In this example there is a dense inflammatory infiltrate immediately below the epithelium and around blood vessels in the deeper corium. The epithelium is separating from the connective tissue, here along the basement membrane, and there is ulceration centrally.

secondary mucosal infection and maintain gingival health while tooth brushing is impossible. Eye lesions require specialist treatment.

Recurrences, usually at intervals of several months, for a year or two are characteristic and are sometimes increasingly severe. An attempt should be made to identify the trigger, though often none is identifiable. It is considered that recurrent *Herpes simplex* infections trigger most cases, and whether or not this can be confirmed, treatment with continuous aciclovir for several months will suppress any triggering infection and confirm the link. In patients who have only oral lesions, mycoplasmal infection should be suspected and suppressed instead.

Web URL 16.1 Treatment: http://emedicine.medscape.com/article/1122915-treatment

Web URL 16.2 Guideline: http://www.pcds.org.uk/clinical-guidance/erythema-multiforme

STEVENS JOHNSON SYNDROME

→ Summary charts 15.2, 16.2 pp. 280, 311

This severe hypersensitivity reaction has many features in common with erythema multiforme but is now considered a separate entity based on its severity, extent and causes. Toxic epidermal necrolysis is the name given to its most severe presentation. The mouth is always involved.

Unlike erythema multiforme, the trigger is usually a drug and sometimes mycoplasmal infection. Many drugs are implicated, but the most frequent causes are sulphonamides, allopurinol, and anticonvulsants. Some genetic predispositions are known for individual drugs.

Skin lesions are erythematous patches, target lesions or raised blisters that break down into ulcers with widespread detachment and loss of epithelium, sometimes in large sheets. Other organs may also be involved. Histopathology shows necrosis of the whole skin thickness by apoptosis with little inflammation.

Treatment is controversial, with immunosuppressants, ciclosporin and antibiotics to control skin infection and cessation of causative drugs. There is a high risk of death when the area of skin involved in toxic epidermal necrolysis is great.

Review PMID: 26769645

Treatment guideline PMID: 27317286

OTHER MUCOSAL ALLERGIC RESPONSES

Oral mucosa is rarely the site of allergic responses. Oral allergy syndrome is discussed in the next chapter.

Allergic stomatitis PMID: 1437060

ORAL SIGNS IN REACTIVE ARTHRITIS

The 'classical' presentation of reactive arthritis, previously known as Reiter's disease, comprises arthritis, urethritis and conjunctivitis. Sexually transmitted *Chlamydia* infection or gut infections such as with *Salmonella sp.* or *Shigella sp.* usually precede arthritis by about 1–3 weeks. Patients are typically males between the ages of 20 and 40 years; 80% of them are HLA-B27 positive. Pain and swelling typically affect the knees, ankles and feet.

Antibiotics are given to eliminate the gut or other triggering infections; non-steroidal anti-inflammatory drugs are frequently effective for controlling joint pain. The disease may be self-limiting or recurrent and progressively debilitating.

Dental aspects

The temporomandibular joints can be involved with erosions but are not a major source of symptoms.

Oral manifestations develop in 15% of patients and are characteristic and consist of scalloped or circinate white lines somewhat resembling erythema migrans but involving all or any part of the mouth and the genital mucosa (Fig. 16.44). In other cases, there may be shallow erosions. Oral lesions are typically painless and frequently unnoticed.

General review: 18436339

Cases PMID: 34391335 and 35620277

KAWASAKI'S DISEASE (MUCOCUTANEOUS LYMPH NODE SYNDROME)

Kawasaki's disease is a self-limiting necrotising systemic vasculitis of children with a particular propensity to attack the coronary arteries. It presents with stomatitis and cervical lymphadenopathy.

Kawasaki's disease is endemic in Japan, Taiwan, Korea and adjacent countries and affects patients with these genetic backgrounds living elsewhere. It is increasingly recognised in European Caucasian populations and is the leading cause of childhood-acquired heart disease in Europe since the decline of rheumatic fever. It affects 8 in every 100,000 children in the UK.

The aetiology remains unknown. An infection is thought to trigger an immune reaction in people who are genetically predisposed, but many infections are implicated. Small and medium-sized arteries are involved, infiltrated by neutrophils that destroy the elastic lamina and endothelial lining. Inflammation weakens the arteries, which dilate to produce aneurysms, thrombose and may rupture.

The features are summarised in Box 16.17.

In a dental setting, presentation mimics childhood viral illnesses but the involvement of lips and diffuse erythema of tongue without ulcers are characteristic. The tongue is bright red with prominent papillae, producing the 'strawberry' appearance (Fig. 16.45). The cervical lymphadenopathy is obvious, with nodes palpable and distinctively affecting only one side of the neck anterior to sternomastoid muscle.

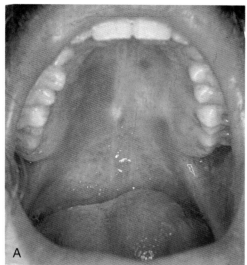

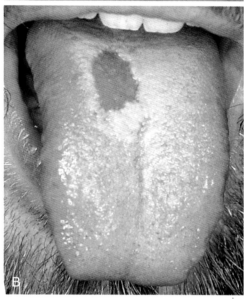

Fig. 16.44 **Reactive arthritis oral signs.** There is erythema and patches of depapillation on the tongue, which when multiple resemble erythema migrans. *(From Fehrnbach, M.J., Phelan, J.A., 2004. Immunity. In: Ibsen, O.A.C., Phelan, J.A. [Eds.], Oral Pathology for the dental hygienist, fourth ed. St Louis, Saunders.)*

Box 16.17   Typical features of Kawasaki's disease

- Children under 5 years old affected
- Fever persisting for more than 5 days
- Marked irritability and malaise ('extreme misery')
- Generalised rash of variable type
- Red, swollen and peeling palms and soles
- Erythematous stomatitis with 'strawberry tongue'
- Swelling and cracking of the lips and pharynx
- Unilateral mass of swollen cervical lymph nodes
- Abdominal symptoms frequently
- Heart involvement in approximately 20%

Almost every kind of rash except blisters can occur, but involvement of the soles and palms with peeling of skin from the tips of fingers and toes is a characteristic, but late, sign (Fig. 16.46).

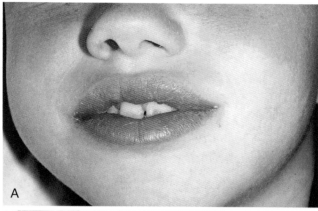

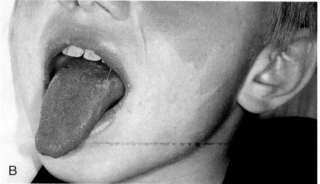

Fig. 16.45 **Kawasaki's disease.** Hyperaemia, crusting and cracking of the lips (A), bright red tongue with prominent papillae (strawberry tongue, B) and facial rash. *(From Paller, A.S., Mancini, A.J., 2016. Vasculitic disorders. In: Paller, A.S., Mancini, A.J. Hurwitz clinical pediatric dermatology. Elsevier, Amsterdam, pp. 495-508.e3.)*

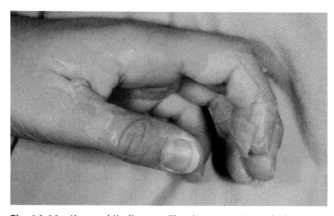

Fig. 16.46 **Kawasaki's disease.** The desquamative rash that characteristically affects the fingers and toes and perineum 7–10 days after onset of fever. The fingers are red and swollen before peeling starts. *(From Baselga, E., Hernandez-Martin, A., Torrelo, A., 2015. Immunologic, reactive, and purpuric disorders. In: Eichenfield, L.F., Frieden, I.J., Mathes, E.F., Zaenglein, A.L. [Eds.], Neonatal and infant dermatology. Saunders, Philadelphia, pp. 303-335.e10.)*

Oral changes arise early in the disease. Suspected cases should be referred to hospital urgently without waiting to see whether the fever persists more than 5 days, usually considered a required diagnostic criterion. Some patients have incomplete presentations with no fever, so a high index of suspicion is required as cardiac vessel damage occurs a week after onset.

There is no diagnostic test and the diagnosis must be based on clinical features. Intravenous immunoglobulin and steroids are the main treatment. Aspirin is still used despite the risk of Reye's syndrome but without evidence of effect. Tumour necrosis factor blockade with infliximab is experimental but shows promise. Oral lesions are treated symptomatically. Recovery takes many weeks or months, and the significant complications are coronary artery aneurysms and myocardial infarction. Treatment significantly reduces these complications, and early recognition and referral could be life-saving. The overall mortality is around 1%.

General review: 30619784

Dental presentation PMID: 10230100 and 2717153

Treatment PMID: 35403975 and 35257507

MULTISYSTEM INFLAMMATORY SYNDROME IN CHILDREN

A clinically similar condition to Kawasaki disease increased in incidence during and after the COVID-19 pandemic. It has identical oral signs, lacks the lymphadenopathy and hand skin signs of Kawasaki disease and has variable additional features including abdominal pain and diarrhoea, headache and vomiting. Initially considered to be Kawasaki disease, it is now called multisystemic inflammatory syndrome in children (MIS-C) and recognised as a sequela of multisystem infection by SARS-CoV-2 virus, often after asymptomatic infection. It carries similar risks of cardiac damage to Kawasaki disease and additional neurological risks. In the dental setting, MIS-C can be recognized by the same oral signs as Kawasaki disease and, similarly, urgent medical referral is indicated. Unlike Kawasaki disease, this condition also affects adults, usually young adults.

Review PMID: 35631077 and oral signs 34792813

Oral reactions to drugs

A great variety of drugs (see Box 16.9, Table 43.1) can cause mucosal reactions, either as local effects or through systemic mechanisms that are often obscure. Systemically-mediated reactions include ulceration, lichenoid reactions and erythema multiforme.

More uncommon mucocutaneous diseases

In many of these conditions, the oral lesions are rare or insignificant in comparison with the skin disease (Table 16.5).

Table 16.5 Some uncommon mucosal diseases

Disease	Cause	Oral features	Treatment
Epidermolysis bullosa **PMID: 19945630 and 34838879**	Autosomal recessive – gravis type due to type VII collagen defect (junctional type usually lethal at birth)	Subepithelial bullae leading to severe intraoral scarring after minimal trauma especially in recessive types	None wholly effective. Protect against any mucosal abrasion
Pyostomatitis vegetans **PMID: 14723710 and 19242389**	Complication of inflammatory bowel disease particularly ulcerative colitis	Yellowish miliary pustules in thickened erythematous mucosa release pus, leaving shallow ulcers. Suprabasal clefting and intraepithelial vesiculation or abscesses containing eosinophils. Peripheral eosinophilia up to 20% of white cells	Control of inflammatory bowel disease or systemic prednisolone
Gonorrhoea **PMID: 806627**	N. gonorrhoeae sexually transmitted	Oropharyngeal erythema or ulcers, rarely seen	Requires specialist referral
Leprosy **PMID: 17223587 and 17119765**	Mycobacterium leprae	Oral ulcers or nodules. Seen mainly in Asia	Dapsone
Keratosis follicularis (Darier's disease; warty dyskeratoma) **PMID: 1931295**	Genetic. Autosomal dominant	Intraepithelial bullae containing granulocytes and acantholytic cells Pebbly lesions mainly of palate due to hyperkeratosis, acantholysis with 'corps ronds' and 'grains' (dyskeratosis) May affect posterior buccal mucosa around the parotid papilla, causing bilateral parotid duct stenosis at the opening	Oral lesions not troublesome but respond to retinoids

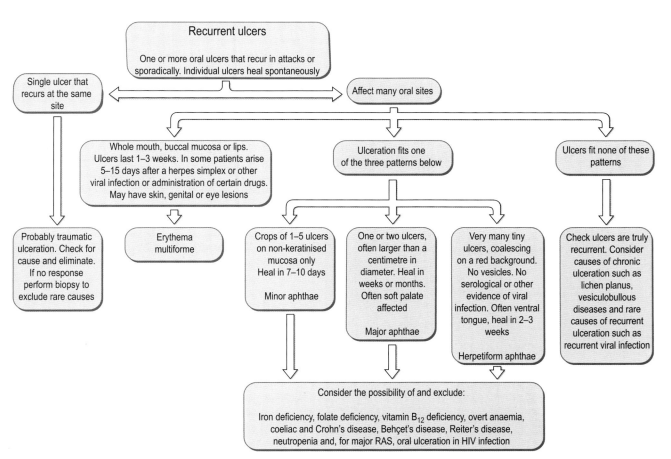

Summary chart 16.2 Differential diagnosis of the common causes of recurrent oral ulceration.

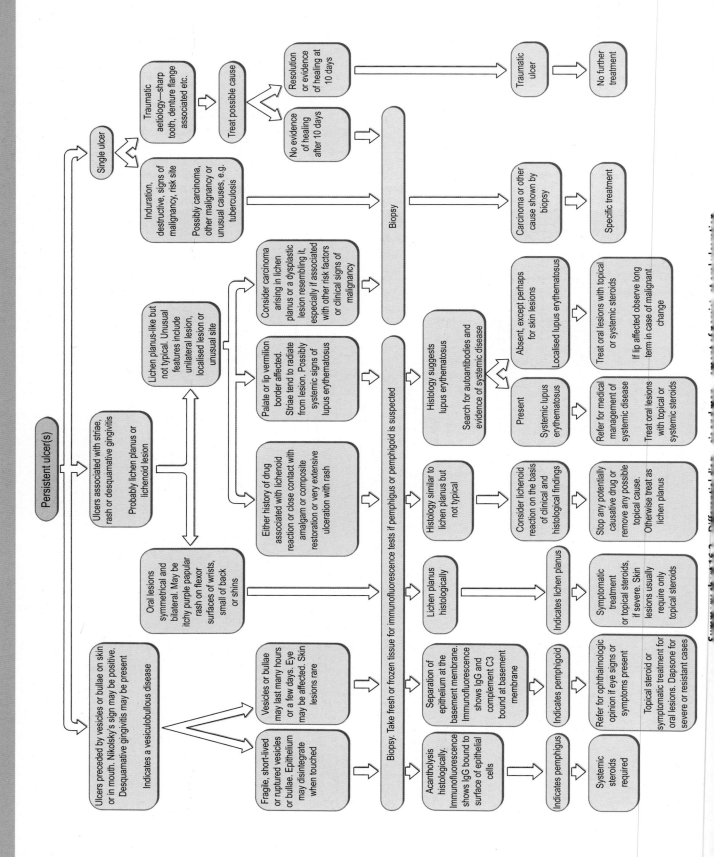

Persistent ulcer(s)

Single ulcer

Traumatic aetiology—sharp tooth, denture flange associated etc.

Treat possible cause

Resolution or evidence of healing at 10 days → Traumatic ulcer → No further treatment

No evidence of healing after 10 days

Induration, destructive, signs of malignancy, risk site

Possibly carcinoma, other malignancy or unusual causes, e.g. tuberculosis

Biopsy → Carcinoma or other cause shown by biopsy → Specific treatment

Ulcers associated with striae, rash or desquamative gingivitis

Probably lichen planus or lichenoid lesion

Lichen planus-like but not typical. Unusual features include unilateral lesion, localised lesion or unusual site

Consider carcinoma arising in lichen planus or a dysplastic lesion resembling it, especially if associated with other risk factors or clinical signs of malignancy

Palate or lip vermilion border affected. Striae tend to radiate from lesion. Possibly systemic signs of lupus erythematosus

Histology suggests lupus erythematosus

Search for autoantibodies and evidence of systemic disease

Absent, except perhaps for skin lesions

Localised lupus erythematosus

Treat oral lesions with topical or systemic steroids

If lip affected observe long term in case of malignant change

Present

Systemic lupus erythematosus

Refer for medical management of systemic disease

Treat oral lesions with topical or systemic steroids

Either history of drug associated with lichenoid reaction or close contact with amalgam or composite restoration or very extensive ulceration with rash

Histology similar to lichen planus but not typical

Consider lichenoid reaction on the basis of clinical and histological findings

Stop any potentially causative drug or remove any possible topical cause. Otherwise treat as lichen planus

Oral lesions symmetrical and bilateral. May be itchy purple papular rash on flexor surfaces of wrists, small of back or shins

Lichen planus histologically

Indicates lichen planus

Symptomatic treatment or topical steroids, if severe. Skin lesions usually require only topical steroids

Ulcers preceded by vesicles or bullae on skin or in mouth. Nikolsky's sign may be positive. Desquamative gingivitis may be present

Indicates a vesiculobullous disease

Vesicles or bullae may last many hours or a few days. Eye may be affected. Skin lesions rare

Biopsy. Take fresh or frozen tissue for immunofluorescence tests if pemphigus or pemphigoid is suspected

Separation of epithelium at the basement membrane. Immunofluorescence shows IgG and complement C3 bound at basement membrane

Indicates pemphigoid

Refer for ophthalmologic opinion if eye signs or symptoms present

Topical steroid or symptomatic treatment for oral lesions. Dapsone for severe or resistant cases

Fragile, short-lived or ruptured vesicles or bullae. Epithelium may disintegrate when touched

Acantholysis histologically. Immunofluorescence shows IgG bound to surface of epithelial cells

Indicates pemphigus

Systemic steroids required

Appendix 16.1

Treatment for aphthous stomatitis

- Exclude underlying causes, e.g. iron, vitamin B_{12} and folate deficiency. Treat these first
- Exclude possibility of Behçet's disease; if likely, refer to specialist centre
- Select treatments appropriate to severity and patients' expectations of treatment. Patients may need to try several treatments before they find one that works well for them
- Before drug treatment, reassure patients that aphthous stomatitis is common, not serious but troublesome with no significance for general health. Advise to avoid spicy, sharp and salty food and acid and carbonated drinks (or use a straw) when ulcers are present. Such reassurance and advice may be sufficient for those with only occasional ulcers
- Select a treatment from those discussed in the following table. Those in the darker shaded boxes are not suitable for treatment in general dental practice because of the need to monitor for adverse effects but could be prescribed in conjunction with the patient's medical practitioner
- Preparations marked * are available without prescription in the UK
- Note that children less than 6 years old cannot rinse and expectorate effectively

Treatment	Instructions	Indication/problems
Covering agents, e.g. carboxymethylcellulose paste (Orabase)*, carmellose sodium*	Apply QDS* to dried areas around ulcer with moist finger. Allow film to hydrate before contact with adjacent mucosa. Use as required	Infrequent ulcers anteriorly in sulci, ideally single ulcers. Handling is difficult, patient must be dextrous. Unpleasant texture and taste Symptomatic treatment only by protecting ulcer
Topical gels, e.g. Carbenoxolone (Bioral)*, choline salicylate (Bonjela)*, dyclonine, aminacrine and lignocaine (various)*	Use according to manufacturer's instructions	Ulcers must be accessible. Carbenoxolone is claimed to speed healing, but the others are symptomatic treatments only. Choline salicylate is not associated with Reye's syndrome and may be used in children. Large amounts can cause salicylate poisoning in small children
Mouthwashes, e.g. obtundents (benzydamine)* or antiseptics (chlorhexidine)*	Use according to manufacturer's instructions Hold in mouth for 1–2 minutes for maximum effect	Infrequent ulcers or crops of ulcers (recurring 6-weekly), useful when ulcers are widely separated around the mouth or inaccessible to pastes and gels. Benzydamine is a symptomatic treatment only. Antiseptics may shorten healing time, presumably by reducing bacterial colonisation of the ulcer surface. Benzydamine may sting and chlorhexidine has unpleasant taste and causes staining
Low-potency steroid, e.g. hydrocortisone adhesive mucosal tablets 2.5 mg	Hold pellet on ulcer and allow to dissolve in contact, QDS	Single ulcers or crops of clustered ulcers. Ulcer must be accessible, usually in sulcus. No significant adverse effects, safe in children. If used regularly have slight therapeutic effect and may reduce recurrence Apply as soon as prodromal symptoms start if possible
Tetracycline mouthwash	Dissolve *soluble* tetracycline capsule contents (very few preparations available) 250 mg in 5–10 mL water and rinse for 2–3 minutes QDS 5 days	Only useful for herpetiform ulceration. Not for those aged less than 16 years. Long courses predispose to candidosis
Steroid aerosols, e.g. beclomethasone dipropionate (100 micrograms/puff)	1 puff per ulcer QDS max, maximum 8 puffs per day	Useful to deliver potent steroids to inaccessible areas, e.g. oropharynx. Spreads dose fairly widely and therefore more useful in widespread ulceration from lichen planus than in RAS. Risk of steroid adverse effects with prolonged use
Steroid mouthwash, e.g. betamethasone sodium phosphate	Dissolve 0.5 mg in 5 mL water and rinse for 2–3 minutes QDS from onset of prodrome and while ulcer or symptoms present. For severe ulceration may be used six times daily	Useful for widespread ulcers and when severity merits potent therapeutic treatment, e.g. crops of ulcers 6-weekly or more frequently, RAS major or severe pain. Significant risk of steroid adverse effects with prolonged use – important to spit out after use. In severe cases, dose may be swallowed for a short period for additional systemic effect
Systemic drugs, e.g. steroids, azathioprine, colchicine, thalidomide, intralesional steroid injection (major RAS only)	Various regimes	Reserved for the most severe minor RAS, major RAS and ulcers refractory to other treatments. Colchicine and thalidomide are particularly effective in Behçet's disease and RAS major Significant risk of adverse effects – reserved for treatment in specialist centres

* *QDS, Quater in die sumendus*, meaning take four times a day.

Tongue disorders | 17

The tongue can be involved in generalised stomatitis, as discussed in the previous chapter, but is also the site of lesions or the source of symptoms peculiar to itself. Soreness limited to the tongue has few causes (Box 17.1). Patterns of tongue fur, fissures, indentations of the teeth and other tongue markings have many associations with systemic disease in folklore and traditional medicine, but without a good evidence base.

Odd tongues, epidemiology PMID: 3466199

NORMAL STRUCTURES

The tongue is easily visible, and normal structures may concern patients and healthcare professionals.

Furred tongue

Some degree of furring is normal, caused by the filiform papillae and is more intense near the midline and posteriorly. Filiform papillae elongate continually from the base and are abraded by the diet. Bacteria adhere to the keratinised tips much more easily than to other parts of the mucosa, so that increased furring may be associated with a bad taste or halitosis.

Furring is increased in smokers, in many systemic upsets, especially of the gastrointestinal tract, in infections in which the mouth becomes dry and little food is taken, and with age. A furred tongue is often seen in the childhood fevers. Many of these causes are reversible, but a tongue scraper is an effective intervention.

Filiform papillae also become long in black hairy tongue, discussed later.

Foliate papillae

These bilateral, pinkish soft ridges on the lateral borders of the tongue contain taste buds and minor oral tonsils forming part of Waldeyer's ring. They lie at the junction of the anterior two-thirds and the posterior third and sometimes become hyperplastic or inflamed and sore (see Figs 1.1 and 1.2).

Sublingual varices

Dilated tortuous veins are considered almost normal along the ventral surface of the tongue, affect almost two-thirds of adults and become more prominent with age (Fig. 17.1). They lie superficially and raise the covering thin mucosa into soft sessile nodules and generally cause no problems, being only extremely rarely the site of thrombus formation. They are almost never the origin of significant bleeding.

However, development of varices is probably related to increased central venous pressure and there is an association between the presence of varices and hypertension, diabetes, hyperlipidaemia, obesity and smoking.

Case series PMID: 19540027

Disease associations: PMID: 35498559

HAMARTOMAS AND DEVELOPMENTAL ANOMALIES

The tongue is the site of many developmental anomalies due to its complex embryology. These usually present in early childhood as a mass and may interfere with feeding or the airway. Some are partly or completely cystic. The most frequent site is the posterior dorsum, followed by the ventral and mid tongue inferiorly. These lesions may include salivary tissue, smooth muscle, blood vessels, gastric mucosa, respiratory or squamous epithelium and very occasionally cartilage. Some are true hamartomas and others choristomas.

The superficial muscle and mucosa of the tongue is a common site for lymphangiomas (Ch. 25). The thyroglossal tract descends through the tongue and may leave ectopic thyroid tissue on or in the tongue (Ch. 37) or epithelial residues that form thyroglossal cysts (Ch. 10). The sublingual dermoid is a developmental cyst below the tongue (Ch. 10). Cysts with gastric or other intestinal mucosal lining are called lingual foregut cysts and those with respiratory

---

Box 17.1   Clinical presentations of sore tongue

- Glossitis
  - Anaemia
  - Candidal infection
- Burning tongue and burning mouth 'syndrome'
- Erythema migrans
- Lingual nerve injury, usually after third molar surgery
- Neurological pain affecting lingual nerve (Ch. 39)

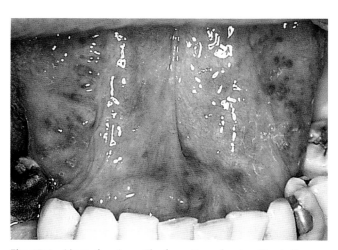

Fig. 17.1   Lingual varices. The formation of varicosities in the vessels of the undersurface of tongue and floor of mouth is a common finding with age. These are relatively small varices.

epithelium are called respiratory cysts, though in practice these rare cysts are often mixed in type.

All these developmental lesions can be excised conservatively and do not recur.

Review lingual hamartomas PMID: 36241602

Lingual respiratory cyst PMID: 29929866

Foregut cyst PMID: 28595986

ERYTHEMA MIGRANS

→ Summary charts 19.1 and 19.3 pp. 347, 349

This common benign condition usually affects only the tongue, producing an appearance likened to a map of the world on the dorsum, hence its alternative common name of *geographic tongue*.

The cause is unknown, and the condition is very common. Approximately 2% of the population are affected at any one time, but more than 20% will have an episode at some time in their life. It is seen at all ages but seems more frequent in young and middle age. There is a familial tendency.

The condition has been postulated to be a manifestation of twenty or more diseases, but no association withstands scrutiny. One that is widely accepted in medical circles is that erythema migrans may be a subclinical manifestation of psoriasis, partly based on histological similarities. This remains unsubstantiated, and several lines of evidence suggest this is incorrect.

Clinically, there are irregular, smooth, red areas on the dorsal tongue caused by loss of filiform papillae. Each patch starts as a small area on or near the lateral border and extends for a few days before healing, only to appear again in another area forming a moving pattern of white lines. The patches have a curved or semicircular shape centred on the lateral margin, a red rim and an enhanced white line around the edge. Several of these areas often coalesce to form a scalloped or geographic pattern (Figs 17.2 and 17.3). While lesions expand, they heal by regrowth of filiform papillae from the centre, and the moving pattern over a period of weeks confirms the diagnosis.

Histologically, the centre of the patch shows thinning of the epithelium with loss of filiform papillae. At the periphery the epithelium has a zone of hyperplasia with long rete ridges and dense infiltration by neutrophils forming microabscesses in the superficial layers (Fig. 17.4). This keratin is seen clinically as the white line around the margin. The superficial layers of epithelium die and desquamate, enlarging the central atrophic zone and enlarging the patch.

Most patients have no symptoms, but some complain of soreness, probably a result of epithelial thinning and inflammation. In such cases reassurance and precautionary exclusion of subclinical anaemia is prudent. Because there is no effective treatment, avoidance of spicy or astringent foods and toothpaste during the active phase is usually all that can be suggested. After a period, the condition usually resolves, sometimes for long periods, but in most patients it is transient but recurs intermittently for decades.

In a small minority of patients, other oral mucosae can be affected. The changes are not so obvious because there are no filiform papillae to lose, but the annular pattern of slowly moving white lines is the same. Buccal and labial mucosa are the typical unusual sites and the tongue is not necessarily involved synchronously.

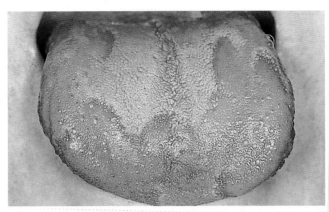

Fig. 17.2 Erythema migrans. Typical appearance with irregular depapillated patches centred on the lateral border of the tongue. Each patch has a narrow red and white rim.

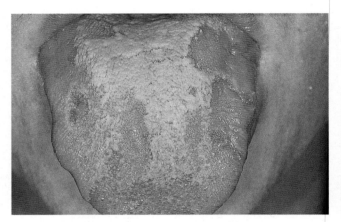

Fig. 17.3 Erythema migrans. The change of pattern can be seen, on a later occasion, in the same patient as in Fig. 17.2.

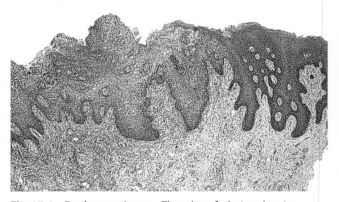

Fig. 17.4 Erythema migrans. The edge of a lesion showing normal mucosa to the right and, to the left, the zone of epithelium densely infiltrated by neutrophils that is visible clinically as the white line. This epithelium heaped up superficially at the advancing edge will be shed, leaving the depapillated red patch.

Erythema migrans is unrelated to the rash of Lyme disease called *erythema chronicum migrans*. A very similar pattern of circinate lines is seen throughout the mouth in reactive arthropathy (Ch. 16).

Features PMID: 1804987

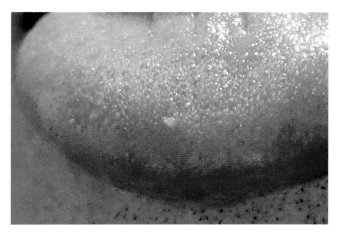

Fig. 17.5 Lingual papillitis. One fungiform papilla appears white and is intensely painful.

LINGUAL PAPILLITIS

This condition, also known as *transient lingual papillitis* or *fungiform papillitis*, is very common in the population, but patients rarely seek treatment. One or a cluster of fungiform papillae become slightly swollen, white and intensely painful to touch (Fig. 17.5). The condition resolves spontaneously after a few days, sometimes after only one, and without an ulcer developing. The cause is unknown, but trauma and certain foods are usually blamed. An association with atopy is not confirmed. A few patients have more diffuse involvement.

Biopsy does not aid diagnosis and shows non-specific inflammatory changes.

Description PMID: 8899785 and 28149482

HAIRY TONGUE AND BLACK HAIRY TONGUE

The filiform papillae can become long and hair-like, forming a thick fur on the dorsum of the tongue. The filaments may be several millimetres long.

There is no clear distinction between a furred tongue and hairy tongue; this is a matter of degree. Hairy tongue is quite common, affecting as much as 1% of the population, and is commoner in heavy smokers and adults. No cause is known, but some patients report acute onset after radiotherapy, a stressful life event, debilitating illness or one of a variety of drugs, often chemotherapy drugs.

The condition is more marked down the centre of the anterior tongue. The colour of the 'hairs' ranges from pale brown to black in colour (Fig. 17.6). When the papillae are dark brown or black, the cause is colonization by adherent pigment-producing bacteria. Onset of dark colour can follow antibiotic treatment that disturbs the normal ecology of the oral flora, allowing overgrowth of pigmented species. Like a furred tongue, trapping of food particles and adherent bacteria may produce halitosis and a bad taste. Otherwise, the condition is asymptomatic, although papillae may be long enough to trigger gagging in susceptible patients.

Treatment is difficult. Pale hairy tongue may be mistaken for candidosis, but treatment with antifungals is inappropriate and ineffective. Tongue scraping is the best solution, with measures to reduce predisposing causes such as smoking or xerostomia.

Review PMID: 25152586

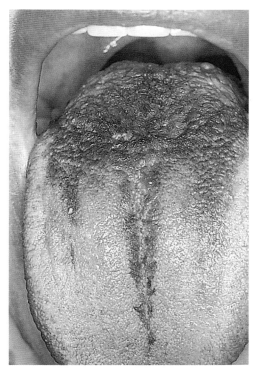

Fig. 17.6 Hairy tongue. In this patient there are numerous elongate papillae but a brown rather than black pigmentation.

Black tongue

The dorsum of the tongue may sometimes become black without overgrowth of the papillae. This may be staining due to drugs, such as iron compounds used for the treatment of anaemia or bismuth from antacid preparations, but is then transient. Occasionally, the sucking of antiseptic lozenges causes the tongue to become black through overgrowth of pigment-producing organisms. Chlorhexidine mouthwash, coffee and other extrinsic agents also stain the dorsal tongue papillae preferentially.

GLOSSITIS

Glossitis means no more than inflammation of the tongue, but the term is confusingly applied to many conditions, not all of which are inflammatory in origin or particularly inflamed.

Glossitis is used to describe erythematous changes, pain or burning, but these can also result from epithelial atrophy and several specific diseases.

Causes of glossitis are listed in Box 17.2, and anaemia is discussed in Chapter 28.

ANAEMIC GLOSSITIS

A red, smooth and sore tongue is particularly characteristic of anaemia, but anaemic patients may also have an asymptomatic red tongue or a normally appearing but sore tongue. A high index of suspicion for anaemia must therefore be maintained when dealing with tongue symptoms.

The cause of symptoms is atrophy of the epithelium, which becomes thin and loses its filiform papillae, and therefore the only keratinised parts of its surface. It then appears smooth and red.

The possibility that candidosis, predisposed to by anaemia, might cause some of the oral symptoms should also be considered. Patchy red zones suggest candidosis; the atrophy of anaemia is more widespread.

Iron deficiency

Three-quarters of patients with established iron deficiency have a painful tongue, and about a quarter have an atrophic tongue. Conversely, only 15% of patients with glossitis or soreness of the tongue are iron deficient when assessed by haemoglobin levels and reduced mean red cell volume. More sensitive measures of iron deficiency such as ferritin levels reveal deficiency before anaemia develops, and such subclinical deficiency is commonly found when the tongue is sore or atrophic. It is also common in the healthy population without symptoms, but individuals with a sore tongue are likely to benefit from supplementation.

The glossitis is mild, with minimal redness and loss of papillae around the outside of the dorsal surface (Fig. 17.7). There is often angular cheilitis associated.

Treatment is by supplementation. In severe cases there is rapid resolution of signs and symptoms with regrowth of papillae in a month, but mild cases require several months supplementation and respond slowly.

Though dietary deficiency is common, all patients with these signs or confirmed deficiency should be investigated for a cause of blood loss. The sore tongue may herald no more than menstrual loss or haemorrhoids, but occasionally signals loss from an intestinal carcinoma or other significant cause. Blood loss is a more likely cause in adult males.

Pain and iron deficiency PMID: 10555095 and 15583540

Paterson Kelly (Paterson Brown-Kelly) syndrome

This combination of iron deficiency, dysphagia and a post cricoid oesophageal stricture is known as Plummer-Vinson syndrome in the United States. It affects middle-aged women. Glossitis and angular cheilitis and obvious systemic signs of anaemia are usual.

Several decades ago the syndrome was found in 7% of patients with overt iron deficiency, but it has reduced in incidence dramatically and is now extremely rare. Its main significance is the association with subsequent carcinoma of the pharynx and oesophagus.

Review PMID: 16978405

B group vitamin deficiency

Glossitis of vitamin B_{12} deficiency is particularly florid, and the tongue is described as 'beefy' (Fig. 17.8). However, as with iron, subclinical deficiency can cause burning and

lingual discomfort and often there are no obvious signs (Fig. 17.9). More than half of patients with a new diagnosis of pernicious anaemia have glossitis on presentation, but less than 10% of patients with glossitis have B_{12} deficiency. Patients may have macrocytosis without overt anaemia. If macrocytosis or deficiency are proven, symptoms usually

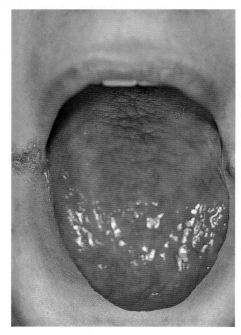

Fig. 17.7   Glossitis in iron-deficiency anaemia. The tongue is smooth, due to atrophy of the papillae, and is red and sore. Anaemia is the most common diagnosable cause of glossitis and must always be looked for by haematological examination. Note also the angular cheilitis, which is also associated with iron deficiency (Ch. 15).

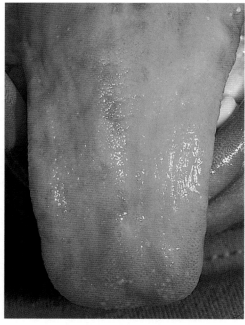

Fig. 17.8 B_{12} deficiency. The tongue has generalised depapillation and toward the tip the typical 'beefy' appearance of severe deficiency. *(From Tersak, J.M., Malatack, J.J., Ritchey, A.K., 2002. Haematology and oncology. In: Zitelli, B.J., Davis, H.W. [Eds.], Atlas of Pediatric Physical Diagnosis, fourth ed. Mosby, St Louis.)*

Box 17.2   Causes of glossitis

Common causes

- Anaemia
- Vitamin B group deficiencies (especially B_{12})
- Erythema migrans
- Candidosis and median rhomboid glossitis (Ch. 15)
- Lichen planus (Ch. 16)

Rare causes

- Bacterial infection or commensal overgrowth
- Scarlet fever (streptococcal infection)
- Kawasaki disease (Ch. 16)
- Glucagon secreting pancreatic tumours
- Syphilitic glossitis of tertiary syphilis (Ch. 15)

resolve on supplementation by injection, pain rapidly and filiform papillae in a month or so.

The underlying cause is usually an absorption defect rather than dietary deficiency. B_{12} deficiency is a particular risk after stomach bypass or other bariatric surgical procedures that remove stomach mucosa, reducing intrinsic factor production. Other causes include proton pump inhibitors such as omeprazole, because they reduce stomach acidity, metformin, many antibiotics used long-term, atrophic gastritis, small intestinal disease such as Crohn's disease, alcoholism and autoimmune diseases such as Grave's disease. The most common cause is lack of intrinsic factor in pernicious anaemia.

An increasing cause of deficiency in younger people is recreational nitrous oxide inhalation.

Folic acid ('folate', vitamin B_9) deficiency is the third most common deficiency to be associated with glossitis, affecting 2%–4% of patients. Again, subclinical deficiency can cause the signs and symptoms, and overt anaemia may not be present. Serum folate levels indicate the deficiency; red cell folate level reflects total body stores and is a second-line test. Treatment is by dietary adjustment, it being difficult to be folate deficient in developed countries as many foods are supplemented. Deficiency tends to affect people who are very old or have alcoholism. Folic acid supplementation may be useful in these cases of overt anaemia, provided B_{12} deficiency is excluded first because folate supplementation in B_{12} deficiency could precipitate significant neurological damage.

Riboflavin (vitamin B_2) deficiency classically causes glossitis with angular stomatitis and these may also be seen less frequently in **nicotinic acid** (Niacin, vitamin B_3) deficiency, but both are rare.

Blind prescribing or self-medicating with B vitamins for oral symptoms in an otherwise healthy patient is virtually invariably ineffective, and investigation is required for all cases with these signs or symptoms.

General review nutritional deficiency PMID: 2693058, 19735964 and 15583540

B_{12} case report PMID: 17209796

Subclinical B_{12} deficiency PMID: 8600284

GLOSSODYNIA AND THE SORE, PHYSICALLY NORMAL TONGUE

The presentation of burning tongue creates some of the most difficult problems in diagnosis and treatment. The symptoms are frequently part of the spectrum of burning mouth syndrome and atypical facial pain, but it is essential to exclude organic disease, particularly a haematological deficiency. These conditions are dealt with together in Chapter 39.

MACROGLOSSIA

Important causes of an enlarged tongue, as opposed to a mass within or on the tongue, are summarised in Box 17.3. In many syndromes and in patients with poor neuromuscular control or muscle tone, the tongue may appear large, but be of normal size with a forward posture.

AMYLOIDOSIS

Amyloidosis is the deposition in the tissues of an abnormal protein with characteristic staining properties. Several different proteins can deposit as amyloid, which requires the molecules to align closely together and bind to form an insoluble and undegradable mass.

The amyloid protein may deposit at the site of its production or circulate to deposit in remote sites, usually the kidneys, around nerves, joints and in some organs. This interferes with function and can lead to organ failure.

In the head and neck, amyloid of AL type (formed from immunoglobulin light chains) is commonly deposited in the tongue where it almost always signifies myeloma or a pre-myeloma plasma cell disorder (Ch. 12). Small deposits form asymptomatic nodules, usually along the lateral borders, but more extensive amyloidosis makes the tongue enlarged and stiff, affecting speech and eating (Figs 17.11 and 17.12). The tongue then feels firm and the mucosa appears pale and yellowish as surface blood flow is reduced by

---

Box 17.3   Important causes of macroglossia

- Congenital haemangioma or lymphangioma (Fig. 17.10 and Ch. 25)
- Down's syndrome (Ch. 40)
- Congenital hypothyroidism (Ch. 37)
- Acromegaly (Ch. 37)
- Amyloidosis
- Lingual thyroid (Ch. 37)
- Mucopolysaccharidoses

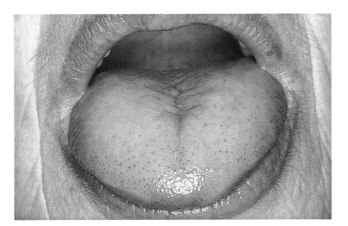

Fig. 17.9   A largely normal-looking but slightly smooth and persistently sore tongue in a patient who had repeated but inadequate haematological investigations that failed to detect early pernicious anaemia.

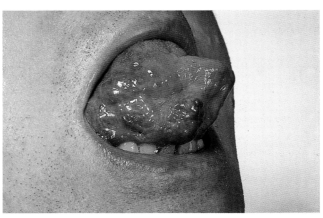

Fig. 17.10   Macroglossia due to a congenital haemangioma.

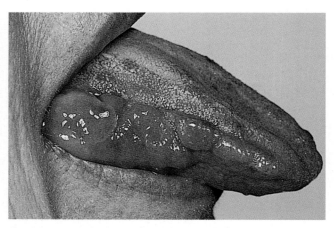

Fig. 17.11 Amyloidosis. These slightly yellow nodules on the lateral border of an enlarged tongue are characteristic of amyloidosis.

deposition around vessels. Vessels cannot constrict properly, and petechiae and ecchymoses are seen in involved mucosa.

Amyloid deposition in salivary glands produces xerostomia.

Management

Biopsy is diagnostic. Amyloid appears as weakly eosinophilic, hyaline homogeneous material replacing the collagen and muscle of the mucosa and tongue and surrounding vessels. Amyloid stains with Congo Red and has a characteristic, usually apple-green, birefringence under polarised light (see Fig. 17.12). Various specialised techniques are used to distinguish the various types of protein that form amyloid (Table 17.1).

Treatment is for the underlying condition, if that is possible. Surgical reduction has been required for massive macroglossia caused by amyloid.

Reviews PMID: 23715681 and 26556575

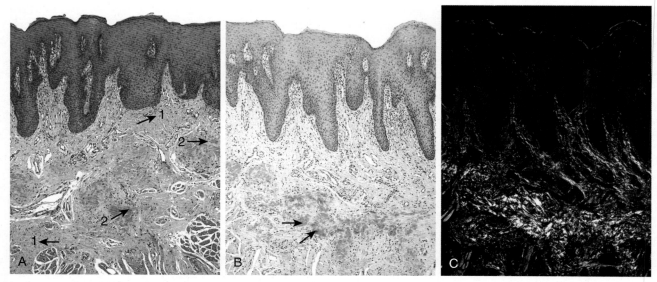

Fig. 17.12 Amyloid deposited in tongue mucosa. (A) The haematoxylin and eosin–stained section shows a broad band of amorphous tissue between the epithelium and underlying muscle (1). This stains bright red with eosin where it is densest (2). (B) Congo Red stain also stains the densest deposits red (arrows). (C) When the Congo Red section is viewed under polarised light, the amyloid shows green birefringence.

Table 17.1   Selected types of amyloids*

Type	Protein	Source	Effect / significance
AL	Immunoglobulin light chains	The usual source is neoplastic plasma cells in myeloma	Deposition mainly in kidneys, but common in the tongue, affecting about a third of patients
SAA	Serum 'amyloid A' protein, an acute phase serum protein	Produced in chronic infections and inflammatory conditions such as rheumatoid arthritis, Crohn's disease or tuberculosis	Rarely affects tongue, deposits mostly in liver and kidney
ATTR	Transthyretin, a serum protein	Usually a familial form associated with mutant protein	Deposits in muscle, kidney and heart, but rarely in tongue
AM	$\beta 2$ microglobulin, a cell surface protein	Serum levels rise dramatically during renal haemodialysis	Deposits mostly in joints and occasionally in tongue. Lingual deposits affect about 2% of patients on long-term dialysis
ACal	Calcitonin	Secreted in excess by medullary thyroid carcinoma	Deposited only in the tumour, aids diagnosis
ODAM	Odontogenic ameloblast-associated protein	Odontogenic epithelium in the calcifying epithelial odontogenic tumour (Ch. 11)	Deposited only in the tumour, aids diagnosis, mineralises focally to produce radiopacities

*Many more are known, but these are more common or more relevant.

OTHER DISEASES AFFECTING THE TONGUE

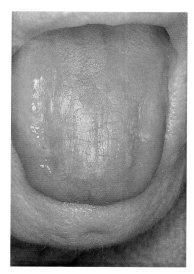

Fig. 17.13 **Smooth atrophic tongue due to lichen planus.** This is a late change due to longstanding disease. There is slight increase in keratinization producing some milky white appearance anteriorly (Ch. 16.).

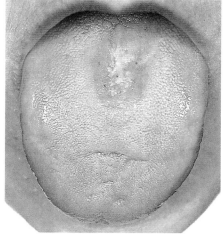

Fig. 17.14 **Median rhomboid glossitis.** This is either an active candidal infection or evidence of past infection. (Ch. 15.).

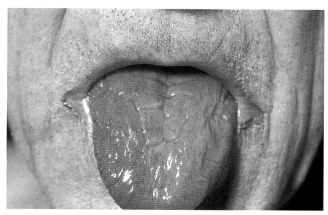

Fig. 17.15 Glossitis in antibiotic sore tongue, a candidal infection. (Ch. 15.).

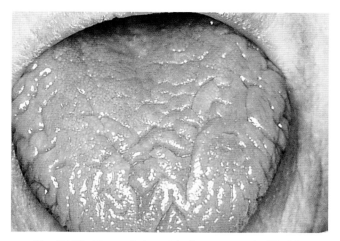

Fig. 17.16 Tongue in longstanding xerostomia. (Ch. 22).

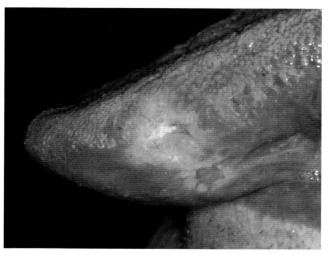

Fig. 17.17 **Traumatic ulcer.** The tongue is a common site, here due to biting.

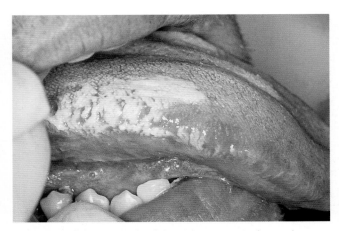

Fig 17.18   Oral hairy leukoplakia. The tongue is almost always involved, often bilaterally on the lateral border. (See Ch. 18).

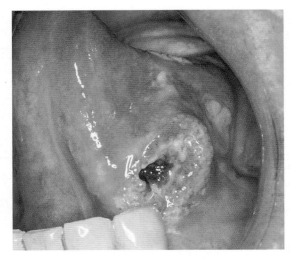

Fig. 17.19   Squamous carcinoma. The lateral tongue is a common site. (See Ch. 20.)

Benign chronic white mucosal lesions | 18

There are many causes of white patches or diffuse whitening of the oral mucosa, and a small minority are potentially malignant, that is squamous carcinoma may develop within them. When confronted with a white lesion in the mouth, every clinician needs a list of oral white lesions in their mind for diagnosis so that the few with significant risk are identified quickly and accurately.

The appearance of most mucosal white lesions is due to hyperkeratosis. Keratin absorbs moisture from saliva and then appears white. Apart from the lingual filiform papillae and leukoedema, visible keratinisation of any significant degree is abnormal in the mouth.

Many white lesions are associated with red areas and some conditions causing white lesions are included in Chapters 15, 16, 17 and 19.

Review oral white lesions PMID: 23600041 and 30671762

Diagnosis PMID: 29274164 and 30736423

Leukoplakia

A *leukoplakia* is a clinical term for a white patch. Understanding how this term is used and avoiding misuse is important. A leukoplakia is a predominantly white patch of the oral mucosa that cannot be characterised clinically or pathologically as any other definable lesion. This states clearly that leukoplakia is idiopathic – no cause is known or can be found after investigation.

Previous definitions included the fact that a leukoplakia cannot be wiped off, but the importance of this finding has been overemphasised. The intention is to exclude thrush (Ch. 15) in which the surface white pseudomembrane can be wiped off. However, not all types of *Candida* infection produce loosely adherent plaques, and this feature is of minimal diagnostic value.

Unfortunately, the term leukoplakia is widely misused. To many it means a white patch that has a risk of malignant transformation to squamous carcinoma. This is true of only a tiny minority, but a patient searching the internet with the term could easily become very frightened. The term also appears in the names of many specific diseases, such as *oral hairy leukoplakia* or *candidal leukoplakia* where the cause is known. Some prefer not to use the term at all, and simply saying 'white patch' instead avoids much of the confusion.

Leukoplakia is only a clinical description, and it can be a useful label for a white patch on first presentation. However, once investigations and biopsy are complete, either a specific cause is known, or a histological diagnosis can be given. The term is then redundant, unless used in the name of a specific entity.

The majority of white patches, without malignant potential, are discussed here (Table 18.1).

Current definition PMID: 17944749 and 33128420

Table 18.1 Important causes of benign mucosal white lesions

Prevalence	Lesion	Cause
Common	Leukoedema	Normal variation
	Frictional keratosis	Friction
	Cheek biting	Cheek biting
	Fordyce's granules	Developmental
	Stomatitis nicotina	Pipe smoking
	Thrush	Candidal infection
	Lichen planus	Unknown
Uncommon	Chemical trauma	Caustic chemicals
	Hairy leukoplakia	Epstein–Barr virus
	White sponge naevus	Genetic
	Oral keratosis of renal failure	Uncertain
	Verruciform xanthoma	Uncertain
	Skin grafts	Iatrogenic

FORDYCE SPOTS → Summary chart 19.2 p. 348

Fordyce spots or granules are sebaceous glands in the oral mucosa. They are normal rather than ectopic, appearing in at least 80% of adults, but perform no function in mucosa.

They are soft, symmetrically distributed, creamy white spots from 0.5–2 mm in diameter, and grow in size to become more prominent with age (Fig. 18.1). The buccal and labial mucosa are the main sites, but sometimes the lips and, rarely, even the tongue are involved. Fordyce spots are more or less evenly spaced, but in some patients they are very prominent and can form a creamy white slightly raised plaque that is mistaken for a leukoplakia. However, they do not show the bright white colour of keratin, and the light yellow colour of the fat in the gland can be seen to be below the surface.

Patients can be reassured that they are of no significance. If a biopsy is carried out, it shows normal sebaceous glands with two or three lobules but no hair follicle, as would be present with sebaceous glands on the skin (Fig. 18.2).

And other oral sebaceous lesions PMID: 8355222

And other yellow mucosal lesions PMID: 30693453

LEUKOEDEMA → Summary chart 19.2 p. 348

Leukoedema is a bilateral, diffuse, translucent white greyish thickening of the surface layers of the epithelium with an increase in thickness of parakeratin at the surface. The characteristic feature for diagnosis is that it disappears on stretching the mucosa. The buccal and labial mucosae are affected.

Leukoedema may be normal rather than a disease, one end of a spectrum of epithelial differentiation; it is present to some degree in 90% of Black people. It is also sometimes seen in other populations but is rarely as obvious. It has been claimed to be caused by some unknown environmental insult, such as smoking, but is seen in non-smokers and children.

Histologically, there is thickening of the surface layers of the epithelium with irregular parakeratinisation and the upper prickle cells show an enhanced 'basket weave' pattern caused by vacuolation of their cytoplasm. There is no oedema, intracellular or otherwise, and no inflammation.

Treatment is unnecessary. The main significance is not to overreact and perform a biopsy without good reason. A biopsy might be indicated only if the leukoedema were in the mouth of a patient who smoked or had other risk factors for oral carcinoma.

Review PMID: 1460680

Epidemiology and causes PMID: 3926975

FRICTIONAL KERATOSIS

→ Summary charts 19.1 and 19.2 pp. 347, 348

White patches can be caused by prolonged mild abrasion of the mucous membrane by such irritants as a sharp tooth or dentures causing the epithelium to develop a layer of protective keratin.

At first, the patches are pale and translucent (Fig. 18.3), but with prolonged friction become dense and white, usually with a smooth surface. Common sites are buccal mucosa and edentulous alveolar ridge, particularly behind the last standing molar (Fig. 18.4). The buccal *linea alba* is a normal mild frictional keratosis.

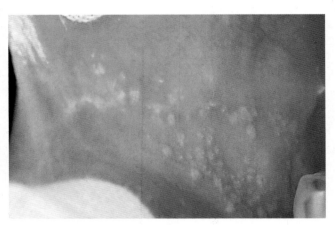

Fig. 18.1 Fordyce's spots. Clusters of creamy, slightly elevated papules on the buccal mucosa.

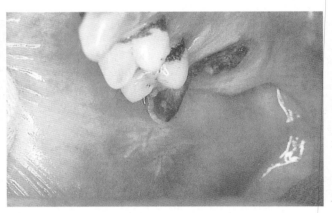

Fig. 18.3 Frictional keratosis. A poorly defined patch of keratosis on the buccal mucosa is due to friction from the sharp buccal cusp of a grossly carious upper molar.

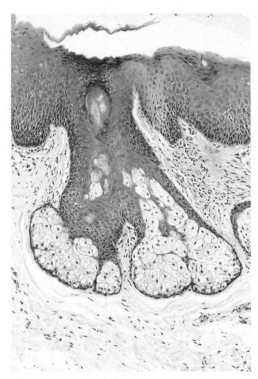

Fig. 18.2 Fordyce's spots. Each spot is a histologically normal superficial sebaceous gland without a hair follicle. The creamy colour clinically is caused by the fatty secretion in the pale cells at the base of the gland.

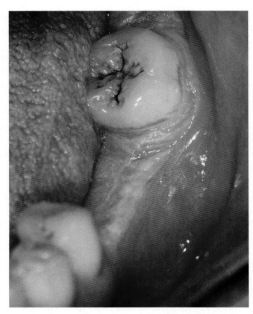

Fig. 18.4 Frictional keratosis. Some degree of frictional keratosis is almost universal on edentulous alveolar ridges when teeth are not replaced.

Excessive trauma will cause an ulcer, and the margins of a traumatic ulcer are often surrounded by a zone of frictional keratosis where the degree of trauma is less.

Diagnosis and management

The diagnosis is usually obvious from the cause. The patch fades gradually into surrounding normal mucosa without sharply defined margins.

Frictional keratosis is completely benign and removal of the irritant causes the patch to disappear. Biopsy is necessary only if the patch persists or there are other clinical indications, such as smoking. If performed, the epithelium shows hyperplasia, thickening of the prickle cell layer and para- or ortho-keratosis but no dysplasia (Fig. 18.5). More intense friction may be associated with mild inflammation, but often there is none.

Ridge keratosis PMID: 32180128

General review white lesions PMID: 23600041 and 30671762

CHEEK AND TONGUE BITING

→ Summary charts 19.1 and 19.2 pp. 347, 348

Habitual biting is very common. Like nail biting, it is one of the most common repetitive behaviours, and is undertaken by a third of undergraduate students and often over several years. The trauma is distinct from frictional keratosis and traumatic ulceration. Unlike the smooth surface of frictional keratosis, biting produces small indentations and shredded tags where small pieces of the superficial epithelium are nipped off. The background epithelium undergoes even keratosis in response.

Biting causes an area of mucosa to appear patchily red and white with a rough surface (Fig. 18.6). The margin of the bitten zone is well demarcated as only a limited amount of the oral mucosa can be interposed between the teeth. The damage is very superficial and usually along the occlusal line, on the lips or lateral tongue.

The diagnosis should be obvious from the clinical appearance and history of the habit, which is rarely unconscious.

Biopsy is not indicated. If performed on a tongue lesion, care must be taken not to mistake the histological features for those of oral hairy leukoplakia as both conditions induce enlarged pale epithelial cells in the prickle cell layer.

Review PMID: 19070760

Epidemiology and psychology PMID: 30300869

STOMATITIS NICOTINA

→ Summary chart 19.1 p. 347

Previously known as *smokers' palate*, or *pipe smoker's keratosis*, this condition has become rare now that pipe and cigar smoking have declined in popularity. It appears to be a reaction to the heat of smoking, which in these habits is directed at the posterior palate. Changes take many years to develop. Only the heaviest of cigarette smokers can produce similar alterations.

Clinical features

The appearances are distinctive in that the palate is affected, but any part protected by a denture and the gingival margins are spared. There is diffuse whitening caused by hyperkeratosis and inflammatory swelling of minor mucous glands. The openings of the minor gland ducts are seen as red spots against the white, and in marked cases they form umbilicated swellings with red centres and a distinct line of keratosis around them (Fig. 18.7). The white plaque is sometimes distinctly tessellated ('cracked' or crazy paving appearance).

Diagnosis and management

The clinical appearance and history are distinctive. If the patient can be persuaded to stop smoking, the lesion resolves within a few weeks or months.

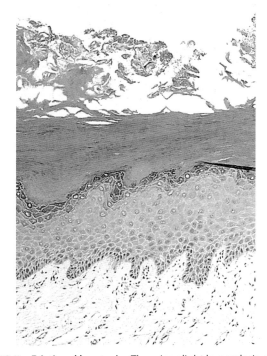

Fig. 18.5 Frictional keratosis. There is a slight hyperplasia of the basal cells and a thick layer of orthokeratin at the surface.

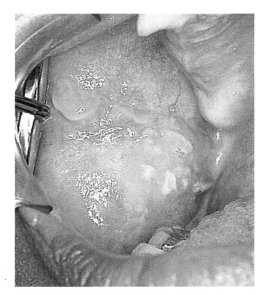

Fig. 18.6 Cheek biting. There is whitening of the buccal mucosa and a shredded surface.

Unlike other oral white lesions associated with smoking, stomatitis nicotina carries no risk of malignant transformation. Management can therefore be conservative, and no biopsy is usually taken unless there are other concerning features.

If performed, biopsy shows hyperorthokeratosis and acanthosis of the epithelium with a variable inflammatory infiltrate in underlying glands and around ducts but no dysplasia (Fig. 18.8).

Although the condition is benign, its presence indicates prolonged heavy smoking and the possibility of carcinoma developing at another site in the mouth, pharynx, larynx or lung should be considered. The predictable healing on stopping smoking is a useful aid in helping patients cease. The changes must not be confused with similar but more marked changes in the high-risk carcinogenic habit of reverse smoking (Ch. 19).

Key features are summarised in Box 18.1.

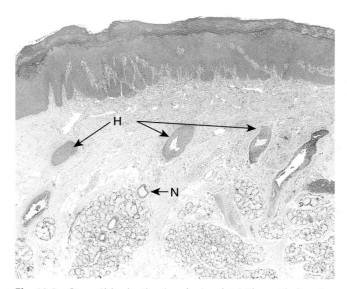

Fig. 18.7 Stomatitis nicotina (smoker's palate). There is a generalised whitening with sparing of the gingival margin. The inflamed openings of the minor salivary glands form red spots on the white background.

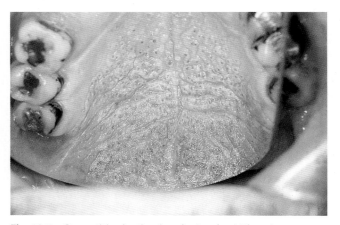

Fig. 18.8 Stomatitis nicotina (smoker's palate). The epithelium is hyperplastic and hyperkeratotic, especially around the orifice of the duct where there is inflammation.

Reverse smoking PMID: 9081765

Similar changes caused by hot drinks PMID: 2234881

ORAL HAIRY LEUKOPLAKIA

→ Summary chart 19.2 p. 348

This Epstein–Barr virus infection of oral mucosa was originally considered to develop only in HIV infection. However, it is now recognised in others who are immunosuppressed and in a small number of healthy individuals. The name causes some confusion. The lesion is not hairy and, having a known cause, is not a leukoplakia.

Clinical features

In HIV infection, hairy leukoplakia is usually a late sign and is 'strongly associated' (Ch. 30). Men who have sex with men are predominantly affected, and antiretroviral treatment reduces the incidence. Hairy leukoplakia is occasionally the presenting sign in unsuspected HIV infection. Renal transplant patients are also predisposed.

Hairy leukoplakia produces an asymptomatic vertically corrugated or shaggy soft keratosis of the lateral borders of the tongue (Fig. 18.9). It may also rarely affect the buccal mucosa, soft palate and pharynx, but tongue lesions will then also be present. The vertical ridging is enhancement of the normal epithelial morphology on the posterolateral tongue and is not a useful feature for diagnosis.

Box 18.1   Stomatitis nicotina

- Affects palatal mucosa exposed to smoke and heat
- Areas protected by denture unaffected
- Gingival margin often spared
- Palate is white from keratosis
- Umbilicated swellings with red centres are inflamed salivary ducts
- Responds rapidly to abstinence from pipe smoking
- Benign despite being tobacco-induced

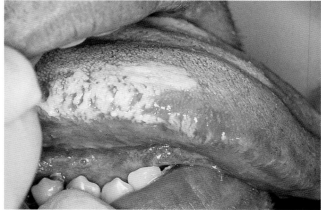

Fig. 18.9   Hairy leukoplakia in a patient with early symptomatic HIV infection. The surface of the lesion is corrugated, accentuating the normal anatomy of the lateral border of the tongue.

Diagnosis

Biopsy is required for diagnosis even when a cause of immunosuppression is known because diagnosis affects HIV staging, may reveal candida infection or an unsuspected diagnosis. Hairy leukoplakia shows hyperkeratosis or parakeratosis, or both, with a ridged or irregular surface. Koilocyte-like cells are the site of the infection. They are vacuolated and ballooned prickle cells with shrunken, dark (pyknotic) nuclei, chromatin pushed to the nuclear rim, and surrounded by a clear halo in the cytoplasm (Fig. 18.10). The infected cells form bands parallel with the surface in alternating layers with parakeratin. The presence of Epstein–Barr virus is demonstrated by using either immunohistochemistry to detect virus particles or in situ hybridisation to demonstrate their DNA (Fig. 18.10).

Secondary infection of the surface by candidal hyphae is common in examples from patients who are HIV-positive; fungal hyphae are then very numerous and not accompanied by an inflammatory response because of the immunosuppression.

Management

No treatment is required. Hairy leukoplakia has a remittent course and can regress when immunosuppression improves. Antiviral drugs are effective only while being taken, but these, and topical podophyllin, have been used in HIV infection when the lesions become very extensive.

Hairy leukoplakia in HIV infection indicates advanced immunodeficiency and a more rapid progression. Patients with a known HIV diagnosis who develop it should be referred to their HIV clinic for reassessment of their anti-HIV medication.

In those few patients without known immunosuppression, it often has a more localised distribution and resolves spontaneously.

Key features are summarised in Box 18.2.

Original description and update PMID: 1312689 and 27109280

Non-HIV cases PMID: 25600979 and 34030995

Box 18.2   Hairy leukoplakia: key features

- Usually in males
- Often a sign of immunosuppression, particularly HIV infection
- In HIV infection indicates advanced immunodeficiency
- Occasionally causes more limited disease in healthy individuals
- Not potentially malignant
- Typically forms soft, corrugated, painless plaques on lateral borders of tongue
- Diagnosis by biopsy
- Histologically, koilocyte-like cells in prickle cell layer are typical
- Epstein–Barr virus antigens detectable in epithelial cell nuclei by in-situ hybridisation
- May regress spontaneously or with treatment of immunosuppression (Ch. 30)

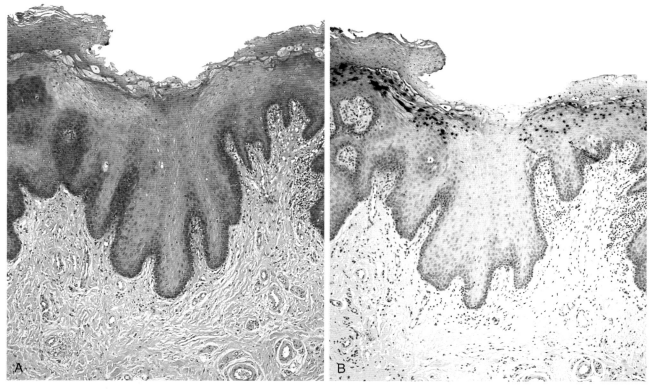

Fig. 18.10   Hairy leukoplakia. (A) There is thickening of the epithelium and a thick superficial layer of parakeratin, below which the pale-staining layer of 'koilocyte-like' cells lies. Because this patient is severely immunosuppressed, there is no inflammatory reaction to the numerous candidal hyphae which are present in the surface layers of the epithelium. (B) In situ hybridisation using probes complementary to the Epstein–Barr virus. The presence of viral DNA is shown by the dark brown staining in the nuclei of upper prickle cells and koilocyte-like cells. Details of this technique are found in Chapter 1.

WHITE SPONGE NAEVUS

➡ Summary chart 19.2 p. 348

White sponge naevus is a developmental anomaly inherited as an autosomal dominant trait, caused by mutation in the gene for either keratin 4 or 13. These keratin molecules are only expressed in the upper layers of non-keratinised mucosal epithelium.

Clinical features

The lining mucosa becomes white, soft and irregularly thickened (Fig. 18.11). The abnormality is usually bilateral on the buccal mucosa, and changes become more prominent with age, often presenting in the second or third decade. There are no defined borders, and the edges fade imperceptibly into normal tissue. Any non-keratinised mucosa can be affected; involvement of multiple sites such as nose or vagina constitutes Cannon's syndrome.

Pathology

The epithelium is very thick, with uniform acanthosis and shaggy hyperparakeratosis. The upper prickle cells are vacuolated with prominent epithelial cell membranes producing an enhanced basket-weave appearance (Fig. 18.12). The abnormal keratin cytoskeleton can sometimes be seen collapsed around the nucleus in scattered cells. Occasional dispersed apoptotic cells may also be found as the cytoskeleton plays a role in initiating and controlling apoptosis. There is no dysplasia or nflammation.

Management

The family history and appearance are virtually diagnostic, but biopsy can confirm the diagnosis if required. The condition requires no treatment.

Key features are summarised in Box 18.3.

And other keratin diseases review PMID: 12688839

Web URL 18.1 Genetics: http://omim.org/entry/193900

OTHER KERATIN DISEASES

Several other diseases strongly resemble white sponge naevus in their oral manifestations but have additional features. Pachyonychia congenita is caused by mutation in keratins 6 and either 16 or 17 and has additional nail abnormalities, palmar-plantar keratosis and skin cysts. Hereditary benign intraepithelial dyskeratosis is an extremely rare autosomal dominant disease affecting mostly native Americans in which the additional features are that the eyes develop gelatinous plaques and the cornea becomes opaque.

CANDIDOSIS

Three types of candidal infection cause white patches and are relatively common.

Thrush (acute candidosis) is readily distinguishable from other white lesions. The patches can easily be wiped off, and the condition is sore (Ch. 15).

Chronic hyperplastic candidosis and **chronic mucocutaneous candidosis** form discrete white plaques similar clinically to other types of leukoplakia (Ch. 15).

ORAL KERATOSIS OF RENAL FAILURE

Leukoplakia-like oral lesions are an unexplained complication of longstanding and severe renal failure. However,

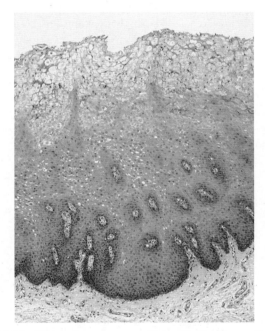

Fig. 18.12   White sponge naevus. The epithelium is acanthotic, and the prickle cell layer is composed of large vacuolated cells.

Box 18.3   White sponge naevus: key features
• Genetic – autosomal dominant trait
• Shaggy whitish thickening can involve all lining mucosa
• White areas lack sharp borders
• Histologically, epithelial thickening
• Defective parakeratinisation
• No dysplasia or inflammation
• No treatment other than reassurance

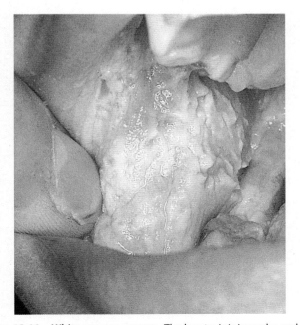

Fig. 18.11   White sponge naevus. The keratosis is irregular and folded and extends into areas which are not subject to friction.

this complication is almost never seen when patients have access to renal dialysis and so is rarely seen now outside terminal renal failure. The condition is therefore poorly described, sometimes described as keratosis and sometimes as ulceration or stomatitis. It is possibly an epithelial reaction to high levels of ammonia or urea, as can be seen in the skin. However, the presentation could be accounted for by several conditions that have been described since the disease became rare, particularly oral hairy leukoplakia.

Clinically, the plaques are soft and are typically symmetrically distributed (Fig. 18.13). Biopsy is useful to exclude adherent plaques of bacteria and desquamated epithelium and debris, which also form in late renal failure (Fig. 18.14). Candidosis, drug reactions and oral hairy leukoplakia must be excluded to make the diagnosis.

Review oral findings PMID: 15723858

SKIN GRAFTS

Split skin grafting is relatively rarely used in current surgical practice, and only to cover relatively small excision sites.

Skin grafts typically appear sharply demarcated, smooth and paler than the surrounding mucosa and occasionally grow hairs (Fig. 18.15). After many years grafts change in appearance and are less easy to differentiate from a leukoplakia (Fig. 18.16). If the history is not known and a biopsy is performed, the graft usually retains some epidermal features to aid diagnosis. These include orthokeratinisation, a high elastin content in the dermis and possibly residual superficial adnexae or erector pili muscles, though the depth of dermis included in the graft can be minimal and exclude these last structures.

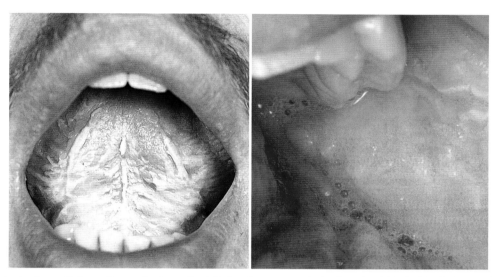

Fig. 18.13 Keratosis of renal failure. Two patients, on the left showing symmetrical soft and wrinkled white lesions and on the right showing patchier less marked keratosis. *(Right image courtesy Dr. S Muller)*

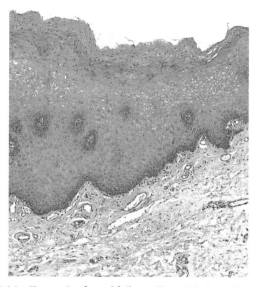

Fig. 18.14 Keratosis of renal failure. The epithelium shows little more than thickening of the prickle cell layer and an increased layer of poorly organised parakeratin at the surface.

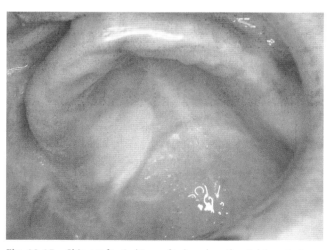

Fig. 18.15 Skin graft. A skin graft placed on the right posterior hard palate appears as a scar-like, pale patch. Hair follicles occasionally survive transplantation to the mouth.

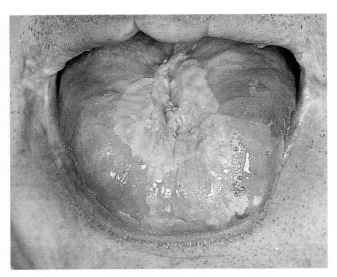

Fig. 18.16 Skin graft. This graft placed on the anterior dorsum of the tongue has contracted to produce an irregular margin and surface and might be mistaken for leukoplakia.

PSORIASIS

Psoriasis is a very common skin disease estimated to affect 2% of the population, but cases with convincing oral lesions are extremely rare and some doubt their existence. A relationship with erythema migrans is often stated but unproven.

The diagnosis should only be considered when there is cutaneous psoriasis and lesions wax and wane in severity with them. The appearance of the oral lesions is reported to vary from translucent plaques, mild stippled erythema to that of erythema migrans. Biopsy appearances are not specific.

OTHER WHITE LESIONS

A number of other conditions can cause localised white lesions. These include lichen planus (Ch. 16), chemical burns (see Fig. 16.2), verruciform xanthoma (Ch. 24) and papillomas (Ch. 24).

Potentially malignant disorders 19

Various oral mucosal lesions indicate that a patient is at risk of developing an oral squamous cell carcinoma. Such lesions are usually red or white in appearance. Their risks of developing into cancer vary considerably.

Terminology

The current preferred term for these conditions is *oral potentially malignant disorders*. This is meant to emphasise that the risk is only potential and may never materialise. 'Premalignancy' and 'precancer' imply that cancer will definitely develop, and these terms are best avoided, although they are widely used.

Current understanding also makes the difference between a premalignant lesion and a premalignant disease redundant. It used to be thought that some conditions indicated a risk of carcinoma at the site of the lesion itself ('premalignant lesion'), whereas others might indicate a risk elsewhere in the mouth ('premalignant disease'). We now understand that all potentially malignant disorders are indicators of genetic 'field change'. They indicate a risk not just at the site of the lesion itself but throughout the mouth and, in smokers, more widely in the upper aerodigestive tract.

Other useful definitions for this chapter are shown in Table 19.1.

The oral potentially malignant disorders

In general, the oral white lesions have the lowest risk of malignant transformation and red and speckled lesions the highest risk, but there are completely benign white and red lesions.

It is the role of the dentist to recognise these lesions, assess their risk and refer when that risk is significant. The process of identifying 'at risk' lesions is fundamental to diagnosis and treatment planning.

The oral potentially malignant disorders are listed in Table 19.2, with their risk and causes, as far as is known.

Nomenclature and classification PMID: 33128420

Lesions versus disorders PMID: 18674954

Table 19.1 **Key definitions for potentially malignant disorders**

Erythroplakia	A predominantly fiery red patch of the oral mucosa that cannot be characterised clinically or pathologically as any other definable disease
Leukoplakia	A predominantly white plaque of questionable risk having excluded other known diseases or disorders that carry no increased risk for cancer
Precursor lesion	Any identifiable lesion or altered mucosa with a risk of transformation. A relatively non-specific term

Field change

Potentially malignant disorders are the visible manifestation of field change or field cancerisation. This is a process whereby a wide area of tissue becomes genetically unstable, making it prone to develop cancer anywhere within the field. In heavy smokers, mutations predisposing to cancer can be found throughout a large field including the mouth, pharynx, larynx and lung. Examples are loss of function of cell cycle control proteins or DNA repair enzymes.

Defects are not limited to individual genes. The cells in the field also show gross chromosome abnormalities, usually amplifications or duplications of whole or part chromosomes. This results from chromosomal instability, a continuous process in which cells develop more genetic damage with every cell division. The genetic changes in the altered field are not in themselves sufficient to cause cancer, but they increase the likelihood of cancer developing.

It is often assumed that the genetic changes in potentially malignant disorders are the beginning of a pathway towards cancer, in which mutations, gene deletions and other genetic changes are progressively collected until a full complement of cancer changes is present and one cell becomes malignant. Many references include diagrams showing genetic changes accruing with time and specific changes developing early or late. However, the genetic basis of potential and actual malignant disease is much more complex. The genetic changes in potential malignancy are generally inhibitory to cancer pathways, the cells are collecting largely irrelevant mutations and deletions. These are not themselves cancer forming but contribute to continuing chromosomal instability. The cells are thus constantly gaining DNA abnormalities and eventually, at random, may become malignant. In molecular terms the cells accumulate 'passenger' mutations and not the 'driver' mutations that promote carcinogenesis.

Within an area of field change in the mouth, not all the epithelial cells have the same DNA defects. There are overlapping areas of slightly different changes making up the field. Each patch is a clone of cells that can survive despite its genetic damage. Some of these clones may have a growth advantage over normal cells and gradually spread, but most grow too slowly to replace surrounding tissue. The area of field change is therefore a patchwork of cells with different genetic changes, possibly interdependent on each other for survival, and each continually developing more genetic damage with each cell division. Different parts of the field will therefore have different risks for developing into cancer.

Field change has several implications. The first is that the extent of the field may or may not be visible clinically or histologically depending on the particular combination of genetic changes present. The size of the field at risk, therefore, cannot be easily determined. Second, the size of the field affects the possibility of surgical treatment because excision could only be effective for a small field. Third, patients at risk of one carcinoma are at risk of multiple potentially malignant lesions and genetically unrelated cancers at different sites in the field.

Table 19.2   Oral potentially malignant disorders

Disorder	Aetiology	Risk of malignant change*	Prevalence in UK
Leukoplakia	Idiopathic/smoking	Varies with dysplasia grade	Common
Proliferative verrucous leukoplakia	Unknown	Very high but long term	Uncommon
Erythroplakia	Idiopathic/smoking	Very high	Rare
Speckled leukoplakia	Idiopathic/smoking	Very high	Rare
Oral submucous fibrosis	Betel quid chewing	High	Uncommon
Dyskeratosis congenita	Genetic	High	Very rare
Pipe smoker's keratosis (stomatitis nicotina")	Pipe smoking	Minimal or none in mouth	Now uncommon
Snuff-dippers' keratosis	Smokeless tobacco	Low	Uncommon
Chronic candidosis	Candida albicans	Low	Uncommon
Lichen planus	Idiopathic	Very low	Common
Oral lupus erythematosus	Autoimmune	Unclear (mainly lip vermillion)	Uncommon
Oral graft versus host disease **	Autoimmune transplant reaction	Unclear	Rare
Oral 'lichenoid lesion' **	Idiopathic	Low	Uncommon
Palatal lesions in reverse smokers	Smoking	Very high	Not seen
Tertiary syphilis	Treponema pallidum	Very high	No longer seen

*Risks of malignant change are difficult to determine accurately and vary with many factors discussed later in this chapter. If more than 25% of patients with a specific disorder develop carcinoma in 10 years, this is considered an exceptionally high risk. Malignant change in 1% of lesions in 10 years is considered a relatively low risk. High-risk disorders are uncommon. Common disorders affect between 1% and 5% of the population.
**Added in WHO 2022 revision
Actinic keratosis is often included in the list but only predisposes to vermillion border carcinoma, not oral (Ch. 21)

When a biopsy is taken, the task for the pathologist is to exclude that carcinoma is already present and, if not, make a histological assessment of the risk of future transformation. This is done by recognising dysplasia, the features of abnormal growth that reflect the underlying genetic changes as discussed later. Dysplasia is the best predictor of risk. It is not necessarily detectable throughout the area of field change, but it often is. Dysplasia is recognised by seeing changes in cell proliferation, differentiation or overall architecture of the epithelium. It is usually graded as mild, moderate or severe, sometimes low or high risk, and the degree is proportional to the risk of developing carcinoma.

In tobacco users PMID: 12949809

'Mapping' fields PMID: 16757199

Genetics of potential malignancy PMID: 28580171

Genetic pathway to cancer PMID: 34418233

ERYTHROPLAKIA

➔ Summary charts 19.1 and 19.3, p. 347, 349

An erythroplakia is a predominantly red lesion of the oral mucosa that cannot be characterised clinically or pathologically as any other definable lesion. The term *erythroplasia* is sometimes used to indicate that these lesions are often not raised plaques like leukoplakias, but flat or slightly depressed (Fig. 19.1).

Pure red lesions are rare and usually affect the floor of mouth, lateral and ventral tongue and soft palate of older people, often smokers. The surface is frequently velvety in texture and ranges from dull matt red to bright scarlet. The margin may or may not be sharply defined. Erythroplasia

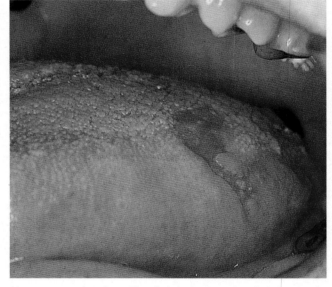

Fig. 19.1 Erythroplasia. This slightly depressed, well-defined red patch on the dorsolateral tongue showed microscopic, clinically occult, squamous carcinoma on biopsy.

is uncommon in the mouth but carries the highest risk of malignant transformation.

Almost half of lesions turn out to contain carcinoma on first biopsy, and the remainder show some degree of dysplasia, often severe. The epithelium is atrophic and non-keratinised, and these features, together with underlying inflammation and vascular dilatation, account for the red colour seen clinically. Dysplasia is discussed later in the chapter.

Review PMID: 15975518 and 35488780

SPECKLED LEUKOPLAKIA

→ Summary chart 19.1, p. 347

Also known as *erythroleukoplakia*, this term applies to lesions with both red and white areas, usually white flecks or nodules on an atrophic erythematous base (Fig. 19.2). They can be regarded as a combination of leukoplakia and erythroplakia.

The clinical features otherwise resemble erythroplakia, and there is a similar risk of finding carcinoma in a first biopsy. Speckled leukoplakia more frequently shows dysplasia than pure white lesions. The histological characteristics are a combination of those in leukoplakia and erythroplasia.

Some cases of chronic candidosis have a similar appearance, but no dysplasia and carry no risk of developing carcinoma.

LEUKOPLAKIA → Summary chart 19.2, p. 348

Leukoplakia is defined as a predominantly white plaque having excluded other known diseases or disorders. Like erythroplakia and speckled leukoplakia, the diagnosis is therefore by exclusion of other diseases. Many completely benign conditions form similar white patches (Ch. 18).

Leukoplakia is common, accounting for over three-quarters of all potentially malignant conditions and being present in 1%–5% of the population, more in India and other countries with many tobacco users.

In the UK, the risk of a leukoplakia undergoing transformation to carcinoma is approximately 0.3% each year if no dysplasia is present and 6% each year if severe dysplasia is present. Homogeneous, flat leukoplakias have a lower risk than those with a nodular or verrucous surface clinically. Large patches, those on the lateral or ventral tongue and floor of mouth, and those in older patients have a higher risk. Nevertheless, the malignant transformation rate of leukoplakia is relatively low, and, even in smokers, the vast majority of leukoplakias show mild or no dysplasia histologically and carry no risk of malignant transformation.

Current definition and diagnosis PMID: 33128420

Definition difficulties in use PMID: 26449439

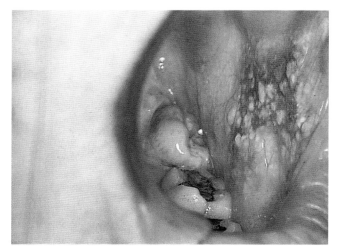

Fig. 19.2 Speckled leukoplakia. A poorly-defined speckled leukoplakia on the cheek of an old female patient. Severe dysplasia and microscopic, clinically occult, squamous carcinoma were present at the first biopsy. See also Fig. 19.11.

Clinical features

Idiopathic leukoplakias, with or without dysplasia, do not have any specific clinical appearance but are tough and adherent white plaques whose surface is slightly raised above the surrounding mucosa. The surface is usually rough or irregular, sometimes with a tessellated or 'crazy paving' pattern criss-crossed by thin lines of normal mucosa. Small and innocent-looking white patches are as likely to show epithelial dysplasia as large and irregular ones (Figs 19.3 and 19.4). However, lesions with red, nodular or verrucous areas (Fig. 19.5) should be regarded with particular suspicion. The most common sites are the posterior buccal mucosa, retromolar region, floor of mouth and tongue.

Pathology

The histopathology is highly variable, but there is always keratinisation, which gives the lesion its white appearance (Figs 19.6 and 19.7). Features of dysplasia and its assessment are considered later in this chapter.

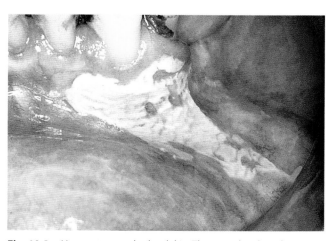

Fig. 19.3 Homogeneous leukoplakia. There is a bright, white, sharply defined patch extending from the gingiva on to the labial mucosa. The surface has a slightly rippled appearance.

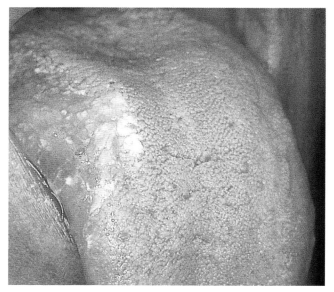

Fig. 19.4 An innocent-looking, poorly-defined inconspicuous white patch which showed dysplasia on biopsy. Despite excision, malignant transformation followed several months later.

Most leukoplakias, 85%, show no dysplasia histologically, whereas 8% show mild dysplasia, 5% moderate and 2% severe dysplasia.

Sublingual keratosis

The term 'sublingual keratosis' is sometimes applied to leukoplakia on the floor of mouth and ventral tongue, a high-risk site for malignant change. Sublingual keratosis is not a specific entity, but white patches at this site do show some unusual features; they are often extensive, form a soft plaque with a finely wrinkled surface and often show a low grade of dysplasia despite having significant risk of developing carcinoma (see Figs 19.6 and 19.7). The histology and treatment are as for leukoplakia.

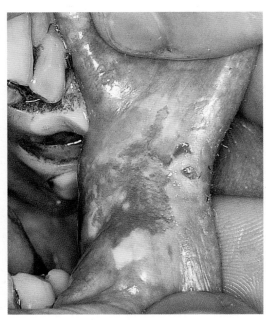

Fig. 19.5 White patch with red areas. This post-commissural lesion is poorly defined. Lesions at this site are frequently due to candidosis, but this example is much more extensive than typical commissural candidosis and showed dysplasia on biopsy.

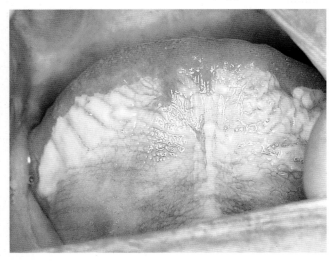

Fig. 19.6 Sublingual keratosis. This white patch involving the entire ventral tongue and floor of mouth has a uniformly wrinkled appearance. No red areas are associated, but the site alone may indicate a high risk of malignant transformation.

PROLIFERATIVE VERRUCOUS LEUKOPLAKIA

This is a distinctive presentation of multiple white lesions with a very high risk of transformation and has recently been accepted as a separate disease from other types of leukoplakia. Patients are older than 55 years of age, mostly female, and most are non-smokers.

They develop flat leukoplakias that, over a period of decades, enlarge, develop a nodular or verrucous surface and progress inexorably to verrucous or squamous carcinoma. Common sites affected are buccal mucosa, gingiva and tongue (Fig. 19.8). Many patches may be present, each at a different stage in its evolution. The progression from flat to verrucous signifies increasing risk, but verrucous patches may persist for many years while carcinoma develops elsewhere in a flat innocuous patch. Patients can develop several separate carcinomas over many years. The leukoplakias are difficult or impossible to eradicate surgically and recur or develop in new sites.

The histological features of the lesions are those of leukoplakia, with or without dysplasia, but it is striking that these lesions often display an apparently innocuous lack of cytological atypia or only mild dysplasia that can lead to underestimation of the risk, especially in the early stages. Their features of dysplasia are primarily architectural and easily underdiagnosed or misdiagnosed histologically, particularly as lichen planus.

For the diagnosis to have any value, it is important that the criteria are strictly applied. Not all verrucous leukoplakias and not all multifocal leukoplakias are proliferative verrucous leukoplakia, regardless of how verrucous they become or how much they enlarge. It is usually said that the ultimate diagnostic criterion is that all cases develop carcinoma. However, recognition must be much earlier to benefit the patient, and identifying the unusual clinical presentation allows close monitoring and targeted intervention.

Patients with proliferative verrucous leukoplakia often have a surprisingly good long-term prognosis. They tend to develop well-differentiated carcinomas, often on the gingiva or buccal mucosa that are detected early and are amenable to surgical excision.

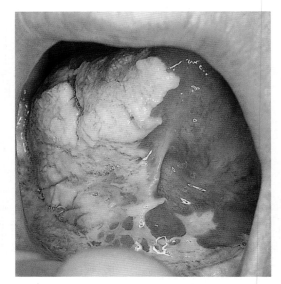

Fig. 19.7 Sublingual keratosis. This more irregular white patch is associated with some reddening in the floor of the mouth.

Review PMID: 17448134

Malignant transformation PMID: 34009718 and outcome 35199416

Is it a distinct entity? PMID: 34763117

STOMATITIS NICOTINA

➜ Summary chart 19.2, p. 348

Palatal keratosis due to pipe-smoking is itself benign (Ch. 18) but may be an indicator of risk elsewhere in the aerodigestive tract.

SMOKELESS TOBACCO-INDUCED KERATOSES

The majority of tobacco used worldwide is dried, cured and then smoked in cigarettes or cigars. However, many cultures have traditional tobacco habits that use snuff, crude tobacco or commercial preparations topically on the oral mucosa. These may be 'dipped', chewed or dissolved in the mouth and are termed smokeless tobacco habits. A dedicated

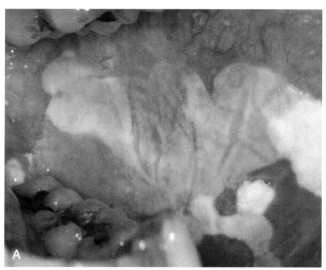

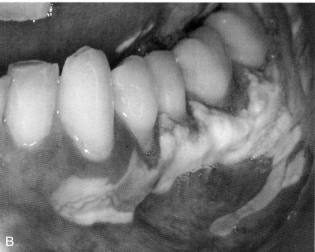

Fig. 19.8 Proliferative verrucous leukoplakia. There are multiple large white patches affecting the typical sites, with areas ranging from flat to nodular on the lower gingiva.

smokeless tobacco user can consume several kilogrammes of tobacco each year in this way. Most smokeless tobacco habits have a limited geographic spread, but international travel and emigration have brought them to new populations and use is increasing dramatically in the United States, with 6% of males being users.

Betel quid is widely used in the UK and other countries by immigrant communities, and further details are given in the section on oral submucous fibrosis. Some smokeless tobacco habits are listed in Table 20.1 and are discussed further in the next chapter.

Web URL 19.1 Review habits and carcinogenicity: https://publications.iarc.fr/107

Clinical features

Application of pure tobacco to the mucosa induces hyperkeratosis and inflammation. Changes are limited to the site where the tobacco is held, usually in the buccal sulcus, and lesions do not have sharply defined margins. These changes seem to take prolonged periods to develop and, in the early stages, there is only erythema and mild, whitish thickening of the epithelium. Later there is extensive white thickening and wrinkling of the mucosa. Before developing carcinoma, the mucosa will usually show varying degrees of dysplasia on biopsy, but even a non-dysplastic lesion at a site of tobacco application signifies a risk of carcinoma.

Betel quid users show distinctive features from the various other components of the quid. In addition to the features mentioned previously, frequent users may develop erythematous areas or erythroplakia. There is often also some localised fibrosis that need not signify submucous fibrosis (discussed later), but makes the lesion firm on palpation. Areca nut in the quid produces a dark red stain on the teeth and, in heavy users, of the mucosa too.

Carcinoma develops at the site of tobacco placement but only after many years of use. Most habits induce squamous cell carcinoma, but snuff dippers develop verrucous carcinomas (Ch. 20) much more frequently and after a longer exposure. If these remain untreated, invasive squamous carcinoma may develop.

Lesions associated with *snus*, Swedish moist snuff, are characteristic. This habit appears to carry a very low or minimal risk. Snus is sold as a loose powder and in a small paper pouch like a teabag that is placed in the sulcus and is popular in Sweden and the United States. Unlike other habits, the site used is often the anterior buccal sulcus. The mucosa is greatly thickened, wrinkled and appears oedematous with a keratotic surface (Fig 19.9). No dysplasia is present on biopsy.

Smokeless tobacco products have other adverse effects including gingival and alveolar bone recession at the site they are placed. The oesophagus and pharynx are also exposed to carcinogens, and carcinoma may also develop there. Betel quid use has also been linked to diabetes and exacerbation of asthma.

Pathology

The main changes in all types are thickening of the epithelium with varying degrees of hyperorthokeratosis or parakeratosis. Regular and heavy users develop a thickened basement membrane and superficial fibrosis in the area where the tobacco is held and atrophy of underlying salivary glands. Later, there may be epithelial atrophy and the features of dysplasia may eventually develop.

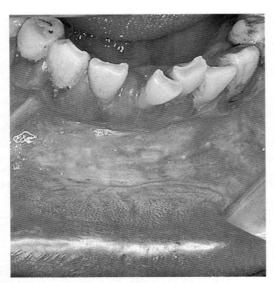

Fig. 19.9 Tobacco pouch or snus lesion. Keratosis with wrinkling of the sulcus mucosa where the pouch is held. Although this type of tobacco has a very low risk of cancer, note the inflammation and recession of the gingiva in contact with the pouch. *(From Pediatric Dentistry, 2005, 'Examination, Diagnosis, and Treatment Planning for General and Orthodontic Problems')*

Management

Diagnosis is based on the history of smokeless tobacco use and the lesion in the area where the tobacco is held. It is important to ascertain exactly what type of tobacco is used and how it is prepared to assess the risk. Biopsy is required to exclude dysplasia or early malignant change.

The most effective and important intervention is to stop the tobacco habit by patient education. Lesions that are dysplastic may then resolve completely or may regress, although there is a risk of delayed progression and malignant transformation. Non-dysplastic lesions in snuff dippers will resolve on stopping the habit even after 25 years of use. If the habit continues, regular follow up and biopsies are required. Most smokeless tobacco users also smoke, and this also needs to be addressed with smoking cessation advice.

Harm reduction for smokers. Scandinavian moist snuff sachets (snus) have a lower carcinogen content than other tobacco products. This is because the tobacco is cured in steam and is not fermented, unlike the kiln-dried tobacco used in cigarettes. The risk of developing carcinoma from these products appears negligible, some claim non-existent.

This has led to the proposal that smokers could reduce their risk of smoking-induced disease by switching to this type of smokeless tobacco. Statistically this makes some sense. The risk of lung and laryngeal carcinoma, of cardiovascular disease and other risks of inhaled tobacco are abolished and replaced by a low risk that affects a more readily examined site. Smokers also find this type of tobacco more acceptable than nicotine patches (and even nicotine patches have adverse health effects).

Opponents of this view point out that no tobacco product is safe, no use should be encouraged and that this is not a safe alternative to smoking. They worry that children and adolescents will develop this habit and progress to become smokers or nicotine addicts, although the Swedish experience suggests the opposite. There is no doubt that these products are still addictive and should never be recommended outside a smoking cessation programme with regular oral

examination. Evidence suggests use is not associated with significant smoking cessation and may have systemic adverse health effects.

The concept of promoting a harmful product as an alternative to an even more harmful one has generated intense argument, similar to that which still surrounds the use of methadone for heroin users. This is a difficult ethical area, and the interpretation of the evidence is still a matter of debate. Medically logical strategies can be confounded by unexpected public behaviours and there is a risk of sending conflicting messages to the public. Use of such products is rising dramatically in the United States, but they are banned, although readily available, in Europe outside Sweden. This harm reduction strategy has been largely overtaken by the introduction of vaping (Ch. 20), to which similar arguments apply.

Topical tobacco lesions review PMID: 17238967

Snuff dipping PMID: 6808102

Snus PMID: 24314326 and snus lesions PMID: 16470839

Use in smoking cessation PMID: 35197366 and 35597944

CHRONIC HYPERPLASTIC CANDIDOSIS

A detailed description of this condition is in Chapter 15, and the difficulty of distinguishing a 'pure' chronic candidal infection from a leukoplakia with superimposed candidosis was noted. If a white plaque is suspected from its clinical presentation to be caused by candida but fails to respond to treatment, or if there is dysplasia on biopsy, the lesion must be treated as a leukoplakia.

The clinical appearance of chronic hyperplastic candidosis can be very worrying, with a florid speckled appearance.

Whether candida itself is a carcinogen is controversial, but it can produce known chemical carcinogens, induce hyperplasia and activate epithelial cells. Leukoplakia infected by candida has an increased risk of transformation, and it is usual to try to treat the infection. However, any risk of transformation is very low.

The chronic candidosis of autoimmune polyendocrine syndrome 1 and the forms of mucocutaneous candidosis are different and have significant risk (Ch 37 and 15).

Is candidal infection oncogenic? PMID: 21523221

ORAL SUBMUCOUS FIBROSIS

Oral submucous fibrosis is an important and readily recognised condition in which the oral mucosa becomes fibrotic and immobile causing progressive limitation of mouth opening. More significantly, oral submucous fibrosis undergoes malignant transformation in 4%–8% of cases and makes a significant contribution to the high incidence of oral cancer in the Indian subcontinent, SE Asia, the Western Pacific and in Asian emigrant populations.

The cause of oral submucous fibrosis has long been known to be the chewing of betel quid (*paan* or *pan*), and its primary ingredient areca nut is the causative agent. The relative risk for users is almost 100 times that of non-users, and betel quid is an extremely potent carcinogen. The basic quid comprises chopped or grated areca nut mixed with slaked lime (CaOH) and wrapped in a leaf from the betel vine. There are enormous regional variations in additional ingredients, which include tobacco, spices and flavourings. The quid is folded tightly, held over molar teeth and chewed and occasionally parked in the buccal sulcus.

Areca nut contains alkaloids and the habit is addictive. However, it also has cultural significance, is associated with tradition and religious rituals and is regarded by many users as a general health tonic with beneficial medicinal effects. Similar ingredients can also be found in toothpastes. For these reasons, the habit is often acquired young, between the age of 5 and 12 years in India and 10–20 years in the UK. In the UK, between 13% and 30% of Asian immigrant children chew betel quid, more in lower socioeconomic classes, and half of adults use it daily though rarely with tobacco included. A heavy adult user may consume at least 20 or 30 quid each day, up to 100, and some will sleep with a quid in the mouth. Betel quid use is prevalent throughout the Indian subcontinent, Southeast Asia, Malaysia, the Philippines, Taiwan and parts of China, as well as among emigrants from these regions. Different combinations of ingredients are used in these different countries.

The two main adverse effects of betel quid use are oral cancer and submucous fibrosis. However, other risks include carcinoma of the pharynx and oesophagus and possibly diabetes. Quid containing tobacco carries the highest risk for carcinoma. Areca nut alone carries the highest risk for submucous fibrosis, but also causes carcinoma at a lower rate.

In the United Kingdom and United States, it appears that most users add tobacco to the quid, even though they develop the habit using tobacco-free quid. Particularly worrying is the emergence of cheap commercially prepared quid preparations *paan masala* and *gutka*, the latter a flavoured and sweetened product aimed at children that contains smokeless tobacco but can be imported legally into the UK.

Clinical features

Clinically, users of all types of quid show some common features. The teeth are typically stained dark brown by a dye extracted from the nut by the lime. At the site of quid placement there is usually erythema, keratosis and a flaking surface ('betel chewer's mucosa'), and sometimes erythroplakia or leukoplakia. Long-term users have periodontitis and recession of the gingiva next to where the quid is habitually held. These features affect regular users but are independent of the development of submucous fibrosis.

If submucous fibrosis develops, there is symmetrical fibrosis in the buccal mucosa, soft palate or inner aspects of the lips. In the earliest stages, there may be a burning sensation and scattered small vesicles. Loss of lingual filiform papillae resulting in a smooth glazed tongue is characteristic. Later, denser fibrosis and loss of vascularity cause extreme pallor or blanching of the affected area, which then appears almost white and marble-like. The fibrosis starts immediately below the epithelium but extends to deeper tissues until eventually the mucosa becomes so hard that it cannot be easily indented with a finger (Fig. 19.10). At this stage, the epithelium appears thin and atrophic. Muscles of mastication are eventually involved and shorten as the fibrosis within shrinks. Ultimately, mouth opening may become so limited that eating and dental treatment become difficult, and liquid feeding may become necessary.

Erythroplakia and leukoplakia may develop in oral submucous fibrosis (Fig. 19.11), and the epithelium may show dysplasia on biopsy. Later, there is a very high risk of carcinoma and, if these changes develop when opening is limited, they may easily be missed.

Pathology

The minority of areca users that develop submucous fibrosis are genetically predisposed. Occasionally, there is a familial incidence. People that are most susceptible can develop the disease in childhood, but most cases follow years of exposure to areca.

An alkaloid component of areca nut, arecoline, can induce fibroblast proliferation and collagen synthesis through stimulation of transforming growth factor beta release and can penetrate the oral mucosa to cause progressive cross-linking of collagen fibres.

The cause of the carcinomas and dysplastic lesions is presumed to be the carcinogens from the tobacco and nitrosamines from the areca nut. Similar molecular changes have been identified in the DNA of epithelial cells in quid users and smokers. The epithelial atrophy, relative avascularity and inflammation may also play a role.

Histologically, the subepithelial connective tissue becomes more collagenous, hyaline and avascular and there may be infiltration by modest numbers of chronic inflammatory cells. The epithelium usually becomes thinned, and the atrophy with superficial inflammatory cells produces a

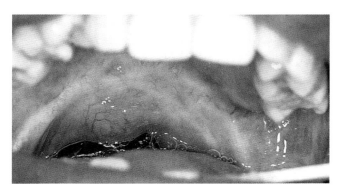

Fig. 19.10 Oral submucous fibrosis. Typical appearance in a relatively advanced case with pale fibrotic bands of scarring running across the soft palate and down the anterior pillar of the fauces. Similar fibrous bands were present in the buccal mucosa bilaterally. Mouth opening is limited.

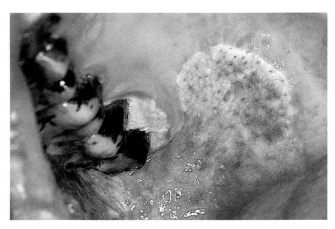

Fig. 19.11 **High-risk potentially** malignant lesion in a betel quid chewer. The classical appearance of a speckled leukoplakia such as this is almost always associated with either severe dysplasia or invasive carcinoma. Note also the brown betel quid staining on the teeth.

lichen planus-like histological appearance that can lead to misdiagnosis. Varying degrees of dysplasia may be superimposed. Underlying muscle fibres undergo progressive atrophy and replacement by dense fibrous tissue (Fig. 19.12).

Management

Treatment is largely ineffective. Patients must stop the causative habit, but no regression usually follows; only stabilisation of the trismus can be expected. Intralesional injections of corticosteroids may be tried in association with muscle stretching exercises or a 'trismus screw' used between the teeth to forcibly stretch the bands of scar tissue, but these require dedication in use and the benefit is not usually great in advanced disease. Wide surgical excision of the affected tissues including the underlying buccinator muscle together with skin grafting or various flap procedures can be carried out, but are likely to be followed by relapse.

The most important measure is to slow progression and reduce the risk of malignant progression by stopping the betel quid habit. Regular follow-up and biopsy of red or white lesions is essential but, even so, the risk of malignant change is reported to be about 5%–8%. Carcinomas also arise in the posterior tongue and pharynx, and in severe cases these sites can only be examined under anaesthetic, using endoscopy or by imaging.

Submucous fibrosis review PMID: 23107623

Oral lesions in betel users PMID: 9890449

Gutka hazards PMID: 20382045

Risks internationally PMID: 24302487

Betel quid use UK PMID: 11309868

Risk of transformation PMID: 33205543 and 35459408

LICHEN PLANUS

Lichen planus is widely, though not universally, accepted as a potentially malignant disorder, but the risk must be extremely low. Some of the problems in proving this controversial association are discussed in Chapter 16.

Occasionally, patients develop carcinoma in a background of keratosis and atrophy that either is lichen planus or is indistinguishable from it, but the overall transformation rate in lichen planus seems unlikely to exceed 0.05% in 10 years on epidemiological grounds. This is lower than often

reported but research studies are performed on hospital referral patients who are likely to have severe or unusual disease.

Review of cases of carcinoma developing in lichen planus often reveals the presence of mild dysplasia or unusual clinical features from the outset, either of which should have favoured an initial diagnosis of leukoplakia or erythroplakia rather than lichen planus. The presence of dysplasia should exclude a histological diagnosis of lichen planus. A significant contribution to the difficulty is that dysplasia is recognised by the immune system, which mounts a cell-mediated host response against the abnormal epithelium. At least a quarter of dysplastic lesions show this feature to some degree. Histologically, it is characterised by T cells migrating into the basal cells and killing them by inducing apoptosis, exactly the same process as causes lichen planus (Fig. 19.13). Some have called this process *lichenoid dysplasia*, but it is not a specific condition, and any lesion that shows dysplasia is best diagnosed as such, and not as lichen planus, however convincing the clinical picture.

Apparent lichen planus with unusual features, such as lesions in the floor of mouth or soft palate, late onset or unusual red areas should be regarded with suspicion, submitted for biopsy and followed up closely. Many cases of proliferative verrucous leukoplakia are initially misdiagnosed as lichen planus as the histological appearances are almost identical in its early stages.

ORAL LICHENOID LESION

The definition of an oral lichenoid lesion is a disease resembling lichen planus but without a full complement of diagnostic features clinically or histologically. This is an attempt to prevent misdiagnosis of dysplastic lesions as lichen planus and it has been proposed that carcinoma only arises in such lesions, not in classical lichen planus. The oral lichenoid lesion is therefore not necessarily a disease entity and its existence is disputed.

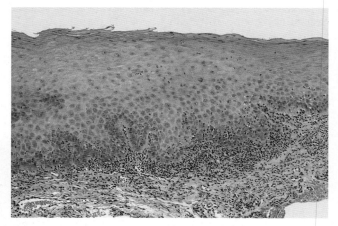

Fig. 19.13 Dysplastic lesion mimicking lichen planus. This sample comes from a lesion described as being a white patch with striae, suggesting lichen planus, and the histological appearances superficially suggest lichen planus, with a well-defined infiltrate of lymphocytes below the epithelium and lymphocytes in the basal cell layer inducing apoptosis. However, note that the basal cell layer survives for the most part. The lichen planus-like features arise from a cell-mediated immune response against the abnormal epithelial cells. Such lesions are good mimics of lichen planus and easily misdiagnosed.

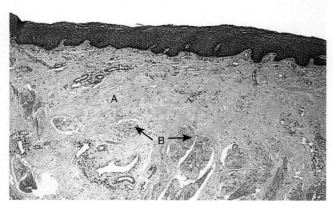

Fig. 19.12 Oral submucous fibrosis. There is fibrosis *(A)* extending from the epithelium down into the underlying muscle *(B)*, which is replaced by hyalinised fibrous tissue.

Unfortunately lichen planus has no absolute diagnostic criteria and those for lichenoid lesion are also rather wide and could include other red and white patches. Further confusion arises because the term lichenoid lesion is also applied to drug reactions and topical reactions to restorations. However, the concept that a lichen planus-like presentation that is not typical should be treated with extra suspicion is valid and prudent.

Lichenoid lesion concept PMID: 17112770

Lichen planus is not potentially malignant PMID: 35858493

LUPUS ERYTHEMATOSUS

Lupus erythematosus, discussed in Chapter 16, is associated with a small risk of malignant change, especially in lesions of the lower lip vermillion.

DYSKERATOSIS CONGENITA

Dyskeratosis congenita is a rare disease with several inheritance patterns caused by loss of chromosomal telomeres. The main oral feature is dysplastic white or red lesions of the buccal mucosa, tongue and soft palate (Fig. 19.14). Other features include cutaneous pigmentation, dystrophies of the nails and haematological abnormalities. Oral carcinoma develops in up to a third of cases and may arise in childhood.

Causes of death include cancers of the mouth or other sites, bleeding (gastrointestinal or cerebral), but in 50% from infections resulting from bone marrow failure.

General review PMID: 23782086

Oral features review PMID: 18938267

HPV-ASSOCIATED DYSPLASIA

During the early years of the AIDS epidemic, oral white patches caused by infection with human papillomavirus were recognised, but these became very rare following introduction of antiretroviral treatment. These were originally called *koilocytic dysplasia*.

More recently, the same white patches have been increasingly recognised in individuals who are not immunocompromised. They are indistinguishable clinically from other leukoplakias but histologically distinctive (Fig. 19.15). Almost all are infected by the same high-risk HPV subtypes that cause oropharyngeal and cervix carcinomas (Ch. 21) and the routes of transmission are probably similar. The viral DNA may be in the cytoplasm or integrated into the host DNA, and there is also low-level viral replication. There have been insufficient cases reported to understand the natural history of this new disease, but it is clear that at least some cases develop carcinoma, and from first principles this is to be expected.

Although it might be expected that papillomavirus infection in dysplastic lesions would produce a papillomatous appearance, clinically this is not so, although some appear slightly stippled clinically. HPV is not associated with proliferative verrucous leukoplakia or the other leukoplakias that are verrucous.

Lesions range from small milky white circumscribed leukoplakias to extensive involvement of the mouth. Most arise on tongue, floor of mouth or buccal mucosa. They are

not usually suspected clinically and biopsy is required for diagnosis.

Description PMID: 28799537 and 34418233

SYPHILITIC LEUKOPLAKIA

Leukoplakia of the dorsum of the tongue is a characteristic complication of tertiary syphilis but is so rare now as to be of only historical interest in the UK. Few patients reach the tertiary stage in developed countries but a few do so in some parts of the world. In the past, syphilitic leukoplakia was a feared complication because of its very high malignant transformation rate of 50% or more.

Syphilitic leukoplakia has no distinctive features but typically affects the dorsum of the tongue and spares the margins. The lesion has an irregular outline and surface. Cracks, small erosions or nodules may prove on histology to be foci of invasive carcinoma.

On biopsy there is hyperkeratosis, dysplasia and the characteristic late syphilitic chronic inflammatory changes with plasma cells, granulomas and endarteritis of small arteries.

The diagnosis depends on serological findings. The presence of syphilitic endarteritis may be a contraindication

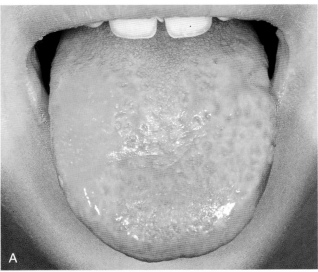
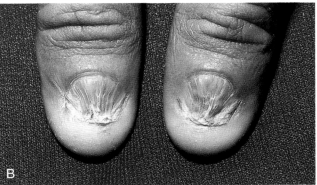

Fig. 19.14 Dyskeratosis congenita. A young patient with diffuse keratosis of the dorsum of the tongue (*A*) and another patient showing the typical nail dystrophy (*B*). *(From Paller, A.S., Mancini, A.J., 2011. Hurwitz clinical pediatric dermatology: a textbook of skin disorders of childhood and adolescence. Saunders, Philadelphia.)*

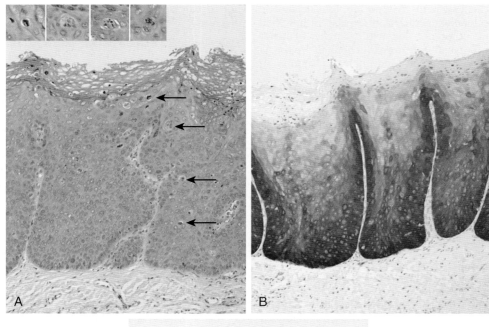

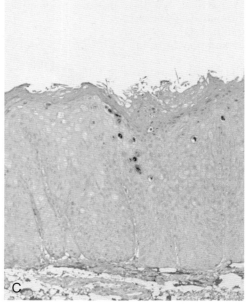

Fig. 19.15 Human papillomavirus–associated dysplasia. There are numerous mitoses and unusual degenerate and apoptotic cells at all levels including the upper prickle cell layers (*A*). These cells often have a chromatin pattern suggesting that they are degenerate mitoses (*inset*). Immunohistochemistry for p16 cell cycle regulatory protein is positive (*B*, brown stain), indicating that the virus is transcribing its oncogenic E6/E7 proteins (see Ch. 21). DNA in situ hybridisation reveals high-risk viral DNA in some of the cells (*C*, blue stain is positive).

to radiotherapy, making treatment of any carcinoma that develops difficult.

Treatment of syphilis does not cure the leukoplakia, which persists and can undergo malignant change many years later.

MANAGEMENT OF POTENTIALLY MALIGNANT DISORDERS

As will be noted in Chapter 20, the prognosis for oral carcinoma is good only when the diagnosis is made early and the tumour is small. The principles of management of potentially malignant disorders are therefore to prevent carcinoma developing, or if already present, to detect it when small.

Red or white lesions in the mouth should never be ignored. Have a high index of suspicion that an oral lesion may be potentially malignant and investigate appropriately. It may turn out to be innocuous but must be assessed with the possibility of future carcinomatous change borne in mind.

The management of dysplastic oral lesions remains controversial because very large numbers must be treated to prevent malignant transformation in a small minority. For all practical purposes, dysplasia seen on biopsy has to be considered a possible early stage in the development of carcinoma, even though carcinoma may develop over ten years later and often not at all. Detecting dysplasia provides an opportunity to treat before carcinoma at an exceptionally early and potentially curative preinvasive stage. Unfortunately, the assumption that surgical removal will prevent carcinoma is not well supported by clinical evidence.

The principles of the management of dysplastic lesions are summarised in Box 19.1. The first step is to assess the risk of malignant transformation.

Review PMID: 17257863

Risk assessment

Clinical

The patient should be questioned, and the lesion should be examined for the features in Box 19.2. Risk habits, tobacco use, betel quid and alcohol should be recorded by type amount and frequency.

Potentially malignant disorders indicate field change so a full and detailed examination of the entire mouth is required, with an attempt made to visualise the pharynx. All cervical lymph nodes should be palpated in case carcinoma is already present and has metastasised. Any additional lesions found must be managed in the same way as the initial lesion.

The size of the lesion, colour, homogeneity, any areas of nodular or verrucous change, ulceration, redness or speckling and whether or not it lies in a high-risk site for developing carcinoma (see Fig. 20.9) must be recorded. A photographic or diagrammatic record is very useful for monitoring changes during follow up. Large and longstanding lesions are at higher risk, and those in older people. A change in nature of a lesion is a worrying sign.

Induration, a feeling of firmness on palpation caused by fibrosis of the underlying connective tissue, is an early sign of carcinoma, signifying invasion into underlying tissues. If induration is present a carcinoma is likely and the patient should be referred directly to a cancer centre for further investigation. Apart from induration and ulceration, the features of carcinoma in its earliest stages may be identical to those of red, white and speckled patches (see Fig. 20.6).

Size is important PMID: 23521625 and 12945594

Several adjuncts to clinical diagnosis are available that are claimed to either identify lesions more effectively, identify higher risk lesions or aid diagnosis of carcinoma. Tolonium chloride rinsing and brush biopsy are considered in Chapter 20 with oral cancer screening. Some 'visualisation' techniques claim to make dysplastic lesions more readily identifiable on examination. Some illuminate the mucosa with a wavelength of light that is normally absorbed but reflected by abnormal epithelium. Others use autofluorescence patterns or more complex laser reflectance. These techniques are sometimes used in conjunction with dyes. All occasionally identify lesions missed in routine examination, but none has yet been proved cost effective in appropriately designed trials, either for screening in primary care or for hospital-based treatment.

Biopsy

Biopsy is the key investigation. It excludes or confirms whether carcinoma is already present and, if not, allows dysplasia to be detected and graded. The term dysplasia (literally, abnormal growth) is the single best indicator of risk of transformation to carcinoma.

It is often said that every red or white patch in the mouth should be subject to biopsy, and this is certainly a logical precaution. In practice, some red and white lesions do not merit biopsy because their clinical features allow confident diagnosis as benign lesions. Examples would be median

rhomboid glossitis or stomatitis nicotina. In further cases a response to treatment may avoid biopsy, for instance a suspected chronic hyperplastic candidosis may resolve on antifungal therapy. However, in most other cases, biopsy is accepted best practice.

Selection of the correct site is critical to obtaining the most informative report. Biopsy must include the highest risk areas, those with erythema or speckling, verrucous or nodular change or induration. The centre of ulcers should be avoided. A biopsy from the margin rather than the centre avoids ulcer slough and non-specific inflammation and aids

---

Box 19.1 Principles of management of dysplastic lesions

- Stop any associated habits, e.g., betel quid or smoking
- Dietary intervention
- Treat candidal infection and/or iron deficiency if present
- Biopsy to assess dysplasia
- Assess risk of transformation on clinical (Box 19.2) and histological findings (Table 19.3)
- Consider ablation of individual lesions (see Box 19.3)
- Maintain observation for signs of malignant change for a prolonged period

---

Box 19.2 Clinical risk factors for malignant change in erythroplakia and leukoplakia

History
- Betel quid use
- Tobacco smoking or topical tobacco habit *
- High alcohol intake
- Specific but very rare genetic disorders

Clinical aspects
- Advanced age
- Female sex †
- Areas of reddening in the lesion
- Areas of speckling in the lesion
- Nodular or verrucous areas or ulceration
- High-risk site:
  - posterolateral tongue
  - floor of mouth
  - retromolar region
  - anterior pillar of fauces
- Large lesions
- Lesions present for long periods
- Enlargement or change in character of pre-existing lesion

---

* Nevertheless, surveys indicate that the risk of malignant change in white lesions is higher in non-smokers, because tobacco induces very many low-risk lesions. Thus, both non-smokers and heavy smokers with red and white patches are at risk.
† Surveys indicate that malignant change in white lesions is more frequent in women. This is partly accounted for by the fact that women have many fewer lesions, smoke less, but develop proliferative verrucous leukoplakia in which the risk is high. Male heavy smokers and female non-smokers with red and white patches thus both carry a relatively high risk.

recognition of dysplasia when it is mild. When several areas in the lesion appear at risk, or when several lesions are present, more than one biopsy may be necessary.

Techniques for biopsy are discussed in Chapter 1.

Dysplasia grading

Epithelial dysplasia is the combination of architectural and cytological abnormalities seen in tissues that indicate a risk of developing carcinoma (Table 19.3). Architectural features are those that describe the structure of the epithelium, such as thickness, differentiation and rete process pattern while cytological features are abnormalities shown by individual cells. Any combination of features may constitute dysplasia but most dysplastic epithelium will show at least four. Dysplasia can be diagnosed on the basis of just architectural or just cytological features.

The features of dysplasia are also those of carcinoma, the only difference between the two is the way the tissues are arranged. In dysplasia the epithelium still forms a covering layer but structure is deranged. In a carcinoma, epithelial cells no longer form a covering layer but invade the underlying connective tissue.

Note that dysplasia means only growth disturbance, and is used in the names of other completely benign conditions such as fibrous dysplasia and cemento-osseous dysplasia. It is only epithelial dysplasia that indicates potential malignancy.

The more abnormal the epithelium, the higher is the risk of carcinoma developing. The features seen in individual specimens vary, but there are common themes.

Mild dysplasia is diagnosed when the basal cells show slight disorganisation. There is increased proliferation with several layers of basaloid cells with large nuclei, and among them are scattered cells with very abnormal shape or size (Fig. 19.16). There is often increased keratin formation and premature keratinisation compared to normal epithelium at the site and a change in rete process pattern. Overall the appearance can be very close to normal and mild dysplasia is often underdiagnosed.

Moderate dysplasia has more layers of basaloid cells and usually increased intercellular spaces as a result of reduced cohesion. There is a disorganised higgledy-piggledy appearance in the basal layers. Mitotic figures and very abnormal cells may be seen not only in the basal cells but in the middle of the epithelium where basal cells proliferate upward

Table 19.3	Epithelial dysplasia: histological features
Architectural features	**Cytological features**
These are changes in the organisation of maturation and normal layering of the epithelium	*These are changes in individual cells reflecting abnormal DNA content in the nucleus, failure to mature and keratinise correctly and proliferation*
Irregular epithelial stratification	Abnormal variation in nuclear size
Loss of polarity or disorganization of basal cells	Abnormal variation in nuclear shape
Drop-shaped rete ridges	Abnormal variation in cell size
Basal cell clustering or nesting	Abnormal variation in cell shape
Increased number of layers of basal-type cells	Increased mitotic activity
Increased number of mitotic figures	Increased nuclear-cytoplasmic ratio
	Increased nuclear size
Abnormally superficial mitotic figures	Atypical mitotic figures
Generalised premature keratinisation	Increased number and size of nucleoli
Premature keratinisation in single cells	Nuclear hyperchromatism
Keratin pearls within rete ridges	Single cell keratinisation
Reduced epithelial cell cohesion	Nuclear hyperhromasia
Altered keratin pattern for oral subsite	Apoptotic mitoses
Verrucous or papillary architecture	
Extension of changes from the surface into minor gland ducts	
Sharply defined margin to changes	
Multiple different patterns of dysplasia in one lesion	
Multifocal or skip lesions	

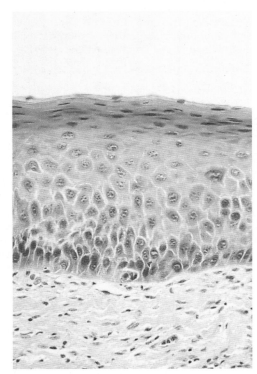

Fig. 19.16 Mild dysplasia. In this lesion there is a very thin layer of parakeratin and the structure, maturation and orderly differentiation of the epithelial cells is largely unaffected. However, there is a degree of irregularity of basal cells with variation in size and hyperchromatism.

at the expense of prickle cells (Fig. 19.17). The surface may be irregular, nodular or verrucous rather than flat and rete processes may disappear, become longer or bulbous. Sometimes cytological changes are absent and dysplasia only architectural, with budding or minimal changes in basal cells, loss of cohesion and premature keratinisation. Changes do not have to extend to the middle third of the epithelium for dysplasia to be moderate in severity.

Severe dysplasia contains cells with the most marked abnormalities and loss of the normal layered structure of the epithelium. There are usually many basal-type cells, few prickle cells or organised keratin layer, but individual cells may keratinise at any level (dyskeratosis). Reduced cohesion is usually marked. The overall epithelial structure and rete process pattern can be very irregular. The features are almost those of carcinoma; only invasion is missing. The term *carcinoma in situ* is sometimes used for this most severe dysplasia ('top-to-bottom change'; Fig 19.18 and 19.19).

Any degree of dysplasia may be accompanied by an immune response against the abnormal cells. Potentially, this could kill the dysplastic cells, but in practice seems to have no protective effect. However, it does produce a histological resemblance to lichen planus, causing misdiagnosis of mild dysplasia and confusing the issue of whether lichen planus is truly a potentially malignant disorder.

Even though dysplasia is the best indicator of transformation, the exact relationship between grade and transformation is ill defined. Any grade signifies some risk.

Whether different grades provide further useful information has been a matter of considerable debate. The histological assessment of oral epithelial dysplasia is notoriously unreliable because it is subjective, there are no well-defined grading criteria and it is therefore not very reproducible. It also depends on the correct high-risk area being biopsied. Several large studies from different countries have shown

no difference in malignant transformation rates between the grades, but this may be because they are performed on hospital patients who all tend to have relatively high risk.

In a recent UK study of 1401 patients with red or white lesions referred to hospital, 49 developed an oral carcinoma in 15 years. The value of dysplasia in predicting this is shown in Table 19.4.

Dysplasia grading works PMID: 34418233

Dysplasia grade not useful PMID: 24388536

Problem of sampling error PMID: 17448135

Patients with severe dysplasia are at higher risk and also at risk of carcinoma developing more quickly, and many patients with severe dysplasia develop a carcinoma in months (Fig. 19.20). This may be partly due to sampling

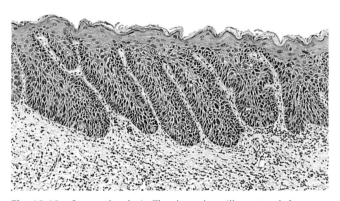

Fig. 19.18 Severe dysplasia. The dermal papillae extend close to the surface, and there are elongate rete processes, some of which are lightly bulbous. Enlarged and hyperchromatic cells are visible at this low power in rete processes and in most of the prickle cell layer.

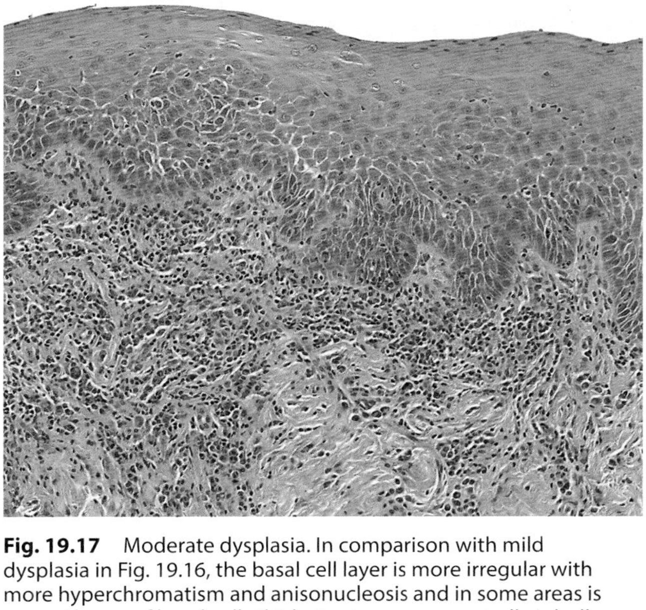

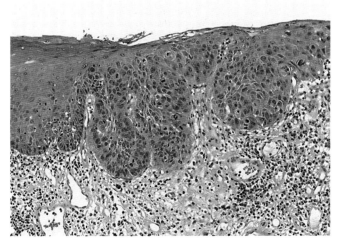

Fig. 19.17 Moderate dysplasia. In comparison with mild dysplasia in Fig. 19.16, the basal cell layer is more irregular with more hyperchromatism and anisonucleosis and in some areas is several layers of basal cells thick. A rete process centrally is bulbous and above that the lower prickle cells show loss of cohesion with increased intercellular space. However, overall the stratification of the epithelium is retained and prickle cells mature to a thin layer of parakeratin at the surface. There is inflammation in the connective tissue below. Compare this with the complete loss of epithelial structure in severe dysplasia in Fig. 19.19.

Fig. 19.19 Severe dysplasia. To the left is a short zone of mild dysplasia with an abrupt transition to a zone of severe dysplasia in the centre and right of the image. To the right cell pleomorphism is much more marked, there are mitoses and abnormal mitoses in the basal cell layer and loss of stratification, with no maturing prickle cells visible. A few flattened keratinising cells remain at the surface but essentially the full thickness of the epithelium has been replaced by disorganised basaloid cells.

Table 19.4 Proportion of the grades of dysplasia in oral red and white lesions in 1401 patients and the number developing carcinoma during 15 years follow up

Grade	Number with each grade	Number developing carcinoma	Predictive value of the grade %
No dysplasia	1182	14	1
Mild dysplasia	105	6	6
Moderate dysplasia	76	14	18
Severe dysplasia	38	15	39

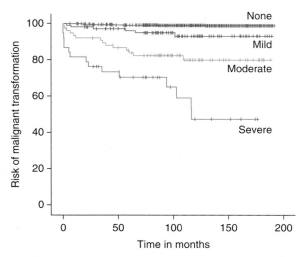

Fig. 19.20 Risk and time course of developing carcinoma in patients with mild, moderate, severe or no dysplasia in white lesions referred to hospital.

error, that is, the carcinoma was present at the time of biopsy, but the invasive areas were not sampled. However, the diagnosis of severe dysplasia successfully identified that risk. Note that even some patients with no dysplasia develop oral carcinoma, so clinical risk assessment is still important. It can take many years to develop carcinoma, even after severe dysplasia.

What happens to the dysplastic lesions that do not transform to cancer? Some resolve, some stay unchanged and others may remain and constitute a risk over an even longer period.

Transformation risk UK PMID: 12945594 and Europe 16316774

Transformation risk United States PMID: 31860085

Transformation risk Taiwan PMID: 17181738

Transformation risk India PMID: 1056293

Metanalysis PMID: 33606345 and 32249069

Other investigations

As dysplasia grading is an imperfect risk assessment, there is interest in molecular investigations that might be better predictors. Detecting abnormalities in chromosome numbers and loss or gain of function of genes is relatively easy, but no marker has yet proved a strong predictor. Loss of heterozygosity (reflecting loss of a gene copy, probably a tumour suppressor gene due to a deletion) at various chromosomal loci is often found in oral carcinoma and potentially malignant epithelium. A panel of molecular markers identifying loss at 12 sites on chromosomes 3, 4, 8, 9, 11, 13 and 17 can be used to divide samples into low, medium and

high-risk groups from which 2%, 15% and 64% of lesions transformed to carcinoma. These results are slightly better than for dysplasia grading, but the test is not yet available outside a research environment.

DNA ploidy analysis, a measure of total nuclear DNA content, is also a good predictor of malignant transformation. Nuclei from the biopsy are stained with a DNA binding dye that allows the total DNA content of each cell to be measured (Fig. 16.21). It is well known that dysplastic and malignant cells show chromosomal instability; their chromosomes have numerous deletions and duplications, sometimes of whole chromosomes. These changes can even be detected in epithelium that does not show dysplasia on routine light microscopic examination. Tissue with abnormal DNA content (aneuploidy) has a risk of transformation of 34% in 15 years, about the same risk as a diagnosis of severe dysplasia.

The value of both tests is that they can often detect risk when dysplasia is not present, so a combination of both assessments produces the most useful result. Unfortunately, both techniques are relatively complex and are not available outside a few specialist centres.

Review diagnostic aids PMID: 17825602

Predictive biomarkers PMID: 33290585 and 35338320

Cochrane review diagnostic tests PMID: 26021841 and update

DNA ploidy analysis and loss of heterozygosity PMID: 33577101

An area of current research is whether artificial intelligence or machine learning algorithms could detect risk better than the human eye. Microscope slides can be digitised and software systems can identify areas for the pathologist to examine in detail or provide a dysplasia grade or risk assessment. Such systems are showing promise but are not yet tested against a sufficiently wide range of diseases to be used routinely.

Experimental systems PMID: 36126604 and 32674040

Treatment

The management of potential malignancy is controversial. Although transformation has serious consequences for the patient, often culminating in death, the vast majority of such lesions will never transform and treatment can cause significant morbidity.

After biopsy, the clinical features, dysplasia grade and any other information (Box 19.2) are compiled into a risk estimate.

Low-risk lesions can be managed conservatively. Patients' risk factors must be addressed, usually by smoking cessation advice or other habit intervention. Any candidal infection should be eliminated and follow up instituted, ensuring a detailed and complete oral examination at every visit. Change in lesions is suspicious, and comparison with photographs or diagrams aids detection of changes.

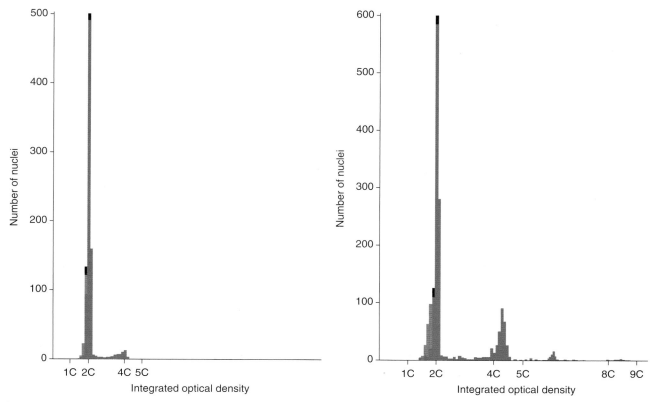

Fig. 19.21 DNA ploidy analysis of normal and dysplastic epithelium. Each graph shows the number of cells on the Y axis and the DNA content of each cell on the X axis. In normal mucosa (*left graph*) epithelial cells (*blue*) almost all have a normal diploid DNA content (called 2c, equivalent to 2 sets of chromosomes or diploid) with a few cells having doubled their DNA content because they are about to divide (small peak at 4c). Lymphocytes (*red*) and fibroblasts (*black*) act as a normal control. Dysplastic epithelium (*right graph, blue*) has peaks at abnormal DNA content (main peak between 4c and 5c) and many cells with grossly abnormal DNA content, up to 9c. Such a lesion may carry a high risk of malignant transformation.

Box 19.3 Options for ablating high-risk potentially malignant lesions

- Surgical excision, with grafting if required
- Laser excision
- Laser vaporisation
- Photodynamic therapy

Multiple interventions may be required to render some patients disease-free. Cryotherapy is generally considered inappropriate.

Many patients, particularly those with heavy tobacco and alcohol intakes, have diets deficient in fruit and vegetables, a known risk factor for oral carcinoma. Dietary intervention to establish a balanced diet is known to reduce cancer development. It has been estimated that each portion of fruit or vegetables consumed each day reduces the risk of oral cancer by around 50%, and diet supplements induce regression of as many as 30% of oral white lesions. Dietary intervention is potentially valuable but not widely used.

High-risk lesions should receive all the aforementioned interventions, but in addition may be ablated, by one of several methods (Box 19.3).

If lesions are of manageable size, it is tempting to excise them. However, evidence that disease eradication can prevent carcinoma is very limited, and surgical removal of large lesions carries morbidity. Visible mucosal changes are seen in only parts of the genetically altered field, making excision of the entire potentially malignant area impossible. Only areas of highest risk can be removed. Lesions in the highest

risk areas in the posterior floor of mouth are technically difficult to excise.

Nevertheless, an attempt is usually made to excise all small lesions with moderate dysplasia and any lesions with severe dysplasia. Removal by laser surgery is well tolerated and heals well with limited scarring. Surgical excision provides a specimen that can be examined for the extent of dysplasia and for possible early clinically unsuspected carcinoma. Such 'occult' microscopic carcinoma may be found in 5%–10% of lesions with severe dysplasia when the whole lesion is excised.

Laser vaporisation, photodynamic therapy and medical treatments such as topical chemotherapeutic agents or systemic retinoids have proved unsuccessful and provide no specimen to detect unsuspected carcinoma, worsening the outcome.

After excision and reassessment of the risk following pathological examination, long-term follow up is required because carcinoma may not develop for 10 years or more (see Fig. 19.20). Three monthly appointments for 2 years are usual, gradually extending appointment intervals if lesions remain unchanged, habits and diet are addressed and the patient is educated about the risk.

An alternative approach for high-risk lesions is not to intervene but to observe closely for signs of deterioration, in the hope of detecting carcinoma as early as possible. Once carcinoma develops, the treatment options are much more clear-cut. Such watchful waiting appears neglectful but avoids morbidity of treatment of little value and is supported by the natural history of the disease. However, the evidence that excision does have some benefit makes this difficult to justify, and patients need to be well informed if this path is to be chosen. Though surgical trials are small, meta-analysis shows that patients who have surgical treatment reduce their risk of malignant transformation from 15% to 5% independent of dysplasia grade.

In the absence of alternative treatments, surgical excision remains the treatment of choice for high-risk lesions, but recurrence of as many as 30% is reported.

Treatment effect PMID: 16316774

Treatment review PMID: 23159193 and 34324758

Treatment has some effect PMID: 19455705

Laser excision PMID: 12102411

Cochrane review PMID: 27471845

SMOKING CESSATION

Approximately 12% of adults in the UK smoke, a dramatic fall from the 50% that smoked in the 1970s. The number of smokers continues to decline slowly, and most are in low socio-economic or disadvantaged groups. However, this reduction is mostly among older smokers; the number of young new smokers has remained stable, and two-thirds start the habit as teenagers. As half of cigarette smokers will eventually be killed by their habit, it is not surprising that almost three-quarters would like to stop.

Nicotine is powerfully addictive, having dopaminergic effects similar to cocaine. Even patients who have had a laryngectomy or are dying of lung cancer will continue to smoke. Only 3% of smokers can quit smoking by willpower alone, and smokers are encouraged to seek professional support to help them quit.

Dentists are well placed to help. They screen a large proportion of the UK population, and oral adverse effects of smoking enable them to raise the issue with patients (Box 19.4). Smoking cessation in dental practice is as effective as in medical primary care. Three minutes' advice will help an additional 2% to quit and 10 minutes' advice a further 6%. These may seem small proportions, but they represent a significant health benefit for individuals.

Smoking cessation advice must be provided as part of a structured programme to be effective. A simple approach is

> **Box 19.4   Oral adverse effects of smoking**
> - Lip, oral and oropharyngeal squamous carcinoma
> - Oral potentially malignant lesions
> - Predisposition to periodontitis
> - Increased risk of implant failure
> - Predisposition to candidal infection
> - Predisposition to osteomyelitis
> - Staining of teeth
> - Taste impairment
> - Halitosis
>
> Recurrent aphthous stomatitis may worsen on smoking cessation, but not when nicotine replacement is used.

to *Ask* about smoking at every consultation, *Advise* on oral and health effects, *Assist* with health promotion material and offer support and *Arrange* follow up or referral for specialist advice. A team approach is most effective at reinforcing the message. Smoking cessation literature should be available in the waiting room, but referral to a specialised cessation service has the highest success rate.

Some patients find nicotine replacement helpful in weaning themselves off tobacco. Chewing gum, skin patches, nasal spray, inhaler, tablets, lozenges and electronic cigarettes are available. When used as part of an individualised cessation plan, nicotine replacement increases the success rate to 1 in 6. Such products are available over the counter and may be provided in dental surgeries. Bupropion (Zyban) may also help some patients.

See also the section on oral cancer aetiological factors in Chapter 20.

Cochrane review role in dentistry PMID: 33605440

Dental patients' views PMID: 26609892 and 33448485

Web URL 19.2 UK NHS guidance dentistry: https://www.gov.uk/government/publications/smokefree-and-smiling

or, WEB search 'NHS smokefree smiling'

Web URL 19.3 US ADA guidance: https://www.ada.org/resources/research/science-and-research-institute/oral-health-topics/tobacco-use-and-cessation

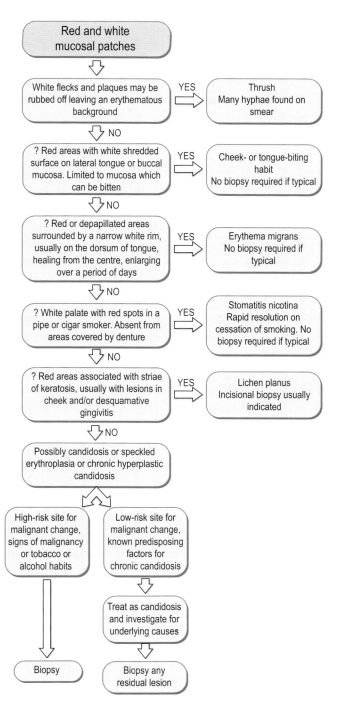

Summary chart 19.1   Differential diagnosis and management of the common causes of red and white patches of the oral mucosa.

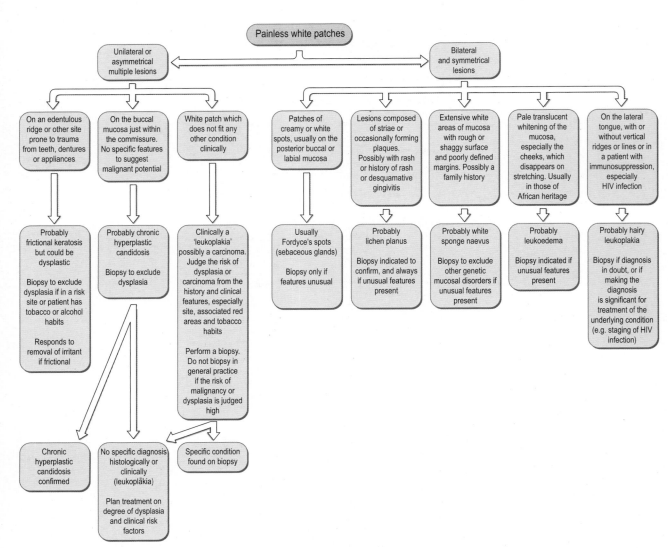

Summary chart 19.2   Summary of the key features of the common and important oral white patches.

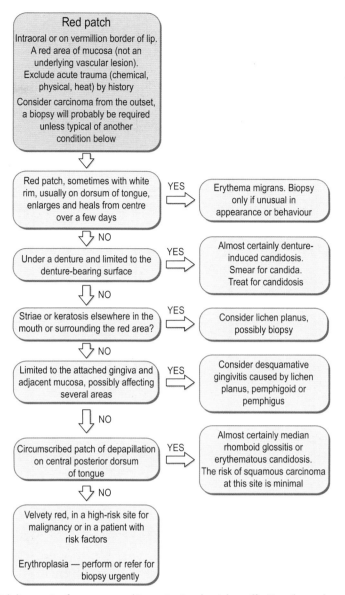

Red patch

Intraoral or on vermillion border of lip. A red area of mucosa (not an underlying vascular lesion). Exclude acute trauma (chemical, physical, heat) by history

Consider carcinoma from the outset, a biopsy will probably be required unless typical of another condition below

⬇

Red patch, sometimes with white rim, usually on dorsum of tongue, enlarges and heals from centre over a few days → **YES** → Erythema migrans. Biopsy only if unusual in appearance or behaviour

⬇ NO

Under a denture and limited to the denture-bearing surface → **YES** → Almost certainly denture-induced candidosis. Smear for candida. Treat for candidosis

⬇ NO

Striae or keratosis elsewhere in the mouth or surrounding the red area? → **YES** → Consider lichen planus, possibly biopsy

⬇ NO

Limited to the attached gingiva and adjacent mucosa, possibly affecting several areas → **YES** → Consider desquamative gingivitis caused by lichen planus, pemphigoid or pemphigus

⬇ NO

Circumscribed patch of depapillation on central posterior dorsum of tongue → **YES** → Almost certainly median rhomboid glossitis or erythematous candidosis. The risk of squamous carcinoma at this site is minimal

⬇ NO

Velvety red, in a high-risk site for malignancy or in a patient with risk factors

Erythroplasia — perform or refer for biopsy urgently

Summary chart 19.3   Differential diagnosis of common and important red patches affecting the oral mucosa.

Oral cancer 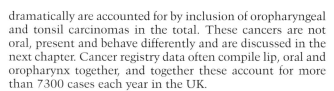 20

More than 90% of malignant neoplasms in the mouth are squamous cell carcinomas arising from mucosal epithelium. Most of the remainder arise in minor salivary glands (Ch. 23), and a few are metastases. The term *oral cancer* is therefore used loosely to mean oral squamous carcinoma. Carcinomas of tonsil, pharynx and lip are considered in the next chapter.

EPIDEMIOLOGY

Oral carcinoma accounts for only approximately 2% of all malignant tumours in such countries as the United Kingdom and the United States. In most countries where reliable data are available, the incidence of cancer of the mouth, although variable, is low. India, Pakistan, Bangladesh and Sri Lanka are, however, exceptional, and cancer of the mouth accounts for approximately 40% or more of all cancer there, although the incidence varies widely in different parts of this subcontinent. Relatively high rates are found in parts of China, Southeast Asia, France, Brazil and Eastern Europe. This variation is largely due to tobacco and other habits, and incidence is rising in these areas. People who neither drink alcohol nor smoke, such as Mormons and Seventh Day Adventists, have very low rates of oral carcinoma.

Approximately 4000 cases of intraoral carcinoma are registered each year in the UK. This equates to an incidence of 4.8 and 7.3 cases per 100,000 population for females and males respectively. For the last 50 years, the incidence of oral cancer has been falling in many developed countries such as the United States and in Europe. In the United Kingdom, unusually, oral carcinoma incidence has been slowly rising (Fig. 20.1 and 20.2). Claims that oral carcinoma is increasing

dramatically are accounted for by inclusion of oropharyngeal and tonsil carcinomas in the total. These cancers are not oral, present and behave differently and are discussed in the next chapter. Cancer registry data often compile lip, oral and oropharynx together, and together these account for more than 7300 cases each year in the UK.

Web URL 20.1 International epidemiology https://gco.iarc.fr/

Web URL 20.2 US epidemiology: http://www.oralcancerfoundation.org/cdc/

India epidemiology PMID: 23410017

Web URL 20.3 UK incidence, mortality: https://digital.nhs.uk/ and enter 'cancer registration' in search bar

UK epidemiology PMID: 30412558

Age and sex incidence

Oral cancer is an age-related disease, and 95% of patients are older than 40 years, with median age at diagnosis of just older than 60 years. There is a sharp and virtually linear rise in mouth cancer with age, as with carcinoma in many other sites, and oral cancer will become more common with an ageing population, though incidence in the UK is rising fastest in the 50–59 years age group (Fig. 20.2). The increased number in the oldest age groups is explained by their increasing total population.

Cancer of the mouth is considerably more common in men than women in most countries, but this is tobacco and alcohol related. In the UK the male:female ratio has sunk to 1.5:1, and figures for southeast England show little difference in incidence between the sexes. The change is the result of the progressive decline in oral cancer in men, but a low rate

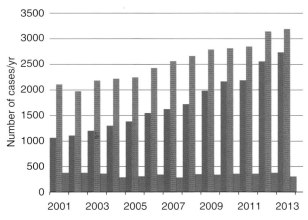

Fig. 20.1 Incidence of oral (*red*), oropharyngeal (*blue*) and lip carcinoma (*green*) for the UK until 2013, to show the dramatic rise in oropharyngeal carcinoma (Ch. 21) relative to oral and lip carcinoma at that time. *(Data from National Cancer Intelligence Network [England], Information Services Division [Scotland], Welsh Cancer Intelligence Surveillance Unit and Northern Ireland Cancer Registry.)*

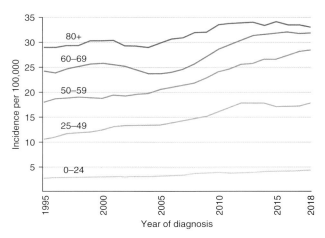

Fig. 20.2 Age-standardised incidence rates for oral carcinoma (including lip) in different age groups with lines marked to show age groups in years. There is an increase overall, but the youngest and oldest age groups are relatively stable and people aged 50–69 years show the greatest increase. *(Data from the UK National Cancer Registration Service Cancer Analysis System at 2021.)*

Box 20.1 Cancer of the mouth: key features

- Accounts for approximately 2% of all cancers in the UK
- One of the most common cancers in the Indian subcontinent
- Males more frequently affected
- Most patients are older than 40 years and incidence rises with age
- Posterolateral tongue is the most common site within the mouth
- Some arise in pre-existing white or red lesions
- Tobacco and alcohol are the main causes
- In the Indian subcontinent and Southeast Asia, betel quid is the main cause
- Oral cancer carries a relatively high mortality

Box 20.2 Possible aetiological factors for oral cancer

- Major factors
  - Tobacco smoking
  - Smokeless tobacco
  - Betel quid habit and oral submucous fibrosis
  - Alcohol
  - Sunlight (lip only, Ch. 21)
- Low risk factors
  - Diet
  - Candidosis
  - Human papillomavirus*
  - Lichen planus
- Rare, but significant
  - Dyskeratosis congenita
  - Fanconi's anaemia
  - Syphilis (historic)
- Speculative factors
  - Radiation
  - Immunodeficiency

* Human papillomavirus infection seems to carry a low risk in the oral cavity but is a high-risk infection in the oropharynx (Ch. 21) and nose.

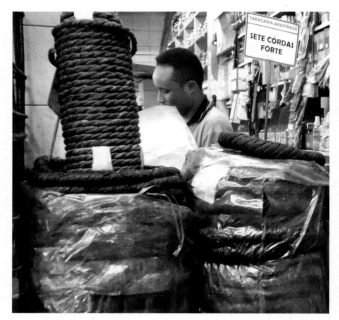

Fig. 20.3   Tobacco for sale in Brazil. Thick ropes of tobacco leaves for smoking and chewing. Such tobacco has been hardly processed, and carcinogenicity varies with the origin of the tobacco and the way the leaf is cured and processed. *(Courtesy Dr C Gomes.)*

in women. However, there is a worrying but relatively small increase in rates in young people, particularly women.

Key epidemiological features of cancer of the mouth are summarised in Box 20.1.

Health inequality and oral cancer PMID: 21490236

AETIOLOGY

Defining the contributions of different causative factors is difficult; the disease is complex and multifactorial, and patients must be exposed to causative factors for a prolonged period to develop cancer. Risk factors for oral squamous cell carcinoma are summarised in Box 20.2. Worldwide, tobacco is by far the most important cause.

Tobacco use

The earliest recorded tobacco-related death, although unsuspected at the time, was in 1621 when Thomas Herriot, who introduced clay pipe smoking to England, died of lip cancer. It has taken many years to finally establish beyond doubt that tobacco is the major aetiological factor for oral carcinoma.

Tobacco may be smoked or used in various smokeless tobacco habits and effects of each are different. Methods of processing tobacco before use also vary widely and affect its carcinogenicity (Fig. 20.3). Nearly 6 trillion cigarettes are smoked each year worldwide, and consumption continues to rise, with the highest intakes in Russia, China, Central Asia, Southern and Eastern Europe. In much of the world, smokeless tobacco predominates. On a slightly more optimistic note, the proportion of the world population that smoke has been declining for 40 years, but the reduction is more than compensated for by population growth. Though use in the UK has reduced, smoking still kills almost 80,000 people each year and many more have smoking-related morbidity.

Tobacco use should always be included in a medical history, and the best way to express cumulative tobacco exposure is in pack years (units of 1 pack (of 20 cigarettes or equivalent) smoked every day for 1 year; multiply packs per day by years smoked).

Web URL 20.4 Pack year calculator: http://smokingpack-years.com/

Cigarette smoking

Smoking is the major aetiological factor, particularly in association with alcohol, and its importance is that it is preventable. Large epidemiological studies of over 1 million individuals in the United States reveal that smokers' risk of cancer is proportional to the amount smoked and years spent smoking. Smokers overall have 30 times the risk of oral cancer versus people who never smoked. It is estimated that 80%–90% of all oral cancers can be attributed to smoking.

Smoking continues to be more common in men than women but the gap is not that large, about 3%. Until recently, one in five adults in the UK smoked, and the level

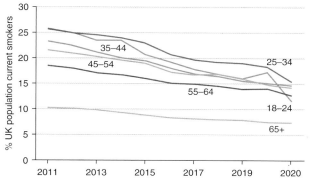

Fig. 20.4 Smoking prevalence in the UK by age. The line for each decade age cohort is labelled with age in years. Note the recent marked reductions in smoking in the 18–34 year old age group. *(Data from UK Office for National Statistics Annual Population Survey.)*

had been in only a slow decline. However, vaping and the disproportionate effects of Covid-19 infection on smokers have promoted smoking cessation, particularly in younger age groups, and in 2022 only 12% of the UK population smoke (Fig. 20.4). The average smoker smokes 31 cigarettes a week. The higher risk habit of hand-rolled cigarettes has doubled in incidence and carries a higher risk of lip than intraoral carcinoma. Over 2 million smokers have switched to electronic cigarettes in just a few years with potential risk reduction.

Smoking is also in decline in the United States, Australia and northern Europe. Improvement in cancer incidence lags behind changes in smoking habits, and it will take decades for these changes to take effect. In the meantime, consumption is increasing in the developing world.

Unlike pipe smoking or smokeless tobacco use, there are no specific oral lesions related to cigarette smoking, although cigarette smokers develop patchy mucosal pigmentation and light keratosis if they smoke heavily.

Marijuana smoking is widespread, and the smoke contains many of the carcinogens and co-carcinogens as tobacco smoke. It is suspected that it may be a more potent carcinogen than tobacco alone, but this has proved difficult to separate from the effects of alcohol and tobacco smoking.

Tobacco-induced cancers and deaths are preventable. Smoking cessation is discussed in Chapter 19 with management of potentially malignant disorders but is equally important in managing patients who already have a carcinoma.

It is unclear how much the risk reduces after quitting smoking. There are substantial reductions in risk of 50% after stopping smoking for 5 years, but data on lung cancer suggest that the risk will never drop back to that of someone who has never smoked. Nevertheless, stopping smoking significantly reduces risk, reduces comorbidity that can impact on treatment outcome, and reduces the risk of a second primary cancer.

Smoking and alcohol PMID: 17647085

Smoking and smokeless tobacco review PMID: 20361572

Pipe smoking

Pipe smoking has steadily declined in most Westernised countries and has never become popular with women. The risk of pipe smoking a Western-type pipe is statistically equal or slightly less than cigarette smoking due to less deep inhalation. The lip is considered at high risk. Other types of pipe used with different tobacco products in developing

countries carry a higher risk. Heavy pipe smokers may also develop stomatitis nicotina of the palate (Ch. 18), a white patch with no malignant potential.

Risks of pipe and cigar smoking PMID: 20162568

Water pipe smoking

Until recently, smoking water pipe (shisha, hookah or narghile) was a habit practiced largely by older people in Asia and the Middle East and was in decline. However, shisha smoking has become popular with adolescents and young adults in the UK and other Westernised countries. Popularity is driven by the social context in which the pipe is smoked, the use of flavoured tobacco (moassel) and a mistaken belief that bubbling the smoke through water reduces its toxicity. Most carcinogens are aromatic hydrocarbons or other water insoluble compounds that are not absorbed by the water and the cooled smoke is inhaled more deeply to exert greater effects. When this is considered with the long duration for which water pipes are smoked, one pipe session using a tobacco mixture could be equivalent to smoking between 50 and 60 cigarettes.

Unfortunately, like vaping, regulation lags years behind widespread adoption. In both the UK and US it is estimated that around 11% of the population have tried the habit. Only 2%–3% are regular users. Use often starts in childhood and is much more frequent in young people from minority ethnic backgrounds.

The risks of water pipe use vary with the combustion method and the smoked material, traditionally charcoal and tobacco. Inhaling charcoal smoke carries an acute risk of carbon monoxide poisoning. Pure tobacco was used traditionally but most young users smoke flavoured tobacco mixtures, which are about a third tobacco with honey or sugar and flavourings. These additional components also produce carcinogens on combustion or electrical heating so that tobacco-free smoking mixtures cannot be considered risk-free.

Charcoal combustion produces aromatic hydrocarbons as well as carbon monoxide, and electronic shisha, a vaping-like alternative, avoids this but often contains nicotine. Based on limited data, e-hookah is highly damaging in terms of lung inflammation and cardiovascular changes, as well as being highly addictive. All types of shisha may be more damaging than cigarettes, though research is sparse and the time required for cancer to develop is long. Any habit that involves inhaling combustion products must be considered carcinogenic.

UK water pipe epidemiology PMID: 24550183

US water pipe epidemiology PMID: 34637482

Water pipe smoking and dentistry: PMID: 27932840

Smokeless tobacco

Much of the world's tobacco consumption is in smokeless form. Tobacco habits and their risks are shown in Table 20.1, and Chapter 19 describes these habits' effects on mucosa in relation to potentially malignant lesions.

The risk varies with the habit but can be extremely high. In the southern United States, the habit of 'snuff dipping' causes extensive hyperkeratotic plaques and, after decades of continuous use, may lead to verrucous carcinoma (discussed later), as well as squamous carcinoma. This is a very slow process, and the relative risk of developing carcinoma arises to about ×12 after 15 years and ×50 after 50 years use. Conversely, Scandinavian moist snuff (snus) appears to carry a very low risk.

Table 20.1 Some common smokeless (topical) tobacco habits, many more exist but are more geographically restricted

Name	Habit	Where used	Risk of carcinoma in oral mucosa
Chewing tobacco ('spit' tobacco)	Chewing a damp plug of cured leaf tobacco or loose strips of leaf. Often flavoured or sweetened	Historically widely used in Europe and United States, now mainly in the United States	Moderate to low for oral cancer
Snuff dipping with dry snuff	Placing a pinch of dry snuff in the buccal sulcus	Southeastern United States and Scandinavia	Relatively low, associated with verrucous rather than squamous carcinomas
Betel quid (and pan masala; supari, paan) with tobacco	Areca nut, slaked lime, betel vine leaf with or without tobacco, sweeteners, flavourings and spices, rolled freshly or produced commercially as premixed dry powder sachets	Indian subcontinent, Southeast Asia, Philippines, New Guinea and China	Very high when tobacco is included. Areca nut is associated with submucous fibrosis in addition
Nass	Tobacco, ash, cotton oil quid held in sulcus	Central Asia and Pakistan	High
Khaini	Tobacco and lime quid placed in sulcus	India and Pakistan	High
Dry (nasal) snuff	Dry snuff inhaled through nose	Historically widespread in Europe but now used mainly in Africa	Low, associated with nasal and sinus carcinoma
Gutka	Commercially prepared powder of areca nut, tobacco, lime and other flavourings and sweeteners	Indian subcontinent, Southeast Asia	Probably high, also risk of submucous fibrosis
Toombak	Rolled ball of tobacco and sodium bicarbonate placed in sulcus or floor of mouth	Sudan	High
Snus (moist snuff sachets; Scandinavian snuff)	Teabag-like pouch of moist unfermented snuff, sometimes with flavouring. Also some rolled leaf products	Originally Scandinavia but now prevalent in the United States	Thought to be very low or absent. See section on harm reduction (Ch. 19)
Dissolvable tobacco	Tablets, strips or sticks of completely dissolvable tobacco for oral use, usually sucked, contains flavourings	A novel product	Unknown, carcinogen content variable, a relatively new product

For all smokeless tobacco habits, carcinomas tend to arise at the site in the mouth where the tobacco is habitually held and carcinomas are often preceded by red or white lesions or dysplasia. However, carcinogens are also swallowed, and the pharynx and oesophagus are also at risk.

Most smokeless tobacco users also smoke.

Smokeless tobacco review PMID: 15470264 and 34863207

Smoking and smokeless tobacco review PMID: 20361572

Snus PMID: 17920914

Electronic cigarettes and 'vaping'

Use of e-cigarettes and other electronic nicotine delivery devices has become very widespread in just a few years. In 2018, 15% of adults in the US had used them once but in most countries the proportion of the population who use them on a regular basis is between 3% and 6%. The attitude of health legislators to e-cigarettes varies between countries. In the UK they are promoted for smoking cessation but they are banned, though widely available, in India. Most countries regulate use and, in the US, UK and Europe the maximum nicotine content of vaping liquids is set at 20 mg/mL and flavoured fluids, likely to be favoured by young adopters of the habit, are no longer available. Use increased further following the introduction of disposable devices, especially among children and adolescents, to the extent that some countries are proposing a ban.

Vaping liquids may or may not contain nicotine, but all are complex mixtures that have propylene glycol or vegetable glycerin as a vehicle and flavourings and preservatives. Over 200 flavourings may be used, usually 10–15 in any one fluid. Many of these compounds have not been assessed for safety by inhalation or after combustion. Tobacco flavoured vape fluids contain known tobacco carcinogens, volatile organic compounds and heavy metals. The ingredients are vapourised in the e-cigarette and not burned, but this still produces breakdown products and generates novel chemicals, such as formaldehyde, some known to be carcinogenic or to have biological effects. The final product depends on the temperature at which the vapour is generated. This complexity makes it very difficult to determine whether vaping might be a risk for oral cancer and research lags far behind the population's adoption of the habit.

Though vaping is safer than smoking it is not harmless. Nicotine is highly addictive, causes tachycardia, hypertension, and vasospasm, risking cardiac arrhythmias and ischemia. Even without nicotine, vapour causes lung inflammation, fibrosis and remodelling of lung vasculature with secondary cardiac effects. Even young short-term users experience increased asthma severity, cough and bronchitis.

An outbreak of a new condition E-cigarette, or Vaping, product use-Associated Lung Injury (EVALI) in 2019 in the US that caused over 60 deaths was most closely linked to fluids containing vitamin E acetate, though other constituents may also have been contributory. Hypersensitivity to ingredients is recognized and also potentially fatal given that the reaction would be centred in the lungs. Many of these adverse effects can affect bystanders in a similar way to passive smoking.

One positive effect of vaping might be that its use as a tobacco cessation aid would lead to a reduction in oral cancer. It has been estimated that the lifetime cancer risk of vaping is 0.5% that of smoking, so vaping has potential as a harm reduction strategy, as adopted in the UK. Unfortunately, though the devices have this potential they are often adopted by non-smokers or young people in whom the adverse effects will dominate. Evidence to date suggests e-cigarettes are no more effective than other smoking cessation strategies that carry lower risks. Promoting them outside a structured cessation programme may simply induce permanent nicotine dependence.

No evidence yet exists to indicate that vaping might cause oral cancer but given the potent carcinogens present in vapour, it would be surprising if there was no risk of lung and oral cancer. DNA changes have been described in the buccal mucosa of users. Anecdotal evidence has linked vaping to an oral carcinoma death in a young patient but it may take decades to prove any association, particularly as many who vape also smoke.

Other oral effects of vaping appear minimal and, to date, no distinctive oral lesion appears to be linked to vaping. Smoking, primarily through the action of nicotine, is known to predispose to gingival inflammation, periodontitis and peri-implantitis. There is insufficient evidence yet to link vaping in the same way though the findings are suggestive of a link.

Oral symptoms self-reported by e-cigarette users include oral dryness, burning, stomatitis, halitosis and bad taste. These have been linked to flavourings menthol and cinnamonaldehyde but seem less prominent than the same symptoms caused by smoking.

Chemistry and toxicology of vaping PMID: 33753133

Use in smoking cessation PMID: 35321930

Oral cancer associated with vaping PMID: 33926987

Vaping and periodontitis PMID: 33274850

Vaping summary for dentists PMID: 33428774

Oral health impact PMID: 32043402

Betel quid

Betel quid habit is practised widely in the Middle East, Indian subcontinent, Southeast Asia and parts of China. The composition of the quid (Table 20.1) varies geographically and between users, changing the risk, but overall, this habit is one of the most carcinogenic known. Addition of tobacco carries the highest risk, but areca nut without tobacco is also carcinogenic. In Thailand, where use has recently declined, the rates of oral carcinoma have fallen. Use also causes oral submucous fibrosis and betel quid use is discussed in more detail in that section (Ch. 19).

Web URL 20.5 Betel quid general information: https://mono graphs.iarc.fr/ENG/Monographs/vol85/mono85.pdf

Betel use in Asia PMID: 22995631

Association premalignancy PMID: 22390524

Alcohol

Many oral cancer patients smoke and drink heavily. The relative risks for alcohol and tobacco consumption are shown in Fig. 20.5.

The increasing rates of oral cancer in the UK despite reduction in smoking have increased interest in alcohol

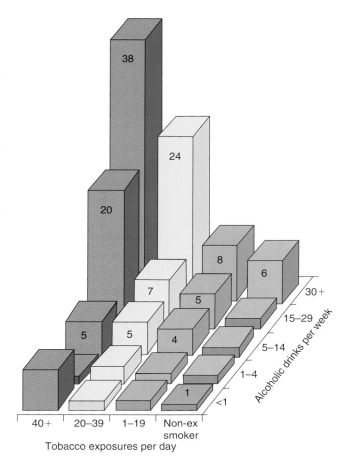

Fig. 20.5 Relative risks of developing oral cancer in consumers (males in a Western population) of tobacco and alcohol. The relative risk for a non-smoker and non-alcohol consumer is taken as one. A smoker consuming 30 cigarettes a day and 20 alcoholic drinks a week is seven times more likely to develop carcinoma.

as a cause. In Denmark, there is good epidemiological evidence to link alcohol intake with oral carcinoma, and in the Bas Rhin area of France, alcohol is responsible for the highest oral and pharyngeal cancer incidence in Europe.

Drinks with the highest content of congeners, such as raw home-brewed spirits, have the closest association with carcinoma in some countries, whereas in others beer-drinking is implicated. As with smoking, total consumption is probably a critical factor. Recommended maximum intakes relate primarily to liver disease, and no safe limit for oral cancer is recognised.

In the UK, alcohol consumption had doubled in 50 years to an average intake of 8 litres pure ethanol each year in 2005 but has shown recent decline. The highest intakes are in older people and in low socioeconomic groups. One in five individuals older than 65 years of age drink alcohol five times or more each week, more frequently if male. People aged 16–25 years drink most, and there is no sex difference in the younger drinkers, but even in the binge drinking population there is a definite decline in intake since 2005. Despite this, alcohol consumption remains the leading cause of ill-health, disability, and death in middle age in the UK.

Alcoholic drinks do not reside in the mouth for long, and there is no specific alcohol-related oral lesion. The mechanisms by which alcoholic drinks might cause carcinoma are unclear but include direct damage and increasing permeability to other carcinogens.

Some mouthwashes contain more than 25% alcohol, but any link to oral cancer remains speculative, with a possible weak association only in heavy users. However, continuing alcohol use after oral carcinoma is associated with a risk of a second primary carcinoma.

Alcohol effect review PMID: 20679896

Alcohol and potential malignancy PMID: 16614123

Smoking and alcohol PMID: 17647085

Infections and immunosuppression

Human papillomavirus (HPV) types 16 and 18 are now well-established causes of tonsil and oropharyngeal carcinomas (see next chapter), but their role in oral carcinomas remains poorly understood. Approximately 5% of oral carcinomas contain DNA from high-risk HPV subtypes and show p16 expression to suggest this is biologically active and potentially oncogenic. However, p16 expression is not specific and HPV DNA alone may be a contaminant or otherwise irrelevant to the carcinoma.

Currently, it seems that HPV is a minor factor in oral carcinoma. A few cases may arise in minor oral tonsils and be analogous to the HPV-associated carcinomas arising in palatine tonsil and oropharynx, with a similar good prognosis. HPV does not account for the recent increase in oral carcinoma in younger individuals.

Chronic candidosis causes hyperkeratotic plaques or speckled leukoplakias (Ch. 15), but outside the mucocutaneous candidosis syndromes carries a very low risk, possibly none.

Immunosuppression is not a significant factor for intra-oral carcinoma; incidence is not increased in HIV infection. However, lip carcinoma is more frequent in people who are immunosuppressed (Ch. 21).

Syphilitic leukoplakia is no longer a significant risk factor (Ch. 19).

Diet and malnutrition

Oral carcinoma is more frequent in those with low intake of fruit and vegetables. Vitamin A, C and carotenoids and other antioxidants are protective factors, together with zinc and selenium. Though these are epidemiologically linked, evidence that dietary intervention could prevent carcinoma is limited, though it can induce regression of some red and white potentially malignant lesions.

In India malnutrition is widespread and may contribute, together with betel quid chewing, to the high incidence of carcinoma.

Diet and oral cancer PMID: 24937666

Folate and oral cancer PMID: 24974959

Diet in Sri Lanka and oral cancer PMID: 23601045

Other habits

Mate, or chimarrão, is an herbal tea made from the *Yerba mate* plant, a species of holly. It is drunk mostly in South and Central America, traditionally through a metal straw at a very high temperature. Use is weakly associated with carcinoma of the oesophagus, pharynx and palate, probably largely as a result of the high temperature, though it also contains known carcinogens.

Mate PMID: 20036605 and 22915329

Poor oral health

Oral sepsis, trauma from teeth, tooth loss and poor oral health have traditionally been regarded as contributing factors but are interrelated in complex ways with habits and socioeconomic factors. Chronic trauma has an effect in animal studies, probably by promoting constant proliferative activity, but in humans, such links remain speculative.

Genetic predisposition

Dyskeratosis congenita (Ch. 19) is rare, has oral precursor lesions and a distinctive presentation, so diagnosis is usually straightforward and established before any oral carcinoma develops.

Fanconi anaemia is an important but rare cause of oral carcinoma in young individuals, and oral carcinoma may be the presenting feature. Defects in several causative genes that are required for DNA repair are known, and inheritance is recessive. Patients develop aplastic anaemia and leukaemia and have a reduced lifespan. They are also at risk of many types of cancer, and one in three patients surviving till 50 years of age will develop one, even more among patients treated by bone marrow transplantation. Squamous carcinomas of mouth, pharynx and oesophagus are relatively frequent, and any young patient with oral carcinoma should be screened for this condition. Clues for diagnosis include pigmented skin patches, short stature and a range of other developmental anomalies, but these features are very variable and genetic screening is required for diagnosis.

Case series PMID: 18831513

Oral cancer in young patients PMID: 33797696

Potentially malignant disorders

These were discussed in detail in the previous chapter and can be considered to fall into three groups:
- High-risk lesions associated with the same aetiological factors as oral carcinoma, such as speckled leukoplakia, erythroplasia, submucous fibrosis and any lesion with dysplasia.
- Specific high-risk conditions independent of typical risk factors such as proliferative verrucous leukoplakia and dyskeratosis congenita
- Chronic candidosis or lichen planus that are not associated with risk habits and leukoplakia with no dysplasia and are of very low risk

The proportion of carcinomas that arise in clinically recognisable potentially malignant diseases is unknown.

Patients without risk factors

A small proportion of patients appear to have no risk factors. Most are old and female, and they tend to have carcinomas of the buccal mucosa, alveolus and tongue. Many have the clinical presentation of proliferative verrucous leukoplakia (Ch. 19).

For the remainder, random mutation, background radiation, atmospheric pollution and passive smoking remain speculative aetiological factors. There is an increased risk for individuals with a first-degree relative who had oral carcinoma, but the relative risk is very low.

In young patients, those under 35 years of age, one in five have no identifiable risk factor.

Oral cancer in young PMID: 24103389 and 33797696

'EARLY' AND 'LATE' ORAL CARCINOMA

→ Summary charts 19.1, 19.2 and 19.3 pp. 347, 348, 349

It is important to recognise oral carcinomas at their earliest stages because this is the most important factor determining success of treatment.

It is often assumed that small carcinomas are early in their development, but carcinomas vary widely in their aggressiveness and rate of growth. Some very small carcinomas are detected small because they are slow growing and stay small and localised for a prolonged period. Conversely, some large carcinomas may have grown in a few weeks. Thus defining 'early' carcinoma as one at a low Tumour Node Metastasis (TNM) stage is illogical, though it is frequently done.

The smallest carcinomas appear as painless red, speckled or white patches and only a minority are ulcerated (Figs 20.6 and 20.7). They are indistinguishable clinically from potentially malignant diseases, and approximately half of lesions thought to be erythroplasias and speckled leukoplakias clinically are already carcinomas on first biopsy.

After enlarging, a carcinoma may develop into a raised nodule, become ulcerated or both. Induration results from inflammation and fibrosis and infiltration of the tissues. By the time a carcinoma has formed an indurated ulcer with the typical rolled border, it will have been present for some months (Fig. 20.8).

Pain is generally considered of little value in the diagnosis of carcinoma. Certainly, early carcinoma is often painless, but some patients are seen with a burning or sharp stinging pain localised to the carcinoma or an apparently normal site, so unexplained pain should not be discounted. Ulceration may be associated with soreness or stinging pain when sharply flavoured food is eaten. Involvement of nerves by a carcinoma produces neuropathic pain, paraesthesia or anaesthesia in that nerve's distribution. Larger carcinomas may present with referred pain to the ear, through complex cranial nerve pathways. Pain increases with carcinoma size and is typically severe only in the late stages.

Presenting symptoms are diverse. Maintaining a high index of suspicion is critical to early diagnosis, and any unexplained lesion that fails to respond to treatment or does not heal spontaneously should raise suspicion of carcinoma.

The features of early and late carcinoma are shown in Table 20.2.

Clinical features early carcinomas PMID: 20860767

Erythroplakia as early sign PMID: 273632

ORAL CANCER DISTRIBUTION

Overall, the tongue is the most frequently affected site in the mouth and the majority of cancers are concentrated in the lower part of the mouth, particularly the lateral borders and ventral tongue, the adjacent floor of the mouth and lingual aspect of the alveolus and retromolar region, forming a U-shaped area extending back toward the oropharynx (Fig. 20.9).

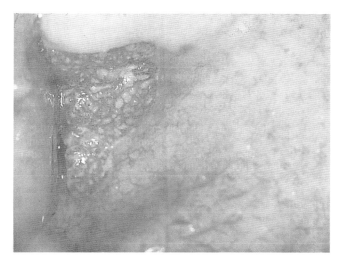

Fig. 20.6 **Squamous carcinoma** of the soft palate and mucosa posterior to the tuberosity appearing as a speckled leukoplakia.

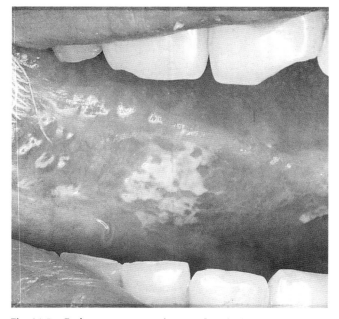

Fig. 20.7 **Early squamous carcinoma.** Despite its inconspicuous appearance, this small white patch on the lateral border of the tongue was found to be a squamous carcinoma on biopsy.

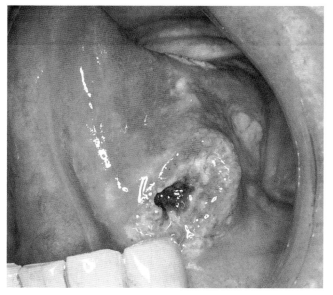

Fig. 20.8 **Advanced squamous carcinoma.** This classical ulcer with a rolled border and central necrosis is a late presentation. Note the surrounding areas of keratosis and erythema which had been present for many years before the carcinoma developed.

Table 20.2   Clinical features of oral squamous carcinoma

Superficially invasive	*Established carcinoma*
Low stage or 'Early'	**High stage or 'Late'**
Red patch	Indurated
Speckled patch	Ulcerated
White patch	Rolled ulcer margins
Soft or minimally firm	Nerve pain
Flat or slightly depressed	Paraesthesia or anaesthesia
Superficial non-healing ulcer	Loose teeth
	Bone loss
	Pain
	Reduced mobility of tissue/ tongue
	Spontaneous bleeding
	Palpable lymph node in neck
	Non-healing tooth socket

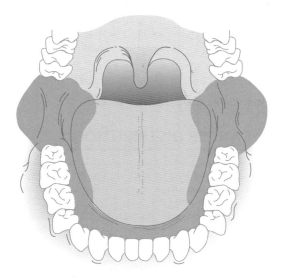

Fig. 20.9   High-risk sites for development of oral carcinoma. The shaded U-shaped area accounts for only approximately 20% of the whole area of the interior of the mouth, but is the site of more than 70% of oral cancers.

This accounts for only approximately 20% of the whole area of the interior of the oral cavity, but 70% of oral cancers arise there. This distribution may be due to pooling of carcinogens in saliva and concentration in the lower mouth before swallowing. Possibly for the same reason, the hard palate and central dorsum of tongue are very rarely affected.

PATHOLOGY

The essential features of carcinoma are invasion and spread to lymph nodes and distant sites.

Oral carcinoma histopathology

The key feature is invasion (Figs 20.10 and 20.11). The epithelial cells lose their organisation into a surface layer of epithelium and grow into the underlying tissues. Invasion is a complex cellular process in which the cells lose their polygonal shape and rigid cytoskeleton and become motile.

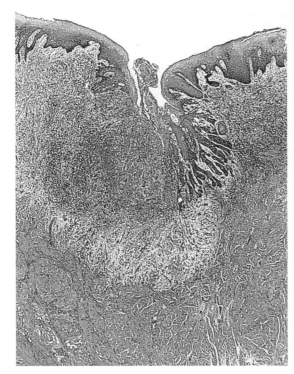

Fig. 20.10   A small squamous carcinoma. At low power, the epithelium is seen to invade deeply into the connective tissue and underlying muscle. At this early stage, there is no ulceration.

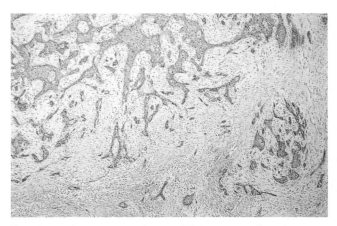

Fig. 20.11   Squamous carcinoma. Higher power of another carcinoma shows strands of malignant epithelium invading the connective tissue.

They induce surrounding fibroblasts and endothelial cells to aid their invasion by producing a fibrous tissue that is rich in proteoglycan ground substance and is easy to migrate through (tumour stroma). Growth of new vessels is induced to supply the increased nutrient requirements of the malignant cells. In late stage poorly differentiated carcinomas almost all cells can show this aggressive invasive nature.

Each carcinoma comprises many genetically different clones of cells coexisting in an ecosystem in which each clone can only survive with nutrients or signals from its neighbouring cells, whether part of the carcinoma or normal cells in the tumour stroma. With time and continuous proliferation of the genetically damaged cells, there is increasing chromosomal instability and development of a more genetically diverse

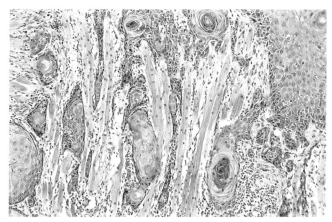

Fig. 20.12   Squamous carcinoma. At high power, groups of tumour cells from the carcinoma above are infiltrating downwards between muscle fibres, seen as pink vertical bands.

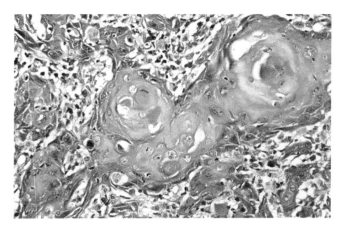

Fig. 20.13   Squamous carcinoma. In this moderately well-differentiated tumour, many of the neoplastic epithelial cells are forming keratin.

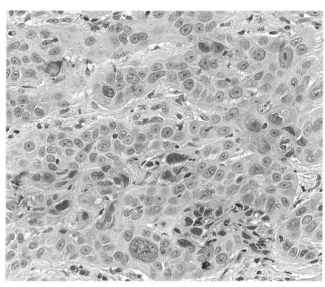

Fig. 20.14   Squamous carcinoma. In this poorly differentiated carcinoma, there is no keratin formation, no organization into basal and prickle cells, and the malignant cells show great pleomorphism with variably sized nuclei, many of which are hyperchromatic.

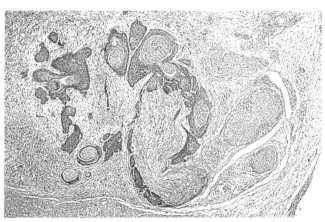

Fig. 20.15   Squamous carcinoma. In this carcinoma, malignant epithelium is invading around nerve sheaths. Although this is infrequent, occasionally carcinoma may spread some distance from the main tumour mass along nerve trunks.

population of clones of cells with slightly different properties and survival abilities. Eventually a clone with metastatic ability emerges. Only a small proportion of cells may eventually do this.

Histologically, the individual cells show the features of malignancy: large and irregularly shaped nuclei, darkly stained nuclei (hyperchromatism), frequent and sometimes abnormal mitoses (Fig. 20.12). These are essentially the same cytological changes as are seen in dysplastic epithelium (Table 19.3); only invasion differentiates the two processes.

Squamous carcinoma is graded according to its degree of differentiation, the degree to which the malignant cells resemble normal epithelium by differentiating to form prickle cells and keratin. In well-differentiated tumours, the cells have cytoplasm that stains palely with eosin or may form concentric layers of keratin (cell nests or keratin pearls; Fig. 20.13). In poorly differentiated tumours, the cells tend to be more irregular and darkly staining and show little evidence of prickle cell differentiation or keratinisation (Fig. 20.14). In the most poorly differentiated carcinomas, the cells have little cytoplasm and, in the least differentiated examples, may be spindle cells not recognisable as epithelial by routine microscopy. Poorly differentiated carcinomas tend to infiltrate more widely at an early stage, are more likely to

metastasise and carry a poorer prognosis. The majority of oral carcinomas are moderately differentiated.

Local spread

The invading cells grow into the tissues by direct extension. Irregular branching processes penetrate the tissue, the tips of which are often cut off in a histological section to give the appearance of separate islands of tumour (see Fig. 20.11). In the more infiltrative, poorly differentiated carcinomas, single cells and small clusters of cells detach along the invasive front of the lesion forming a discohesive invasive front. This carries a higher risk of metastasis than a cohesive invasive front of large islands of epithelium.

Aggressive carcinomas may show perineural infiltration, selective spread along nerves, or vascular invasion (Figs 20.15 and 20.16) both of which are adverse prognostic features. Carcinomas that spread along nerves are less likely to be easily excised and more likely to recur because of their unpredictable

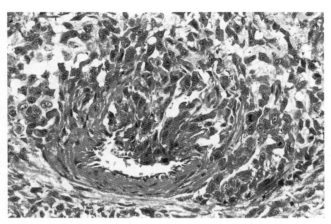

Fig. 20.16 Squamous carcinoma. Less frequent than perineural invasion is vascular invasion. Here a cluster of poorly differentiated malignant epithelial cells have eroded the wall of the vessel and entered the circulation.

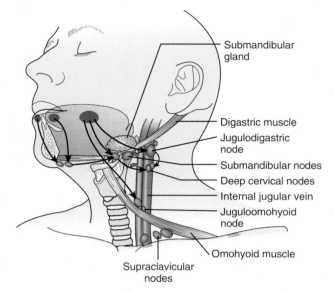

Fig. 20.17 Typical routes of lymphatic spread from lip and intraoral squamous carcinomas (*purple*) to nodes (*green*).

outline. Those with vascular invasion are more likely to metastasise.

Tumour cells invade all tissues (Fig. 20.11). Muscle, fat, nerves and eventually bone are infiltrated and destroyed. Carcinoma induces resorption of the bone by activating normal osteoclasts across a broad front, 'saucerising' the cortex until it can invade the medullary cavity to spread more widely and destroy the bone from within.

Invading cancer cells excite a variable inflammatory and immune reaction and can become surrounded by lymphocytes and plasma cells. Tumour-infiltrating lymphocytes do kill some carcinoma cells, but unfortunately, the immune response provides no significant protection.

Perineural infiltration PMID: 25457832

Pattern of invasion PMID: 23250819 and 8039106

Metastasis

Lymphatic metastasis to the regional lymph nodes is the most likely and earliest form of distant spread. Clones of cells in the tumour eventually acquire the range of abilities required to migrate, penetrate lymphatics, survive as single cells during transit, lodge in a lymph node and proliferate to form a metastasis. For some time before metastasis develops, cancer cells can be detected in the circulation but fail to seed metastases. These cells presumably lack some of the necessary abilities and are killed or die in the circulation.

The specific sites of metastasis depend on the drainage of the tumour site but, because most carcinomas arise posteriorly in the lower mouth, the submandibular and jugulodigastric nodes are those most frequently involved. Lymphatic drainage from the tongue is shown in Fig. 20.17. Floor-of-mouth carcinomas and others involving or crossing the midline may spread bilaterally.

Metastases develop progressively down the jugular lymphatic chain (Fig. 20.18), reaching level IV supraclavicular lymph nodes at a late stage. Although these patterns of spread are relatively predictable overall, there is great difficulty in identifying and predicting metastatic spread to the neck when planning treatment for an individual case. Spread of cancer may be by an abnormal route, and all the lymph nodes of both sides of the neck must be examined and imaged.

Metastatic carcinoma is initially limited to the affected node but, in time, grows through the capsule into the tissues of the neck. This is a marker of an aggressive carcinoma,

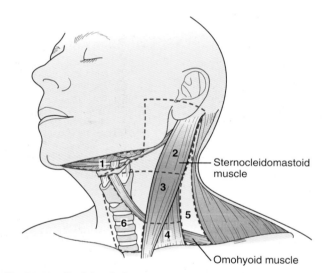

Fig. 20.18 Neck levels for assessing metastasis for TNM staging. The neck is conventionally divided into level 1, the submandibular and submental region nodes, three levels 2, 3 and 4 down the jugular chain, 5 in the posterior triangle and 6 in the anterior neck. Metastasis patterns follow lymphatic drainage, and lower neck levels carry a poorer prognosis. In contrast, thyroid carcinomas metastasise to levels 6 first, then 3 and 4, while metastases in level 5 are usually from the skin or pharynx.

excision is then difficult, and the chances of survival are diminished. Extranodal spread is evident clinically as fixation of the node.

Metastatic carcinoma forms a hard mass when small, but in larger masses the central area can become necrotic. The centre may then break down, so that the metastasis becomes cystic and fluctuant clinically.

Bloodstream metastasis is an uncommon, late feature of the disease and often after several episodes of treatment. Metastases then develop most frequently in lung, followed by liver and bone, heralding a terminal phase.

Key features are summarised in Box 20.3.

- Early cancers appear as white or red patches or shallow ulcers and are painless or only slightly sore
- Later carcinomas appear as ulcers with prominent rolled edges and induration and become painful
- More than 70% of oral cancers form on the lateral borders of the tongue and adjacent alveolar ridge and floor of mouth
- Over 95% are well- or moderately well-differentiated squamous cell carcinomas
- Spread is by direct invasion of surrounding tissues and by lymphatic metastasis
- The submandibular and jugulodigastric nodes are those most frequently involved
- The prognosis deteriorates sharply with lymph node metastasis

Tumour thickness and metastasis PMID: 16240329

Metastasis poor prognosis PMID: 20406474

Site variation

Tongue

The lateral border of the anterior two-thirds of the tongue and the adjacent ventral tongue are common sites. Conversely, a carcinoma arising centrally on the dorsum is extremely rare.

Carcinomas of the tongue must invade only a millimetre or so before they enter muscle, a vascular tissue that seems to promote carcinoma growth. Carcinoma in the tongue is renowned for its unpredictable spread, in part because growth is directed along muscle bundles, which in the tongue radiate all directions. Carcinomas sometimes show selective sarcolemmal spread along muscle fibres and grow out long thin extensions of tumour, often reaching the midline at a relatively early stage. The tongue becomes progressively stiffer and more painful. Eating, swallowing and talking become a challenge.

Carcinoma of the tongue is also known for its unpredictable metastasis. In addition to drainage to lymph nodes around the submandibular gland in level 2, carcinoma of the lateral border will metastasise directly the jugulo-omohyoid or other nodes in level 3. One in five carcinomas generate such 'fast track' metastases, directly to level 3 without involving level 2 first.

Once the midline is reached, metastases may develop bilaterally. Tongue carcinoma develops metastases at an early stage.

Floor of mouth

Unlike tongue carcinomas, floor of mouth carcinomas tend to spread laterally producing broad relatively superficial tumours. If they extend to the alveolar mucosa, they may erode bone, and if they extend up onto the ventral tongue, they may then extend into underlying muscle. Most arise anteriorly.

Treatment is difficult, and this site carries a poor prognosis. More carcinomas here are poorly differentiated, and there are few barriers to spread to deep vital structures. Metastases occur early, in almost half of patients on presentation.

Alveolar ridge and gingiva

This site accounts for approximately 10% of all oral carcinomas. Patients tend to be older people. The carcinomas tend to be well differentiated and more slowly growing than tongue carcinomas but erode bone at an earlier stage, making treatment more complex. However, only a minority invade the underlying bone in a dispersed pattern, and the cortical bone is usually resorbed without penetration far into the medullary cavity. These carcinomas have a lower risk of lymph node metastasis. Metastasis is usually to the relatively easily treated levels 1 and 2.

Unfortunately, despite these good features, gingival carcinoma often shows delayed diagnosis, being mistaken for inflammatory periodontal disease or denture trauma. It is important not to extract teeth adjacent to such a carcinoma because that allows the carcinoma to spread deep into the medullary cavity easily.

Buccal mucosa

At this site, carcinomas erode the soft tissue and eventually penetrate through to the skin. Most arise posteriorly, and some are associated with betel quid chewing.

Retromolar region

This is a common site but difficult to treat because carcinoma may spread into underlying bone, medial to the ramus to the pharynx, laterally into the cheek and up to the tuberosity region and infratemporal fossa, making surgery and reconstruction difficult. Half of cases present with metastases.

MANAGEMENT

Early diagnosis is critical if patients are to be cured because survival is highly dependent on tumour size. Even after diagnosis, the speed of treatment is critical to outcome and patients need to progress rapidly along the treatment 'pathway'. However, this urgency must be balanced with assessment of patients' expectations and understanding of treatment. Surgery and radiotherapy produce significant morbidity, and the quality of life of survivors of large operations and radiotherapy can be poor. Patients will spend a week or two undergoing intensive investigations and planning and may feel rushed into making decisions about their treatment and life after treatment. Good communication and rapport with patients can be as important as good surgery or oncology.

Treatment should be performed in a specialist centre because these have been shown to have superior outcomes. Resources are concentrated to make the widest range of treatment and support available. Patients should follow a defined pathway, as shown in Table 20.3, and be managed by a multidisciplinary team (Box 20.4).

Preoperative assessment

The first stages in management are to identify the type, spread and stage of the carcinoma (Table 20.4) to evaluate comorbidity and patient expectations and resilience.

Palpation is not always effective in delineating the outline of a tumour. Well-differentiated carcinomas containing much keratin are usually firm and readily identified but dispersed poorly differentiated carcinomas may be impalpable. Clinical signs, such as nerve palsies, also indicate extent of spread.

Imaging involves several techniques to delineate the tumour and to provide baseline data to compare post-treatment

Table 20.3 The UK patient 'pathway' for oral squamous carcinoma

Step	Reasons/components
Biopsy and diagnosis, initial examination	May be outside or in the specialist centre. The cancer centre will usually run 'one stop' clinics for suspected cancer allowing patients to access a range of services at one visit. Bad news should be broken by someone with specialist cancer training and the patient should be seen by members of the cancer team as soon as possible, within 2 weeks in the UK.
Imaging	Computed tomography (CT) and magnetic resonance imaging (MRI), possibly with positron emission tomography (PET) scans to assess size, stage and possible spread to lymph nodes. CT of the chest is usually performed to check for lung metastases, which would usually prevent curative treatment, and to exclude a second primary lung carcinoma in smokers. Cone beam CT is useful to detect minor degrees of bone involvement. MRI imaging is useful to detect perineural spread, extension around vessels or to skull base, CT is used for bone involvement. PET is used to detect metastases or exclude a distant primary in suspected metastasis to the mouth or jaws.
Clinical Nurse Specialist review	These advanced specialist nursing staff provide information, assess patients medically and act as a 'key worker' single point of contact for the patient throughout treatment. Arrange smoking cessation and alcohol advice, assess home circumstances, ability to cope at home after treatment and educate the patient's relatives.
Pre-treatment nutritional assessment	Many patients are poorly nourished and need parenteral feeding, either by a nasogastric tube or a gastrostomy to be able to withstand treatment. If feeding after treatment is difficult, gastrostomy feeding may become permanent. Improved diet after treatment improves outcome.
Pre-treatment speech and language therapy assessment	Treatment often results in reduced swallowing ability. If radiotherapy fields include the larynx, the voice may be affected.
Examination of pharynx and larynx	To determine whether smokers have other upper aerodigestive tract carcinoma or potentially malignant disease that would affect treatment.
Pre-treatment dental assessment	Complete examination and eradication of foci of infection and removal of teeth with poor prognosis to prevent osteoradionecrosis. Dentistry after treatment can be difficult with trismus and dry mouth. Aggressive preventive regime.
Ultrasound examination and fine needle aspiration	If lymph node metastases are suspected clinically or on imaging, an ultrasound examination and fine needle aspiration under ultrasound guidance should be performed.
Discussion at multidisciplinary team meeting (or tumour board)	Meeting with members of all specialties in the treatment team, reviewing and confirming pathological diagnosis, extent and staging on imaging, the patient's medical, psychological and home circumstances and proposing an ideal treatment and any options to be presented to the patient.
Surgical treatment	Most patients receive surgical treatment if cure is thought possible.
Post-treatment discussion at multi-disciplinary team or tumour board	Review of success of surgical treatment and any complications. Add pathological data to refine the TNM stage and review completeness of excision, confirm treatment plan or update it.
Radiotherapy and chemotherapy treatment	Most patients receive radiotherapy as well as surgery. Planning starts immediately taking 2 weeks and treatment usually takes a further 6 weeks, and is followed by imaging, often a PET scan at 3 months to assess response.
Post-treatment discussion at multi-disciplinary team or tumour board	Review of success of overall treatment and any complications, confirm treatment plan or update it. If there is incomplete treatment response, decision on palliative treatments.
Follow up	Involves the cancer team and their outreach staff, medical and dental practitioners.

Box 20.4 Members of a head and neck cancer multidisciplinary team should include as a minimum

- Clinical nurse specialist
- Clinical oncologist
- Dietitian
- Palliative care physician
- Pathologist
- Radiologist
- Restorative dentist
- Specialist head and neck cancer surgeons
- Speech and language therapist

scans. Particular attention is paid to extension to the base of skull, prevertebral fascia, large areas of skin or around the carotid sheath as these usually render tumours inoperable. Extension to the posterior tongue is significant as surgical removal of posterior tongue risks aspiration of food and saliva and may necessitate laryngectomy with consequent loss of voice. Imaging includes the neck and chest to identify or exclude lymph node and blood-borne metastases.

Smokers and heavy alcohol users are assessed for cardiovascular or respiratory, neurological or liver disease that will pose an anaesthetic risk or compromise recovery from surgery. Nutritional status may need to be improved before treatment. The patient's psychological fitness for possible disfiguring surgery and future difficulty in speaking and swallowing must also be assessed. These and other complications of surgery

Table 20.4 Tumour Node Metastasis (TNM) staging for oral carcinoma.

T Tumour size	N Lymph node metastasis	M Distant metastasis
Tis Carcinoma in situ, not invasive, dysplasia only	**N0** No regional lymph node metastasis	M0 No distant metastasis
T1: Tumour 2 cm or less greatest dimension and 5 mm or less depth of invasion	**N1** Metastasis in a single ipsilateral lymph node, 3 cm maximum diameter without extranodal extension	M1 Distant metastasis present
T2: Tumour 2 cm or less in greatest dimension and with more than 5 mm depth of invasion <u>OR</u> 2–4 cm in greatest dimension with depth of invasion up to 10 mm	**N2a** as N1 but with extranodal extension <u>OR</u> Metastasis in a single ipsilateral node 3–6 cm diameter without extranodal extension **pN2b** Metastasis in multiple ipsilateral lymph nodes, all less than 6 cm maximum diameter, without extranodal extension **pN2c** Metastasis in bilateral or contralateral lymph nodes, all less than 6 cm in maximum diameter, without extranodal extension	
T3: Tumour more than 4 cm in greatest dimension but with 10 mm depth of invasion or less <u>OR</u> any tumour with depth of invasion greater than 10 mm	**N3a** Metastasis in a lymph node more than 6 cm maximum diameter without extranodal extension **N3b** Metastasis in any combination of lymph nodes with extranodal extension	
T4a: Tumour invades through the cortical bone of the mandible or maxillary sinus, or invades the skin of the face OR Any tumour greater than 4 cm diameter with depth of invasion more than 10 mm **T4b:** Tumour invades masticator space, pterygoid plates, or skull base, or encases internal carotid artery		

Stage 1	T1 N0 M0	
Stage 2	T2 N0 M0	
Stage 3	T3 N0 M0 T1-3 N1 M0	
Stage 4A	T4a N0 or 1 M0 T1-4a N2 M0	
Stage 4B	Any T N3 M0 T4b Any N M0	
Stage 4C	Any T Any N M1	

Note the importance of lymph node metastasis in determining the stage (in the lowest six table rows). Staging after pathological examination, Adapted from UICC TNM version 8 (2017) with corrections (2018).

must be understood by patients if they are to make properly informed choices and consent to treatment.

Actual and potential dental infection in the mouth must be dealt with before starting treatment, particularly if this is to be by irradiation. After treatment, dental infection or extractions may lead to osteoradionecrosis (Ch. 8), which is very resistant to treatment. Extraction sockets should be healed as nearly as possible before radiotherapy is begun. In practice, teeth for which rapid successful treatment cannot be guaranteed are usually extracted because of the need to start treatment quickly.

Treatment

At the multidisciplinary team meeting (or 'tumour board'), the clinical, imaging and pathological features, comorbidities, patient expectations and family or social support are reviewed. The final staging is confirmed according to the TNM classification (Table 20.4). This is the major determinant of possible treatments. Each carcinoma is given a score for size (T),

lymph node metastasis (N) and distant blood-borne metastasis (M). These are combined together to give a score between stage 0 (premalignancy) and IV. Unfortunately, most patients with oral carcinoma present at stage III or IV (Fig. 20.19).

Histopathological features of the carcinoma may indicate additional specific risks for local recurrence or metastasis.

The team will propose either a curative or palliative care plan for the patient to consider. Patients are usually recommended to have the most aggressive treatment that they can tolerate and accept. There is usually only one chance to cure a patient; recurrence is often the start of a prolonged course that ends in death.

Web URL 20.6 TNM staging general principles https://www.uicc.org/resources/tnm

TNM staging oral cavity PMID: 35048052

Histopathology predicts behaviour PMID: 31411752

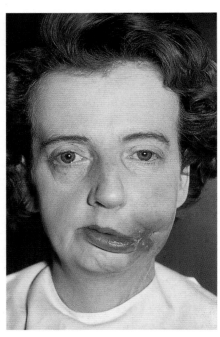

Fig. 20.19 Late-stage presentation of oral carcinoma, ulcerated through the cheek, thus at Stage 4a in TNM staging.

Oral carcinomas are not normally treated according to standardised protocols unlike carcinomas at other body sites. There have been very few large-scale trials of surgical and multimodality treatment, and a sound evidence base for treatment of individual cases is often lacking. Morbidity of treatment is high, and the patient's view of adverse effects is often the major consideration in the final treatment plan. Small differences in site and extent of carcinoma make large differences to the optimum treatment despite equivalent stage, because they affect important structures or practicality of reconstruction. Surgical excision is tailored to the individual tumour rather than its stage alone.

In practice, most intraoral carcinomas are treated by surgery combined with radiotherapy ('multimodality therapy'). Surgery alone is preferred for small carcinomas of the tongue that may be easily excised and for those involving bone because of the risk of later radionecrosis. Irradiation provides a more acceptable cosmetic and functional result than major surgery but involves considerable discomfort during a long course of treatment and has unwanted effects in the long term (Box 20.5).

When surgery is used, it is usually performed first, unless there has been a poor response to, or recurrence after, irradiation (salvage surgery). The aim is to excise the carcinoma with as wide a margin as possible, ideally 1 cm or more. Modern surgical methods allow excision, reconstruction, grafting or bypassing of many structures in the oral regions. However, a margin of more than a few millimetres is rarely achieved in practice because carcinomas have unpredictable irregular outlines or extend close to important anatomical structures. Also, wider excision may make reconstruction difficult.

Reconstructive surgery is normally performed at the same operation as excision, to provide a better cosmetic and functional result, and utilises a range of donor tissue sites. Excision by less than a few millimetres is insufficient to guarantee removal of the carcinoma, which may recur at the original site, and post-operative radiotherapy is, therefore, usually recommended.

Surgery also has adverse effects (Box 20.6).

All oral cancer radiotherapy in the UK is now delivered as intensity-modulated radiotherapy, a technologically complex system of linear accelerators allowing precisely controlled doses accurately conforming to the 3D shape of the tumour determined from imaging. This allows higher doses to be delivered to the carcinoma while reducing dose and adverse effects to surrounding normal tissue, particularly the eye, bone and salivary glands. Damage to surrounding tissues is further limited by fractionating the dose over many visits. A dose in the region of 60 Gy is usual for oral lesions, delivered in 30 daily fractions. A mask is made to fit the patient's head and immobilise it during treatment to allow reproducible beam angulation at each visit. Radiotherapy planning and mask construction are complex and involve a short delay before treatment can start.

Chemotherapy is less widely used in the UK than in Europe. Alone it gives good initial control, but relapse will always occur without surgery or radiotherapy. For best effect, it is carried out *concomitantly* with radiotherapy and gives approximately a 10% improvement in survival at best. The usual agent is cisplatin. All regimens have significant adverse effects, particularly with mucositis and immunosuppression, and these are compounded by radiotherapy. Only the fittest patients are able to tolerate concomitant chemotherapy.

Management of the neck

When surgery is to be recommended and lymph node metastases have been detected, neck dissection will be performed. Neck dissection removes all the cervical lymph nodes along the jugular chain from the base of skull to the clavicle, together with those in the submandibular and submental triangles and posterior triangle of the neck. Depending whether spread beyond the lymph node capsule is present or not, the sternomastoid muscle, internal jugular vein and accessory nerve may also be sacrificed. Neck dissection may also be required to provide access for reconstructive flap surgery, which requires space and suitable blood vessels to anastomose to the transplanted tissue.

When no cervical lymph nodes appear involved, small deposits of carcinoma may already have spread to lymph nodes. If left in place, they will grow during a period of months or years to form a recurrence. A decision must be made whether or not to perform a neck dissection as an elective procedure to ensure any potential microscopic metastases are removed. However, the value is a matter of statistical chance, and many patients have an elective neck dissection and its consequences for no benefit.

Alternatively, a sentinel node biopsy may be performed. In this technique, a radioisotope is injected around the tumour the night before surgery, followed by a blue dye at the time of surgery. These drain via lymphatics to the sentinel lymph nodes, those that are first in the drainage pathway and are most likely to be involved by metastasis. These nodes are identified at surgery by using a radiosensitive probe and by their blue colour (Fig. 20.20), removed and examined histologically. If no metastasis is present, the rest of the neck is almost certainly uninvolved and a neck dissection and its adverse effects can be avoided. If metastasis is present, a neck dissection is performed separately. As metastasis is confirmed in only approximately 80% of therapeutic neck dissections and 33% of elective (apparently metastasis-free) neck dissections, this technique saves many patients from unnecessary neck dissections and the resultant morbidity.

Sentinel node biopsy PMID: 28864148

Outcome

The highest mortality from oral cancer is in the first 2 years after diagnosis and treatment. The disease then continues to claim victims but at a slower rate, and the few patients that survive for 10 years are likely to have been cured. As a guide to survival rates, more than 90% of patients with stage 1 and 2 disease survive the first year and approximately 75% survive for as long as 5 years. Stage 3 and 4 carcinomas will kill almost half of the patients by 2 years and as many as 60% at 5 years (Fig. 20.21).

As to the site of the cancer, the best results are seen in cancer of the lip vermillion, where the 5-year survival rate

A

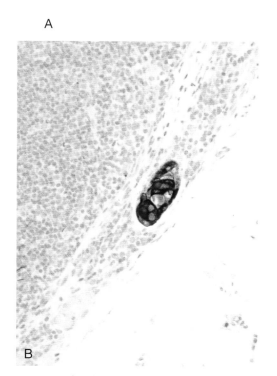

B

Fig. 20.20 Sentinel node biopsy. (A) Lymphoscintigraphy, an image captured by a gamma camera (or scintillation camera) to localise the injected radioisotope. The tongue tumour at the top is the largest signal, where isotope remains at the injection site. Drainage to sentinel nodes can be traced to two nodes in the jugular chain. (B) Biopsy of the sentinel node reveals a microscopic metastasis comprising only a few cells, detected using immunohistochemistry for keratin. The dense brown positive stain aids discovery of single cells and small clusters that could be missed on routine haematoxylin and eosin stains. *(Image A courtesy of Dr G Tartaglione)*

is 85% (Ch. 21). For cancer of the tongue it is 60%, but for late-stage carcinomas in adverse sites, only 20%. In general, the more posterior the tumour is, the poorer the survival.

Duration of survival after treatment depends on many factors (Box 20.7). In comparison with malignant neoplasms at other body sites, oral carcinoma has a poor prognosis. The quality of life in the terminal stages can be poor.

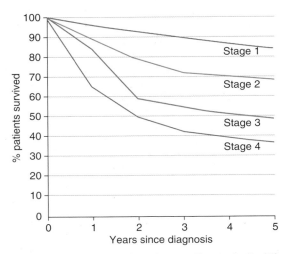

Fig. 20.21   Survival from oral carcinoma. The markedly different survival of stages 1–4 can be seen (see Table 20.4) and therefore the benefit of early diagnosis. These figures are for all oral sites; those in posterior sites have a worse prognosis than shown. *(Data from England until 2013, National Cancer Registration Service Cancer Analysis System.)*

Box 20.7   Some factors adversely affecting survival from oral cancer

- Delay in referral and treatment
- Advanced age
- Male sex
- Poor general health, usually smoking-related diseases
- Large tumour size
- Posterior site in mouth
- Perineural spread
- Lack of histological differentiation (high histological grade)
- Dispersed invasive front
- Lymph node spread
- Blood-borne metastasis

The poorer survival of older people is probably because they are less able to withstand radiotherapy or surgery. The reason for the poorer survival rates for males is uncertain, although later presentation is a possibility.

Development of radiation-induced sarcoma as a complication of treatment is a risk that has been estimated to be 1.6% after 10 years but carries a very poor prognosis.

Web URL 20.7 UK incidence, mortality: https://digital.nhs.uk/ and enter 'cancer registration' in search bar, and then 'national statistics' from the left menu

Second primary carcinomas

About 5% of patients with treated oral carcinoma develop a second primary carcinoma each year somewhere in the upper aerodigestive tract or lung. With better treatment and longer survival, this is an increasing problem. Patients who are young, smokers or treated by radiotherapy alone are at highest risk. Patients with proliferative verrucous leukoplakia (Ch. 19) may develop several primary carcinomas, but the main cause in most oral cancer patients is field change from tobacco smoking. Treatment of a second primary is made more complex by previous surgery or radiotherapy for the first carcinoma.

Treatment failure

Treatment fails in approximately 40% of patients and recurrence develops, either at the primary site, in lymph nodes or in distant sites such as lung, liver or bone.

Primary site recurrence usually signifies a poor prognosis because either a full course of radiotherapy or as large an excision as practical will already have been performed. Recurrence in lymph nodes usually appears within 2 years after treatment. The metastases probably arise from microscopic deposits of carcinoma already in the lymph nodes at the time of initial therapy (occult metastases). Neck recurrences alone may be treated surgically by neck dissection or by radiotherapy and do not necessarily indicate failure of treatment as further treatment is often curative.

Recurrent carcinoma is often less well differentiated and more aggressive. It invades more widely and unpredictably in the tissues than the initial carcinoma, particularly in tissues that have been irradiated, and is difficult to localize clinically and on imaging. Re-excision is often impossible.

Primary and recurrent disease have been treated more aggressively and more successfully in recent years so that more patients than previously now survive but succumb to distant blood-borne metastases later. Distant metastases are usually multiple, and there is no curative treatment.

Metastasis and death PMID: 20406474

Undetected metastasis and treatment failure PMID: 25074731

Distant metastasis PMID: 25883102

Palliative care

Palliative treatment is given to patients who have advanced tumours that cannot be cured, when comorbidity prevents full treatment or for treatment failures. It is an active multidisciplinary treatment, not only pain control, that aims to reduce symptoms of all types and provide psychological, social and other holistic needs. Radiotherapy is the most frequent method for active palliative treatment, but surgery is occasionally used when a large tumour compromises the airway or becomes grossly necrotic.

Causes of death

The combination of pain, infection and difficulty in eating cause loss of weight, anaemia and deterioration of general health. This state (malignant cachexia) is ultimately fatal. In other patients, aspiration of septic material from the mouth causes bronchopneumonia.

In the terminal stages, oral carcinoma recurrent at the primary site can form a large fungating mass that erodes major vessels or the cranial cavity. Extranodal spread from affected lymph nodes may ulcerate through the skin and erode the jugular or carotid vessels.

A small, but possibly growing, proportion of patients survive treatment of the primary carcinoma but die later from distant metastases in the lungs, liver or brain.

Targeted treatments

Malignant neoplasms at other body sites are increasingly treated using targeted treatments, drugs that act specifically on cell signalling pathways or genetic alterations in the individual cancer, or the immune response against it. Targeted therapy avoids damage to surrounding and remote cells, as occurs with radiotherapy or chemotherapy but usually only a proportion of cancers of any type are susceptible.

The agents used in targeted therapy are diverse and include antibodies, enzymes, toxins coupled to molecules or nanoparticles and small molecule inhibitors of receptors and signalling molecules. The first and best-known example is tamoxifen, the oestrogen receptor binding drug used against breast carcinoma.

Targeted therapy for oral carcinoma is in its early development, mostly using single agent therapy. Unfortunately, a general feature of targeted therapy is that single agent treatment, even if initially successful, will eventually induce resistance in the cancer. In future, multiple drug cocktails are likely to be more effective.

Cetuximab and erlotinib are inhibitors of the epidermal growth factor receptor, which controls cell cycle and apoptosis and has indirect effects in invasion and metastasis. The former is an antibody that binds the extracellular portion and the latter a small molecule inhibitor that binds the cytoplasmic portion of the receptor when specific mutations are present. Cetuximab is widely used in combination with cisplatin for recurrent or widespread carcinoma in palliative care and provides approximately 3 months survival advantage but is being supplanted by PD-L1/PD-1 targeted drugs.

Nivolumab is an antibody that binds PD-L1, a cancer cell surface protein that blocks T lymphocyte function, protecting the cancer cell from destruction by the patient's immune response. Pembrolizumab acts similarly by binding to PD-1, the lymphocyte receptor for PD-L1, preventing lymphocyte inactivation. Both drugs reactivate the immune response to kill the cancer cells. Pembrolizumab is given when the tumour is known to express PD-L1, as a second-line treatment for otherwise untreatable carcinoma in a palliative setting providing a mean survival advantage of 6–12 months.

Targeted treatments are also used for benign tumours and the use of BRAF inhibitors and hedgehog pathway inhibitors is discussed with ameloblastoma (Ch. 11) and odontogenic keratocyst (Ch. 10).

PD-L1 treatment PMID: 30866171 and 35395371

Molecular targeted drugs PMID: 34771633

Experimental treatments

Talimogene laherparepvec (T-Vec) is an engineered virus targeting cancer that showed promise in an early trial and awaits full evaluation. A number of molecular targeted immunotherapy approaches are in trial including engineering patients' own lymphocytes to react to their carcinoma. Robotic surgery holds promise to excise carcinomas more accurately with smaller but disease-free margins, avoid large facial and neck incisions and provide a better functional outcome. However, its use is limited to small carcinomas.

Survivorship

At any time, there are approximately 60,000 patients surviving after head and neck cancer treatment in the UK. Improved survival has produced many patients who live long term with the adverse effects of treatment and with a risk of second primary carcinoma. Psychological effects, usually depression, disfigurement and other long-term medical effects can cause poor quality of life. Support for survivors is becoming increasingly important, and their complex medical needs are ideally managed outside cancer centres. Some of these patients are vocal advocates for research, reducing morbidity of treatment and awareness of cancer, but the survivorship agenda is in its infancy. The dentist has important roles to play.

Survivorship PMID: 30552794

Guidelines Europe PMID: 35932637 and US 27002678

ROLE OF THE DENTIST

Early diagnosis is critical. Small carcinomas are more easily excised, less likely to have metastasised and have the best prognosis. Unfortunately, healthcare workers, including dentists, frequently either fail to make the diagnosis or actively delay referral.

Dentists must be alert to the possibility of carcinoma, despite its rarity, perform a risk assessment on any chronic ulcer, white or red lesion, or swelling of the mucous membrane and perform, or refer for, a biopsy. Indecision or trying the effect of local measures or antibiotics can prove fatal. It is better if the biopsy is performed by the cancer management team. Never perform an *excisional* biopsy of a possible small carcinoma. Once the biopsy site has healed, there may be no clue to its site or size, making further treatment difficult. Survival is reduced in such circumstances.

In the UK, every dental practice is within a cancer network that has an urgent referral system for suspected cancer for UK National Health Service (NHS) patients. Referral criteria are published by the NHS of the devolved nations and in England and Wales by the National Centre for Clinical Excellence. In each country, every dentist is expected to be familiar with the relevant criteria. Patients meeting the criteria in Table 20.5 can be referred direct to rapid access clinics and, at least in England, be guaranteed an appointment within 2 weeks. Note that the dentist provides a key 'gatekeeper' role in this referral pathway and is expected to be able to risk assess oral lesions so that patients with trivial or benign lesions are not needlessly referred to hospital. This role is specifically included in the criteria for England, Wales and Northern Ireland. This places great responsibility on all dentists to be able to do this accurately.

The 2-week wait system is for *suspected* cancers, and it is expected that only a small proportion of referred patients will have cancer. Referral criteria are based on having more than a 3% chance of indicating cancer. If you were highly suspicious or confident that a lesion was either a high-risk potentially malignant disorder or already a carcinoma, a direct referral on the same day would be appropriate. For some cancers, even a 2-week wait is too long.

The dental practitioner is likely to see many more patients with white or red mucosal patches than carcinomas. As noted in Chapter 19, the vast majority of such lesions are benign and may be biopsied in a practice setting. However, it is inadvisable to perform a biopsy of a high-risk lesion (for instance, an erythroplasia or speckled leukoplakia) because the practitioner may be forced into the unenviable position of having to tell the patient that they have cancer, a task for which most dentists are not trained.

Although much of a patient's treatment has to be performed in hospital, patients often continue to see their practitioner after treatment.

The dental practitioner is also ideally placed for the prevention of oral cancer and can contribute in other ways (Box 20.8).

Role of dentist in United States PMID: 24192734

Table 20.5 General practice referral criteria in the UK for head and neck cancer (excluding thyroid)

England and Wales 2015 (revised 2021)

Consider a suspected cancer pathway referral (for an appointment within 2 weeks) for oral cancer in people with either:

- Unexplained ulceration in the oral cavity lasting for more than 3 weeks or
- A persistent and unexplained lump in the neck.

Consider an urgent referral (for an appointment within 2 weeks) for assessment for possible oral cancer by a dentist in people who have either:

- A lump on the lip or in the oral cavity or
- A red or red and white patch in the oral cavity consistent with erythroplakia or erythroleukoplakia.

Consider a suspected cancer pathway referral by the dentist (for an appointment within 2 weeks) for oral cancer in people when assessed by a dentist as having either:

- A lump on the lip or in the oral cavity consistent with oral cancer or
- A red or red and white patch in the oral cavity consistent with erythroplakia or erythroleukoplakia.

Scotland 2019*

- Persistent unexplained head and neck lumps for >3 weeks.
- Unexplained ulceration or unexplained swelling/induration of the oral mucosa persisting for >3 weeks.
- All unexplained red or mixed red and white patches of the oral mucosa persisting for >3 weeks.
- Persistent hoarseness lasting for >3 weeks
- Persistent pain in the throat or pain on swallowing lasting for >3 weeks.

Northern Ireland 2012 (issue 2021)

Red Flag referral, patients with:

- An unexplained lump in the neck, of recent onset, or a previously undiagnosed lump that has changed over a period of 3 to 6 weeks
- An unexplained persistent swelling in the parotid or submandibular gland
- An unexplained persistent sore or painful throat
- Unilateral unexplained pain in the head and neck area for more than 4 weeks, associated with otalgia (ear ache) but a normal otoscopy
- Unexplained ulceration of the oral mucosa or mass persisting for more than 3 weeks
- Unexplained red and white patches (including suspected lichen planus) of the oral mucosa that are painful or swollen or bleeding.

For patients with persistent symptoms or signs related to the oral cavity in whom a definitive diagnosis of a benign lesion cannot be made, refer to follow up until the symptoms and signs disappear. If the symptoms and signs have not disappeared after 6 weeks, make an urgent referral.

Red Flag referral to a dentist:

- Patients with unexplained tooth mobility persisting for more than 3 weeks – monitor for oral cancer patients with confirmed oral lichen planus, as part of routine dental examination. Advise all patients, including those with dentures, to have regular dental checkups.

Non-urgent referral:

- A patient with unexplained red and white patches of the oral mucosa that are not painful, swollen or bleeding (including suspected lichen planus).

*Comment in accompanying text: With the changing pattern of disease, age, non-smoking or non-drinking status should not be a barrier to referral.
American Dental Association evidence-based clinical practice guideline is more complex, with a significant triage role for dental practitioners, published in 2017: see *PMID: 28958308*

Box 20.8 Role of the dental practitioner in cancer prevention and diagnosis

Prevention

- Actively discourage all types of smoking, smokeless tobacco and betel quid use
- Encourage moderation of alcohol intake
- Health promotion and education on oral carcinoma
- Provide check-ups for people who are edentulous, older and/or in institutions and other high-risk non-attenders

Early diagnosis

- Be vigilant and suspicious
- Always examine all of the mucosa and the teeth
- Monitor low-risk premalignant lesions
- Refer all high-risk lesions on discovery
- Perform biopsy appropriately

After treatment

- Manage simple denture problems after surgery
- Alleviate the effects of post-irradiation dry mouth, e.g., preventing caries
- Monitor for recurrence, new premalignant lesions and second primary tumours
- Monitor for cervical metastasis
- Maintain morale of, and provide additional support to, patients and their relatives

Dentist in diagnosis PMID: 26682494

Dental team diagnosis PMID: 12973333

Web URL 20.9 NICE referral criteria for all head neck cancers are in the Improving Outcomes document at: https://www.nice.org.uk/guidance/csg6

ORAL CANCER SCREENING

Screening is the process of applying a rapid test or examining a population to identify a group at risk from a disease. This group can then be referred for accurate and earlier diagnosis. Oral carcinoma screening should be possible because the mouth is easily accessible for examination and because those at most risk (older people, smokers) are readily identified. A simple effective screening test is an examination of the mouth for red and white lesions.

Screening is not intended to provide an accurate diagnosis and may be performed by a variety of trained healthcare workers in the community. Such oral cancer screening schemes have proved successful in several countries with a high incidence. In the UK, such a scheme might reach the highest risk individuals who tend to be irregular dental attenders and would provide an opportunity for preventive advice.

The benefits of a national screening scheme for the UK have been evaluated. Such a scheme would be effective in identifying cancers but would not be cost effective, and this conclusion was reaffirmed in 2020. No study has shown that screening improves life expectancy. In the absence of nationally administered schemes, oral cancer screening remains within the remit of general dental and medical practitioners.

Cochrane review screening PMID: 24254989 and methods: 34891214

Narrative review PMID: 34036828

Status screening in United States PMID: 22779205

Patient view screening in dental practice PMID: 23249393

Screening effective in dental practice PMID: 16707071

Screening and detection aids

Several tests are marketed, some without a clear distinction as to whether they are for screening or diagnosis (the latter would demand a much higher predictive value). All require evaluation in properly controlled trials before any could be recommended. In the meantime, all produce significant false-positive and false-negative results. Incisional biopsy is still the correct approach when there is any doubt about a lesion.

Tolonium chloride (toluidine blue) rinsing

Tolonium chloride is a dye that binds to nucleic acids and can be used as an oral rinse in the hope of staining carcinoma and dysplastic lesions blue.

The technique is not an accurate test for either carcinoma or premalignancy and is no more than an adjunct to clinical diagnosis. If used indiscriminately on white lesions, lichen planus and ulcers, the technique has a high false-positive rate. It may be of value when deciding which part of an extensive lesion should be biopsied or when the clinician does not feel confident about a clinical diagnosis. Any suspicious lesion must be subjected to biopsy as soon as possible, regardless of the pattern of staining with toluidine blue.

Brush biopsy

This technique is relatively non-invasive and therefore attractive for screening or long-term follow-up. It uses a round stiff-bristle brush to collect cells from the surface and subsurface layers of a lesion by vigorous abrasion. The brush is rotated in the fingers in one spot until bleeding starts, to ensure a sufficiently deep sample. There is little or no pain, minimal bleeding and no need for sutures. The cells collected are transferred to a microscope slide and the smear is scanned to identify abnormal cells.

Once collected, the cells can be subjected to several different test systems. A high degree of sensitivity and specificity for carcinoma is claimed, but studies have shown widely varying accuracy. It may have a role in follow-up for patients with potentially malignant lesions after definitive diagnosis.

Saliva tests

It is an attractive possibility that oral cancer or potential malignancy might be diagnosed by a simple saliva test. More than 100 different salivary biomarkers have been investigated. Despite claims for high sensitivity, none has yet been proven in a well-designed trial including patients with the many inflammatory and benign conditions with which cancers can be confused.

Review screening aids PMID: 17825602 and 29080605

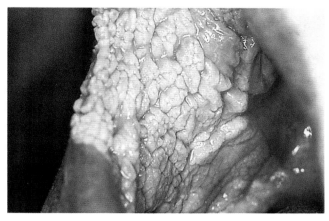

Fig. 20.22 Verrucous carcinoma. An extensive lesion covering most of the buccal mucosa and starting to involve the skin at the commissure. Verrucous carcinoma does not metastasize, but such large and longstanding lesions are likely to develop a focus of invasive squamous carcinoma within them that can metastasise. *(Courtesy Prof. SJ Challacombe.)*

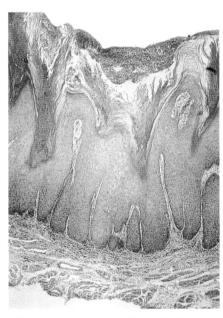

Fig. 20.23 Verrucous carcinoma. The epithelium is thickened and thrown into a series of folds with a spiky parakeratotic surface. Deeply, the carcinoma retains a broad pushing invasive front.

VERRUCOUS CARCINOMA

This variant of squamous cell carcinoma is a low-grade carcinoma. In the UK it is more frequent in older people, particularly males, and has a characteristic white, warty appearance, forming a well-circumscribed mass raised above the level of the surrounding mucosa (Fig. 20.22). If small, it may easily be mistaken for a papilloma. Verrucous carcinoma in some countries is particularly associated with the habit of snuff dipping (mentioned previously).

Pathology

Verrucous carcinoma consists of close-packed papillary masses of well-differentiated squamous epithelium that are heavily keratinised. The lower border of the lesion is well defined and formed by blunt rete processes that indent the underlying tissues (Fig. 20.23), a process called *pushing* invasion.

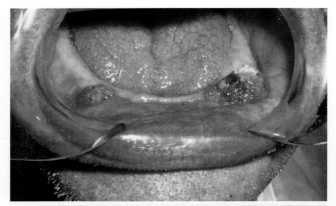

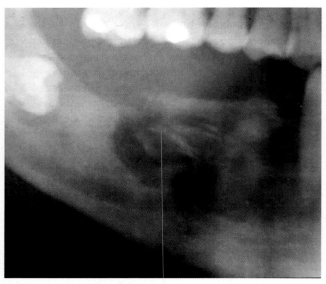

Fig. 20.25 **Carcinoma cuniculatum.** Unlike conventional squamous carcinoma, the bony destruction is better defined, there is little surface destruction and numerous sequestra are visible centrally, resembling osteomyelitis.

CARCINOMA CUNICULATUM

Carcinoma cuniculatum is a very rare variant of squamous carcinoma. It is well-differentiated and forms epithelial lined crypts or burrows that penetrate deeply into underlying tissues, particularly through bone.

Carcinoma cuniculatum arises mostly on the gingiva or alveolar ridge mucosa in older people. Several features cause frequent misdiagnosis as osteomyelitis or abscess. Firstly, there is deep bony destruction and tooth mobility, often without a large mass or ulcer at the surface (Fig. 20.24). Secondly, small sequestra and keratin, resembling pus, discharge from the crypt openings mimicking infected sinuses. Thirdly, the carcinoma resembles osteomyelitis radiologically (Fig. 20.25) and, last, it is difficult to diagnose histologically.

The prognosis is excellent if completely excised as the carcinoma is well delineated and metastasis does not occur.

Cases PMID: 24035112

DIAGNOSTIC CATCHES

A number of conditions resemble oral squamous carcinoma clinically and histologically, and may be misdiagnosed as carcinoma. These lesions are discussed at the end of the next chapter.

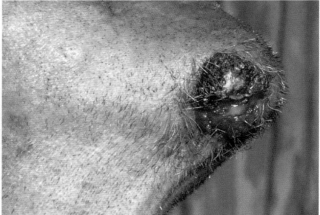

Fig. 20.24 **Carcinoma cuniculatum.** This patient developed a slow growing and apparently innocuous white verrucous nodule on the edentulous alveolar ridge in the lower left canine area. This remained small but was a carcinoma cuniculatum, which burrowed down and across the midline in the mandibular medullary space and back out to the surface both in the opposite alveolar ridge and submental skin.

Verrucous carcinoma is slow-growing and spreads laterally rather than deeply, so it can be excised relatively easily unless it is extensive. If left untreated for a period of years, a focus within verrucous carcinoma may progress to a more invasive squamous carcinoma and must then be treated as a conventional squamous carcinoma.

Review PMID: 18088849

Review and treatment outcome PMID: 11443616

Treatment PMID: 18620896

Other mucosal and lip carcinomas

21

LIP CARCINOMA

Lip carcinoma is much less common than intraoral carcinoma, with approximately 250 cases each year in the UK, but rarely presents directly to a dentist unless it is a chance finding. However, dentists should be able to recognise a sun-damaged lip and the early signs of malignant change.

Aetiology

Exposure to ultraviolet light is the primary cause (Fig 21.1), usually sunlight, because the lip vermillion does not produce protective melanin. Lip cancer is predominantly a disease of outdoor workers and fair-skinned persons are at most risk. The relationship between exposure to sunlight and lip cancer has been clearly shown in Australia and the United States with large immigrant, fair-skinned populations of European origin. In the United States, for example, the risk of lip cancer approximately doubles for every 250 miles nearer the equator of the site of residence.

Sunbed use is also a risk because high doses of ultraviolet light can be achieved. Legal limits on ultraviolet light output are equivalent to tropical sun. Sunbed use is thought to account for 8% of skin cancer in the United States and is more damaging in young people.

Changes due to ultraviolet light are preventable, and dentists should encourage the use of a high-factor sunblock, minimum factor 30, ideally 50, when exposed to strong sunlight and avoidance of sunbeds.

Smoking, particularly of roll-your-own cigarettes without a filter, cigars or pipes, are the next most important factors, supplying heat and carcinogens to the lip.

People who are immunosuppressed, particularly organ transplant recipients, have an increased risk of lip carcinoma.

Pathology

More than 90% of lip carcinomas arise on the lower lip, to one side of the midline. Men are affected twice as frequently as women, and older people are predominantly affected.

An area of thickening, induration, crusting or shallow ulceration of the lip, less than a centimetre in diameter, is a typical early presentation (Fig. 21.2).

All are squamous carcinomas, and most are well differentiated. Spread to lymph nodes tends to be late and is seen in only 10% of patients, usually to the submental nodes. These factors, combined with relatively easy excision, give lip carcinoma a good prognosis, and 90% of patients survive 5 years and are cured. Carcinomas over 2 cm diameter; those that recur, metastasise, occur in young patients or in the upper lip are more likely to be fatal, but this is still infrequent.

Approximately half of cases are preceded by a zone of keratosis with dysplasia seen histologically, equivalent to an intraoral leukoplakia. All keratosis on the lip should be subject to biopsy. A sun-damaged lip may be identified clinically by its loss of elasticity, atrophic epithelium, loss of definition of the vermillion border and telangiectasia (Fig. 21.3).

Lip carcinoma is treated by excision if small; larger tumours may receive multimodality treatment.

Skin cancer for dentists PMID: 24852988 and 10528565

Solar damage for dentists PMID: 8150192

HUMAN PAPILLOMAVIRUS–ASSOCIATED OROPHARYNGEAL CARCINOMAS

Since 1990, an epidemic of carcinoma of the oropharynx has been identified in many countries, particularly Canada,

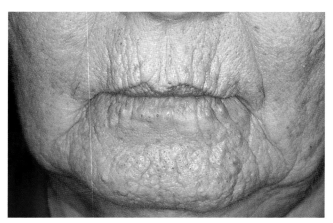

Fig. 21.1 Photoaged skin. Severe sun damage causing leathered wrinkling. Smoking exacerbates solar skin damage independently of any carcinogenic effect on the lip.

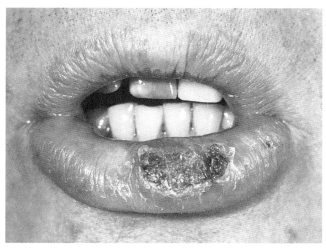

Fig. 21.2 Squamous carcinoma of lip. There is an indurated, crusted ulcer with keratosis at one margin in the centre of the lower lip.

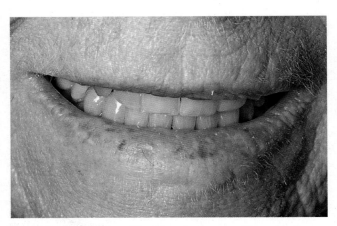

Fig. 21.3 Sun-damaged lip. There is atrophy of the epithelium, producing increased redness, loss of wrinkles and definition of the skin-vermilion boundary and telangiectasia. White flecks or patches of keratosis may also develop. Any keratosis, flaking or crusting, nodule or ulcer developing in this background should be regarded with suspicion.

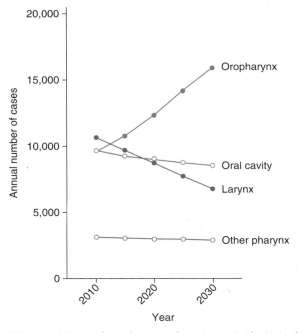

Fig. 21.4 Incidence of oropharyngeal carcinoma in the United States. Observed (until 2007) and projected (till 2030) number of new patients with oropharyngeal, oral cavity, larynx and other pharynx cancers per year. Larynx and oral carcinoma are in slow decline, pharynx cancer rates are stable but oropharyngeal carcinoma is predicted to rise dramatically. See also data from the UK in Fig. 20.1. (*Data from Chaturvedi, A.K., Engels, E.A., Pfeiffer, R.M., et al., 2011. Human papillomavirus and rising oropharyngeal cancer incidence in the United States. J. Clin. Oncol. 29 [32], 4294–4301.*)

Eastern Europe, North America and the UK (Figs 21.4). There is a wave of increasing incidence, led by the US and gradually peaking later in other countries. Oropharyngeal carcinoma is the fastest increasing cancer in parts of the UK, incidence doubled between 1990 and 2006 and doubled again between 2006 and 2010 (see Fig 20.1).

In the UK, 80% or more of these cancers are caused by viral infection. This section describes the virus-induced carcinomas because these differ in many respects from oral carcinoma. The remainder are usually caused by smoking and alcohol and present in a similar fashion to oral carcinoma.

Aetiology

The cause of the dramatic increase in incidence is human papillomavirus (HPV) infection. There are more than 150 subtypes of human papillomavirus, some of which cause warts and benign disease, and others of which can infect and cause carcinoma in the uterine cervix. The most common carcinogenic types by far are types 16 and 18. These viruses are relatively widespread in the population and are the most common sexually transmitted infection with more than 6 million new infections each year in the United States and 20 million people infected at any one time. However, most patients' immune systems clear the infection in under a year, and the overall risk of developing carcinoma is very low.

Genital papillomavirus types can be transmitted to the mouth, primarily through oral sex though transmission across the placenta, during birth or shortly after is also possible. Clearance of oral and pharyngeal infection takes several years and, as in the cervix, infection is common but the risk of carcinoma is very low. It appears that persistent or repeated infection carries the highest risk, and it is possible that the few patients who develop carcinoma have a genetic or immunological predisposition to infection. The current increase in incidence started in about 1990 and appears to be a delayed effect of changes in sexual practices since the 1960s. In the United States, human papillomavirus now causes carcinoma more frequently in the oropharynx than in the cervix.

Worldwide incidence PMID: 35303618

US incidence PMID: 31503300

UK incidence PMID: 32978578

Transmission PMID: 25873485 and 26908748

Pathogenesis

Human papillomavirus–associated carcinomas almost always arise in the oropharynx, specifically in the tonsil and minor tonsils of Waldeyer's ring, around the base of tongue, soft palate and pharynx. Tonsil crypts are lined by non-keratinised and permeable epithelium designed to allow antigens to penetrate into the lymphoid tissue below. HPV infects the epithelium, and the viral DNA either integrates into the DNA of the crypt lining epithelial cells or remains in their cytoplasm. Viral proteins E6 and E7 bind to and inactivate the tumour suppressor proteins p53 and retinoblastoma protein respectively, inhibiting apoptosis, increasing cell proliferation and generating genomic instability. After a prolonged latent period of 20–30 years, carcinoma may result. The mechanisms are slightly different from the way HPV causes cancer of the uterine cervix, but the differences are not yet understood.

HPV carcinogenesis in head and neck PMID: 35105976

Clinical

It is often said that papillomavirus–associated carcinomas arise in young patients. While this was true in the early stages of the epidemic, the age of onset is now almost exactly the same as intraoral cancer. HPV does not account for the increase in intraoral cancers in young people.

The presenting signs of HPV–associated oropharyngeal carcinomas are very different from those of other oral and upper aerodigestive tract carcinomas. Half of patients are first seen with a cervical lymph node metastasis producing a mass in the neck (Figs 21.5 and 21.6) and a third with a sore throat. Only 15% will have a visible lesion because the carcinoma arises inside the tonsil crypts without producing a surface mass (Figs 21.7 and 21.8). This type of carcinoma

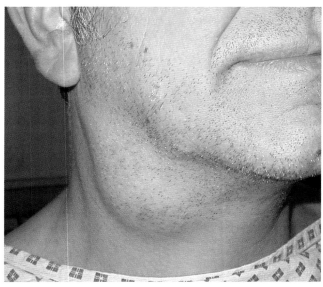

Fig. 21.5 Metastatic tonsil carcinoma in a cervical lymph node. This is often the presenting symptom.

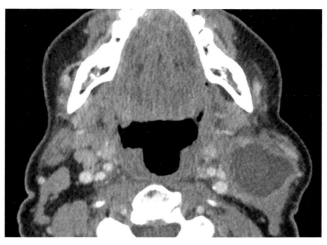

Fig. 21.6 Metastatic tonsil carcinoma in a computed tomography (CT) scan. On the patient's left is a large cystic lymph node metastasis several centimetres in diameter, but there is no mass detectable at the site of primary tumour in the adjacent tonsil. CT with contrast.

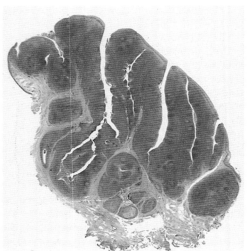

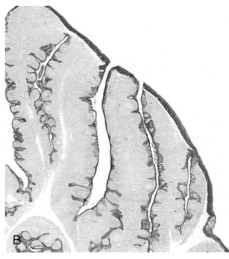

Fig. 21.7 Normal tonsil. (A) Stained with haematoxylin and eosin, the crypts can be seen as deep clefts surrounded by dark blue-stained lymphoid tissue. (B) At slightly higher magnification and stained immunohistochemically for keratin (brown stain positive), the epithelial covering and crypt lining epithelium is highlighted. *(Courtesy Dr S Thavaraj.)*

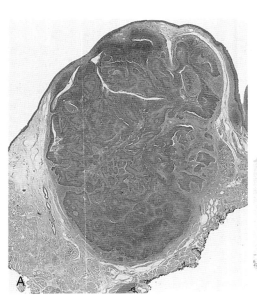

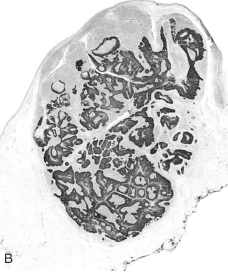

Fig. 21.8 Carcinoma of the tonsil. (A) Stained with haematoxylin and eosin, the carcinoma that has arisen in the crypt; epithelium is difficult to see. (B) Stained immunohistochemically for p16 as a marker of human papillomavirus, the carcinoma is highlighted. Note that the surface epithelium is not involved, not ulcerated and would appear normal clinically. *(Courtesy Dr S Thavaraj.)*

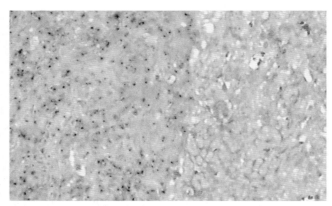

Fig. 21.9   HPV in a carcinoma of the tonsil. DNA in situ hybridisation reveals the presence of viral DNA as blue dots (see Fig. 1.10). HPV DNA is present in the nuclei of the carcinoma cells in an island of carcinoma on the left, but not in the connective tissue on the right. Red counterstain is for orientation, but the process partly degrades the tissue so that cells are not clearly seen.

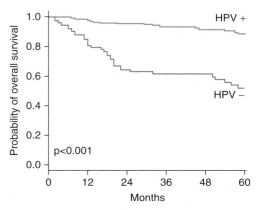

Fig. 21.10   Survival of patients with oropharyngeal carcinoma. Patients with human papillomavirus (HPV)-positive carcinomas survive much better than patients with HPV-negative carcinomas. Kaplan Meier survival curve, drops in the line indicate death of patients in the study population followed up for 5 years. *(Data from De Felice et al. 2020 PMID: 31981964.)*

typically metastasises very early, and the primary tumour may only be a few millimetres across when metastasis becomes evident. Clinical examination is therefore unlikely to detect the primary carcinoma.

The cervical node metastases are unusual. Virus-associated carcinomas produce metastases that are soft, usually single, and often cystic and only become fixed at a late stage, unlike the hard, fixed, multiple lymph nodes caused by other head and neck carcinomas. Metastases are frequently mistaken for branchial or other cysts. They are also often the first sign of the disease.

Review for clinical practice PMID: 25709145

Pathology

The primary carcinoma is often undetected before it metastasises. Fine needle aspiration of the presenting neck mass will show squamous carcinoma and trigger a search for the primary site. If the appearances in the metastasis suggest an oropharyngeal primary, or if papillomavirus is detected in the neck node sample, sites in Waldeyer's ring tonsillar tissue are almost certainly the primary site. If it cannot be detected on clinical examination or imaging, bilateral tonsillectomy, adenoidectomy and biopsies of the posterior tongue are performed to search for it.

The carcinoma comprises sheets, ribbons and islands of pale squamous epithelium with only microscopic foci of keratinisation (see Figs 21.7 and 21.8). There is often central necrosis in the islands ('comedo' necrosis) and infiltration by numerous lymphocytes ('lymphoepithelial carcinoma').

Viral infection is demonstrated by in situ hybridisation for viral DNA (Fig. 21.9) and overexpression of p16 protein, a cell cycle regulatory protein. Inactivation of retinoblastoma protein by the E7 viral protein triggers overexpression of p16 protein by the cancer cells. Demonstration of excess p16 protein indicates that the virus is driving carcinoma growth. Alternatively, in situ hybridisation against the E6 or E7 mRNA indicates both viral presence and activity.

Testing cancers for HPV PMID: 22782227

Treatment

Human papillomavirus–associated carcinomas have a much better prognosis than carcinomas induced by tobacco and

alcohol. However, this link between virus and good prognosis appears limited to oropharynx carcinomas. More than 95% of patients with virus-positive carcinomas survive 3 years compared with only 60% of patients with conventional carcinomas (Fig. 21.10). Chemoradiotherapy is the usual treatment but, if the carcinoma is accessible, surgery is also highly effective. Even very small excision margins may be effective and robotic surgery or laser microsurgery is often performed, avoiding radiotherapy if successful. If patients smoke and drink, they have an additional carcinogenic effect that generates a more aggressive carcinoma, and the response to treatment is slightly worse.

The better prognosis is probably explained by the carcinomas having less DNA damage than smoking-induced carcinomas. The cells retain intact signalling pathways to trigger apoptosis when exposed to chemotherapy or radiation-induced DNA damage.

This type of carcinoma should eventually be prevented by vaccination against human papillomavirus. There are two vaccines, which are very safe and licensed in more than 100 countries. In the UK, a single dose of the quadrivalent vaccine against types 6, 11, 16 and 18 is currently recommended for all children aged 12–13. Vaccine uptake is high, with 91% of people offered the vaccine having at least one course, above the level at which there should be an impact on both cervical and oropharyngeal carcinoma. Vaccine uptake in the United States is much lower. The vaccine is only effective if given before first sexual contact, and it has minimal protective effect in adults.

The concern that this cancer is caused by a sexually transmitted disease has led to considerable confusion and misinformation about the risks, transmission and prevention. Testing patients' saliva for papillomavirus has no value in predicting the risk of carcinoma. The virus does not replicate in the cancer, which is not infectious. By the time a cancer develops, 20–30 years may have passed since the original infection, and it will take this long for vaccination to have an impact on the incidence.

Good outcome PMID: 23606404 and 20530316

Staging is different 31981964

Web URL 21.1 NICE referral criteria all head neck cancers are in the Improving Outcomes document at: https://www.nice.org.uk/guidance/csg6

Robotic surgery PMID: 35419634

HPV cancers for dentists PMID: 32978578

HPV in oral carcinoma

Human papillomavirus can be found in approximately 5% of intraoral carcinomas. However, because infection in the population is so common, the significance is unclear. There is no evidence yet that papillomavirus plays a role in inducing oral carcinomas, and only very early evidence that it may be associated with a better response to treatment, if present.

Key features of human papillomavirus–associated oropharyngeal carcinomas are shown in Table 21.1.

NASOPHARYNGEAL CARCINOMA

Nasopharyngeal carcinoma arises high in the nasopharynx, specifically in the minor tonsil tissue in the fossa of Rosenmüller at the pharyngeal opening of the Eustachian tube. The significance to dentists is that it often presents as an enlarged lymph node in the neck following metastasis, when the primary carcinoma is still unsuspected.

Aetiology

The cause is infection with Epstein–Barr virus in a genetically predisposed individual, often a patient with family origin in China, Southeast Asia or North Africa. Dietary factors may contribute. Patients are usually middle-aged males, except in Africa where they are usually children. A small minority of cases are caused by human papillomavirus types 16 or 18.

Pathology

Presenting symptoms are often vague and include deafness or tinnitus from blockage of the Eustachian tube. Eighty-five per cent of cases present with a cervical lymph node metastasis, almost always to level 2 (see Fig. 20.17). Diagnosis is by fine needle aspiration of the node, aided by identifying Epstein–Barr virus DNA in the carcinoma.

Treatment is usually by radiotherapy, with or without chemotherapy, but only 50% of patients survive 5 years because diagnosis is often late.

Web URL 21.1 NICE referral criteria all head neck cancers are in the Improving Outcomes document at: https://www.nice.org.uk/guidance/csg6

General review PMID: 31178151

Table 21.1 Features of human papillomavirus–associated and other carcinomas of the oropharynx compared

Tobacco and alcohol-induced carcinomas, oral carcinoma and human papillomavirus–negative oropharyngeal carcinomas	Human papillomavirus–associated oropharyngeal carcinomas
Often have precursor dysplastic lesions	No precursor dysplastic lesion known
Present as visible ulcer or mass	Primary carcinoma often invisible
Usually symptomatic	Usually asymptomatic
Late metastasis	Early metastasis
Hard, fixed, multiple lymph node metastases	Soft cystic solitary lymph node metastases
Metastasise to any level in the neck	Usually metastasise to level 2 in the neck
Primary is large	Primary is small
Poor response to treatment	Good response to treatment
Primary prevention smoking avoidance or unknown	Primary prevention by HPV vaccination in adolescence

PSEUDOCARCINOMAS AND DIAGNOSTIC CATCHES

Various conditions can mimic oral malignant neoplasms either clinically or histologically. Those that are both clinical and histological mimics are particularly prone to be misdiagnosed as a cancer, to the detriment of the patient. This is best avoided by being aware of the conditions and always providing full clinical information to the pathologist who reports the biopsy. The fact that many of these conditions are relatively rare only increases the risk of misdiagnosis.

Many oral lesions are heavily inflamed, and others are prone to trauma. These processes may confuse the histological interpretation of a biopsy, and clinicians must always follow up a mismatch between clinical findings and biopsy results in case an error has been made.

The features of these lesions are summarised in Table 21.2.

In addition to these pseudomalignant lesions, the dental follicle can also be mistaken for the benign odontogenic myxoma (see Ch. 11).

Table 21.2   Oral conditions that may resemble malignant neoplasms

Condition	Clinical features	Histological features	Further information
Median rhomboid glossitis	Red and white, sometimes nodular appearance midline dorsum tongue	Usually readily distinguished from carcinoma	See Chapter 15
Traumatic and eosinophilic ulcer (and traumatic ulcerative granuloma with stromal eosinophilia and CD30 positive lymphoproliferative disease of mucosa)	Repeated trauma may prevent ulcers from healing and induce fibrosis mimicking carcinoma.	Simple traumatic ulcers are usually readily distinguished from carcinoma. Eosinophilic ulcers and traumatic ulcerative granuloma with stromal eosinophilia sometimes resemble lymphoma	See Chapter 16
Granular cell tumour	Smooth surfaced nodule, not usually suggestive of carcinoma clinically	Induces pseudocarcinomatous hyperplasia of overlying epithelium in a minority of cases. A biopsy that is superficial risks misdiagnosis.	See Chapter 25
Oral keratoacanthoma	Nodular lesion, usually on gingiva or palate, grows rapidly and ulcerates to form a keratin-filled crater appearing exactly as carcinoma, but usually in child or young adult. May resorb underlying bone	Almost identical to well-differentiated squamous carcinoma	Very rare. Probably not analogous to keratoacanthoma of skin or lip, but a similar self-healing epithelial proliferation. Untreated lesions resolve but are often excised through uncertainty of diagnosis. PMID: 6961343
Epstein–Barr virus ulcers in immunosuppression and acute EBV ulcers in glandular fever	Not usually concerning clinically, except EBV ulcers in immunosuppression, which can be very chronic	Resemble lymphoma	PMID: 26254983
Papillomas	Normally readily identifiable but large lesions resemble verrucous carcinoma	Superficial biopsy may be indistinguishable from verrucous carcinoma	The main risk is misdiagnosis of verrucous carcinoma as papilloma because of inadequate biopsy or clinical information
Necrotising sialometaplasia	Nodular inflamed lesion on palate, becoming ulcerated, rapid enlargement, appears as malignant salivary tumour	Biopsy may resemble squamous or mucoepidermoid carcinoma, although usually readily identifiable.	Eventually heals without intervention. Small or superficial biopsies risk misdiagnosis. See Chapter 22
Lupus erythematosus of vermilion border and gingiva	Ulcers, erythema and keratosis	Resembles dysplasia	Diagnosis aided by skin lesions elsewhere and serology

Non-neoplastic diseases of salivary glands

22

DUCT OBSTRUCTION

➜ Summary charts 12.1 and 22.1 pp. 228, 392

Salivary calculi

A stone can form in a salivary gland or duct. At least 80% of salivary calculi form in the submandibular gland or duct, approximately 8% in the parotid and approximately 2% in the sublingual and minor salivary glands.

Clinical features

Adults are mainly affected, males twice as often as females. Calculi are usually unilateral. Symptoms are absent until the stone causes obstruction. Intermittent obstruction causes the classical symptom of *mealtime syndrome*, pain and swelling of the gland when the smell or taste of food stimulates salivary secretion. Persistent obstruction leads to infection, pain and chronic swelling of the gland.

Otherwise, there are no symptoms unless the stone passes forward and can be palpated or seen at the duct orifice (Fig. 22.1). Alternatively, the stone may be seen in a radiograph. However, approximately 40% of parotid and 20% of submandibular stones are not densely radiopaque, and sialography or ultrasound may be needed to locate them.

Pathology

Saliva is supersaturated, and calcium and magnesium phosphates deposit around a nidus, probably cell debris. Degenerate cells within the gland can also mineralise and may enter the duct system to act as a nidus. Mineralisation proceeds incrementally because the saturation of saliva varies with flow rate so that stones have a layered structure (Fig. 22.2).

An adherent layer of microbial flora often grows on stones and this, their rough surface and obstruction trigger inflammation and fibrosis around the duct.

Calculi are not a cause of dry mouth, but factors increasing the saturation of saliva including dry mouth, dehydration, obstruction and sialadenitis all predispose to stones, producing a vicious cycle in which the effects of a calculus contribute to its further growth. Established stones probably never redissolve. Stones are frequently multiple.

Parotid saliva is less saturated than submandibular and so produces fewer stones. These have a higher organic content, making them less radiopaque and sometimes completely lucent.

Minor gland stones are unusual and present as a hard mass just below the surface of the mucosa or with infection.

Management

The stone should be identified by plain radiography or ultrasound and the degree of damage to the gland from ascending infection and sialadenitis assessed by sialography.

Occasionally, small stones may be manipulated out of the duct orifice. Larger or distally placed stones must be treated starting with the least invasive method likely to succeed. Lithotripsy uses an ultrasonic shock wave applied extraorally and focused on the stone. A series of treatments may fracture the stone into small pieces that will pass out of the duct orifice. If this fails, stones in the duct but outside the gland can be removed using a basket of fine wire manipulated down the duct and around the stone under radiological control. Alternatively, microendoscopy can be combined with laser disruption of the stone. These

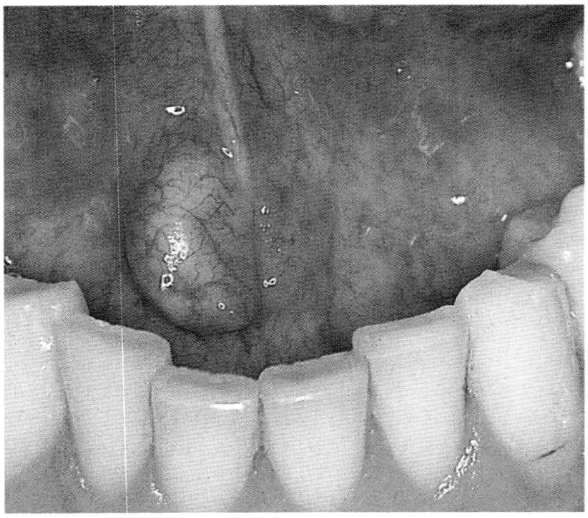

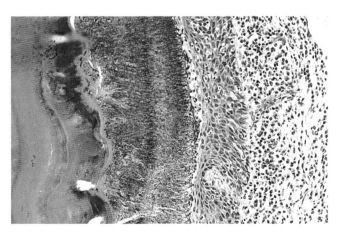

Fig. 22.1 Salivary calculus. This stone has impacted just behind the orifice of the submandibular duct forming a hard nodule. The yellow colour of the stone is visible through the thin mucosa.

Fig. 22.2 Salivary calculus in a duct. To the left is the salivary calculus which has a lamellar structure and an irregular surface. On the surface is a thick layer of microbial flora filling the space between the stone and the epithelial lining. In the surrounding wall, there is an infiltrate of lymphocytes and plasma cells and neutrophils are migrating through the duct epithelium into the lumen.

Key Features

- Adult males mainly affected
- Usually (80%) in submandibular gland or its duct
- Form by accretion of calcium salts round organic nidus
- Typically cause pain by obstructing food-related surge of salivary secretion
- Occasionally asymptomatic until palpable in the mouth or seen in routine radiograph
- Do not cause dry mouth
- Can often be treated conservatively

conservative techniques are often successful and, perhaps surprisingly, the gland will often recover normal function despite a history of repeated attacks of chronic sialadenitis and evidence of damage on imaging.

If conservative measures fail and the stone is within the duct, the duct has to be opened, usually under local anaesthesia. A temporary suture should be put around the submandibular duct behind the calculus to prevent it from slipping backward and the stone released through an incision along the line of the duct. The opening should be left unsutured or sutured to the mucosa to prevent scarring and a fibrous stricture forming.

When stones are within the gland or a sialogram reveals that the gland is severely damaged by recurrent infection and fibrosis, the gland will probably have to be excised.

Stones in minor glands are treated by removal of the gland, stone and duct.

Key features of salivary calculi are summarised in Box 22.1.

Management review PMID: 17957846

Salivary duct strictures

→ Summary chart 22.1 p. 392

The usual cause of strictures at the parotid papilla is chronic trauma (from such causes as projecting denture clasps, faulty restorations or sharp edges of broken teeth) leading to fibrosis round the duct.

Strictures of the duct itself are almost always caused by fibrosis resulting from inflammation round a calculus or scarring following surgery. Stones and strictures are often found together.

Obstruction from strictures presents with mealtime syndrome in the same way as when caused by calculi.

Sialography should show the zone of narrowing with dilatation behind. Once any causative calculus has been removed, no further treatment may be required, but persistent obstruction may require dilatation of the duct with bougies, excision of the narrow segment or the whole gland.

Management review: PMID: 17957846

MUCOCELES AND SALIVARY CYSTS

A mucocele is a cavity filled with mucus. Salivary mucoceles can be of two types, but these cannot be distinguished clinically and the difference is of little practical importance.

Review PMID: 20708324

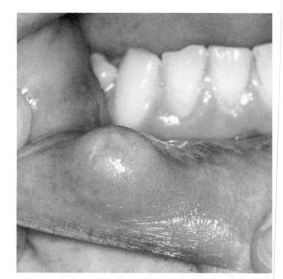

Fig. 22.3   Mucous extravasation cyst. The typical presentation at the commonest site: a rounded bluish, translucent cyst in the lower lip.

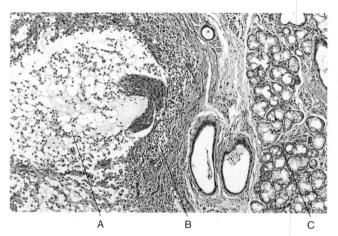

A   B   C

Fig. 22.4   Extravasation mucocele. To the left is a cavity of spilt mucin with the remnants of the ruptured duct lining epithelium at its edge. To the right is the associated minor mucous salivary gland. (A) Saliva and macrophages. (B) Compressed connective tissue wall. (C) Minor salivary gland.

Mucous extravasation

The most common type is the extravasation mucocele of minor glands, often called a *mucous extravasation cyst* even though it has no epithelial lining. The cause is trauma causing duct rupture so that saliva can escape into the tissues. Mucous extravasations most often form in the lower lip because it is more prone to trauma. They are commonest in children and young adults.

The pool of mucin in the tissues is superficial and rarely larger than 1 cm in diameter. In the early stages, they appear as rounded fleshy swellings. Later, they are obviously cystic, hemispherical, fluctuant and bluish due to the thin wall (Fig. 22.3).

The saliva leaking into the surrounding tissues excites an inflammatory reaction (Figs 22.4 and 22.5), the pools of saliva gradually coalesce to form a rounded collection of fluid,

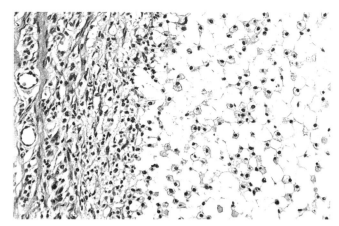

Fig. 22.5   Extravasation mucocele. Higher power showing the lining of the mucin-filled space. Macrophages are migrating into the mucin from the wall on the left and, in phagocytosing it, develop a foamy or vacuolated cytoplasm in the lumen, seen on the right.

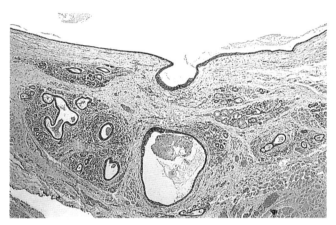

Fig. 22.6   Mucous retention cyst. Remnants of the minor mucous salivary gland are visible, together with its dilated duct, the epithelium of which forms the epithelial lining of the cyst lumen above.

surrounded by compressed connective tissue. Gradually macrophages infiltrate and degrade the mucin, the duct heals and a scar remains. However, extravasation mucoceles often recur at the same site, probably because of recurrent trauma.

In a *superficial mucocele*, the saliva pools just below the epithelium, mimicking a vesicle and potentially presenting similarly to pemphigoid. In this type, the translucent blisters are a few millimetres in diameter and usually affect the soft palate.

Superficial mucoceles PMID: 3174068

Mucous retention cysts

These cysts are less common and have an epithelial lining because they are salivary ducts that become very dilated following obstruction (Fig. 22.6). Retention cysts arise within both major glands, usually the parotid, and minor glands. There is less inflammation because the saliva does not escape into the tissues, and the pool of mucin is surrounded by duct epithelium. The epithelium often shows hyperplasia or oncocytic metaplasia.

Key features are summarised in Box 22.2.

Box 22.2   Mucoceles:

Key Features

- Most frequently on lower lip
- Usually caused by damage to duct and extravasation of saliva
- Saliva leaking into surrounding tissues causes mild inflammation
- Saliva eventually pools to form a mucocele with compressed fibrous wall
- Rarely due to duct obstruction and dilatation forming a retention cyst with epithelial lining
- Almost never in the upper lip – consider alternative diagnosis of salivary gland neoplasm

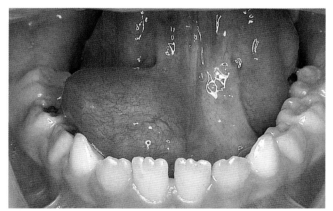

Fig. 22.7   Ranula. A large bluish, translucent swelling in the floor of the mouth caused by a mucous extravasation cyst.

Ranula

A ranula* is an uncommon and distinctive type of mucous extravasation arising in the floor of mouth from the sublingual gland. The structure is the same as other salivary extravasation cysts. The cause is damage to, or obstruction of, one of the several ducts of Rivinius that drain into the submandibular duct or floor of mouth.

Ranulae are usually unilateral and 2 or 3 cm in diameter (Fig. 22.7). Occasionally, they extend across the whole of the floor of the mouth. They are soft, fluctuant and bluish, typically painless but may interfere with speech or mastication.

Sublingual glands secrete continuously, unlike the larger glands, and ranulae can therefore reach a very large size. In addition, no back pressure develops in the loose surrounding tissue. A *plunging ranula* arises when the mucus passes through the mylohyoid muscle, which is a discontinuous sheet in many individuals, or around its posterior margin. Large volumes of mucus can then collect in the submandibular space and extend down into the neck, sometimes with minimal intraoral swelling.

Treatment

Untreated mucoceles rupture, often repeatedly, and some eventually heal spontaneously. Otherwise, they should be

---

* The name ranula means frog and comes from the clinical resemblance of the thin dilated wall to the air sac of a frog, together with the croaking speech that very large ranulae can cause by displacing the tongue.

excised with the associated gland. The latter is usually found to have been removed with the cyst, but if not, recurrence is likely.

Ranulae do not require excision. If the cavity is drained and decompressed by marsupialisation, it will heal spontaneously provided the causative gland, always the sublingual, is removed. The sublingual gland comprises as many as 20 small glands, each with a separate duct, and only the involved segment needs to be removed if it can be identified.

An important diagnostic point is that what appears to be a mucocele in the upper lip is much more likely to be a salivary neoplasm and has a significant chance of being malignant (Ch. 23, Fig. 23.1). Some salivary neoplasms contain mucous-filled cysts, producing a similar appearance. Upper lip nodules should not be excised without this possibility having been investigated.

Review and treatment ranula PMID: 20054853

ACUTE SIALADENITIS

Mumps ➜ Summary chart 22.2 p. 393

Mumps[†] is due to a paramyxovirus (the mumps virus) and causes painful swelling of the parotids and other exocrine glands. It is highly infectious through droplet spread and, though rare, is the most common cause of acute parotid swelling.

In the UK, mumps vaccination (in the MMR (measles-mumps-rubella) combination) was introduced in 1988. Before this there were epidemics every 3 years in schoolchildren. MMR vaccination is given at around 1 and 3–4 years of age and is also available to adults. Concerns over side effects have proved unfounded, and uptake in the UK is now approximately 95%, but small clusters of cases still occur and in 2005 there was an epidemic of more than 70,000 cases. Unvaccinated adults from a period of vaccine hesitancy between 2000 and 2014 in the UK remain at risk. Several hundred cases occur each year. Almost all are 15–30-year-olds, and a quarter will have had at least one dose of vaccine, suggesting it is not as effective as natural mumps immunity (which is lifelong after infection). The mumps component of MMR is known to be less effective than the measles and rubella components.

In other countries with low vaccination rates such as Japan, there are large epidemics every 4-6 years.

Vaccination is with a live virus, and a small minority of recipients develop a mild presentation of mumps with salivary gland swelling 3 weeks after the first dose.

Clinical features

Classically, children were affected in epidemics. The disease is highly infectious and spread by saliva via air borne droplets. Headache, malaise, fever and tense, painful and tender swelling of the parotids follow an incubation period of about 21 days.

Currently, cases are adolescents or young adults, who unlike children may have severe and prolonged malaise and are prone to complications including orchitis, oophoritis (both potentially leading to sterility), deafness, pancreatitis, arthritis, mastitis, nephritis, pericarditis or meningitis.

Classical presentations are easily recognised, but adults may have only one or two glands swollen, raising possible

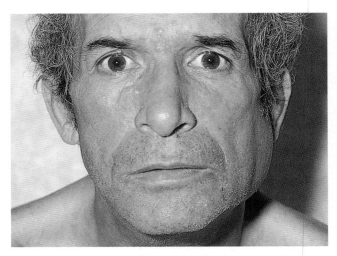

Fig. 22.8   Mumps in an adult. Adults often have atypical presentations such as this patient with unilateral parotitis. *(From General Medical Conditions in the Athlete, Mosby, 2012, Fig. 15-6.Source: Jarvis C: Physical examination and health assessment, ed 5, Philadelphia, 2008, Saunders.)*

misdiagnosis as dental infection, sialadenitis or lymphadenitis. A history of mumps, but not of vaccination, excludes the diagnosis. Immunised adults have reduced disease severity and often atypical presentations (Fig. 22.8). Many are subclinical, with mild non-specific malaise and tender glands without swelling.

If necessary, the diagnosis can be confirmed by a rise in titre of immunoglobulin M (IgM) antibodies in the unvaccinated. Unfortunately, vaccination prevents development of the IgM antibodies in 90% of cases, and laboratory diagnosis is then difficult.

There is no specific treatment, and supportive care maintaining fluid intake with analgesia is provided, monitoring for complications, particularly neurological complications that require inpatient care.

Mumps review PMID: 18342688

Complications despite vaccination PMID: 20517181

Acute bacterial parotitis

Acute suppurative parotitis historically affected debilitated patients, particularly post-operatively, as a result of dehydration. This should now be effectively prevented. Currently, suppurative parotitis is more commonly seen in patients with severe xerostomia, particularly Sjögren's syndrome, as an uncommon complication of drugs causing severe xerostomia or, in the newborn. Low flow allows bacteria to enter the gland from the mouth through the duct.

Important bacterial causes include *Staphylococcus aureus*, streptococci and oral anaerobes. Typical clinical features are pain in one or both parotids with swelling, redness and tenderness, malaise and fever. The regional lymph nodes are enlarged and tender, and pus exudes or can be expressed from the parotid duct (Fig. 22.9). The progress of the infection depends largely on the patient's underlying physical state. Biopsy plays no role in diagnosis, but shows abscess formation, pus in ducts and acute inflammation.

In view of the potentially virulent pathogenic organisms involved, aggressive antibiotic treatment is required, usually with flucloxacillin, but only after pus has been obtained for culture and sensitivity testing because of the wide range of possible causative organisms. The antibiotic can be changed if necessary. Drainage is rarely necessary.

[†]Mumps comes from an old English word meaning to look miserable, describing well the marked malaise induced.

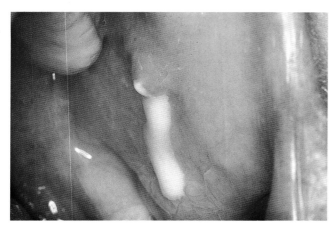

Fig. 22.9 Suppurative parotitis. Pus is exuding from the parotid papilla.

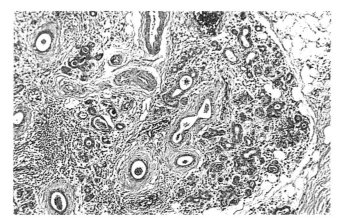

Fig. 22.10 Chronic sialadenitis resulting from obstruction. The ducts contain casts of mucin and neutrophils and are surrounded by a layer of fibrosis. There is severe acinar atrophy, and the space previously occupied by acinar cells now contains infiltrates of lymphocytes and plasma cells.

Acute parotitis case series PMID: 3468465

Salivary gland infection review PMID: 19608046

Tuberculous sialadenitis is very rare and seen mostly in the parotid gland in HIV infection and immunosuppression. It presents clinically as a mass resembling a tumour or as a slowly and diffusely enlarging gland over many years. Fine needle aspiration will usually be diagnostic. Involvement of the gland probably follows spread from an intraparotid lymph node.

CHRONIC SIALADENITIS

➔ Summary chart 22.1 p. 392

Chronic sialadenitis is usually a complication of duct obstruction, and the commonest cause by far is calculi. It is usually unilateral and asymptomatic or with intermittent painful swelling of one gland. Sialography may show the effects of past infection and inflammation, dilatation of ducts behind the obstruction, with tortuous distorted ducts compressed by fibrosis.

Pathology

There are varying degrees of destruction of acini, duct dilatation and a scattered chronic inflammatory cellular infiltrate, predominantly lymphoplasmacytic (Fig. 22.10). Extensive interstitial fibrosis and, sometimes, squamous metaplasia in the duct epithelium follow.

Untreated, sialadenitis progresses over many years until the gland is almost completely fibrotic. This terminal fibrosis produces a hard gland, easily mistaken for a lymph node metastasis or neoplasm[‡].

Once any obstruction is removed, mild sialadenitis may resolve and the gland recover. If extensively damaged, the gland has to be excised.

Salivary gland infection review PMID: 19608046

XEROSTOMIA

Xerostomia is dry mouth. There are many causes, as summarised in Box 22.3. Medication is by far the commonest cause, though in most patients the effects are not severe. Some drugs act on the gland, others on the sympathetic or parasympathetic secretory pathways and others on general hydration. Some may alter the saliva quality rather than its amount. In many cases the cause is not known. Dry mouth is not associated with ageing itself but is common in older people because of their disease burden and medications.

Though the mouth is dry and saliva sparse, stringy or frothy, many patients with mild xerostomia make no complaint of dry mouth, but rather of difficulty eating or speaking. Some complain of an unpleasant taste in the mouth. Most find severe dryness almost unbearable.

Conversely, some with a subjective sensation of dry mouth have normal salivary flow rates on objective testing. Mucosal diseases that cause roughening, particularly lichen planus, are often interpreted as dryness. Such patients are said to have *false xerostomia*. Before detailed investigation for xerostomia, a measurement of salivary flow is required to differentiate true from false xerostomia (see Sjögren's syndrome in the following section). Alternatively, a clinical assessment is reasonably accurate (Table 22.1).

Xerostomia, calculi and ascending infection are related in some patients, as shown in Fig. 22.11.

Significant sequelae of xerostomia are caries, often root caries, and candidosis. Treatment is discussed under Sjögren's syndrome.

Review PMID: 20887509 and 25463902

Medication induced xerostomia PMID: 25994331

SJÖGREN'S SYNDROME

➔ Summary chart 22.2 p. 393

In 1933, Sjögren noticed the association of dryness of the mouth and dryness of the eyes. Later, he found that there was a significant association with rheumatoid arthritis. These combinations of complaints are caused by two closely related but distinct diseases.

Primary Sjögren's syndrome comprises dry mouth and dry eyes that is not associated with any connective tissue disease but does have other extraglandular manifestations. *Sicca syndrome* is a poorly defined term that is best avoided because it can be used for any cause of dry eyes and mouth, as well as primary Sjögren's syndrome.

[‡] This end stage of chronic sialadenitis with sclerosis is sometimes called a *Küttner tumour*, although it is not neoplastic. However, this term has also been incorrectly and confusingly applied to other causes of fibrosis in the gland, such as IgG4 disease. ***See PMID: 21707715***

Box 22.3 Causes of xerostomia

Organic Causes

- Sjögren's syndrome
- Irradiation
- Mumps (transient)
- HIV infection
- Hepatitis C infection
- Sarcoidosis
- Amyloidosis in salivary glands
- Iron deposition in salivary glands (haemochromatosis, thalassaemia)

Functional Causes

- Dehydration
  - Fluid deprivation or loss
  - Haemorrhage
  - Persistent diarrhoea and/or vomiting
- Psychogenic
  - Anxiety states
  - Depression

Drugs

- Diuretic overdosage
- Drugs with antimuscarinic effects
  - Atropine, ipratropium, hyoscine and other analogues
  - Tricyclic and some other antidepressants and antipsychotics, selective serotonin reuptake inhibitors (SSRI) drugs
  - Antihistamines
  - Antiemetics (including antihistamines and phenothiazines)
  - Neuroleptics, particularly phenothiazines and oxepines
- Some older antihypertensives (ganglion blockers and clonidine), Verapamil
- Drugs with sympathomimetic actions
  - 'Cold cures' containing ephedrine, etc.
  - Decongestants
  - Bronchodilators
  - Appetite suppressants, particularly amphetamines
- Anti-obesity drugs that act centrally
- Medications for urinary incontinence

Table 22.1 The Challacombe scale for assessing dry mouth clinically*

Feature	Total score
• Mirror sticks to buccal mucosa • Mirror sticks to tongue • Saliva frothy	Total score of 1–3 indicates mild dryness. May not need treatment or management. Sugar-free chewing gum for 15 mins, twice daily and attention to hydration is needed. Many drugs will cause mild dryness. Routine checkup monitoring required.
• No saliva pooling in floor of mouth • Tongue shows generalised mild depapillation • Gingival architecture is smooth	Total score of 4–6 indicates moderate dryness. Sugar-free chewing gum or simple sialogogues may be required. Needs to be investigated further if reasons for dryness are not clear. Saliva substitutes and topical fluoride may be helpful. Monitor at regular intervals especially for caries and symptom change.
• Glassy appearance of oral mucosa, especially palate • Tongue lobulated / fissured • Cervical caries in more than two teeth • Debris on palate or sticking to teeth	Total score of 7–10 indicates severe dryness. Saliva substitutes and topical fluoride usually needed. Cause of hyposalivation needs to be ascertained and Sjögren's syndrome excluded. Refer for investigation and diagnosis. Patients then need to be monitored for changing symptoms and signs, with possible further specialist input if worsening.

*Features often appear in sequence as the mouth becomes dryer, but the sequence is not important for scoring. Each feature in the first column scores 1 and the significance of the total score, regardless of specific features, is shown on the right.

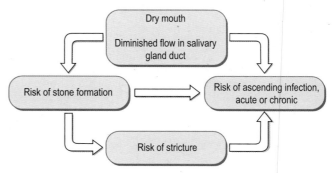

Fig. 22.11 Interrelationships between dry mouth, calculi and their complications. Note: dry mouth may promote stone formation, but stones do not cause dry mouth.

Secondary Sjögren's syndrome comprises dry mouth and dry eyes associated with a connective tissue disease, usually rheumatoid arthritis or lupus erythematosus.

Primary Sjögren's syndrome causes more severe oral and ocular changes and has a higher risk of complications than secondary.

Clinical features

Females are affected nearly 10 times as frequently as males. Sjögren's syndrome affects 10%–15% of patients with rheumatoid arthritis, possibly 30% of patients with lupus erythematosus and a variable proportion of patients with other connective tissue diseases. Sjögren's syndrome is therefore relatively common.

Major oral effects of Sjögren's syndrome are summarised in Box 22.4.

Onset is usually in middle age, around 50 years of age, but even children are affected occasionally. In the early stages, the mucosa may appear moist, but salivary flow measurement shows diminished secretion. In established cases, the oral mucosa is obviously dry, often red, shiny and parchment-like (Fig. 22.12). The tongue is typically red, the papillae characteristically atrophy, and the dorsum becomes lobulated with a cobblestone appearance (Fig. 22.13). With diminished salivary secretion, the oral flora changes, and

Box 22.4 Oral effects of Sjögren's syndrome

- Discomfort
- Difficulties with eating or swallowing
- Disturbed taste sensation
- Disturbed quality of speech
- Predisposition to mucosal infection

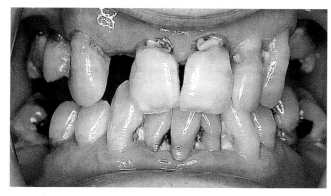

Fig. 22.14 Sjögren's syndrome. Extensive cervical caries is a frequent complication of dry mouth. In addition to the lack of saliva, patients may attempt to stimulate salivary flow with sweets or chewing gums.

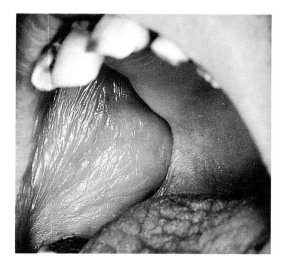

Fig. 22.12 Sjögren's syndrome. The mucosa is dry, red, atrophic and wrinkled and sticks to the fingers or mirror during examination. These changes are common to all causes of xerostomia.

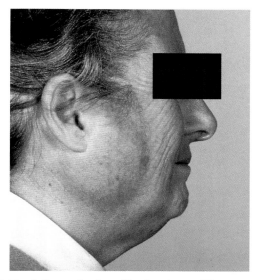

Fig. 22.15 Salivary gland swelling in primary Sjögren's syndrome. The outline of the parotid gland is clearly demarcated.

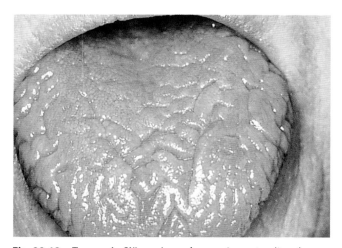

Fig. 22.13 Tongue in Sjögren's syndrome. Longstanding dry mouth and repeated candidal infection produce this depapillated but lobulated tongue.

candidal infections are common. The latter are the main cause of soreness of the mouth in Sjögrens syndrome and cause generalised erythema of the mucosa, often with angular stomatitis. Plaque accumulates, and there may be rapidly progressive dental caries (Fig. 22.14). The most severe infective complication is acute bacterial sialadenitis, usually of the parotid gland. These oral changes are not specific and are seen in severe xerostomia with other causes.

Parotid swelling is found at some stage in about 30% of patients but is not a common finding because it is often intermittent. Swollen glands are not inflamed clinically and are rarely painful (Fig. 22.15). A hot, tender parotid swelling with red, shiny overlying skin would indicate acute bacterial parotitis. Bilateral persistent parotid swelling strongly suggests lymphoma or its earliest stages (discussed later).

People with Sjögren's syndrome have increased incidence of allergy to antibiotics, particularly allergy to trimethoprim which causes fever, headache, backache and meningeal irritation.

Sjögren's syndrome can have serious ocular effects (Box 22.5). Dryness leads to keratinisation, splitting and inflammation of the conjunctiva and cornea. Ulceration, corneal scarring and induction of blood vessel ingrowth can lead to visual impairment.

Primary Sjögren's syndrome is not just a localised form of the disease. Although patients lack a connective tissue disorder, they have other extraglandular manifestations including involvement of all exocrine glands, hypergammaglobulinaemia and features such as Raynaud's phenomenon.

General review PMID: 16039337

Review causes and prognosis PMID: 23993190

Extraglandular features primary disease PMID: 26231345

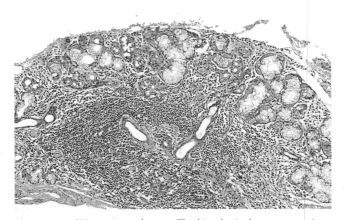

Fig. 22.16 Sjögren's syndrome. The histological appearance is typical. A dense, well-defined focus of lymphocytes surrounds the larger ducts in the centre of the gland lobules. In the area occupied by the lymphocytes, there is complete acinar atrophy and a rim of residual salivary parenchyma remains around the periphery of the lobule.

Aetiology and pathology

The cause is unknown, but genetic predisposition exists and environmental triggers, possibly viral, are suspected. These may act directly on the salivary acinar cells, which show changes in the earliest stages. Acinar cells secrete cytokines that recruit inflammatory cells and promote antigen presentation. Either dysregulation of the immune response or a continual stimulation causes B cell hyperreactivity and polyclonal activation. The outcome is an autoimmune attack on all exocrine glands, including those of the skin, vagina, lung and pancreas, though these other sites rarely cause significant problems clinically.

Histological changes are shown in Box 22.6. Initially, T lymphocytes infiltrate the glands, cluster around small ducts, and proliferate to form focal infiltrates. Later B lymphocytes are recruited, proliferate and come to predominate and lymphoid follicles develop in the gland indicating persistent immune activity. The infiltrates enlarge at the expense of, and gradually replace, acinar cells (Fig. 22.16). The mechanisms of acinar cell destruction are unclear but may be via apoptosis, cytokine secretion or disruption of the normal replacement mechanisms. Over many years, the lymphocytic infiltrates enlarge and replace most of the gland. The ductal cells proliferate, possibly in response to cytokines released by the lymphocytes, to form islands and sheets of cells around the ducts that become infiltrated by lymphocytes. Although myoepithelial cells are not a feature, the islands are called *epimyoepithelial islands* (Fig. 22.17), and the overall appearance is sometimes called *myoepithelial or lymphoepithelial sialadenitis*.

The final result is complete destruction of acini and replacement of the whole gland by a dense lymphocytic infiltrate (Fig. 22.17). However, the infiltrate remains confined within the gland capsule and by the intraglandular septa.

There is systemic polyclonal B cell activation, producing a variety of autoantibodies (Table 22.2) that aid diagnosis.

Pathogenic mechanisms PMID: 34660815

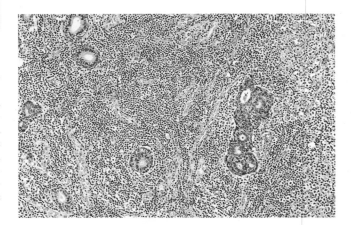

Fig. 22.17 Sjögren's syndrome. In late disease no salivary acini remain and the gland is replaced by a confluent infiltrate of lymphocytes. A few ducts remain and proliferate to form the epimyoepithelial islands. Such extensive changes suggest that there is a risk of progression to low-grade lymphoma.

Table 22.2 Typical patterns of autoantibodies in primary and secondary Sjögren's syndromes

Autoantibodies	Primary SS	Secondary SS
Salivary duct antibody	10%–36%	67%–70%
Rheumatoid factor	50%	90%
SS-A (Ro) antibodies	5%–10%	50%–80%
SS-B (La) antibodies	50%–75%	2%–5%
Rheumatoid arthritis precipitin	5%	75%

Diagnosis

No test is definitive; many may be required in early disease (Box 22.7). The least invasive tests are used first.

Salivary secretion should be assessed by testing unstimulated whole saliva flow by the patient drooling into a graduated container over 10 minutes. Normal salivary flow is between 1 and 2 mL/min but may be reduced to 0.2 mL/min or less. Reduction to or below this level confirms a true

Box 22.7 Diagnostic tests in Sjögren's syndrome

- Diminished total salivary flow rate
- Diminished tear secretion and ocular effects
- Raised immunoglobulin levels and erythrocyte sedimentation rate
- Autoantibodies, especially rheumatoid factor and SS-A and SS-B
- Circulating CD4+/CD8+ lymphocyte ratio altered
- Sialectasis on sialography or ultrasound
- Labial salivary gland biopsy showing periductal lymphocytic infiltrate

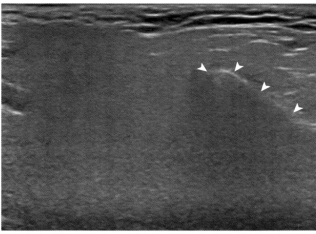

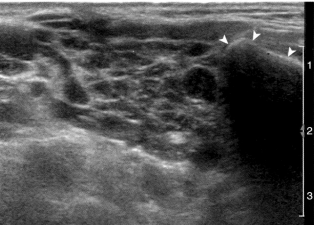

Fig 22.19 Sjögren's syndrome. This ultrasound shows two images of parotid gland at the same scale labelled in centimetres, with skin at the top of each image and the outline of the ramus of the mandible arrowed. The upper panel shows normal parotid to the left of the ramus, which is of homogeneous echo density. The lower panel shows a gland in late Sjögren's syndrome with numerous foci of reduced echodensity producing a non-homogeneous multicystic or reticular appearance. *(Courtesy Dr J Brown.)*

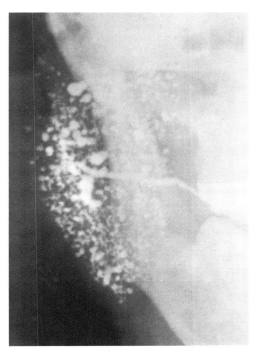

Fig. 22.18 Sjögren's syndrome. The sialogram in anterior-posterior view shows the typical snowstorm appearance of blobs of contrast medium that have leaked from the duct system in the parotid. Emptying and clearance of the contrast medium are also much delayed because of the reduced salivary flow.

xerostomia. Alternatively, dryness can be scored relatively accurately from clinical features (Table 22.1). Specialist centres may use a Lashley cannula to measure exact flow rates from individual parotid glands, with or without stimulation by citric acid applied to the tongue. If xerostomia is present, other causes must be excluded (Box 22.3).

Specialist ophthalmic examination is the best way to detect corneal drying and its effects. The Schirmer test, in which a filter paper strip tucked under the lower eyelid is used to measure tear production, is considerably less informative, extremely variable, uncomfortable for the patient and best avoided.

Serological support for the diagnosis should be sought next, using the tests in Table 22.2 while noting that none are specific to the disorder. A sialogram will usually show the snowstorm appearance, due to leakage of contrast material through the terminal duct walls (Fig. 22.18). Ultrasound examination may reveal similar features and is less invasive and more tolerable for the patient (Fig 22.19).

If no definitive diagnosis is yet possible, a labial gland biopsy may be performed. Pathological changes in labial salivary glands correlate closely with those in the parotid glands, and lip biopsy avoids the risks of damage to the facial nerve inherent in parotid gland biopsy. However, this test is considerably overrated. A harvest of 6–8 glands is required. The usual method for assessment is to count the number of foci of lymphocytes per 4 mm^2 of tissue. Although a score of 1 or more is highly suggestive, it is easy to misinterpret non-specific inflammation and normal age changes. The predictive value is probably no higher than 80% when correctly interpreted, and often much less.

Several sets of international diagnostic criteria exist but are not completely accurate, do not identify the same cases and fail to identify early and subclinical cases.

Because there is no specific treatment for the underlying disease process, the effort, expense and morbidity of investigations have to be weighed against the certainty of diagnosis required.

Labial gland biopsy PMID: 21480190

Diagnostic criteria PMID: 27789466

Box 22.8 Principles of management of Sjögren's syndrome

- Salivary gland damage is largely irreversible
- Give reassurance and help with dry mouth
- Ophthalmological investigation for keratoconjunctivitis sicca
- Refer to specialist if connective tissue disease is untreated
- Check for any associated drug treatment contributing to dry mouth
- Alleviate dry mouth
  - Frequent small sips of water
  - Prescribe saliva substitutes
- Control caries and plaque accumulation in dentate patients
  - Avoid sweets (e.g., lemon drops)
  - Suggest sugar-free gum
  - Check diet for excess sugary foods
  - Maintain good oral hygiene
  - Fluoride applications
  - Chlorhexidine (0.2%) rinses
- Monitor for mucosal candidosis
  - Give antifungal mixtures (not tablets) as necessary
- Treat difficulties with dentures symptomatically
- Observe regularly for possible development of ascending parotitis or lymphoma

---

Box 22.9 Types of artificial saliva currently available in various countries

- **Aequasyal oral spray** (prev. Aquoral). Glycerolesters of fatty acid
- **Bioextra gel**. Lactoperoxidase, lactoferrin, lysozymes and immunoglobulins*
- **Caphosol solution.** Supersaturated calcium phosphate rinse
- **Glandosane spray.** Carboxymethyl cellulose, sorbitol and electrolytes*
- **Luborant spray.** Carmellose solution with electrolytes
- **Oasis spray.** Glycerin solution
- **OralBalance gel.** Lactoperoxidase, glucose oxidase and xylitol*
- **Oralieve spray and gel.** Glycerin, xylitol and vegetable gum*
- **Saliva Orthana spray.** Gastric mucin, xylitol, sodium fluoride with preservatives and flavouring*
- **Saliva Orthana lozenges.** Gastric mucin with xylitol in sorbitol base*
- **Saliva stimulating tablets.** Citric and malic acids and sorbitol*
- **Salivasure lozenges.** Xylitol and carboxymethyl cellulose
- **Salivace spray.** Carmellose with xylitol and electrolytes
- **Saliveze spray.** Carboxymethylcellulose*
- **Salivix pastilles.** Gum acacia and malic acid*
- **Xerotin.** Sorbitol, carboxymethylcellulose, electrolytes*
- **Xylimelt dissolvable disks.** Xylitol and cellulose gum

Saliva secretion may also be stimulated by chewing gums or electrostimulation. Availability and prescribing varies between countries, those available currently for prescription in the UK are marked *. Not all ingredients shown.

Management

Many aspects need to be considered (Box 22.8).

Ophthalmological review is important to exclude or treat keratoconjunctivitis sicca, which is symptomless in its early stages. Dryness of the eyes is treated with artificial tears, such as methyl cellulose solution.

Anaemia should be excluded, particularly when there is rheumatoid arthritis, because it contributes to candidosis.

Dryness of the mouth can be relieved to some degree by providing artificial saliva (Box 22.9), although these preparations are not very pleasant to use. Patients usually need to try several to find one they are happy with. Acid products should generally be avoided as they may contribute to caries risk, as should coffee and smoking. Patients must conserve what little mucin they have in the mouth by sipping liquid, not rinsing and swallowing. Alcohol containing mouthwashes have a drying effect and should not be used.

The natural cholinesterase inhibitor pilocarpine has been used to stimulate salivary secretion but has unpleasant side effects such as nausea, diarrhoea and bradycardia. Newer selective agonists of the M3 muscarinic receptor such as Cevimeline are effective with less marked adverse effects and also stimulate tear secretion.

Residual salivary secretion can be enhanced using sugar-free chewing gum. An electrostimulation device that contacts the mucosa over the lingual nerve in the third molar region bilaterally has been shown to increase saliva secretion and may also promote gland regeneration.

In dentate patients, an aggressive preventive regime is required with topical fluorides and chlorhexidine mouth rinses to reduce plaque formation. Soreness of the mouth due to infection by *Candida albicans* can be treated with fluconazole or nystatin.

A dry and sore mouth and eyes, perhaps with pain from rheumatoid arthritis persisting over many years, is deeply distressing. Depression is a common consequence, and patients need support and reassurance.

Systemic treatment PMID: 34951923

Oral treatment PMID: 20664046

Ophthalmic assessment PMID: 20035924

Increasing salivary flow PMID: 22161442 and 29956369

Electrostimulation PMID: 20882668

Review xerostomia and treatment PMID: 25463902

Complications → Summary chart 22.2 p. 393

The risk to the eyes has been noted previously (Box 22.5). Ascending acute bacterial parotitis should be treated as described earlier.

Primary Sjögren's syndrome carries a relative risk of developing lymphoma of ×16, equivalent to 5% of patients, and more among severely affected cases. The lymphomas are of B cell type, usually of the low-grade MALT (**M**ucosa-**A**ssociated **L**ymphoid **T**issue) type (Ch. 28), which are relatively indolent and carry a good prognosis. They arise in the affected glands and respond well to treatment while still localised there. Persistent swelling, particularly in long-standing disease, is suggestive, as is sudden enlargement of previously swollen glands, especially with cervical lymph node enlargement. Higher disease severity, a low $CD4^+$ lymphocyte count or $CD4^+/CD8^+$ ratio and high density of lymphocytes in the gland are strong predictors for lymphoma. High-grade B cell lymphomas also arise and sometimes develop from the low-grade lymphomas.

Key features are summarised in Box 22.10

Lymphoma in Sjögren's PMID: 25316606 and 32631601

HIV-ASSOCIATED SALIVARY GLAND DISEASE → Summary chart 22.2 p. 393

This disease affects primarily children and young adults with HIV infection, causing chronic soft parotid enlargement of one or both parotid glands, sometimes painful. It is discussed in detail in Chapter 30. Immunosuppression also leads to enlargement of intraparotid lymph nodes, which may be mistaken for parotid neoplasms.

IgG4 RELATED DISEASE

This relatively recently recognised disease[§] causes chronic focal inflammation and dense fibrosis. It affects particularly pancreas and lung and in the head and neck, salivary and lacrimal glands and the soft tissues. Either a single or multiple sites may be involved. Onset is after middle age. The disease is usually asymptomatic, and recurrent periods of activity are characterised by raised levels of serum IgG_4 in about half of cases. This subclass of immunoglobulin normally has a low serum concentration.

Fibrosis produces a firm enlarging mass, often mimicking a neoplasm, and the gland is progressively destroyed.

Diagnosis is by biopsy showing fibrosis with obliteration of small veins, fibrosis and a dense lymphoplasmacytic infiltrate with numerous IgG_4 secreting plasma cells (Fig. 22.20). Diagnosis is difficult as the exact number of IgG_4 secreting plasma cells required for diagnosis is unclear and small numbers may be found in non-specific inflammation. Initial misdiagnosis appears relatively common. Measuring

serum IgG_4 levels may aid diagnosis but has low sensitivity and specificity.

When one salivary gland is affected, a search must be made for other sites, both other salivary glands and remote sites. The condition responds well to steroids and other immunosuppressants, but if untreated, fibrosis will extend beyond the gland to adjacent tissues.

Review IgG4 head and neck PMID: 23068303

Salivary gland PMID: 34024478 and oral sites 35347770

Is a rare cause of salivary fibrosis PMID: 23692045

EOSINOPHILIC (ALLERGIC) SIALADENITIS

This under-recognised condition has been called eosinophilic sialodochitis (implying inflammation centred on the ducts), sialodochitis fibrinosa, and Kussmaul disease. The presentation is distinctive, with intermittent painful salivary gland swelling of parotid glands, submandibular glands or both, mealtime syndrome and sometimes itching of the overlying skin. Inflammation around and in the ducts is dominated by eosinophils. The salivary glycoproteins become denatured and precipitate as mucous plugs that fill and obstruct the larger ducts. Sometimes patients are able to pull long strands of stringy 'fibrous' mucus out of the duct opening. Repeated attacks cause secondary changes of obstruction, with inflammation and fibrosis of the gland. Eosinophilic sialadenitis seems to be more common in patients of Japanese and African heritage and affects people in middle age.

The cause is an allergic reaction and most patients are atopic. Triggering antigens are unknown. Most patients have hay fever, much less commonly food allergy and attacks are not usually related to diet. There is raised serum IgE and numerous eosinophils infiltrate the glands, collect around, and migrate into the ducts (Fig 22.21). Their degranulation releases numerous enzymes presumed to damage the acinar and ductal cells and denature the mucin.

Diagnosis is made by the clinical history and microscopic examination of mucous plugs, either pulled from the duct or washed out, revealing very numerous eosinophils. Imaging or ultrasound reveals a dilated duct system. Without specific investigation the condition is easily misdiagnosed as chronic sialadenitis. No treatment is established, but antihistamine and anti-inflammatory drugs used in severe atopy are usually used and sometimes effective.

Eosinophilic sialadenitis/sialodochitis PMID: 33660371 and 27748012

NECROTISING SIALOMETAPLASIA
→ Summary charts 23.1 and 23.2 pp. 409, 410

This tumour-like lesion affects mainly the minor glands of the palate and probably results from infarction or ischaemia triggered by thrombosis or trauma. The condition is commoner in males and in cigarette smokers and in middle aged or older people. Occasionally is it bilateral.

Typically, a relatively painless swelling 15–20 mm in diameter forms on the hard palate at the site of the minor glands (Fig. 22.22), growing rapidly. The surface becomes ulcerated, and the ulcer margins are irregular and heaped up or everted. Clinically, it resembles a salivary gland carcinoma.

[§] Footnote: This disease is now recognised to be the common cause of several previously different diseases including lung pseudotumours, autoimmune pancreatitis and retroperitoneal fibrosis. However, it is not equivalent to Küttner tumour, the terminal fibrotic stage of chronic sialadenitis. Nor does it explain so-called *Mikulicz's disease*, which was probably MALT lymphoma. These confusing historical eponyms are frequently misapplied and best avoided. *See PMID: 21707715*.

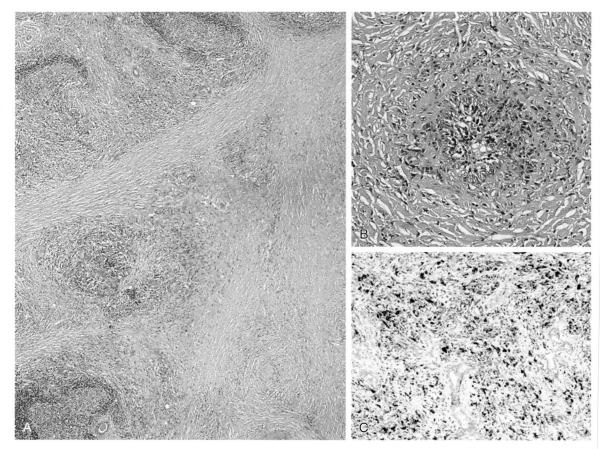

Fig. 22.20   IgG4 related disease in a submandibular gland. The gland is destroyed by intersecting bands of *storiform fibrosis* (an appearance of interwoven and radiating bands of fibrosis) and inflammatory infiltrate including lymphoid follicles (*A*). Small veins are obliterated by inflammation (*B*). Immunohistochemistry against IgG4 class immunoglobulin produces a brown positive reaction on numerous cells secreting IgG4 (C). In a typical non-specific sialadenitis, such cells are rarely present in any numbers.

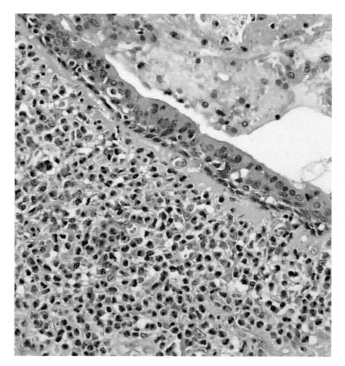

Fig. 22.21   Allergic sialadenitis. Wall of a salivary gland collecting duct showing a dense inflammatory infiltrate around it, in which numerous bright red-stained eosinophils dominate. Eosinophils are migrating through the duct epithelium into the lumen at the top where there are thickened mucin deposits.

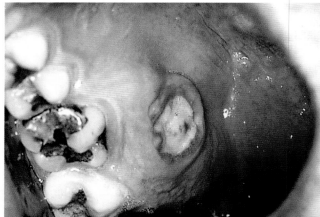

Fig. 22.22   Necrotising sialometaplasia. The clinical appearances are similar to those of a malignant salivary neoplasm, with ulceration over a palatal salivary gland.

There is necrosis of the gland acini, inflammation and, after a short period, a hyperplastic healing response of the duct epithelium. The duct epithelium forms squamous islands so that the condition can mimic a carcinoma histologically as well as clinically (Fig. 22.23).

Biopsy is often performed for diagnosis, although the clinical presentation is distinctive. Untreated, it heals in 6–8 weeks and no intervention speeds recovery.

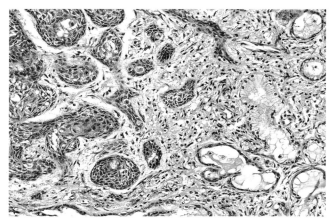

Fig. 22.23 Necrotising sialometaplasia. The histological features may also be mistaken for malignancy. There is necrosis of all the acinar cells and the islands of epithelium on the left are hyperplastic ducts showing squamous metaplasia.

Similar histological changes can be seen in major glands following surgical trauma

Review and case series PMID: 1923419 and 22921832

NODULAR ONCOCYTIC HYPERPLASIA

Oncocytes are cells expanded by large abnormal mitochondria that give the cell a granular eosinophilic appearance in H&E stains. Oncocytes are an age change caused by mitochondrial DNA mutations and are found particularly in thyroid, kidney and salivary glands and neoplasms arising from them. Microscopic foci of oncocytic change are relatively common.

The term nodular or multifocal oncocytic hyperplasia is given when small nodules of oncocytes develop throughout one or several salivary glands, almost always the parotid glands of older people. When the change is extensive, the gland becomes swollen and soft, multiple nodules are visible on imaging and the largest nodules may be palpable. Initially the foci are microscopic, unencapsulated and irregularly shaped but as they enlarge they form lobular encapsulated masses (Fig 22.24). Oncocytosis is otherwise asymptomatic and often a chance finding on imaging or histologically in a gland excised for other reasons. Similar changes can develop in the mucous glands in the mucosa of the upper aerodigestive tract.

No treatment is required but nodules may be subjected to fine needle aspiration (FNA) or biopsy to make the diagnosis.

Large nodules resemble oncocytoma, a benign salivary neoplasm composed of oncocytes, for which multifocal oncocytosis appears to be a precursor lesion (Ch. 23).

Case series PMID: 2361662

SARCOIDOSIS

This disease causes bilateral parotid enlargement with destruction of the gland and replacement by granulomatous inflammation (Fig. 22.25). It is discussed in detail in Chapter 31.

SIALADENOSIS → Summary chart 22.2 p. 393

Sialadenosis is a non-neoplastic, non-inflammatory soft enlargement of salivary glands, most noticeably of the parotids. There are many causes (Box 22.11). Enlargement is slow, and the process is usually bilateral (Fig. 22.26).

Histologically, there is hypertrophy of serous acini and the enlarged cells contain excess large secretory granules. The myoepithelial cells are atrophic. Both these effects are probably mediated by autonomic neuropathy caused by the underlying disease. There is no specific treatment and often none is required, but the underlying cause needs to be identified and addressed if possible.

Cases and review PMID: 7551515

Minor gland involvement in anorexia PMID: 15250838

Histological features PMID: 20580282

Box 22.11   Important causes of sialadenosis

- Alcoholism
- Diabetes mellitus
- Other endocrine diseases
- Pregnancy
- Bulimia
- Malnutrition
- Idiopathic

OTHER SALIVARY GLAND DISORDERS

Irradiation Salivary tissue is highly sensitive to ionising radiation, which causes irreversible destruction of acini and fibrous replacement of glands in the irradiated field. Xerostomia is immediate in onset, severe, and recovers poorly. Management is as for Sjögren's syndrome. Radioiodine, used to treat thyroid carcinomas, is concentrated in salivary glands but causes minimal problems with dry mouth unless repeated doses have been used.

Salivary fistula is a communication between the duct system or gland with the skin or mucous membrane and is uncommon. Internal fistulae drain into the oral cavity and cause no symptoms. By contrast, parotid fistula on the skin is troublesome and often persistent. It may be the result of an injury to the cheek or a complication of surgery. Infection often becomes superimposed, and persistent leakage of saliva prevents healing. The treatment is primarily by surgical repair but is difficult. Greater success is achieved if the tissue surrounding the fistula and adjacent gland is injected with botulinum toxin before surgery, to dry secretion and aid healing.

Sjögren's-like syndrome in graft-versus-host disease develops in approximately one-third of all cases of graft-versus-host disease, particularly when severe, and mimics primary Sjögren's.

Juvenile recurrent parotitis is rare and poorly understood, possibly a low-grade recurrent infection or allergic condition.

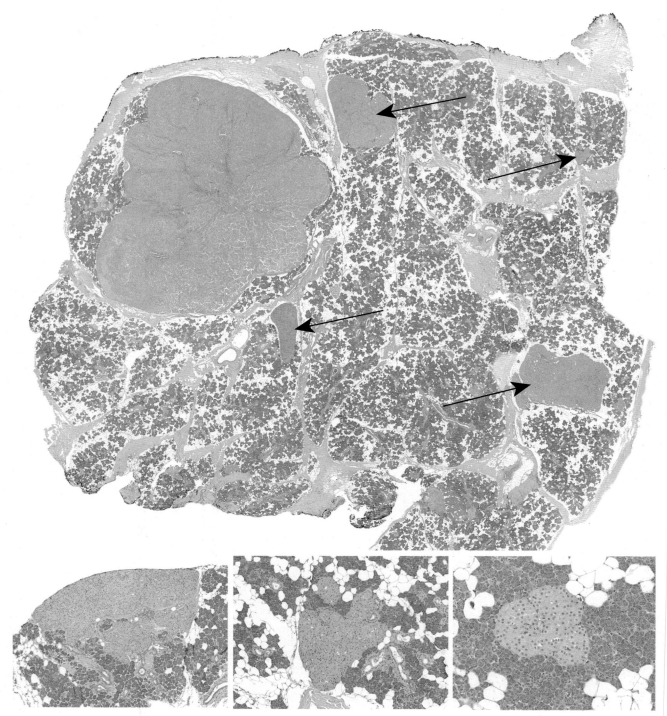

Fig 22.24 Nodular oncocytic hyperplasia. The upper panel shows a section through a parotid gland containing a large oncocytic nodule (upper left) and several smaller nodules in the background (arrowed). Below are three smaller nodules, the smallest not visible at the magnification in the upper image and comprising small cluster of oncocytes with an irregular outline.

It starts before the age of 6 years and causes recurrent episodes of acute swelling lasting a few days with fever and malaise, usually unilaterally. It resolves around the time of puberty.

Cytomegalovirus infection in the newborn causes parotid gland swelling and the gland acinar cells are directly infected by the virus, but infection in adults with immunosuppression does not appear to cause salivary disease.

Sodium retention syndrome is a poorly understood condition that has been identified as a possible cause for otherwise unexplained xerostomia but can only be diagnosed by detecting reduced sodium concentration in the saliva. As well as dry mouth, it is associated with intermittent short-lasting unilateral salivary gland swelling.

Hepatitis C infection causes salivary gland swelling and lymphocytic inflammation with dry mouth as a relatively

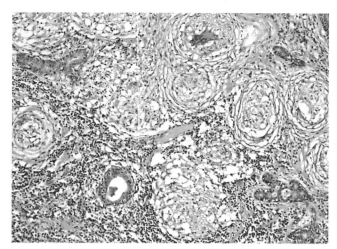

Fig. 22.25   Sarcoidosis of salivary gland. The acinar cells are completely effaced and only a few ducts remain, surrounded by fibrosis and pale staining rounded granulomas of loosely cohesive macrophages. The granuloma near the top in the centre contains a small multinucleate cell.

common extra-hepatic manifestation and is occasionally associated with development of lymphoma in the gland. Though these signs are similar to Sjogren's syndrome, there is no causal link between the two diseases.

Cystic fibrosis is discussed in Chapter 34 and **Frey's syndrome** in Chapter 23.

HYPERSALIVATION AND DROOLING

True hypersalivation, also known as ptyalism, is rarely a significant complaint because excess saliva is swallowed.

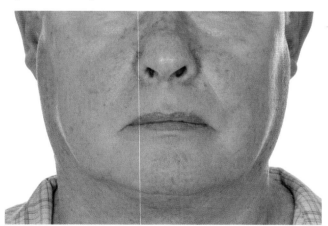

Fig. 22.26   Sialadenosis. Typical appearance of bilateral swelling of parotid glands.

Box 22.12   Causes of ptyalism

Local Reflexes

- Teething
- Oral infections (e.g., acute necrotising ulcerative gingivitis)
- Oral wounds
- Dental procedures
- New dentures

Systemic Reflexes

- Nausea
- Oesophageal disease and reflux oesophagitis
- Rare effect of pregnancy

Medication

- Clozapine and some other antipsychotics
- Cholinergic agents for myasthenia gravis and dementia
- Drugs associated with oesophagitis and gastric irritation

Toxins

- Iodine
- Heavy metals: mercury, thallium, copper, arsenic
- Acetylcholinesterase insecticides

False Ptyalism And Drooling

- Psychogenic
- Bell's palsy
- Parkinson's disease
- Stroke

However, it is a symptom increasingly considered to merit medical investigation given its many causes (Box 22.12). Idiopathic paroxysmal sialorrhea, known to patients as *waterbrash*, is reflex secretion caused by oesophagitis, peptic ulcers, infections and other gastrointestinal irritation, usually during the night. There is a rush of saliva, sometimes waking the patient because their mouth is suddenly full of saliva.

False ptyalism, a sensation of excess saliva, is more common than true ptyalism and is either delusional or results from failure to swallow.

Drooling of saliva from the mouth does not usually indicate increased secretion, though it may be contributory. It is common in neurological disorders, or in people with syndromic presentations such as Down's syndrome, due to weak neuromuscular control, often with a forward head and tongue posture and weak swallowing. Drooling is often associated with angular cheilitis (Ch. 15).

Drooling PMID: 19236564 and 15202698

Botulinum toxin treatment PMID: 23112272

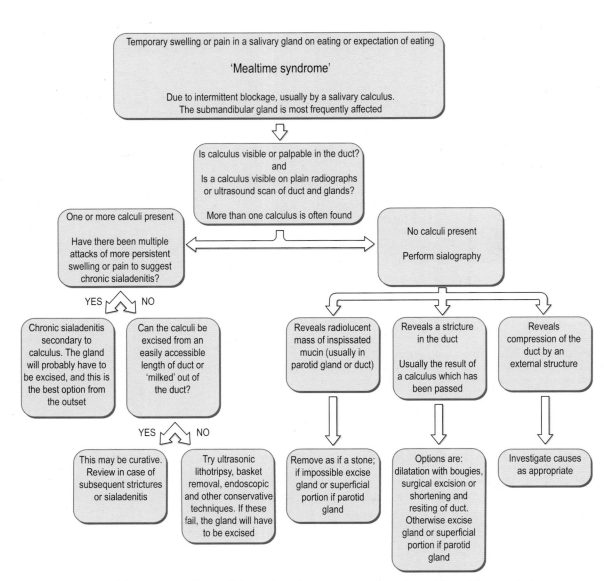

Temporary swelling or pain in a salivary gland on eating or expectation of eating

'Mealtime syndrome'

Due to intermittent blockage, usually by a salivary calculus.
The submandibular gland is most frequently affected

Is calculus visible or palpable in the duct?
and
Is a calculus visible on plain radiographs
or ultrasound scan of duct and glands?

More than one calculus is often found

One or more calculi present

Have there been multiple attacks of more persistent swelling or pain to suggest chronic sialadenitis?

No calculi present

Perform sialography

YES   NO

Chronic sialadenitis secondary to calculus. The gland will probably have to be excised, and this is the best option from the outset

Can the calculi be excised from an easily accessible length of duct or 'milked' out of the duct?

Reveals radiolucent mass of inspissated mucin (usually in parotid gland or duct)

Reveals a stricture in the duct

Usually the result of a calculus which has been passed

Reveals compression of the duct by an external structure

YES   NO

This may be curative. Review in case of subsequent strictures or sialadenitis

Try ultrasonic lithotripsy, basket removal, endoscopic and other conservative techniques. If these fail, the gland will have to be excised

Remove as if a stone; if impossible excise gland or superficial portion if parotid gland

Options are: dilatation with bougies, surgical excision or shortening and resiting of duct. Otherwise excise gland or superficial portion if parotid gland

Investigate causes as appropriate

Summary chart 22.1 Differential diagnosis and management of a patient with mealtime syndrome.

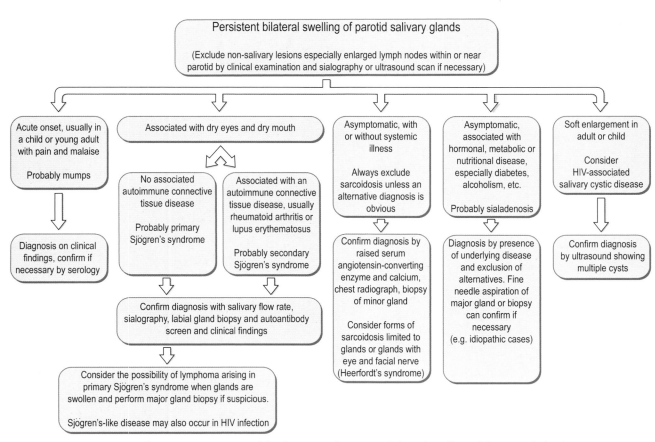

Summary chart 22.2 Summary of the diagnosis of persistent bilateral swelling of the parotid glands.

Salivary gland tumours 23

SALIVARY GLAND NEOPLASMS

Most salivary gland neoplasms arise in the parotid glands, but they are also frequent in intraoral minor glands, making them the second most common neoplasms of the mouth after squamous cell carcinoma. Neoplasms of salivary glands arise from the stem cell population that resides in the ducts and gives rise normally to duct lining epithelium, secretory acinar cells and myoepithelial cells. The histology of the tumours is therefore complex because all these lines of differentiation may appear in different proportions. Many tumours are *biphasic*, that is they comprise more than one cell type, usually duct lining and myoepithelial cells.

Occasionally, lymphomas arise in the intraparotid lymph nodes and other soft tissue neoplasms can develop from the supporting connective tissue of the gland. Although within the gland, these are not considered primary salivary gland neoplasms.

Mucous-secreting glands in the nose and nasal sinuses, pharynx, larynx and lung can also give rise to many of the same types of neoplasms that develop in salivary glands.

Epidemiology and aetiology

The total incidence of salivary gland tumours is difficult to determine because the majority are benign tumours and are not recorded by cancer registries. Taken together, benign and malignant tumours arise in at least 10 per 100,000 of the population so that several thousand cases arise in the UK each year. *Malignant* salivary neoplasms have a relatively stable prevalence of approximately 0.8 per 10,000 in the UK, and approximately 700 new salivary gland cancers are registered in England each year. Women are slightly more frequently affected, and the peak incidence for all types is in the fifth decade, although both benign and malignant neoplasms have a very broad age distribution. Although the numbers are small, the incidence of *malignant* salivary gland tumours in the UK is increasing slowly.

The aetiology of most salivary gland tumours remains obscure. They can result from irradiation to the head and prevalence increased in survivors of the atomic blasts at Hiroshima and Nagasaki. Salivary tumours can also follow therapeutic irradiation for other head and neck cancers, especially when irradiated in childhood. It has also been suggested that multiple dental diagnostic radiographs may play a role. Studies on association with mobile phone use suggest no risk of malignant tumours, but there are no good data to analyse for benign tumours.

Several salivary tumours are known to be caused by specific fusion genes. These arise through chromosomal breakage during mitosis, the fragments rejoining incorrectly as chromosomal translocations, deletions or inversions. Where the fragments rejoin, a new fusion gene is formed, a hybrid that links together parts of two previously unrelated genes. Such fusion genes are often oncogenic and in salivary gland are mostly associated with low grade or slow growing cancers. An important consequence of the presence of a

fusion gene is that some can be targeted by drugs, providing an additional line of treatment. Fusion genes can be detected by fluorescence in situ hybridisation (Ch. 1, Fig. 1.11), DNA or RNA sequencing to aid diagnosis of difficult cases. Other salivary gland tumours are associated with specific gene mutations. A summary of established important genetic changes in salivary gland tumours is shown in Table 23.1.

There are large differences in the incidence of individual tumour types worldwide. In the United Kingdom, mucoepidermoid and acinic cell carcinomas are rarer than in the United States, and lymphoepithelial carcinomas are much more common in the Eastern countries.

US incidence PMID: 19861510

UK incidence PMID: 23103239

Presentations worldwide PMID: 35622296

Tumour genetics treatment significance PMID: 27101980

Fusion genes in salivary tumours PMID: 34913211

Presentation of salivary gland tumours

Salivary neoplasms almost always present as a mass, sometimes with added symptoms of obstruction if the excretory duct is compressed. Often the lump may be longstanding, but that does not necessarily indicate that it is likely to be benign. Key symptoms to elicit in the history are those of

Table 23.1 Molecular changes in salivary gland neoplasms

Salivary Gland Tumour	Molecular changes
Pleomorphic adenoma	*PLAG1* or, less frequently, *HMGA2* fusions or amplification
Basal cell adenomas	*CTNNB1* or *CYLD* mutations
Mucoepidermoid carcinoma	Fusion gene between *MAML2* and either *CRTC1* or *CRTC3*
Adenoid cystic carcinoma	*MYB* fusion/activation/amplification
Acinic cell carcinoma	*NR4A3* fusion or activation
Secretory carcinoma	Fusion gene between *ETV6* and usually *NTRK3*
Microsecretory adenocarcinoma	Fusion gene between *MEF2C* and *SS18*
Polymorphous adenocarcinoma	*PRKD1* mutations or fusions
Hyalinising clear cell carcinoma	Fusion gene between *EWSR1* and either *ATF1* or *CREM*
Salivary duct carcinoma	*HER2* amplification, *TP53* mutation, *AR* copy gain, *PTEN* deletion
Myoepithelial carcinoma	Fusion gene involving *PLAG1*
Epithelial-myoepithelial carcinoma	*HRAS* mutation

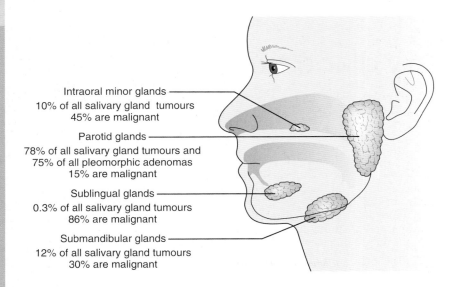

Intraoral minor glands
10% of all salivary gland tumours
45% are malignant

Parotid glands
78% of all salivary gland tumours and
75% of all pleomorphic adenomas
15% are malignant

Sublingual glands
0.3% of all salivary gland tumours
86% are malignant

Submandibular glands
12% of all salivary gland tumours
30% are malignant

Fig. 23.1 The distribution of salivary gland neoplasms showing the approximate overall frequency of tumours in different sites and the relevant frequency of benign and malignant tumours by site.

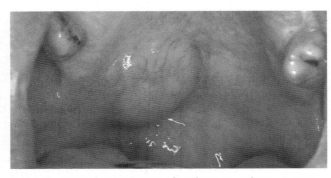

Fig. 23.2 Typical presentation of a salivary neoplasm. A mass lies at the junction of hard and soft palate, a common intraoral site. This particular example is a pleomorphic adenoma, which usually feels rubbery and firm on palpation.

Table 23.2 Typical clinical features of salivary gland tumours

Benign salivary gland tumours	Malignant salivary gland tumours
Slow-growing	Some are fast-growing and painful, but many are slow growing and asymptomatic
Soft or rubbery consistency	Sometimes hard consistency
Comprise 85% of parotid tumours	Comprise 45% of minor gland tumours
Do not ulcerate	May ulcerate and invade bone
No associated nerve signs	May cause cranial nerve palsies, usually lingual, facial or hypoglossal depending on the site

nerve involvement. Facial nerve signs almost certainly indicate that a parotid mass is a malignant neoplasm. Adenoid cystic carcinoma has a particular propensity to spread along nerves and give rise to symptoms of facial palsy, pain or paraesthesia. At a late stage, malignant neoplasms will ulcerate into the mouth or to the skin and may seed metastases, usually to adjacent cervical lymph nodes, but occasionally to lung or other distant sites.

It is critically important to recognise the relationship between the gland of origin and risk of a neoplasm being malignant (Fig. 23.1) before planning a biopsy or excision. About 75% of salivary gland tumours develop in the parotid gland, most in the superficial lobe, and about 10% in the submandibular glands. These produce a visible or palpable mass. Tumours in the deep lobe of parotid present as a mass in the lateral wall of the pharynx, close to the tonsil, or are not noticed. Tumours in the sublingual glands are rare but usually malignant. The usual intraoral site is the palatal glands at or near the junction of the hard and soft palate (Fig. 23.2), followed by the buccal mucosa or labial minor glands.

Typical clinical features of benign and malignant salivary gland tumours are shown in Table 23.2. However, in their early stages, benign and malignant salivary gland tumours usually cannot be distinguished clinically (Summary chart 23.2).

Most major gland tumours are unlikely to present to the dentist and are more likely to be incidental findings in primary care. Conversely, minor gland tumours are likely to be noticed first in a dental setting.

Minor gland tumour incidence and outcome PMID: 26632951

Minor gland diagnostic difficulties PMID: 34042205

Types and classification

The classification of salivary gland tumours is complex. The numerous types of cells in salivary glands give rise to many neoplasms, with diverse origins, appearances and behaviours. The current World Health Organization scheme lists 21 malignant and 15 benign tumours, but still more have been described. However, many are rarities, and a simplified classification of the commoner and more important entities is shown in Box 23.1. The full classification, with a brief note on the rarer entities, is shown in Appendix 23.1.

Investigations

Treatment depends on tumour type and extent, and either a definitive diagnosis or categorisation into benign or malignant is needed to plan surgery. The key investigation is fine needle aspiration (FNA). For pleomorphic adenoma, Warthin's tumour, adenoid cystic carcinoma and many common neoplasms, fine needle aspiration almost always gives the correct diagnosis. For other tumours, it can often determine whether neoplasms are benign or malignant, low or high grade, or can be used to narrow down a differential diagnosis. Neoplasms in the superficial parotid gland are amenable to fine needle aspiration, and ultrasound guidance can be used to target more deeply seated tumours.

Imaging for suspected salivary neoplasms is best performed by magnetic resonance imaging (MRI), which is capable of detecting perineural spread and base of skull invasion by palatal and parotid cancers. Cone beam computed tomography (CBCT) or conventional thin slice CT is useful to detect palatal bone perforation below palatal tumours. Sialography no longer has any role in investigation of salivary neoplasms, and ultrasound scanning is the best way to differentiate salivary neoplasms from enlarged intraparotid lymph nodes. The thought processes underlying investigation and diagnosis are shown in Summary charts 23.1 and 23.2.

Diagnosis of minor gland tumours

The diagnosis and management of minor gland tumours is beset by several difficulties that do not apply to the major glands. This is of particular importance in the dental context because minor gland neoplasms are much more likely to present to the dentist, who is often responsible for initial biopsy. Some of problems reflect the complexity, small size and superficial location of minor gland tumours, and others the different biology and tissue anatomy of minor glands. A summary of these problems is shown in Table 23.3.

To ensure these potential problems do not cause misdiagnosis, under- or overtreatment the clinician needs to allow for them in the management strategy. Ideally, when a minor gland tumour is suspected, the initial biopsy and definitive treatment should be in one treatment centre. The biopsy must be of a sufficient size and include lateral, and ideally some deep, margin of the tumour. If a biopsy fails to provide a specific diagnosis, it should not be repeated, the entire tumour should be removed to prevent repeat biopsy disrupting the remaining tumour and causing inflammation that confuses histological diagnosis. If the clinical picture is benign, fine needle aspiration is inconclusive and the tumour is very small (10 mm diameter or less), it may be a better diagnostic procedure to avoid incisional biopsy and go direct to excision, ensuring a complete margin of a few millimetres of normal tissue. In the event of an unexpected diagnosis of a low-grade malignant neoplasm, the tumour will have been adequately treated. Each possible salivary tumour needs a tailored investigation strategy based on its location, size, and clinical and imaging features.

Review PMID: 34042205

Treatment

Salivary gland neoplasms are generally treated by surgery, with radiotherapy reserved for high-grade malignant tumours, those that are incompletely excised or have recurred after treatment. Treatment is often tailored to individual tumour types, the stage at presentation and, for some, histological grading. Treatment details are given later with each type and in the introduction to malignant tumours. Additional treatment options may also be effective when specific targetable molecular changes are present in the tumour. Such treatments have variable success and adverse effects and are usually reserved for recurrent tumour after surgery or disseminated metastases in the palliative setting. Most are still experimental and may only be available in clinical trials.

Surgery of salivary glands carries potentially significant morbidity. Parotid gland surgery risks facial paralysis from damage to the facial nerve. Branches of the nerve may need to be resected and grafted if involved by a malignant tumour. Submandibular tumours lie close to important structures and removal of even a small tumour in the lip can result in disfigurement through deep scarring in the easily distorted soft tissues.

A particular complication of parotid surgery is Frey's syndrome or gustatory sweating caused by surgical damage to the auriculotemporal nerve. This carries parasympathetic secretomotor supply to the parotid gland and during healing severed fibres may reconnect inappropriately with the sweat glands in the skin over and around the parotid gland. Eating and thought of food will then trigger sweating in the affected skin (Fig. 23.3). Frey's syndrome also occurs in diabetes and following facial trauma, including forceps delivery trauma sustained during childbirth. The condition can be treated with botulinum toxin injection into the affected skin (Ch. 27).

BENIGN TUMOURS

→ Summary charts 23.1 and 23.2 pp. 409, 410

Pleomorphic adenoma

Pleomorphic adenomas, or pleomorphic salivary adenomas, are benign salivary tumours characterised microscopically by an unusually broad range of types of tissue. The neoplastic cells are epithelial but differentiate to a connective tissue cell type and secrete connective tissue ground substance, collagen, form cartilage and sometimes bone. This mixture

Table 23.3   Complications in diagnosis and treatment of salivary tumours in minor glands

Feature of minor gland neoplasms	Problems arising
A higher proportion are malignant than in major glands	Malignant salivary neoplasms are in any site more difficult to diagnose than their benign counterparts Many malignant neoplasms in minor glands are low grade, with minimal cytological atypia. Diagnosis of a malignant neoplasm therefore requires a biopsy of its lateral or deep periphery to identify invasion Minor gland neoplasms tend to be of rarer types, of which surgeons and pathologists may have little experience
Biopsy is frequently performed	In major glands fine needle aspiration usually provides either a diagnosis or sufficient information to proceed to treatment and diagnosis is easy when the whole tumour is available for examination. However, biopsy is the usual strategy for minor glands. Many problems then result from inadequate or inappropriate biopsy.
The easily accessible area for biopsy is superficial	Many malignant tumours in minor glands are of low grade and diagnosis as malignant requires finding invasion. This tends to occur laterally and deeply and so is not seen in a biopsy of the 'top' of the lesion Perineural spread is also rarely evident in superficial tissue
Benign minor gland tumours are often unencapsulated and lack a well-defined periphery	A potential cause of overdiagnosis of invasion, and thus of malignancy
Those on the palate lie deeply in the mucoperiosteum	The dense fibrous tissue forms a major barrier to growth and so even benign tumours grow deeply, causing pressure resorption of the adjacent bone. When seen on imaging, this may lead to incorrect assumption of malignancy.
Those in other areas of mucosa lie superficially	These tumours come into contact with overlying epithelium early in growth and may fuse with it, producing a hyperplastic and sometimes papillary surface change. This reaction is evident clinically and may be misconstrued as the primary lesion, resulting in a superficial biopsy that contains too little of the underlying tumour. Malignant tumours often ulcerate early and the inflammation that results makes microscopic diagnosis difficult Superficial benign tumours may ulcerate due to trauma or denture pressure, mimicking a malignant neoplasm
Malignant tumours extend beyond the small glands very early	This makes malignant tumours more difficult to excise in a compartment of tissue in the way that parotid tumours can be removed by excising the gland. Minor gland tumours spread unpredictably and irregularly into surrounding muscle, fibrous tissue and bone at an early stage

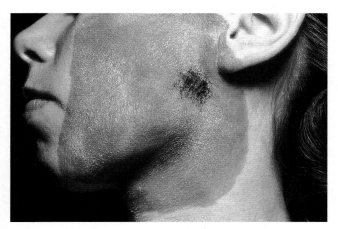

Fig 23.3   Frey's syndrome. Gustatory sweating as a consequence of parotid surgery. The skin has been painted with iodine solution and then dusted with starch powder. A salivary stimulus such as citric acid has then been applied to the tongue. Moisture from reflex sweating combines the iodine and starch to produce the dark blue colour seen on the patch of skin just below and anterior to the ear lobe. This test can be used for diagnosis and to monitor the area for treatment and the response to it.
(Source: Reproduced from Hurley HJ. Hyperhidrosis. Curr Opin Dermatol. 1997;4:105–14. Philadelphia: Rapid Science Publishers)

of epithelium and connective tissue accounts for the old name of mixed tumour.

These benign tumours are the commonest salivary tumours and account for about 75% of parotid tumours, and a further 20% are distributed equally between the submandibular gland and intraoral minor glands, usually on the palate (see Fig. 23.2). They can arise at any age but are most common in middle age.

Pleomorphic adenomas grow slowly and take several years to reach 2 cm in diameter. They are rubbery, firm swellings (see Figs. 23.2 and 23.4), smooth when small but often very lobulated when large (Fig. 23.5). The overlying skin or mucosa is mobile over the lump, although in the palate the more inflexible mucoperiosteum may appear fixed.

The cause of most pleomorphic adenomas is a chromosomal translocation that activates one of two genes, *PLAG1* or *HMGA2*, by forming fusion genes with one of several possible partner genes. *PLAG1* and *HMGA2* encode transcription factors important in normal development. Their constitutive activation results in cell proliferation and abnormal differentiation, explaining the varied tissues formed. In addition to these causative translocations, pleomorphic adenomas can have many other chromosomal abnormalities involving oncogenes and tumour suppressor genes. These additional changes increase with time and probably

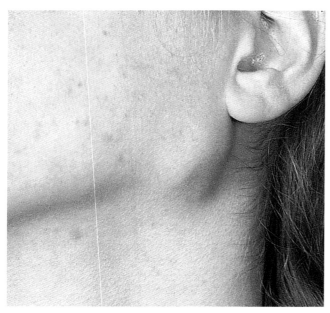

Fig. 23.4 **Pleomorphic adenoma.** This slowly enlarging lump in the lower pole of the parotid gland is caused by a pleomorphic adenoma, but the appearance is not specific and any benign and some low-grade malignant neoplasms could appear the same.

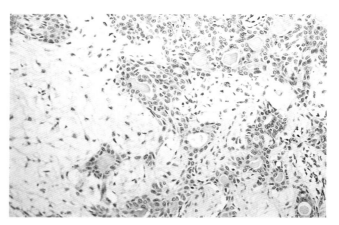

Fig. 23.6 **Pleomorphic adenoma.** The histological appearances are very varied. In this typical area, there are clusters of ducts containing eosinophilic material surrounded by stellate cells lying in a myxoid stroma.

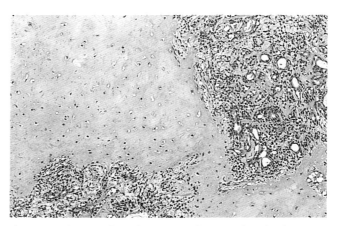

Fig. 23.7 **Pleomorphic adenoma.** In this area, there has been maturation of the mucinous stroma to form a cartilage-like material around which there are more cellular islands with ducts.

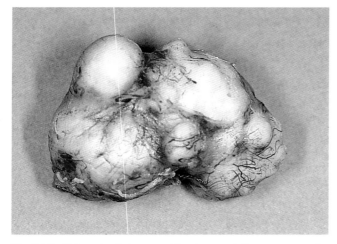

Fig. 23.5 This excised pleomorphic adenoma is 3 cm across, and the lobular shape is clearly seen.

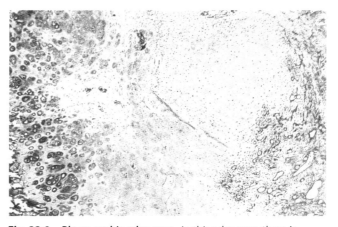

Fig. 23.8 **Pleomorphic adenoma.** In this adenoma, there is formation of true cartilage which is undergoing calcification.

account for the risk of malignant transformation in long-standing tumours.

Each adenoma is circumscribed, and there is usually a capsule around most of the periphery. While it grows, the tumour pushes out large finger-like extensions or bulges through the capsule to form a lobulated outline. Inside, there is a disorganised arrangement of tissues (Figs 23.6–23.9). The epithelial cells form ducts and small cysts and sheets. Around the ducts and detaching and migrating from them are cells that show partial differentiation into myoepithelial cells. These cells can be identified immunohistochemically by their expression of cytokeratins and contractile proteins such as actin, but unlike normal myoepithelial cells around acini, they have no useful contractile function. Rather they take on the shapes and functions of connective tissue cells. Most are spindle or stellate in shape, secrete excess

proteoglycan ground substance and become dispersed in it to form a myxoid (gelatinous) tissue. Some are rounded and look like plasma cells microscopically, and others form collagen or cartilage that may mineralize and become bone (Box 23.2). The proportion of these tissues varies widely

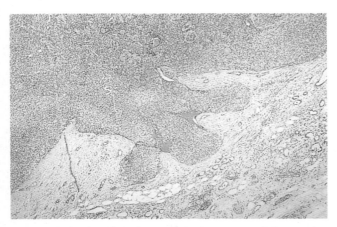

Fig. 23.9 Pleomorphic adenoma. At the margins of pleomorphic adenomas there are often extensions of the tumour into and beyond the capsule, rendering enucleation a risky treatment that is likely to be followed by recurrence.

Box 23.2   Histological features of pleomorphic adenomas

- Capsule, can be thick but is almost never complete
- Ducts
- Sheets and strands of dark-staining epithelial cells
- Cells at the periphery of sheets detach and secrete matrix proteoglycans
- Dispersed cells in matrix form 'myxoid' stroma
- Myxoid stroma may develop into cartilage
- Cartilage may ossify to form bone
- Other parts of the stroma may be densely collagenous and hyalinised
- Sometimes there are foci of keratin formation
- Bulging lobular growth through the capsule

---

between tumours producing a confusing range of histological appearances.

Pleomorphic adenomas are treated by excision with a margin of normal tissue; without this, recurrence is likely. The reputation of the pleomorphic adenoma for recurrence is due a combination of its structure and anatomical location. In the parotid gland, the facial nerve in particular makes dissection hazardous. Tumours in the deep lobe require complete parotidectomy, and it is not unusual for tumours to have to be peeled off nerves to preserve them.

The risk of recurrence also depends on the tumour. Those comprising almost exclusively the gelatinous myxoid tissue can burst at operation, if not gently handled, and even a small disruption of the capsule can allow the semisolid contents to seed widespread recurrence in the tissues. Recurrence is most problematic for parotid tumours, where spillage of gelatinous tumour into the fascial planes of the neck can seed very numerous nodules of tumour in tissues from the base of skull down to the clavicle. Unfortunately, almost all pleomorphic adenomas contain at least some of this myxoid component.

The strategy to avoid recurrence is to remove tumours intact with a margin of normal tissue. In the superficial parotid gland, this is normally considered to require removal of the whole superficial lobe. For those in the submandibular gland, the whole gland is removed. Tumours in minor glands

are excised with a few millimetres of normal tissue margin and rarely recur.

Recently it has been shown that pleomorphic adenomas can be effectively treated by more conservative surgery, *extracapsular dissection*, removing a minimal amount of tissue beyond the capsule. This remains controversial and risks both puncture of the capsule or failure to gain clearance in areas without a capsule. Nevertheless, it seems to have a low recurrence rate when performed by those skilled in the procedure.

When recurrence develops, it is often multifocal and difficult or impossible to eradicate by surgery. Although the recurrent nodules are benign, there may be a hundred or more microscopic 'seedlings' and radiotherapy is sometimes used as a last resort to control surgically unresectable spread in the infratemporal fossa or neck.

If neglected, pleomorphic adenomas can grow to a great size, over 10 cm diameter is not unusual. Longstanding examples, regardless of size, occasionally undergo malignant change as described later in the section on carcinoma ex pleomorphic adenoma.

Review treatment PMID: 18376235

Treatment by extracapsular dissection PMID: 34697837

Warthin's tumour

This is the second commonest type of salivary tumour worldwide. Almost all arise in the parotid glands, usually the lower pole, and account for approximately 10% of parotid tumours. Although previously considered much more common in males, this is not supported by current evidence. Almost all patients are aged older than 40 years, and there appears to be a close association with heavy smoking, particularly in multifocal tumours. In countries with ageing populations, Warthin's tumour incidence is increasing and in some countries it has overtaken pleomorphic adenoma to become the commonest salivary neoplasm.

Warthin's tumours develop not only in salivary glands but also in the lymph nodes around the lower pole of the gland and in the upper third of the deep cervical lymphatic chain. The lymph node tumours are not metastatic but arise from developmental rests of salivary gland ducts that are commonly found in lymph nodes at these sites.

Approximately 15% of patients will have a second Warthin's tumour, and 10% of patients have bilateral tumours. Histologically there are often multifocal microscopic foci of developing Warthin's tumours in surrounding gland or lymph nodes.

The nature of this unusual multifocal tumour is unclear. Molecular analysis shows that the tumours are not clonal, suggesting that they are not true neoplasms despite findings of chromosomal translocations in some. The cause may be defects of mitochondrial genes.

The tumour is a cyst or part solid part cystic mass with a thin capsule and a highly characteristic histological appearance with a lymphoid and an epithelial component. The lymphoid tissue resembles lymph node, with many lymphoid follicles and germinal centres. The epithelial cells are tall, eosinophilic columnar cells that form a much-folded cyst lining epithelial with papillary projections into the cystic spaces (Figs 23.10 and 23.11). The bright pink appearance of the epithelial cells' cytoplasm is caused by abnormal large, distorted mitochondria that almost completely fill the cell. Cells showing this change are referred to as *oncocytic* (see also oncocytoma later in this chapter and oncocytosis in Ch. 22).

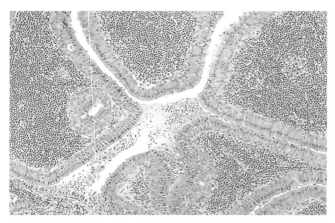

Fig. 23.10 Warthin's tumour. Tall columnar cells surround lymphoid tissue and line a convoluted cystic space.

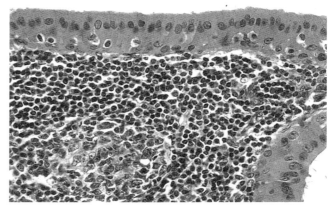

Fig. 23.11 Warthin's tumour. At higher power, the tall columnar epithelial cells are readily identified and beneath them the lymphoid tissue.

Warthin's tumour is benign and cured by simple excision but may appear to recur because new tumours develop elsewhere in the gland. Preoperative diagnosis by FNA is accurate, and it has been suggested that, after FNA diagnosis, surgery can be avoided and the lesion managed conservatively, monitored by repeated imaging. This may be an attractive option in a very old or debilitated patient. However, Warthin's tumours can reach several centimetres diameter, and FNA results can be incorrect because oncocytic cells are found in many salivary tumours, including a variant of mucoepidermoid carcinoma that is a very close mimic histologically. In practice, most are excised.

The older name of adenolymphoma should not be used as it risks confusion with lymphoma and other types of tumour.

Review PMID: 3458128

Conservative management PMID: 34441400

Infarcted Warthin's: PMID: 2743609

Salivary gland myoepithelioma

This benign neoplasm of myopepithelial cells arises in parotid, palatal glands and submandibular gland at almost any age. 'Salivary gland' is included in the name because myoepitheliomas also develop in other glands.

Salivary myoepitheliomas are circumscribed, encapsulated cellular tumours in which the cells express contractile proteins of myoepithelium. Many patterns are possible - sheets or strands of epithelium, plasmacytoid cells or spindle cells dispersed in myxoid or hyalinised stroma – but any one tumour only has one pattern. This uniformity and lack of ducts differentiate myoepithelioma from pleomorphic adenoma, though in the past they have been considered to be related and this is supported by shared genetic changes in some.

Myoepithelioma does not usually recur after excision.

Canalicular adenoma

Canalicular adenomas affect particularly the upper lip and buccal mucosa, and some are multifocal in origin. They have a uniform cellular structure, comprising strands and trabeculae or duct-like rings of basaloid epithelial cells. They lack myoepithelial cells and do not form the myxoid or cartilaginous tissues of pleomorphic adenoma and do not recur on simple excision.

Basal cell adenoma

These adenomas arise mostly in the parotid glands of older people. They are encapsulated and comprise basaloid cells arranged in ducts, strands, trabeculae and solid sheets (Fig 23.12). Like canalicular adenomas, they do not form myxoid tissue or cartilage. Several histological patterns exist, and these seem to have different genetic causes.

Basal cell adenomas do not recur on excision, but because they can be difficult to confidently differentiate from pleomorphic adenomas on FNA, they are often diagnosed only after a superficial parotidectomy undertaken for an assumed pleomorphic adenoma.

Oncocytoma

Oncocytoma is a rare benign tumour that almost always affects the parotid gland, particularly in older people. It consists of large eosinophilic cells with small compact nuclei (*oncocytes*), arranged in solid cords, nests or sheets (Fig. 23.13). Oncocytes stain a granular bright pink in haematoxylin and eosin stains because their cytoplasm is packed with enlarged mitochondria. The cause is mutation of genes encoded by mitochondrial DNA controlling mitochondrial synthesis.

Some oncocytomas arise in a background of multinodular oncocytic hyperplasia (Ch. 22). Oncocytomas do not recur after complete excision.

Sclerosing polycystic adenoma

Sclerosing polycystic adenoma was until recently considered a condition of uncertain nature but has now been renamed as an adenoma to reflect its acceptance as a benign neoplasm caused by mutations in the *PTEN* gene or elsewhere in the PI3-kinase signalling pathway. The process is analogous to sclerosing adenosis in the breast. It affects adults in middle age and usually develops as a slow growing firm mass in the parotid gland, occasionally in the nasal and lacrimal glands.

There is a fibrotic mass containing proliferating ducts and small cysts lined by epithelium with apocrine differentiation, mixed with acinar cells containing bright red secretory granules. Treatment is by excision and about 10% recur. The main significance is that this benign condition can be misdiagnosed as a malignant neoplasm because it is dense and firm clinically and histologically resembles an infiltrative tumour.

Review PMID: 33526220

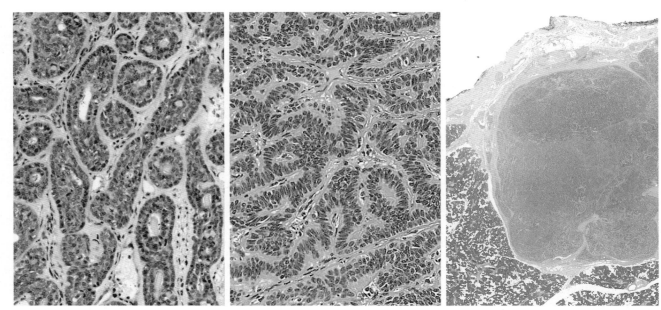

Fig 23.12 Basal cell adenoma. On the right is a typical well circumscribed encapsulated tumour in parotid tissue with a lobular outline, similar to most benign salivary neoplasms. The basal cells can be organised in various ways, on the left they form ducts and tubules and in the centre trabeculae of two rows of cells back-to-back.

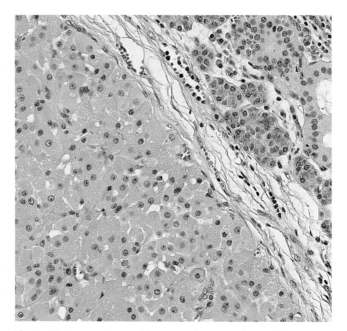

Fig 23.13 Oncocytoma. The oncocytoma, centre and lower left is separated from normal gland, top right, by a thin capsule. The tumour cells are large and rounded and have pink cytoplasm as a result of their numerous large mitochondria. Note now the same appearance is seen in the cytoplasm of the epithelial cells in Warthin's tumour (Fig. 23.10) and the normal striated ducts in the top right corner of the image, all of which contain numerous mitochondria.

MALIGNANT SALIVARY GLAND TUMOURS

→ Summary charts 23.1 and 23.2 pp. 409, 410

Malignant salivary gland neoplasms are rarer than benign neoplasms. More than 21 different types are recognised

and many have several variants. No one type stands out as particularly frequent. The average age of patients with malignant neoplasms is almost the same as those with benign neoplasms; malignant salivary neoplasms can be found in very young as well as in older individuals.

Many are low-grade carcinomas, with slow growth, local infiltration and only a low risk of metastasis. Their clinical presentation can be identical to that of benign neoplasms. Appreciating that these tumours are malignant preoperatively is critical to providing the correct treatment and achieving a good outcome. A key clue to malignancy is recognising how the risk of a salivary neoplasm being malignant varies between sites, as shown in Fig. 23.1. Most types present as an unremarkable firm mass. Conversely, some are aggressive and present with classical signs of malignancy: fixation to adjacent tissues, nerve signs, ulceration, bleeding, bone erosion or metastasis to regional lymph nodes. Trismus may result from infiltration of muscles of mastication when carcinomas arise in the parotid, soft palate and retromolar area.

The risk of metastasis varies widely between different types, but those that do metastasise usually spread to cervical lymph nodes and less frequently via the blood to lungs and other distant sites.

Diagnosis depends on histological examination. High-grade neoplasms are readily recognised on FNA, which can often provide an accurate diagnosis. However, many of the lower grade types are not amenable to diagnosis in this way and are only diagnosed after excision. For this reason, excision of any salivary mass without a diagnosis after FNA and imaging must be undertaken on the assumption that it may turn out to be a low-grade malignant tumour.

Malignant salivary gland tumours are treated by surgical excision, followed by radiotherapy if excision is incomplete or margins close. Recurrence is often difficult to manage; minor gland re-excision may require resection of facial skin, and parotid gland recurrences may involve the base of skull and infratemporal fossa. The prognosis depends on the

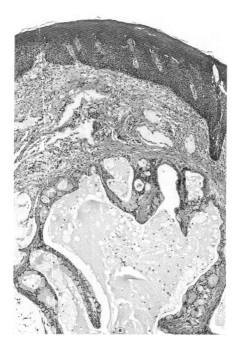

Fig. 23.14 Mucoepidermoid carcinoma. Palatal mucosa overlying a multicystic poorly defined lesion.

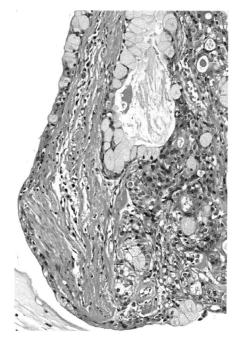

Fig. 23.15 Mucoepidermoid carcinoma. Higher power showing cysts lined by pale mucous cells and lower right a solid area of epidermoid and mucous cells.

site, size and extent of the carcinoma, its histological type and, for some types, its histological grade. Some types have specific causative genetic changes, and some of these can be targeted specifically by drugs. Others may express hormone receptors, making them suitable targets for the types of hormone therapy used for breast or prostate carcinomas.

UK incidence PMID: 23103239

US epidemiology PMID: 10613342

Mucoepidermoid carcinoma

Mucoepidermoid carcinoma is the most common single type of malignant salivary neoplasm, yet it accounts for less than 10% of salivary gland neoplasms. About half arise in a parotid gland, but all glands including minor glands can be affected. The carcinomas usually contain mucin-filled cysts and when they develop in minor glands they are easily mistaken clinically for mucous extravasation or retention cysts.

The cause is a t(11;19) translocation that brings the *CRTC1* gene together with the *MAML2* gene, producing a novel fusion gene that activates the notch signalling pathway, an important developmental pathway that is deregulated in several types of cancer. This accounts for low-grade and intermediate-grade mucoepidermoid carcinomas but only half of high-grade tumours.

The diagnosis requires histological examination and can be aided by identifying the translocation if required. Most contain numerous cysts lined by epithelium that resembles skin epithelium and is therefore called *epidermoid*. It has basal and prickle cells but does not keratinise. Scattered in the epidermoid sheets and cyst linings are variable numbers of mucus-secreting goblet cells, the two cell types explaining the name mucoepidermoid (Figs 23.14 and 23.15). Either mucous or epidermoid cells may predominate.

The tumour usually grows slowly and infiltrates into surrounding tissues and so treatment is by wide excision. Mucoepidermoid carcinomas occasionally metastasise, and

the risk is predicted fairly accurately, by histological grading, dividing the carcinomas into high-, intermediate- and low-grade types. Approximately 40% of high-grade carcinomas metastasise and approximately 30% of patients with high-grade carcinomas die of the disease. Conversely, low-grade and intermediate-grade carcinomas metastasise in only a few percent of patients and are almost never fatal. The prognosis of carcinomas with the *CRTC1::MAML2* translocation is better than for those without.

Review PMID: 21371076

Genetics PMID: 23459841

Adenoid cystic carcinoma

The adenoid cystic carcinoma is distinctive among salivary carcinomas and must be appreciated for its unusual behaviour and poor outcome.

This carcinoma is almost as frequent as mucoepidermoid carcinoma and can affect any gland. Most arise in major glands, usually the parotid, but it accounts for almost a third of minor gland carcinomas (Fig. 23.16). They also arise in mucous glands in the nose and antrum and throughout the mucosa of the aerodigestive tract. Most arise in older individuals, but the age range is broad.

The cause of most cases is a t(6;9) translocation that fuses the proto-oncogene *myb* with a transcription factor gene *NFIB*, producing a novel fusion protein. Several different gene break points produce multiple different fusions all of which increase expression of the myb protein, which in turn activates genes controlling proliferation and cell survival. The translocation can be identified by fluorescence in situ hybridisation or RNA sequencing to aid diagnosis. Higher grade carcinomas have additional genetic changes.

Adenoid cystic carcinomas grow slowly and have a peculiar propensity to invade along nerves - *perineural spread*. In some cases, the carcinoma can extend several centimetres along nerves beyond the clinically apparent mass (Fig. 23.17).

Carcinomas in palatal glands or parotid are sometimes found to have reached the brain at presentation. Perineural spread can produce unusual sensory symptoms, pain or facial weakness, and occasional patients present with these symptoms rather than a mass. Suspicion of adenoid cystic carcinoma may arise when nerves are seen to be thickened on magnetic resonance imaging.

The diagnosis can be made accurately by FNA, biopsy or after excision. There is a highly characteristic histological pattern consisting of rounded groups of small darkly staining cells of almost uniform size, surrounding multiple small clear spaces (cribriform or 'swiss cheese' pattern) (Fig. 23.18). Small ducts lie in the sheets of epithelium, and the carcinoma islands are widely infiltrative.

The prognosis in adenoid cystic carcinoma is poor. Although some small or well-circumscribed tumours are effectively excised, larger tumours and those with perineural spread and diffuse infiltration through bone and soft tissues are difficult or impossible to excise despite extensive surgery. Post-operative radiotherapy is usually given but cannot be relied on to kill this radio-resistant tumour. The slow growth means that a third of patients survive 5 years, but the outcome is ultimately fatal in most cases, although patients may live 15 years after diagnosis. Lymph node metastasis is unusual, but about a third of patients eventually develop blood-borne metastases in lung, liver or bone. Drugs targeting myb overexpression are being tested in clinical trials.

Review PMID: 25943783

Molecular genetics review PMID: 23821214

Acinic cell carcinoma

Acinic cell carcinomas are less common in Europe than in the United States. They arise almost always in the parotid gland and have an unpredictable behaviour despite their slow growth. All ages may be affected. The cause is a t(4;9) translocation that links the *SCPP* gene enhancer to the *NR4A3* gene, activating the latter causing altered proliferation, cell differentiation, energy production and cell survival.

Histologically, they show an almost uniform pattern of large cells similar to serous cells, with granular basophilic cytoplasm. These are often arranged in acini (Fig. 23.19), though a variety of different histological patterns are recognised. Despite apparently benign histological appearances, even sometimes including encapsulation, acinic cell carcinomas can be invasive and occasionally metastasise. Most are low grade; high grade carcinomas frequently recur and metastasise in about half of cases. If left untreated, low-grade acinic cell carcinomas may undergo high grade transformation to aggressive carcinomas.

Review: PMID: 33455041

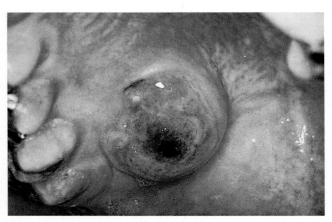

Fig. 23.16 Adenoid cystic carcinoma. There is an ulcerated mass arising from a minor gland in the palate. The clinical appearance would be the same as other malignant salivary neoplasms.

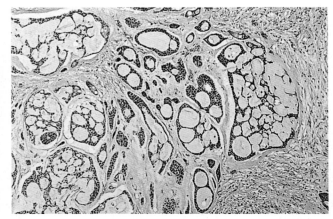

Fig. 23.18 Adenoid cystic carcinoma. The small darkly staining cells of the adenoid cystic carcinoma form cribriform islands with large holes which have been likened, rather inappropriately, to Swiss cheese.

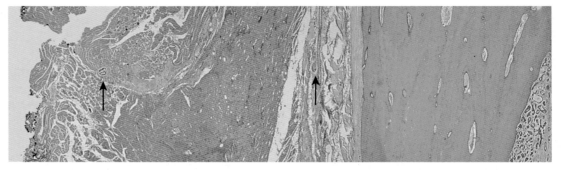

Fig. 23.17 Adenoid cystic carcinoma. In this low power photomicrograph taken from a resection, an adenoid cystic carcinoma in the floor of the mouth has infiltrated into the medullary cavity of the mandible and can be seen in the lower right corner. The extremely infiltrative nature of this carcinoma is demonstrated by the two small islands of dispersed carcinoma that have penetrated the intact cortical bone and now infiltrate the buccal muscle over 10 mm from the main tumour (arrowed).

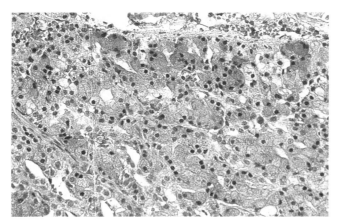

Fig. 23.19 Acinic cell carcinoma. The tumour is composed of granular acinar-type cells, sometimes arranged in acinus-like clusters and sometimes forming irregular sheets. Cytological atypia is uncommon.

Secretory carcinoma

Secretory carcinoma arises in all glands but usually in the parotid during middle age. It is caused in almost all cases by a t(12;15) translocation between the *ETV6* and *NTRK3* genes, activating the latter. *NTRK3* encodes a membrane receptor that activates proliferation, differentiation, and cell survival through the MAP kinase and PI3-kinase pathways.

The carcinoma is well circumscribed, solid and cystic, with papillary areas, and contains many ducts and cysts filled with secretory material (Fig. 23.20).

Most secretory carcinomas are relatively indolent and respond well to excision. Approximately 20% of cases metastasise. Larotrectinib and entrectinib are *NTRK* inhibitors that have been effective in other cancers with similar fusion genes and are undergoing clinical trials for secretory carcinoma.

Polymorphous adenocarcinoma

Polymorphous adenocarcinoma arises almost exclusively in minor glands, particularly of the palate. It is the commonest or second commonest carcinoma in minor glands and, though most cases arise in people older than 50 years of age, it can develop over a broad age range. The cause is either activating mutations or activating fusion of one of the three *PRDK* genes that have roles in cell differentiation, apoptosis and migration through the MAP kinase and Ras cell signalling pathways.

The name derives from the presence of its many histological patterns, with sheets of cells, ducts, narrow strands and cysts, the last sometimes containing papillary projections (Figs 23.21 and 23.22). Despite the diversity of pattern, there is only one cell type, small and bland epithelial cells with very infrequent mitoses. Only infiltration of surrounding tissues may indicate that these are malignant neoplasms. Polymorphous adenocarcinomas are mostly low grade, but they do metastasise in about 10% of cases, although the outcome is almost never fatal. Treatment is by complete local excision. Tumours with gene mutations have a better prognosis than those with fusion genes, which are more likely to metastasise.

The many patterns can cause histological misdiagnosis, particularly confusing it with adenoid cystic carcinoma because both may contain cribriform islands and show perineural spread. Despite the histological similarity, the behaviour of the two carcinomas is very different. Perineural

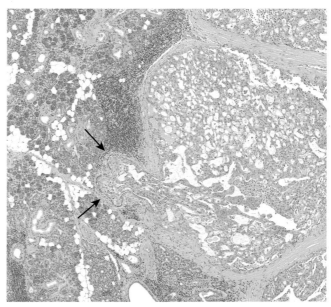

Fig 23.20 Secretory carcinoma. The carcinoma (right) has a lobular structure of pinkish cells forming many small ducts and spaces filled with mucin. A projection of the carcinoma (arrowed) is invading adjacent parotid gland (left).

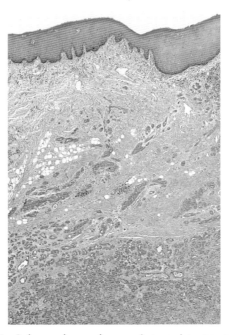

Fig. 23.21 Polymorphous adenocarcinoma. Low power showing a poorly circumscribed tumour with small islands invading upward into the overlying mucosa.

spread in polymorphous adenocarcinoma is very limited in extent, unlike in adenoid cystic carcinoma. To prevent histological misdiagnosis, it is important to obtain a good-sized incisional biopsy that includes part of the periphery for all minor gland neoplasms. Punch and needle core biopsies are often used on palatal tumours but are often inadequate to make a confident diagnosis.

Review PMID: 20403856

Genetics PMID: 34913211

Salivary duct carcinoma

This aggressive high-grade carcinoma is so called because it resembles ductal carcinoma of the breast microscopically. It develops mainly in people older than 50 years of age, is significantly commoner in males and carries a poor prognosis. Most arise in the parotid gland but can develop in other major and, occasionally, minor glands. This carcinoma

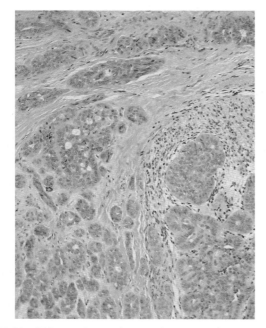

Fig. 23.22 Polymorphous adenocarcinoma. High power showing the cytologically bland cells organised as sheets, ducts and strands.

usually presents as an obviously malignant tumour with rapid growth.

Many genetic changes are present, none clearly causative. One important change is gene amplification or gene fusion of the *AR* androgen receptor gene leading to overexpression.

Perineural spread and lymphatic invasion are common, the latter accounting for the fact that many patients have lymph node metastases on presentation. The cells of the carcinoma are large and show apocrine differentiation, with very pink oncocytic cytoplasm and form ducts and cysts with the cribriform pattern known as 'Roman bridging'.

Salivary duct carcinoma is the most aggressive salivary carcinoma and more than half of patients die in less than 5 years from diagnosis as a result of metastasis to lungs, liver and bone. Perineural and dispersed infiltration are frequent and make excision difficult. Overexpression of androgen receptor raises the possibility that blocking drugs might be useful in late stage disseminated disease, but they frequently fail. Many carcinomas ex pleomorphic adenoma (discussed below) have this histological pattern.

Review PMID: 26939990

Epithelial-myoepithelial carcinoma

Epithelial-myoepithelial carcinoma is a low-grade carcinoma affecting mostly the major glands and older people. It has a striking microscopic pattern of ducts or small islands of epithelium, each with an outer layer of clear myoepithelial cells and a small duct centrally (Fig. 23.23). This type often presents as a benign tumour clinically and, although most are effectively treated by local excision, local recurrence is frequent but metastasis is rare. The cause is unknown. Mutations in the *HRAS* gene are frequent but not found in those that arise in pleomorphic adenomas. A range of rare histological subtypes can complicate microscopic diagnosis.

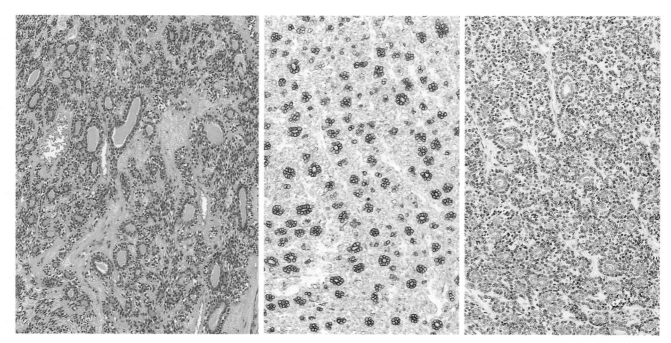

Fig 23.23 Epithelial myoepithelial carcinoma. The carcinoma consists of epithelium forming ducts with an inner lining cell layer and an outer layer of myoepithelial cells. In routine stains the myoepithelial cells are just visible as partly clear cells with vacuolated cytoplasm around the outside of the ducts. The pattern is much clearer on immunohistochemistry. In the centre a keratin stain that identifies duct lining cells shows tiny clusters and small lumina and a stain for the myoepithelial cells (right) shows the mirror image pattern with rings of cells around the duct lining, which is not stained using this antibody.

Review PMID: 17197918

Lymphoepithelial carcinoma

This carcinoma is commoner in in Japan, Southeast China and in Inuit ethnic groups but rare elsewhere. It almost always develops in major glands. These have the same histological features as non-keratinising carcinomas arising in the nasopharynx and tonsil, with diffuse sheets of large pleomorphic and mitotically active cells. As with nasopharyngeal carcinoma, most cases are caused by Epstein–Barr virus infection.

Rapid spread and metastasis is typical but there is a good response to radiotherapy.

Carcinoma ex pleomorphic adenoma

Pleomorphic adenoma is one of the few benign tumours that can undergo malignant change. It is estimated that as many as 5% of pleomorphic adenomas show some progression to carcinoma, but the process seems to take many years, so the diagnosis is usually made in older individuals. However, because pleomorphic adenomas may arise at any age, occasional carcinomas can present in young adults and the middle aged. As noted above, pleomorphic adenomas harbour a surprising range of genetic abnormalities for benign neoplasms. It seems that these lead to chromosomal instability, and the cells progressively become genetically more and more damaged until carcinoma develops.

The history is usually of a slow-growing mass that enlarges suddenly and rapidly and may develop the classical signs of malignancy, usually facial nerve palsy because most arise in the parotid gland. However, the initial adenoma may be small or deeply situated and unsuspected until carcinoma develops.

Histologically, the original pleomorphic adenoma may be detectable as a circumscribed benign tumour, but more often it is destroyed by the carcinoma and only a nodule of hyaline stroma or cartilage may remain. The carcinoma cells have obviously malignant features, infiltration is usually extensive and there is often necrosis (Fig. 23.24). The carcinoma that develops may be of a recognisable type, such as a salivary duct, mucoepidermoid, epithelial-myoepithelial type, multiple types or be an unclassifiable carcinoma. Salivary duct carcinoma is the commonest type to develop.

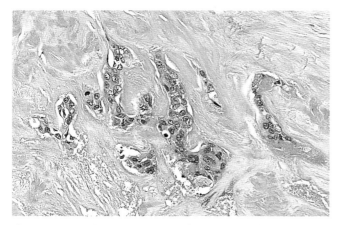

Fig. 23.24 Carcinoma arising in a pleomorphic adenoma. In longstanding pleomorphic adenomas, the stroma may become hyalinised, dense and acellular. In such tumours, there is a risk of transformation to carcinoma, as shown here by clusters of cells showing cytological atypia.

Carcinoma ex pleomorphic adenoma is an aggressive carcinoma, and over half of carcinomas produce distant metastases to lung, bone or brain. The further the carcinoma has invaded beyond the capsule of the original pleomorphic adenoma (not always easy to define histologically), the worse the prognosis. There is disagreement about exactly how far is critical, but those that invade more than a few millimetres require aggressive surgery and radiotherapy.

A minority of cases are termed *non-invasive carcinoma ex pleomorphic adenoma* (in a confusing oxymoron) meaning that the carcinomatous changes are detected histologically but remain confined within the capsule of the old pleomorphic adenoma. This is analogous to the concept of an *in situ* carcinoma or a pleomorphic adenoma with dysplasia. Such cases can be removed in the same way as a benign pleomorphic adenoma and carry no risk of recurrence or metastasis. Accurate histological assessment of any carcinoma ex pleomorphic adenoma is therefore essential to plan whether post-operative radiotherapy may be required.

Review PMID: 21744105

Salivary carcinoma NOS

Sometimes a salivary carcinoma cannot be classified into a specific type histologically. Under these circumstances it is classified as NOS (not otherwise specified) and graded as low, intermediate or high grade to plan treatment.

METASTATIC NEOPLASMS

Metastatic neoplasms account for at least 1 in 20 lumps in salivary glands and almost all occur in an older age group, matching the age distribution of the common malignant neoplasms at other body sites. Almost all metastases develop in the parotid gland by lymphatic spread to the intraparotid lymph nodes, and only involve the gland itself if they invade beyond the lymph node capsule. The primary carcinoma is usually in the sites drained by these nodes so that squamous carcinomas or melanoma of the scalp are likely primary tumours.

Very occasionally the parotid or submandibular gland is the site of a blood-borne metastasis from a more distant primary. The commonest example is renal cell carcinoma, which has a particular tendency to spread through central veins to the head and neck. Usually these tumours are readily recognised as metastases microscopically, though renal cell carcinoma can resemble some types of salivary carcinoma histologically. Diagnosis is usually suspected on the basis of the known cancer elsewhere.

Metastases to salivary glands are indistinguishable from primary salivary neoplasms in their clinical presentation and diagnosis is histological.

NON-EPITHELIAL TUMOURS

Haemangioma of the parotids

Haemangiomas are easily recognised hamartomas that may present at birth or in childhood. Almost all salivary examples arise in the parotid gland, and they are relatively common causes of a salivary gland enlargement in children but rare in adults. Girls are more frequently affected.

Haemangiomas are soft, sometimes bluish, swellings. The salivary gland may be involved by localised lesions or as part of a more extensive vascular malformation of the head and neck.

Histologically, the parotid parenchyma is largely replaced by lobular sheets of endothelial cells and small blood vessels of capillary type with a few clusters of residual acini and ducts scattered through (Fig. 23.25). Sometimes there are larger vessels or even an arteriovenous fistula, the higher blood throughput then making the lesion feel warm or producing a bruit.

Despite their dramatic appearance, especially if the skin is involved, these tumours are hamartomas not neoplasms. They grow initially but gradually regress in the first 5 years of life and may almost vanish by 10 years of age. Corticosteroids may delay their growth and facilitate later surgery but propanolol is currently the preferred treatment and is highly effective. Unless the eye or other important structures are threatened, most are treated conservatively depending on site and appearance.

Review PMID: 19910858

Lymphoma

The most common non-epithelial neoplasms in salivary glands are lymphomas and there are two distinct presentations. The first type arise in the lymph nodes that lie within the parotid gland and are identical to lymphomas arising in the cervical or other lymph nodes. They are usually a high-grade non-Hodgkin lymphoma of B-cell origin or Hodgkin's disease. Salivary gland involvement is sometimes the first sign of these systemic diseases.

The second scenario is the extranodal marginal zone lymphoma of Mucosa-Associated Lymphoid Tissue or MALT lymphoma that arises in the gland parenchyma rather than the nodes. These are described in more detail in Chapter 28. MALT lymphomas are a complication of chronic antigen stimulation in infection or autoimmunity and salivary MALT lymphomas arise as a complication of Sjögren's syndrome. The development of lymphoma is indicated by a persistent painless swelling or sudden enlargement of the gland, particularly in patients with longstanding disease.

MALT lymphomas are usually low grade and indolent with an excellent prognosis, but more aggressive high-grade variants can also arise in salivary glands.

INTRAOSSEOUS SALIVARY GLAND TUMOURS

Salivary gland tumours can develop within the medullary cavity of the mandible or maxilla, so-called *central* or *intraosseous salivary tumours*. This is extremely rare and also difficult to explain. It is suggested that there are developmental rests of salivary tissue within the bone, although origin in odontogenic epithelium would appear a more likely explanation. Odontogenic epithelium lining dentigerous and other cysts often undergoes mucous metaplasia to form goblet cells, and so it is surmised that odontogenic epithelium might be able to undergo salivary differentiation if it became neoplastic. This is supported by the fact that most of these tumours are mucoepidermoid carcinomas, a type that includes many mucous cells.

Radiographically, intraosseous salivary tumours produce cyst-like or poorly circumscribed areas of radiolucency. The diagnosis can only be made histologically, and a metastasis from a carcinoma elsewhere must be excluded before the rarer central tumour diagnosis is accepted. Wide excision is required.

Intraosseous salivary neoplasms do not arise in Stafne bone cavity (salivary inclusion 'cyst') at the angle of the mandible because this is merely submandibular gland in a depression or indentation of the cortex; the salivary tissue does not extend into the medullary cavity.

Case series PMID: 11149964 and 18940488

TUMOUR-LIKE SALIVARY GLAND SWELLINGS

Necrotising sialometaplasia and **IgG4 sclerosing disease can** mimic salivary gland tumours, both clinically and histologically. They are described in Chapter 22.

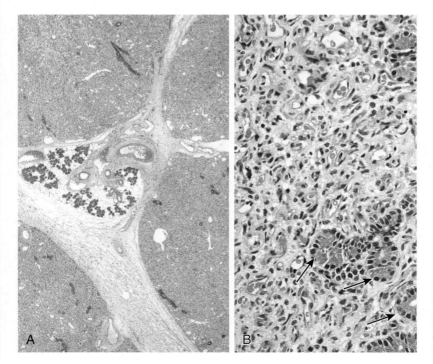

Fig. 23.25 Haemangioma of the parotid.
(A) The lobular structure of the gland is seen to be preserved, with a small lobule of normal parotid centrally. (B) The tissue that replaces the lobules, closely packed small capillary vessels with a few scattered residual serous acini (arrowed).

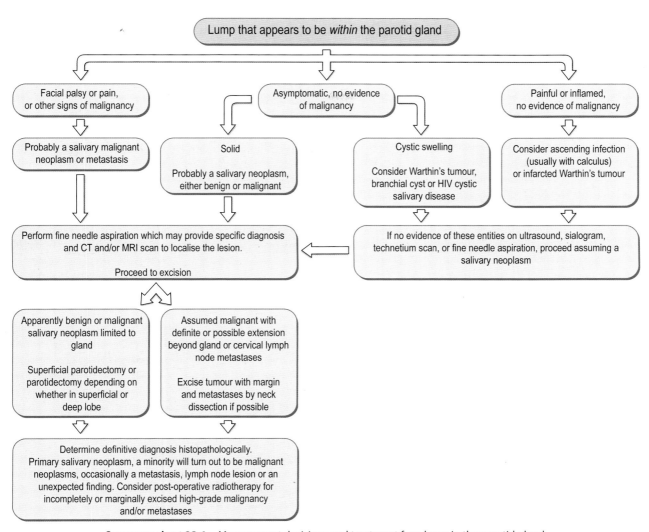

Summary chart 23.1   Management decisions and treatment for a lump in the parotid gland.

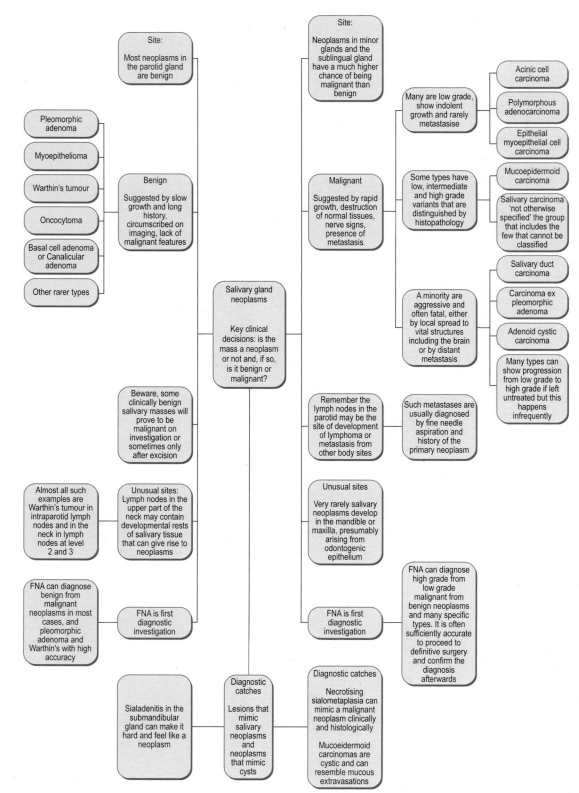

Summary chart 23.2 Considerations in differentiating salivary neoplasms. A mind map.

Appendix 23.1

Salivary gland neoplasms

Benign epithelial tumours

Pleomorphic adenoma	See text of Chapter 23
Metastasising pleomorphic adenoma	Very rare. An apparently benign pleomorphic adenoma that metastasises, to bone, lung or lymph node. Arise in the parotid, submandibular and palatal glands and seem to spread into vessels after surgical manipulation or to the lungs by aspiration of disrupted tumour rather than by true metastasis. Most cases spread after multiple local recurrences. The distant deposits behave as benign tumours, grow slowly, but may eventually prove fatal after a prolonged course, depending on their location. ***PMID:*** 25958295
Basal cell adenoma	See text of Chapter 23
Warthin's tumour	See text of Chapter 23
Oncocytoma	See text of Chapter 23
Myoepithelioma	See text of Chapter 23
Canalicular adenoma	See text of Chapter 23
Cystadenoma	Rare lesion of numerous duct-like cysts, arise in any gland and in the middle aged and older age groups. In minor glands present like mucocoeles. Rarely recur after local excision
Ductal papillomas, inverted, intraductal	Develop in or at the opening of minor gland ducts, usually in lip, buccal or palatal glands, wide age range, usually near the distal end of minor gland ducts and are readily excised without recurrence
Sialadenoma papilliferum	Neoplasm of the excretory duct, usually of glands in the palate or buccal mucosa in the older individuals. The surface appears papillary. Rarely recurs after local excision
Lymphadenoma	Two types, both very rare. Sebaceous lymphadenoma arises in parotid glands and less frequently the submandibular gland, and in older people. Non-sebaceous lymphadenoma arises in the parotid glands of young patients. They comprise ducts and islands of epithelium in dense lymphoid stroma, with or without sebaceous cells and do not recur on local excision
Sebaceous adenoma	Circumscribed tumour of nests of sebaceous cells, do not recur on excision
Intercalated duct adenoma and hyperplasia	These small proliferations of ducts are probably neoplastic since they contain alterations in the *CTNNB1* or *HRAS* genes. Most are in the parotid and only a few millimetres in diameter. They never reach a size that can be detected clinically, being found usually as incidental findings on imaging or in glands removed for other reasons. No treatment is required
Striated duct adenoma	Adenomas composed of numerous closely packed striated ducts. Can arise in any gland and in middle and old age, but are very rare. Caused by alterations in the *IDH2* gene
Sclerosing polycystic adenoma	See text of Chapter 23
Keratocystoma	Very rare tumour of the parotid gland that can arise at any age. It consists of numerous cysts of keratinising epithelium. Its main significance is that it must not be mistaken histologically for metastasis of a well-differentiated squamous carcinoma to an intraparotid lymph node, a much more frequent occurrence

Malignant epithelial tumours

Mucoepidermoid carcinoma	See text of Chapter 23
Adenoid cystic carcinoma	See text of Chapter 23
Acinic cell carcinoma	See text of Chapter 23
Secretory carcinoma	See text of Chapter 23
Microsecretory carcinoma	Recently described very rare carcinoma arising in minor glands and caused by a *MEF2C::SS18* translocation. Histologically it is composed of many small ducts resembling intercalated ducts and containing mucin. Behaviour is low grade with limited infiltration peripherally
Polymorphous adenocarcinoma	See text of Chapter 23
Hyalinising clear cell carcinoma	Composed of clear cells and with no features of other tumours. Usually intraoral minor glands, especially the palate. Low-grade malignancy, prognosis good. Almost all have a translocation involving the *EWSR1* and *ATF-1* genes, a few with *EWSR1* and *CREM* that us useful for diagnosis. Behaviour is low grade, with slow growth and rarely metastasis
Basal cell adenocarcinoma	Appear clinically and histologically like basal cell adenomas but infiltrative. Recur locally but rarely metastasise
Intraductal carcinoma	Previously known as low-grade salivary duct or cribriform cystadenocarcinoma, a mostly cystic carcinoma that is almost always in the parotid gland, has a very low-grade behaviour and responds well to excision. Caused by rearrangements of the *RET* gene. Histologically composed of cysts resembling large ducts with a lining of ductal cells and an outer layer of myoepithelial cells, both of which are neoplastic. Not located within ducts despite the name
Salivary duct carcinoma	See text of Chapter 23
Myoepithelial carcinoma	The malignant variant of myoepithelioma, high grade with recurrence and frequent distant metastases. Arise in parotid, submandibular and palatal glands in any age group. May develop as a pattern of carcinoma ex pleomorphic adenoma

Epithelial-myoepithelial carcinoma	See text of Chapter 23
Mucinous adenocarcinoma	A very rare carcinoma that forms extensive pools of mucin in which islands of malignant epithelium appear to float. Arises in minor glands in older people. Carries a consistent mutation in the *AKT1* gene. Behaviour varies with histological pattern, from low to high grade
Sclerosing microcystic adenocarcinoma	A low-grade carcinoma arising in minor glands in older people. Histologically composed of small ducts, nest and strands of epithelial cells compressed in a densely collagenous hyalinised stroma. Rarely recurs and does not metastasise
Carcinoma ex pleomorphic adenoma	See text of Chapter 23
Carcinosarcoma	A very rare highly malignant neoplasm containing both carcinoma, of any pattern, with a sarcoma, usually chondrosarcoma or osteosarcoma. Almost all are in major glands in older individuals and about half arise in pre-existing pleomorphic adenomas. Survival is very poor with frequent local and distant metastasis
Sebaceous adenocarcinoma	Very rare, usually in parotid but can arise in any gland and in young adults or older people. High grade, recur after surgery but rarely metastasise. Some develop as part of the Muir-Torre syndrome
Lymphoepithelial carcinoma	See text of Chapter 23
Squamous cell carcinoma	Very rare, resemble mucosal squamous carcinomas. Parotid and submandibular glands, wide age range. Any squamous carcinoma in the parotid must be assumed to be a metastasis to an intraparotid lymph node and this possibility excluded, because this is a much commoner occurrence than a primary squamous carcinoma
Sialoblastoma	Very rare, often congenital or in first 2 years of life. Histologically resembles embryonal salivary gland. Respond well to excision but can recur and 10% may metastasise. Most are in the parotid gland
Salivary carcinoma NOS*	A category comprising all the salivary carcinomas that do not fall into defined categories and those not yet fully characterised. Includes carcinomas that resemble intestinal adenocarcinomas and other types. Prognosis varies with type, ranging from low to high grade
Non-neoplastic epithelial lesions	
Nodular oncocytic hyperplasia	See text of Chapter 22
Lymphoepithelial lesions	See text of Chapter 22 Sjogren's syndrome
Soft tissue lesions	
Haemangioma	See text of Chapter 23
Lipoma / sialolipoma	Lipomas of salivary glands usually develop in the parotid glands and may contain salivary ducts and acinar cells dispersed in the fat (sialolipoma)
Lymphoma	
Extranodal marginal B-cell lymphoma	See text of Chapter 22 Sjogren's syndrome and Chapter 28 ('MALT lymphoma')

* NOS indicates 'not otherwise specified'.

Benign mucosal swellings | 24

FIBROEPITHELIAL POLYP, EPULIS AND DENTURE-INDUCED GRANULOMA

➔ Summary chart 24.2 p. 418

Although different names are given to these lesions, they are similar in origin and nature and are the commonest oral swellings. They develop in sites of chronic minor injury or low-grade infection. Irritation of the gingival margin by a carious cavity, calculus or a plaque trap, irritation of mucosa by a denture, and biting trauma are common initiating factors. The resulting lesions are hyperplastic reactions involving both the epithelium and the fibrous tissue below, producing a mass. On the gingiva this is called a fibrous epulis. The term *epulis* means only 'on the gingiva' and many other lesions can present as an epulis but almost all epulides are fibrous epulides. Those induced by a denture are called denture-induced granulomas and those caused by biting are fibroepithelial polyps. Although all these fibrous hyperplasias are sometimes called *fibromas*, they are not benign neoplasms.

Key points are shown in (Box 24.1).

Clinical features

A fibrous epulis is most common near the front of the mouth on the gingiva between two teeth (Fig. 24.1), where teeth are imbricated, or other plaque traps are present. Fibroepithelial polyps (fibrous polyps) usually form on the buccal mucosa along the occlusal line, on the lateral tongue, or on the lip at sites of biting (Fig. 24.2). Denture-induced granulomas often form in alveolar or sulcus mucosa at the edge of dentures (Fig. 24.3) and are usually long and thin. All these swellings are pale and firm but may be abraded and ulcerated, and then inflamed. They are usually up to 10 mm in diameter, but the largest examples reach 5 cm across.

Leaf fibroma is denture-induced granuloma which forms under a denture and becomes flattened against the palate (Fig. 24.4). It may be difficult to see until lifted away from its bed.

Pathology

In their early stages, these nodules consist of hyperplastic, lightly inflamed, slightly myxoid fibrous tissue, but they grow, sometimes rapidly, and mature to a dense uninflamed collagenous mass. The surface is covered by epithelium, which is usually also hyperplastic (Fig. 24.5).

Box 24.1   Fibrous nodules: practical points

- The most common oral tumour-like swellings
- Most frequently form at gingival margins (fibrous epulis) or on the buccal mucosa
- They are hyperplastic responses to chronic irritation
- Should be excised complete
- Histological examination confirms diagnosis and excludes unsuspected causes

---

Bone formation is sometimes seen in a fibrous epulis (Fig. 24.6). In American usage, this combination is termed a *peripheral ossifying fibroma*, but this lesion has no relation to the ossifying fibroma of bone and is not a fibroma. Some consider that those containing bone are more likely to recur after excision, but there is little evidence for this. Ossifying fibrous epulis is a better name.

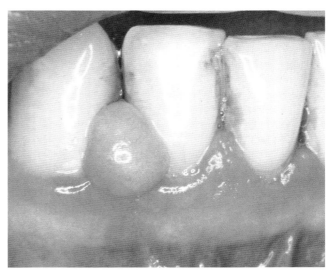

Fig. 24.1   Fibrous epulis. This lesion, arising from the gingival margin between the lower central incisors, is firm, pink and not ulcerated.

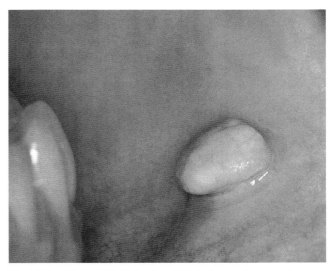

Fig. 24.2   Fibro-epithelial polyp. This lesion on the buccal mucosa has arisen as a result of cheek biting and is a firm, painless polyp covered by mucosa of normal appearance.

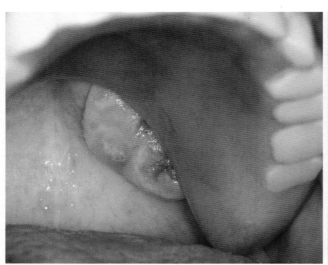

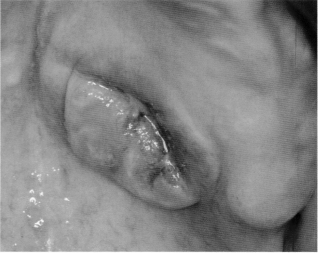

Fig. 24.3   Denture-induced granuloma. Fibrous hyperplasia at the posterior border of this upper complete denture has resulted in a firm mucosal swelling ridged by pressure from the posterior border.

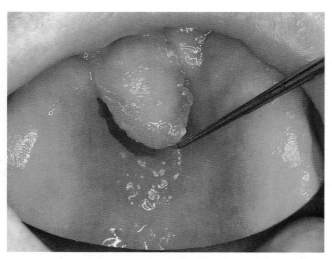

Fig. 24.4   Leaf fibroma. Flat lesions formed between the denture and mucosa are often termed leaf fibromas because of their flat shape. Raising this example with a probe reveals its pedunculated shape.

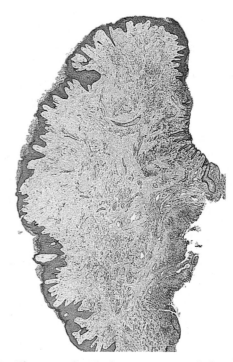

Fig. 24.5   Fibrous epulis. The lesion is composed of mature fibrous tissue covered by hyperplastic epithelium with spiky rete processes. A few inflammatory cells are present near the base and along the surfaces in contact with the teeth and plaque.

All these fibrous nodules should be excised together with the small base of normal tissue from which they arise. In the case of a fibrous epulis, the underlying bone should be curetted. There should be no recurrence if this is done thoroughly and the source of irritation is removed.

Histological examination is needed to confirm that an epulis is fibrous and not an unsuspected diagnosis. Several different types of lesions occasionally form on the gingival margin and simulate a fibrous epulis, including pregnancy epulis, pyogenic granuloma, giant cell epulis, odontogenic tumours and even metastases from distant cancers.

The giant cell fibroma is a variant distinguished microscopically by scattered large, stellate, darkly staining multinucleate fibroblasts. Clinically, giant cell fibromas are typically pedunculated and usually arise from the gingivae or tip of tongue.

Review gingival lesions PMID: 6936553 and 2120653

All fibroepithelial hyperplasias PMID: 26355878

PAPILLARY HYPERPLASIA OF THE PALATE

Nodular overgrowth of the palatal mucosa is occasionally seen, particularly under complete dentures in older persons (Fig. 24.7). The exact cause is unclear, but a poor denture fit and poor denture hygiene are usual. Although candidosis is sometimes superimposed, it is not the cause. Mild palatal papillary hyperplasia is also occasionally seen in non-denture wearers.

Histologically, palatal papillary hyperplasia shows close-set nodules of vascular fibrous tissue with a variable chronic inflammatory infiltrate and a covering of hyperplastic epithelium (Figs 24.8 and 24.9).

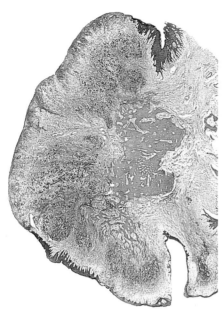

Fig. 24.6 Fibrous epulis with ossification. Much of the surface of this pedunculated nodule is ulcerated, and hyperplastic epithelium covers the margins. Centrally, the lesion is very cellular, partly because of inflammatory infiltrate. Trabeculae of woven bone are being formed and maturing into lamellar bone in the deeper uninflamed tissue.

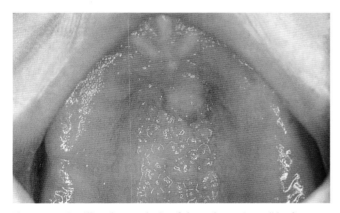

Fig. 24.7 Papillary hyperplasia of the palate. A small leaf fibroma is also present in the anterior palate.

Conservative treatment of denture hygiene, cessation of night wear, and treatment of any superimposed candidal infection is usually sufficient. In the most florid cases, with deep clefts between nodules or when new dentures are to be constructed, surgical removal may be considered. After surgery, a temporary soft lining must be placed to prevent the healing tissue proliferating back into the space below the denture.

Case series PMID: 4917113

Cause PMID: 6938680

PYOGENIC GRANULOMA AND PREGNANCY EPULIS

➔ Summary chart 24.2 p. 418

These are hyperplastic lesions of granulation tissue, proliferating masses of endothelial cells and fibroblasts. Clinically, they are usually painless, pedunculated, red and relatively

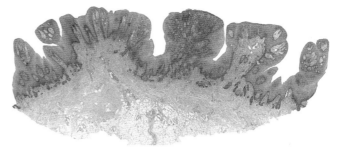

Fig. 24.8 Papillary hyperplasia. There are nodules, each similar to a fibrous polyp, and the subepithelial inflammatory infiltrate indicates either probable candidal infection or poor denture hygiene.

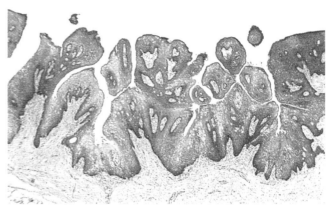

Fig. 24.9 Papillary hyperplasia. Higher-power view after antifungal treatment. The mucosa is now uninflamed, but the papillary structure remains.

soft (Fig. 24.10) and on the gingiva or at sites of recent trauma. Microscopically, they consist of many dilated blood vessels in a loose oedematous connective tissue stroma (Fig. 24.11) that matures with time to become more fibrous and less vascular. No true granulomas are present. Inflammation is variable, often scanty or absent. A pregnancy epulis can only be distinguished by the patient's pregnancy and, usually, associated pregnancy gingivitis (see also Fig. 37.8). Treatment is as for fibrous epulis or fibroepithelial polyp. Excision of pregnancy epulis may be delayed as they tend to regrow if removed during pregnancy. Improved oral hygiene may halt or slow growth until parturition.

Pyogenic granuloma pregnancy PMID: 1923399

GIANT-CELL EPULIS

➔ Summary chart 24.2 p. 418

The giant-cell epulis, like the fibrous epulis, is considered a hyperplastic lesion. Despite this, they contain the same activating mutations in the gene *KRAS* and show the same MAPK/ERK pathway activation mutations seen in the giant cell granuloma of bone (Ch. 12). This indicates a shared pathogenesis but does not indicate that either lesion is a neoplasm.

Giant cell epulis arises only on the gingival margin, usually interdentally and anterior to the permanent molars. There is a female predilection. The swelling is rounded, soft, typically maroon or purplish and as large as 2 cm in diameter (Figs 24.12 and 24.13). There is often an inflammatory

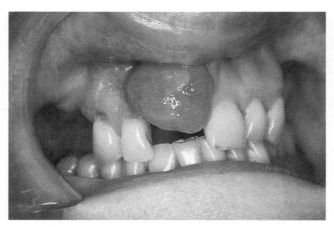

Fig. 24.10 Pyogenic granuloma. A bright-red polypoid swelling. The gingiva is a common site.

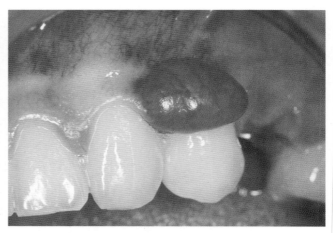

Fig. 24.13 Giant-cell epulis. Larger lesion showing the characteristic blue-purple colour.

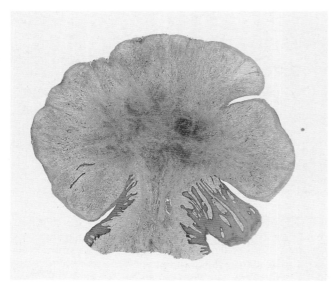

Fig. 24.11 Pyogenic granuloma. Lobular nodule of granulation tissue. Differences from a fibrous polyp (Fig. 24.5) include the ulcerated surface, dominance of proliferating vessels and lack of collagen.

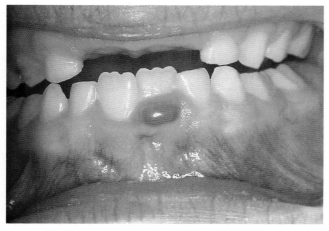

Fig. 24.12 Giant-cell epulis. Small lesion with a maroon colour in a child. *(Courtesy Mrs H Pitt-Ford.)*

stimulus at the site of origin, such as a retained primary root fragment, plaque trap, periodontitis or implant.

Histologically, numerous multinucleate cells lie in a vascular stroma of plump spindle-shaped cells. The appearance is similar to that of a giant cell granuloma of the jaw, but the epulis is superficial and outside the cortical bone (Fig. 24.14).

Untreated, the mass eventually becomes less vascular and shrinks, but a giant-cell epulis is normally excised, together with its gingival base, and the underlying bone curetted. Adjacent teeth need not be extracted if they are healthy and, if treatment is thorough, there should be no recurrence. A radiograph should be taken to exclude the possibility that the lesion is the superficial part of a central giant cell granuloma (see Ch. 12) that has perforated through the cortex into the gingiva. Very rarely, histologically similar lesions are a sign of hyperparathyroidism (see Ch. 13) or Noonan syndrome (Ch. 12).

Review PMID: 29569293

PAPILLOMAS → Summary chart 24.1 p. 417

These benign lesions have spiky exophytic or rounded cauliflower-like shapes as large as a centimetre or so in diameter. Probably all are caused by human papillomavirus (HPV) even though it cannot be detected in some lesions.

Human papillomaviruses are ubiquitous, and almost all individuals harbour some of the more than 170 well-characterised types as commensals. In the mouth most papilloma lesions are associated with types 6, 7, 11, 16 and 32.

HPV types tend to infect specific anatomical sites. However, this is not absolute, and types 6 and 11 are more frequently associated with cervical and genital infection. Genital types 16 and 18 are rarely found in the mouth and are associated with oral HPV-associated dysplasia as well as papillomas. Papillomas with a rounded non-keratinised shape (condylomas) are not necessarily infections transmitted from genital warts, though they often are. Genital types of HPV can be transmitted at birth, in utero and vertically and horizontally in families without direct sexual contact.

Oral papillomas are not premalignant, regardless of the HPV type that caused them. Dysplastic oral lesions containing low-risk or high-risk HPV are increasingly recognised, but they present as white patches, sometimes with a velvety surface and are not papillomatous (Ch. 19).

All oral papillomas are painless and of extremely low infectivity. All types respond to simple excision, including a small amount of normal mucosa at the base.

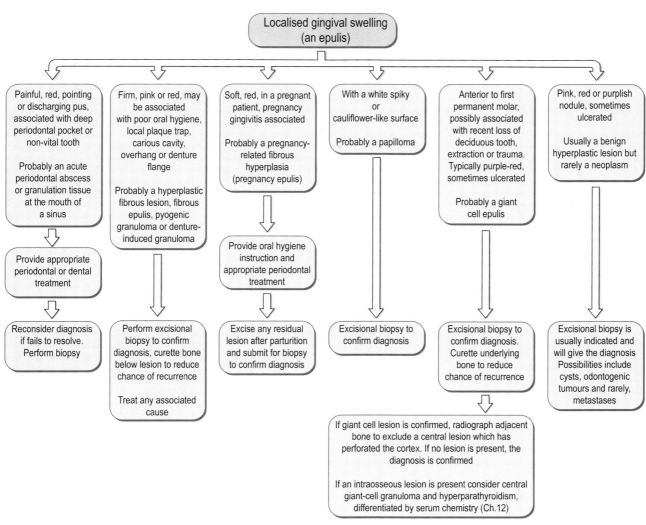

**Localised gingival swelling
(an epulis)**

**Painful, red, pointing
or discharging pus,
associated with deep
periodontal pocket or
non-vital tooth**

Probably an acute
periodontal abscess
or granulation tissue
at the mouth of
a sinus

↓

Provide appropriate
periodontal or dental
treatment

↓

Reconsider diagnosis
if fails to resolve.
Perform biopsy

**Firm, pink or red, may
be associated
with poor oral hygiene,
local plaque trap,
carious cavity,
overhang or denture
flange**

Probably a hyperplastic
fibrous lesion, fibrous
epulis, pyogenic
granuloma or denture-
induced granuloma

↓

Perform excisional
biopsy to confirm
diagnosis, curette bone
below lesion to reduce
chance of recurrence

Treat any associated
cause

**Soft, red, in a pregnant
patient, pregnancy
gingivitis associated**

Probably a pregnancy-
related fibrous
hyperplasia
(pregnancy epulis)

↓

Provide oral hygiene
instruction and
appropriate periodontal
treatment

↓

Excise any residual
lesion after parturition
and submit for biopsy
to confirm diagnosis

**With a white spiky
or
cauliflower-like surface**

Probably a papilloma

↓

Excisional biopsy to
confirm diagnosis

**Anterior to first
permanent molar,
possibly associated
with recent loss of
deciduous tooth,
extraction or trauma.
Typically purple-red,
sometimes ulcerated**

Probably a giant
cell epulis

↓

Excisional biopsy to
confirm diagnosis.
Curette underlying
bone to reduce
chance of recurrence

↓

If giant cell lesion is confirmed, radiograph adjacent
bone to exclude a central lesion which has
perforated the cortex. If no lesion is present, the
diagnosis is confirmed

If an intraosseous lesion is present consider central
giant-cell granuloma and hyperparathyroidism,
differentiated by serum chemistry (Ch.12)

**Pink, red or purplish
nodule, sometimes
ulcerated**

Usually a benign
hyperplastic lesion but
rarely a neoplasm

↓

Excisional biopsy is
usually indicated and
will give the diagnosis
Possibilities include
cysts, odontogenic
tumours and rarely,
metastases

Summary chart 24.1 Differential diagnosis and management of the common localised gingival swellings.

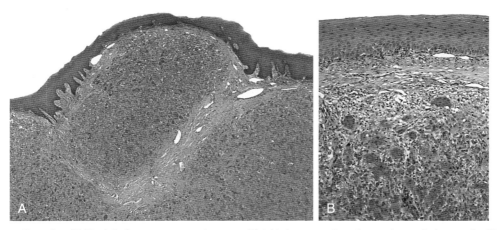

Fig. 24.14 Giant-cell epulis. (A) The lobular structure can be seen. (B) A high-power view shows giant cells in vascular fibrous lying immediately below the covering epithelium.

Oral papillomas of all types are occasionally multiple but, if numerous or confluent, HIV infection or other cause of immunodeficiency should be suspected. Extensive lesions in people who are immunosuppressed are difficult or impossible to eradicate and, counterintuitively, can become larger and more numerous when immunosuppression is treated, especially in HIV infection.

Review PMID: 6154913

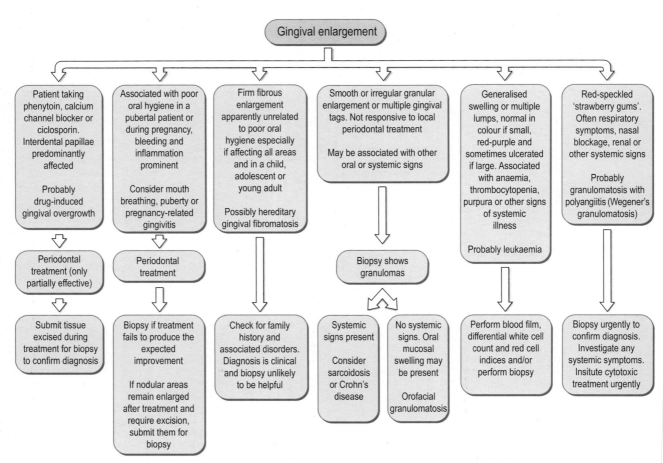

Gingival enlargement

Patient taking phenytoin, calcium channel blocker or ciclosporin. Interdental papillae predominantly affected

Probably drug-induced gingival overgrowth

Associated with poor oral hygiene in a pubertal patient or during pregnancy, bleeding and inflammation prominent

Consider mouth breathing, puberty or pregnancy-related gingivitis

Firm fibrous enlargement apparently unrelated to poor oral hygiene especially if affecting all areas and in a child, adolescent or young adult

Possibly hereditary gingival fibromatosis

Smooth or irregular granular enlargement or multiple gingival tags. Not responsive to local periodontal treatment

May be associated with other oral or systemic signs

Generalised swelling or multiple lumps, normal in colour if small, red-purple and sometimes ulcerated if large. Associated with anaemia, thrombocytopenia, purpura or other signs of systemic illness

Probably leukaemia

Red-speckled 'strawberry gums'. Often respiratory symptoms, nasal blockage, renal or other systemic signs

Probably granulomatosis with polyangiitis (Wegener's granulomatosis)

Periodontal treatment (only partially effective)

Periodontal treatment

Biopsy shows granulomas

Submit tissue excised during treatment for biopsy to confirm diagnosis

Biopsy if treatment fails to produce the expected improvement

If nodular areas remain enlarged after treatment and require excision, submit them for biopsy

Check for family history and associated disorders. Diagnosis is clinical and biopsy unlikely to be helpful

Systemic signs present

Consider sarcoidosis or Crohn's disease

No systemic signs. Oral mucosal swelling may be present

Orofacial granulomatosis

Perform blood film, differential white cell count and red cell indices and/or perform biopsy

Biopsy urgently to confirm diagnosis. Investigate any systemic symptoms. Insitute cytotoxic treatment urgently

Summary chart 24.2   Differential diagnosis of common and important causes of gingival enlargement.

Squamous cell papilloma

Squamous papillomas mainly affect adults and have a distinctive, clinically recognisable, cauliflower-like or branched structure of finger-like processes (Fig. 24.15). They may be soft or firm and spiky.

Histologically, the papillae consist of stratified squamous epithelium supported by a vascular connective tissue cores (Fig. 24.16). Most are keratinised and so appear white.

Human papillomavirus (HPV) of various subtypes is the cause, but koilocytes (infected keratinocytes producing virus and with crumpled nuclei, perinuclear space and condensed cytoplasm) are seen in only a minority. Probably either HPV is present at very low level or has been eliminated from the lesion in its later stages. When present, it is usually of types 6 and 11.

Infective warts (verruca vulgaris)

Lesions caused by autoinoculation from warts on the hands are uncommon but seen particularly in children. The lesions may appear identical to squamous papillomas, be more rounded or even only slightly raised.

Histologically, the structure is generally similar to that of papillomas, but there are typically obvious koilocytes indicating active viral infection, which can be confirmed with immunohistochemistry. The causative HPV type is usually type 2 or 4.

Multifocal epithelial hyperplasia

Multifocal epithelial hyperplasia or Heck's disease is numerous rounded mucosal papillomas as large as a centimetre across,

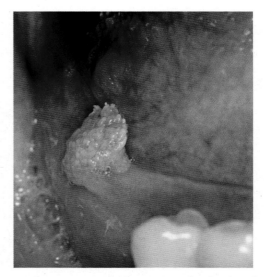

Fig. 24.15   Squamous papilloma arising on the alveolar ridge. Note the spiky white surface.

usually clustered on the labial, buccal mucosa and tongue mucosa (Fig. 24.17). These may be confluent, producing raised plaques or a cobblestone appearance.

Children, adolescents and young adults are affected, often in familial clusters. The condition is an infection by human papillomavirus types 13 or 32, which spreads easily between family members under close living conditions. The condition is endemic in some parts of the world.

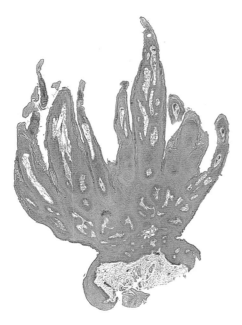

Fig. 24.16 Papilloma. The lesion consists of thickened fingers of epithelium. Slender vascular cores of connective tissue support each frond. The fronds are keratinised and so appear white clinically.

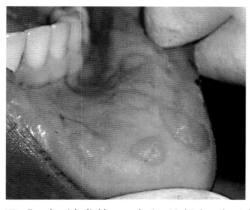

Fig. 24.17 Focal epithelial hyperplasia. Multiple pale pink slightly raised rounded soft nodules on the labial mucosa. *(Courtesy Dr Braz Campos Durso.)*

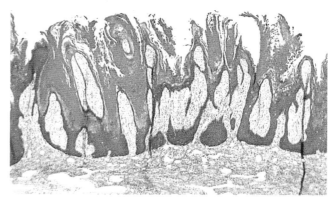

Fig. 24.18 Verruciform xanthoma. The epithelium is thin and parakeratotic and forms a series of spiky folds.

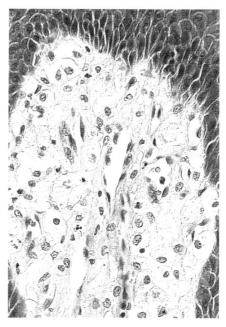

Fig. 24.19 Verruciform xanthoma. At higher power, dermal papillae within the folded epithelium can be seen to contain many large, rounded cells with foamy or vacuolated cytoplasm.

Unlike most other papillomas, the surface is smooth or slightly nodular without keratin so that the lesions appear pink rather than white. Histologically, the papillomas have a characteristic feature that the infected cells resemble mitotic figures (mitosoid bodies). No treatment is required and there is usually resolution, although only after many years. If appearance dictates, individual lesions are readily excised or removed by laser.

Description and series PMID: 8065729

Review PMID: 23061874

VERRUCIFORM XANTHOMA

Verruciform xanthoma is a rare hyperplastic lesion that can have a white, hyperkeratotic surface resembling a papilloma.

Verruciform xanthoma is most common in the fifth to seventh decades. It is usually found on the gingiva but can form in almost any site in the mouth. Its colour can be white (because it is keratinised) or yellow (because of its high fat content). Lesions are usually sessile, with a flat but slightly nodular or warty surface and range in size from one to several centimetres across. They may be mistaken for a papilloma, leukoplakia or carcinoma clinically, but are readily recognisable histologically. Verruciform xanthoma is benign and has no known associations with diseases such as hyperlipidaemia or diabetes mellitus that are associated with cutaneous xanthomas, and the cause is unknown.

Pathology

The warty surface is due to the much-infolded epithelium which, in most, is hyperkeratinised or parakeratinised. In haematoxylin and eosin-stained sections, the parakeratin layer stains a distinctive orange colour. The elongate rete ridges are of equal length and extend to a straight, well-defined lower border (Fig. 24.18).

The diagnostic feature is the large, foamy, xanthoma cells that fill the connective tissue papillae but extend only to the lower border of the epithelium (Fig. 24.19). These cells are

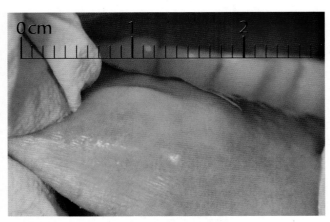

Fig. 24.20 Calibre-persistent artery. This example forms a raised linear firm and pulsatile swelling just below the 1 on the scale. *(From Awni, S., Conn, B., 2016. Caliber-persistent artery. J. Oral MaxFac. Surg. 74, 1391–1395.)*

macrophages containing lipid and periodic acid–Schiff (PAS) positive granules.

Simple surgical excision is curative.

Review PMID: 12676251

Yellow mucosal lesions PMID: 30693453

CALIBRE-PERSISTENT ARTERY

Calibre-persistent artery is a loop or tortuosity of the labial artery that pushes superficially from its normal site deep in the lip to lie just below the vermilion border or labial mucosa. It appears to be an age change seen in older people. It may be palpable, or if superficial, visible and forms a nodule or linear curved firm mass, sometimes pulsatile (Fig. 24.20). Some appear bluish, and they are frequently mistaken for mucoceles despite the site on the vermilion border (where mucoceles never form). Those on the lower

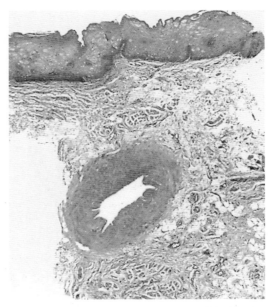

Fig. 24.21 Calibre-persistent artery. A loop of the labial artery ascends high into the mucosa, almost to the overlying epithelium.

lip are usually to one side of the midline, whereas those in the upper lip are usually near the midline.

Histology shows normal labial artery (Fig. 24.21), but ideally the condition should be recognised clinically as biopsy will cause considerable haemorrhage and produces no benefit.

The name comes from the fact that the lumen of the artery does not narrow while it passes up into the superficial tissues, as a normal artery would at the site. A similar vascular anomaly of the same name occurs in the stomach where it is a cause of gastric bleeding, but lip lesions do not cause this problem.

Cases and review PMID: 20646912 and 26868184

Soft tissue tumours 25

BENIGN TUMOURS

Benign nerve sheath tumours

Several types of benign neoplasm arise from peripheral nerve. All present as firm, mobile lumps, are treated by excision and are differentiated histologically. Recurrence is very rare for all types.

Traumatic neuromas are hyperplastic healing responses at the site of damage to a nerve and comprise a tangled mass of regrowing normal nerve bundles.

Neurilemmomas or schwannomas are benign neoplasms of Schwann cells. Histologically, they comprise an encapsulated mass of elongate spindle cells with palisaded nuclei (Antoni A tissue – Fig. 25.1) and a variable amount of myxoid loose connective tissue (Antoni B tissue). 'Ancient' schwannomas are long standing tumours with degenerate nuclear changes that look worrying histologically but are of no significance.

Solitary circumscribed neuromas are of uncertain nature and could be either neoplasms or reactive lesions composed of Schwann cells and neurites. They are the most common oral nerve sheath tumour and present usually on palate or gingiva, forming mucosal nodules, usually 5–20 mm in diameter.

Mucosal neuromas are hamartomatous malformations often associated with syndromes, particularly multiple endocrine neoplasia (Ch. 37). They are superficial convoluted large nerves.

Neurofibromas are rarer than other nerve sheath tumours, and if seen in the mouth, neurofibromatosis should be suspected. Histologically, neurofibromas are cellular masses of spindle cells with plump nuclei separated by fine, sinuous collagen fibres among which mast cells can usually be found.

Lingual nerve traumatic neuromas PMID: 15772589

Schwannomas PMID: 10748827

Solitary circumscribed neuroma PMID: 20237984

Mucosal neuromas PMID: 21552134

Neurofibromatosis type 1 is a syndrome of skin pigmentation, multiple neurofibromas and various bone distortions, usually scoliosis but also of the sphenoid bone. The condition is relatively common, affecting 1 in 3000 births and the cause is mutation, deletion or mis-splicing of the *NF1* gene that encodes neurofibromin, causing loss of function and dysregulation of cell proliferation and differentiation.

Neurofibromatosis 1 is inherited in an autosomal dominant fashion and is evident in childhood but there is considerable variation in signs between patients. The skin café-au-lait pigmented macules have smooth rounded borders and are mainly on the trunk, may affect the face and neck, but are rarely intraoral. Neurofibromas may develop on any nerve and form slow growing lumps that occasionally affect the oral mucosa, usually on the tongue or gingiva. Superficial neurofibromas usually form discrete nodules but deeply seated and larger examples cause diffuse enlargement and can result in significant disfigurement. Gingival lesions may cause a relatively diffuse enlargement rather than a discrete lump. Over two-thirds of patients have oral signs.

Neurofibromin regulates the RAS signalling pathway, and patients with neurofibromatosis type 1 are predisposed to develop malignant tumours, including malignant nerve sheath tumours, leukaemias, sarcomas and breast carcinomas.

Neurofibromatosis type 2 is less common, genetically distinct and characterised by hearing loss caused by neurofibromas on the vestibular nerve. It may sometimes also produce the skin features of type 1 disease.

Neurofibromatosis PMID: 1545973 and 30092804

Lipoma

Lipomas, benign neoplasms of fat, are rare in the mouth and occur in middle aged and older people. They are smooth, soft, sometimes yellowish, asymptomatic, slow growing swellings, which may be deeply sited or superficial and pedunculated (Fig. 25.2). Tongue, lips and buccal fat pad are common sites.

Histologically, lipomas consist of apparently normal fat (Fig. 25.3) with a variable amount of supporting fibrous tissue and a partial fibrous capsule (Fig. 25.4). When fibrous tissue is prominent, the lesion is called a fibrolipoma, and other variants include types with cartilage and prominent

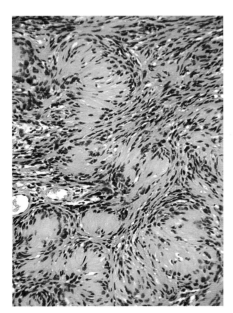

Fig. 25.1 Neurilemmoma. Antoni A tissue showing striking palisading of nuclei.

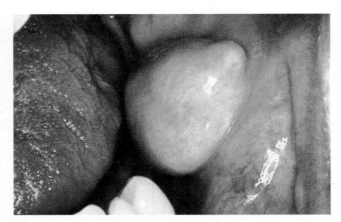

Fig. 25.2   Lipoma of the cheek. The tumour forms a pale, very soft yellowish swelling.

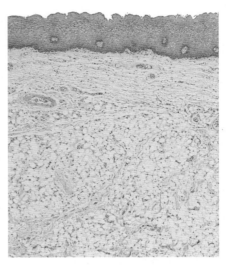

Fig. 25.4   Lipoma. A lipoma immediately below the oral mucosa; the fat appears normal and is often only partially encapsulated at the margin.

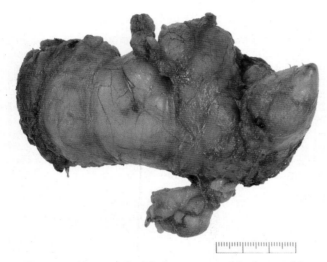

Fig. 25.3   Lipoma. The lobular structure of the fat is visible.

blood vessels. Lipomas should be excised and recurrence is rare, even if incompletely excised.

Oral lipoma review PMID: 21447447

Granular cell tumour

Clinically, granular cell tumours typically form painless domed smooth swellings. The dorsum of tongue and buccal mucosa are the commonest sites. They are occasionally multiple.

Histologically, large granular cells form the bulk of the lesion. Their origin is unclear, but they probably arise from Schwann cells of small nerves, although they appear to merge with muscle around the periphery (Fig. 25.5). The granular cells are large, with clearly defined cell membranes, and the granular cytoplasm is explained by large eosinophilic lysosomes containing cell debris, mitochondria and degenerate cell membrane. The cause is mutational inactivation of genes that control lysosomal pH, disturbing lysosomal function.

The granular cell tumour can induce striking proliferation of the overlying epithelium that mimics carcinoma histologically and is often called pseudocarcinomatous (or pseudoepitheliomatous) hyperplasia (Figs 25.6 and 25.7). This is present in between a quarter and half of cases and has resulted in misdiagnosis as carcinoma, with resulting

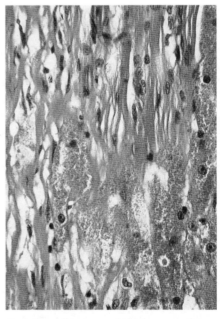

Fig. 25.5   Granular cell tumour. At high power, the granular cells indicate the diagnosis and characteristically apparently merge with surrounding muscle fibres.

overtreatment. Such misdiagnosis is likely in an insufficiently deep biopsy that shows only the superficial tissue.

Simple excision is curative, often even when incomplete.

Granular cell tumours are occasionally seen in LEOPARD, Cowden's and Noonan's syndromes

Review PMID: 31898368 and treatment 29661274

Congenital granular cell epulis

The rare congenital epulis is typically present at birth as a smooth soft nodule a few millimetres in diameter, usually on the upper alveolar ridge (Fig. 25.8) and very occasionally the tongue. A very large majority are in females.

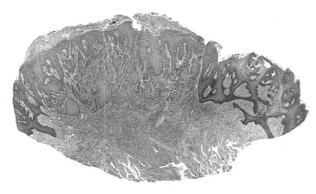

Fig. 25.6 Granular cell tumour. The irregular proliferation of the overlying epithelium (pseudocarcinomatous hyperplasia), which is very florid in this example, is a good mimic of a squamous carcinoma.

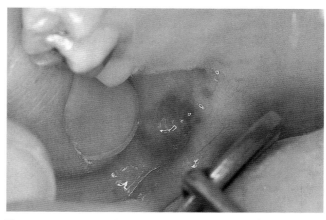

Fig. 25.9 Cavernous haemangioma of the cheek. The colour is deep purple, and the structure, a mass of thin-walled blood sinuses, is visible through the thin epithelium. A mass engorged with blood and as prominent as this is liable to trauma and to bleed profusely.

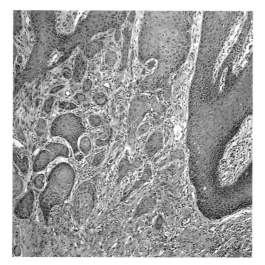

Fig. 25.7 Granular cell tumour. High power of a superficial area in Fig. 25.6 showing the small irregular islands of epithelium that appear to bud off the covering epithelial layer and invade the fibrous tissue and superficial muscle. Some show keratin formation similar to keratin pearls in squamous carcinoma. Granular cells are only present along the lower edge of the figure, so that a superficial biopsy might lead to misdiagnosis as carcinoma.

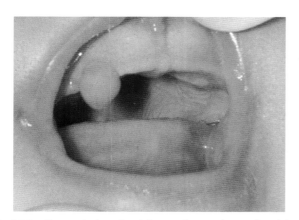

Fig. 25.8 Congenital epulis. A firm pink non-ulcerated nodule on the alveolar ridge of a neonate is the typical presentation. *(From Oda, D. 2005. Soft-tissue lesions in children. Oral Maxillofac Surg Clin North Am, 17:383, pp. 402.)*

Histologically, the mass comprises large pale granular cells that resemble those of granular cell tumour. Pseudocarcinomatous hyperplasia is not seen. If small, spontaneous resolution is likely. If large, interfering with feeding or respiration, conservative excision is curative even if incomplete.

Cases and review PMID: 21393037 and 26712684

Haemangiomas → Summary chart 26.1 p. 435

Haemangiomas are difficult to classify. Some are developmental anomalies, some are hamartomas and others are benign neoplasms. A further group are vascular ectasias, developmental conditions in which the number of vessels is normal, but they are constantly dilated. Few types are common, and the only frequent true vascular neoplasm is Kaposi's sarcoma (later in this chapter).

Capillary and cavernous haemangiomas form purple, flat or nodular superficial lesions of skin or mucosa that blanch on pressure (Fig. 25.9). The capillary type consists of innumerable minute blood vessels and vasoformative tissue – mere rosettes of endothelial cells (Fig. 25.10). The cavernous type consists of large blood-filled sinusoids. Some show both histological patterns. In infancy these will usually resolve without treatment but will often recur if excision is attempted. In adults they can usually be excised easily if required as they have low blood flow. Cryosurgery can be used to destroy a haemangioma without excessive bleeding. The parotid gland is a common site in children and adolescents (Ch. 23), and intraoral lesions usually affect gingiva and lips of people in middle age.

Arteriovenous and venous malformations have higher blood flow, are hamartomas that are present from birth and grow with the patient. Thrombosis is common, causing pain. They affect deep and superficial tissues, and excision carries significant risks depending on blood flow. Embolisation is the first line of treatment.

Haemangiomas of bone are discussed in Chapter 12.

Port wine stains are non-inherited congenital vascular ectasias caused by mutation in a G-signalling protein gene. Vessels in the lesions are normal in number, but their walls cannot contract, so they are constantly dilated (Fig. 25.11). This causes prolonged bleeding on surgery. Port wine stains in the distribution of the trigeminal nerve, including intraoral haemangiomas, together with meningeal angiomas, epilepsy and sometimes learning disability constitute the

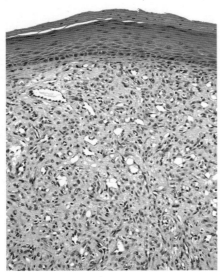

Fig. 25.10   Capillary haemangioma. Numerous large and small closely packed capillary vessels extend from just below the epithelium into the deeper tissues.

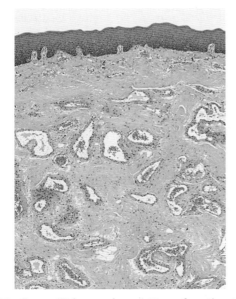

Fig. 25.11   Sturge-Weber syndrome. Biopsy from the gingiva affected by an intraoral port wine stain. The number of vessels and their distribution is normal, but all are markedly dilated, producing the appearance of many extra vessels.

Sturge-Weber syndrome. In this syndrome, the intracranial lesions often cause epilepsy in later life.

Pyogenic granulomas are not haemangiomas but hyperplastic nodules of endothelial cells and granulation tissue (Ch. 24). However, they are often confusingly called lobular capillary haemangiomas.

Hereditary haemorrhagic telangiectasia is discussed in Chapter 29.

Head and neck vascular lesions review PMID: 25439548

Infantile haemangiomas PMID: 23338947

Arteriovenous malformations PMID: 20115972

Oral port wine stains PMID: 22226814

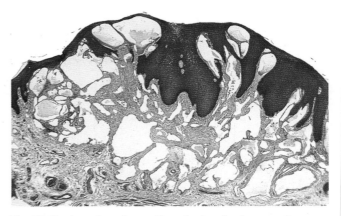

Fig. 25.12   Lymphangioma. There is a localised aggregation of cavernous lymphatics which form a pale superficial swelling. Bleeding into these lesions causes them suddenly to become purple or almost black.

Lymphangiomas

These are uncommon malformations of lymphatic vessels arising before birth or in infancy. They form pale, translucent, smooth or nodular elevations of the mucosa in which the superficial dilated lymphatics can often be seen clinically. The commonest site is the tongue and, if large and diffuse, lymphangiomas cause generalised macroglossia. They are normally asymptomatic but may present due to bleeding into the lymphatic spaces.

Histologically, lymphangiomas consist of thin-walled lymphatics containing lymph, seen as a pinkish amorphous material in sections (Fig. 25.12).

Localised lymphangiomas can be excised if necessary, but larger and diffuse types are difficult to remove. Injection of sclerosing agents is then the first line of treatment.

Cystic hygroma is a large diffuse lymphangioma of very dilated lymphatics, each several millimetres in diameter, usually in the neck in a young child.

Lymphatic malformations PMID: 24157637

Oral lymphangiomas PMID: 31823215

MALIGNANT CONNECTIVE TISSUE TUMOURS

Sarcomas of virtually any type can affect the oral soft tissues, but most are rare. Sarcomas grow rapidly, are invasive, destroy surrounding tissues and metastasise via the bloodstream. Most present as destructive masses that cannot be identified as sarcomas clinically. Occasional sarcomas are late complications of therapeutic irradiation.

Many sarcomas are caused by relatively limited genetic changes, often chromosomal translocations that produce activating fusion genes. This sometimes allows targeted drug therapy.

Osteosarcomas and chondrosarcomas are described in Chapter 12 and lymphomas in Chapter 28.

General review PMID: 19216845

Rhabdomyosarcoma

Rhabdomyosarcomas show striated muscle differentiation and are the most common oral sarcomas in children or adolescents. They form rapidly growing soft swellings, usually centred around the maxilla or in the orbit. Two main forms affect the head and neck, alveolar and embryonal.

Embryonal rhabdomyosarcomas consist of cells of variable shape and size, often strap- or tadpole-shaped, like rhabdomyoblasts in the early embryo. Sometimes muscle cross-striations can be seen in their cytoplasm to indicate their muscle nature.

Alveolar rhabdomyosarcomas consist of slit-like spaces into which hang tear-shaped, darkly staining cells attached to the walls. These alveoli are separated by a fibrous stroma. Muscle-like cells are not seen.

Diagnosis of both types can be difficult and relies on immunostaining for markers of muscle differentiation such as desmin or myogenin and on molecular analysis. The alveolar type has a characteristic chromosomal translocation t(2;13).

TFCP2-translocated rhabdomyosarcoma is a recently described type that often develops in the jaws and is discussed in Chapter 12.

Treatment is by excision and combination chemotherapy, but the prognosis is poor.

In children PMID: 26231745

Mixed case series PMID: 12001077

Sarcomas of fibroblasts

Fibrosarcomas and myofibroblastic sarcomas are the second commonest sarcomas in the head and neck after rhabdomyosarcoma, but are still rare. Some are cellular, others contain abundant collagen and yet others are myxoid; several different types are recognised. In general, treatment is by radical excision. Local recurrence and spread are common, but metastasis is rare. These sarcomas may follow radiotherapy to the head and neck after an interval of 10 years or so.

Kaposi's sarcoma → Summary chart 26.1 p. 435

Kaposi's sarcoma is a low-grade and relatively indolent malignant multifocal tumour of lymphatics or blood vessels caused by infection of endothelial cells by human herpesvirus 8 (HHV-8). Its status as a true malignant neoplasm is unclear as it shows a range of behaviours.

Most affected people are immunosuppressed. Therapeutic immunosuppression with ciclosporin and tacrolimus can be associated with Kaposi's sarcoma, but by far the main predisposing condition is HIV infection, and almost all oral Kaposi's sarcoma is in people infected by HIV. Among HIV-infected individuals, Kaposi's sarcoma affects mainly men who have sex with men in Western populations. It has equal sex incidence in Africa. Antiretroviral therapy for HIV has greatly reduced the incidence of Kaposi's sarcoma, but it remains the most common type of intraoral sarcoma.

The HHV-8 virus is endemic in sub-Saharan Africa, common around the Mediterranean and rare elsewhere. In endemic regions it is transmitted vertically and elsewhere sexually, through saliva. After infection the virus remains latent, suppressed by the immune system, probably for life. While latent, HHV-8 inhibits the p53 and retinoblastoma tumour suppressor genes causing cell proliferation, although the full mechanism of sarcomagenesis is still unclear. HIV infection has an additive effect, probably mediated by the tat protein that promotes viral gene transcription. The HHV-8 virus also causes some lymphomas and types of Castleman's disease.

In the mouth, the palate and gingiva are the most frequent sites, and the tumour appears initially as a flat purplish area and enlarges rapidly into a nodular mass that may ulcerate and bleed readily (Fig. 25.13). The clinical differential

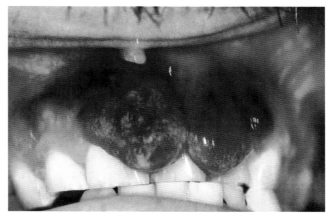

Fig. 25.13 Kaposi's sarcoma. Lesions are red, maroon or bluish and highly vascular. They may be flat or form tumour masses, and the gingivae or palate are characteristic sites. *(Courtesy Prof WH Binnie.)*

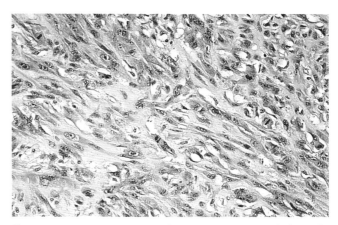

Fig. 25.14 Kaposi's sarcoma. The tumour is composed of spindle and plump cells with cytological atypia and frequent mitoses. Many of the small holes visible are the result of formation of capillaries by the tumour cells.

diagnosis is from oral purpura, bacillary angiomatosis and pyogenic granulomas, from which it can be distinguished by microscopy. The colour is usually maroon or purple, rather than the bright red of haemangiomas or pyogenic granulomas. Associated HIV infection is usually suggested by other clinical and oral manifestations, notably candidosis or hairy leukoplakia.

Histologically, Kaposi's sarcoma is a proliferation of endothelial cells and poorly organised vessels. In the early stages these are capillary-size blood vessels and resemble granulation tissue, particularly in the mouth where traumatised superficial lesions become secondarily inflamed. Later, the vessels are slit shaped and compressed in a densely cellular mass of spindle cells that show mitotic activity and ultimately dominate the picture (Fig. 25.14). Leakage of blood from the poorly formed vessels results in haemosiderin pigment that contributes to the colour seen clinically. Diagnosis is aided by immunostaining for podoplanin, a lymphatic endothelial cell marker, and confirmed by immunohistochemical staining for the HHV-8 virus (Fig. 25.15).

Management

Any patient with such a presentation must have Kaposi's sarcoma excluded since, in the absence of immunosuppressive

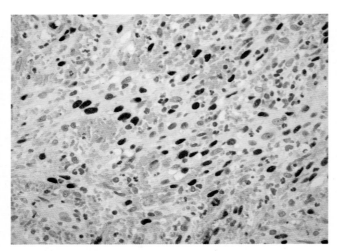

Fig. 25.15   Kaposi's sarcoma. Immunocytochemistry for human herpesvirus 8 reveals numerous infected cell nuclei (dark brown stain) confirming the diagnosis.

treatment, it is pathognomonic of the symptomatic stage of HIV infection. Kaposi's sarcoma is occasionally the presenting complaint in HIV infection.

Many Kaposi sarcomas are relatively indolent and may not require aggressive treatment, but this depends on extent. Localised oral lesions may be amenable to excision. However, disease is always multifocal, and chemotherapy is required for more widespread involvement. Radiation is widely used in other parts of the body but is usually avoided in the mouth because of adverse effects. Late-stage sarcomas can become widely infiltrative. Currently, the most effective chemotherapy regimens are interferon alpha with Didanosine for slowly progressing disease or Doxorubicin and Paclitaxel with antiretroviral treatment. Antiretroviral treatment alone will induce remission in approximately one-half of cases. With other treatments, remission can usually be induced in 90% of cases, but Kaposi's sarcoma remains a disease that is controlled rather than cured.

Box 25.1   Kaposi's sarcoma: key features

The most common type of oral sarcoma

In developed countries most common in HIV-infected men who have sex with men

Equal sex incidence in countries with endemic HIV infection

Due to human herpesvirus 8

Appears clinically as a flat or nodular purplish area

Histologically consists of proliferating blood vessels

Good response to antiretroviral treatment, but long-term control is difficult

Multifocal and often widespread when oral lesions appear

Most patients with skin Kaposi sarcoma also have at least one oral lesion

In immunosuppression, death from Kaposi sarcoma is rare and more frequently from associated opportunistic infections

Endemic Kaposi sarcoma without immunosuppression found in sub-Saharan Africa and in countries around the Mediterranean

Oral Kaposi sarcoma PMID: 3059252

Histological diversity PMID: 23312917

General review and treatment PMID: 25843728

Classical and endemic forms

The original description of Kaposi's sarcoma among older persons of Mediterranean or Jewish origin in Central Europe was in 1872, long predating HIV infection. This classical or sporadic form affects the skin, mainly the lower extremities and hardly ever the head and neck and not the mouth. Kaposi's sarcoma with broadly similar characteristics is also common as an endemic form in Africa, particularly in Zaire, where it formed approximately 12% of all malignant tumours in the pre-AIDS era.

Key features of Kaposi's sarcoma are summarised in Box 25.1.

Oral pigmented lesions 26

There are many causes of colour change in the mucosa, but the significant causes are melanin, superficial blood vessels, haemorrhage and blood pigments, and extrinsic agents (Box 26.1).

Melanin pigmentation is the most common, and oral pigmented lesions are more frequent and more darkly pigmented in people with darker skin colour. Pigmentation caused by extrinsic agents and drugs is often limited to the mouth, but some cause additional pigmentation of skin and nails.

Box 26.1   Oral pigmented lesions

Usually brown or black

Melanin pigmentation

- Physiological pigmentation
- Melanotic macules
- Melanoacanthoma
- Naevi
- Lichen planus (Ch. 16)
- Malignant melanoma
- Addison's disease (Ch. 37)
- HIV infection (Ch. 30)
- Peutz–Jeghers and other syndromes
- Melanotic neuroectodermal tumour (Ch. 12)
- Heavy smoking

Extrinsic agents

- Amalgam tattoo
- Black hairy tongue (Ch. 17)
- Chlorhexidine staining
- Some systemic drugs (Box 26.2)
- Heavy metal poisoning

Usually purple or red

Superficial, enlarged or numerous blood vessels

- Erythroplasia (Ch. 19)
- Haemangiomas (Ch. 25)
- Kaposi's sarcoma (Ch. 25)
- Telangiectases and lingual varices (Chs 28 & 1)
- Pyogenic granuloma (Ch. 24)
- Pregnancy epulis (Ch. 24)

Haemorrhage or blood pigments

- Purpura (Ch. 29)
- Other blood blisters
- Giant-cell epulis (Ch. 24)

Inflammation

- Geographical tongue (Ch. 17)
- Erythematous candidosis (Ch. 15)
- Median rhomboid glossitis (Ch. 15)

Review oral pigmentation PMID: 24034073, 15530266 and 32892857

DIFFUSE MUCOSAL PIGMENTATION

➔ Summary chart 26.1 p. 435

Addison's disease is the most important cause of diffuse pigmentation (Ch. 37), but it is rare and a sign of late disease in an obviously debilitated patient.

Drugs, including non-steroidal anti-inflammatory drugs, phenothiazines and antimalarials, may increase melanin formation (Fig. 26.1). Examples are listed in Box 26.2 by cause, but many more drugs have this effect, either more rarely or less prominently.

Remote carcinomas can occasionally cause diffuse oral melanin pigmentation, usually around the soft palate, as a paraneoplastic syndrome.

Heavy smoking is a common cause, increasing pigmentation in a patchy distribution and causing melanin 'drop out' into the connective tissue.

General review pigmentary disorders PMID: 16631966

LOCALISED MELANIN PIGMENTATION

➔ Summary chart 26.1 p. 435

Melanin in epidermis functions as a protective sunshade for the DNA of basal cells. The oral mucosa contains equivalent numbers of melanocytes to the skin, but they are usually inactive, and melanin in the mouth has no function. However, it is synthesised by oral melanocytes

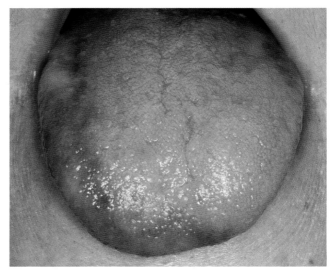

Fig. 26.1   Drug-induced melanin pigmentation. This example was caused by chemotherapy. *(From Alawi, F. 2013. Pigmented lesions of the oral cavity. Dent Clin North Am, 57, pp. 699–710.)*

Box 26.2 Drugs causing oral discolouration

Topical stains
- Chlorhexidine
- Bismuth
- Iron salts

Metal deposition
- Gold*
- Cisplatin

Binding of coloured drug or product or binding to melanin
- Chloroquine and hydroxychloroquine
- Minocycline (through staining underlying bone)
- Amiodarone
- Chlorpromazine

Increased melanin formation
- Non-steroidal anti-inflammatory drugs
- Oral contraceptives

Mechanism unclear
- Haloperidol
- Various chemotherapy agents

* Largely obsolete

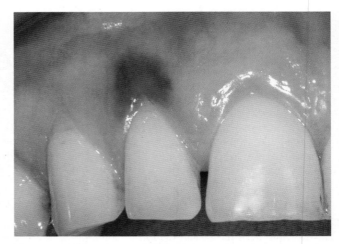

Fig. 26.3 Melanotic macule. This pigmented patch on the gingiva has no specific clinical features to aid diagnosis, other than that is unchanged for many years. *(Courtesy Mr R Saravanamuttu.)*

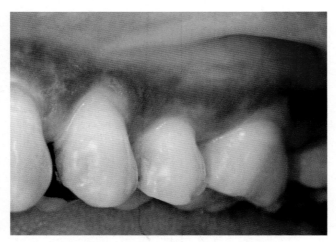

Fig. 26.2 Physiological pigmentation. The symmetrical distribution of melanotic mucosa around the gingival margin is characteristic.

at a very low level and passed to adjacent keratinocytes by phagocytosis in the same way as in the skin. Increased melanin pigmentation can arise from increased synthesis or by increase in the number of melanocytes.

The colour of melanin varies with its depth in the mucosa. When superficial, it appears black or brown, and when deeply sited, it can appear dark blue.

Light-skinned individuals have an average of 30 cutaneous local pigmented lesions of various types, and occasionally one will be present in the mouth.

Physiological pigmentation

This is the most common cause of oral pigmentation. The gingivae are the commonest site (Fig. 26.2). The inner aspect of the lips is typically spared. Intraoral pigmentation

is commoner in people with a dark skin and has previously been called *racial* or *ethnic pigmentation*. Although pigmentation may be widespread, it is in well-defined symmetrical zones. Melanocyte numbers are normal, and activity is increased.

Physiological pigmentation PMID: 24661309

Melanotic macules

These are well-defined flat brown or black pigmented patches a few millimetres in diameter caused by increased melanocyte activity. They are unusual, but still the commonest intraoral localised melanotic lesions.

Lip, gingiva, buccal mucosa and palate are the favoured sites (Fig. 26.3). The lesions are completely benign. However, as the appearance is indistinguishable from early melanoma and because they are infrequent, they are usually excised for confirmation of diagnosis unless a long history is obtained.

Case series review PMID: 8351123

Oral melanotic macules associated with HIV infection

Oral and labial melanotic macules may develop in as many as 6% of patients with HIV infection, approximately twice the frequency seen in HIV-negative persons. Oral melanotic macules may appear before infection is recognised and become more numerous while HIV infection advances.

Histologically, the patches are the same as conventional melanotic macules.

Excision biopsy of melanotic macules is necessary for diagnosis. Unlike those in HIV-negative persons, these macules are more likely to enlarge and to recur after excision, giving a clue to the HIV infection.

Case series and review PMID: 27006825 and 2175872

Oral melanocytic naevi

→ Summary chart 26.1 p. 435

Acquired melanocytic naevi are otherwise known as moles. These are common developmental conditions in which melanocytes proliferate and form a mass between the epithelium and connective tissue (melanocytes outside the epithelium are called *naevus cells*). Moles appear in childhood,

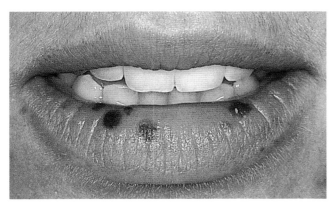

Fig. 26.4 Melanocytic naevi. These flat, pigmented patches are occasionally found on the lip and intraorally but can only be differentiated from other pigmented lesions by biopsy.

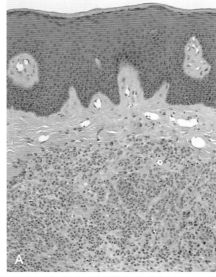

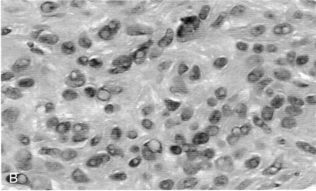

Fig. 26.5 Intramucosal naevus. In this late lesion (A), the naevus cells have migrated down into the underlying tissue and are separated from the epithelium by a band of fibrous tissue, the intramucosal stage of development. The naevus cells at higher power (B) are pale staining, often have vacuoles in their nuclei and occasionally form a small amount of dark melanin pigment, as in a cell near the top.

grow until adolescence and then regress until the age of approximately 30 years. While they regress, the naevus cells produce less melanin and migrate deeper into the underlying tissue and become inactive. Intraoral lesions are unusual and form circumscribed brown to black patches, usually flat, approximately 5 or 6 mm across (Fig. 26.4). Palate and gingiva are favoured sites.

Histologically, the cluster of naevus cells is seen below the epithelium (Fig. 26.5).

Blue naevus is a deeply sited cluster of pigmented naevus cells, appearing blue from light scattering in the intervening tissue. They are almost always on the palate of children or young adults. A focus of spindle-shaped pigmented melanocytes lies deeply.

Congenital naevi cannot be distinguished from acquired naevi when they arise in the mouth.

All these naevi are asymptomatic but are rare and, unless in children or having a long unchanged course, should be excised and sent for microscopy to exclude early malignant melanoma. This is the opposite of the situation in the skin where naevi are much commoner and excision cannot be justified as the chance of discovering melanoma is so much lower.

Case series PMID: 2359037

Melanoacanthoma

Oral melanoacanthoma is rare lesion, poorly understood and considered to be a reaction to an unknown insult. People affected are almost always of African heritage and in middle age.

Buccal mucosa is the common site, but any intraoral site may be involved. The lesions are asymptomatic flat or domed brown-black patches with an ill-defined periphery (Fig. 26.6). They enlarge during several weeks, remain stable for a variable period and then slowly regress. The rapid growth usually triggers either a biopsy or excision of the whole lesion, if small, to exclude melanoma . Multiple and extensive multifocal patches are sometimes found.

Histologically, there is an increase in melanocytes, increased melanin production and the melanocytes migrate up from the basal layers to all levels in the epithelium (Fig. 26.7).

Confusingly, oral melanoacanthoma is a different lesion from skin melanoacanthoma.

Case series PMID: 12544093

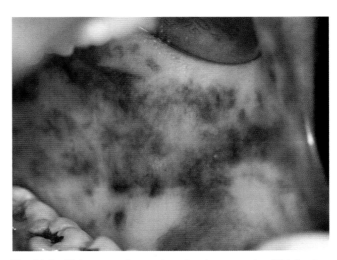

Fig. 26.6 Melanoacanthoma. An extensive example of this benign condition that would raise the concern of melanoma. *(From Alawi, F. 2013. Pigmented lesions of the oral cavity. Dent Clin North Am, 57, pp. 699–710.)*

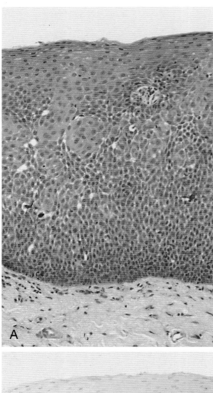

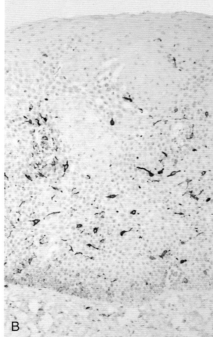

Fig. 26.7 Melanoacanthoma. In routine stains the increased number of melanocytes is difficult to see. A few contain melanin and appear brown, but many are seen as clear spaces (A). An immunohistochemical stain for melanocytes reveals very many more than normal and shows them to have migrated upwards throughout the prickle cell layer (B). Normally, melanocyte cell bodies are limited to the basal cell layer.

Post-inflammatory pigmentation

Inflammation interferes with both melanin synthesis by melanocytes and its transfer to keratinocytes. During transfer, melanosomes can escape from the epithelium into the underlying connective tissue, a process known as melanin 'drop out'. There the melanin granules are phagocytosed

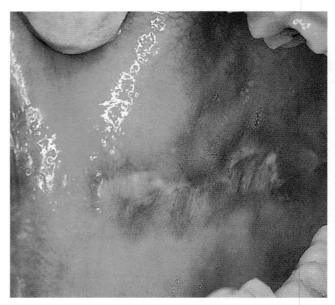

Fig. 26.8 Post-inflammatory pigmentation in lichen planus. Inflammatory conditions may become pigmented, especially in dark-skinned ethnic groups. Here, melanin delineates mucosa affected by lichen planus. See also Figs. 16.15 and 16.19.

by macrophages, which migrate outwards into the tissues, spreading the melanin.

Accumulation of this subepithelial melanin gives rise to post-inflammatory pigmentation. The process is commoner in dark-skinned individuals.

Intraorally, the most common inflammatory condition to become pigmented is lichen planus (Fig. 26.8), and it can become very dark. Pigmentation may also develop in other inflamed sites and scars.

This type of pigmentation is also seen patchily throughout the mouth of heavy cigarette smokers.

Case series PMID: 20526252

Syndromes with oral pigmentation

→ Summary chart 26.1 p. 435

Peutz–Jeghers syndrome

Peutz–Jeghers syndrome is a rare disease characterised by multiple mucocutaneous pigmented macules and intestinal polyposis. The cause is mutation or inactivation of the *STK11* gene that encodes a signalling kinase with functions in energy metabolism and growth regulation.

The pigmented patches typically develop during the first decade of life and can be widespread, affecting the hands and feet and perioral skin, as well as the oral mucosa. Cutaneous patches usually fade after puberty, but the oral macules persist. The oral patches resemble melanotic macules and affect the lips, buccal mucosa, tongue and palate (Figs 26.9 and 26.10). They are often the first feature.

The intestinal polyps affect mainly the small intestine, are regarded as hamartomatous and rarely undergo malignant change, but can cause obstruction and recurrent pain. However, patients are at risk of pancreatic, breast, ovarian and other cancers. This includes bowel cancers, even though they do not arise in the polyps.

Histologically, the oral lesions show slight acanthosis and increased numbers of melanocytes in the basal layer,

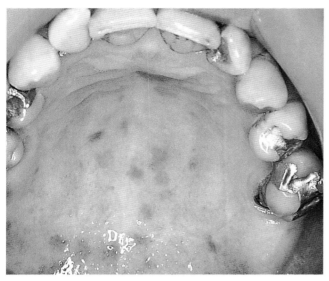

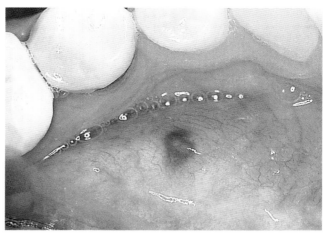

Fig. 26.11 Amalgam tattoo. Typical appearance and site; however, the lower second premolar, from which the amalgam probably originated, has been crowned.

Fig. 26.9 Peutz–Jeghers syndrome. There are multiple flat, pigmented patches on the palate. Those on the lips are most characteristic but fade with age.

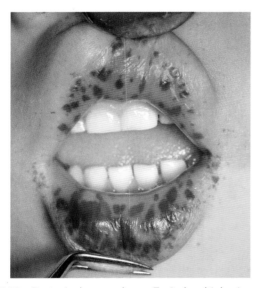

Fig. 26.10 Peutz–Jeghers syndrome. Typical multiple pigmented patches on the labial mucosa. *(From Alawi, F. 2013. Pigmented lesions of the oral cavity. Dent Clin North Am, 57, pp. 699-710.)*

so technically these lesions are lentigos and not melanotic macules (which have normal melanocyte numbers).

No treatment is required, but patients should be referred for genetic diagnosis and follow-up.

Web URL 26.1 Genetics and description: http://omim.org/entry/175200

Review PMID: 20581245 and 33394507

Other syndromes with pigmentation

Several rare syndromes include oral lentigos or other pigmented patches, including LEOPARD and Laugier–Hunziker syndromes, neurofibromatosis type I, Albright's syndrome and Carney complex.

Laugier-Hunziker case and review PMID: 23562360

Oral syndromic pigmentation review PMID: 33394507

OTHER LOCALISED PIGMENTED LESIONS

➜ Summary chart 26.1 p. 435

Amalgam and other tattoos

Fragments of amalgam frequently become embedded in the oral mucosa and form the most common intraoral pigmented patches. Amalgam is usually traumatically implanted close to the dental arch, and tattoos are typically 5 mm or more across and dark grey or bluish (Fig. 26.11). The amount of implanted amalgam necessary to produce a tattoo is very small. Initially they are sharply defined, but the amalgam becomes dispersed and lesions slowly enlarge and develop irregular outlines, as components dissolve, diffuse outwards and reprecipitate on nearby collagen. Particles are also phagocytosed and then dispersed by migrating macrophages, some reaching the draining lymph nodes.

Early after implantation, there is a foreign body reaction with macrophages or giant cells, but this fades with time. Histologically, amalgam is seen as brown or black granules with fine particles deposited along collagen bundles and around small blood vessels (Fig. 26.12) because of the affinity of silver for collagen. Any free mercury solubilises in a few weeks and is excreted, remaining in the tissues only if complexed in amalgam.

Amalgam, being radiopaque, is visible in radiographs provided the amount implanted is large. If radiographs fail to show metal and there is no record of implantation in the patient's records, excision is often necessary to exclude a melanocytic or other lesion.

Corundum, other dental materials, traumatically implanted pencil lead fragments (usually in children) and cosmetic tattoos are occasionally seen.

Fate of implanted amalgam PMID: 6752362

Case series PMID: 6928285

Lead line and heavy metal poisoning

Heavy metals such as mercury, bismuth and lead can cause black or brown deposits in the gingival sulcus. The metals pass in solution from serum into the crevice, where they are reduced to sulphides by bacterial products and are visible through the thin gingival margin as a dark line running along the floor of the crevice or pocket (Burton's line). The blue line caused by lead (*lead line*) may be particularly prominent and sharply defined and is a good indicator of chronic exposure and still an important sign for diagnosis (Fig. 26.13).

Mercury and bismuth are no longer used in medicine, and lead is no longer a major industrial hazard. However, platinum released from cisplatin, a cytotoxic drug, can cause a blue line, and unintentional toxicity can develop in hobbyists and others using metals or their salts without sufficient protection. Older houses may still have lead piping, lead can be inhaled during battery recycling and a cluster of cases in Germany was due to contamination of marijuana.

Case report PMID: 108646

Surface staining

Topical antibiotics and antiseptics may cause dark pigmentation, particularly of the dorsum of the tongue, due to overgrowth of pigment-forming bacteria. Chlorhexidine stains the mucosa directly, as does bismuth in antacids.

MELANOMA → Summary chart 26.1 p. 435

Melanomas are malignant neoplasms of melanocytes, and though intraoral melanomas are rare they are important. They have a long asymptomatic period, are diagnosed late and have an appallingly poor prognosis. As noted previously, many other pigmented lesions cannot be distinguished clinically from melanoma, making biopsy of oral pigmented lesions mandatory in almost all cases.

Ultraviolet light exposure, fair complexion and sun sensitivity cause cutaneous melanoma, but no aetiological factors are known for mucosal melanoma. Very few melanomas are intraoral, 1% in Europe and the United States, but a much higher proportion of 12% in Japan. Mucosal melanomas are also common in India and Africa and in individuals from these areas. The peak age incidence is between 40 and 60 years.

Key features are summarised in Box 26.3.

Clinical

The most frequent sites are the palate and upper alveolar ridge (Fig. 26.14). Early oral melanomas are asymptomatic dark brown, gray or black flat patches. Pigment may be so readily shed that rubbing the surface with gauze stains the latter black or dark brown. Symptoms only develop in the late stages with nodular growth, pain, ulceration, bleeding or loosening of teeth.

Melanomas grow in a predictable fashion. Initially, the malignant melanocytes grow only in a thin superficial layer about a millimetre thick, spreading laterally. This preinvasive or in situ stage is called the *radial* or *horizontal growth* phase, and lesions at this stage rarely metastasise. Later, the melanocytes extend more deeply into the connective tissue in the vertical growth phase. This stage is associated with a very high risk of metastases. In the mouth, almost all melanomas are diagnosed late and are invasive on diagnosis. Because of their rapid growth, most oral melanomas are at least a centimetre across before being noticed, and approximately 50% of patients have metastases at presentation,

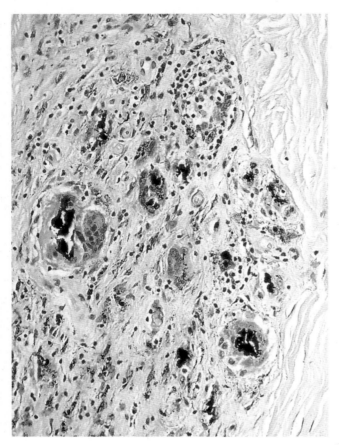

Fig. 26.12 Amalgam tattoo. There are large fragments of amalgam surrounded by foreign body giant cells and macrophages and smaller particles dispersed in fibrous tissue. Silver leaching from the smaller fragments has stained the adjacent collagen brown.

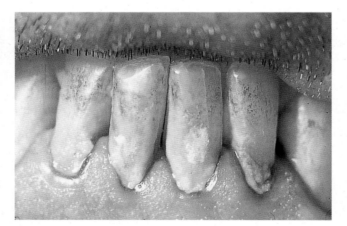

Fig. 26.13 Lead line. The lead line is the bluish grey darkening of the gingival crevice. *(From Forbes, C., and Jackson, W. 2003. Color atlas and text of clinical medicine. 3rd ed. St Louis: Mosby.)*

Box 26.3   Malignant melanoma: key features

- Peak incidence between 40 and 60 years
- Usually appear as black, gray or brown patches
- Commonest site is palate
- Amelanotic melanomas appear red
- Later cause soreness and bleeding
- Biopsy required for diagnosis
- Very variable histological features
- Treated by wide excision
- Median survival probably not longer than 2 years

most commonly in cervical lymph nodes. In addition to the regional lymph nodes, metastases can involve the lungs, liver, brain and bones.

Approximately 30% of melanomas are preceded by an area of hyperpigmentation, often by many years. These preceding lesions are either dysplasia of melanocytes or melanoma in the radial growth phase. Early diagnosis by biopsy at this stage may allow surgical removal before metastasis.

Pathology

Malignant melanocytes invade both epithelium and connective tissue. In the radial growth phase, they grow within the

epithelium, in nests along the basement membrane and in the most superficial connective tissue (Fig. 26.15). In the invasive vertical growth phase, melanoma spreads deeply into the connective tissue. The neoplastic melanocytes range from round to spindle-shaped cells with hyperchromatic and angular nuclei and usually granules of melanin (Fig. 26.16). However, melanoma is highly variable and cells can be plasmacytoid, epithelioid or small clear cells, and mitotic activity and pigment may or may not be prominent.

Diagnosis is greatly helped by immunohistochemistry, which is often essential for confident diagnosis. The cells are positive for the immunohistological markers S-100, MelanA and SOX10.

Amelanotic melanomas

Approximately 15% of oral melanomas produce so little pigment that they appear red or reddish brown rather than grey, brown or black, causing difficulties in clinical

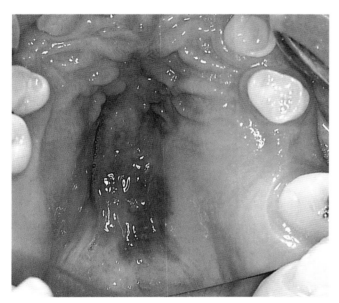

Fig. 26.14 Melanotic patch. There is poorly demarcated pigmentation of varying density in the palate. All pigmented lesions such as this should be treated with the utmost suspicion and biopsied to exclude melanoma.

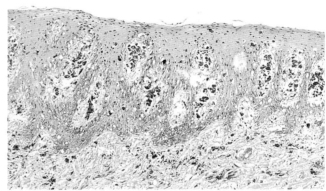

Fig. 26.15 Superficial spreading melanoma. Numerous pigmented and atypical melanocytes form nests and clusters along the basement membrane and are present within the epithelium and superficial connective tissue.

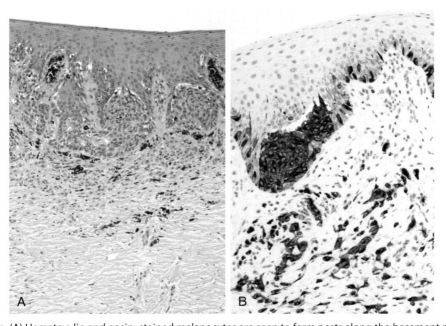

Fig. 26.16 Melanoma. (A) Hematoxylin and eosin–stained melanocytes are seen to form nests along the basement membrane. Invading melanocytes are difficult to see, but melanin is present in the deep connective tissue giving a clue. (B) At slightly higher magnification, immunohistochemistry for a melanocytic marker reveals numerous dispersed melanocytes invading deeply, indicating the vertical growth phase and a poor prognosis.

diagnosis. Probably because of greater delay in diagnosis, the prognosis is appreciably worse than for these non-pigmented or amelanotic melanomas. In such cases, the diagnosis is rarely made until a biopsy and immunohistochemistry have been carried out.

Treatment

Oral melanomas are highly invasive, metastasise early and have a high mortality. Early diagnosis is critical to survival so that early biopsy of all oral pigmented lesions is essential.

As many as 50% of oral melanomas involve regional lymph nodes at presentation, and 20% have distant metastasis. Wide excision with, if possible, a 2–5 cm margin (often with a simultaneous neck dissection) followed by radical radiotherapy or chemotherapy or both is recommended.

The 5-year survival for node-negative patients may be 30%, but as low as 10% after metastasis. Many experimental treatments are in trial including chemotherapy, immunotherapy, immunostimulatory antibodies and novel biological agents targeting genes and signalling pathways.

Case series PMID: 7633281

Review PMID: 21540752 and 12744608

Treatment and survival PMID: 22349277

Oral Amelanotic melanoma PMID: 34309791

Novel treatments for melanoma PMID: 35849287

Oral discoloration, pigmentation or pigmented lesion

Black, dark brown or bluish-brown pigment, radiopaque, usually adjacent amalgam restorations, lesions usually in gingivia or hard palate

Pigment is amalgam or other foreign material. Biopsy is diagnostic but clinical and radiographic diagnosis may be adequate

Decorative tattooing

Chlorhexidine staining

Exclude extrinsic causes of pigmentation

Black or dark brown/blue line around gingival margin and periodontal pockets

Pigment may be lead or other heavy metal sulphides. Check for occupational exposure, drugs such as cisplatin. Analysis of serum or biopsy may be helpful

Black or dark brown pigment localised to the dorsum of the tongue with or without overgrowth of filiform papillae

Pigment probably bacterial in origin (black hairy tongue). Check history for possible associations: radiotherapy, drug treatment, recent period of ill-health. Biopsy and microbiology unhelpful, diagnosis clinical

Haemangioma or varix. Check for haemangiomas elsewhere and exclude extension into bone radiographically if overlying jaw. Consider risks of haemorrhage before biopsy or excision. Cryotherapy, arteriography and embolisation may be of value

Localised lesion which blanches on pressure

Discoloration is due to blood in vessels

Consider blood and blood-derived pigmentation

Red, blue, brown or yellow-brown pigmentation or vascular appearance but no blanching on pressure

Pigment is extravascular blood-derived pigment and/or blood in very small vessels

Consider a bruise or haemorrhage, Kaposi's sarcoma (check for other signs of immunosuppression), pyogenic granuloma, capillary haemangioma, benign and malignant vascular neoplasms. Biopsy indicated. Consider risk of haemorrhage before biopsy or excision

Physiological pigmentation

Dark-skinned individuals, gingiva especially involved. Diagnosis clinical. Biopsy not indicated unless diagnosis unclear

Inflammatory pigmentation

Pigmentation follows the distribution of an inflammatory condition, e.g. lichen planus and is in a dark-skinned patient. Biopsy usually required for pigmentation and underlying condition

Generalised diffuse or patchy pigmentation

Melanin pigment

Black, brown or bluish-grey discoloration

Associated with a tumour mass

Pigmented neuroectodermal tumour of infancy

Pigmented swelling on the gingiva of a neonate. Biopsy indicated

Melanoma

Most likely cause of pigmented tumour. Check for signs of malignancy. Consider possibility of a metastasis, search for a primary lesion and check history for pre-existing lesion. Biopsy indicated

Addison's disease

Neither inflammatory nor racial pattern. Check for history, signs and symptoms of Addison's disease. Biopsy will require steroid cover

Drug-induced pigmentation

Increased mucosal pigmentation due to smoking

Diagnosed by excluding other causes. Biopsy may be helpful

Discrete flat pigmented patches

Benign melanotic macule

Single or a few. No signs of malignancy. Often freckles also on the facial skin. Impossible to differentiate from melanoma (much less likely) clinically. Biopsy indicated

Multiple lentigenes syndromes

Very large numbers of melanotic macules on face periorally or possibly intraorally. Often diagnosed in child or adolescent. Consider Peutz-Jehgers, LEOPARD and other syndromes and investigate for other signs and family history. Biopsy a lesion to exclude other causes

Melanoma and melanoma in situ

Most frequently on the palate. May be signs of malignancy. Early lesions are unremarkable pigmented patches that cannot be distinguished from benign pigmentation. Be suspicious of enlargement, ulceration and in older patients. Biopsy all suspicious intraoral pigmented patches

Summary chart 26.1   The common and significant causes of oral pigmented lesions.

Cosmetic procedures 27

There is an increasing demand for cosmetic dental procedures and in developed countries with low caries rates many dentists are practising at the interface between conventional dentistry and the cosmetic industry. Regulation varies between countries. Some prohibit certain activities that can be performed elsewhere by therapists, hygienists or nurses. In many countries these procedures are performed by unregistered individuals, sometimes with minimal training.

Unlike conventional dentistry, in which procedures are intended to restore a state of oral health, cosmetic procedures are intended to enhance appearance when no disease is present. This alters the balance between the risks and benefits of procedures; doing no harm becomes paramount. Adverse outcomes are more likely to be unacceptable to patients leading to complaints and litigation.

Cosmetic procedures are often not taught in dental schools and postgraduate specialisation is often not recognised or regulated. It is also argued that dentists also do not have the necessary psychology or psychiatric skills necessary to evaluate patients' wishes properly. Beauty is in the eye of the beholder, but many patients' desires are driven by social media concepts of beauty and celebrity endorsement. Failing to recognise that a patient has a distorted body image is likely to lead to inappropriate and possibly harmful interventions and difficulty meeting patient expectations.

Ethics and marketing cosmetic dentistry PMID: 22852509 and 22928452

Ethics US perspective PMID: 16737066

Body dysmorphic disorder and aesthetic dentistry PMID: 21500621

Body dysmorphic disorder in facial treatments PMID: 31758136

How to identify body dysmorphia in dentistry PMID: 30579858

Social media and body image PMID: 35030460

Dentists offering cosmetic procedures in the UK must adhere to medical guidance at Web URL 27.1 https://www.gmc-uk.org/ and enter 'cosmetic interventions' in the search box

TOOTH WHITENING

Tooth whitening is a largely safe procedure and adverse effects usually result from improper materials or poor technique, often performed by patients themselves or those without training. In the UK, whitening is regulated. Bleaching reagents must contain less than 6% hydrogen peroxide, can only be supplied to registered dental practitioners. The first cycle of use can only be performed by, or under the supervision of, a registered dentist. Tooth whitening products are considered cosmetics in the UK and EU but in the US may be considered drugs or cosmetics depending on formulation and use. Use in children is not recommended and, in the UK, whitening for cosmetic purposes on healthy teeth is not permitted on patients aged under 18 years.

The commonest adverse effects are tooth sensitivity and gingival irritation and pain. Sensitivity is usually mild and short-lived and is more frequent with higher peroxide concentrations, prolonged exposure and application in close fitting trays. It is likely that the effect is mediated mostly through exposed dentine, but peroxide can pass through both enamel and dentinal tubules to the pulp causing pulpitis and high concentrations of peroxide (30%+) can cause pulpal necrosis. This effect is greatest in lower incisors where the dentine thickness is least. Standard concentrations and milder peroxide releasing agents such as carbamyl peroxide are not considered to affect the pulp directly when used correctly. Up to two-thirds of patients experience tooth sensitivity and the effect is greater in early use than in subsequent cycles. Reagents for home bleaching can also cause tooth sensitivity.

Gingival irritation is caused by direct oxidative damage causing surface epithelial sloughing and subsequent inflammation. It is normally prevented by relieving application trays or covering with various barrier materials, should not occur with correct technique and is more frequent with home bleaching. The effects are peroxide concentration dependent and caused by both hydrogen and carbamyl peroxide. Irritation is generally considered mild and short-lived, but attempts to bleach with improper reagents or without gingival protection can cause chemical burns of the mucosa (Fig 27.1). Most such burns are superficial and the gingiva will recover well if an antiseptic mouthwash such as chlorhexidine is prescribed until healed. Concentrations over 5% peroxide cause mucosal irritation. Repeated use has been associated with gingival recession, roughening of enamel and discolouration of restorations. The surface of

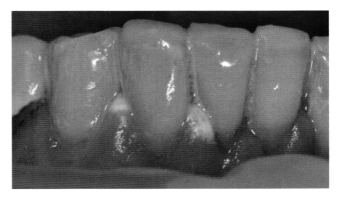

Fig 27.1 Gingival burn following leaking of high concentration hydrogen peroxide onto the gingiva. This superficial epithelium sloughs off quickly leaving a red, painful ulcerated area. Considerably larger and deeper burns can be found on social media, posted by people using higher concentrations of peroxide or materials incorrectly. *(From Banerjee A, Millar B, 2015. Minimally Invasive Esthetics: Essentials of Esthetic Dentistry. Oxford: Mosby Ltd)*

Box 27.1 Dermal filler materials

- Bovine and avian collagen
- Human cadaveric collagen
- Gelatin
- Hyaluronic acid
- Hydroxyapatite
- Polymethylmethacrylate
- Poly-L lactic acid
- Alkyl-imide polymer
- Expanded polytetrafluoroethylene
- Autogenic fat
- Cultured fibroblasts
- Combination agents

enamel develops microcracks and reduced hardness at 7% peroxide, but at lower concentrations in acidic formulations.

Cervical resorption (Ch. 6) is associated with internal bleaching of discoloured root filled teeth but appears not to be a significant risk in external bleaching.

Whitening is often performed in multiple cycles rather than in prolonged exposures in an attempt to reduce adverse effects but whether this is effective is unproven.

'Alternative' tooth whitening agents used by patients such as charcoal, bicarbonate, coconut oil and others have no proven whitening ability and other adverse effects. Some methods use abrasive compounds or citrus fruits that abrade or erode enamel.

There has not yet been time to determine the long-term effects of repeated bleaching, which is concerning as many patients are young, expect unrealistically white teeth and may demand whitening throughout their life.

Review PMID: 32615235

Adverse effects PMID: 23846062 and 19543926

TISSUE FILLERS

Dermal or tissue fillers are materials injected into the superficial fat planes of the face between muscles to reduce wrinkles and fill out areas of tissue deficiency. Fillers may be used in a therapeutic or cosmetic setting, depending on the defect and its cause. Fat is lost through aging, less frequently in genetic lipodystrophy diseases and can be an effect of drugs, particularly antiretroviral drugs. Many fillers are available (Box 27.1) and they vary in the time for which they remain in the tissues, their consistency and likelihood of causing adverse reactions. Fillers can be selected to last a few months, years or be permanent.

Applications in dentistry include both facial, enhancing lip volume and removing deep folds at the angles of the mouth, and intraoral, for interdental gingival recession. Placement requires considerable skill for good cosmetic results.

Although many of these fillers are normal tissue components, none is ideal. Apparently biologically compatible agents like collagen or hyaluronic acid are often of animal origin or biochemically modified and thus recognised as foreign material and are allergenic. It seems that almost all fillers can induce an inflammatory reaction, a foreign body reaction or fibrosis in some patients. Some, such as poly-L-lactic acid and silicone, are intended to stimulate mild inflammation and induce collagen formation (Fig 27.2). Hyaluronic acid, cross linked to slow degradation, is currently

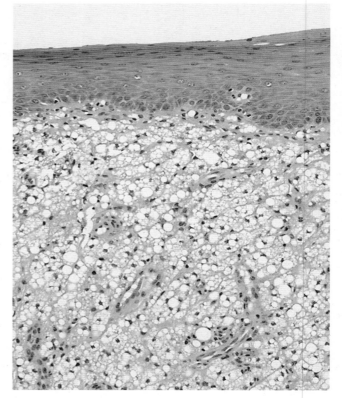

Fig. 27.2 Silicone cosmetic filler. All of the connective tissue visible is infiltrated by macrophages that have phagocytosed multiple small droplets of silicone. More deeply, the macrophage infiltrate had induced extensive fibrosis and the lower lip was hard and distorted by scarring. No history of cosmetic procedure was elicited, even after the diagnosis was made and the clinical appearance of an enlarged firm lip was interpreted initially as orofacial granulomatosis.

considered closest to ideal but is not free of adverse effects. Hyaluronic acid is often used in preparations containing hydroxyapatite or other solid filler particles. However, patients still present with bad outcomes from older materials that are now considered obsolete.

Immediate adverse outcomes include injection into the wrong site, overinjection and movement of material after injection producing lumps and bumps. If the filler is hyaluronic acid, these can be reversed by injecting hyaluronidase, though this is also allergenic and carries risks of thrombosis in some patients. Otherwise, bruising, redness and discomfort are the effects of multiple injections rather than the material itself.

Necrosis of the skin is a severe early adverse effect, caused by injection of filler into a blood vessel, causing occlusion and ischaemia. Even in the face, with its good collateral blood supply, necrosis of the overlying skin is likely to follow if hyaluronidase reversal is not possible.

The main irreversible and longer-term adverse event is fibrosis, producing hard inflexible skin, puckering, nodules and tethering, worse if infection develops (Fig 27.3). In a minority of patients, solid fillers can induce a foreign body reaction, causing persistent inflammation and worsening fibrosis. If the patient is allergic to the material, the inflammation is more florid, oedematous and of early onset (Fig 27.4).

Filler complications can be mistaken for a variety of lesions depending on the site. In the lip, discrete nodules of filler or fibrosis may be mistaken for salivary gland neoplasms or

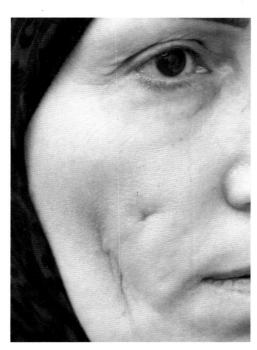

Fig 27.3 Infection and drainage from previous permanent filler producing depressions and scars *(From Niamtu J, 2023. Cosmetic Facial Surgery, 3rd ed. Philadelphia: Elsevier Inc.)*

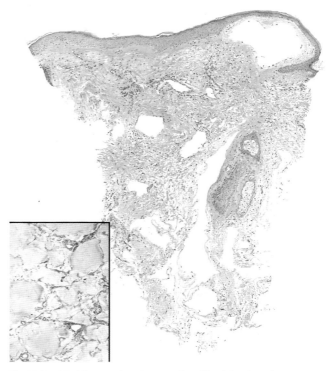

Fig 27.5 Lip biopsy taken 2 years after filler injection, the spaces in the tissue were filled with hyaluronic acid, only faint blue wisps of which remain after section preparation. The filler is lying too superficially and appeared blue clinically. Inset, a high power from deeper tissue in another patient showing how the filler is supposed to be distributed in small droplets lying between collagen fibres.

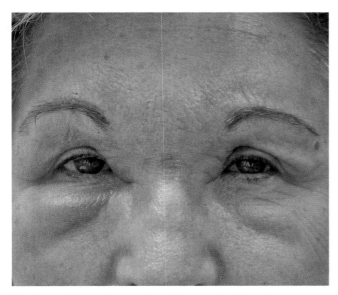

Fig 27.4 Urticaria-like reaction with severe facial oedema caused by dermal filler injection *(From Fay A, Dolman PJ, 2018. Diseases and Disorders of the Orbit and Ocular Adnexa. Oxford: Elsevier Inc.)*

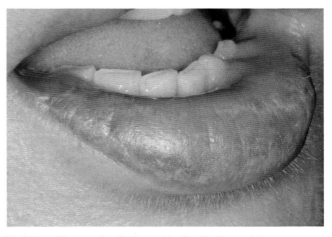

Fig 27.6 Firm swollen lip caused by liquid silicone injection resembling orofacial granulomatosis *(Courtesy Dr L Collins.)*

cysts. Hyaluronic filler lying near the surface gives the skin a bluish tint (from the Tyndall effect). Large collections form a swelling suggesting mucous extravasation and may also track to the surface to exude, resembling mucin (Fig 27.5). Diffuse fibrosis with swelling and inflammation can mimic orofacial granulomatosis or Crohn's disease (Fig 27.6) and be very disfiguring. Superficial hydroxyapatite can be palpated as a hard mass and can be seen as a white patch through mucosa (Fig. 27.7). On the skin, superficial inflammation caused by filler may alter the normal pigmentation pattern.

Surgical removal of fillers in the event of allergic response, foreign body reaction or fibrosis is difficult or impossible. If there are focal areas of foreign body reaction or inflammation that can be localised by ultrasound, it may be possible to surgically expose and extrude filler, but scarring is likely to follow.

Filler materials may also be detected radiographically, hydroxyapatite being strongly radiopaque. Some radiolucent materials may be detected on ultrasound and magnetic resonance imaging if a history is not forthcoming (Fig 27.8). Such chance findings can be puzzling initially.

As filler complications are frequently mistaken for other diseases and lesions, biopsy is often performed and most materials can be readily identified histologically as cosmetic fillers, often the individual type (Fig. 27.9).

Interdental papilla augmentation PMID: 31520457

Fillers resembling lesions PMID: 31444444 and 22727099

Histology of implanted materials PMID: 23021056

Web URL 27.1 Identify implanted materials: http://www. aaomp.org/atlas/

Long term adverse effect hyaluronic acid PMID: 18225451

Radiographic features PMID: 35799966

BOTULINUM TOXIN

Therapeutic botulinum toxin ('Botox') preparations are variants of the type A bacterial neurotoxin, the most potent and longest lasting. Several preparations are available with slightly different properties and the most used are onabotulinumtoxinA, abobotulinumtoxinA and incobotulinumtoxinA. Their primary action is to inhibit cholinergic transmission at the neuromuscular junction leading to muscle weakness or, at higher dose, paralysis. A secondary effect is to interfere with muscle spindle function to reduce muscle tone.

Muscles inhibited by toxin induce sprouting of their motor nerves to form new motor end plates. This eventually limits the action of the toxin, after about 2 to 6 months for most cosmetic doses but with considerable variability between patients. Type 1 fibres recover fastest and the proportion of type 1 fibres varies dramatically between facial muscles. If repeated doses are given before recovery, the muscle is effectively denervated and will atrophy, the muscle fibres becoming replaced with fat.

Botulinum toxin also has remote effects and after injection can spread via the blood stream and by neuronal transport, reaching the central nervous system. The toxin also affects the release of nociceptive transmitters and this, acting locally and centrally, may account for its activity against pain, migraine and some headaches. Effects are also seen on functions as diverse as inflammation and hair growth.

The medical uses of the toxin are legion and constantly increasing but many are 'off label' uses without regulatory approval to date (Table 27.1). Use in temporomandibular joint pain dysfunction is controversial and not yet of proven effectiveness. When mandibular dislocation is caused by excessive protrusive muscle activity rather than a small articular eminence, the muscle can be weakened.

Botulinum toxin appears a very safe drug when used in small doses and with good technique. Adverse effects are primarily those of increased activity from misplaced injection, high dose or repeated use. The toxin is a small diffusible protein and spreads rapidly in the tissues (Fig 27.10). Spread to unwanted sites, particularly around the eye, can cause brow or eyelid ptosis, diplopia and eyelid eversion leading to dry eye. Altered facial expression, facial asymmetry and altered facial appearance with loss of expressivity may follow cosmetic use with high doses diffusing into adjacent muscles or repeated use. When used for cosmetic purposes, 1%–2% of patients experience such effects. Hoarseness and dysphagia may follow diffusion of toxin injected into the neck and difficulty with speech may follow use in and around the lips and mentalis muscle.

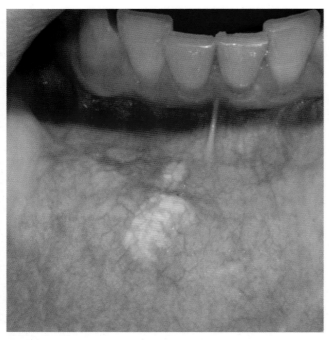

Fig 27.7 Filler containing hydroxyapatite particles visible through mucosa *(Courtesy Dr L Collins.)*

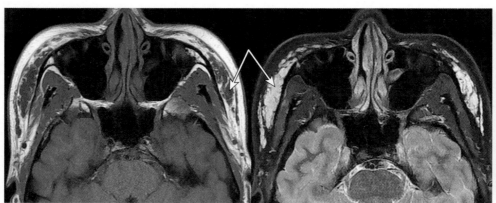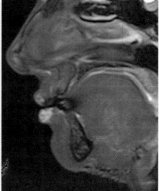

Fig 27.8 Hyaluronate is visible on MRI scanning because of its high water content (arrowed), appearing dark in T1-weighted images and bright white on T2-weighted images (left). On the right in a T2-weighted image, the lips are seen to contain considerable hyaluronic acid filler. *(Courtesy Dr S Connor and Dr P Richards)*

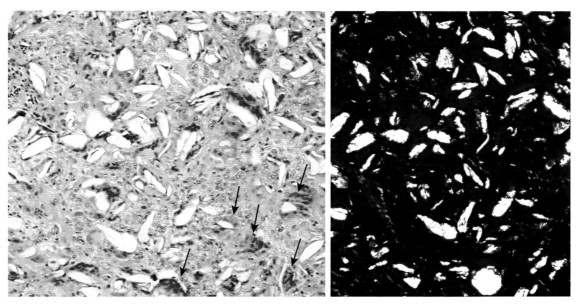

Fig 27.9 Poly-L-lactic acid, multiple crystalline fragments surrounded by giant cells (arrowed) and macrophages in a florid foreign body reaction. Viewing under polarised light shows bright birefringence of the material.

Table 27.1 Therapeutic and cosmetic uses of botulinum toxin in the head and neck

Action	Possible indication
Reduce muscle tone and contraction	Masseter muscle hypertrophy Muscle asymmetry Bruxism Tremor, dystonia, and dyskinesia in various diseases Recurrent dislocation Cosmetic wrinkle reduction
Inhibit parasympathetic secretomotor activity in salivary gland	Sialadenosis Ptyalism and drooling
Inhibit parasympathetic secretomotor activity in skin glands	Frey's syndrome, craniofacial hyperhidrosis
Interference with pain pathways	Scar pain Postherpetic neuralgia Chronic idiopathic facial pain Neuropathic pain
CNS actions	Migraine Some types of headache
Unclear, possibly multiple	Temporomandibular pain dysfunction syndrome

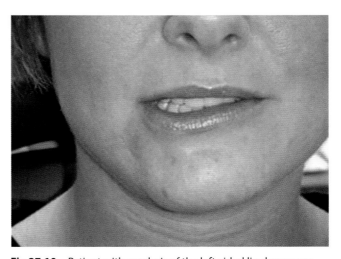

Fig 27.10 Patient with paralysis of the left-sided lip depressors (likely the depressor labii inferioris) after botulinum toxin injection of the left depressor anguli oris *(From Niamtu J 3rd. Complications in fillers and Botox. Oral Maxillofac Surg Clin North Am. 2009;21:13–21.)*

For bruxism PMID: 35779974

For chronic neuropathic pain PMID: 35293078

In temporomandibular joint pain dysfunction PMID: 34743162 and 35775414

Migraine treatment 20487038 and 34078259

Ptyalism/drooling PMID: 23112272

Adverse effects of cosmetic use PMID: 34456155

Use in muscles of mastication can lead to temporary difficulty with jaw movement, reduced occlusal force and masticatory fatigue. Masseter muscle has poor regenerative ability and is prone to atrophy, an effect purposefully used to reduce masseteric hypertrophy using the toxin. Alteration of contraction force in temporalis and masseter changes the forces transmitted to the mandible and changes in condyle and ramus and reduced bone density have been detected radiographically.

Botulinum toxin pharmacology PMID: 33466571

Use for movement disorders of mouth PMID: 35448891

THREAD FACELIFTS

Thread facelifts use threads or wires threaded in the dermis to lift and support tissue. Some also induce fibrosis to maintain the new tissue position. 'Contour threads' are usually made of resorbable materials such as polydioxanone

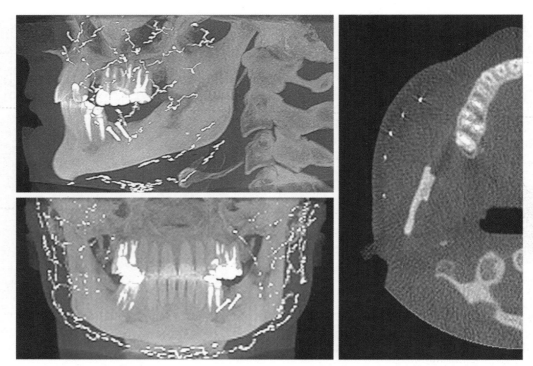

Fig 27.11 Gold wire facelift seen on axial and CT reconstruction. There is a mesh of fine wires in the superficial dermis and subcutaneous tissues *(Courtesy Dr J Brown.)*

or poly-L-lactic or lactic-co-glycolic acid and are placed in the dermis through a long needle. The threads may have a barbed or shaped structure to stop the thread slipping and hold the tissue up more effectively. Though usually used for cosmetic procedures, therapeutic uses include restoring appearance of tissue that has sagged through facial nerve palsy or surgical damage to the facial nerve.

Resorbable threads resorb slowly, maintaining their integrity for up to 4–6 months before breaking up, considerably longer in some patients. The cosmetic effects usually last longer and may be long lived if threads induce scarring. Complications are more likely with older non-resorbable polypropylene threads and wires but are generally minor and resolve spontaneously.

As with all implanted materials, newer resorbable threads can cause inflammation, foreign body reaction, and infection with subsequent scarring. Nerves and vessels can be damaged by incorrect placement. As the threads lie superficially in the dermis, they occasionally dehisce, may be visible or cause skin wrinkles.

A variation and forerunner of the technique is using gold wire. Pure gold is used in an attempt to reduce tissue reaction. The wires are 0.1 mm diameter and induce mild scarring. Unlike the polymeric threads, the gold wires are radiopaque and potentially interfere with imaging (Fig. 27.11).

Thread complications PMID: 35265439

Gold wire artefact PMID: 24701463

SUSUK NEEDLES

Susuk or charm needles are short needles made of gold or silver implanted into the tissues for a variety of cultural beliefs; to prevent or treat disease, slow ageing, or as a cosmetic or good luck charm. They are most frequently found in women from Southeast Asia, particularly Malaysia. Susuk

are usually placed by traditional medicine practitioners, the face and around the jaws are common sites and the needles are frequently multiple. As part of the belief system, patients will often not acknowledge their presence.

The significance of susuk is that they may be mistaken for a variety of metallic objects depending on the tissue over which they are superimposed on radiographs. They may be misdiagnosed as fractured endodontic instruments or needles, restorative pins, or surgical clips on blood vessels from previous surgery (Fig 27.12). Most susuk are about 0.5 mm in diameter and up to 10 mm in length but may become distorted and appear larger on panoramic radiography, depending on orientation. Aside from these misdiagnoses and the generation of metallic artefact on imaging, complications appear limited to infection and movement in the tissues.

No treatment is usually required.

Susuk PMID: 17082343 and 2036281

BODY ART

Body art in the oral cavity includes decorative restorations, intraoral tattooing, tooth shaping, piercing, and more extreme procedures such as tongue splitting. Tooth shaping was widespread in some countries, notably in central Africa and Southeast Asia, in the past century for spiritual or cultural reasons but is now limited to a few indigenous peoples. These practices usually involved filing the anterior teeth into pointed or other shapes. Such procedures obviously risk pulpal exposure and the sequelae of pulpal infection unless performed incrementally over a long period to allow reactionary dentine to form.

Piercings involving the oral cavity are common. In the US, one survey found that 4% of males and 16% of females had had a tongue piercing.

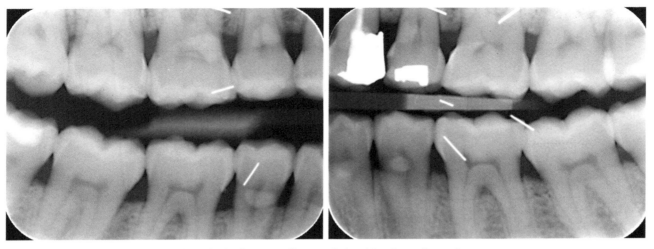

Fig 27.12 Susuk. Multiple charm needles revealed on bitewing radiographs *(Courtesy Dr J Brown.)*

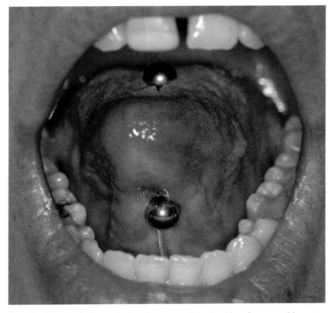

Fig 27.13 An intraoral piercing associated with a fractured lower left first permanent molar cusp *(From Nowak A, Christensen J, Mabry T et al, 2019. Pediatric Dentistry, 6th ed. Philadelphia: Saunders.)*

Piercing the oral tissues carries risks, some potentially fatal. Because the procedures are often performed by unregulated individuals, there is a risk of blood-borne virus transmission, bleeding and infection.

Tongue piercing carries the greatest risks. There is a chance of rupture of large high-pressure arteries and damage to the lingual and hypoglossal nerves. The tissue path pierced is long and haemorrhage or infection can spread quickly, both deeply into the body of the tongue and to the floor of mouth, risking the airway. It takes more than 6 weeks to epithelialise a vertical tongue piercing tract, possibly up to 3 months, during which time it is prone to infection, estimated to occur in 6% of patients though data is sparse. Local infection involves typical oral pathogens and spread to systemic infection, cerebral abscess and bacterial endocarditis have occurred. Piercings in people who are immunosuppressed or have diabetes should be strongly discouraged.

Intraoral jewellery requires meticulous oral hygiene, and some recommend regular antiseptic mouthwash. Persistent inflammation can induce a pyogenic granuloma at the ends of the piercing tract.

Allergy to nickel or other metals in the jewellery is also possible, and loose items may be inhaled or swallowed.

Longer term complications of oral piercings include gingival recession, chipping of enamel on incisors and tooth fracture (Fig 27.13). It is estimated that approximately 20%–25% of oral piercings become infected at some time. After removal, a scar will be present.

Dentists should discourage oral piercings. Individuals that choose to have them need to be properly advised on care and should remove them for contact sports.

Adverse effects review PMID: 35339940

Case series PMID: 16244618

Infective complications PMID: 21358880

Anaemias, leukaemias and lymphomas

28

Haematological disease is common and can cause serious complications or oral symptoms (Box 28.1).

ANAEMIA

Causes and important types are summarised in Table 28.1.

Haemoglobin estimation and routine indices should be carried out when any patient has signs suspicious of anaemia in the mouth, must undergo significant oral surgery or receive a general anaesthetic.

Iron deficiency (microcytic) anaemia is the most common type, commoner in women and then usually results from chronic menstrual blood loss. Males are more likely to have a cause such as peptic ulcer, haemorrhoids or bowel carcinoma.

Pernicious anaemia chiefly affects women of middle age or over and is the main cause of macrocytic anaemia. Unlike other anaemias, it can cause neurological disease. B_{12} deficiency is also seen in older people, vegans and vegetarians.

Folate deficiency also causes a macrocytic anaemia, often in younger patients, particularly in pregnancy. It must be accurately differentiated from pernicious anaemia because administration of folate to the latter can worsen neurological disease.

Leukaemia is an uncommon cause of anaemia but should be suspected in an anaemic child.

Sickle cell anaemia and trait are most common in people of African heritage.

Thalassaemia is mainly seen in ethnic groups from the Mediterranean area.

Clinical features

The skin complexion is a poor indicator of anaemia. The conjunctiva of the lower eyelid, the nail beds and, sometimes, the oral mucosa, are more reliable.

Anaemia, irrespective of cause, produces essentially the same clinical features (Box 28.2), particularly if severe, but some anaemias have distinctive features.

Glossitis and oral diseases (Box 28.3) can be the earliest signs.

Box 28.1   Important effects of haematological diseases

- Anaesthetic complications
- Oral infections
- Prolonged bleeding
- Mucosal lesions

Table 28.1   Types and features of important anaemias

Type of anaemia	Causes or effects
1. Iron deficiency (microcytic, hypochromic anaemia)	Usually due to chronic blood loss
2. Folate deficiency (macrocytic)	Pregnancy, malabsorption, alcohol*, phenytoin-induced, etc.
3. Vitamin B_{12} deficiency (macrocytic anaemia)	Usually due to pernicious anaemia, occasionally to malabsorption or, in older people or vegetarians, dietary lack
4. Leukaemia and aplastic anaemia (normochromic normocytic)	Reduced erythrocyte synthesis, susceptibility to infection and bleeding tendency often associated
5. Sickle cell disease (normocytic anaemia)	Genetic. Haemolytic anaemia. Deformed sickle cells seen in low oxygen tension, sickling crises
6. Beta-thalassaemia (hypochromic, microcytic)	Genetic. Haemolytic anaemia. Many misshapen red cells
7. Anaemia of chronic inflammatory disease (normochromic, normocytic)	Rheumatoid arthritis is a common cause
8. Liver disease (usually normocytic)	Haemorrhagic tendency may be associated

*Alcoholism should always be excluded when macrocytosis in the absence of anaemia is found – it is a characteristic sign of alcohol-mediated bone marrow damage.

Box 28.2   General clinical features of anaemia

- Pallor
- Fatigue and lassitude
- Headaches
- Breathlessness
- Tachycardia and palpitations
- In acute onset anaemia, confusion

Box 28.3   Features of anaemia important in dentistry

Mucosal disease

- Glossitis
- Angular stomatitis
- Recurrent aphthous stomatitis
- Infection, particularly candidosis

Risks from general anaesthesia

- Reduced blood oxygen carrying capacity

Lowered resistance to infection

- Apart from candidosis, this is seen only in severe anaemia or when due to leukaemia

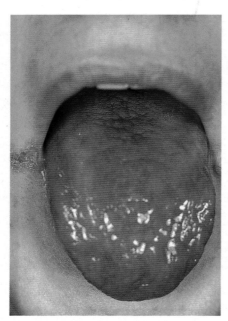

Fig. 28.1   Iron deficiency anaemia causing glossitis. Note the accompanying angular cheilitis. See also Chapter 17.

Mucosal disease

Glossitis

Anaemia is the most important, though not the most common, cause of a sore tongue. It is discussed in detail in Chapter 17. Soreness *can precede a fall in haemoglobin levels*, particularly when resulting from vitamin B_{12} or folate deficiency, and can be their first sign. Later, there may be lingual epithelial atrophy with loss of filiform papillae (Fig. 28.1). Sore tongue always requires careful haematological investigation, by means of haemoglobin indices, serum iron, ferritin and folate levels. If any deficiency is found, the underlying cause must be investigated.

General nutritional deficiency PMID: 2693058 and 19735964

Pain and iron deficiency PMID: 10555095

Subclinical B_{12} deficiency PMID: 8600284

Recurrent aphthae

Aphthous stomatitis is sometimes worsened by haematological deficiency, as discussed in Chapter 16.

Candidosis and angular stomatitis

Iron deficiency, in particular, is a predisposing factor for candidosis (Ch. 15). Angular stomatitis is also a classical sign of iron deficiency anaemia.

Dangers of general anaesthesia

Reduction of oxygenation in severe anaemia can precipitate brain damage or myocardial infarction. General anaesthesia, particularly in sickle cell disease, requires special precautions.

Lowered resistance to infection

Oral candidosis is the main example. Osteomyelitis can follow extractions in severe anaemia. Sickle cell disease is most important in this context.

Box 28.4   Factors that can precipitate sickling crises
- Hypoxia, particularly during anaesthesia
- Dehydration
- Infections (including odontogenic infection)
- Acidosis and fever

Box 28.5   The main types of sickling crises
- Painful or vaso-occlusive crises, acute onset, localised, usually in bone marrow, caused by ischaemia resulting from sickling
- Aplastic crises, often virally induced, red cell formation inhibited
- Sequestration (splenic) crises, often infection induced, increased trapping and haemolysis of red cells in an enlarged spleen
- Haemolytic crises, often infection or drug induced, increased haemolysis

---

SICKLE CELL DISEASE AND SICKLE CELL TRAIT

Sickle cell anaemia, caused by mutations in the *HBB* gene encoding beta-globin, mainly affects people of African, Afro-Caribbean, Indian, Mediterranean or Middle Eastern heritage. Approximately 15,000 persons in Britain are estimated to have sickle cell disease (homozygous mutation), and 250,000 sickle cell trait (heterozygous mutation), making it one of the commonest genetic diseases. In sickle cell disease, abnormal haemoglobin (HbS) causes haemolysis, anaemia and other effects. In heterozygotes, sufficient normal haemoglobin (HbA) is formed to allow unaffected life.

Sickle cell disease

Deoxygenated HbS is less soluble than HbA and precipitates into long polymeric fibres that deform the red cells into sickle shapes* and make them vulnerable to haemolysis. Chronic haemolysis causes anaemia. Periodic exacerbation of sickling raises blood viscosity, causing blocking of capillaries and tissue ischaemia, called *sickling crises* (Boxes 28.4 and 28.5).

Patients, under normal circumstances, typically feel well but are predisposed to infection, particularly pneumococcal or meningococcal, and osteomyelitis.

Painful crises are caused by blockage of blood vessels and bone marrow infarcts. Painful crises can affect the jaws, particularly the mandible, and mimic acute osteomyelitis clinically and radiographically. The infarcted tissue forms a focus susceptible to infection.

Sequestration crises result from sickle cells pooling in the spleen, liver or lungs. Spleen infarction requires splenectomy, and this renders the patients prone to infection with encapsulated organisms for life; *Salmonella* osteomyelitis in bone infarcts is a recognised hazard.

---

* Sickling was first identified in 1910 in the blood of a student from Grenada called Walter Clement Noel, who was studying dentistry in Chicago.

Managing infection PMID: 26018640

Web URL 28.1 Description and genetics: http://omim.org /entry/603903

General review PMID: 15474138 and disease burden 35472249

Dental aspects

Enquiries should be made about family members with sickle trait when anyone in a predisposed genetic group requires anaesthesia or sedation. If the haemoglobin is less than 10 g/dL, the patient probably has sickle cell disease. Rapid screening tests show erythrocyte deformation when a reducing agent is added to blood, and haemoglobin electrophoresis confirms the diagnosis.

Sedation and general anaesthesia must be carried out with haemoglobin over 10 g/dL, full oxygenation and hydration.

Radiographic changes were discussed in Chapter 13.

Occasionally, crises may be precipitated by dental infections such as acute pericoronitis. Prompt antibiotic treatment is therefore important, and facial cellulitis should prompt hospital referral for patients with sickle cell disease.

Painful bone infarcts should be treated with non-steroidal anti-inflammatory analgesics, and fluid intake should be increased, with hospital referral if unresponsive.

Rigorous dental prevention is necessary because of the susceptibility to infection. Prophylactic antibiotics for dental interventions are not recommended. Sickling in pulpal blood vessels can cause sterile pulp necrosis.

Sedation relevance PMID: 22046909

Treatment, complications, review PMID: 7676364 and 31841224

Oral complications PMID: 8863314 and 34721900

THE THALASSAEMIAS

Alpha-thalassaemias mainly affect people of Asian or African heritage, whereas beta-thalassaemias mainly affect ethnic groups from Mediterranean countries. Screening for the causative mutations in some Mediterranean countries has considerably reduced the incidence of these diseases. Mutation diminishes synthesis of one or more of the globin chains of haemoglobin, causing the other alpha or beta globin chains to precipitate in erythrocytes. Haemolysis can result.

The severity of the disease depends on the numbers of alpha- or beta-globin genes affected. *Thalassaemia minor* or *trait* (in heterozygotes) causes mild but persistent microcytic anaemia but is otherwise asymptomatic apart, sometimes, from splenomegaly. Anaemia in mild alpha-thalassaemia is easily mistaken for iron deficiency.

Thalassaemia major (usually homozygous beta-thalassaemia) causes severe hypochromic, microcytic anaemia, great enlargement of liver and spleen and skeletal abnormalities (Ch. 13). Regular blood transfusions are lifesaving and prevent the development of bony deformities. However, progressive iron deposition in the tissues leads to dysfunction of glands and other organs, including salivary glands, causing xerostomia.

Frequent blood transfusions carry a risk of blood-borne virus infection if these have been performed in countries without blood screening. Sedation and anaesthetic management is as for sickle cell disease.

Craniofacial features PMID: 26219152

Dental implications PMID: 9161189

Box 28.6   Major effects of acute leukaemia

- Anaemia due to suppression of erythrocyte production
- Raised susceptibility to infection due to deficiency or abnormalities of granulocytes
- Bleeding tendency (purpura) due to suppression of platelet production
- Organ failure due to infiltration by leukaemic cells

LEUKAEMIA

These malignant neoplasms of bone marrow overproduce one type of white cell and that population expands to replace the normal marrow, suppressing production of normal cells and platelets (Box 28.6). The excess white cells circulate in the blood (leukaemia means white blood). There are approximately 10,000 cases each year in the UK and 61,000 in the US and incidence is higher in developed countries.

Acute leukaemia → Summary chart 24.2 p. XXX

Acute lymphoblastic leukaemia is the most common leukaemia in children (usually between 3 and 5 years old), whereas acute myeloblastic anaemia is the most common type in adults. Diagnosis depends on the peripheral blood picture and marrow biopsy and is complex, requiring immunohistochemical characterisation and molecular analysis. The following signs should raise suspicion of acute leukaemia (Table 28.2).

Management

Being suspicious about features in Table 28.2 is key for early diagnosis. Gingival swelling unresponsive to conventional treatment requires a biopsy.

Any patient having cytotoxic treatment requires dental review and preventive treatment. Meticulous oral and dental hygiene control the bacterial population and prevent infectious complications (see Fig. 7.36).

During treatment, chlorhexidine mouthwash will often control severe gingival changes and superficial infections. Mucosal ulceration by Gram-negative bacilli or anaerobes may need specific antibiotic therapy. Oral ulceration caused by methotrexate may be controlled by folinic acid. Extractions and oral surgery must be deferred until remission, other than in an emergency, because of the risks of severe infections and bleeding.

Chronic leukaemia

Chronic lymphocytic leukaemia is a slowly progressive disease of adults, can be asymptomatic and may not shorten life. Conversely, myeloid leukaemia becomes acute after a few years and necessitates chemotherapy or bone marrow transplantation.

Oral manifestations (Box 28.7) are relatively uncommon or mild.

Management

Dentistry can usually be carried out with routine care. If there is significant anaemia, bleeding tendency or susceptibility to infection, similar precautions need to be taken to those for acute leukaemia.

Paediatric leukaemia dental considerations PMID: 1831649 and 10895145

Table 28.2 Features and causes for clinical features of leukaemias

Sign	Notes
Lymphadenopathy	Usually present, particularly in lymphocytic leukaemia. Nodes are expanded by the neoplastic cell population, but lymphadenopathy may also be secondary to infections.
Anaemia	Mucosal pallor is an important sign in children, among whom anaemia is otherwise uncommon.
Abnormal gingival bleeding	In a child, without other cause, strongly suggests acute leukaemia. Caused by thrombocytopaenia. Worse with poor oral hygiene.
Gingival swelling	The gingivae become packed and swollen with leukaemic cells, particularly in acute myeloid leukaemia in adults (Fig. 28.2). Worse when oral hygiene is poor. The gingivae are often purplish and may become necrotic and ulcerate (Fig. 28.3)
Leukaemic deposits	Tumour-like masses of leukaemic cells which may occasionally form in the mouth or salivary glands (Fig. 28.4)
Mucosal ulceration	Immunodeficiency caused by leukaemia predisposes to herpetic infections and thrush. Also caused by cytotoxic drugs given for leukaemia
Purpura	Purplish mucosal patches, blood blisters, or prolonged bleeding after surgery result from thrombocytopaenia
Delayed healing	Caused by lack of normal white cells and leukaemic infiltration of the wound. For dental extractions gingiva and adjacent bone marrow may be involved (Fig. 28.5) and acute osteomyelitis can result.

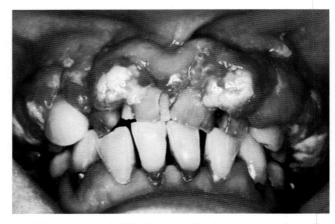

Fig 28.3 Acute myeloid leukaemia. The gingiva are grossly swollen and purplish-red with white areas of fibrin indicating ulceration, worst in areas of pre-existing periodontitis. This florid presentation is a late change and only likely to be seen after treatment relapse.

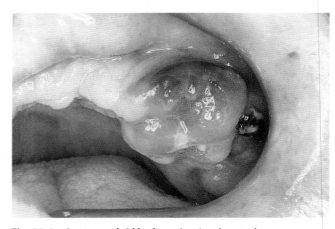

Fig. 28.4 Acute myeloid leukaemia. An ulcerated tumour mass formed by leukaemic cells emigrating into tissues and proliferating there.

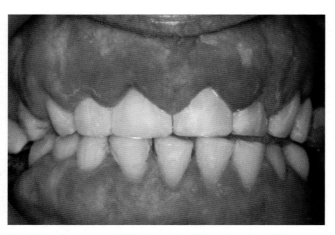

Fig. 28.2 Acute myeloid leukaemia. This patient has diffuse gingival enlargement, slightly more swollen in places previously inflamed by periodontitis, with leukaemic cells infiltrating beyond the mucogingival junction in places. The patient's myeloid leukaemia was first diagnosed after this appearance triggered a gingival biopsy.

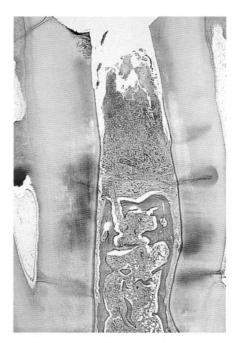

Fig. 28.5 Acute leukaemia. The gingiva, bone marrow and interdental bone contain a confluent infiltrate of leukaemic cells, which would prevent socket healing.

Dental manifestations children PMID: 9177429

Dental management adults PMID: 25784937 and 25189149

LYMPHOMAS

Lymphomas are malignant neoplasms of lymphocytes that remain localised in bone marrow, lymph nodes and other organs. Classification is complex; only common and key types are discussed here.

Lymphomas often present with enlarged cervical lymph nodes and are rare in the mouth except those in HIV infection (Ch. 30). Most lymphomas in the head and neck arise from B lymphocytes. Their inappropriate cytokine secretion causes 'B symptoms', which are common features of Hodgkin's lymphoma and many B-cell lymphomas: intermittent fever, severe night sweats and weight loss.

The risk of developing a lymphoma is raised in the following conditions:
1. some of the primary immunodeficiency diseases
2. cytotoxic immunosuppressive treatment
3. HIV infection
4. connective tissue diseases, especially rheumatoid arthritis and Sjögren's syndrome
5. obesity

Review head and neck lymphoma PMID: 20374502

Hodgkin's lymphoma

Patients are either adolescents or young adults, or older people. About half of cases are caused by Epstein-Barr infection and incidence is increased in people who are immunosuppressed. Three-quarters of patients present with, or have, enlarged cervical lymph nodes. Nodes are rubbery and mobile and often very large. The mouth is almost never involved.

Diagnosis is made on fine needle aspiration or node biopsy. Excision of cervical nodes for diagnosis is best avoided because of scarring.

Permanent cure of some types is possible, and the overall 5-year survival rate is 90% using irradiation and chemotherapy. Patients treated with radiotherapy when young are at increased risk of thyroid and salivary gland tumours in later life.

Oral manifestations Hodgkin's lymphoma PMID: 11885430

Oral complications Hodgkin's lymphoma PMID: 10687450

Non-Hodgkin lymphomas

Adults are predominantly affected and, within the mouth, lymphomas form non-descript, usually soft, painless swellings, which may ulcerate and resorb adjacent bone. Many patients present with enlarged cervical lymph nodes as in Hodgkin's lymphoma.

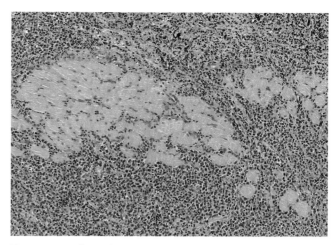

Fig. 28.6   High-grade non-Hodgkin lymphoma. Small darkly staining lymphoma cells infiltrating diffusely through muscle and destroying it.

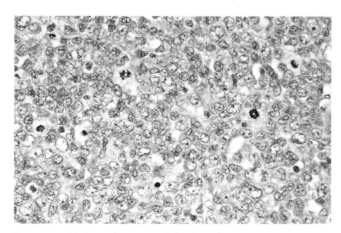

Fig. 28.7   High-grade non-Hodgkin lymphoma. Neoplastic lymphocytes with large vesicular nuclei are packed in a confluent sheet. Mitotic figures are numerous.

There are many types classified by histology, expression of various lymphocyte cell surface marker proteins, proliferation rate and genetic changes, with considerable variation in presentation and aggressiveness.

The tissues contain sheets of diffusely infiltrative atypical lymphocytes (Fig. 28.6), sometimes arranged in a follicular pattern like normal lymph nodes. The presence of necrosis, high mitotic activity and cytological atypia indicate high-grade lymphomas with a poorer prognosis (Fig. 28.7).

Lymphoma diagnosis is aided by immunohistochemistry (Ch. 1) revealing production of kappa or lambda light chains only, indicating the infiltrate to be monoclonal, and markers to identify the type of lymphocyte (Fig. 28.8).

In general, localised disease is treated by irradiation, whereas disseminated disease (the majority of patients) is treated by combination chemotherapy. Oral ulceration and infection are common complications.

Diagnosis in dental setting PMID: 2114452

Medical treatment review PMID: 19101479

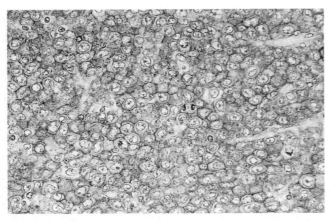

Fig. 28.8 High-grade lymphoma. Immunohistochemistry for a B-cell marker produces a ring of positive brown stain around the membrane of virtually every tumour cell, indicating their B-cell origin, allowing correct classification and treatment selection.

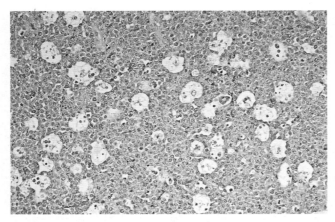

Fig. 28.9 Burkitt's lymphoma. Small darkly staining neoplastic lymphocytes form a sheet in which macrophages containing cellular debris form round pale holes, producing the 'starry sky' appearance.

Burkitt's lymphoma

Burkitt's lymphoma is a B-cell lymphoma caused, in almost all cases, by Epstein–Barr virus infection in an immuno-compromised host. It may be endemic, sporadic (rare) or immunodeficiency-associated. All are caused by chromosomal translocations that deregulate the c-myc transcription factor controlling cell proliferation and inhibiting apoptosis.

In its endemic form, onset is in childhood, and incidence is high across a belt of tropical Africa, paralleling the incidence of malaria. Immunodeficiency-associated lymphoma usually arises in individuals who are infected by HIV or immunosuppressed after transplants, an older age group.

Burkitt's lymphoma is predominantly extranodal. In the endemic form, the jaw is the single most common initial site and spread to the parotid glands is common.

Histologically, Burkitt's lymphoma comprises sheets of small lymphocytes containing scattered pale macrophages, which produce a so-called *starry sky* appearance (Fig. 28.9).

More than 95% of endemic cases respond completely to single-dose chemotherapy. Immunosuppression-associated cases have a poorer prognosis.

Presentation PMID: Africa 23661887 US 6697316 Brazil 23986017

MALT lymphoma

MALT (mucosa-associated lymphoid tissue) lymphomas, or extranodal marginal zone lymphoma of MALT, develop from the marginal zone B lymphocytes that normally circulate through tonsils, Peyer's patches and other gut-associated lymphoid tissue to generate mucosal immune responses. Thus, these lymphomas usually arise in the stomach and small intestine rather than in lymph nodes. MALT lymphomas account for 8% of all non-Hodgkin lymphomas.

MALT lymphomas are unusual. They are mostly low grade and indolent, and survival is excellent even in disseminated disease. Some are associated with infectious causes. MALT lymphomas of the stomach are triggered by chronic immune response to *Helicobacter pylori* infection, and elimination of infection can lead to regression of the lymphoma.

MALT lymphomas also arise in autoimmune diseases as a result of continuous antigenic stimulation, in the thyroid in Hashimoto thyroiditis and in salivary glands as a complication of Sjögren's syndrome.

Salivary MALT lymphoma usually presents as persistent painless swelling, sometimes with enlarged lymph nodes. MALT lymphoma complicates primary rather than secondary Sjögren's syndrome, and most patients are 50–65 years old at diagnosis. Almost all cases arise in parotid gland, though any salivary gland may be affected (see also Sjögren's syndrome Ch. 22).

Histologically, the salivary gland is replaced by sheets of small lymphocytes, many of which appear like monocytes and have a thin rim of clear cytoplasm. These neoplastic cells destroy the gland and infiltrate the residual ducts, which proliferate in response to form much larger epithelial islands (see Fig. 22.17). The islands of epithelium containing numerous lymphocytes are called *lymphoepithelial* ('epimyoepithelial') lesions. The MALT lymphoma is centred on these islands, which resemble Peyer's patches, the MALT tissue in the small intestine. The remainder of the gland is replaced by non-neoplastic lymphocytes and lymphoid follicles, so that the gland comes to resemble a huge lymph node histologically, with its glandular structure completely destroyed.

Management

Any patient with primary Sjögren's syndrome and persistently swollen glands must be followed up and investigated with MALT lymphoma in mind.

Diagnosis is difficult, as Sjögren's syndrome itself causes replacement of the gland by lymphocytes. A biopsy of the tail of parotid is usual because fine needle aspiration is not reliable for diagnosis of low-grade lymphomas. Even histologically, the diagnosis is not always obvious and definitive diagnosis requires molecular analysis. Polymerase chain reaction analysis of the immunoglobulin chain gene rearrangements can identify that the lymphocytes are a clonal population. However, clones of cells can also develop in Sjögren's syndrome, as in all autoimmune diseases. Identifying early MALT lymphoma with certainty remains difficult.

The management of MALT lymphoma is also highly controversial. Patients tend to be treated by radiotherapy or chemotherapy, even though evidence suggests that the low-grade lymphomas progress very slowly, with a 100% 5-year survival. Some untreated patients have remained well for 30 years after diagnosis. Despite this indolent behaviour, MALT lymphoma can spread to other mucosal sites and a minority progress to high-grade lymphoma. All patients require long-term follow-up because high-grade transformation requires much more aggressive treatment.

Key features are shown in Box 28.8.

Box 28.8   Mucosa-associated lymphoid tissue lymphomas

- In the head and neck affect primarily parotid glands
- Almost all patients have primary Sjögren's syndrome
- Histologically a difficult diagnosis requiring molecular tests
- Most are low grade and have excellent prognosis
- A minority are high grade or progress to a higher grade after some years
- Treatment controversial, survival usually excellent

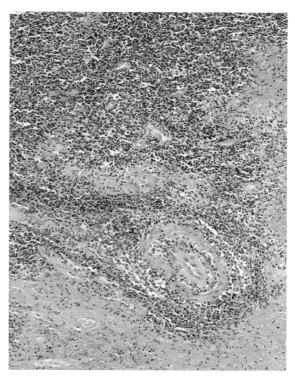

Fig. 28.11   Natural killer/T cell angiocentric or nasopharyngeal type lymphoma. A dense infiltrate of lymphocytes, within which are smaller numbers of the neoplastic cytotoxic T cells or natural killer cells, has infiltrated a vessel wall causing thrombosis and thus tissue necrosis, seen along the lower and right edges.

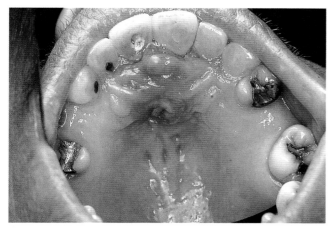

Fig. 28.10   Natural killer/T cell angiocentric or nasopharyngeal type lymphoma. Typical ulcer with minimal swelling in the midline of the palate caused by perforation through from the nasal cavity, where these lymphomas usually originate.

Lymphoma in Sjögren's syndrome PMID: 25316606

Salivary MALT lymphoma PMID: 26268740

Nasopharyngeal extranodal NK/T-cell lymphoma

These rare and very aggressive lymphomas start in the upper respiratory tract. They are commoner in people of Asian and Central and South American heritage and are strongly associated with, and probably caused by, Epstein–Barr virus infection. Some arise in the setting of immunosuppression. Presentation is usually after the age of 50 years.

The malignant cells resemble both natural killer and cytotoxic T cells, and they cluster around and within blood vessels in a dense mixed inflammatory infiltrate with many eosinophils. Obliteration of blood vessels leads to extensive ischaemic necrosis of the tissues of the nasal wall, septum, sinuses, base of skull and palate, sometimes perforating the palate (Fig. 28.10). Symptoms are minimal initially, perhaps only stuffiness or epistaxis, but it is not unusual to discover a very large bony defect on imaging at presentation (see midfacial destructive lesions, Ch. 34).

In their early stages, they can be indistinguishable clinically from Wegener's granulomatosis. However, they are anti-neutrophil cytoplasmic autoantibody-negative on serology.

Diagnosis requires biopsy and immunohistochemical stains to identify the relatively small numbers of malignant cells present. Histological diagnosis is difficult because of the extensive

Box 28.9   Nasopharyngeal T-cell lymphoma: key features

- Onset symptoms typically indistinguishable from Wegener's granulomatosis
- Early disease is in the nasal cavity or sinuses
- Downward extension may cause central ulceration or necrosis of the palate
- Histologically a difficult diagnosis, avoid necrotic tissue on biopsy
- Necrosis results from destruction of blood vessels
- Immunohistochemistry for T-cell or natural killer–cell markers confirm the diagnosis
- Treatment by chemoradiotherapy but with poor outcome
- One cause of midfacial destructive lesions (Ch. 34)

necrosis, and several biopsies may be required to find affected vessels (Fig. 28.11).

Treatment is with radiotherapy combined with chemotherapy, and initial response rates are good, but the lymphoma eventually recurs and disseminates. Median survival may be only 1 year, and only a third of patients are disease free at 2 years, and many of them relapse later.

Key features are shown in Box 28.9.

Oral presentations PMID: 9049909

Other types of lymphoma

Myeloma affects primarily bone and is discussed in Chapter 12.

Dental needs of lymphoma survivors PMID: 20059589

LEUKOPENIA AND AGRANULOCYTOSIS

Leukopenia is a deficiency of white cells (fewer than 5000/μL) with many possible causes (Box 28.10). It is a peripheral blood manifestation of actual or incipient immunodeficiency and may result from destruction of bone marrow or loss of either the myeloid or lymphoid stem cells. Leukopenia requires adjustments to dental management (Box 28.11). Agranulocytosis typically presents with oropharyngeal ulceration.

Aplastic anaemia

Aplastic anaemia is rare, a failure of production of all bone marrow cells (pancytopenia). The systemic and oral effects are not unlike those of acute leukaemia (purpura, anaemia and susceptibility to infection). Aplastic anaemia may be autoimmune, caused by viral infection, or an effect of drugs.

Patients develop anaemia, infections from lack of neutrophils and bleeding from lack of platelets. Without successful marrow stimulation, treatment of the cause or a bone marrow transplant, approximately 50% of patients die within 6 months, usually from infection or haemorrhage.

Agranulocytosis

Agranulocytosis is lack of granulocytes (neutrophils, eosinophils and basophils). Severe neutropenia causes fever, rigors, lethargy and mucosal ulceration, particularly of the gingivae and pharynx, and bacterial infections. Periodontitis is accelerated; candidosis is frequent.

Cyclic neutropenia

In cyclic neutropenia, there is a fall in the number of circulating neutrophils at regular intervals of 3–4 weeks. The cause is mutation in the neutrophil elastase gene. This is a rare disease; undue emphasis has been placed on the fact

---

Box 28.10   Important causes of leukopenia

- Leukaemia replacing the marrow
- Aplastic anaemia
- Drugs
  - Chloramphenicol
  - Phenothiazines
  - Antithyroid drugs such as thiouracil
  - Cytotoxic drugs
  - And many others, though infrequently
- Autoimmune reactions, as in lupus erythematosus
- HIV infection
- After bone marrow transplantation

Box 28.11   Leukopenia: principles of general and dental management

- Refer for medical investigation if discovered in a dental setting
- Optimise oral hygiene
- Control oral infections (as for acute leukaemia)
- Avoid extractions
- Antibiotic cover and transfusions, if necessary, when surgery is unavoidable

---

that cyclic neutropenia occasionally, but not necessarily, causes oral ulceration or rapidly progressive periodontitis. Patients with mild disease are healthy but treatment with granulocyte-colony stimulating factor is effective for those who develop infections. The latter should be treated as immunosuppressed and infection prone.

Haemorrhagic disorders 29

PREOPERATIVE INVESTIGATION

When a patient gives a history of excessive bleeding, a careful history (Box 29.1) is essential.

The most common causes of bleeding for up to 24 hours after an extraction are local and should be manageable by local measures.

The majority of patients with more prolonged bleeding have acquired medical conditions, most are not severe, and the medical history will normally reveal a cause. Conversely, the severe haemorrhagic diseases are mostly hereditary, and the cause also needs to be sought in the family history.

Prolonged bleeding is significant. Even a patient with *mild* haemophilia can bleed for weeks after a simple extraction, and minor oral surgery is often the first sign of these diseases.

Signs of anaemia and purpura should be looked for. Any extractions should be carried out at a single operation and preoperative radiographs taken to anticipate possible difficulties.

Laboratory investigations

Details of investigations are decided by the haematologists but summarised in Box 29.2.

It is essential to look for anaemia. It is a result of repeated bleeding, increases the risks of general anaesthesia and is a feature of some haemorrhagic diseases.

Blood grouping is required in case transfusion is needed during or after operation, if blood loss is severe.

MANAGEMENT OF PROLONGED DENTAL BLEEDING

Some oozing is to be expected for 24 hours after extraction. Patients returning with prolonged bleeding from an extraction socket are a relatively common problem. It is not usually a real emergency, though concerning to patients and accompanying friends or relatives. A small amount of blood diluted with saliva can appear significant and engender worry in patients and onlookers.

Bleeding re-starting a few hours after surgery is probably secondary to vasoconstriction wearing off. If no clot ever formed, and bleeding has been continuous, a coagulation defect is likely. Onset after a few days is likely to indicate infection.

If bleeding stopped and has restarted, do not waste time reapplying pressure, which is unlikely to be a definitive treatment. After local anaesthetic, clean the mouth and identify the source of bleeding, usually soft tissue. Any rough edges of the socket should be tidied up, the margins squeezed together, and the soft tissue neatly sutured over it. A small piece of Surgicel, fibrin gauze or other proprietary haemostatic agent can be put in the socket mouth beforehand, but suturing is the essential measure, compressing the soft tissue against the socket margins and reducing the size of the opening. Soft tissue bleeding may also be reduced with electrocautery, laser or tranexamic acid if other methods fail. If there is a bleeding point in bone, it can be crushed with an instrument first. If this fails, a socket pack is required.

Take the pulse and blood pressure and, if significant blood loss is suspected, assess for shock.

Once this is done, enquiry should be made about the information in Box 29.1.

The patient should be kept under observation to ensure that bleeding has been completely controlled. Continued

---

Box 29.1   Information required about haemorrhagic tendencies

- Results of previous dental operations. Have simple extractions led to prolonged bleeding?
- Has bleeding persisted for more than 24 hours?
- Has admission to hospital ever been necessary for dental bleeding?
- Have other operations or injuries caused prolonged bleeding?
- Is there a family history of prolonged bleeding?
- Are anticoagulants or other drugs being taken?
- Is there any medical cause such as leukaemia or liver disease?
- Does the patient carry a warning card or hospital letter about bleeding tendencies?

Box 29.2   Investigations in haemophilia and bleeding tendency

Diagnosis

- Haemoglobin level to assess anaemia
- Cell and platelet counts
- Platelet aggregometry to assess possible non-coagulation defects
- Prothrombin time (expressed as the International Normalised Ratio)
- Activated partial thromboplastin time (APTT)
- Factor specific assays if required
- Targeted genetic testing
- Genetic testing and counselling for female close relatives if haemophilia suspected

Management

- Individual factor level monitoring
- Blood grouping and cross-matching if surgery is planned

For diagnostic investigation of coagulation defects, laboratory tests need to be performed slightly differently to routine testing and should be performed in a specialised coagulation laboratory.

Box 29.3 General precautions to prevent bleeding after dental procedures

- Ensure the medical history information on bleeding is correct and up to date
- Consult the patient's haematologist or coagulation clinic to plan treatment
- If medication is time limited, delay treatment until it ceases
- If factor supplements are to be used, check they have been administered
- Have a plan to deal with any unexpected haemorrhage locally
- If required, organise for tranexamic acid preparations to be available
- Treat early in the day
- Use infiltration and intraligamentary analgesia if possible
- Use atraumatic surgical technique
- Use haemostatic pack in sockets and suture if required
- Ensure haemostasis before discharge
- Provide written instruction on what to do if bleeding starts
- Reinforce postoperative instructions – no rinsing or pressure on the site
- Avoid aspirin and non-steroidal anti-inflammatory drugs for postoperative analgesia
- Afterwards monitor, provide intensive oral disease prevention

oozing of blood suggests some haemorrhagic disease and this, or a family history of this, is an indication for referring the patient to hospital, because prolonged dental bleeding is a recognised way in which haemophilia is sometimes first identified.

Prevention of bleeding complications is key (Box 29.3)

Post-extraction bleeding PMID: 24930250

BLOOD VESSEL ABNORMALITIES

Hereditary haemorrhagic telangiectasia

This is an uncommon autosomal dominant disorder caused by mutation in one of several different genes that weaken the walls of small blood vessels. Superficial telangiectases develop, particularly around the lips and in the nose and mouth and on the hands (Fig. 29.1). Significant haemorrhage is rarely a problem, but intracranial or visceral bleeding can be dangerous, and intestinal bleeding causes anaemia. Nosebleeds are often the presenting sign. Cerebral abscesses may result from circulatory shunting, compromising bacterial clearance in bacteriaemia.

Oral surgery is generally safe, but regional anaesthetic blocks should be avoided because of the risk of deep bleeding into the soft tissues.

Cryosurgery or laser can obliterate superficial vessels that have bled significantly.

Hereditary haemorrhagic telangiectasia can occur alone or as part of a syndrome with intestinal polyposis, and similar mucosal changes may be present in patients with CREST syndrome (Ch. 14).

Genetics and diagnosis PMID: 25674101

Dental relevance PMID: 18230376

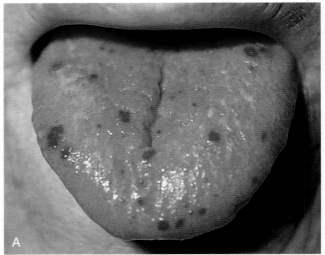

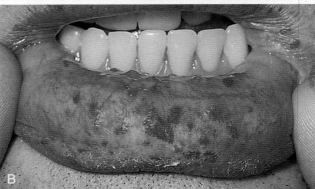

Fig. 29.1 Hereditary haemorrhagic telangiectasia. Two patients with multiple telangiectasias on tongue and lips. The distribution can vary between patients, not all have lip or perioral lesions. *(From Textbook of Physical Diagnosis: History and Examination, 'The Oral Cavity and Pharynx', 2006)*

Angina bullosa haemorrhagica

Angina bullosa haemorrhagica* causes apparently spontaneous blood blisters in the oral mucosa, probably after minor trauma, but there is no haemostatic defect. Rupture of the blood blisters leaves an ulcer that heals without scarring (Figs 29.2–29.4). Older adults are affected, and blisters are usually on the soft palate. They last a few hours or 2 days; patients often burst them to be rid of the discomfort. The condition has been suggested to be linked to diabetes and steroid inhaler use, but the majority of cases remain unexplained.

The condition can be confused clinically with an immunobullous disease, usually pemphigoid.

Case series PMID: 25386327 and 34564682

Ehlers–Danlos syndrome

The vascular presentation of this syndrome is noted in Chapter 14.

PURPURA AND PLATELET DISORDERS

Purpura is typically the result of platelet disorders (Box 29.4) and relatively rarely caused by vascular defects. Platelet aggregation, with vascular contraction, is a major factor in initial haemostasis, but platelets also contribute to coagulation.

---

* The name comes from the fact that blisters may form in the throat and cause a choking sensation. Angina historically meant choking or pain in the throat.

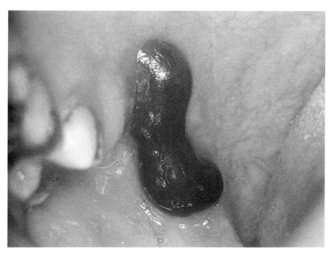

Fig. 29.2   Angina bullosa haemorrhagica. An intact blood blister on the soft palate and fauces.

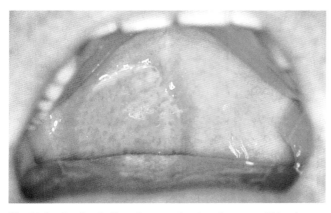

Fig. 29.3   Angina bullosa haemorrhagica. A ruptured blood blister has formed a large superficial ulcer on the soft palate.

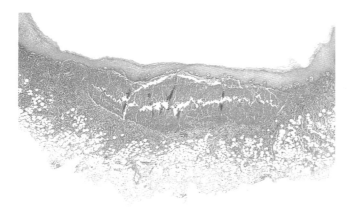

Fig. 29.4   Angina bullosa haemorrhagica. A blood-filled space lies immediately below the epithelium in this intact bulla.

General features of purpura

Purpura is bleeding into the skin or mucous membranes, causing petechiae or ecchymoses, usually caused by platelet deficiency but it may be an age change. It predicts prolonged bleeding after injury or surgery. Unlike haemophilia, haemorrhage immediately follows the trauma but, usually, bleeding in purpura ultimately stops spontaneously because coagulation is normal.

> **Box 29.4   Causes of purpura**
>
> **Platelet disorders**
> - Idiopathic thrombocytopaenic purpura
> - Conditions with splenomegaly
> - Antiphospholipid syndrome
> - Connective-tissue diseases (especially lupus erythematosus)
> - Acute leukaemias
> - Drug-associated
> - HIV infection
>
> **Vascular disorders**
> - Von Willebrand's disease
> - Corticosteroid treatment
> - Ehlers–Danlos syndrome
> - Infective
> - Nutritional
> - Hereditary haemorrhagic telangiectasia
> - Scurvy
> - Vasculitis, often allergic types
> - Weakened small vessels with aging

The bleeding time is prolonged and is the most informative test; clotting is normal. Platelet function tests and counts are a second step. Thrombocytopenia is defined as fewer platelets than $100,000/mm^3$, but spontaneous bleeding is uncommon until the count falls below $50,000/mm^3$.

Purpura forms at any site subjected to minor trauma, and the gingival margin is the most common site for bleeding (Fig. 29.5).

Causes of purpura

Idiopathic thrombocytopaenic purpura is caused by autoimmune destruction of platelets. Both children and middle-aged adults are predominantly affected. The first sign is usually purpura on the skin but it may be profuse gingival bleeding or post-extraction haemorrhage.

Some cases resolve spontaneously, with steroids to dampen the immune response, with thrombopoietin receptor agonist drugs eltrombopag or romiplostim that stimulate platelet production, or with splenectomy, which reduces platelet destruction. Treatment is only indicated if bleeding is a problem, reduced platelet numbers alone does not require intervention.

AIDS-associated purpura Autoimmune thrombocytopenia can complicate HIV infection and can be an early sign. Purpuric patches in the mouth may need to be distinguished from oral Kaposi's sarcoma by tests of haemostasis and, if necessary, biopsy.

Drug-associated purpura Many drugs, particularly aspirin, interfere with platelet function (Box 29.5). Others act as haptens and cause immune destruction of platelets or suppress marrow function causing aplastic anaemia, of which purpura is typically an early sign.

Fibrinolytic drugs, such as streptokinase, used in the acute treatment of myocardial infarction, are potential causes of bleeding tendencies.

The antiplatelet drugs listed in Box 29.5 at therapeutic doses extend the bleeding time but do not cause purpura unless in overdose or idiosyncratic reaction. If purpura develops, the drug should be stopped but, in the case of aplastic anaemia, the process may be irreversible and fatal.

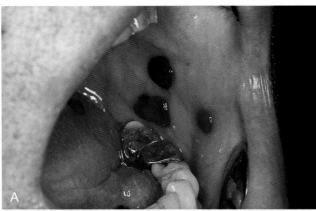

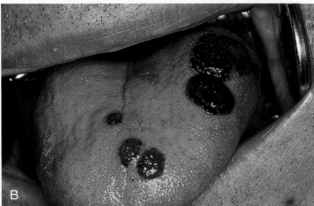

Fig. 29.5 Systemic purpura on the buccal mucosa (A) and tongue (B). The lesions are due to spontaneous bleeding into the tissues and often form at sites of trauma.

Box 29.5 Some drugs causing thrombocytopenia or reduced platelet function

Drugs used for antiplatelet effect

- Aspirin
- Clopidogrel
- Dipyridamole
- Prostacyclines (epoprostenol)
- Prasugrel
- Ticagrelor
- Anti-platelet receptor antibodies (abciximab) and peptides (eptifibatide)

Platelet effects as an adverse reaction

- Glycoprotein inhibitors
- Non-steroidal anti-inflammatory drugs
- Loop and thiazide diuretics
- Colloidal gold
- Penicillins
- Quinine and quinidine
- Chemotherapy agents
- Sulphonamides
- Statins

Tropical haemorrhagic fevers These rare diseases – Ebola, Lassa, Marburg and other fevers – are highly infectious, frequently fatal and a risk to healthcare workers. Extensive bleeding from orifices and internally is caused by infection of vessels causing their lysis. Guidance to healthcare workers is provided during outbreaks.

Scurvy is now of little more than historical interest in developed countries, but sporadic cases are seen in individuals who are disadvantaged, older, malnourished or living in institutions. Defective collagen synthesis weakens blood vessels, and platelet function is impaired.

Extractions in thrombocytopaena PMID: 23932116

Dental treatment bleeding in HIV PMID: 18841624

Management

For urgent operative treatment, platelet numbers frequently increase after systemic corticosteroids. Transfusion of platelet concentrate is usually reserved for emergency situations and patients with very low counts, below 30,000/mm³. At levels between 50,000/mm³ and 100,000/mm³ oral surgery is safe, and local haemostatic measures alone are usually sufficient, although hospital-based care is prudent. Block analgesia carries risks at platelet levels below 50,000/mm³ and must be avoided below 30,000/mm³.

Tranexamic acid 5% mouthwash, four times per day, started just before surgery and continued for 2 days, is effective for most oral surgery, but is not available in most primary care settings. In the UK it is only recommended when prescribed by the patient's medical team.

As with other platelet disorders, aspirin and other anti-inflammatory analgesics should be avoided.

Anti-platelet medication

Platelet aggregation inhibitors prevent the platelet reaction in early haemostasis. Unlike anticoagulants that function in venous, slow flowing or extravasated blood, antiplatelet drugs prevent arterial thrombosis and so are used for prevention of stroke, myocardial infarction or pulmonary embolus.

The most common treatment is low dose aspirin, sometimes used in combination with ADP receptor blocking drugs such as clopidogrel or dipyridamole (Box 29.5).

Aspirin alone is of little significance for dental extraction, but precautions should include limiting the number of extractions in one episode, avoidance of complex procedures and using enhanced haemostasis as described above routinely. Dual therapy or a single other antiplatelet drug cause prolonged bleeding and socket suturing and packing is required, and surgery must be minimised. Bleeding is not problematic if precautions are taken. Drug cessation would be dangerous and is not indicated.

Web URL 29.1 UK Guideline antiplatelet drugs: http://www.sdcep.org.uk/ and then enter 'anticoagulants' into search box.

Web URL 29.2 US guidance https://www.ada.org/ and then enter 'antiplatelet medication' into search box.

Case series PMID: 34522658

Evidence review PMID: 28936297

INHERITED CLOTTING DISORDERS

Important causes are shown in Box 29.6.

Haemophilia A

Haemophilia is the most common and severe clotting disorder. Haemophilia A (factor VIII deficiency) affects approximately 1 in 5000 males and is approximately 10 times as common as haemophilia B (Christmas disease, factor IX deficiency). Extractions in haemophiliac patients have been fatal.

Box 29.6 Important causes of coagulation disorders

Heritable deficiencies of plasma factors

- Haemophilia A (by far the most important cause)
- Haemophilia B
- Von Willebrand's disease with low factor VIII levels

Acquired clotting defects

- Liver disease
- Vitamin K deficiency
- Anticoagulant medication (by far the most common cause)
- Disseminated intravascular clotting

Clinical features

Severity varies with the level and function of any factor VIII produced. Some patients have bleeding into muscles or joints after minor injuries in childhood. Others are asymptomatic and unrecognised until an injury, surgery or a dental extraction in adult life. The majority of patients with haemophilia are undiagnosed and diagnosis often follows dental extraction.

Typically, bleeding starts after a short delay as a result of normal platelet and vascular constriction, which provide the initial phase of haemostasis. There is then persistent bleeding which, if untreated, can continue for weeks or until the patient dies. Pressure packs, suturing, or local applications of haemostatics are ineffective.

Frequent use of blood and blood products place people with haemophilia at risk of blood borne viral infections if the donations have not been screened. Formation of antibodies to administered factor VIII is another complication, and it reduces the effectiveness of treatment.

Principles of management

Patients must be identified by their history. Inheritance is an X-linked recessive trait, thus affecting mostly males. However, a third of cases are spontaneous mutations and have no family history. Severity in females is less than in males. A positive family history is always significant. By contrast, a patient who has had extractions without serious bleeding is not haemophiliac.

Patients require aggressive prevention and carefully planned treatment to minimise the number of admissions to hospital and episodes of factor VIII replacement. Treatment plans must emphasise prevention to minimise the risk of emergency treatment being required. Any dental intervention must be discussed with the patient's haematologist or coagulation specialist to devise an individualised plan.

Severe and prolonged bleeding can follow local anaesthetic injections. Inferior dental blocks are most dangerous because of the rich plexus of veins in this area from which blood can leak down to the glottis. Even a submucous infiltration can occasionally have severe consequences (Fig. 29.6). Intraligamentary analgesia is without risk. Gingival bleeding in periodontitis is increased, but must not inhibit oral hygiene.

Patients with mild (5%–40% factor VIII level) or moderate haemophilia (1%–5% level) can be managed routinely in dental practice. Extractions or treatment requiring inferior dental or lingual block analgesia or subgingival scaling of 6 mm pockets require factor VIII supplementation. Current treatment recommends continuous prophylactic therapy, not intermittent administration for dentistry or other interventions. This may allow treatment without additional

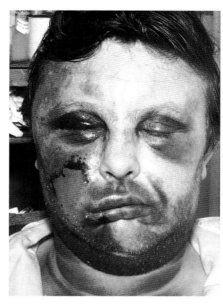

Fig. 29.6 Haemophilia. This patient had mild and unsuspected haemophilia and had never had any previous serious bleeding episodes. This enormous haematoma developed after infiltration analgesia for extirpation of an incisor pulp. *(Courtesy Mr AJ Bridge.)*

factor VIII supplementation but may not be available in resource-poor countries and depends on the effectiveness of home dosing and the surgical challenge.

The timing of any supplemental coagulation factors can be adjusted to be at the same time as any prophylactic cover given routinely, or patients may self-administer from their own stock. Severe haemophilia (less than 1% level) or individuals with antibodies or inhibitors require hospital care. Tranexamic acid mouthwash can be used but, in the UK, must be prescribed in hospital; a –10-day regime is recommended for haemophilia A. Desmopressin can be used to release body stores of factor VIII, reducing the requirement for supplementation.

Extraction should always be atraumatic, avoid block analgesia and be followed by socket packing and suturing. Patients must return immediately in the event of haemorrhage as bleeding into the neck is potentially fatal.

Recently treatment for many patients has been revolutionised by use of the bispecific monoclonal antibody emicizumab, which binds factor IXa and Xa and acts to simulate factor VIII. This can be administered subcutaneously and has a long half-life. It is used prophylactically and continuously, producing a similar effect to approximately 15% factor VIII. It has no role in managing acute bleeding and its role in surgery is not defined. Haemostatic 'rebalancing' is a further new treatment using agents such as fitusiran, which suppresses antithrombin production in the liver by RNA interference.

As in all bleeding disorders, local measures must be followed, and aspirin and other platelet inhibiting drugs must be avoided.

Principles for management in dentistry are shown in Box 29.7.

References are included below with haemophilia B.

Haemophilia B (Christmas disease)

Haemophilia B is caused by deficiency of factor IX, is an autosomal trait and has equal sex incidence. The bleeding disorder is clinically similar to haemophilia A, but milder.

Factor IX fraction, fresh frozen plasma, tranexamic acid and desmopressin are all used, depending on severity, which is unpredictable from serum factor level. Haemostatic rebalancing, as for haemophilia A, is also effective.

Factor IX remains active in the blood for more than 2 days; replacement therapy can be given at longer intervals than for haemophilia A. Otherwise, management is similar.

References for Haemophilia A and B:

International guideline, medical and dental PMID: 32744769

Dental management childhood PMID: 35088637

Conventional management PMID: 24279214 and 24264665

Novel treatments PMID: 35869698

ACQUIRED CLOTTING DEFECTS

Overall, these are more common than the inherited disorders (Box 29.8).

Dental management anticoagulation PMID: 24120910

Web URL 29.3 UK Guideline antiplatelet drugs: http://www.sdcep.org.uk/ and then enter 'anticoagulants' into search box.

Web URL 29.4 US guidance https://www.ada.org/ and then enter 'anticoagulation' into search box.

Web URL 29.5 NICE guide and drug information: http://cks.nice.org.uk/anticoagulation-oral

Vitamin K antagonist anticoagulants

Vitamin K antagonists include the coumarins and the older indandiones, of which the coumarin Warfarin is by far the most frequently used. Coumarin anticoagulants are used to prevent thromboembolic disease in atrial fibrillation, for deep vein thrombosis, pulmonary embolism and prosthetic heart valves. The underlying condition may therefore influence dental management more than the treatment.

Vitamin K is required for activation of clotting factors II, VII, IX and X by carboxylation and coumarins prevent recycling of the vitamin to its active form.

Anticoagulation is checked regularly to maintain the prothrombin time, and the patient should have a record card of the results. Many patients now self-test at home, and some adjust their own drug dose. If a practice has its own testing machine, it must follow a quality assurance scheme to ensure the accuracy of results.

The INR (International Normalised Ratio) prothrombin test is not highly reproducible to decimal places, and the overall trends and level of anticoagulation are more important than small changes in decimal places of the result. INR is maintained at 2–3 in most cases, but at 3–4 for people with prosthetic valves or recurrent embolism. Dental extractions can usually be carried out safely with an INR of 2–3, but the INR alone is not a completely reliable guide to haemostatic function. Adjusting the INR downward for treatment carries significant risks of thrombosis.

Current UK recommendations for treatment are shown in Box 29.9.

If serious bleeding starts, tranexamic acid can be given but, if otherwise incontrollable, vitamin K may be needed or fresh frozen plasma for a more rapid response, depending on the INR.

Drugs prescribed in dentistry can enhance warfarin anticoagulation, notably antibiotics (erythromycin, metronidazole, ciprofloxacin) and azole antifungals. Significant increased anticoagulation has been reported following use of miconazole gel on a denture surface.

Direct oral anticoagulants

Dabigatran is a direct thrombin inhibitor. **Rivaroxaban** and **apixaban** are inhibitors of factor Xa. These new agents are rapidly acting, have a short half-life and are used for similar indications as warfarin. They do not require close monitoring and regular dose adjustment like warfarin and are not subject to fluctuations in coagulation caused by vitamin K intake, bowel flora changes and drug interactions.

Direct anticoagulants produce approximately the same incidence of postoperative bleeding as warfarin in its normal therapeutic range when correct operative precautions are taken. All these drugs appear to carry similar risks.

Little evidence base yet exists for oral surgery or dentistry for these agents. Being short-lived, it is possible to adjust dose before surgery. Currently in the UK, recommendations are conditional pending better data. For dental procedures with a low risk of bleeding, patients may be treated without change to medication but with the general precautions for haemostasis (Box 29.3). When there is a risk of persistent bleeding, after extraction or surgery the advice varies with the drug. Doses are normally taken in the morning and for apixaban and dabigatran it is advised to omit the dose on the day of surgery. For rivaroxaban and edoxaban it is recommended to delay the morning dose until later in the day. For all drugs, surgery should be performed early in the day, limited in extent or staged and socket packs and sutures should be considered. As these recommendations are not yet evidence based it is important to inform the patient when consenting for treatment.

The INR cannot be used to monitor these drugs' effects, and tests to monitor levels are only available in specialised laboratories. Until recently they were not reversible, but new antagonists are in trial, although they are unlikely to be used in a dental environment and are currently reserved for life-threatening haemorrhage.

Routine treatment in primary care is unaffected, including extractions of up to three teeth and scaling, using precautions as for warfarin.

Direct anticoagulants and dentistry PMID: 26386350 and 32110759

Web URL 29.6 UK Guideline antiplatelet drugs: http://www.sdcep.org.uk/ and then enter 'anticoagulants' into search box.

Web URL 29.7 US guidance https://www.ada.org/ and then enter 'anticoagulation' into search box.

Heparin

Short-term anticoagulation with heparin is given before renal dialysis and is effective only for about 6 hours. Extractions or other surgery can therefore be delayed for 12–24 hours after the last dose, when the benefits of dialysis are also maximal. Patients with renal failure also have mild anticoagulation and compromised platelet function as a result of their disease.

Otherwise, heparin will have been prescribed because of a high risk of thrombosis and dental treatment is best avoided until anticoagulation is stabilised on another drug.

Liver disease

Viral hepatitis, alcoholism and obstructive jaundice are important causes of liver failure that result in inability to absorb and metabolise vitamin K, inhibiting synthesis of clotting factors. Thrombopoietin production also reduces, leading to reduced platelet production. Haemorrhage can be severe and difficult to control. In severe cases vitamin K is valueless, but tranexamic acid and fresh plasma infusions may control bleeding.

A clotting screen is required before minor surgery in any patient with a history of alcoholism or liver failure. Those with jaundice may require vitamin K. Local measures should always be used.

Vitamin K deficiency

Causes include obstructive jaundice (usually from hepatitis, gallstones or carcinoma of the pancreas) or, less commonly, malabsorption. Long-term antibiotics can reduce the bowel flora, a significant source of vitamin K. The INR may fluctuate dramatically after only a week or two of wide spectrum antibiotic, disturbing Warfarin dosing and causing marked bleeding tendency.

Extractions or other surgery should preferably be delayed until haemostasis recovers. Oral supplementation is effective, provided there is not significant liver disease.

COMBINED BLEEDING DISORDERS

Von Willebrand's disease

Von Willebrand's disease is a complex group of inherited disorders with both a prolonged bleeding time and deficiency of factor VIII. It is usually inherited as an autosomal dominant: both males and females are therefore affected. Though incidence is high when all types are included, up to 1 in 100 individuals, significant effects are only seen in less than 1% of them, so that most cases are undiagnosed and asymptomatic until revealed by dental extraction.

Von Willebrand factor circulates bound to factor VIII, which it protects from degradation. It also binds to activated platelets, enhancing aggregation and activation. Lack of von Willebrand factor causes primarily a platelet functional defect, so that purpura, prolonged menstrual bleeding and nosebleeds are the more common manifestations. Some patients have factor VIII levels low enough to cause a significant clotting defect.

Oral signs are seen in only the most severely affected, most frequently gingival bleeding and less often oral soft tissue bleeding and haematoma formation.

Desmopressin nasal spray is effective, stimulating release of pre-formed Von Willebrand factor from endothelium, but cannot be used in some rare types of the disease. Tranexamic acid and factor VIII may be required depending on severity and medical advice. As bleeding is mostly platelet mediated, aspirin and non-steroidal anti-inflammatory drugs must be avoided.

Diagnosis and management PMID: 25113304

Review PMID: 24762277

Disseminated intravascular coagulation

This disorder, also known as consumption coagulopathy, is an uncommon and complex acute disorder of haemostasis triggered by incompatible blood transfusions, severe sepsis, burns and trauma. A chronic form is seen in patients with cancer or large aortic aneurysms, and no clinical features may be evident.

There is a complex mixture of enhanced and inhibited coagulation. Initially, spontaneous coagulation occurs within vessels and circulating blood. Consumption of platelets and clotting factors in the circulation, and activation of the fibrinolytic system, cause subsequent failure of clotting and then result in purpura and internal bleeding. Clotting in capillaries can damage the kidneys, liver, adrenal glands and brain in particular.

Complication of extraction PMID: 15772592

PLASMINOGEN DEFICIENCY

This rare autosomal recessive condition is not a haemorrhagic disorder but causes excessive and abnormal fibrin exudation at sites of inflammation or trauma. Mutations in the plasminogen gene reduce levels of plasmin, fibrin breakdown is inhibited causing loss of control of clot formation and clot maturation. Excess fibrin oozes from sites of chronic inflammation, particularly mucous membranes, forming large masses and also accumulates within the tissues.

In the mouth, the gingival margin is the usual site (Fig. 29.7). Apparently ulcerated masses of soft tissue originate at the gingival margin. Excision is associated with rapid recurrence. The eye is also frequently affected, and the fibrin here, and deposited in other mucosae, becomes hard, producing the condition of ligneous conjunctivitis. Other mucosal surfaces affected include nose, larynx, bronchi and vagina and cervix.

Histologically, the nodules comprise fibrin clot, often with hyperplastic strands of degenerate epithelium partly covering the surface. Fibrin leaks into the tissues and forms a deposit that resembles amyloid histologically. Fresh frozen plasma can be used to supplement plasmin to cover surgical removal and prevent recurrence, but treatment is often unsatisfactory.

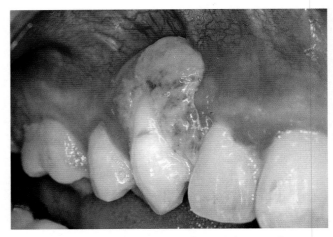

Fig. 29.7   Plasminogen deficiency. Fibrin exudation at the gingival margin forming a soft mass moulded into the sulcus by soft tissue pressure.

The disease is sometimes called *ligneous gingivitis*, but this is a misnomer, as the deposits are not hard and woody in consistency, as they are in the eye.

Many patients are of Turkish heritage.

Review and treatment PMID: 18996031

Case report PMID: 19302964 and 32173395

Nature of lesions PMID: 21993334

Immunodeficiency 30

Immune deficiencies can be primary, developmental and genetically based, or more frequently, acquired (Box 30.1). They may affect B or T lymphocytes, sometimes both, neutrophils, macrophages or the complement system. T lymphocytes regulate B lymphocyte activity; T-cell defects may therefore impair both antibody production and cell-mediated immunity.

Any patient who develops recurrent infections, particularly if they respond poorly to treatment or are caused by opportunistic pathogens, is likely to be immunodeficient.

The main causes of *severe* immunodeficiency are HIV infection and immunosuppressive treatment, particularly for organ transplants (Fig. 30.1). Many cancer patients are also severely immunodeficient as a result of both the neoplasm and cytotoxic drugs used for treatment. The severe primary immunodeficiencies are rare.

Oral manifestations of immunodeficiency

The main oral effect is unusual susceptibility to infections, particularly candidosis or viral infections. Resistance to treatment or recurrences of such infections strongly suggest immunodeficiency, as do opportunistic infections by microbes that rarely affect healthy persons. General oral manifestations of immunodeficiencies are summarised in Box 30.2, but there is some variation in presentation among different causes.

SELECTIVE IgA DEFICIENCY

Selective immunoglobulin (Ig)A deficiency is common and would seem relevant to oral disease because IgA has a key role in mucosal immunity and is the only immunoglobulin secreted in saliva. Selective IgA deficiency affects approximately 1 in 900 people in the UK but as many as 1 in 150 people in Spain and the Middle East (Box 30.3).

Surprisingly, almost all patients are asymptomatic. If symptomatic, bacterial sinusitis, lung infections and intestinal parasite infections are the usual infections.

IgA deficiency may facilitate absorption of allergens. There is predisposition to allergy, particularly asthma and eczema, and autoimmune disease, notably idiopathic thrombocytopaenic purpura and juvenile arthritis. Salivary and serum IgA deficiency appears to have no effect on dental caries or periodontal disease.

General review PMID: 20101521

And autoimmunity 24157629

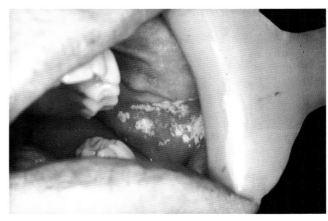

Fig. 30.1 White patches of thrush and erythema in a patient on long-term immunosuppressive treatment.

Box 30.1   Important causes of immunodeficiency

Primary (congenital)

- T or B lymphocyte defects (Swiss-type agammaglobulinaemia, Di George's syndrome, etc.)
- Immunoglobulin A deficiency
- Complement component deficiencies
- Down's syndrome (multiple types of deficiency)

Secondary (acquired)

- Infections (HIV, other severe viral or bacterial infections, malaria, etc.)
- Drug-induced (immunosuppressive and anticancer treatment)
- Malnutrition (worldwide a major cause)
- Cancer (particularly lymphoma and leukaemia)
- Diabetes mellitus
- Aging

Box 30.2   Examples of important oral manifestations of immune deficiency states

Infections

- Candidosis
- *Herpes simplex, Herpes zoster*
- Epstein–Barr virus (including hairy leukoplakia)
- Cytomegalovirus
- Bacterial infections
- Recurrent sinusitis

Neoplasms

- Kaposi's sarcoma
- Lymphomas

Other possible manifestations

- Lymphadenopathy
- Thrombocytopenia
- Autoimmune disease

C1 ESTERASE INHIBITOR DEFICIENCY

The familial form of this disease, hereditary angio-oedema, is, pedantically speaking, an immunodeficiency, but there is no abnormal susceptibility to infection. It is discussed in Chapter 31.

LEUKOPENIA AND AGRANULOCYTOSIS

Deficiency of circulating leucocytes is one cause of immuno-deficiency. Causes and effects are discussed in Chapter 28.

IMMUNOSUPPRESSIVE TREATMENT

Haemopoietic stem cell transplantation

Two main types of haemopoietic stem cell (bone marrow) transplantation are used. For congenital immunodeficiency, a related donor is required (allogenic transplant). In some leukaemias, lymphomas, and myelomas, the patient's own marrow stem cells can be harvested while the disease is in remission and reimplanted (autologous stem cell transplant). In this second type, the marrow stem cells are harvested from blood after drug treatment to induce them to emigrate from the marrow. Bone marrow itself is transplanted infrequently as stem cell transplants are more effective.

During the transplant procedure, there is total immuno-suppression as the marrow is ablated by cytotoxic chemo-therapy. An intensive preventive treatment is required while the immune system recovers during a few weeks or months after autologous transplantation or as long as a year after allogenic transplants.

Preoperatively, oral sources of infection should be eliminated and the mouth should be brought to as near perfect health as possible. Elimination of periodontal disease has a significant effect on lessening post-transplant complications.

Possible complications after transplantation are numerous (Box 30.4), particularly during the initial phase of complete immunosuppression.

The main dental considerations are maintenance of me-ticulous oral hygiene, fluorides to control caries, and prompt treatment of infections. Any oral surgery should be avoided during engraftment.

Oral effects stem cell transplant PMID: 17000279

In children PMID: 10730289

Graft-versus-host disease

This complication of bone marrow transplant is caused by transplanted immunocompetent cells mounting an immune response against tissues in their immunosuppressed host. It is, in effect, a graft rejection reaction in reverse. It most frequently follows bone marrow or haemopoietic stem cell

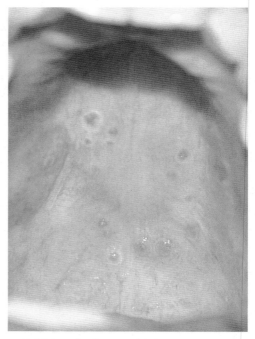

Fig 30.2   Multiple palatal mucocoeles is a common oral manifestation of chronic graft-versus-host disease *(from Bolick B, Reuter-Rice K, Madden MA et al, 2021. Pediatric Acute Care, 2nd ed. St. Louis: Elsevier Inc)*

transplantation, both because of the deep immunosuppression and because of the many immunologically active cells produced by the implanted marrow.

Graft-versus-host disease can be acute or chronic. Acute disease has early-onset and presents with rash, hepatitis, and other manifestations, depending on the organ involved. The mouth is not usually involved though ulceration may develop.

The manifestations of chronic graft-versus-host disease are variable, but bowel inflammation, rash, hepatitis, and infections are usual. Involved sites develop fibrosis as a late complication. The oral effects of chronic graft-versus-host disease closely resemble those in lichen planus (Ch. 16), a Sjögren's-like syndrome with xerostomia (Ch. 22), and a condition resembling systemic sclerosis (Ch. 14) with limited oral opening. The lichen-planus-like disease may be dominated by erythema and ulceration rather than keratosis and may cause desquamative gingivitis (Ch. 16). Salivary enlargement is uncommon, but dry mouth is fre-quent, as are multiple spontaneous superficial mucocoeles on the soft and hard palate (Fig 30.2). All these specific pre-sentations may be accompanied by candidosis as a result of the background immunosuppression and high dose steroid treatment.

Chronic oral graft versus host disease following stem cell transplant for haematological malignancy carries a risk of oral squamous carcinoma.

Review oral lesions PMID: 23107104

Pictorial review for dentists PMID: 33616057

Predisposition to oral carcinoma PMID: 35565303

OTHER ORGAN TRANSPLANTS

Transplantation of other organs, most frequently kidneys, is associated with complications similar to those of bone marrow transplantation. The main differences are that immunosuppression is less complete but has to be maintained indefinitely to prevent rejection. Initial suppression is usually with antibodies against T cells (basiliximab or daclizumab) followed by long-term treatment with ciclosporin, tacrolimus, or mycophenolate.

The chief problems are therefore the enhanced susceptibility to infections and the increased risk of lymphomas. Gingival hyperplasia due to cyclosporin may be difficult to control, particularly after renal transplant when a calcium channel blocking drug is commonly given in addition. Occasionally, Kaposi sarcoma or oral hairy leukoplakia develop.

HIV INFECTION AND AIDS

The most marked acquired immunodeficiency is caused by HIV infection. Oral features are important for diagnosis and staging.

AIDS/HIV infection was first recognised in 1981. It rapidly became a global pandemic that peaked in incidence around 1997 and is now in very slow decline (Fig. 30.3). It has become a disease of two populations.

The vast majority of new infections are in resource-poor countries, particularly sub-Saharan Africa, which accounts for over 70% of cases. There, limited healthcare and lack of education and understanding are associated with high infection rates and high mortality. Concerted efforts to make antiretroviral drugs available to low-income countries have increased the proportion of known cases on treatment to 75% worldwide. In resource rich nations, HIV infection has become almost a treatable chronic disease, but there is evidence of a worrying resurgence in individuals who put themselves at high risk.

The highest incidence areas are now sub-Saharan Africa, Russia, Eastern Europe (concentrated in drug users), and Southeast Asia. In some areas of Africa, 40% of the population is infected. Portugal has the highest incidence in Western Europe. Worldwide, less than 60% of people infected are aware of their status and 40 million lives have been lost.

In 2021, there were just over 100,000 infected individuals in the UK and over 98% of those aware of their infection were receiving antiretroviral treatment. Widespread access to testing may account for part of the fall in incidence, but approximately half of cases are still diagnosed in late disease, potentially having transmitted the infection for a prolonged period. It is hoped that the UK epidemic will continue to decline. The main barriers to this are discrimination, stigma, and lack of knowledge. Although new infections overall are reducing, the number of individuals with HIV infection continues to increase because treatment increases their lifespan. Effective treatment also means that HIV infection now affects all age groups in the UK.

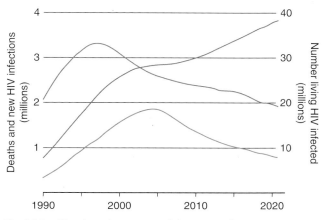

Fig. 30.3   The changing nature of the HIV epidemic worldwide. Total of new infections (*green*), deaths (*red*), and people living with HIV (*blue*).

The main populations at risk in the UK are people of African heritage and men who have sex with men. Drug users are now a very small risk group. Unfortunately, between 10%–25% of infected patients are unaware of their status, the percentage varying in different risk populations. A worrying rise in infection in men who have sex with men has just produced more than 3000 new cases in a year, the highest ever recorded. Just less than half of cases in the UK are transmitted heterosexually, and half are transmitted within the UK.

In the US, approximately 1.2 million are living with HIV and there are just over 32,000 new cases each year, with a disproportionate incidence in African American populations. The main transmission route there remains men who have sex with men, with heterosexual infection reducing and accounting for 25% of new infections.

Web URL 30.1 Global epidemiology: https://www.who.int/health-topics/hiv-aids

Web URL 30.2 HIV in the UK: https://www.gov.uk/government/collections/hiv-surveillance-data-and-management

Web URL 30.3 HIV in the United States: http://www.cdc.gov/hiv/statistics/overview/

Aetiology

Human immunodeficiency virus is an RNA retrovirus. Originally a pathogen of primates, it has successfully jumped species barriers several times and first infected humans early in the 20th century. The HIV-1 species is more virulent and accounts for most of the pandemic; HIV-2 is more or less limited to West Africa, is less infectious, and causes less deep immunosuppression.

The chief mode of transmission is sexual. The risk of sexual transmission is higher in resource-poor countries, probably because of the high incidence of other urogenital infections, particularly those that cause mucosal ulceration.

Direct spread to the baby can occur during pregnancy via the placenta, during birth and afterwards by breast feeding. The risk of vertical transmission is approximately 30%, and this accounts for almost all cases of HIV infection in children.

Saliva is not infectious, unless contaminated with blood.

Life cycle

HIV directly infects cells, using its gp120 surface protein to bind to the cell CD4$^+$ surface protein and chemokine co-receptors. Viral RNA is released into the cytoplasm of the cell, and viral reverse transcriptase generates viral DNA using the host cell synthetic pathways. The viral DNA integrates into the host genome and synthesises viral components that assemble into new virus particles that are released from the cell surface coated in host cell plasma membrane.

It is thought that dendritic antigen–presenting cells are infected first in the mucosa and lymph nodes. These infect lymphocytes and macrophages by cell-to-cell contact during the process of antigen presentation. Free virus is also shed into the blood, but direct cell-to-cell transfer is more efficient in spreading the infection through the body.

Each virus particle contains two RNA strands of slightly different sequence, and during reverse transcription the sequences are recombined to generate virus with a novel sequence. Mistakes in transcription are frequent. These mechanisms generate genetic variation while the virus replicates, and each patient becomes infected with multiple genetic variants of the virus. This genetic variability is important in generating resistance to antiretroviral drugs.

Only a minority of infected cells produce new virus; the majority die through a process called *pyroptosis*. This is a variant of apoptosis, in which the cells detect that their DNA has been damaged and undergo apoptosis mediated by the enzyme caspase 1, rather than the usual apoptotic pathway mediated by caspase 3. Unlike conventional apoptosis, in which the dying cell debris is cleanly disposed of, pyroptosis causes cell lysis and inflammation, attracting further lymphocytes and macrophages that become infected. This cycle of infection and destruction of CD4+ cells slowly reduces the helper T-cell count and reverses the ratio of helper to suppressor T-lymphocytes.

The effect of depletion of helper T-cells is depression of cell-mediated immunity and progressive immunodeficiency.

The humoral immune system is also affected. Apparently paradoxically, polyclonal B-lymphocyte activation results in hypergammaglobulinaemia and autoantibody production. This causes loss of memory B cells and exhausts the humoral immune mechanisms, causing further loss of immunity. Antibody is produced in response to the virus but is not protective initially. After several years, some mildly protective antibodies may develop and slow disease progression, but the main importance of these antibodies is in diagnostic tests to indicate that a patient is infected.

The human immunodeficiency virus also attacks the central nervous system. Virus is carried to the brain in infected macrophages and infects glial cells, which carry receptors for the virus.

Basic biology of HIV PMID: 24162027

Diagnosis of HIV infection

Testing for HIV infection has been surrounded by stigma and previously required formal counselling before testing. However, current practice in the UK is to offer testing as widely as possible and as frequently as necessary in an effort to reduce late diagnosis. In the US, the Centers for Disease Control and Prevention recommends that everyone aged between 13 years and 64 years should be tested once during routine healthcare, and that people with risk factors should be tested every year. The majority of patients who die of HIV infection have been diagnosed late.

The UK national testing action plan suggests that 'opt-in' testing schemes should be replaced with 'opt-out' schemes in which patients are offered HIV testing alongside other routine medical tests and must actively refuse the test. This has proved extremely successful in antenatal testing and is also recommended for all new general medical practice registrations, all surgical hospital admissions, drug dependency

schemes and services for patients with blood-borne viral infection, TB, or lymphoma. HIV testing has become routine.

A range of tests are available. Antibodies appear approximately 6–8 weeks after infection and persist for life. Detection of antibody alone using enzyme-linked immunosorbent assay (ELISA)-based tests requires confirmation with virus-specific Western blotting or immunofluorescence. Tests may detect antibody or viral RNA/DNA and these are used for viral load testing to monitor treatment and progression.

Caution is required in use of some rapid screening techniques and home testing kits based on blood or saliva as these have worrying false-negative rates and may not become positive until three months after infection.

HIV staging

The symptomatic period of HIV infection was previously called AIDS and this term is still widely used. In resource-poor countries, it is defined clinically by the presence of opportunistic infections alone. Elsewhere, countries use the Centers for Disease Control system based on laboratory tests (Table 30.1) and infections (Box 30.5) in which AIDS is equivalent to stage 3. Staging of HIV infection is important for epidemiological studies but is less important for managing an individual patient since treatment is now given early and is so effective. Nevertheless, identifying HIV infection stage 3 is important in monitoring drugs and dosage.

In children, HIV infection is staged N (non-symptomatic infection) or A to C based on specific infections.

CDC AIDS definition PMID: 24717910

Clinical course

After HIV infection there is a short incubation period, followed by an acute disseminated infection and then a long latent period until opportunistic infections develop.

Approximately half of the patients have an acute glandular fever-like illness 2–4 weeks after exposure with fever and headache, tender lymphadenopathy, throat inflammation, and rashes. The features are non-specific and easily misdiagnosed or ignored. Symptoms last 1–2 weeks, and individuals whose illness lasts longer than 14 days progress more rapidly to stage 3. The patient is highly infectious during the acute illness. Antibodies develop, and virus is detectable during the acute phase (also known as *seroconversion illness*).

This is followed by a prolonged latent period during which CD4+ lymphocyte numbers slowly decline but immune responses are sufficient to prevent opportunistic infection. Approximately two-thirds of patients develop persistent lymphadenopathy during this period. Note that the term *latent period* relates to *clinical* latency, and that the patient is infectious during the latent phase. This is different from

Table 30.1   HIV disease stage for adults*

Stage	CD4+ cells/µL	% total lymphocytes CD4+
1	≥500	≥26
2	200–499	14–25
3 (symptomatic infection / AIDS)	<200	<14

*CD4+ absolute counts take precedence over percentage of lymphocytes. Patients must also be positive for HIV infection. Presence of a disease in Box 30.5 overrides laboratory staging.

Box 30.5   In an adult patient with a positive HIV test, the following indicate stage 3 HIV infection*

- Bacterial infections, multiple or recurrent*
- Candidosis of bronchi, trachea, or lungs
- Candidosis of oesophagus
- Cervical cancer, invasive
- Coccidioidomycosis, disseminated or extrapulmonary
- Cryptococcosis, extrapulmonary
- Cryptosporidiosis, chronic intestinal
- Cytomegalovirus disease (other than liver, spleen, or nodes)
- Cytomegalovirus retinitis (with loss of vision)
- Encephalopathy attributed to HIV
- Herpes simplex: chronic ulcers (>1 month's duration)
- Histoplasmosis, disseminated or extrapulmonary
- Isosporiasis, chronic intestinal (>1 month's duration)
- Kaposi sarcoma
- Lymphoma, Burkitt or immunoblastic
- Lymphoma, primary, of brain
- Atypical mycobacterium infection, disseminated or extrapulmonary
- Mycobacterium tuberculosis of any site, pulmonary, disseminated, or extrapulmonary
- Pneumocystis jirovecii (Pneumocystis carinii) pneumonia
- Pneumonia, recurrent**
- Progressive multifocal leukoencephalopathy
- Salmonella septicemia, recurrent
- Toxoplasmosis of brain
- Wasting syndrome attributed to HIV

Simplified Centers for Disease Control criteria. Several of these AIDS-defining illnesses can be detected in the mouth.
* only in children aged less than 6 years
** only in those aged greater than 6 years.

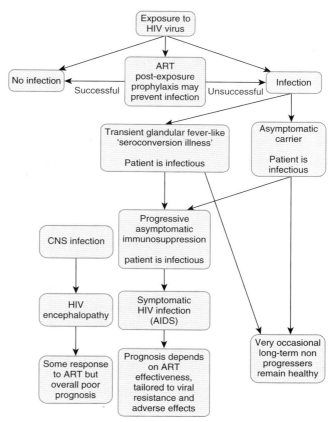

Fig. 30.4   Outcomes of HIV infection.

viral latency, as seen in herpes viruses, during which the patient is not infectious.

The latent phase lasts on average approximately 8 years but is very variable in duration. Some patients, termed *long-term non-progressors,* may remain in the latent phase for 25 years or longer as a result of polymorphisms or mutations in viral receptors or by producing weakly protective antibodies. Only approximately 1 in 300 infected individuals are long-term non-progressors; in the absence of antiviral treatment, the vast majority of infected patients progress to stage 3 symptomatic infection.

Symptomatic HIV infection is characterised by multiple infections by bacteria, fungi, parasites, and viruses. These tend to become symptomatic when the CD4+ cell count falls below 300 cells/µL. Many of these infections, such as *Pneumocystis* pneumonia, are opportunistic and almost unknown in immunocompetent persons. Almost any commensal or pathogenic species can cause infections, including species normally considered environmental organisms. The infections are more severe and more difficult to treat than in immunocompetent patients and often in unusual body sites. Non-specific fever, diarrhoea, and weight loss are common.

Though infections are the main cause of death, there is also a greatly raised incidence of malignant neoplasms, particularly Kaposi's sarcoma and lymphomas because these are caused by infectious agents, notably Epstein–Barr virus. Plasmablastic lymphoma has a predilection for the oral cavity and is virtually only seen in HIV infection.

Neuropsychiatric disease in HIV infection can range from depression to dementia and death.

A less frequent manifestation of HIV infection in some patients is autoimmune disease, particularly thrombocytopenic purpura or, less frequently, a lupus erythematosus-like disease.

Once HIV infection has reached its symptomatic stage, the outcome *without treatment* is death within 2 years, approximately 10 years after initial infection.

The outcomes are summarised in Fig. 30.4.

Treatment

Effective treatment of HIV infection is provided by combination antiretroviral treatment (ART or cART), regimes of combinations of antiretroviral drugs with different modes of action. Such drugs were previously called 'highly active' antiretroviral drugs. These have changed prevention and treatment dramatically since their introduction (Fig. 30.5).

A plethora of antiretroviral drugs is available with different modes of action. Some important oral adverse effects from the drugs mentioned in Box 30.6 are indicated in brackets. New drugs are constantly being introduced.

Treatment should start as early as possible because this is more effective and also reduces transmission of infection to others. The drugs must be changed repeatedly because the high viral mutation rate constantly produces resistant strains. Treatment cannot be stopped without risking emergence of highly resistant strains, which can infect others, and the drugs are best continued for life. The exact combination of drugs used varies from country to country.

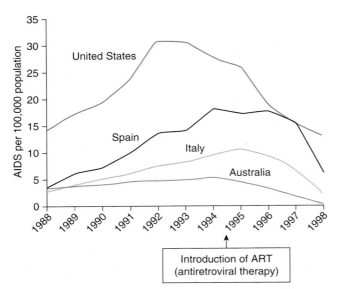

Fig. 30.5 Progress of the HIV epidemic. Before and after antiretroviral treatment in developed nations.

Problems with these drugs include many adverse effects that can limit patient tolerance. For the first decade of ART, adverse effects restricted use to people with low CD4$^+$ cell count. Newer drugs are more effective and can be given earlier. ART can never cure the infection, it only suppresses viral replication and delays onset of immunosuppression. The virus remains integrated into the host cells and currently cannot be eradicated (though a handful of patients worldwide who have unusual genetic lack of co-receptor in their T cells have been cured by bone marrow transplant undertaken for other reasons).

Provided the viral load can be suppressed, patients with HIV can expect to avoid death from opportunistic infection and live a typical life span, but are at risk of adverse drug effects, neurological effects and increased rates of hypertension, heart disease, and diabetes. HIV infection, diagnosed early, is now a medically managed chronic disease.

Key features of HIV infection are summarised in Box 30.7.

ORAL LESIONS IN HIV INFECTION

Although reduced incidence and effective treatment have removed HIV infection from many peoples' consciousness, it remains an important disease that can be diagnosed for the first time in the dental setting. Dentists have an important role as more than 75% of patients with symptomatic HIV infection have characteristic orofacial disease (Box 30.8).

These same signs are also seen in patients in late disease with treatment failure.

The accepted list of oral conditions associated with HIV infection is now old but remains a useful categorisation for clinical use. The conditions strongly associated with HIV infection remain significant. A third of individuals on ART still have oral lesions, mostly oral candidosis. Ulcers affect approximately 5%, and Kaposi's sarcoma and hairy leukoplakia each affect approximately 1%–5% of patients on ART. In resource-poor countries, oral manifestations appear to be more common, even with ART.

Box 30.6 Antiretroviral drugs used for antiretroviral treatment and some oral adverse effects

Entry (fusion) inhibitors
- Enfuvirtide

Receptor blocking drugs
- Maraviroc (CCR5 receptor)
- Fostemsavir (gp120 blocker)

Nucleoside/nucleoside reverse transcriptase inhibitors
- Abacavir (Stevens–Johnson syndrome)
- Lamivudine
- Zidovudine
- Emtricitabine
- Tenofovir
- Stavudine

Non-nucleoside reverse transcriptase inhibitors
- Nevirapine (Stevens–Johnson syndrome)
- Efavirenz (Stevens–Johnson syndrome)
- Etravirine
- Rilpivirine
- Delavirdine
- Cabotegravir

Protease inhibitors
- Indinavir (dry mouth, taste disturbance)
- Nelfinavir
- Ritonavir (taste disturbance, circumoral paraesthesia)
- Saquinavir (oral ulceration)
- Darunavir
- Atazanavir
- Tipranavir
- Lopinavir
- Fosamprenavir

Integrase inhibitors
- Raltegravir
- Elvitegravir
- Dolutegravir
- Cabotegravir
- Bictegravir

Infected cell binding antibody
- Ibalizumab

Not all drugs are available in all countries. In addition, drug boosters such as cobicstat increase effective drug levels of other ART. Most drugs are used in combinations.

Oral manifestations are likely when the circulating CD4$^+$ lymphocyte count falls below 200/mm^3, the viral load exceeds 3000 copies/mL or the patient also has other predisposing factors such as dry mouth. Although oral lesions should be a good marker of the failure of ART, no definite predictors are known. However, it would be prudent to report any increase in, or new, oral manifestations (other than papillomas, see later) to the patient's HIV physician. Onset of signs such as recurrent candidosis or hairy leukoplakia often coincides with a rise in circulating viral copy number as the disease progression accelerates. For a patient on ART, this indicates emergence of a new genetic variant and a need to consider changing drugs to regain control of viral replication.

Although these diseases are strongly associated with HIV infection, all can be found in patients immunocompromised for other reasons and sometimes in immunocompetent individuals. Many are therefore also dealt with in other chapters.

Box 30.7   HIV infection: key features

- Caused by a retrovirus – usually HIV-1
- Transmitted sexually, during pregnancy, at birth or in breast milk
- Acute seroconversion disease like glandular fever
- Long clinical latent period while infectious
- Progressive deterioration mainly of cell-mediated immunity
- Immunodeficiency leads to opportunistic infections
- Common oral lesions include candidosis and hairy leukoplakia
- Kaposi's sarcoma and lymphomas, often in oral regions
- Neurological and psychological disorders
- Effectively treated with antiretroviral treatment
- Risk of occupational transmission in dentistry very low

Box 30.8   Oral disease in HIV infection (EC Clearinghouse 1993)

Lesions strongly associated with HIV infection

- Candidosis, erythematous and pseudomembranous
- Hairy leukoplakia
- Kaposi sarcoma
- Non-Hodgkin's lymphoma
- Periodontal disease
- Linear gingival erythema
- Necrotising periodontitis

Lesions less commonly associated with HIV infection

- Mycobacterial infections
- Melanin pigmentation
- Necrotising (ulcerative) stomatitis
- Xerostomia
- HIV salivary cystic disease
- Thrombocytopenic purpura
- Ulceration, non-specific
- Viral infections
  - Herpes simplex
  - Condyloma acuminatum
  - Multifocal epithelial hyperplasia
  - Papillomas
  - Varicella zoster infections

Lesions seen in HIV infection

- Bacterial infections
  - *Actinomyces israelii*
  - *Escherichia coli*
  - Klebsiella pneumoniae
  - Cat scratch disease
  - Bacillary angiomatosis
- Drug reactions
- Other fungal infections
- Facial palsy
- Trigeminal neuralgia
- Recurrent aphthous stomatitis
- Cytomegalovirus infection
- Molluscum contagiosum

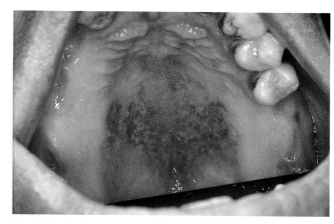

Fig. 30.6   Erythematous candidosis. An extensive red patch on the palate without white flecks, which appears as denture stomatitis but without any denture being worn. Such a presentation is characteristic of immunodeficiency.

Oral manifestations PMID: 8229864

Oral Manifestations controversies PMID: 23517181

Since ART PMID: 12656429 and 33762122

Candidosis

Thrush or other forms of oral candidosis may be seen in more than 50% of patients at some stage, regardless of ART, and candidosis is often the first oral sign. With ART, candidosis is now usually chronic or erythematous in type (Fig. 30.6). Decline in incidence of thrush may be partly an effect of antiretroviral protease inhibitors on the fungi, as well as improved immune status.

Erythematous infections respond to topical antifungals and HIV-infected patients require no longer courses of antifungals than non-HIV infected patients. A single dose of 750 mg fluconazole may be effective, but other factors such as smoking, dry mouth, or denture wearing may need to be taken into account.

Linear gingival erythema, previously thought a bacterial infection or type of gingivitis, is now thought to be candidosis (later in this chapter).

Viral mucosal infections

Herpetic stomatitis is less common than might be expected and causes chronic ulceration unlike the typical infection in immunocompetent patients (Fig. 30.7). People with HIV are at high risk of intraoral secondary herpes infection. Severe orofacial zoster indicates late disease progression.

The Epstein–Barr virus (EBV) is the cause of hairy leukoplakia (Ch. 18), which is highly characteristic of HIV infection (Figs 30.8 and 30.9).

HIV-infected patients have an increased risk of papillomas. Counterintuitively, treatment with ART causes a much higher risk of oral warts of all types, verruca vulgaris, condyloma acuminatum, and focal epithelial hyperplasia. This appears to be an unintended effect of immune reconstitution. After ART, papillomas can be numerous or form large confluent patches that are very difficult to eradicate. Repeated excisions, cryosurgery, or laser ablation may only keep them under control.

Oral hairy leukoplakia is discussed in Chapter 18.

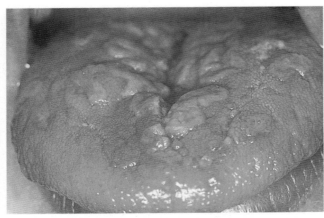

Fig. 30.7 Herpes simplex ulceration in immunodeficiency. Extensive ulceration along the midline of the dorsal tongue and separate ulcers toward the lateral margins is observed. In immunodeficiency, the ulcers may be chronic and their clinical appearance, as here, may not suggest viral infection. Biopsy may be required for diagnosis.

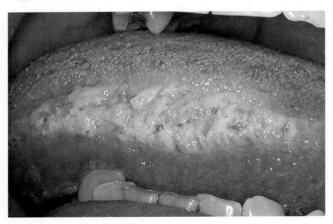

Fig. 30.8 Hairy leukoplakia. Close-up view shows the corrugated surface and suggests the soft texture of the lesion.

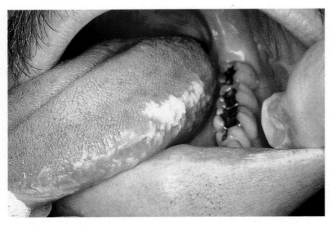

Fig. 30.9 Hairy leukoplakia. The characteristic appearance on the lateral margin of the tongue. Posteriorly, the vertical ridging pattern of the lateral tongue is enhanced. *(Courtesy Prof. WH Binnie.)*

Bacterial infections

Infections by bacteria that otherwise rarely involve the oral tissues, such as *Klebsiella pneumoniae*, *Enterobacter cloacae*, and *Escherichia coli*, can develop but are less frequent than fungal or viral infections. In the later stages, ulcers secondary to systemic infections, particularly mycobacterial may develop.

Bacillary angiomatosis is a vascular proliferative disease caused by *Bartonella henselae* and should respond to antimicrobial therapy. However, it can mimic Kaposi's sarcoma clinically and, to some extent, histologically. It affects the skin more frequently than the oral cavity.

Systemic mycoses

Histoplasmosis or cryptococcosis can give rise to tumour-like masses or ulcerative lesions. Histoplasmosis most frequently affects the palate, gingivae, and oropharynx.

Malignant neoplasms

Kaposi's sarcoma → Summary chart 26.1 p. 435

Kaposi sarcoma is discussed in detail in Chapter 25. In the setting of HIV, Kaposi sarcoma is mainly seen in men who have sex with men. Despite reduced incidence following introduction of ART, this is still the commonest oral malignant neoplasm in HIV infection.

Kaposi sarcoma is also very occasionally seen in HIV-negative immunosuppressed organ transplant patients, but one in the mouth of a young or middle-aged male patient is virtually pathognomonic of HIV infection. It is usually associated with a CD4+ lymphocyte count of less than 200/µl and frequently associated with other effects of HIV infection such as candidosis, hairy leukoplakia, or necrotising periodontitis.

Although oral Kaposi's sarcoma may be the presenting complaint for HIV infection, the tumour is usually multifocal, with lesions affecting skin, lymph nodes, and viscera.

Head and neck sites are typically oropharyngeal, cutaneous, or in the cervical lymph nodes. Within the mouth, the palate is the most frequently affected site and the tumour produces a flat or nodular purplish lesion. The clinical differential diagnosis is from oral purpura, bacillary angiomatosis, and pyogenic granulomas, from which it can be distinguished by biopsy (Ch. 25).

Lymphomas

General features of oral lymphomas are discussed in Chapter 28. Lymphomas develop in intraoral sites or salivary glands far more frequently than in HIV-negative persons. Typical sites within the mouth are the palate or gingiva, causing soft painless swellings that ulcerate when traumatised. Lymphomas have no useful features for diagnosis clinically, biopsy is required.

Most lymphomas in HIV infection are high-grade B-cell lymphomas of large cell or immunoblastic type, and many are caused by EBV infection. Lymphomas are increasingly the first presenting sign of HIV infection but are now overall less frequent since ART has become widespread.

Burkitt's lymphoma is the second commonest lymphoma in HIV-positive persons and carries a poor prognosis.

Plasmablastic lymphoma is seen virtually only in HIV-positive persons and has a strong predilection for the oral cavity. It is caused by coinfection with HIV and EBV and, unlike other lymphomas, has increased since ART introduction.

Lymphomas combined with immunosuppression used to have a dire prognosis, but with ART they have much the same prognosis as in the non-HIV population.

General review PMID: 34469512

Oral plasmablastic lymphoma PMID: 21783402 and 29917262

Lymphadenopathy

Lymphadenopathy is characteristic of symptomatic HIV infection and its prodrome. Cervical lymphadenopathy is probably the most common head and neck manifestation of HIV infection.

The nodes have reduced helper T-cells in the paracortical region and greater numbers of suppressor T-cells there and in the follicles. The nodes are enlarged initially because of hyperplasia but later undergo involution and shrink. HIV infection can be detected in the dendritic antigen-presenting cells in the lymphoid follicles. Untreated, the lymph nodes become virtually or entirely functionless.

Enlarged cervical lymph nodes in HIV infection can also be due to lymphomas and Castleman's disease (Ch. 32).

Autoimmune disease

The most common autoimmune phenomenon in AIDS is thrombocytopenic purpura (Fig. 30.10). This can give rise to oral purple patches that may be mistaken for Kaposi's sarcoma, petechiae, or blood blisters. Other autoimmune diseases reported in AIDS are lupus erythematosus and Sjögren's-like salivary gland disease.

Gingivitis and periodontitis

HIV-related periodontal disease in untreated patients includes necrotising gingivitis and periodontitis and accelerated periodontitis (Ch. 7). Necrotising periodontitis (NUP) indicates marked immunosuppression and a poor prognosis. The causative organisms are as in immunocompetent patients, and there is marked pain with local bone loss, tooth mobility, ulceration, and bleeding (Fig. 30.11). Systemic metronidazole or penicillin with topical povidone iodine, or chlorhexidine are rapidly effective.

Linear gingival erythema is a controversial entity currently considered a manifestation of candidosis in the gingival crevice and attached gingiva. Scaling, improved oral hygiene, and chlorhexidine is usually effective, but antifungals may be required. Linear gingival erythema usually affects the anterior gingiva. Whether candidal infection accounts for all cases is unclear as the diagnostic criteria are not very specific. It may be mistaken clinically for desquamative gingivitis (Ch.16).

Introduction of ART has caused a dramatic fall in the incidence of necrotising periodontitis. In effectively treated individuals, the types and severity of periodontitis are similar to those in immunocompetent individuals. However, the longer lifespan of treated patients may yet reveal some degree of predisposition to conventional periodontitis. Gingival recession appears to be more severe.

Types of gingivitis and periodontitis seen in HIV infection are summarised in Summary chart 30.1.

Review PMID: 22909108 and 23755999

In treated patients PMID: 31850628

Salivary gland disease

→ Summary chart 22.2 p. 393

In adults a Sjögren's-like syndrome with xerostomia may develop, but with lack of characteristic autoantibodies (particularly SS-A and SS-B).

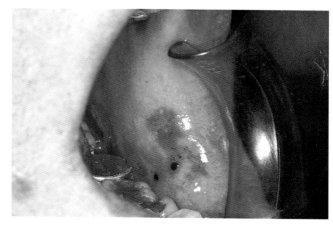

Fig. 30.10 Purpura. Patches such as these in late HIV infection can be mistaken for Kaposi's sarcoma.

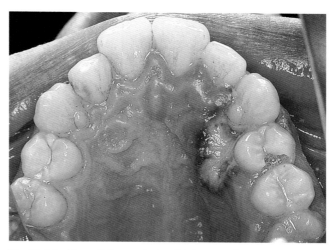

Fig. 30.11 Necrotising periodontitis in HIV infection. Soft tissue and bone are lost virtually simultaneously, and tissue destruction of the degree shown here can take only a few months. A low CD4⁺ cell count and poor prognosis are typically associated. *(Courtesy Prof. WH Binnie.)*

A specific HIV-associated salivary gland disease (previously HIV salivary cystic disease) primarily affects children and young adults with HIV infection, causing chronic soft parotid enlargement of one or both glands, usually asymptomatic but sometimes painful. As many as 20% of HIV-positive children are affected. The disease has increased in incidence since ART introduction, suggesting it is an infection, and the BK virus has been proposed as the cause. Lymphocytes infiltrate the glands, form lymphoid follicles, and cause the ducts to expand into large cysts, which are easily seen on ultrasound.

In diffuse CD8⁺ lymphocytosis syndrome, a disease of adults, the glands are infiltrated by CD8⁺ T cells, mostly memory T cells. This HIV effect affects many organs. The T cells localise around ducts, kill and replace the acini, and cause fibrosis in a manner similar to that in Sjögren's syndrome. Salivary secretion is reduced. There may also be new lymphoid tissue with lymphoid follicles and cysts. These various salivary gland diseases are not clearly defined and show clinical and histological overlap. Ultrasound scans and the clinical presentation are usually sufficient for diagnosis, but if HIV infection is not suspected, biopsy

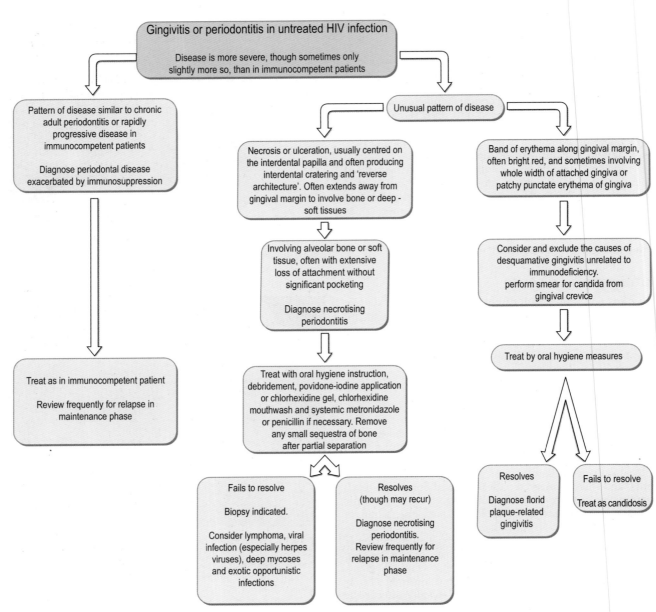

Summary chart 30.1 Types of gingivitis and periodontitis seen in HIV infection.

shows the typical features and HIV p24 protein can be identified using immunohistochemistry in the lymphoid follicles.

Lymphoma is a risk, developing in 1% of patients.

Review PMID: 30827854

Diffuse CD8⁺ lymphocytosis syndrome
PMID: general 25660200 salivary 9619675

Miscellaneous oral lesions

Mucosal ulcers

Major aphthae (Figs. 30.12 and 30.13) can be troublesome, interfere with eating, and accelerate deterioration of health. They become frequent and severe with declining immune function. Necrotising oral ulceration of an ill-defined nature and aphthae-like ulcers are common oral signs.

Persistent ulcers that might be left to assess healing in a non-HIV infected person require biopsy in HIV infection to assess them for possible infectious causes: *herpes simplex*

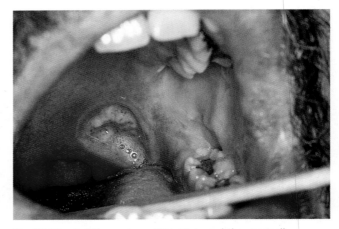

Fig. 30.12 Aphthous stomatitis. Major aphthae typically become more frequent and severe while immune function deteriorates and can add considerably to the patient's disabilities. Note the deep ulceration.

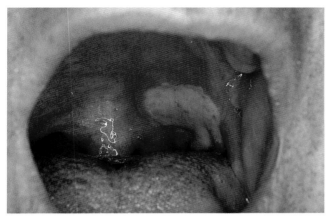

Fig. 30.13 Major aphthous ulcer. A shallower ulcer with surrounding erythema, in an earlier stage than that in Fig. 30.12.

virus, cytomegalovirus or mycobacteria, and also for lymphoma.

Major aphthae usually respond dramatically to thalidomide, but this should only be used when other possible causes of ulcers have been excluded. The possibility that oral ulceration may be an adverse effect of drugs used in ART needs to be borne in mind.

Diagnosis and treatment PMID: 14507229

Oral hyperpigmentation

→ Summary chart 26.1 p. 435

Pigmentation in HIV infection is of unknown cause. It may also be a complication of treatment with zidovudine (see Ch. 26).

Oral adverse effects of ART

Most of the protease inhibitors can cause xerostomia, disturbed taste sensation, and perioral paraesthesia. Many of these and other components of ART can also cause erythema multiforme, other allergic responses, and ulcers. Allergic responses to all drugs are increased in HIV infection as a result of immune dysregulation. Atrophy of facial fat is an unusual complication of nucleoside reverse-transcriptase inhibitors that can be treated with dermal fillers (Ch. 27).

ART is extremely complex and consultation with the patient's HIV physician is likely to be required if any oral manifestation fails to respond to initial treatment or when the diagnosis is in doubt.

Oral adverse effects ART PMID: 23530806

RISKS OF TRANSMISSION OF HIV INFECTION TO HEALTHCARE WORKERS

It is normal practice to regard all patients as potentially infective and treat them with universal precautions. These are effective against HIV transmission, so infection in a healthcare setting is very rare. The usual cause has been a needle-stick injury causing accidental injection of a significant amount of infected blood. By contrast, many other needle injuries in which little blood has been transferred have failed to transmit the virus. Most healthcare workers who have developed HIV infection have not acquired it as a result of their occupation.

Almost all documented cases of transmission to healthcare workers in the United States occurred before 1999. ART reduces infectivity.

General aspects of dental management

Attitudes to the risks of managing patients with HIV infection have changed dramatically during the epidemic. In the 1990s there was considerable fear that HIV infection was an unstoppable pandemic. Currently is it managed as any other infection risk and it is understood that other infectious diseases carry greater risks. These changes have come about with reduced stigmatization, better identification, effective treatment, post-exposure prophylaxis, and better understanding of the risks.

At the time of writing, there are just under 100,000 antibody-positive, potentially infective persons in Britain, but most are on ART and of low infectivity. A greater risk is posed by patients unaware of their HIV-positive status, but there are estimated to be only 6500 such individuals, a number that is in decline. It would be unethical and unprofessional to refuse to treat an HIV-infected patient regardless of the possibilities of acquiring the infection or transmitting it to other patients. No special precautions are necessary but the operator should take particular care to avoid accidental self-injury with an instrument that may have been contaminated with serum or blood. The possibility of transmitting HIV infection during dental treatment inevitably causes anxiety, but the risk is considerably lower than that of acquiring viral hepatitis.

References for infection control are with hepatitis in Chapter 35.

Post-exposure prophylaxis and sharps injury

Any healthcare worker receiving a needle-stick or other sharps injury exposure to potentially HIV infected body fluids should be assessed to determine whether anti-retroviral drugs should be prescribed. This reduces the risk of transmission of HIV. All UK national health service employers including dental practices are required to have a procedure in place that allows post-exposure prophylaxis to be given within 24 hours. After that time, its effectiveness is much reduced.

Whether or not post-exposure prophylaxis with ART is appropriate depends on the risk of transmission as assessed by the type of injury and infectivity of the patient. Although there is a general acceptance that benefits generally outweigh risks, it is generally not recommended in occupational injury unless the index patient has a detectable HIV viral load or the viral load is unknown. If required, the drugs selected take into account any drug-resistant HIV strains known in the donor. The adverse effects of current post-exposure prophylaxis are significant but not problematic, and treatment is usually continued for 4 weeks.

The immediate action for any injury potentially contaminated with infectious body fluids is to wash liberally with soap and water and encourage free bleeding. Wounds should not be sucked, squeezed, or scrubbed but may be cleaned with an antiseptic if desired. Splashes to the mucous membranes, including conjunctivae, should be irrigated copiously with water. This should be done before and after removal of contact lenses. Saliva is considered infectious in the context of a dental surgery because it is almost certainly contaminated with small amounts of blood.

HIV infection is transmitted by 0.3% of medical sharps injuries and 0.1% of exposures to mucous membranes, including the eye if the patient is not on ART. Transmission by splash injury is considered very rare and always follows splashes with blood, but only eight cases are accepted worldwide. HIV cannot be transmitted through intact skin.

Post-exposure prophylaxis is considered more than 90% effective in preventing transmission, but these data come from sexual transmission and the evidence base is weak. It may be even more effective in healthcare exposure for a variety of reasons. The current UK recommendation is that prophylaxis should be given if the risk of transmission exceeds 1:1000. Pregnancy is not a contraindication. Prophylaxis is not generally recommended for bite injuries unless the risk is high.

UK post exposure prophylaxis 2021 PMID: 35166004

Web URL 30.4 US occupational prophylaxis 2018 https://stacks.cdc.gov/view/cdc/20711

RISKS OF TRANSMISSION OF HIV TO PATIENTS

Although transmission to healthcare workers is exceedingly rare, transmission to patients has occurred. A dentist in Florida infected six patients, and three other healthcare workers have been documented to have infected a single patient each. However, all these cases occurred many years ago in the early years of the epidemic, before ART. There has been no documented case of transmission to a patient in the UK.

Current regulations require that dental clinicians who have become or think that they have become infected by HIV, hepatitis, or other blood-borne viruses should seek appropriate medical supervision.

HIV-positive dentists, who are receiving effective treatment, have a viral load less than 200 copies/mL and are regularly monitored, are allowed to undertake exposure-prone procedures. The decision on fitness to practice is made by the patient's HIV consultant physician, and the dentist will need to be listed on a confidential register. Individuals may be subject to restrictions on a case-by-case basis. A list of 'exposure prone procedures' is provided in which there would be a risk of contamination of the patients open tissues by blood from an injured dentist.

Web URL 30.5 UK guidance for dentists infected by blood borne viruses: https://www.gov.uk/government/publications/bbvs-in-healthcare-workers-health-clearance-and-management

Allergy, autoimmune and autoinflammatory disease

31

Abnormal immune reactions against environmental antigens (allergy), self-antigens (autoimmunity) and diseases associated with abnormal control of inflammation (autoinflammatory) are common (Box 31.1). They cause specific diseases, adverse drug reactions, and can affect dental management.

ALLERGIC OR HYPERSENSITIVITY REACTIONS

Epidemiology and presentation

Allergy has complex epidemiology. Allergic dermatitis is more frequent in people of African heritage than in Europeans, who have a greater incidence of hay fever, but within these groups there are large differences in incidence between countries. People of African heritage also appear more susceptible to some, but not all, types of food allergy and anaphylactic reactions. It is important to be aware of this as rashes may be significantly difficult to identify on dark skin. Inflamed oedema of a skin anaphylactic reaction is less obvious, often a darker purple colour than is usually described, sometimes without colour or detectable only by swelling. These differences could be critical in an emergency.

Atopy

Atopy is a genetic predisposition to multiple allergic responses, usually of the immunoglobulin (Ig) E-mediated or type 1 reaction type. Patients who are atopic may have several of the conditions listed in this chapter and usually have more pronounced responses than those with a single allergy. The main atopic diseases are atopic dermatitis (eczema), hay fever, and asthma. Incidence of atopic disease rose dramatically in Western countries after the 1960s but has now peaked; it continues to increase in prevalence in developing countries. In the UK and US between 5% and 10% of adults are atopic and the incidence is twice as high in children.

The cause(s) of atopy are unknown. Mutations in the filaggrin protein that contributes to the epithelial permeability barrier are very frequent.

Atopy presents in the first year of life with dermatitis. Asthma and hay fever develop in later childhood or adolescence. In late adulthood the severity wanes.

There are no oral manifestations of atopic disease itself, and there is no such entity as oral eczema. Food allergies affect 30% of atopic individuals, usually to cow's milk, wheat, soya or fruits, and those with hay fever may also experience oral reactions in the pollen-food syndrome (discussed later). Atopic individuals are likely to develop latex allergy, and atopic dentists need to take extra precautions against hand eczema. Contrary to previous belief, atopy does not predispose to penicillin allergy, but people with atopy tend to have severe reactions if they do develop this allergy.

Drugs (Box 31.2) used to treat atopic diseases may complicate dental treatment.

Box 31.1 Important immunologically mediated diseases

Atopic disease and related allergies (reactions to exogenous antigens)

- Asthma; eczema; hay fever; urticaria
- Food allergies: nuts, wheat, shellfish, milk, eggs
- Insect stings
- Latex allergy
- Some drug reactions, especially to penicillins
- Anaphylaxis and acute allergic angio-oedema
- Contact dermatitis
- Exercise-induced/food anaphylaxis

Autoimmune diseases (reactions to self-antigens)

Autoimmune connective tissue diseases

- Rheumatoid arthritis
- Sjögren's syndrome*
- Lupus erythematosus*
- Systemic sclerosis*

Autoimmune diseases with specific autoantibodies

- Pernicious anaemia (chronic atrophic gastritis)*
- Idiopathic and drug-associated thrombocytopenic purpura*
- Drug-associated leukopenia*
- Autoimmune haemolytic anaemia
- Addison's disease*
- Hashimoto's thyroiditis
- Hyperthyroidism
- Idiopathic hypoparathyroidism*
- Pemphigus vulgaris*
- Mucous membrane pemphigoid*

Mixed autoimmune/autoinflammatory diseases

- Behçet's disease
- Reactive arthritis*

Autoinflammatory diseases (abnormal inflammatory response)

- Crohn's disease* and ulcerative colitis
- Orofacial granulomatosis*
- Sarcoidosis *
- PFAPA (**P**eriodic **F**ever, **A**phthous stomatitis, **P**haryngitis, cervical **A**denitis) syndrome
- SAPHO (**S**ynovitis, **A**cne, **P**ustulosis, **H**yperostosis, **O**steitis) syndrome (Ch. 8)
- A20 haploinsufficiency

* Can give rise to characteristic oral changes

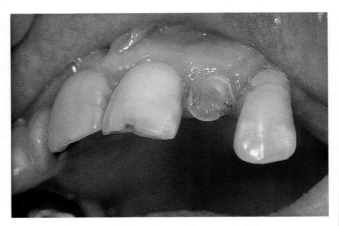

Fig. 31.2 Hypersensitivity to impression material. The same patient as in Fig. 31.1, showing the site of the impression photographed at the same time. No allergic response is evident intraorally.

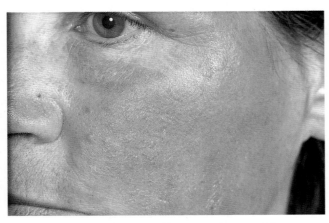

Fig. 31.1 Allergic rash triggered by impression material. Generalised facial erythema and slight oedema can be observed.

Contact dermatitis

Contact dermatitis resembles eczema clinically but is a cell-mediated (type 4) reaction. It affects only the region where the allergen contacted the skin, appears after 24–72 hours and persists for several weeks after exposure. It causes an erythematous rash, with blisters in severe cases. Nickel is the most common cause. The oral equivalent to contact dermatitis is, however, exceedingly rare (Figs 31.1 and 31.2).

Contact dermatitis is an occupational hazard in dentistry. Nurses and technicians are at higher risk than dentists. Latex, soaps, and detergents, the aromatics they contain and methyl methacrylate are the most common occupational allergens. X-ray processing chemicals were potent sensitisers, but now are little used. Chlorhexidine has recently become a frequent cause of contact allergy. Volatile disinfectants and methacrylate fumes can be inhaled to cause respiratory symptoms, both allergic and through direct irritation.

The UK dentist has a legal obligation to protect the dental team against contact dermatitis (Box 31.3).

Chlorhexidine reactions PMID: 23222325

Oral contact reactions PMID: 23010830

Occupational risks PMID: 15884321

Latex and glove allergy

Latex allergy is the main allergic occupational disease affecting healthcare workers.

The necessity for gloving for all clinical work resulted in a dramatic rise in latex allergy in medicine and dentistry since 1980. In a survey in one UK dental school, the prevalence

of latex allergy was 9%, and 22% complained of chronic glove dermatitis. In the past, powdered latex gloves were particularly dangerous because the starch powder spread latex proteins into the environment.

There is no completely satisfactory alternative to latex gloves. Low protein content ('low NRL') latex gloves are available, and these are recommended when a latex glove is considered best, but they cannot be used if there is a risk of triggering asthma in the workplace. Once latex allergy

> **Box 31.4 Individuals at risk of latex allergy**
> - Healthcare professionals
> - Atopic patients
> - Patients with spina bifida
> - Patients with urogenital anomalies
> - Latex industry workers
> - Patients subject to multiple surgical procedures before the age of 7 years

Table 31.1 Some reactions to local analgesics in dentistry

Reaction	Cause
Failed analgesia	Usually poor technique
Pain on injection	Poor technique
Persistent anaesthesia or paraesthesia	Direct toxic effect of agent on nerve, not necessarily following intraneural injection. Most common with articaine, possible with lidocaine
Post-operative trismus	Injection into medial pterygoid muscle, resulting in inflammation or haematoma. Haematoma from the venous plexus distal to nerve may cause trismus for several days
Syncope	Stress of injection, anxiety. By far the most common adverse reaction. See Box 44.3.
Diplopia, blanching of skin of face, loss of vision, ptosis	Intra-arterial injection or venous injection with retrograde flow. Effects mostly related to vasoconstrictor
Facial palsy or weakness	Intraparotid injection
Neuralgic pain on injection, prolonged analgesia	Intraneural injection or injection close to nerve
Methaemoglobinaemia. Cyanosis, tachycardia and, at high dose, sedative effect 1–3 hours after administration	Non-allergic pharmacological effect of prilocaine metabolite. Recommended dose exceeded. Increased risk in glucose-6-phosphatase deficiency
Muscle twitching and tremors with increasing dose, epileptiform seizures. At high doses central nervous system depression drowsiness, tinnitus, respiratory depression, bradycardia and arrhythmias	Lidocaine toxicity. Recommended dose exceeded. Other particular agents may have specific effects.
Angio-oedema	Could be non-allergic angio-oedema, but consider allergic reaction first.
Oedema, urticarial or erythematous rash and itching	Likely allergic reaction.

to gloves has been acquired, reactions to all natural rubber products are observed, which may include rubber tubing, anaesthetic masks, catheters and tourniquets, prophylaxis cups, and alginate mixing bowls.

Latex allergy is important because it most frequently manifests as a type 1 urticarial contact reaction. In dentistry, this has the potential to put the airway at risk. Rarely, reactions to latex can be severe and fatal. Latex also triggers contact dermatitis. Different patients and dental team members have different risks and require different avoidance strategies and treatment.

It is not always obvious that a medical or dental device may contain natural rubber. For instance, bungs in local anaesthetic cartridges may contain latex. Even covered latex, such as a sphygmomanometer cuff, can shed latex proteins and trigger a reaction. For severe cases, it may be necessary to refer patients to a centre with a latex-free surgery. Premedication with antihistamines or steroids to prevent reactions remains controversial. This may reduce the severity of a reaction but does not prevent it. Avoidance is a better strategy.

Prevention requires identifying people at risk (Box 31.4). Patients allergic to latex often have cross reactions with foods including banana, pineapple, kiwi, avocado, chestnut, and mango that contain related latex-type molecules. Food allergy must always be included when taking a medical history. Patients may report lip swelling on blowing up balloons.

Each dental practice should have a policy for latex allergy, its management, and the safe treatment of allergic patients. The majority of allergic patients can be safely treated in general practice with suitable precautions.

Most UK dentists now use non-latex gloves and rubber dam, usually nitrile or vinyl gloves though hypoallergenic latex remains available. Unfortunately, allergic dermatitis and localised urticarial reactions can still be triggered by these alternative materials, though much less frequently. The causative agents are thiurams and dithiocarbamate accelerators. Accelerator-free nitrile gloves are available. Contact hand dermatitis cannot automatically be blamed on gloves since all are permeable to some degree to other sensitising agents.

General review PMID: 14616859

Dental implications review PMID: 9927072

Latex-free anaesthetics PMID: 23094572

Allergy to local anaesthetic

Allergic reactions to local anaesthetics are rare but possible, affecting 1% or less of patients who claim to be affected. The vast majority of patients referred for testing have developed other recognised complications of analgesia, either expected pharmacological reactions to high doses of the analgesic or vasoconstrictor, intravascular injection, intraparotid injection, intraneural injection, or similar adverse events. These are normally readily recognised by their clinical signs and symptoms (Table 31.1).

True allergic reactions may be to latex in the cartridge (unlikely), analgesic agent or other components such as preservative (metabisulphite antioxidant in adrenaline containing preparations), or to some unrelated dental material to which the patient was exposed at the same time. Amide agents used in dentistry are the least likely type to cause allergy. Unfortunately, determining the exact cause of a reaction is not always possible with confidence. Nevertheless, it is important to investigate potential reactions as genuine allergy could cause a medical emergency. The dentist should be able to screen out the non-allergic reactions listed in Table 31.1 by questioning the patient and, if necessary, contacting the dentist who administered the analgesic to check which agent was given.

Features suggesting a true allergy are facial swelling or other peripheral oedema, hypotension, and itchy erythematous or urticarial rash, which indicate a possible type 1 reaction. A few patients develop delayed reactions, usually with a rash and sometimes delayed oedema. Reactive patients are also likely to have multiple allergies or atopy.

The common allergens appear to be metabisulphite preservative and bupivacaine, whereas lidocaine allergies are rare. Prilocaine causes more reactions overall, but these are rarely allergic. Referral for testing is indicated when no definite alternative explanation is found or multiple reactions are developed.

Local anaesthetic testing

Testing is difficult because a definitive result requires a challenge injection and thus carries some, albeit small, risk. Skin patch tests may reveal a delayed reaction but are of little value. Skin scratch tests, allowing a minute amount of various solutions to penetrate to the dermis, are usually performed, followed by a small intradermal (very superficially placed) injection of agents that produce no reaction on a scratch test. Control saline injections are required to identify patients with an exaggerated inflammatory response that might be misconstrued as allergy. If allergy appears likely before testing, the solutions may be diluted to reduce the challenge. A positive reaction is identified by a wheal and erythematous flare around the agent, but not the control. A negative result makes allergy extremely unlikely, but a full-dose injection is required to exclude other types of pharmacological or idiosyncratic reaction. The whole procedure must be performed in an environment equipped to deal with a severe anaphylactic reaction, even though this is very unlikely.

Allergy to both ester and amide types of analgesic is extremely rare, so an effective safe analgesic can usually be found. Most other adverse reactions can be reduced in frequency using good technique and management of anxiety.

Review PMID: 20831929 and 32090398

Diagnosis & management reactions PMID: 21905354

Adverse reactions in general PMID: 34909470

Asthma

Asthma can carry significant risks in dentistry and is dealt with in Chapter 34.

Other type 1 reactions

Many prescribed drugs and materials used in dentistry can trigger type 1 allergic or anaphylactic reactions. Penicillins are the most frequent trigger prescribed by dentists. Chlorhexidine has recently been recognised to cause type 1 reactions, two of which have been fatal following irrigation of extraction sockets.

Chlorhexidine allergy PMID: 27439274

MUCOSAL ALLERGIC RESPONSES

Many patients claim mucosal allergic responses to foods, toothpastes, and other agents, but do not distinguish allergic from irritant effects. The oral mucous membrane is an unusual site and normally is unable to mount contact dermatitis reactions. There is no such condition as oral eczema.

The oral mucosa has some features of an 'immunologically privileged site' such as the brain or placenta, where external antigens induce tolerance rather than immune responses.

Oral allergy 'syndrome'

This name is given to a mild type 1 hypersensitivity reaction in the oral mucosa caused by cross-reacting food allergens and affects approximately 2% of the UK population, mostly individuals with hay fever. Typical allergens are raw, but not cooked, apples and fruits, nuts and vegetables. Most patients are atopic and have a primary diagnosis of hay fever or other allergies, particularly in Europe and North America to birch pollen, but react to 'class 2' food allergens that often have a particular protein fold domain structurally similar to the sensitising pollen. This is a recently recognised condition and appears to be increasing in incidence in parallel with the increase in childhood hay fever.

Individuals allergic to pollens may have cross reactions with a wide range of raw foods (pollen food syndrome) with specific cross reactions recognised. The most common allergen in the UK is birch pollen, and people allergic to it, and particularly those allergic to grass pollens in addition, have more than 75% chance of developing pollen food syndrome. Birch pollen is suggested to cross react with almonds, apples, apricots, avocados, celery, hazelnuts, kiwi (Chinese gooseberry), nectarines, and many other foods. Different pollens and cross reactions occur in different countries depending on their different environmental challenges. People allergic to latex may react intraorally to apple or avocado (latex food syndrome) as noted previously.

Reactions are mild and localised, start shortly after allergen exposure with an itching or burning sensation followed by localised swelling in site where the mucosa is lax: lips, floor of mouth, and soft palate. Diagnosis is based on signs, symptoms on exposure, and history of allergy.

Similar reactions are seen in children and adolescents who use pollen desensitisation as a treatment for hay fever. Short-lived swelling appears when the pollen suspension is held under the tongue. Unfortunately, this desensitisation treatment seems to have little effect on the severity of any associated oral allergy syndrome.

Oral allergy can be used in reverse to treat hay fever. Desensitisation with the oral allergen, such as dietary apple can reduce the reactivity to some tree pollens. Oral allergy syndrome is normally managed by avoiding allergens but can be treated with conventional antiallergic medications if required. Severe anaphylactic reactions are extremely rare, but concentrated allergens in foods could be a risk and patients should be referred for specialist advice.

Oral allergy syndrome must be distinguished from simple type 1 hypersensitivity reactions in which the primary allergen is placed on the mucosa. These are more severe.

Review PMID: 25887974 and 25757079

Role of dentist 31478696

Web URL 31.1 Management guideline UK: https://www.bsaci.org/ and enter 'pollen food syndrome' in the search box

Allergy to metals
Nickel and chromium

Nickel is the most common metal causing skin and mucosal allergy, and this affects 10% of women. It usually causes

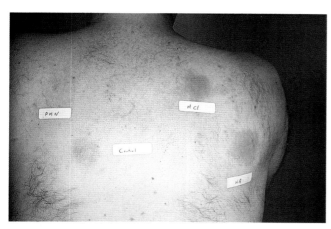

Fig. 31.3 Patch testing for dental materials. Four panels of 12 patches impregnated with different dental materials were kept in contact with the skin for 48 hours. Erythema, oedema and a palpable nodule indicate reaction to mercury but amalgam restorations provoked no intraoral reaction.

contact dermatitis as described previously. Skin patch testing is diagnostic. Nickel is ubiquitous and present in foods, as well as cobalt-chromium and other dental metal alloys. However, patients with known allergy can tolerate these in the mouth. In a few it may then cause a characteristic rash but not oral lesions. Indeed, it may even be therapeutic as oral dosing with nickel salts has been shown to induce tolerance and can be used to desensitise patients.

Chromium in dental alloys does not sensitise, because in its metallic state the metal is immunologically inert.

Nickel dental allergy PMID: 21439867

Dental allergens PMID: 19489970

Mercury

Mercury hypersensitivity

Reactions to mercury might be either allergic or toxic. By far the greatest danger from mercury is systemic absorption of toxic doses of organic mercury compounds such as methyl mercury, from the diet or environment. Diets containing fish and other marine products provide the greatest doses of mercury to humans by far. This mercury comes from environmental pollution concentrated in marine organisms. Otherwise, high intake is likely to be occupational. Organic mercury salts are powerful neurotoxins, but not the metal.

Metallic mercury, with an oxidation state of zero, is almost completely inert and non-toxic other than by inhalation of vapour. Mercury in dental amalgam is either in this metallic form or has reacted to form inorganic salts.

Hypersensitivity to mercury or its salts causes an inflammatory and sometimes vesiculating reaction on contacting skin. Allergy can be confirmed using skin patch testing. The incidence of mercury allergy is difficult to assess because testing has, in the past, often been performed with high concentrations of mercury salts that are directly irritant to skin. It appears that only a few per cent of the population claiming to be allergic actually are. Even those with proven sensitivity can usually tolerate mercury amalgams in the mouth (Fig. 31.3), but care must be taken during removal and placement that no amalgam touches the patient's skin. In practical terms, it is usually simpler to use composite materials.

Topical amalgam lichenoid reactions are discussed in Chapter 16. These have a moderately strong relationship to mercury hypersensitivity and are usually associated with corroded amalgams that leach component metals. Allergy to silver, copper or tin components can account for amalgam sensitivity but is rarer. Those who are demonstrably allergic and show the closest physical relationship between mucosal inflammation and the amalgam gain the best response on removal of the offending restoration(s).

There appears to be no adverse reaction to amalgam tattoos, even in those allergic to mercury.

Mercury toxicity

Systemic mercury toxicity remains a possible occupational hazard of dentistry, but widespread use of encapsulated amalgam has rendered this risk of only historical interest. Practices must include risk assessments and procedures for dealing with potential spillage. Dentists have had decades of exposure to mercury and absorbed significant amounts, but do not appear to have been significantly harmed. Some evidence suggests association with minor neurological changes, but the exact cause of these is unclear.

The possibility of chronic mercury toxicity caused by release of mercury from amalgam fillings has given rise to public anxiety and been promoted by some practitioners with vested interests. While mercury, and particularly its organic compounds, are undoubtedly toxic, exposure to vapour or soluble inorganic salts from amalgams provide infinitesimally small doses. Vapour levels in the mouth have been overestimated and incorrect assumptions made about its efficient absorption in the lungs. Most is exhaled and doses do not exceed exposure to environmental levels. The vapour released by removing an amalgam far exceeds the amount it could release in situ in the patient's lifetime, even though oral bacteria are able to convert metallic mercury to organic mercury salts.

It is unfortunate that the potential symptoms of chronic low-level mercury toxicity are so vague. People opposed to amalgam list many diseases they say are caused by mercury toxicity. These are often chronic relapsing conditions in which disease activity is unpredictable and difficult to monitor making any possible association with amalgam difficult or impossible to investigate. To date, no official body considers amalgam restorations to cause any harm to patients, indeed most actively declare it safe. Reactions can also occur to the composite synthetic alternatives and such substitute restorations require replacement twice as frequently.

Using the precautionary principle, some countries have made restriction on the placement of amalgam restorations in individuals who are potentially more sensitive, usually those with proven allergy, children, pregnant and breast-feeding women, and those with severe kidney disease. There is no evidence that these groups are at risk but avoiding amalgam in deciduous teeth reduces environmental pollution on shedding. Such environmental and political concerns often drive regulation. In 2021 the World Dental Federation (FDI) updated and confirmed its policy of phasing down amalgam use despite the lack of evidence to link amalgam with chronic and degenerative diseases. This conclusion must remain under constant review as currently some studies have suggested links between amalgam restorations and multiple sclerosis, Alzheimer's disease, and Parkinson's disease, but these require further evaluation.

As caries is an entirely preventable disease and reducing in most countries, the need for amalgam may disappear before these contentious disease linkages can be proven or disproven.

Nevertheless, dentists have a duty to avoid environmental pollution with mercury. Eventually amalgam may be phased out for environmental reasons, but in the meantime amalgam separators in wastewater outlets and safe waste disposal (including extracted teeth) are required of every UK dentist.

It is beyond the remit of dentists, but amalgam released into the environment from crematoria also has to be controlled and generates significant metallic mercury environmental contamination unless process to trap the emissions are in place.

Mucosal reactions to amalgam PMID: 18350847

Mercury toxicity PMID: 9231518 and 9391753

Amalgam versus composite toxicity PMID: 35308016

Amalgam versus composite restoration life PMID: 34387873

FDI phase down information PMID: 35074198 and 35074199

Neurological disease PMID: 30909378

ANGIO-OEDEMA → Summary chart 35.1 p. 518

Allergic angio-oedema

Allergic angio-oedema is an IgE-mediated or type 1 acute hypersensitivity reaction. It is directly equivalent to an urticarial rash but affects deeper tissues and may arise in conjunction with an urticarial rash. The head and neck, particularly around and in the mouth, are the most common site, followed by the hands. Angio-oedema can cause gross swelling of the lips, face and neck over a period of minutes to hours and, when severe, can threaten the airway. Patients may have a history of allergic disease or atopy.

Treatment is same as for any acute type 1 hypersensitivity reaction (Ch. 44).

Hereditary angio-oedema

Hereditary angio-oedema is due to deficiency or mutational inactivation of the complement factor C1 esterase inhibitor, and is thus, pedantically speaking, an immunodeficiency. However, this complement deficiency produces no abnormal susceptibility to infection. Since C1 esterase inhibitor is an inactivator of the first complement component, its absence leads to uncontrolled spontaneous complement activation via the classical pathway. The result is excessive bradykinin production, causing vasodilation, increased permeability, and pain. In the process, C4 is consumed, and its persistently low level in the serum during asymptomatic periods is a useful diagnostic test, together with assay for C1 esterase inhibitor itself.

Inheritance is autosomal dominant, but 25% of cases are new mutations and have no family history. Episodes of gross but localised oedematous swelling follow stimuli such as minor injuries and, particularly, dental treatment (Fig 31.4). The attacks last several days unless treated and can cause respiratory obstruction. There is a significant mortality.

Similar angio-oedema may also be an effect of angiotensin-converting enzyme inhibitor drugs, and some patients have alterations in other genes affecting function of C1 esterase inhibitor.

Treatment of an acute attack requires purified C1 esterase inhibitor concentrate or fresh frozen plasma, kallikrein inhibitors or bradykinin receptor antagonists. These drugs can

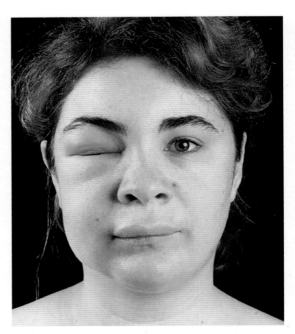

Fig. 31.4 Typical facial swelling in a patient with hereditary angioedema due to C1 inhibitor deficiency *(from Bork K, Barnstedt S-E, 2003. Laryngeal oedema and death from asphyxiation after tooth extraction in four patients with hereditary angioedema. In: The Journal of the American Dental Association, 134 (8): 1088–1094.)*

be used prophylactically if dental treatment triggers attacks or when intubation is required.

The most important point is not to mistake an attack for an allergic reaction. Angio-oedema does not respond to epinephrine, steroids or antihistamines.

Case series PMID: 1518394

Dental complications 18063242 and fatality 12956349

Causes PMID: 24484972

Management PMID: 25605519

AUTOIMMUNE DISEASES

Autoimmune diseases result from immune reactions against host antigens ('self' antigens). They may be mediated by antibodies (humoral response) or T cells (cell-mediated) or both. In many cases the exact mechanisms are unknown. Autoimmune diseases are one end of a spectrum of diseases that extends to auto-inflammatory disease (Box 31.1) and tissue damage in some autoimmune diseases is caused partly by a degree of dysregulation of inflammation.

To develop a host-targeted immune response requires breakdown of immunological tolerance. Possible mechanisms include extrinsic agents inducing a cross-reacting response ('molecular mimicry', e.g., rheumatic fever), release of self-antigens normally held sequestered in protected sites (e.g., sympathetic ophthalmia) or exposure of internally concealed antigens when proteins are denatured in inflammatory foci. It is thought that most autoimmune disease results from loss of B-cell tolerance. When T-cell reactions are involved, they appear to be secondary to changes in control by B cells.

Many autoimmune diseases trigger polyclonal B-cell activation, resulting in random activation of many B lymphocytes with antigen specificity unrelated to the disease itself.

Box 31.5   Typical features of autoimmune disease

- Significantly more common in women
- Onset often in middle age
- Levels of immunoglobulins usually raised
- Family history frequently positive
- Circulating autoantibodies frequently also detectable in unaffected family members
- Multiple circulating autoantibodies to several different and possibly unrelated antigens
- Often a higher risk of developing a second autoimmune disease
- Immunoglobulin and/or complement often detectable at sites of tissue damage
- Often associated with human leukocyte antigen-B8 and DR3
- Immunosuppressive or anti-inflammatory treatment frequently limits tissue damage

Box 31.6   Types and examples of autoimmune disease

Organ or cell-specific autoantibodies

- Hashimoto's thyroiditis
- Chronic atrophic gastritis (pernicious anaemia)
- Addison's disease
- Idiopathic hypoparathyroidism
- Pemphigus
- Pemphigoid
- Idiopathic thrombocytopenic purpura
- Autoimmune haemolytic anaemia
- Myasthenia gravis

Non-organ-specific autoantibodies (the connective tissue diseases)

- Lupus erythematosus
- Rheumatoid arthritis
- Sjögren's syndrome
- Systemic sclerosis
- Primary biliary cirrhosis
- Dermatomyositis
- Mixed connective tissue disease

These secrete large amounts of antibody, raising the plasma immunoglobulin concentration. This explains why these diseases often have many other different and apparently anomalous autoantibodies. For example, anti-thyroid antibodies are common in Sjögren's syndrome despite autoimmune thyroiditis having no apparent connection to salivary gland disease. Similarly, rheumatoid factor, an autoantibody against immunoglobulin Fc is found in many autoimmune and connective tissue diseases without arthritis as a component.

The autoimmune diseases have many features in common (Box 31.5). By no means are all of their mechanisms are clearly understood (Box 31.6). Others with particular dental relevance have been discussed in other chapters, and only the connective tissue diseases are described here.

Oral manifestations autoimmunity PMID: 23040353

The connective tissue diseases

The connective tissue diseases used to be thought of as autoimmune diseases directed against connective tissue components such as collagen, proteoglycan and elastin. In reality the targets and mechanisms of immune damage are unclear. The main examples are rheumatoid arthritis, lupus erythematosus, systemic sclerosis, primary biliary cirrhosis and Sjögren's syndrome. The last can be associated with any of the others or develop in isolation. Many patients have mixed connective tissue disease or overlap diseases.

Rheumatoid arthritis

Rheumatoid arthritis is by far the most common connective tissue disorder and an example of a disease with both autoimmune and autoinflammatory components. It affects at least 1% of the population and is three times more common in women than men. The general features of arthritis and temporomandibular joint involvement are discussed in Chapter 14.

The implications of rheumatoid arthritis for dentistry are shown in Box 31.7.

Sjögren's syndrome

See Chapter 22.

Box 31.7   Features of rheumatoid arthritis of importance in dentistry

- Association with Sjögren's syndrome
- Chronic anaemia and its sequelae (Ch. 28)
- Fatigue
- Reduced manual dexterity, challenges with oral hygiene
- Access to dental care may be problematic
- Reduced mobility, difficulty lying supine, or still for long periods
- Atlantoaxial weakness in severe cases
- Joint replacement (currently not thought to merit antibiotic cover for dentistry)
- Drug treatment
  - Aspirin (bleeding, anaemia)
  - Non-steroidal anti-inflammatory drugs (bleeding, anaemia, lichenoid reactions)
  - Corticosteroids (adrenal suppression, immunosuppression, infections)
  - Antimalarials, gold (lichenoid reactions, oral and skin pigmentation)
  - Penicillamine (lichenoid reactions, taste loss)
  - Methotrexate (poor healing, oral ulcers, folate deficiency)

Systemic lupus erythematosus

Systemic lupus erythematosus (SLE) is caused by autoantibodies against DNA and its associated proteins. Antibodies against double-stranded DNA are almost diagnostic of SLE. There are also genetic predispositions affecting genes involved in non-specific immune mechanisms and complement producing an autoinflammatory element to the disease. Circulating autoantibody-antigen complexes lodge in small vessels where they trigger complement and activate neutrophils and macrophages, damaging the tissue. This happens particularly in the kidney.

Table 31.2 Organs and tissues affected in systemic lupus erythematosus

Organ/tissue	Clinical feature
Joints	Joint pains and arthritis
Skin	Rashes, erythema nodosum
Mouth	Stomatitis, Sjögren's syndrome
Serous membranes	Pleurisy, pericarditis
Heart	Endocarditis, myocarditis, pericarditis
	Libman-Sacks endocarditis of valves
Lungs	Pneumonitis
Kidneys	Nephritic syndrome, kidney failure
Central nervous system	Neuroses, psychoses, strokes, cranial
	Nerve palsies
Eyes	Conjunctivitis, retinal damage
Gastrointestinal tract	Hepatomegaly, pancreatitis
Blood	Anaemia, purpura

Box 31.8 Features of lupus erythematosus of importance in dentistry

- Association with Sjögren's syndrome
- Painful oral lichen-planus-like lesions
- Chronic anaemia and its sequelae (Ch. 28)
- Bleeding tendencies (antiplatelet antibodies or anticoagulants)
- Cardiac disease and risk of endocarditis
- Lower lip vermillion border involvement is a low risk potentially malignant disorder
- Drug treatment
  - Non-steroidal anti-inflammatory drugs (bleeding, anaemia, lichenoid reactions)
  - Corticosteroids (adrenal suppression, immunosuppression, infections)
  - Antimalarials (lichenoid reactions, oral and skin pigmentation)
  - Methotrexate (poor healing, oral ulcers, folate deficiency)
  - Belimumab (anti-B cell cytokine, immunosuppressant)

SLE affects approximately 0.05% of the UK population. People of Asian or African heritage are prone, and women are eight times more frequently affected than men. It is a disease of early adulthood and middle age. SLE can affect almost any body system, and the features vary according to the main organ systems affected (Table 31.2).

Clinically, joint pains and rashes are the most common manifestations, but the classical picture of a young woman with a butterfly rash across the midface is uncommon and not peculiar to SLE. Some patients have mild disease affecting only the skin; in others severe and debilitating disease can be fatal.

Approximately 20% of patients with SLE develop oral lesions. These somewhat resemble lichen planus (Ch. 16) but are more difficult to treat. The discoid form that affects the skin is also associated with oral lesions. Otherwise, it is the individual manifestations rather than the disease process itself that affect dental management (Box 31.8).

General review PMID: 17307106

Oral manifestations PMID: 15567365 and 17576335

Systemic sclerosis (scleroderma)

Systemic sclerosis is rare but has a poor prognosis. Clinically, the most common early signs are Raynaud's phenomenon and joint pains. Later, the skin becomes thinned, stiff and pigmented and the facial features become smoothed-out and mask-like. Opening of the mouth may become limited. This condition is discussed in detail in Chapter 14.

AUTOINFLAMMATORY DISEASES

Autoinflammatory diseases are caused by changes in genes that control inflammation, triggering spontaneous inflammation to damage the tissues without an activating immune reaction. Interleukin-1 pathways, tumour necrosis factor receptors and the cytokine and immune signalling pathway NF-κB are often involved.

The majority of such diseases recognised to date are rare and many are associated with single gene defects that produce unusual manifestations. Some are somatic mutations

affecting only myeloid stem cells in the bone marrow. Examples of pure autoinflammatory diseases with dental relevance include periodic fever with aphthous stomatitis pharyngitis and adenitis (PFAPA) (Ch. 16), synovitis, acne, pustulosis, hyperostosis and osteitis syndrome (SAPHO) (Ch. 8) and A20 haploinsufficiency disease. Oral ulcers and periodic fever are common features of several.

More significant for dentistry are diseases that have autoinflammatory and autoimmune components such as Crohn's disease (Ch. 35), sarcoidosis, Behçet's disease (Ch. 16) and ankylosing spondylitis.

Autoinflammatory concept PMID: 33609798

Oral manifestations, role of dentist PMID: 23040353

Sarcoidosis

→ Summary charts 22.2, 24.2 and 35.1 pp. 393, 418, 518

Sarcoidosis has an autoinflammatory component though it may be triggered initially by an immune reaction. An extrinsic trigger remains suspected but unknown. Microorganisms, pollens and environmental antigens have all been proposed. A number of genes are linked, and there is sometimes a familial predisposition. Mutations in the *NOD2* gene, that regulates recognition of bacterial peptidoglycan and induces inflammation, are known to cause childhood sarcoidosis. This gene is also linked to Crohn's disease, a similar granulomatous disease. Inflammation is enhanced, and immune reactions are suppressed.

The disease is more frequent in people of African heritage and those from Scandinavia, and the age of onset is usually 20–40 years. Almost any tissue can be affected. Common effects include fever, loss of weight, fatigue, breathlessness, cough and arthralgia. Erythema nodosum is the most common skin manifestation. Hypercalcaemia can lead to nephrocalcinosis.

Pathology

Affected tissues contain numerous small non-caseating granulomas that often contain multinucleate giant cells and

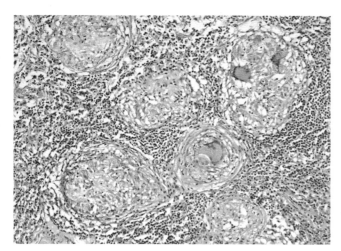

Fig 31.5 Sarcoidosis. Microscopically, the granulomas are small and round with occasional small multinucleate cells and no caseation. Microscopically, sarcoidosis can be difficult to distinguish from tuberculosis and additional tests must be performed.

> **Box 31.9   Important granulomatous diseases**
>
> **Infections**
> - Tuberculosis and atypical mycobacterial infections
> - Systemic mycoses
> - Cat-scratch disease
> - Toxoplasmosis
> - Syphilis
>
> **Reactive**
> - Foreign body reactions
>
> **Unknown causes**
> - Sarcoidosis
> - Crohn's disease
> - Melkersson–Rosenthal syndrome
> - Orofacial granulomatosis
> - Wegener's granulomatosis

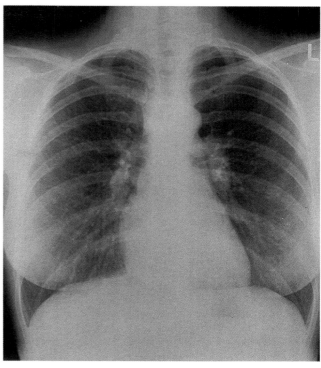

Fig. 31.6   Sarcoidosis. Prominent hilar lymphadenopathy is the main radiological finding. Granuloma formation may be widespread in the lungs but not visible radiographically.

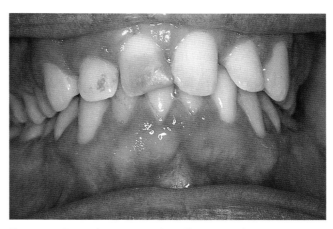

Fig. 31.7   Sarcoidosis. Gingival swelling is not clinically distinguishable from several other possible causes. In this case changes are relatively mild and easily overlooked, but biopsy showed granuloma formation.

are surrounded by lymphocytes (Fig. 31.5). Granulomas and the fibrosis they induce around them spread to destroy the tissues. Cells in the granulomas produce vitamin D3, causing hypercalcaemia, and angiotensin converting enzyme, aiding diagnosis. The granulomas are not distinguishable from those of other diseases histologically. Tuberculosis and other granulomatous diseases must therefore be excluded by specific investigations (Box 31.9).

Lung and lymph node involvement

Sarcoidosis is primarily a disease of lungs and lymph nodes. Over 90% of patients have lung damage, but only in a minority is there diffuse fibrosis and a risk of death. Most patients have a dry cough and a few have breathlessness on exertion. In some patients it is an asymptomatic chance finding on imaging.

Lymphadenopathy is usually hilar or mediastinal, bilateral and associated with lung lesions (Fig. 31.6). Other sites are involved in 40% of patients, including cervical lymph nodes (Ch. 32).

Oral involvement

The most frequently affected oral sites are the gingivae (Fig. 31.7) and lips, followed by palate and buccal mucosa. Gingival involvement produces a lumpy multifocal or diffuse gingival enlargement identical to that in Crohn's disease or orofacial granulomatosis. Granulomas are present on biopsy.

Other lesions include ulcers and swellings. Although they are uncommon overall, oral lesions frequently precede other manifestations and are the presenting sign in two-thirds of patients.

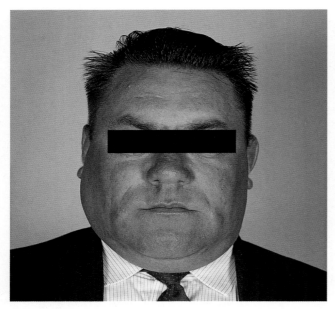

Fig. 31.8 Bilateral parotid swelling in a case of sarcoidosis.

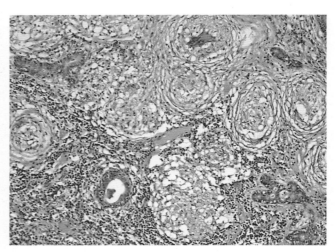

Fig. 31.9 **Sarcoidosis of salivary gland.** The acinar cells are completely effaced, and only a few ducts remain, surrounded by fibrosis and pale staining rounded granulomas of loosely cohesive macrophages. The granuloma near the top centre contains a small multinucleate cell.

Salivary gland involvement

Sarcoidosis causes bilateral diffuse swelling of major salivary glands, almost always parotid glands (Figs 31.8 and 31.9). This is uncommon but can occasionally be the first manifestation of sarcoidosis. The disease also affects minor glands, and in more than 50% of patients with bilateral hilar lymphadenopathy, biopsy of a labial salivary gland shows typical granulomas and is a valuable, minimally invasive diagnostic aid. Concurrent lacrimal gland involvement produces a Sjögren's syndrome-like clinical presentation with both dry eyes and mouth.

Heerfordt's syndrome is the combination of parotid swelling, xerostomia, uveitis and, often, facial palsy due to sarcoidosis in salivary gland, eye and facial nerve. It is now recognised as one of several neurological sarcoid presentations and patients with facial or other cranial nerve involvement should be referred for exclusion of more widespread brain and nerve involvement. Patients with Heerfordt's syndrome are at risk of aseptic meningitis.

Diagnosis and management

Diagnosis depends on chest radiography (Fig. 31.6) and, if necessary and depending on symptoms, biopsy of affected

tissue. In the active stages of the disease, plasma levels of angiotensin-converting enzyme and calcium are frequently raised. Tuberculosis must be excluded by other tests.

The great majority of patients require no treatment and spontaneous resolution follows in a few years. When required, non-steroidal anti-inflammatory drugs are usually sufficient. However, patients with extrapulmonary or extensive lung involvement may be given corticosteroids, methotrexate or azathioprine, other immunosuppressants, or tumour necrosis factor-alpha antagonists. Many novel targeted agents are in trial.

The mortality rate is 5%, usually from lung or central nervous system disease. Lung transplants may be used in severe cases. Sarcoidosis carries a risk of lung cancer and leukaemia in later life.

General review PMID: 24090799

Orofacial manifestations PMID: 18953304

Literature review PMID: 15888103

Cervical lymphadenopathy 32

There are so many potential causes of enlargement of the cervical lymph nodes that differential diagnosis is complex and requires knowledge of many diseases. Dental causes are common (Fig. 32.1), and the primary role of the dentist is to exclude them. Cervical lymphadenopathy without an obvious local cause is a warning sign that must not be ignored, and no dental examination is complete without an examination of the cervical lymph nodes.

Important causes of cervical lymphadenopathy are summarised in Box 32.1. Many have been discussed in other chapters.

INVESTIGATION

The first step in diagnosis is not to investigate the node, but to examine the sites draining to it. This may involve checking all the head and neck skin, oral cavity, visualising tonsil and pharynx and asking about nasal symptoms. If a lesion is found, biopsy of it with fine needle aspiration (FNA) of the node will usually be diagnostic. If nothing is found and the node is single or suspicious of malignancy, imaging to examine deeper sites would be the next step. If nodes are multiple or bilateral and no lesion is present, attention turns to the nodes themselves.

Lymphadenopathy of acute onset and with tender or painful nodes bilaterally is the easiest type to diagnose. The causes are mostly acute viral or bacterial infections, and spontaneous resolution follows. It is persistent enlargement without such a history that causes diagnostic problems. Various clinical features provide important guides as to the likely cause of lymphadenopathy (Box 32.2), but there is no simple algorithm for diagnosis; the diseases are simply too diverse and individually variable.

A soft lymph node in an otherwise healthy child is unlikely to be of great significance. It is usually due to a recent viral infection and typically resolves spontaneously after a month or so. It is estimated that up to a half of children have one or more enlarged nodes at any time and those less than 15 mm

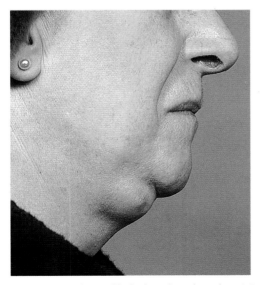

Fig. 32.1 Enlarged submandibular lymph node with incipient drainage to the skin resulting from a dental abscess.

Box 32.1 Some important causes of cervical lymphadenopathy

Infections

- Bacterial
  - Dental
    - apical and facial abscess
    - cellulitis
    - periodontitis
    - pericoronitis
  - Tonsil, face or scalp infections
  - Tuberculosis
  - Syphilis
  - Cat-scratch disease
  - Lyme disease
- Viral
  - Herpetic stomatitis
  - Infectious mononucleosis
  - HIV infection
  - Childhood fevers
- Parasitic
  - Toxoplasmosis
- Possibly infective
  - Mucocutaneous lymph node syndrome (Kawasaki's disease)

Neoplasms

- Primary
  - Hodgkin's disease
  - Non-Hodgkin lymphoma
  - Leukaemia – especially lymphocytic
- Secondary
  - Carcinoma – oral, tonsil, salivary gland, thyroid, oro- or nasopharyngeal
  - Malignant melanoma
  - Metastases from gastric and abdominal cancers

Miscellaneous

- Sarcoidosis
- Drug reactions
- Connective tissue diseases
- Recent surgery or trauma to mouth or face
- 'Normal' enlarged nodes in children

in diameter are so common they are often considered normal, but resolution needs to be confirmed.

Cervical lymphadenopathy associated with generalised lymphadenopathy in a child or young adult with acute onset, a sore throat and fever is likely to be due to infectious mononucleosis as discussed later in this chapter. By contrast, persistent lymphadenopathy raises the possibility of leukaemia.

In the older patient with a hard lymph node, a carcinoma must be suspected. Thyroid carcinomas and human papillomavirus (HPV)-associated oropharyngeal and base of tongue carcinomas often present with lymph node metastases before the primary is evident, and in these cases the nodes may be cystic or soft. Conversely, oral carcinomas are usually obvious by the time they metastasise.

Various patterns of involvement of cervical lymph nodes can be produced by metastasis of carcinoma of the mouth (Ch. 20).

In a patient with Sjögren's syndrome, enlargement of cervical lymph nodes may be due to infection secondary to the dry mouth, but alternatively may be due to the development of lymphoma – a recognised hazard of this disease (Ch.s 22 & 28).

Investigations for cervical lymphadenopathy where the cause is not obvious are summarised in Box 32.3. The first-line investigation should always be FNA. This will provide an accurate diagnosis of most lymphomas, metastases, and many infections including tuberculosis. Inadequate specimens or failed diagnosis should trigger a re-aspiration in the first instance.

In difficult cases, or when FNA fails, biopsy provides the most reliable diagnosis. Biopsy is only justified if all other investigations have proved inadequate and must be done by an expert. Biopsy may spill infectious material or malignant cells into the neck and produce unsightly scarring. Needle core biopsy is usually preferred, but surgical excision of a node may be required depending on the likely diagnosis. When lymphoma is present, a lymph node may be required for definitive classification but sites other than the neck are preferred.

Approach to lymphadenopathy in dentistry
PMID: 15954248

TUBERCULOUS CERVICAL LYMPHADENOPATHY

One-third of the world's population is infected by *Mycobacterium tuberculosis*, but only 10% will develop clinical disease. In the UK, infection rates for tuberculosis (TB) can reach 1% in high incidence areas, and incidence is increasing. This is mostly accounted for by latent disease that has been contracted outside the UK, or is in low socioeconomic or marginalised social groups.

Cervical lymph node enlargement indicates spread beyond the lungs. Extrapulmonary spread is seen in 10% of cases with active disease and is much more likely in people who are immunosuppressed, particularly from HIV infection. The hilar nodes are involved first, but in 5% of cases, the cervical nodes are the presenting sign. Infection by *Mycobacterium tuberculosis* accounts for 95% of cases with enlarged cervical nodes. Patients are mostly adults, in the risk groups noted previously. Non-tuberculous (*atypical*) mycobacteria account for the remaining 5%. The clinical features are summarised in Box 32.4.

Cervical disease always accompanies pulmonary disease, and other sites may be involved. Treatment with anti-tuberculous drugs remains highly effective in developed countries, but multiple drug-resistant strains are becoming widespread, especially in Southeast Asia.

Pathology

A tuberculin skin test (Mantoux test) or interferon gamma release assay will usually be positive, unless the patient is immunosuppressed. However, these measure the immune response to the organisms, not active disease. It is usually easier, faster and more specific to perform fine needle aspiration to detect granulomas in the node (Fig. 32.3) and provide material for culture or polymerase chain reaction (PCR)–based detection. Ideally, mycobacteria should be demonstrable by Ziehl–Neelsen or other special staining techniques, but the organisms are sparse and often not found. Similarly, positive cultures are often not obtained, and patients may have to be treated regardless of whether granulomas are found, the clinical picture fits and sarcoidosis and other granulomatous disease is excluded. Open biopsy and incision of a cold abscess must be avoided at all costs as this would spread the infection widely.

Affected tissues contain numerous well-organised non-caseating granulomas with frequent Langhans-type giant cells in a background of fibrosis. After many years, fibrotic nodes may calcify and be seen radiographically (Fig 32.2).

ATYPICAL MYCOBACTERIAL INFECTION

Non-tuberculous (or *atypical*) mycobacteria, particularly *Mycobacterium avium intracellulare* or *Mycobacterium scrofulaceum*, account for only 5% of mycobacterial cervical lymphadenitis in adults but 95% in children (Fig. 32.4). This infection is very different from TB, and the organisms are environmental or spread from pets such as birds and not spread person to person. It is thought that children contract these infections through oral contact, developing the equivalent of a tuberculous primary infection. A further difference is that the treatment for this disease is often surgical. Features are shown in Box 32.5.

Case series PMID: 18312877

SARCOIDOSIS

Multiple cervical lymph nodes are firm, and the hilar nodes and lung are affected, producing a clinical picture like that of tuberculosis, but the numerous small granulomas seen on biopsy show no caseation. Sarcoidosis is discussed in detail in Chapter 31.

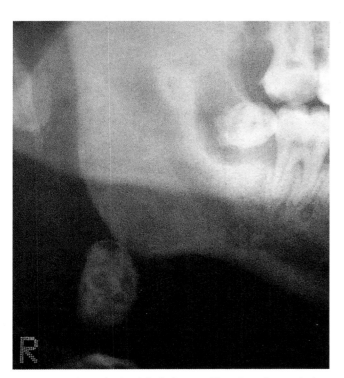

Fig. 32.2 Tuberculosis. Calcified cervical lymph node seen below the angle of mandible in a panoramic tomogram. Calcified nodes are often multiple and indicate past rather than active infection. *(Courtesy Mr EJ Whaites.)*

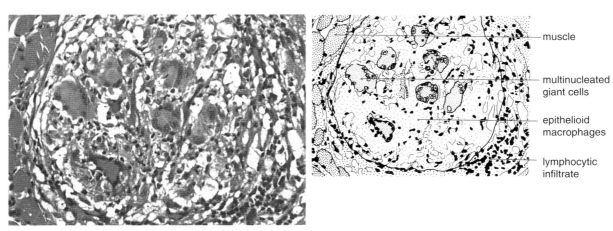

muscle

multinucleated giant cells

epithelioid macrophages

lymphocytic infiltrate

Fig. 32.3 Tuberculosis. Numerous multinucleate Langerhans giant cells are conspicuous in this granuloma.

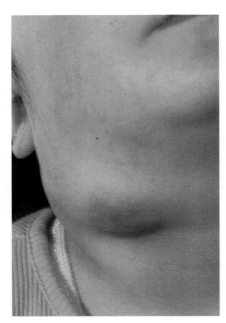

Fig. 32.4   Atypical mycobacterial infection in a child. Typical single large node, slightly tender and with mild erythema of the overlying skin. *(From Hambleton, L., Sussens, J., Hewitt, M., 2016. Lymphadenopathy in Children and Young People. Paediatr. Child Health 26, 63–67.)*

Box 32.5   Typical clinical features of atypical mycobacterial lymphadenitis

- Firm swelling, usually one large node
- Most frequently in a child
- No systemic symptoms
- Incomplete response to antituberculous drugs
- Histologically poorly formed granulomas and no caseation
- Surgery is curative, combined with drug treatment

SYPHILIS

The cervical lymph nodes are enlarged, soft and rubbery when the primary chancre is in the mouth or on the lip. Cervical nodes are also involved in the widespread lymphadenopathy of the secondary stage. Features are discussed in Chapter 15.

CAT-SCRATCH DISEASE

This infection is common in the US and is increasingly frequently found in the UK. Ticks spread the causative organism *Bartonella henselae*, a small Gram-negative bacillus, among cats, particularly kittens, and cats transmit the infection to humans through scratches or saliva. Though named after cats, the disease may also be spread by dogs, rabbits, guinea pigs and probably other pets.

Typical features are summarised in Box 32.6.

Pathology

Young adults and children develop signs and symptoms 1–3 weeks after infection. An ulcer or nodule forms at the site of infection, usually on the skin, that lasts a few weeks. Lymphadenopathy develops and usually persists for

---

Box 32.6   Typical features of cat-scratch disease

- Children frequently affected
- Frequently a history of a scratch by a cat or other animal
- Formation of papule, which may suppurate, at the site of inoculation
- Mild fever, malaise and regional lymphadenitis 1–3 weeks after exposure
- Lymph nodes soften and typically suppurate
- Conjunctivitis may be associated
- Encephalitis is a rare complication

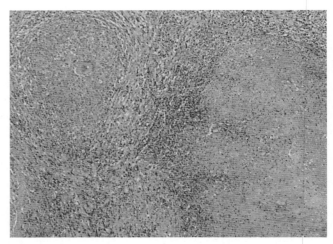

Fig. 32.5   Cat-scratch disease. There is a large area of necrosis on the bottom right, surrounded by macrophages, and a separate granuloma top left with a giant cell centrally.

up to three months. The skin overlying the nodes may be inflamed.

Adults and the immunocompetent may clear the infection without signs in a month or two. Sometimes the disease is discovered as a cause of unexplained fever with no other signs. Rare complications include neurological and ocular involvement.

If infection persists, the site of infection usually heals but infection persists in lymph nodes. There is destruction of lymph node architecture, necrosis and lymphocytic infiltration, formation of histiocytic granulomas and central suppuration (Fig. 32.5).

The organisms cannot be cultured for diagnosis. When cat scratch fever is suspected, diagnosis may be made on serological tests or by PCR on an FNA sample from the node. As a last resort, or when the disease is unsuspected and lymph node biopsy is performed, the organisms may be seen on silver (Warthin–Starry) stain or immunohistochemistry and the histological features are then diagnostic.

When symptoms are mild, no treatment is required once other conditions are excluded. Otherwise, a short course of azithromycin is used, and subsequent immunity is lifelong.

Active treatment is always required in patients who are immunosuppressed. The infection may spread to cause bacillary angiomatosis, a nodular infection of blood vessels that presents like Kaposi sarcoma but is unrelated to it. The risk of a debilitating prolonged course with complications is then much higher.

Review PMID: 23654065

- A rash spreading outwards from the insect bite
- Enlarged regional lymph nodes
- Fever, malaise, other systemic symptoms
- Arthritis (the main chronic effect) particularly of the knees, rarely of the temporomandibular joints
- Neurological complications (in about 15% of patients) include facial palsy, pain or other cranial nerve lesions
- Diagnosis by serological tests for antibody or polymerase chain reaction for the organism

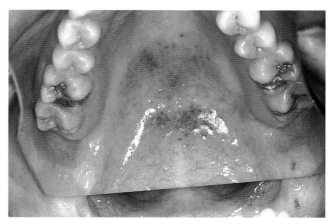

Fig. 32.6 Petechiae on the palate are frequently seen in infectious mononucleosis.

LYME DISEASE

Lyme disease is caused by a spirochaete, *Borrelia burgdorferi*, which is transmitted by insects, particularly deer ticks. The disease is found in the temperate northern hemisphere but is far more common in the US than in the UK. However, the disease is under recognised in the UK and increasing with global warming throughout the US, UK and Europe. UK incidence has doubled in 20 years.

Though less common presentations, facial pain mimicking dental pain or temporomandibular pain dysfunction are recognised.

Diagnosis is by the history and clinical picture. It is confirmed serologically or, sometimes, by demonstration of the spirochaete by silver staining of a skin biopsy. Antibiotics are effective. However, joint pains may recur or destructive arthritis may develop later, apparently an immunologically mediated reaction to the treated infection. Note that erythema migrans in Lyme disease is a rash, unrelated to lingual erythema migrans.

Typical features are summarised in Box 32.7.

Review PMID: 21903253

INFECTIOUS MONONUCLEOSIS

The Epstein–Barr virus (EBV) is the main cause of this self-limiting lymphoproliferative disease. Infection is by saliva, but with relatively low infectivity. The virus replicates in pharyngeal epithelium and tonsils, from where it disseminates by infection of B lymphocytes. By early adulthood, almost all individuals are immune through subclinical infection.

The clinical features are usually distinctive but, rarely, there is more persistent lymphadenopathy that may mimic a lymphoma both clinically and histologically. Patients with severe sore throat, palatal petechiae (Fig. 32.6), enlarged tonsils with exudate and pharyngeal oedema are said to have the anginose form, which may compromise the airway. Almost all patients make a full recovery; a few develop chronic fatigue.

Typical features are summarised in Box 32.8.

General review PMID: 20505178

Oral manifestations PMID: 5255344

Management

The diagnosis is confirmed by a peripheral blood picture showing the atypical (monocyte-like) lymphocytes. A heterophil antibody (Paul-Bunnell) test and, if necessary, demonstration of a raised titre of EBV antibodies are confirmatory. If these tests are negative in an otherwise typical case, cytomegalovirus infection, toxoplasmosis and acute HIV infection (seroconversion disease) should be considered.

There is no specific treatment, but infection is self-limiting.

Ampicillin or amoxicillin should be avoided during the disease as they cause irritating non-allergic macular rashes.

Box 32.8 Typical features of infectious mononucleosis
- In children especially
  - Generalised lymphadenopathy, typically with conspicuous enlargement of the cervical nodes
  - Sore throat
  - Fever
- In adolescents
  - Lymphadenopathy often less conspicuous
  - Vague illness with fever
  - Fatigue
- In adults
  - Greater risk of complications: anaemia, jaundice, encephalitis

HIV INFECTION

Lymphadenopathy is one of the most frequent manifestations of HIV infection and is discussed in detail in Chapter 30. Soon after infection there may be a transient glandular fever-like illness. Later, there may be widespread and persistent lymphadenopathy. Lymphadenopathy in HIV infection may also be due to lymphomas and infections.

TOXOPLASMOSIS

Toxoplasma gondii is a common intestinal parasite of many domestic animals, particularly cats. *T. gondii* is a low-grade pathogen in humans but can affect previously healthy persons, particularly young women. Infection is acquired by ingestion of parasites in poorly cooked foods or contact with cat litter, and three main types of disease can result (Box 32.9). Chorioretinitis is a complication that can lead to loss of sight and more often follows congenital infection.

Acute toxoplasmosis produces enlarged lymph nodes, often asymptomatic, but usually with mild malaise and fatigue. In adults only a single node may be enlarged; in children they are usually multiple. Node enlargement gradually resolves during several months, often 6 months. In immunosuppression, toxoplasmosis can be a severe infection with spread to the brain.

The diagnosis is confirmed serologically by a high or rising titre of antibodies or by other immunological methods. The enlarged lymph nodes are reactive to the infection and contain small granulomas that contain the parasites around and within the germinal centres (Fig. 32.7). If the diagnosis is not suspected or confirmed, a node may have to be removed for diagnosis.

Antimicrobial treatment is required only for severe infections.

Toxoplasma lymphadenopathy PMID: 3326123

MUCOCUTANEOUS LYMPH NODE SYNDROME (KAWASAKI'S DISEASE)

Kawasaki's disease is discussed in detail in Chapter 16. It causes an acute disease with fever, malaise, stomatitis, a characteristic rash and lymphadenopathy. Vasculitis of coronary arteries is a common feature. The disease is usually in a child younger than 5 years.

Box 32.9   Possible effects of toxoplasmal infection

Acute toxoplasmosis in healthy children or adults

- Cervical lymphadenopathy in a disease resembling infectious mononucleosis
- Atypical lymphocytes present in the blood but heterophil (Paul Bunnell) antibody production is absent
- Infection usually self-limiting

Toxoplasmosis in immunodeficient patients

- Disseminated disease
- Risk of complications including encephalitis

In pregnant women

- Transmission across placenta, an important cause of foetal abnormalities

---

The lymphadenopathy is seen in three-quarters of cases and can be the main presenting feature. There is either a single large node or cluster of adjacent nodes. They are soft asymptomatic or minimally tender and usually unilateral. There may be erythema of the overlying skin.

Fine needle aspiration of nodes may show necrosis but is not diagnostic. Diagnosis is based on multiple features; there are no specific tests (Ch. 16).

LANGERHANS CELL HISTIOCYTOSIS

Cervical lymph nodes can be enlarged, sometimes massively, in multisystem types of Langerhans cell histiocytosis, which is discussed in detail in Chapter 12. Occasionally lymphadenopathy is the presenting or only feature, and then the neck is the usual site. Fine needle aspiration is usually diagnostic, otherwise node excision or biopsy of another involved body site may be required.

SINUS HISTIOCYTOSIS WITH MASSIVE LYMPHADENOPATHY

This condition, also known as Rosai-Dorfman disease, is rare and causes extensive grossly enlarged lymph nodes, almost always cervical nodes bilaterally. It may also develop in the salivary glands, soft tissues, the respiratory sinuses and many other sites without concurrent lymphadenopathy. The name comes from the sinuses of the lymph nodes that are packed with large macrophages or histiocytes containing cell debris, and not the respiratory sinuses. The cause is unknown.

Key features are shown in Box 32.10.

In cervical nodes PMID: 24412136 and 16618918

CASTLEMAN'S DISEASE

This uncommon disease is also known as angiofollicular lymph node hyperplasia and occurs in three forms, unicentric, multicentric and one caused by human herpes virus 8 (HHV-8). These forms have different presentations and require different treatment

Viral infection, either by HHV-8 (Kaposi-sarcoma associated virus) or HIV infection, accounts for half of cases. The remainder are probably caused by unknown viral infections.

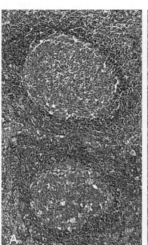
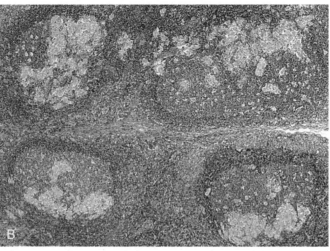

Fig. 32.7   Toxoplasmosis. *(A)* Two normal lymphoid follicles from a normal reactive node for comparison, showing the paler germinal centres surrounded by the dark mantle zones of immature lymphocytes. *(B)* Four lymphoid follicles from a lymph node in toxoplasmosis showing granulomas formed by pale clustered macrophages around the edges of, and within, the germinal centres.

Box 32.10 Features of sinus histiocytosis with massive lymphadenopathy

- Most cases in children in first decade
- Occasional young adults affected
- Markedly enlarged cervical nodes bilaterally
- May be very high levels of circulating immunoglobulin
- Sinonasal tract, salivary gland and deep organs sometimes involved
- Cause unknown
- Lymph node biopsy or fine needle aspiration diagnostic
- Most cases resolve spontaneously
- Otherwise, treatment by steroids, methotrexate or chemotherapy, rarely surgery

Box 32.11 Complications and disease associations of multicentric Castleman's disease

- Anaemia
- Kaposi sarcoma in human herpesvirus 8–positive disease
- Paraneoplastic pemphigus
- Autoimmune and connective tissue diseases
- Infection due to neutropaenia or immunosuppression
- Amyloidosis
- POEMS syndrome*
- Lymphoma of Hodgkin's and non-Hodgkin's types

* *POEMS*, **P**olyneuropathy, **O**rganomegaly, **E**ndocrinopathy, **M**onoclonal gammopathy and **S**kin abnormalities syndrome.

Adolescents or young adults are most frequently affected, rarely children. The extent of lymphadenopathy is very variable.

Review both types PMID: 25310208

Unicentric Castleman's disease

This is the most common type, causing enlargement of a group of nodes, often in the mediastinum or neck, and consisting of a single large mass of nodes. Occasionally parotid nodes are involved, mimicking a parotid gland enlargement. Many cases are asymptomatic, but some develop the systemic features of the multicentric form. The prognosis is excellent. Surgical removal is curative, but if not possible, steroids or rituximab will control symptoms and the mass may remain for many years without progression or remission.

Multicentric Castleman's disease

In this type, nodes at many sites are affected and there are systemic features including fever, night sweats, weight loss and rash. Most cases are associated with HHV-8 or HIV infection. HHV-8 produces a homologue of interleukin 6 (vIL6) which mediates some of the systemic features. These features mimic lymphoma closely.

Multicentric disease is aggressive. In cases not caused by these viruses, treatment with monoclonal antibodies directed against IL-6 or its receptor are effective. When HIV or HHV-8 infection are present, treatment is by antiretroviral treatment for HIV or rituximab or ganciclovir for HHV-8 in conjunction

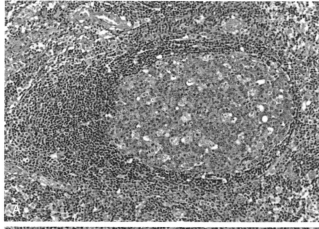

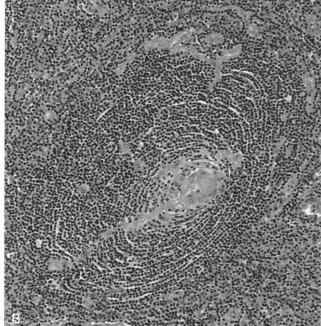

Fig. 32.8 Castleman's disease. Hyaline vascular-type histological pattern. *(A)* For comparison, a normal lymphoid follicle, with a germinal centre surrounded by a normal mantle of small dark lymphocytes. *(B)* Atrophic follicle in Castleman's disease with a prominent swollen vessel entering the follicle from lower left. The vessel is surrounded by concentric rings of lymphocytes, mimicking the mantle zone of the normal follicle.

with chemotherapy. Treatment is complex, evolving and not always successful. Death can result from several complications. Only 30% of patients positive for both HIV and HHV-8 survive 3 years versus 75% of those who are HHV-8-positive-but HIV-negative.

Complications of multicentric Castleman's disease are shown in Box 32.11.

Pathology

The node is enlarged by proliferation of either plasma cells or lymphocytes. Almost all cases in the head and neck are the lymphocyte-rich pattern (hyaline vascular type). Lymph node follicles are atrophic and shrunken leaving prominent epithelioid blood vessels and proliferating dendritic cells, surrounded by concentric rings of lymphocytes (Fig. 32.8). Conversely, in the plasma cell pattern the lymphoid follicles are active and enlarged. Diagnosis is usually based on lymph

Box 32.12 Some drugs that can cause lymphadenopathy

- Phenytoin
- Carbamazepine
- Allopurinol
- Sulphasalazine
- Phenobarbital
- Lamotrigine
- Nevirapine
- Isoniazid
- Iodine
- Penicillin
- Captopril
- Tetracycline
- Atenolol

node biopsy, and the specimen can be tested for HHV-8 by immunohistochemistry.

Multicentric disease review PMID: 33505874

DRUG-ASSOCIATED LYMPHADENOPATHY

Lymphadenopathy is an occasional adverse effect of long-term treatment with the antiepileptic drug phenytoin. Phenytoin lymphadenopathy is not associated with systemic symptoms and frequently first affects the neck before becoming widespread. Substitution of phenytoin with an alternative usually leads to resolution.

Many other drugs can cause lymphadenopathy (Box 32.12) but do so very rarely. Lymphadenopathy caused by these drugs is typically associated with fever, rashes, eosinophilia and joint pains, and they are thought to be drug hypersensitivity reactions (DIHS, drug-induced hypersensitivity syndrome or DRESS, drug reaction with eosinophilia and systemic symptoms). Other organ damage may be associated, making these potentially fatal drug reactions. Other drugs cause

node enlargement by inducing a sarcoidosis-like disease, probably also a hypersensitivity reaction. Cervical nodes are often the most frequently affected.

VIRCHOW'S NODE

A single firm or hard node in the lower left side of the neck immediately above the medial end of the clavicle should raise suspicion of a Virchow's node presentation[*]. Lymphatic drainage from the chest, abdomen and pelvis flowing in the thoracic duct regularly flows in a retrograde manner into the lymphatics of the lower neck rather than into the central venous circulation in the thorax. This is because of either the neck lymphatics low pressure or variations in lymphatic and venous anatomy. Cells from cancers in the thorax and abdomen can thus seed a metastasis in a lymph node low in the neck. Any single enlarged supraclavicular lymph node has a 75% chance or greater of harbouring a metastasis.

The left side is more frequently the site of metastases, and these usually originate from the stomach, abdomen and pelvis. Although classically described on the left, the right side may develop metastases from the oesophagus, chest and lungs.

DELPHIAN NODE

A Delphian node is a single midline level VI lymph node (Fig. 20.18) anterior to the cricothyroid membrane of the larynx that is often the first involved by carcinoma of the larynx or thyroid. It is named after the mythical oracle of Delphi, because historically enlargement was known to predict that cancer would subsequently become apparent at one of these sites.

---

[*] Rudolf Virchow, a German pathologist (1821–1902) from what is now Poland, working in Berlin, described this sign. Contrary to some reports he did not actually suffer it himself. Although renowned as the father of modern pathology and cellular theories of disease, he is perhaps more widely remembered for choosing sausages as a duelling weapon when challenged by Bismarck, the first Chancellor of Germany. Sadly, this story is also apocryphal.

Cardiovascular disease | 33

Cardiovascular disease is commonly encountered in dental practice. Heart disease becomes more frequent and severe in later life and is the most frequent single cause of death in Britain in males, with only dementia slightly more common in females. Younger patients can also be affected, and many children have congenital heart disorders. Infective endocarditis is one of the few ways in which dental treatment could lead to death of a patient.

The nature of the relationships between periodontitis, atheroma and diabetes remains unclear, although these conditions are associated.

Acute angina and myocardial infarction are discussed with medical emergencies (Ch. 44).

In terms of dental management, patients with cardiac disease provide no significant barriers to treatment. Patients in ASA groups 3 and 4 (American Society of Anaesthesiologists Physical Status score) for cardiac reasons can still be managed with intravenous sedation, provided the treatment is individually assessed and provided by a person with specialist training and in a specialist centre. It is important to be aware of each patient's disease type, medication (Table 33.1) and severity to assess the likelihood of a cardiac emergency, but the main risks are for general anaesthesia.

General review PMID: 11060950

Table 33.1   Some dental implications or adverse effects of drugs used for heart disease

Drugs	Implications for dental management
Diuretics	Dry mouth
Angiotensin-converting enzyme (ACE) inhibitors, captopril, perindopril, etc.	Burning mouth symptoms, lichenoid reactions, angio-oedema
Angiotensin II receptor blockers, losartan, disopyramide, etc.	Taste disturbance, dry mouth
Calcium channel blockers, amlodipine, diltiazem, etc.	Gingival overgrowth (especially with diltiazem and nifedipine – Fig. 33.1)
Beta-adrenergic blockers, labetalol, propranolol, etc.	Dry mouth, lichenoid reactions, theoretical interaction with epinephrine
Antihypertensives (as above)	Potentiated by general anaesthetics
Direct anticoagulants	Risk of prolonged post-operative bleeding
Warfarin anticoagulation	Risk of prolonged post-operative bleeding Potentiated by topical miconazole
Antianginal drug Nicorandil	Oral ulceration (Ch. 16)

GENERAL ASPECTS OF MANAGEMENT

Patients at risk of cardiac events are usually severe hypertensives, have severe angina or have had a previous myocardial infarct. Anxiety or pain can precipitate a dangerous increase in cardiac load and dysrhythmias through the action of epinephrine. To die of fright may be a figure of speech but can sometimes result from severe dysrhythmia and a prolonged period of stress can induce myocardial failure. The first essential element for these patients is therefore to ensure painless dentistry and to alleviate anxiety.

Consideration may be given to providing an anxiolytic before treatment (a benzodiazepine at low dose on the preceding night and again before treatment) in very anxious patients. If sedation is required, inhalational sedation is safe because nitrous oxide has no cardiorespiratory depressant effects and is more controllable, but it should be administered by an expert and not given within 3 months of a heart attack or angina attack requiring hospitalisation.

Patients with severe or longstanding hypertension are at risk from ischaemic heart disease. Medical advice should be sought before treating anyone with a resting systolic blood pressure over 160 or a diastolic over 95 mmHg.

Lingual varices and hypertension PMID: 26163474

Treatment in heart failure PMID: 23444163

Dentistry in heart disease PMID: 20527501 and 12085723

Local analgesia

Over many decades, different precautions have been recommended for combinations of local analgesics and vasoconstrictors with various drugs. Concern often arose with what were newly introduced classes of drugs at the time. None of these theoretical interactions have ever proved significant in a dental setting with normal doses of drugs. Patients with

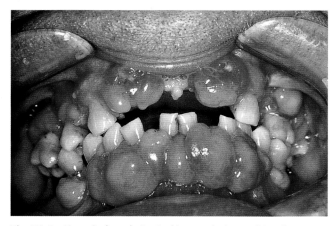

Fig. 33.1   Drug-induced gingival hyperplasia resulting from treatment of hypertension with nifedipine. These swellings are centred on the interdental papillae.

cardiovascular disease need to be treated with care, but the risks of adverse reactions are very low indeed.

The most effective analgesic agent is 2% lidocaine with epinephrine and, after more than half a century of use, no local anaesthetic has been shown to be safer. The epinephrine content can *theoretically* cause a hypertensive reaction in patients receiving beta-blocker antihypertensives, because of an unopposed alpha-adrenergic effect. This interaction is only likely if doses of epinephrine are considerably larger than used routinely in dentistry.

In view of the risk of dysrhythmias, it is important to reduce anxiety and achieve good analgesia. Doses of local anaesthetics should be kept to the minimum necessary and treatment split into several sessions if extensive. Good injection technique is essential. If larger doses have to be given, for example for multiple extractions, then continuous cardiac monitoring is prudent and hospital treatment probably wise if cardiac disease is severe.

If general anaesthesia is unavoidable, it must be given by a specialist anaesthetist in hospital, especially as some of the drugs used for cardiovascular disease increase the risks. Cardiovascular disease is the chief cause of sudden death under general anaesthetic.

Cardiac effects LA PMID: 19893562

Vasoconstrictor safety review PMID: 10332135

Adrenaline effects PMID: 19330241

Anxious patient PMID: 19023307

Cardiac transplant PMID: 11863154

INFECTIVE ENDOCARDITIS

If there is a cardiac defect that can be colonised by organisms circulating in the blood, infective endocarditis can develop. Patients at risk have mainly congenital anomalies, such as valve or septal anomalies, or prosthetic heart valve replacements and often an additional risk factor (Box 33.1). Most of these patients have no symptoms and some congenital valve anomalies, such as a bicuspid aortic valve, cause no symptoms to signal their presence.

Damaged valves are infected by bacteria passing through the lumen of the large vessels, when turbulent flow around a damaged valve brings bacteria in contact with the endothelium.

There are many causes of bacteraemia. Bacteria can spread into the blood from tissue infections, during surgery, colonoscopy and, particularly, from infection of peripherally inserted central catheters ('PICC' lines), cannulae and traditional central lines. Intravenous drug users risk bacteraemia by using contaminated needles. Mucosal surfaces are potent sources of bacteraemia because they are heavily colonised by bacteria, as in the bowel. Oral organisms were responsible for 10%–25% of all cases of infective endocarditis, but this proportion has reduced in the last 20 years.

Bacteraemias can be detected in more than 80% of persons after tooth extraction and even after tooth brushing or chewing, but the numbers of bacteria released by the latter are much lower. Although a larger number of bacteria in the circulation appears to pose a higher risk, it is unclear whether chronic low-grade bacteraemia may be as dangerous as a short high-level bacteraemia.

Normally, bacteria entering the bloodstream are rapidly cleared by the phagocytic cells lining the sinusoids in the liver or spleen, or by circulating leucocytes, aided by complement. These are largely non-specific mechanisms that do not depend on an immune response or the virulence of the organism. Almost all circulating bacteria are cleared within a few minutes to an hour, and even in a patient with a heart lesion, infective endocarditis does not necessarily follow.

The main sources of oral bacteria causing bacteraemia are the gingival crevice and periodontal pockets. The risk is high when oral hygiene is poor. At these sites, large numbers of bacteria are in close contact with inflamed tissue containing dilated, thin-walled blood vessels (Fig. 33.2). The chance of bacteria entering vessels is increased by movement of teeth, even just during mastication. When teeth are mobile, movement repeatedly compresses and stretches the periodontium so that bacteria can be pumped into the tissues, and possibly the bloodstream.

Infection of cardiac valves may cause either an acute or subacute endocarditis. Acute endocarditis is not linked to bacteraemia of dental origin and is usually associated with species of high virulence such as *Staphylococcus aureus*, fungi or unusual organisms.

Bacteraemias of oral organisms are associated with subacute infective endocarditis and are of low virulence organisms such as viridans streptococci. These bacteria adhere to the valve using fibronectin and other carbohydrate receptors to bind to platelets and fibrin on the damaged surface, similar to the mechanisms by which they adhere to plaque matrix. The more virulent obligate anaerobes of the periodontal pocket rarely survive long enough in the blood to cause endocarditis.

Once bacteria adhere to the damaged valve, platelets and fibrin deposit over them. Lumpy 'vegetations' of bacteria and fibrin form on the free edges of the valves, which are progressively destroyed by inflammation and immune response against the bacteria, rendering the valves incompetent. Cardiac failure is the main cause of death if untreated, but infected emboli and bacteria released into the bloodstream can also cause renal or cerebral damage.

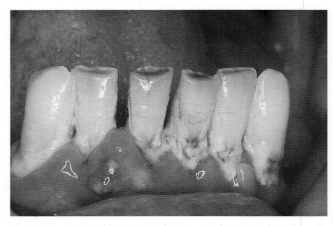

Fig. 33.2 Poor oral hygiene and severe pocketing such as this constitutes a risk to life, particularly in an older patient with a cardiac valve anomaly.

> **Box 33.1 Additional non-cardiac risk factors for infective endocarditis**
>
> - Age
> - Prior severe kidney disease
> - Diabetes mellitus
> - Poor oral hygiene (although the relative risk is very low)

More than 2800 cases arise each year in the UK, and a quarter of patients die within 1 year. Attributing infective endocarditis to a bacteraemia caused by dental procedures is difficult. Fewer than 15% of cases of infective endocarditis can be associated with (but not necessarily caused by) a dental operation. When dental procedures are linked to endocarditis, the most common likely precipitating factor is dental extraction, found in more than 95% of cases.

General review PMID: 26341945

Clinical features

It is important to appreciate that the onset of subacute infective endocarditis is typically very insidious. Symptoms are vague, variable among patients and may not be related to the heart valve damage itself. The descriptions that follow relate to subacute bacterial endocarditis caused by oral organisms, almost always streptococci, and not to acute or other types of endocarditis in intravenous drug users or other groups at risk.

The mitral valve is most frequently affected but, surprisingly, congestive heart failure due to valvular insufficiency is a very infrequent presenting sign.

The most common signs and symptoms are all non-specific: fever, malaise, headache, night sweats, shortness of breath, joint pains and, over the longer term, anorexia and weight loss. Although association with a dental procedure is rarely if ever proven, when it appears likely, the onset is usually between 2 weeks and 2 months after it.

The valve vegetations shed small emboli into the systemic circulation. Classically, these cause distant effects such as splinter haemorrhages and damage to various organs. These embolic phenomena are rare in oral streptococcal endocarditis, but nevertheless a range of rare complications such as stroke, osteomyelitis, meningitis and renal infarcts may be seen. Similar complications can arise from sterile emboli of immune complexes in the kidney and joints.

These variable and non-specific symptoms make it important that patients at risk understand that they should report any mild, unexplained, febrile illness within 3 months of dental treatment. Delay in diagnosis is the main factor affecting survival in infective endocarditis and death results within one year in approximately a quarter to one third of patients. Treatment is by high-dose antibiotics often followed by urgent valve replacement, either by open heart surgery or placed via a catheter.

PREVENTION OF ENDOCARDITIS

Principles of antibiotic prophylaxis

The principle of antibiotic prophylaxis is that high doses of antibiotic given before a dental or medical intervention will achieve a sufficiently high blood level to kill any bacteria that enter the circulation before they adhere to the heart valves. In the past, all patients at risk were given antibiotics such as amoxicillin before any procedure that might cause bacteraemia.

This approach remains sound and antibiotic prophylaxis is used before procedures such as colonoscopy or barium enema that displace large numbers of bacteria into the circulation.

However, it has never been possible to prove that the previously recommended prophylactic measures used for dentistry were effective. It was estimated that in the UK, in a year, no fewer than 670,000 at-risk patients may have been undergoing high-risk dental procedures without antibiotic prophylaxis. Despite this, only a tiny minority of all cases of endocarditis might have been associated with dentistry. The incidence of infective endocarditis does not appear to have been significantly reduced by the introduction of antibiotic prophylaxis.

It has always been accepted that there is little evidence that prophylaxis is effective. It is known that infective endocarditis may develop despite appropriate prophylaxis, and also that bacteraemia from mastication and tooth brushing may constitute a significant risk because of the frequency with which it occurs.

In the absence of clear evidence, antibiotic prophylaxis has previously been provided on the precautionary principle.

Current guidance on antibiotic prophylaxis

The evidence on antibiotic prophylaxis has been reviewed by several groups in different countries, including the European Cardiac Society and the American Heart Association, who have produced guidance for their countries. Over the years the complexity of prophylaxis and the number of patients considered at risk have reduced.

In the UK there has been a significant move away from routine antibiotic prophylaxis. The definitive UK guidance is that of The National Institute for Health and Care Excellence (NICE). The guidance was issued in 2008, updated in 2015, 2016 and 2018 and remains current at time of publication. Initially, it was suggested that all prophylaxis cease, but updates have since clarified this and guidance now states that antibiotic prophylaxis is 'not recommended *routinely*' for dental procedures. This decision was a judgement based on the lack of evidence to support prophylaxis for dental procedures balanced against potential harm from allergic reactions and antibiotic resistance. A randomised controlled trial to define the benefit of routine prophylaxis is unlikely to be performed, and the low-level evidence used to support the guidance is open to different interpretations.

Making a risk benefit analysis for dentistry is, therefore, difficult. If the benefit is small, the risk of anaphylaxis and antibiotic resistance become more significant. It is noteworthy that anaphylactic reactions against amoxicillin used for prophylaxis in dentistry are vanishingly rare because the allergy history is known, most patients will have received previous doses and there is time to confirm any suspected allergy before administration. Single-dose amoxicillin prophylaxis has not caused a single fatal reaction in the UK for several decades, and its immediate adverse effects in the dental context may have been overestimated. Similarly, the risk of community antibiotic resistance from antibiotic prophylaxis is probably very low, though individual patients may become colonised by resistant strains after repeated use. Clindamycin, used for individuals allergic to penicillins, even in single dose, carries a risk of *Clostridium difficile* colitis, which is potentially fatal.

Since the near complete discontinuation of antibiotic prophylaxis in the UK in 2008, the number of cases of infective endocarditis in the UK has shown a dramatic increase (Fig. 33.3). This has caused some consternation, but review of this additional evidence by NICE has not changed the guidance. Epidemiological studies cannot make a causative link between the increasing incidence and discontinuation of antibiotic prophylaxis, although the temporal association is striking. Similar increases have been seen in other countries but are less marked and incidence of endocarditis is stable or falling in the US, where guidance on antibiotic prophylaxis is similar. The proportion of cases associated

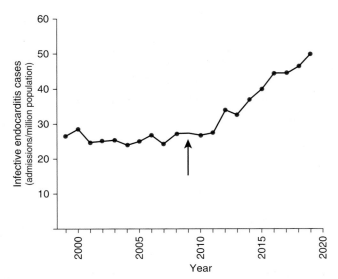

Fig. 33.3 UK hospital admissions for infective endocarditis before and after the 2008 NICE guidance that recommended cessation of routine antibiotic prophylaxis. (***Data from Thornhill et al. 2020 PMID:*** 32334690.)

with prior dental treatment and oral bacteria appears to remain stable and low. There are other reasons to expect an increase, including the ageing population, increasing use of artificial valves and implanted cardiac devices, injecting drug use, and increase in predisposing conditions such as diabetes mellitus and renal dialysis.

Routine management

It is critical to understand that the discontinuation of routine antibiotic prophylaxis does not absolve the dentist from responsibility for preventing and detecting endocarditis.

The first step is to identify patients at risk through their medical history (Box 33.2) and, if necessary, by consulting the relevant medical consultant.

Patients who have become accustomed to receiving antibiotic prophylaxis may not always feel happy without it, given the emphasis that was previously placed on its administration. Guidance therefore includes an important element of patient education. The recommendations are that dentists should offer patients at risk 'clear and consistent information about prevention, including the benefits and risks of antibiotic prophylaxis, and an explanation of why antibiotic prophylaxis is no longer routinely recommended'. Patient advice should also include general health advice such as the risks of undergoing other medical invasive procedures, body piercing or tattooing as well as oral health education. Ensuring patients are informed and involved in any decision is paramount for valid consent to *not* provide cover. Discussion of this information should be recorded in the patient's notes.

Any foci of oral infection should be addressed and eliminated promptly. Current guidance refers to infection, but this should be taken to include any foci of periodontitis or gingivitis, as well as overt tissue infection. There needs to be a good preventive regime in place to prevent development of caries and odontogenic infection, as well as gingival inflammation. All patients at risk must maintain the highest standards of oral health.

Some patients will continue to demand antibiotic prophylaxis. Similarly, some cardiologists will request prophylaxis even though a patient may not be in a high-risk group. The recommendations are guidance rather than mandatory so

that clinical judgement may allow a different course of action provided it can be justified.

All patients at risk need to be reminded of the signs and symptoms and the need to return if unwell, after all types of dental treatment.

Patients requiring special consideration

Though the great majority of patients previously considered at risk after dental procedures no longer receive antibiotic prophylaxis, it may need to be considered and advice sought from the patient's cardiologist. Patients requiring special consideration are shown in Box 33.3, a relatively limited subset of those theoretically at risk and the same group identified in European and US guidelines. Not only are these patients at higher risk but they are more likely to have severe endocarditis and greater complications. To this list should be added patients not in a high-risk category but who request antibiotic prophylaxis after discussion of the risks and benefits.

Treatment of this group must include all the measures discussed above for routine treatment. If antibiotic prophylaxis is required, the dentist needs to assess the proposed treatment as 'invasive' or 'non-invasive'. Invasive procedures are those in which gingival margins, pockets, or periapex are manipulated and those in which the oral mucosa is perforated by an instrument (but not local anaesthetic needle) and are thus likely to cause a bacteraemia. Antibiotic cover is not required in the management of soft tissue trauma or for exfoliating deciduous teeth. Invasive and non-invasive procedures are shown in Table 33.2.

If cover is required, UK guidelines are shown in Appendix 33.1.

The use of chlorhexidine mouthwash prior to procedures to attempt to reduce the bacterial flora or around teeth before extraction is not recommended.

Table 33.2 Invasive and non-invasive dental procedures for prevention of infective endocarditis

Non-invasive dental procedures	Invasive dental procedures
Infiltration or block local anaesthetic injections in non-infected soft tissues	Placement of matrix bands
Basic periodontal examination screening	Placement of subgingival rubber dam clamps
Supragingival scale and polish	Subgingival restorations including fixed prosthodontics
Supragingival restorations	Endodontic treatment before an apical stop has been established
Supragingival orthodontic bands and separators	Preformed metal crown placement
Removal of sutures	Full periodontal examinations (including pocket charting in diseased tissues)
Radiographs	Root surface instrumentation/ subgingival scaling
Placement or adjustment of orthodontic or removable prosthodontic appliances	Incision and drainage of abscess
	Dental extractions
	Surgery involving elevation of a mucoperiosteal flap or in the mucogingival area
	Placement of dental implants including temporary anchorage devices and mini-implants
	Uncovering implant substructures

Review PMID: 26794105

Web URL 33.1 NICE guidance: https://www.nice.org.uk/guidance/cg64

Web URL 33.2 UK Implementation guide: www.sdcep.org.uk and enter 'antibiotic prophylaxis' into search box

IE increasing UK PMID: 32334690

Causes of IE in Europe PMID: 31504413

European Soc Cardiol Guidelines PMID: 26320109

Dental IE in Taiwan PMID: 26512586

US guidelines PMID: 26373316 and 34711348

US and European guidelines compared PMID: 29923105

Case reports PMID: 26992086

Web URL 33.3 UK medicolegal advice: http://www.dentalprotection.org/uk/ and enter 'antibiotic prophylaxis' into search box

Risks from oral piercings PMID: 21358880

Web URL 33.4 Patient advice: https://www.bhf.org.uk/ and enter 'endocarditis' into search box

IMPLANTED CARDIAC DEVICES

Increasing numbers of patients have either pacemakers or implantable cardioverter defibrillators to treat bradycardia, arrhythmias, tachycardia, fibrillation and heart block. Similar electronic pulse generators are also used as vagus nerve stimulators to treat epilepsy.

Some types of ultrasonic scalers (the magneto-constrictive and not the piezoelectric type) and electrosurgical equipment produce a pulsating magnetic field that potentially interferes with their function, and use should be avoided as a precautionary measure even though the risk appears largely theoretical. Pulp testers and apex locators are safe. In the absence of a good evidence base, following the advice from the manufacturer is appropriate and use of the magnetic type of ultrasonic scaler should be avoided for these patients.

There is no indication for antibiotic prophylaxis.

Cardiac devices and dentistry PMID: 30188858 and 27269668

Appendix 33.1

UK Guideline for antibiotic prophylaxis for infective endocarditis

For further advice on implementing UK guidelines see https://www.sdcep.org.uk/media/qvpj2kfb/sdcep-antibiotic-prophylaxis-implementation-advice.pdf

Regimen	Patient	Dose and route of administration	Notes
Standard	Adult	Amoxicillin, 3 g oral powder 60 minutes before procedure	Equivalent to one oral powder sachet. Warfarin interaction requires monitoring after administration
	Child 6 months to 17 years of age	Amoxycillin 50 mg/kg with maximum dose 3 g 60 minutes before procedure	Doses less than 3 g can be made up using Amoxycillin oral suspension 250 mg/5 ml
Allergy to penicillins	Adult	Clindamycin capsules 600 mg 60 minutes before procedure	Usually provided as 300 mg capsules. Avoid if patient has diarrhoea. Risk of antibiotic colitis.
	Child 6 months to 17 years of age	Clindamycin 20 mg/kg with maximum dose 600 mg 60 minutes before procedure	As for adult
Allergy to penicillins and unable to swallow capsules, or when a child requires a dose of Clindamycin that cannot be provided using 300 mg capsules	Adult	Azithromycin 500 mg 60 minutes before procedure	Usually provided as Azithromycin oral suspension 200 mg/5 ml. Can cause abdominal pain, nausea and vomiting
	Child 6 months to 17 years of age	Azithromycin 12 mg/kg with maximum dose 500 mg 60 minutes before procedure	As for adult
Intravenous	Adult	Amoxicillin 1 g just before the procedure or at induction of anaesthesia	As for oral dosing
	Child 6 months to 17 years of age	Amoxicillin 50 mg/kg; maximum dose 1 g just before the procedure or at induction of anaesthesia	As for oral dosing
Intravenous for individuals allergic to penicillins	Adult	Clindamycin 300 mg just before the procedure or at induction of anaesthesia	As for oral dosing
	Child 6 months to 17 years of age	Clindamycin 20 mg/kg with maximum dose 300 mg just before the procedure or at induction of anaesthesia	As for oral dosing

Respiratory tract disease | 34

MAXILLARY ANTRUM DISEASE

The maxillary antrum is prone to develop infection and inflammation. Both ventilation and drainage are required to maintain health and the antrum has a narrow, convoluted and upward drainage pathway to the nose (Fig. 34.1). Continuous mucociliary clearance moves a mucous layer from the inferior sinus upwards over all its walls to converge on the ostium. This opens into the lower part of the ethmoid sinuses, which drain together with the antrum through the narrow hiatus semilunaris, then through the ostium into the nose. Inflammatory oedema in either sinus blocks the narrow exit, raising the internal pressure. Inflammation in the sinus also inhibits the mucociliary clearance mechanism and produces exudate that quickly overwhelms its capacity and collects in the lower sinus.

ACUTE SINUSITIS

➡ Summary chart 39.1, p. 552

Acute maxillary sinusitis is a very common condition that often presents with pain suggesting a dental cause. However, almost all acute sinusitis is a sequela of viral infection in the nasal passages and sinuses, blocking the sinus opening.

Clinical features

Onset almost always follows a respiratory viral illness. Infection of the lining mucosa is by the same virus that caused the respiratory infection and usually resolves with the main infection in 7–10 days. Symptoms lasting longer probably indicate bacterial infection.

There is sudden onset of pain from the sinus, often poorly localised, with tenderness of the overlying skin. Teeth with roots in or close to the antrum are painful on pressure. Symptoms also include nasal congestion, weakened sense of smell and sometimes referred pain to the ear. Fluid will often discharge into the nose on tilting the head or lying down and movement of the head worsens pain. Additional involvement of ethmoid or sphenoid sinuses is often perceived by patients as headache.

Diagnosis and management

The diagnosis may usually be made on the history and examination. Radiography of the sinuses provides little additional information in acute sinusitis. Computerised tomography (CT) is the method of choice if radiographs are required (Fig. 34.2), mainly to detect the inflammatory polyps that can develop after repeated attacks rather than for diagnosis.

Acute sinusitis is self-limiting. No active treatment may be required, but nasal decongestants aid drainage, speed recovery and provide symptomatic relief. Many patients manage well with non-prescription steam inhalations containing menthol or eucalyptus oils. More severe cases benefit from ephedrine or oxymetazoline nose drops, but these should not be continued for more than 7 days.

The inflamed sinus is prone to additional bacterial infection. Even when bacterial infection is present, antibiotic treatment is not indicated, at least initially. Persistence or worsening of symptoms after 10 days or presence of pus suggest bacterial infection, and the usual organisms are aerobes such as *Streptococcus pneumoniae*, *Haemophilus influenzae* and beta-haemolytic streptococci. *Staphylococcus aureus* is a more frequent isolate from the sphenoid sinus. These pathogens are beta-lactamase positive in half of cases, and either high-dose amoxicillin or amoxicillin with clavulanic acid are appropriate empirical first-line drugs. If these fail, a pus sample for sensitivity testing must be obtained by puncture of the sinus.

Dental causes need to be excluded but are present in only 5% of cases, being much more likely to be identified in chronic sinusitis.

Although most cases resolve, sinusitis may become recurrent or chronic.

US guideline PMID: 25832968

European guideline PMID: 32077450

UK guideline PMID: 18167126

Web URL 34.1 NICE guidance: http://cks.nice.org.uk/sinusitis

CHRONIC SINUSITIS

➡ Summary chart 39.1, p. 552

Chronic sinusitis may develop with or without a preceding acute sinusitis.

The clinical features are those of the acute disease but milder and without the generalised symptoms of upper respiratory tract viral infection. When pain is poorly localised, radiographic examination of the sinuses may reveal mucosal thickening, mucosal polyps or a fluid level. Computerised tomography is the examination of choice for all sinuses (Fig. 34.3), but the maxillary antrum is also well visualised on panoramic tomography or occipitomental view.

Chronic sinusitis in some patients produces oedematous thickenings and pedunculated polyps of the antral mucosa. These can fill the lumen, block drainage and cause persistence of sinusitis. Rarely, after longstanding disease, bone may form in them, obliterating the sinus.

Management

When no dental cause is present, the bacteria are initially those found in acute sinusitis, but the flora gradually shifts to an anaerobic population after 3 months and *S. aureus* is often present.

Patients with chronic sinusitis without a dental cause must be referred to a specialist. Polyps, allergic and fungal causes must be excluded by endoscopy. Antibiotic treatment alone usually fails and a combined approach with improving drainage, saline irrigation, reducing inflammation with topical steroids and tackling infection is required. It is suggested

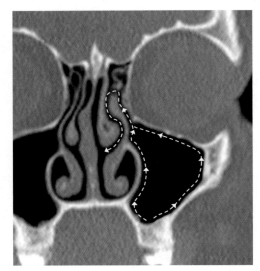

Fig. 34.1 The convoluted drainage and ventilation pathway of the maxillary antrum.

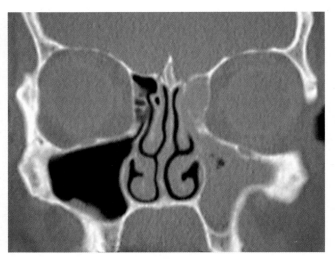

Fig. 34.2 **Acute sinusitis involving maxillary antrum and ethmoid sinuses unilaterally.** The affected sinuses are completely filled by oedematous sinus lining mucosa and inflammatory exudate, seen radiographically as opacified sinuses. *(Courtesy Mr EJ Whaites.)*

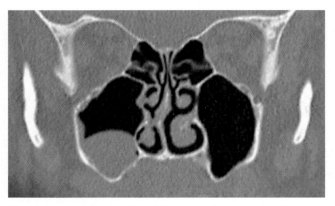

Fig. 34.3 **Chronic sinusitis with an antral polyp**, a localised area of mucosal oedema and thickening. Mucosal thickening or polyps on the floor of the antrum indicate a need to exclude dental and periodontal causes. (See also Fig. 34.6.) *(Courtesy Dr S Connor.)*

that the bacteria in chronic sinusitis exist in a biofilm, resistant to antimicrobials and the host response. Endoscopic sinus surgery may be required if there is no improvement in a few weeks.

US guideline PMID: 25832968

European guideline PMID: 32077450

UK guideline PMID: 18167126

Web URL 34.1 NICE guidance: http://cks.nice.org.uk/sinusitis

Odontogenic sinusitis

Potential dental causes are relatively frequent in chronic sinusitis but may not necessarily be the primary cause. Dental contributing factors are often poorly diagnosed in medical management and the role of the dentist in identifying and treating possible causes is important for success of treatment. Odontogenic sinusitis is usually unilateral.

The roots of the maxillary molar teeth lie close to or within the antrum. In some patients, the root apex perforates the cortex and socket lamina dura so that only mucous membrane covers it. The most common dental causes of sinus inflammation are therefore periapical periodontitis from a non-vital molar, extraction, root treatment or severe periodontal disease. An iatrogenic cause is excessive sinus lift graft material placed for implants. These causes are best identified by vitality testing, clinical examination and dental radiography, particularly cone beam computed tomography (CT).

When dental infection is a factor, additional anaerobic oral bacteria such as *Prevotella* spp. and *Fusobacterium* spp. are found. Antibiotic treatment is only effective in conjunction with removal of the cause. Appropriate regimens are amoxicillin with clavulanic acid or a penicillin with metronidazole or as guided by culture and sensitivity but integrated with the timing of medical and endoscopic treatments. An odontogenic cause indicates a risk of infectious complications beyond the sinuses, including orbital and intracranial infection.

Odontogenic sinusitis PMID: 25732329, 35619928 and 33384837

Fungal sinusitis

Fungal sinusitis results from inhalation and germination of air-borne fungal spores that are not cleared by mucociliary transport, usually because of pre-existing sinus inflammation. The causative fungi originate in soil and their spores are widespread in the environment.

The most common type is a 'fungus ball' or mycetoma, a tangled mass of fungal hyphae bound together with mucus and inflammatory exudate. The ball may grow to fill the sinus and is commonly *Aspergillus* spp. Radiographic diagnosis is aided by the frequent presence of spotty mineralisation in the fungus ball (Figs. 34.4 and 34.5).

Mycetoma formation has been associated with particles of zinc-containing root filling material. These presumably enter the sinus after root treatment and may sometimes be seen on radiographs. Inflammation from apical periodontitis would prevent clearance of spores from the sinus and zinc encourages fungal growth.

Mycetomas are treated by surgical, usually endoscopic, removal of the fungus followed by irrigation and sometimes topical or systemic antifungal treatment.

Sinus mycetoma PMID: 17361410

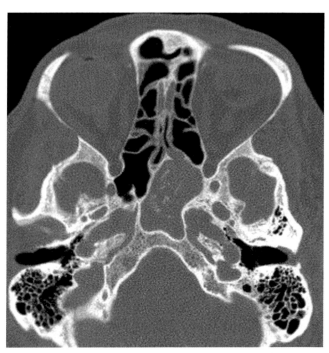

Fig. 34.4   A fungus ball or mycetoma in the sphenoid sinus. The sinus is opacified and faint spotty mineralisation can be seen in the centre of the fungus ball, which has grown to expand and distort the sinus. Maxillary sinus lesions appear identical.

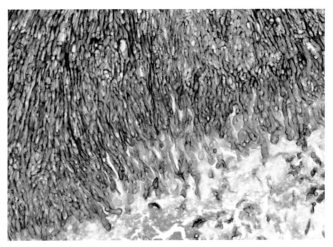

Fig. 34.5   A fungus ball or mycetoma from the maxillary sinus. Grocott stain has a green background and stains the cell walls of the fungal hyphae black. At the top the tubular hyphae are densely packed together in a single huge colony, and at the edge individual hyphae can be seen growing outwards.

Allergic fungal sinusitis

Some patients mount a florid type 1 hypersensitivity reaction to fungus in the sinuses. Serum immunoglobulin (Ig) E is usually raised. The inflammatory reaction produces thick putty-like masses of dense mucin containing numerous eosinophils and a few fungal hyphae. Mucosal polyps are usually present. Previously considered rare, allergic fungal sinusitis has increasing incidence.

Some studies have suggested that almost all cases of chronic sinusitis refractory to treatment are caused by allergy to fungi. Many species are identified, usually environmental species such as *Alternaria sp.*, *Aspergillus sp.* or *Bipolaris sp.*

Allergic fungal sinusitis requires endoscopic surgical removal of the thick 'allergic mucin'. Antifungal drugs are sometimes used but of limited value. In those with recurrent disease, drugs to damp down the allergic response may be required, topical antihistamines, steroids or biological anti-inflammatory drugs such as dupilumab, an interleukin signalling inhibitor, or omalizumab, an IgE binding antibody.

Allergic fungal sinusitis can produce worrying signs radiographically. The chronic inflammation may cause resorption of the sinus wall, mimicking a malignant neoplasm.

Allergic fungal sinusitis PMID: 19330659 and 30996535

Invasive fungal sinusitis

In individuals who are immunocompromised, fungi may invade the sinus wall, cause rapid extensive destruction and often a fatal outcome. Such cases are caused by more virulent environmental fungi such as *Mucor sp.* and require aggressive surgical and antifungal treatment (Ch. 9).

SURGICAL DAMAGE TO THE MAXILLARY ANTRUM

The floor of the antrum may be damaged during dental extractions that cause an oroantral communication. If the antrum is opened during an extraction, a displaced root or bacteria from the mouth can introduce infection. There is also damage to the ciliated lining and loss of normal mucociliary transport that carries foreign material out of the cavity. If sinusitis becomes established and the fistula has not been closed, the walls of the passage may become epithelialised, polyps develop in the sinus mucosa and the opening becomes a permanent fistula to the mouth.

Displacement of a root or tooth into the maxillary antrum

A tooth or root can be driven into the antrum if excessive force has been used during extraction or in attempting to elevate fragments, particularly in a pneumatised sinus when a thin antral floor extends down into the alveolar ridge.

Displacement of a tooth or root into the antrum can give rise to signs (Box 34.1), partly depending on the size of the opening.

Management

The position of the root or tooth should be confirmed. Sometimes it is still within the alveolar process or between the mucosal lining and bony floor. If the fragment is not visible on a periapical radiograph and occlusal view, cone beam CT provides the best localisation. Plain films taken with the head in two different positions will reveal whether the tooth is mobile.

A root displaced into the antrum usually causes sinusitis, but it may cause no more than mucosal thickening. Severe sinusitis is less common. The root should be removed from the antrum as soon as possible and any oroantral opening closed. Several measures are important (Box 34.2).

After any acute sinusitis has been treated, the surgical approach depends on the position of the root and whether there is a wide oroantral opening. The classical method is to reflect a mucoperiosteal flap in the labiobuccal sulcus, open the antrum in the canine fossa (Caldwell–Luc approach)

- The root or tooth suddenly disappears during the extraction
- Blowing the nose may force air into the mouth or cause frothing of blood from the socket
- The patient may notice air entering the mouth during swallowing, or fluid from the mouth escapes into the nose
- Bleeding from the nose on the affected side, occasionally
- Later, a salty taste or unpleasant discharge
- Facial pain if acute sinusitis develops
- Rarely, antral lining or polyps may prolapse into the mouth

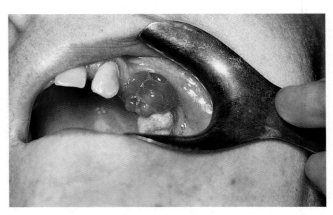

Fig. 34.6   Antral polyp. A polyp of inflamed antral mucosa has prolapsed through an oroantral fistula left untreated after the extraction of an upper first permanent molar.

**Box 34.2   Principles of management of a root
             displaced into the antrum**

- Explain to the patient how the accident has happened and give the necessary reassurance
- Do not to try to retrieve the lost root immediately by digging through the socket opening and damaging the antral floor and lining further
- Localise the fragment using cone beam CT or plain views at right angles
- If a root or tooth has been displaced into the antrum, it should be removed by elective open or functional endoscopic sinus surgery
- If the tip of a root causes a minimal antral reaction or lies between the bony floor and the mucosal lining, removal may not be essential but there is a risk of infection later

infection, persistent discharge and proliferation of granulation tissue or sinus polyps.

Occasionally, the opening may be blocked by prolapsed oedematous sinus lining or antral polyp which is purplish red (Fig. 34.6). If the opening is large enough, these may sometimes be pushed gently back into the antrum to confirm their origin, but need to be removed surgically.

Principles of management are summarised in Box 34.3.

Review PMID: 20591776 and 33685787

PNEUMATISATION OF THE SINUS

Pneumatisation is the process by which the maxilla is progressively hollowed during sinus formation and enlargement. Pneumatisation progresses through childhood until the permanent dentition is fully erupted. The floor of the sinus reaches the level of the palate by about 9 years of age, and of the developing permanent teeth at around 12 years of age but there is considerable variation in rate of enlargement and final size. In about half the population the sinus extends to and around the apices of the molar teeth and a degree of asymmetry is normal.

The term *pneumatisation of the sinus* is also applied to enlargement of the sinus in adults. This is a poorly understood process and is linked to molar tooth extraction, sinus inflammation and increased sinus pressure. Loss of molar teeth leads to reduction in alveolar bone mass and, in most patients, this is accounted for almost exclusively by loss of bone from the alveolar ridge. However, in a minority of patients, extraction allows the sinus to expand down into the space previously occupied by the roots. Pneumatisation is more likely when the extracted teeth had roots that extended into the sinus and when more than one molar is extracted. The most likely cause is loss of physiological forces to maintain alveolar bone mass and organisation.

In extreme cases the cortical bone layers of the antrum and alveolar ridge fuse (Fig 34.7). Even mild degrees of pneumatisation predispose to traumatic oroantral communication, fracture of the tuberosity and difficulty placing implants.

Pneumatisation of the antrum in adults may also extend into the zygoma or the palatal shelf.

All the respiratory sinuses may undergo pneumatisation, particularly the sphenoid and frontal. An even greater expansion occurs in pneumocoele, when consistently increased sinus air pressure caused by a valve effect in the

and find the root by direct vision or endoscopy. The tooth or fragment may then be removable on a sucker nozzle. A better conservative approach without the need for wide external surgical access is by functional endoscopic sinus surgery, which preserves the sinus ciliary transport, improves drainage after the operation and causes less morbidity.

Oroantral communication

The usual test for communication is to ask the patient to blow gently against pinched nostrils. Air (detectable with a tuft of cotton wool held in tweezers), blood, pus or mucus will then be expelled from the possible opening into the mouth. However, if the communication is small, or only suspected, this can cause more damage or even produce a communication. In such cases it is better to pack and suture the socket and allow a period of healing during which the patient must avoid nose blowing and use nasal decongestants and antibiotics. Definite or large communications are best closed immediately surgically.

Unrepaired communications undergo epithelialisation to form a fistula, which is thereby prevented from healing spontaneously. Usually, a large oroantral fistula gives adequate drainage, but a pinhole fistula is often associated with recurrent attacks of sinusitis. If the patient is not seen until late after the accident, there is typically chronic antral

Box 34.3 Principles of management of an oroantral communication

The communication (non-epithelialised)

- If small or only suspected, treat conservatively by socket pack and suturing
- Or, reflect a mucoperiosteal flap and suture it over to give an air-tight seal over the opening

Post-operatively

- Give penicillin for 5 days and a 10-day course of decongestant nose drops and inhalations
- Warn the patient against blowing the nose

The established fistula (epithelialised communication) with infection

- Control chronic sinusitis by removal of any polyps, ideally by liaison with ENT surgeons to perform endoscopic surgery, otherwise via a Caldwell–Luc approach, or through the oral opening if the fistula is sufficiently large
- Excise the entire epithelialised fistula
- Close the opening by reflecting a mucoperiosteal flap over it

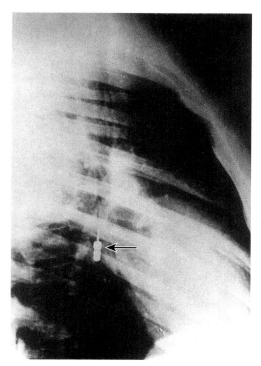

Fig. 34.8 Radiograph of the chest used to localise an inhaled reamer.

If left, infection from a tooth in a bronchus can cause collapse of the related lobe and a lung abscess. Prevention by good technique is key.

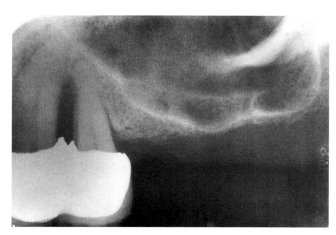

Fig. 34.7 Radiograph of edentulous maxillary molar and tuberosity area showing severe pneumatisation of the maxillary sinus. The cortices of the expanded antrum and alveolar ridge have fused into a single layer separating the sinus from the oral cavity
(From Newman M, Takei H, Carranza F et al, 2012. Carranza's Clinical Periodontology, 11th ed. St. Louis: Elsevier Inc).

ventilation pathway causes slow but uniform gross expansion and thinning of the bony walls.

Sinus variations PMID: 28578369

Sinus septa PMID: 19767706

ASPIRATION OF A TOOTH, ROOT OR INSTRUMENT

A tooth or root that slips from extraction forceps is more frequently swallowed than inhaled. Small instruments such as reamers can also occasionally be inhaled if rubber dam is not used (Fig. 34.8). The patient should be reassured but should be sent for a chest radiograph and, if necessary, bronchoscopy.

TUBERCULOSIS

Dentists and dental personnel in the UK previously all received a BCG (Bacillus Calmette–Guérin) vaccination, but routine vaccination of healthcare workers has now ceased, although all students and dentists should be offered vaccination. Prevention now relies on screening patients and contacts using newer sensitive indicators of infection such as the interferon gamma release assay. An individual decision on the need for vaccination is made and may vary depending on practice in a high incidence area, with high-risk patients or the dentist's origin in a high incidence area.

BCG vaccination reduces only slightly the risk of infection but prevents progression to active tuberculosis in 70% of those immunised in the UK. Protection rates are lower in tropical countries. Infection control and other precautions must therefore be maintained, particularly while the incidence of tuberculosis is rising.

Tuberculous cervical lymphadenopathy is discussed in Chapter 32 and oral tuberculous ulcers in Chapter 15.

CHRONIC OBSTRUCTIVE AIRWAYS DISEASE

Chronic obstructive airways disease (COAD) is typically caused by smoking and recurrent respiratory infections, environmental pollution, or genetic α1-antitrypsin deficiency. Patients are hypoxic and may be cyanotic. COAD is a contraindication to intravenous sedation because of its respiratory depressant effect and to general anaesthesia except in hospital. Dental treatment must often be provided in an upright position, and severely affected patients may be taking corticosteroids.

Dental significance PMID: 25213520

ASTHMA

Asthma is a common respiratory disease characterised by paroxysmal wheezing on expiration due to bronchospasm. Cough and variable degrees of dyspnoea may be associated. Many cases are mild with only minor wheezing but, at the opposite extreme, it can be a lethal disease. In the UK 12% of the population are affected. Asthma is increasingly diagnosed in older patients.

Asthma is common in atopy (Ch. 31), but only so-called *extrinsic asthma* is a response to allergens such as house-dust mites, feathers or animal dander and is IgE mediated. *Intrinsic asthma* is non-allergic and is a result of mast cell degranulation and a hyperresponsive airway. Attacks of either type of asthma can be triggered by inhaled irritants such as tobacco smoke, respiratory infections, exercise and food additives. Emotional stress can also precipitate episodes.

Management is by identification and avoidance of allergens and respiratory irritants. The medical history should include specific questions about triggers and allergies. Many patients respond well to beta-2 agonists such as salbutamol by inhaler. Longer-term control may require steroid inhalers such as beclomethasone, leukotriene receptor antagonists or mast cell stabilisers, such as cromoglycate.

The mortality from asthma is mainly due to under treatment, and use of anti-asthmatic drugs is increasing.

The medical emergency of status asthmaticus is dealt with in Chapter 44. Other dental aspects of asthma are shown in Box 34.4.

Dental treatment asthmatic children PMID: 27012346

Review and dental relevance PMID: 11709681

MIDFACIAL DESTRUCTIVE LESIONS

This is not a group of related diseases, rather a list of disparate diseases with a common presentation: variable degrees of necrotic destruction of the central facial tissues. Improved diagnosis and treatment have made the previous term 'midline lethal granuloma' inappropriate.

All these conditions start in the upper respiratory tract, sinuses, skin around the nose or oral cavity, and they are not clinically distinguishable in their early stages. All cause extensive necrosis, and this makes diagnosis by biopsy difficult. The most common and most important in the UK are granulomatosis with polyangiitis, nasopharyngeal T/natural killer (NK) cell lymphoma (Ch. 28) and mucormycosis (Ch. 9).

Causes of midfacial destructive lesions are shown in Box 34.5.

Granulomatosis with polyangiitis

→ Summary chart 24.2, p. 418

Granulomatosis with polyangiitis, widely known as Wegener's granulomatosis, is a potentially lethal and uncommon systemic vasculitis with a predilection to present in the nose and sinuses. It is thought that the vasculitis is an anomalous, probably cross-reacting, immune reaction to an infection or environmental agent. There is a strong genetic

---

Box 34.4 Dental significance of asthma

- Steroid inhalers predispose to candidosis
- Potential triggers of attack in dental surgery: acrylic, colophony, aspirin, stress
- Dry mouth
- Adverse effects of systemic steroid therapy, adrenal suppression and infection
- Status asthmaticus is a medical emergency
- Increased frequency of allergy to a variety of drugs
- Some antibiotics interact with theophylline
- Some patients have difficulty lying supine
- Ensure patients bring inhalers to appointments in case of attack

---

Box 34.5 Causes of necrotic midfacial destructive lesions

Infectious

- Rhinoscleroma, bacterial infection by *Klebsiella* sp.
- Mucormycosis and similar deep mycoses
- Noma/cancrum oris
- Gumma of tertiary syphilis

Inflammatory disease

- Granulomatosis with polyangiitis (Wegener's granulomatosis)
- Severe systemic lupus erythematosus

Malignant neoplasms

- Nasopharyngeal natural killer/T cell lymphoma
- Poorly differentiated and undifferentiated carcinoma
- Carcinoma associated with *NUT* gene rearrangements
- Adenoid cystic carcinoma
- Rhabdomyosarcoma

Other

- Cocaine use

---

association with genes that modulate immune responses. All ages are affected.

Circulating antibodies (antineutrophil cytoplasmic antibodies or ANCA) against neutrophil granule proteinase 3 bind to the enzyme when it is secreted onto the surface of neutrophils in an inflammatory focus or during emigration through vessel walls. Binding activates the neutrophil and triggers a positive feedback loop of acute inflammation. ANCA-producing autoreactive B cells migrate into granulomas in the lesion and produce the antibody locally to further sustain the inflammation.

Damage to small arterioles causes kidney damage, focal lung lesions, a rash, and characteristic nasal lesions.

Biopsy of affected tissue shows a dense inflammatory infiltrate, small, dispersed granulomas and collections of giant cells (Fig. 34.9). In deeper tissues, vasculitis with destruction of small arteries is seen. Circulating ANCA antibodies are present in approximately 85% of cases and aid diagnosis but are not completely specific. Autoantibodies directed against proteinase 3 (PR3) are highly specific.

The features are summarised in Box 34.6.

General review PMID: 25149391

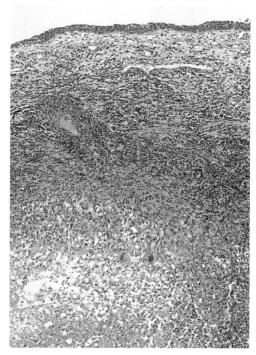

Fig. 34.9   Granulomatosis with polyangiitis (Wegener's granulomatosis). In the deepest tissues, near the bottom of the image, there is necrosis with a few small multinucleate giant cells at the periphery. Superficially there is intense inflammation with numerous eosinophils (not visible at this magnification) around a blood vessel, a focus of vasculitis.

> **Box 34.6   Granulomatosis with polyangiitis (Wegener's granulomatosis): key features**
>
> - Granulomatous inflammation of nasal tract
> - Vasculitis, small vessel destruction and tissue necrosis
> - Potentially fatal glomerulonephritis
> - Proliferative gingivitis occasionally
> - Oral mucosal ulceration occasionally
> - Antineutrophil cytoplasmic autoantibodies (ANCAs) circulate
> - Biopsy diagnosis often difficult, may require several biopsies

Oral and nasal lesions

In the nose, granulomatous inflammation with discharge and crusting is typically the first sign. Untreated, necrosis will destroy the nasal septum producing a saddle nose deformity and may perforate the palate, appearing in the mouth as a large ulcer. Signs and symptoms are very similar to NK/T cell lymphoma.

In the mouth, a characteristic proliferative gingivitis is the first sign in a minority of patients. The changes initially resemble pregnancy gingivitis, but the gingivae become swollen with a granular surface and dusky or bright red colour ('strawberry gums' – Fig. 34.10). The changes can be widespread or patchy (Fig. 34.11) and may be so florid as to cover the teeth (Fig. 34.12). Alternatively, superficial mucosal ulceration can be widespread but appears at a later stage.

Parotitis is an uncommon but early manifestation of Wegener's granulomatosis.

Oral features PMID: 1995819 and 17332039

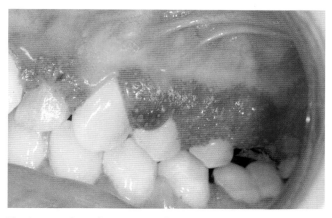

Fig. 34.10   Granulomatosis with polyangiitis (Wegener's granulomatosis). In this florid presentation, the typical stippled appearance is well shown. *(From Staines, K.S., Higgins, B., 2009. Recurrence of Wegener's granulomatosis with de novo intraoral presentation treated successfully with rituximab. Oral Surg. Oral Med. Oral Pathol. Oral Radiol. Endod. 108, 76–80.)*

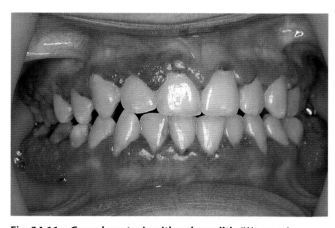

Fig. 34.11   Granulomatosis with polyangiitis (Wegener's granulomatosis). There is irregular gingival hyperplasia affecting a few teeth and redness extending the full depth of the attached gingiva. The distribution is not related to plaque.

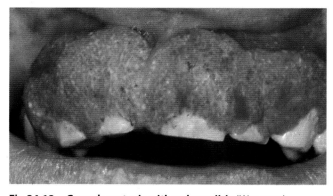

Fig 34.12   Granulomatosis with polyangiitis (Wegener's granulomatosis). This florid case has gingival enlargement to almost cover the teeth. As with some patients, in this case disease was limited to the gingiva.

Management

The diagnosis must be established by biopsy at the earliest possible moment to initiate treatment and prevent renal damage. Haematuria suggests glomerulonephritis and a poor prognosis. Treatment until recently has been with cyclophosphamide and corticosteroids, switching to azathioprine or methotrexate for long-term control. On these drugs, 80% of patients survive 5 years but without treatment almost all die in a few months. More recently, targeted biological agents have proved even more effective, including the anti-B cell antibody rituximab, avacopan, a complement C5a receptor inhibitor, and mepolizumab, an anti-interleukin 5 monoclonal antibody.

Patients with oral and nasal lesions but no systemic signs have a much better prognosis.

CARCINOMA OF THE ANTRUM

Carcinoma of the maxillary antrum is rare. Pain is not an early symptom, and a large size can be attained before presentation. Later, pain and anaesthesia in the distribution of adjacent nerves develop. Most are squamous in type and often poorly differentiated; some are adenoid cystic carcinomas arising in the mucosal glands. Many rare types of carcinoma may arise in the antrum and the sinuses are also frequently involved by metastasis of renal cell carcinoma. Spread through the posterior wall of the maxilla to involve vital structures around the base of the skull is often present on diagnosis.

Oral and dental symptoms from carcinoma of the antrum result from involvement of its floor. It may cause pain in the teeth or under a denture. As the disease advances, teeth may become loose and a swelling becomes obvious (Fig. 34.13).

Any dental radiograph from a person older than 40 years showing an opaque maxillary antrum or erosion of the antral wall without obvious underlying dental or nasal disease indicates a need for further urgent investigation.

CYSTIC FIBROSIS (MUCOVISCIDOSIS)

In this autosomal recessive disease caused by mutation in the *CFTR* gene, there is failure of water and chloride transport across epithelium in exocrine glands. Saliva and sputum are viscid, airways become blocked and recurrent respiratory infections develop in childhood.

There is reduced growth and malabsorption from pancreatic failure. Eruption of the teeth may be delayed, and repeated infections and other sequelae cause chronological hypoplasia.

Salivary gland swelling is frequent, but mild and significant salivary obstruction is surprisingly rare. The saliva is high in sodium and calcium, and slightly reduced in amount, but this seems to be a problem only rarely, though it probably predisposes to stones.

Chronic sinusitis and sinonasal polyps are present in most patients.

Dental surgical treatment PMID: 18201621

SLEEP APNOEA SYNDROME

In sleep apnoea syndrome, there is recurrent spontaneous obstruction of the airway during sleep. Approximately 2%–4% of the middle-aged population are affected, particularly obese males. Fragmented sleep patterns and poor-quality sleep cause daytime drowsiness and difficulty in concentrating, with a consequently raised risk of impaired work performance and of road traffic accidents for drivers. Depression and irritability may be associated. In the longer term, there

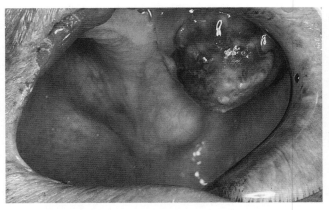

Fig. 34.13   Antral carcinoma. Occasionally, an antral carcinoma will present intraorally, either after eroding the alveolus or through an extraction socket.

is a significantly raised risk of hypertension, ischaemic heart disease and stroke.

During sleep there are snoring and breathing pauses. The cause is recurrent occlusion or partial occlusion at the back of the throat, partly due to relaxation of the palatoglossus and genioglossus which, during wakefulness, maintain the patency of the airway. Most patients have several areas of narrowing in their airway. A deviated nasal septum, a high arched palate, large tonsils or long soft palate are among other contributing factors. The apnoea causes lowered oxygen saturation and risk of dysrhythmias.

Snoring does not itself indicate sleep apnoea.

General review PMID: 23910433

Management

Medical treatment involves weight loss, forcing sleeping on one side and avoiding evening alcohol and sedatives.

The primary medical treatment is positive pressure ventilation using a mask. This is highly effective.

Alternatively, intraoral appliances that hold the mandible 2–5 mm anteriorly can be worn at night. These increase the size of the airway by pulling the soft palate forward; long-term compliance is good, and they are highly effective in mild obstructive sleep apnoea. Alternative designs can be used that are intended to hold the tongue forward. Compliance with use of these large and uncomfortable appliances is surprisingly good, but they may trigger temporomandibular joint pain-dysfunction or occasionally worsen apnoea in some patients. Use of appliances is preferred if patients do not tolerate ventilation, or if it fails to improve sleep.

Trials have found that oral appliances can be as effective for improving oxygenation as continuous positive pressure ventilation, but only the latter has been shown to improve mortality in the long term.

In the event that the mandible cannot be held sufficiently forward with an appliance and pressure ventilation fails, surgery may be required. Several different operations are available depending on the site of airway narrowing. This may seem drastic, but failure to control symptoms in severe cases may necessitate a tracheostomy, which can bring other complications.

A novel approach is use of electrical stimulators that act on the hypoglossal nerve bilaterally to increase tone in the genioglossus muscle. Previous systems used implanted electrodes but new devices provide transmucosal stimulation with simple hand-held devices. These have been shown effective to increase airway patency and reduce symptoms and seem likely to become used increasingly

Dental treatment for snoring or apnoea in the UK falls outside the practice of dentistry because a full medical assessment and diagnosis are required before any treatment. Dentists should work in a multidisciplinary team with an integrated treatment plan.

Dental treatment PMID: 31702942

Dental appliances US guideline PMID: 26094920

Dental appliances Australia guideline PMID: 24320895 and review 31810332

Electrostimulation PMID: 26380757 and 36217095

Web URL 34.2 UK guideline: http://cks.nice.org.uk/obstructive-sleep-apnoea-syndrome

VIRAL PNEUMONIA

Viral infections of the lungs are common and the usual causes include influenza and parainfluenza viruses and respiratory syncytial virus. From time to time, new viruses emerge to cause significant infections, notably Middle East respiratory syndrome–related coronavirus (MERS-CoV) and severe acute respiratory syndrome coronavirus 2 (SARS-CoV-2). Many other viruses can infect the lungs less frequently.

Influenza

Influenza is caused mostly by variants and subtypes of influenza A virus, new types emerging annually and spreading in seasonal epidemics and pandemics. Disease is usually mild, with a cough, sore throat, myalgia and fatigue and resolves in 7–10 days without significant complications. However, more virulent strains emerge sporadically and may have significant mortality. Exceptionally, the 1918–20 pandemic had a mortality of approximately 15%. Typical flu pandemics have a much lower mortality of approximately 0.1%–0.2% and are most dangerous to neonates and people who are older, obese, immunosuppressed, or pregnant. Death results from extent of pneumonia, with oedema and failure of gas exchange, secondary bacterial infection, systemic inflammation from cytokine release and infection of other organs such as the heart.

Formal laboratory diagnosis is not usually required as most patients self-diagnose their symptoms, but viral RNA sequencing and immunoassays are available for those in hospital.

Effective vaccination is available with new vaccines tailored to each year's strains.

COVID-19

COVID-19 is caused by SARS-CoV-2 virus, a new virus that emerged in 2019 and caused a pandemic lasting several years. The virus is spread by small respiratory droplets and has an incubation period of 1–10 days, longer after a low dose inoculum. As the epidemic progressed, variants of higher infectivity but generally lower severity appeared in succession.

The virus enters cells using the angiotensin 2 converting enzyme receptor, which is expressed by epithelial cells throughout the respiratory tract and mouth. Infection triggers inflammation, respiratory oedema and pneumonia. Up to a third of people infected have completely asymptomatic disease, and most of the remainder develop mild flu-like symptoms, but all are highly infectious in the early stages and less so for up to 3 weeks.

A minority of patients develop a florid cytokine response that produces life-threatening pneumonia. The fatality rate is approximately 1% and people with early onset severe disease, older individuals and those with pre-existing lung disease, those who smoke, are obese, or have diabetes or immunosuppression are at higher risk of dying. The cause of death is usually secondary bacterial infection with sepsis and multiorgan failure, less frequently respiratory failure or cytokine 'storm'. By 2022, over 6.5 million individuals had died of COVID-19 worldwide.

Symptoms include fever, headache, loss of smell and taste, cough and blocked or runny nose, myalgia and sore throat. Breathing difficulty develops in more severe disease. Loss of taste and smell is discussed in Chapter 39. Multisystem inflammatory syndrome in children, which causes a Kawasaki-like disease in children with COVID-19 is discussed in Chapter 16. Mucormycosis is a frequently fatal complication in diabetic patients (Ch. 9).

Patients with COVID-19 carry a high risk of neurological complications that may affect subsequent management in dentistry. Most significant is dementia, which may affect up to 70% of those infected by early strains and is more frequent in older patients. While more severe infection carries higher risk, many patients with mild disease may be affected. Other post-COVID-19 neurological complications include stroke, seizures, migraine, motor changes and polyneuritis in approximately 7% of people infected.

Whether there are distinctive oral signs of COVID-19 remains unresolved. The virus is detectable in saliva, and oral epithelium may be infected. Whether this accounts for oral ulcers is unclear but some patients report oral ulcers developing in early disease. Some appear as aphthae and may be exacerbations of aphthous stomatitis. In patients with more severe disease requiring hospitalisation, necrotic ulcers sometimes develop and these appear more likely to result from direct mucosal viral infection. Haemorrhagic patches resembling purpura or blood-stained ulcers are also reported resembling angina bullosa haemorrhagica (Ch. 29). Both these types are most commonly on the tongue and palate. However most of the reported signs and symptoms including xerostomia, dysphagia and gingival bleeding appear to be non-specific results of acute illness, secondary haemorrhagic effects or result from intubation of severely ill patients.

Oral manifestations PMID: 34886241 and 35648785

Dental significance

The main significance of influenza pandemics, COVID-19 and similar diseases to dentists is their role in prevention of spread. In the UK, seasonal influenza vaccination is recommended for all dentists and dental care professionals involved in direct patients care, but not yet for reception and other staff. SARS-CoV-2 vaccination during the 2020 pandemic was initially mandatory for all dental team members involved in direct patient care but has now been designated a recommended vaccination. These vaccines are effective in reducing disease severity but have limited effect on transmission so that these diseases can be passed on in the early asymptomatic but infectious stages.

Unfortunately, patients do not always stay at home when they experience respiratory symptoms, risking spread to other patients in waiting rooms. They should be identified, and treatment deferred. Outside high-risk epidemics, emergency treatment can be provided using the additional precautions in Box 34.7.

Box 34.7   Additional precautions for patients with minor respiratory disease

If possible, defer treatment in acute illness, otherwise:

- Isolate patient in a closed room
- Provide a mask to the patient while waiting
- Provide tissues and clinical waste disposal
- Use a closed surgery
- During treatment, clinical staff should wear a FFP2/N95 mask, gown and eye protection
- Minimise aerosol generation and spread
- Hand hygiene with plain soap or alcohol-based hand rub, or antiseptic handwash
- All staff involved should monitor themselves carefully for symptoms after the treatment

---

Additional precautions may be required for infections with high infectivity or high risk of complications, such as COVID-19. During the 2020 pandemic different countries introduced differing control procedures, many of which had major impact on the ability to practice dentistry and patient access. Dentists suffered excess mortality in the early pandemic before vaccination was available. Universal infection control precautions were not effective because the virus spread primarily through air by respiratory droplets rather than by direct contact and contaminated objects. Precautions were sometimes overcautious until this was understood.

Disposable masks used routinely in dentistry are not sufficient and fit-tested masks to the FFP2 standard (N95 in the US) are required, must be worn correctly and replaced after the appropriate period. However, these and numerous other possible precautions need to be balanced against the risk of severe disease which, in the case of COVID-19 in vaccinated individuals, is now very low. In the UK, specific mandatory regulations were issued during the early stages of the pandemic. Now that vaccine coverage (one dose) is 94% and the incidence of disease is falling, these mandatory precautions are removed and responsibility lies with dentists to make a risk assessment and take their own decisions about treatment precautions. COVID-19 is likely to become a seasonal epidemic managed similarly to influenza.

Potential additional precautions to be considered in the risk assessment and when drawing up practice procedures are shown in Box 34.8.

A final consideration is the possible redeployment of dentists and other staff, either voluntarily or mandated, during epidemics of respiratory and other diseases. During the early COVID-19 pandemic many dentists worked in a medical environment, including in intensive care, and in vaccination centres, contributing to the saving of many lives.

COVID aerosols PMID: 35574425

Redeployment in epidemics PMID: 32710053

BRONCHOGENIC CARCINOMA

With reduction in smoking, lung cancer has been in decline for 40 years but is still the second most common cancer in the UK, after breast carcinoma. There is now almost equal incidence in males and females, but the proportion in other countries follows smoking habits.

Box 34.8   Additional precautions that may be adopted after risk assessment for treatment of patients with high-risk respiratory pathogens

- Staff lateral flow testing for SARS-CoV-2 if symptomatic, or asymptomatic during periods of high incidence
- Staff must not work if they have respiratory symptoms or test positive for a respiratory virus
- Assess risk individually for staff in contact with suspected or confirmed disease. Consider the role of pregnant, immunocompromised or staff at particular risk
- Staff vaccination
- Facemasks for those with respiratory symptoms, or all during periods of high incidence
- Clinical staff to wear facemask during treatment, FFP2/N95 during periods of high incidence or known risk
- Use of fit-tested facemasks
- Patient symptom screening before appointment and on arrival
- Defer treatment if patient symptomatic or has been in contact with disease
- Patient to attend without accompanying persons
- Maintain physical distancing before and after treatment
- Avoid aerosol generating procedures
- Personal protective equipment: fluid resistant surgical masks, gowns, gloves, eye protection
- Ensure effective ventilation in surgeries and waiting rooms
- Antiviral hand scrub available at entrance
- Regular surface disinfection and general cleaning
- Allowing a 10 minute 'droplet settling time' after treatment
- Possible 'fallow time' after aerosol generating procedures depending on ventilation efficiency
- Environmental decontamination after treating infected or at-risk patients
- Information posters and visual reminders of precautions
- Management of emergency situations in infected patients by conservative means until recovery when possible
- Patients with known or suspected disease requiring emergency treatment to be referred to specialist centres with safe treatment facilities

Adapted from Recommendations for UK from Dental framework – Supporting Guidance for Primary and Community Care Dental Settings, 1 June 2022

Clinically, recurrent cough is the most common feature and often ignored as 'smoker's cough'. Later manifestations include haemoptysis, chest pain and dyspnoea. Loss of weight and anorexia may also develop. The diagnosis is confirmed by radiography, CT and magnetic resonance imaging, sputum cytology, bronchoscopy and endoscopic biopsy.

Only approximately 25% of patients present at a stage suitable for surgery. Treatment is frequently therefore by radiotherapy or palliative chemotherapy. The overall 5-year survival rate is around 15% and has improved only slightly in decades. Lung cancer is the most common cause of cancer death.

Dental aspects

Management depends greatly upon the stage of the cancer when the patient is seen. In the early stages, dental treatment can be carried out as usual, but conscious sedation should preferably be avoided.

Metastases to the jaw or cervical lymph nodes are usually a late manifestation, and an uncommon manifestation is diffuse pigmentation of the soft palate, as a paraneoplastic syndrome.

Patients with lung carcinoma are at risk of a second primary carcinoma in the upper aerodigestive tract and must be screened for potentially malignant changes in the oral mucosa.

Gastrointestinal and liver disease | 35

GASTRO-OESOPHAGEAL REFLUX AND GASTRIC REGURGITATION

Gastro-oesophageal reflux and consequent oesophagitis are a common cause of the symptoms of dyspepsia and 'heart burn'. Smoking, excessive alcohol consumption, obesity, frequent stooping, and overlarge meals are frequent precipitating factors. If persistent, the oesophageal lining may undergo metaplasia to a more resistant gastric-type mucosa (Barrett's oesophagus). Acid rarely reaches the mouth in any quantities and, unless severe, reflux alone is not a potent cause of dental erosion, though it may contribute to it. Inhibition of acid secretion by protein pump inhibitors, such as omeprazole, is highly effective in controlling it.

By contrast, chronic vomiting or regurgitation of gastric acid contents, due to causes such as hypertrophic pyloric stenosis, rumination syndrome or in bulimia, can lead to marked dental erosion, often, but not always, worse on the palatal and occlusal aspects of the anterior teeth (Fig. 35.1).

Erosion intrinsic causes PMID: 24993266 and 29389338

Rumination syndrome PMID: 36046491

COELIAC DISEASE

Coeliac disease is a common and important cause of malabsorption affecting 1% of the population. The cause is hypersensitivity to gluten in wheat and other cereal products. Almost all patients have the predisposing human leukocyte antigen (HLA) DQ2. Specific degradation products of gluten trigger ileal mucosal inflammation and cause loss of villi, which results in failure of absorption.

The disease is frequently asymptomatic, and it may not be recognised until adult life as a result of its complications. It can also have a great variety of effects. Malabsorption, stunting of growth, fatty diarrhoea, and abdominal pain or discomfort are typical consequences. The malabsorption can lead to vitamin and mineral deficiencies resulting in anaemia or bleeding tendencies.

Oral aspects

Anaemia can have a variety of oral effects such as glossitis or recurrent aphthae as discussed in Chapter 28. As many as 5% of patients with coeliac disease may have recurrent aphthae, even in the absence of anaemia.

Enamel hypoplasia is common in coeliac disease, seen as spotty hypoplastic mottling, localised opacities, chronological banding, pitting, or discolouration. These probably result from malabsorption and are not specific to the disease. Usually only permanent teeth are affected.

Enamel hypoplasia in a child of short stature and with bowel symptoms should raise suspicion of coeliac disease, recognising that many cases are diagnosed late.

Review PMID: general 23496382 and oral 27173708

CROHN'S DISEASE

→ Summary chart 35.1 and 24.2, p. 518, 418

Crohn's disease is an inflammatory bowel disease of unknown aetiology. However, it shares many features with the autoinflammatory diseases, and some cases are known to be associated with mutations in the *NOD2* gene that controls inflammatory responses to bacteria. Mutations cause failure of the formation of the mucin and defensin antimicrobial barrier lining the bowel and may also inhibit degradation of phagocytosed bacteria. Changes in bowel flora are probably also important. Bacteria normally kept separate in the lumen adhere to the bowel wall and penetrate through the mucous layer to the crypts to cause inflammation.

Granulomatous inflammation affects the ileocaecal region, causing thickening and ulceration. Symptoms vary with the severity of the disease, but effects can include abdominal pain, variable constipation or diarrhoea and, sometimes, obstruction and malabsorption. Repeated bowel resections may ultimately be needed. Many other sites can be affected including any part of the bowel, joints and occasionally the skin.

Treatment controls symptoms but is not curative. Dietary adjustment, corticosteroids, antibiotics, sulfasalazine, or mesalazine are used to induce remission with addition of immunosuppressants and tumour necrosis factor (TNF)-alpha blockers such as infliximab and adalimumab, if required. Severe or refractory disease may be treated with a range of biological agents such as interleukin blocking drugs ustekinumab or T cell receptor blocking drugs such as vedolizumab. Remission may be controlled with low-dose methotrexate or azathioprine. Surgery is required for strictures and fistulas.

General review PMID: 22914295

Oral effects

Most patients have no oral signs, although aphthous ulcers and candidosis may be associated with anaemia.

When the disease process itself affects the mouth, the signs and symptoms are the same as those in orofacial granulomatosis (discussed later).

Non-caseating granulomas resembling those in the intestine develop in the oral mucosa. The common sites of involvement are lips and buccal mucosa. These show prominent oedema with folds tethered by fibrosis to the underlying deeper tissues, producing the characteristic cobblestone mucosa appearance (Figs 35.2–35.3). Linear ulcers often run along the buccal sulci, particularly the lower sulci, and have hyperplastic folds of inflamed mucosa along their margins. The gingiva (Fig. 35.4) may show an erythematous nodular gingivitis with hyperplastic tags.

The granulomas are typically small, loose, and contain few multinucleate giant cells and are often sited deeply in underlying muscle. They may be few, and a biopsy needs to extend unusually deeply to increase the chance of finding

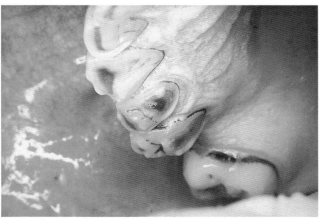

Fig. 35.1 Erosion of the palatal surfaces of the upper teeth due to repeated vomiting.

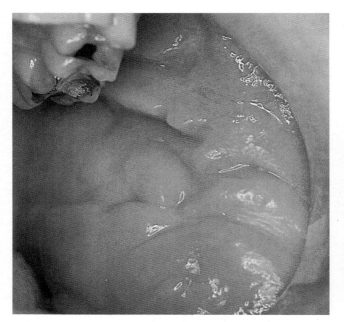

Fig. 35.2 **Crohn's disease.** Soft nodular thickening of the oral mucosa is a typical feature and, in this case, was associated with facial swelling and intermittent diarrhoea.

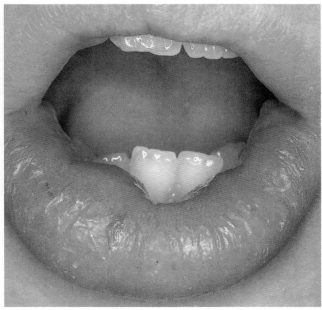

Fig. 35.3 **Crohn's disease.** Gross labial swelling and intraoral mucosal oedema with typical histological changes led to the finding of extensive intestinal involvement.

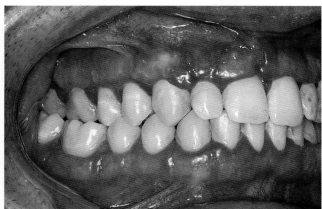

Fig. 35.4 **Crohn's disease.** The gingivae are hyperplastic and irregular and erythematous. These changes are obvious, but more subtle signs are easily missed. The appearances are identical to those in orofacial granulomatosis and sarcoidosis in the gingivae.

them because only by identifying granulomas can the diagnosis be made (Figs 35.5–35.6). The granulomas are associated with vascular dilatation and tissue swelling in early disease. Later, dense fibrosis is observed that fixes the tissues in their distorted shape.

These features can be the presenting features of Crohn's disease, and occasionally oral lesions precede gastrointestinal symptoms by a long period. Oral disease is much more likely to progress to bowel disease in children than when diagnosed in an adult.

Oral lesions may lessen in severity with treatment of systemic disease. Aggressive treatment is merited in the early stages to prevent fibrosis and permanent disfigurement. The drugs listed above for bowel disease are used, together with steroid injections of swollen mucosa.

Key features are shown in Box 35.1.

Oral features PMID: 2007740 and 31090144

In children PMID: 11343060

Treatment PMID: 26593695

OROFACIAL GRANULOMATOSIS

→ Summary chart 35.1 and 24.2, p. 459, 373

Orofacial granulomatosis is used to describe oral mucosal granulomatous inflammation without an identifiable cause. The clinical features are very similar to oral lesions of Crohn's disease, but this is probably a distinct disease. However, distinguishing these conditions is difficult, and some patients considered to have orofacial granulomatosis will subsequently prove to have Crohn's disease when bowel symptoms appear after several years. The chances of eventual rediagnosis as Crohn's disease are higher if orofacial granulomatosis is diagnosed in childhood.

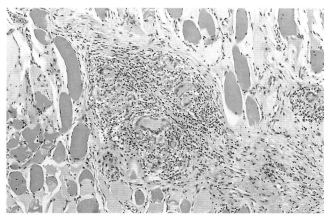

Fig. 35.5 Crohn's disease. The granulomas are frequently deep in the mucosa and widely dispersed. Here granulomas are present in muscle, showing the importance of adequate biopsy depth.

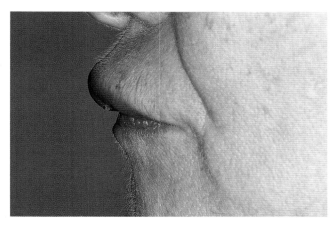

Fig. 35.7 Orofacial granulomatosis. There is conspicuous swelling of the upper lip with eversion of the vermilion border. The lip is thickened and tense.

in Crohn's disease, a deep biopsy is required to give the best chance of finding granulomas (Figs 35.8 and 35.9).

The cause of orofacial granulomatosis is related to food allergy. The patients often have subclinical bowel disease, a higher-than-average risk of allergy to a range of common allergens and react to common food additives, such as cinnamon, benzoates and phenolic compounds. Both type 1 and type 4 hypersensitivity mechanisms are implicated.

Treatment is initially by exclusion diet, and nearly two-thirds of patients respond. Intralesional steroid injections, immunosuppressants such as tacrolimus or ciclosporin, methotrexate or TNF-alpha inhibitors such as infliximab may be used depending on severity.

Differences from Crohn's PMID: 21910172 and 31090144

Treatment by diet PMID: 23574355 and 21815899

MALABSORPTION SYNDROMES

Malabsorption syndromes (Box 35.2) can cause haematological deficiencies that can contribute to development or exacerbation of recurrent aphthae, glossitis, candidosis, or other symptoms.

ULCERATIVE COLITIS

Ulcerative colitis is an inflammatory disease of the large intestine causing ulceration and fibrosis. Patients typically age between 15 years and 50 years. The cause is similar to Crohn's disease, failure of the mucin and defensin layer protecting the bowel lining from the flora in the lumen. The main effect is intractable diarrhoea with blood and mucus in the stools. Abdominal pain, fever, anorexia, and weight loss are seen in severe cases.

Oral aspects

Anaemia can have its usual effects on the oral mucosa (Chapter 28).

There is no direct oral involvement, but the oral condition of pyostomatitis vegetans is a closely associated rare complication. This causes diffuse mucosal oedema and erythema on which there are slightly raised multiple tiny pustules just below the surface (Figs 35.10 and 35.11). Histologically, the epithelium contains clusters of neutrophils and eosinophils (Fig. 35.12). The lesions often resolve with treatment of the

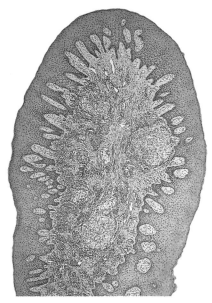

Fig. 35.6 Crohn's disease. A hyperplastic tag of gingiva contains several large round granulomas.

Box 35.1 Typical orofacial features of Crohn's disease

- Diffuse soft or tense swelling of the lips, or mucosal thickening
- Cobblestone thickening of the buccal mucosa, with fissuring and hyperplastic folds
- Gingivae may be erythematous and swollen
- Sometimes, painful mucosal ulcers, linear in sulci or resembling aphthae
- Mucosal tags in sulcuses
- Glossitis due to iron, folate or vitamin B_{12} deficiency can result from malabsorption
- Orofacial granulomatosis shares many features

Orofacial granulomatosis presents mainly in young adults, and lip and buccal mucosa are the main sites involved (Fig. 35.7), with marked oedema and a cobblestone appearance. Linear sulcus ulcers and gingival lesions are less frequent than in Crohn's disease. Diagnosis requires biopsy and, as

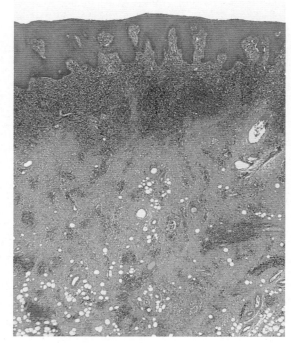

Fig. 35.8 Orofacial granulomatosis. Low power showing the dense inflammation and scarring extending deeply several millimetres into fat. These changes are common to both Crohn's disease and orofacial granulomatosis.

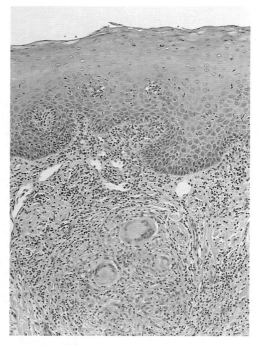

Fig. 35.9 Orofacial granulomatosis. Below the epithelium is a patchy inflammatory infiltrate and scattered poorly organized, and thus difficult to see, granulomas containing large multinucleate giant cells.

bowel disease or with steroids, but occasionally they are the presenting sign of unsuspected bowel disease.

Oral signs inflammatory bowel disease PMID: 25917394

> **Box 35.2 Important causes of malabsorption syndrome**
>
> - Coeliac disease, milk and other allergies
> - Crohn's disease
> - Resection of stomach or ileum, bariatric surgery
> - Pancreatic insufficiency or disease
> - Liver disease (failure of bile secretion into the gut)
> - Bowel damage, fistula
> - Some parasitic and other chronic gut infections

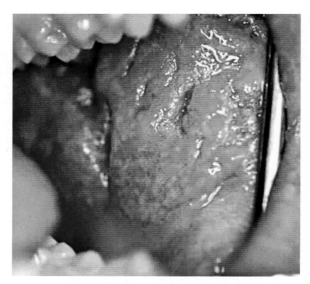

Fig. 35.10 Pyostomatitis vegetans. Diffuse erythema with multiple pinpoint abscesses or ulcers. *(From Markiewicz, M., Suresh, L., Margarone, J. 3rd, et al., 2007. Pyostomatitis vegetans: a clinical marker of silent ulcerative colitis. J. Oral Maxillofac Surg. 65, 346–348.)*

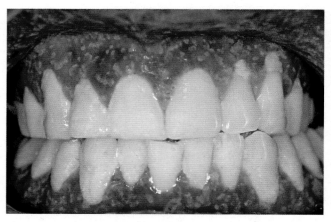

Fig. 35.11 Pyostomatitis vegetans. Florid white flecks of ulcers and abscesses across the alveolar, gingival and labial mucosa.

Pyostomatitis vegetans review PMID: 14723710 and 17236948

INTESTINAL POLYPOSIS SYNDROMES

Gardner's syndrome with polyposis of the colon, multiple osteomas of the jaws and a high malignant potential in the colon is discussed in Chapter 12.

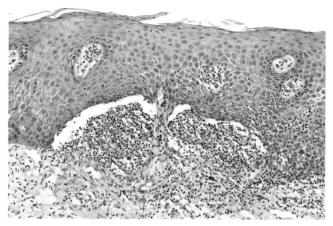

Fig. 35.12 Pyostomatitis vegetans. There are two microabscesses of neutrophils and eosinophils in connective tissue papillae at the lower edge of the epithelium centrally and dermal papillae higher in the epithelium show early collections of these cells.

Peutz-Jeghers syndrome of intestinal polyposis with skin pigmentation is discussed in Chapter 26.

ANTIBIOTIC-ASSOCIATED COLITIS

Mild diarrhoea following prolonged antibiotic treatment results from disturbance of the bowel flora and is often self-limiting.

Pseudomembranous colitis is more severe, with passage of blood and mucus in the stools and sometimes fragments of necrotic bowel mucosa (pseudomembrane). It is typically a complication of prolonged antibiotic therapy, particularly with clindamycin or lincomycin and due to proliferation of toxin secreting *Clostridium difficile* resistant to these antibiotics. Pseudomembranous colitis was traditionally treated with metronidazole and vancomycin but often relapsed and could be fatal in people who were old or debilitated. New bacterial RNA polymerase inhibitor antibiotics such as fidaxomicin are more effective.

Antibiotics prescribed for dental reasons must be used for the shortest courses that are effective and selected according to guidelines or culture and sensitivity and not repeated unnecessarily to avoid such adverse effects.

Pseudomembranous colitis general review PMID: 25875259

Dental prescribing and pseudomembranous colitis PMID: 26404991

Case report in dentistry PMID: 11209501

Clindamycin in dentistry PMID: 16003416

LIVER DISEASE

Common types of liver disease are infections (particularly viral hepatitis), obstructive jaundice, cirrhosis (often due to alcohol) and tumours. There are various aspects of liver disease that are relevant to dentistry (Box 35.3).

Cirrhosis PMID: 34543610

Non-alcoholic fatty liver disease

Also known as metabolic (dysfunction)-associated fatty liver disease, this is the commonest liver disorder, affecting up to

---

> **Box 35.3 Important aspects of liver disease relevant to dentistry**
>
> - Haemorrhagic tendencies (Chapter 29)
> - Impaired drug metabolism
> - Transmission of viral hepatitis
> - Drug-dependent patients are frequently viral hepatitis carriers
> - Cutaneous manifestations (purpura, telangiectasia, finger clubbing)
> - Sialadenosis
> - Sjögren's syndrome (in primary biliary cirrhosis)

25% of populations worldwide, with high incidence in developed countries, in Asian populations and older people. The cause is metabolic, primarily obesity, and type 2 diabetes, with contributions from hypertension and hyperlipidaemia, all related to overeating. The liver becomes enlarged and replaced by fatty tissue. Almost all individuals with obesity and most individuals with type 2 diabetes have some degree of fatty liver disease. It is common in children with obesity.

Mild and early non-alcoholic fatty liver disease causes few problems because the simple fatty replacement is not associated with cirrhosis (fibrosis). However, 10% of cases develop liver inflammation and then frequently progress to cirrhosis, liver failure, and liver cancer making fatty liver disease a common cause for liver transplantation.

Once cirrhosis is established, patients with non-alcoholic fatty liver disease have the same significance to dentistry as those with other causes of liver failure (Box 35.3) and may have associated diseases of relevance to dental treatment.

Review PMID: 33894145

Impaired drug metabolism

Most drugs are metabolised in the liver, and no drugs should be given to patients with liver disease without first consulting the British National Formulary, other national references or drug datasheet. Drugs of dental relevance metabolised by the liver include local anaesthetics, aspirin, intravenous sedatives, penicillin, and metronidazole.

Causes of parenchymal liver disease and liver failure are shown in Box 35.4. Cirrhosis is frequently the result of alcoholism but often of unknown cause.

VIRAL HEPATITIS

The main types of hepatitis, relevant here, are B, C and D. Hepatitis B is the chief risk to dental personnel, but hepatitis C can also be transmitted during dentistry. The hepatitis B virus can also carry within it the delta agent that can cause a particularly virulent combined infection (hepatitis D).

All types in dentistry PMID: 10203901

Hepatitis A

Hepatitis A is the common form of infectious hepatitis. In the UK it is frequently acquired from contaminated food or water during a holiday abroad in a tropical country. The incubation period is 2–6 weeks, jaundice is usually mild and spontaneous recovery takes 3 months or so. Long-term complications are extremely rare. A vaccine is available.

> **Box 35.5   Special hazards to dental staff from hepatitis B**
>
> - The virus is widespread in developing countries
> - The majority of UK cases are in people from high-risk areas outside the UK
> - A chronic infective carrier state is common
> - Minute traces of body fluids can transmit infection
> - The virus survives well outside the body for short periods
> - The virus is relatively resistant to disinfection
> - Hepatitis B infection can cause serious complications (Box 35.6)

Hepatitis E

Hepatitis E transmission is also by the faecal–oral route, but the reservoir of infection is in animals. Infection is endemic in hot resource-poor countries, particularly India, but the risk to travellers abroad is small. Spontaneous recovery is usual. A vaccine has recently become available but is licensed in only a few countries.

Hepatitis B

Hepatitis B is usually spread vertically at birth or horizontally in families in endemic areas. Where prevalence is low, as in developed countries, transmission is by sexual contact or through infected blood. Before effective vaccination, this was the greatest infective hazard to dental staff (Box 35.5), and there are still risks from blood transfusions and medical procedures in parts of the world. Vaccination may appear to have made hepatitis B in dentistry a historic topic in developed countries, but in many parts of the world there remains a significant risk of transmission through dentistry. The effects of hepatitis B infection vary widely (Box 35.6).

Hepatitis B general review PMID: 24954675

Clinical aspects

The incubation period is at least 2–6 months. The virus replicates in hepatocytes, and the immune response to the virus eventually clears the infection in most patients, damaging the liver in the process. The majority of infections are subclinical and do not cause jaundice, but 5%–10% of patients, particularly those who have had no overt illness, become persistent carriers and can transmit the infection. A minority develop acute hepatitis with loss of appetite, muscle pains, fever, jaundice and often a swollen, painful liver. The illness is often severe and debilitating but usually followed by complete recovery and long-lasting immunity. Overall mortality from clinical infection is probably approximately 1%. In occasional case clusters, it has been as high as 30%, probably because of co-infection by the delta agent.

Biochemical markers of infection are raised serum levels of liver enzymes, bilirubin and often of alkaline phosphatase.

> **Box 35.6   Possible results of hepatitis B infection**
>
> - Complete resolution
> - Asymptomatic carrier state
> - Acute hepatitis (rarely fatal)
> - Chronic active hepatitis
> - Cirrhosis
> - Liver failure
> - Liver cancer

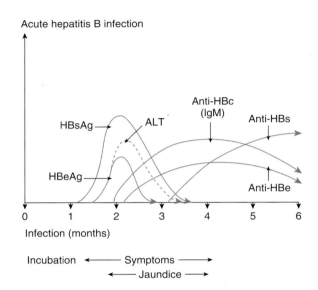

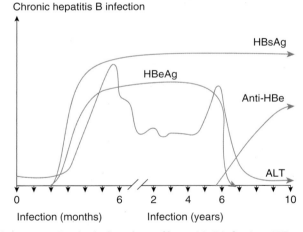

Fig. 35.13   Serological markers of hepatitis B infection. ALT, serum alanine aminotransferase; HBc, hepatitis B core; HBs, hepatitis B surface; HBe, e antigen; Ag, antigen; anti, antibody **against.** *(From Crash course: gastrointestinal system. 2012. In: Kumar, P., Clarke, M. Clinical Medicine. third ed. Saunders, London, pp. 99–133.)*

However, confirmation of the diagnosis is by serology (Fig. 35.13 and Table 35.1).

Serological markers of hepatitis B

The hepatitis B virus (HBV) is a DNA virus termed the *Dane particle*. The Dane particle consists of a central core and an outer shell. The core contains DNA, an enzyme (DNA polymerase – DNA-P) and the hepatitis B core antigen (HBcAg). The protein shell contains the hepatitis B surface antigen

Table 35.1 Serological markers of hepatitis B and their significance

Serological marker	Relation to infection	Significance
The surface antigen (HBsAg)	HBsAg particles detectable in late incubation period and during acute and chronic infections	HBsAg carriage indicates past infection, but indicates a low risk of transmitting infection, unless HBeAg is also present
Antibody to HB surface antigen (HBsAb)	Begins to appear when recovery starts but HBsAg may briefly disappear before anti-HBsAb becomes detectable. Both serological tests then become negative	During recovery, anti-HBs usually appears and rises in titre; it usually implies persistent immunity Anti-HBs also appears after hepatitis B immunisation
Hepatitis B core antigen (HBcAg)	Found only in liver cells, not serum	
Antibody to HB core antigen (HBcAb)	Anti-HBc appears at onset of disease Quickly rises in titre and persists for many years	One of the most sensitive indicators of past infection
Hepatitis B e antigen (HBeAg)	Appears in the serum simultaneously with HBsAg but disappears earlier if there is full recovery	Indicator of high infectivity
Antibody to e antigen (anti-HBe, HBeAb)*	Usually appears in the serum soon after the e antigen and heralds recovery	Failure to develop anti-HBe indicates high infectivity
DNA polymerase (DNA-P)		Indicates high infectivity

*Carriers of both HBsAg and HBeAg but who lack anti-HBe are more likely to develop chronic active hepatitis and serious complications, and to transmit the infection.

(HbsAg). The e antigen is related to the HbcAg but is only expressed by some strains and is only produced during viral replication by alternative transcription. Immune responses to these antigens can be used to track the progression of disease, recovery and infectivity.

Web URL 35.1 Hepatitis B tests: http://emedicine.medscape.com/article/2109144

The carrier state and complications

Most patients with acute hepatitis B recover completely within a few weeks. Approximately 5%–10% fail to clear the virus within 6–9 months and develop chronic infection and become carriers.

Chronic carriage of HbsAg alone indicates a low risk of severe liver damage. Persistent carriage of both HbsAg and HbeAg is associated with chronic active hepatitis and infectivity. These patients have biochemical evidence of liver damage. They are chronically ill and at special risk from cirrhosis and, possibly, carcinoma of the liver because of continued viral replication and damage mediated by the immune response.

Chronic active hepatitis with persistent malaise, and sometimes mild jaundice, is particularly likely to develop in people who are very young, old or immunosuppressed.

Risks to dental staff

The carriage rate of hepatitis B virus in the general population of the UK is 0.3%. The rate in UK dentists used to be double that in the general population, though this should fall now that dentists are vaccinated. There are also high-risk groups (Box 35.7).

In endemic areas in Asia and Africa, carriage rates may be 20% and dental staff there are potentially at high risk.

Transmission of hepatitis B

Blood and blood products can transmit infection in as little as 0.000 000 1 mL fluid, particularly when containing the e antigen. Many cases have followed needle-stick injuries, injections and blood transfusions. Saliva can also contain hepatitis B antigens and, experimentally, can transmit the

Box 35.7 Patients with higher risk of being hepatitis B carriers

In the UK vaccination is now offered to:
- Intravenous drug users and their partners
- Men who have sex with men
- Those with frequent changes of sexual partners
- Babies, family and partners of people infected
- Anyone with chronic liver or renal disease
- Patients who need regular blood transfusions
- Male and female sex workers
- Travellers to endemic areas
- Prison staff and prisoners
- Healthcare staff, including dentists
- Families adopting children from endemic areas

And these are also at risk:
- Patients and staff of institutions for people who are disabled
- Patients who are immunosuppressed or immunodeficient
- Patients who have received unscreened blood or blood products
- Patients who have had acupuncture or tattooing, especially in tropical countries

virus. Saliva is frequently also contaminated with blood and, when splashed on to the conjunctiva, might transmit infection to a dentist.

Hepatitis B can also be transmitted sexually, and carriage rates are high in sex workers and people with HIV infection.

The degree of infectivity is indicated by the serological markers (Fig. 35.13). Infective carriers can only be suspected if they have a history of jaundice or are in a high-risk group. Nevertheless, it must be emphasised that only 1 in 4 carriers gives a positive medical history. Many infectious patients, as in the case of HIV carriers, will therefore be treated unknowingly.

Transmission in dentistry PMID: 23539395

Occupational infection risk dentistry PMID: 22701774

Patient to patient transmission PMID: 17397000

Prevention and management of hepatitis B

In the UK, hepatitis B vaccination is included in the 6 in 1 vaccine recommended for all babies at 8, 12 and 16 weeks of age. Those at particular risk of infection from their mother have booster doses. However, universal vaccination started in 2017 so that most adolescents and adults have not yet been protected. Therefore, the vaccine is available to all adults in risk groups. In the US, the first dose is recommended at birth as a single vaccine.

It is *essential* for dentists to have active immunisation. It is effective, safe and protects against both hepatitis B and delta infection. The vaccine is the HBsAg engineered in yeast and thus contains no complete virus. Three injections should be given at intervals into the deltoid muscle (the vaccine is less effective injected into fatty tissue), but adequate protection may not develop until after 6 months. Side effects are mild and rare, but a few (particularly in individuals with obesity) do not produce adequate antibody levels after a standard course of vaccination and may need it to be repeated.

It is technically possible to measure the resulting antibody levels, but this is no longer considered necessary, either to measure effectiveness or the need for a booster vaccination. Blood tests are offered to the general population and often required for dentists depending on their occupational health service. Immunity does not depend on the circulating antibody level, rather on the cell-mediated response and memory B lymphocytes primed to respond when needed. Although booster doses are no longer recommended in the UK, they are in other countries. The effectiveness of the current vaccines exceeds 95% in adults, near 100% in children, but is not complete and vaccination of the dentist should not lead to complacency.

Vaccine review PMID: 26978406 and 1971874

Booster vaccination PMID: 10683019

Vaccination and cancer prevention PMID: 35632549

Hepatitis D: the delta agent

The delta agent is a defective RNA virus that can only infect and replicate in the presence of HBsAg, which it uses to bind to hepatocyte receptors. Delta infection is, therefore, only transmitted with hepatitis B or to a person already infected by it. It is endemic in the Middle East, Africa and parts of South America, but in the UK and developed countries it is usually spread by intravenous drug users, by blood or blood products. Only 100 patients per year test positive for hepatitis D in the UK, and approximately 2% of patients in the UK with hepatitis B carry the delta agent. However, worldwide 5% of people with hepatitis B carry the delta agent.

Delta infection causes acute hepatitis, and this rarely resolves but causes progressive liver disease with a high mortality rate. Carriage rates are in decline because immunisation against hepatitis B also protects against the delta agent.

Delta agent review PMID: 26568914

Hepatitis C

The hepatitis C virus (HCV) is now more important than the B virus in dentistry because no vaccination is available. It is also a more severe infection and more frequently fatal.

After infection, only approximately 15% of patients have signs or symptoms of hepatitis. Few patients, perhaps 20%, clear the infection despite their immune response. This is because the virus has an extremely high rate of genetic variability (even higher than HIV virus) and each patient becomes infected with many newly generated genetic variants. This genetic heterogeneity and high mutation rate are major factors preventing vaccine development. Most patients become chronically infected without realising it.

Almost all transmission is via direct blood transfer, not transfusion products (which are tested in the UK and many countries), needle sharing by drug users or tattooing. Unfortunately, blood is not screened in many resource-poor countries, and the highest incidences are in China, Africa and parts of South America. Only approximately 260,000 patients are chronically infected in the UK, but around 0.75% of the UK, 2% of the US and 3% of the worldwide populations are infected. Many HIV-positive patients are also positive for hepatitis C.

Once infected, 85% of patients progress to chronic hepatitis, potentially causing cirrhosis and liver failure.

Hepatitis C and B are similar in most respects but have some important differences (Box 35.8).

In some high-incidence countries, particularly in Italy, an association between hepatitis C infection and lichen planus is reported. This has not been confirmed in the UK or US, and a plausible pathological link between the two diseases does not yet exist, although infection is associated with other autoimmune diseases.

Hepatitis C review PMID: 25687730

Hepatitis C in dentistry PMID: 24666473 and 24282263

Management

HCV is detected serologically by anti-viral antibodies for diagnosis, and polymerase chain reaction (PCR) reaction for viral RNA is used to monitor treatment. Liver damage can be assessed by circulating liver enzymes and confirmed by biopsy.

Treatment is improving, and success depends on the strain of virus. Interferon and various hepatitis C specific antiviral drugs such as ledipasvir and glecaprevir can prevent chronic hepatitis in over three-quarters of patients and clear infection in up to 90% if selected based on virus genotype and level of infection and cirrhosis. However, hepatitis C remains a common cause requiring a liver transplant, though even this is not guaranteed to remove the infection

---

Box 35.8 Important differences between hepatitis C and B

Hepatitis C
- is less widespread
- is less readily transmitted by needle-stick injuries
- is more vulnerable to disinfection
- is rarely transmitted during dentistry
- acute hepatitis is uncommon and usually mild

But
- no protective vaccine is as yet available
- infection persists in 80% of infected individuals
- infection more frequently leads to chronic active hepatitis
- there is a higher risk of cirrhosis and liver cancer

as the virus can also replicate in lymphocytes. Those that do not respond to treatment have a high mortality from liver failure, liver carcinoma and a range of unusual extrahepatic complications including encephalopathy, myocarditis or the complications of cirrhosis such as oesophageal varices.

Hepatocellular carcinoma will develop in approximately 2% of patients after 30 years. This complication continues to appear in patients who contracted the disease before screening tests for blood and blood products were available.

Universal infection control is more than adequate to prevent transmission, and sharps injury is the main risk to dentists.

Control of transmission of viral hepatitis

The principles of standard precautions (or 'universal' precautions) should be well understood. Although hepatitis B vaccination and improved infection control have much reduced occupational transmission, the risk remains. There is as yet no vaccine against hepatitis C. Hepatitis B vaccination is not completely effective, immunity may fade with age and it is less effective when given to older individuals. Immunisation is not a substitute for good infection control.

Gloves, masks and eye shields provide only partial protection and must be used correctly. Many infected patients will be treated unknowingly, and hepatitis B can be transmitted by saliva.

In the event of a sharps injury, follow local guidelines. Knowing the patient's medical history may be important in assessing the risk. The average UK dentist gives themselves 2–3 sharps injuries a year, and nurses are at higher risk while clearing away and cleaning instruments.

Standard precautions are summarised in Box 35.9.

Hepatitis B virus is more resistant than HCV, but routine sterilisation and disinfection measures (Box 35.10) apply to both.

Restrictions on dentists who are infected by any bloodborne virus change from time to time. In the UK, advice is available from the UK Advisory Panel for Healthcare Workers Infected with Bloodborne Viruses (UKAP) and working restrictions from the General Dental Council UK, both of which are available on their websites. Almost all dentistry constitutes 'exposure prone procedures', and any potential infection risk to a patient will probably require restriction of practice. Note that it is the *infectivity* of the dentist that is key, not simple serological positivity.

Web URL 35.2 Infection control NICE guidance CG139 primary care: https://www.nice.org.uk/cg139

Evidence-based guidelines infection control
PMID: 24330862

Book: infection control for dental team ISBN: 978-3030163068 and 978-1284220308

Box 35.9 Standard precautions against transmission of viral hepatitis

- Take a good medical history; following a sharps injury you may need details from it
- Treat all patients as infectious ('universal precautions')
- Wear gloves for all clinical dental work and cover exposed skin and abrasions
- Take special care to avoid sharps injuries
- Use safety syringes or needle retraction devices
- Wear goggles for eye protection
- Consider use of rubber dam for more procedures
- Zone work areas, disinfect them and follow good working practice
- Follow hand hygiene protocols
- Use disposable instruments and autoclave all others
- Clean and prepare instruments for sterilisation without risking injury
- Handle saliva contaminated impressions and patient samples as though infected
- Clean saliva and blood contaminated spillages correctly and quickly
- Be immunised against hepatitis B
- Be aware of guidelines for dealing with possible exposure and follow them
- Be aware of legal responsibilities in your country (in the UK the Health and Safety at Work Act 1974 and the Control of Substances Hazardous to Health Regulations 1999 (COSHH)).
- Take precautions with waste disposal

Box 35.10 Sterilisation and disinfection for hepatitis B and C

Sterilisation

- Autoclaving at 134°C for 3 minutes or
- Hot air at 160°C for 1 hour (effective but automatic control necessary; not used in UK)

Disinfectants

- Sodium hypochlorite, 1% of freshly diluted stock solution (0.1% with detergent for surface disinfection) (hepatitis C virus is also susceptible to solvent detergents)

Web URL 35.3 US Infection prevention guidance: http://www.cdc.gov/ and enter 'infection prevention dental settings' into search box

Summary chart 35.1   Causes and treatment of diffuse swelling of the lips and mucosa

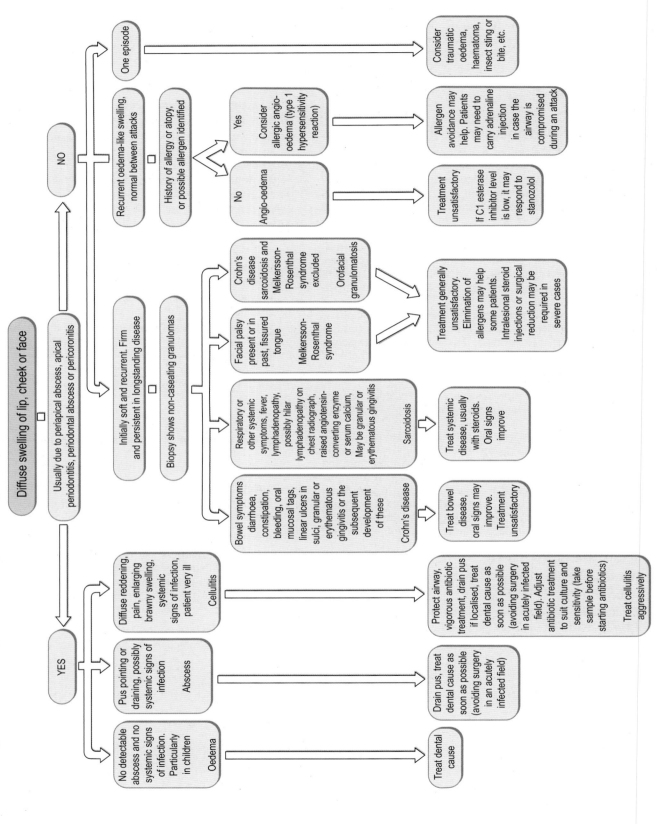

Nutritional deficiencies | 36

Despite the UK population consuming an unhealthy diet high in fat, sugar, and salt, nutritional deficiencies are rarely seen in Britain. Susceptible individuals tend to be older and living on a scanty diet, alcoholic and living on a grossly unbalanced diet or following diets or food fads. On average, dietary intakes of all vitamins are adequate, apart from vitamin D. Intake of some B vitamins is typically too low in individuals who are young or old and female.

Malabsorption syndromes (Ch. 35) are a rare cause of deficiency.

Although several oral conditions are linked to vitamin deficiencies, patients are generally found to be otherwise healthy and well-fed with only a borderline deficiency. Prescribing vitamin preparations brings benefit largely to the multibillion-pound vitamin supplement industry.

However, identifying vitamin deficiencies can be important. Older people with vitamin deficiency are quite likely to be malnourished and the first signs may be noticed in a dental setting.

In older people PMID: 1956659

General oral review PMID: 31940621

VITAMIN DEFICIENCIES

The effects of specific deficiencies are summarised in Table 36.1.

Vitamin A deficiency

Vitamin A has a role in epithelial maturation and retinoids, more potent analogues, have been given for conditions with abnormal keratinisation such as leukoplakia. Lycopene and

Table 36.1 Effects of specific vitamin deficiencies

Deficiency	Systemic effects	Oral effects
Vitamin A	Night-blindness xerophthalmia	None
Thiamin (B$_1$)	Neuritis and cardiac failure	None
Riboflavin (B$_2$)	Dermatitis	Angular stomatitis and glossitis
Nicotinamide/ niacin (B$_3$ family)	Dermatitis, central nervous system disease, diarrhoea	Glossitis, stomatitis and gingivitis
Vitamin B$_{12}$	Pernicious anaemia	Glossitis, aphthae
Folic acid	Macrocytic anaemia	Glossitis, aphthae
Vitamin C	Scurvy (purpura, delayed wound healing, bone lesions in children)	Gingival swelling and bleeding
Vitamin D	Rickets	Hypocalcification of teeth (severe rickets only)

β-carotenes, vitamin A precursors, have also been tried. Changes in keratinisation are reported but are not reproducible, and whether this might reduce the risk of carcinoma is unclear. Adverse effects are significant. Deficiency has no oral significance.

Riboflavin (B$_2$) deficiency

Riboflavin deficiency can occasionally result from a malabsorption syndrome. In severe cases, angular stomatitis is typically observed with painful red fissures at the angles of the mouth and shiny redness of the mucous membranes. The tongue is commonly sore. A peculiar form of glossitis in which the tongue becomes magenta in colour and granular or pebbly in appearance due to flattening and mushrooming of the papillae may be seen but is uncommon. The gingivae are not affected. Resolution follows within days when riboflavin is given.

Riboflavin is ineffective for the commonly seen cases of glossitis and angular stomatitis, which are rarely associated with vitamin deficiency.

Riboflavin has been used to cross-link dentine collagen in an attempt to toughen dentine for adhesion of restorations. This is because it absorbs blue light and not for any nutritional reasons.

Nicotinamide (B$_3$) deficiency (pellagra)

Pellagra, which affects the skin, gastrointestinal tract, and nervous system, is rare in the UK but may occasionally result from malabsorption or alcoholism. Deficiency is often multifactorial and a range of drugs may contribute, particularly the antituberculous drugs isoniazid and pyrazinamide, which compete in the conversion of the precursor niacin into nicotinamide. Weakness, loss of appetite, and changes in mood or personality are followed by glossitis or stomatitis and dermatitis. The tip and lateral margins of the tongue become red, swollen and, in severe cases, deeply ulcerated (Fig. 36.1). The dorsum of the tongue may become coated with a thick, greyish fur with a thick layer of adherent bacteria. The gingival margins also become red, swollen, and ulcerated and generalised stomatitis may develop.

A combination of nicotinamide and tetracycline is sometimes used to treat skin bullous and mucous membrane pemphigoid, particularly in the US, but the evidence base for use in oral disease is weak.

Vitamin B$_{12}$ deficiency

This disease has many oral effects (see Ch. 17).

Folic acid deficiency

Deficiency can result from malnutrition but is more often seen in pregnancy, or as a result of malabsorption or drug treatment (particularly with phenytoin) (Ch. 17). Women are advised to take folic acid supplements preconceptually with the aim of reducing the risk of neural tube defects. It

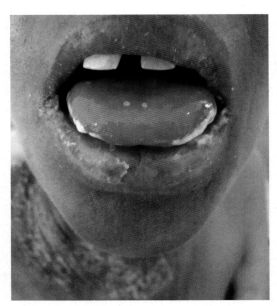

Fig. 36.1 **Pellagra.** Diffuse reddening of the dorsum and lateral tongue. Note also the scaling of the vermillion of the lips *(Courtesy Michelle Weir, MD.)*

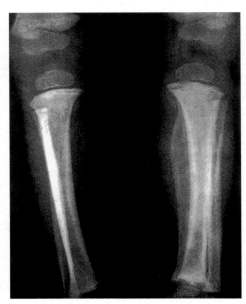

Fig. 36.2 **Scurvy.** In contrast to rickets, calcification is unimpeded and a thick layer of calcified cartilage is observed at the end of the bone. Osteoid formation, on the other hand, is poor, so little bone can be formed. The attachment of the periosteum to the bone is weak, so it is easily separated; haemorrhage beneath it (as here around the tibia on the right of the image) is due to haemorrhage and this becomes calcified.

also appears that multivitamin preparations containing folic acid may reduce the risk of orofacial clefts.

Vitamin C deficiency

Scurvy, once common among crews of sailing ships, is now exceedingly rare. In the UK, scurvy may very occasionally be seen among people who are older, have an inadequate or eccentric diet, or are homeless. In children the causes are usually developmental conditions or restricted diet, particularly in people with autism spectrum disorders. The main features of scurvy are dermatitis and purpura and, in advanced cases, anaemia and delayed healing of wounds. In younger individuals, bone growth is delayed by poor collagen synthesis (Fig. 36.2).

Grossly swollen bleeding gums may develop (Fig. 36.3). The gingival swelling is due to a combination of chronic inflammation and an exaggeration of the inflammatory oedema due to purpura. In children, severe scurvy causes early tooth loss. The diagnosis should only be made on clear evidence of dietary deficiency and of clinical signs. In these cases, treatment with vitamin C and adequate oral hygiene relieves the gingival condition. There is no evidence that deficiency of vitamin C plays any part in periodontal disease except in established scurvy.

Scurvy review PMID: 11838878

In children PMID: 32330999

Case reports PMID: 16301149 and 21462768

Vitamin D deficiency

Deficiency of vitamin D during skeletal development causes rickets (Ch. 13). Dental hypocalcification is a feature only of exceptionally severe rickets (Ch. 2).

In sunlight, vitamin D is synthesised in the skin, and this is the main source of vitamin D, even in the UK. A few foods, notably, fish liver oils, eggs, and butter contain significant amounts of vitamin D. In the UK, fat spreads are fortified with vitamins A and D, but milk is not as in many other countries.

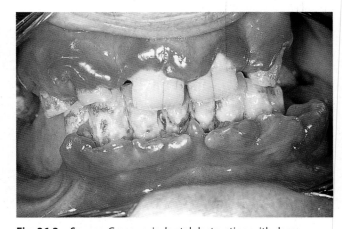

Fig. 36.3 **Scurvy.** Gross periodontal destruction with deep pocketing and mobility of several teeth resulting from the combination of poor oral hygiene and deficiency of vitamin C is observed.

As much as 30% of the UK population has a low serum level at some time, mostly people who are older or very young. Serum levels are lower in winter when as many as 40% of children become temporarily deficient but most of these individuals have only slightly low levels and are considered to have insufficiency rather than deficiency. Requirements are small except during bone growth or pregnancy, and a small reserve is stored in fat.

Use of routine vitamin D_3 supplementation remains controversial and of proven benefit only in people who are very old to reduce the risk of hip fracture.

Rickets is now rare, but immigrants in the north of the UK are at risk. Contributory factors are lack of sunlight, a high-carbohydrate diet and possibly also phytate, flour and other dietary factors that impair calcium absorption.

There is no basis for the idea that dental caries is due to poor calcification of the teeth. Giving vitamin D and calcium for dental caries or 'dental health' is valueless and dangerous, but a widespread urban myth. Hypervitaminosis D causes hypercalcaemia and renal calcinosis.

Mild osteoporosis has been considered to predispose to periodontitis.

Rickets general review PMID: 24412049

Vitamin D and periodontitis PMID: 23574464

Endocrine disorders and pregnancy

37

Endocrine disorders, apart from diabetes mellitus and thyroid disease, are uncommon. They are rare causes of oral disease but, occasionally, oral changes can lead to their diagnosis. Patients with Addison's disease, diabetes mellitus and thyrotoxicosis, in particular, may also need special care for dental surgery.

PITUITARY GIGANTISM AND ACROMEGALY

Overproduction of growth hormone by the anterior pituitary during skeletal growth causes overgrowth of the skeleton and soft tissues to produce gigantism.

Acromegaly arises from excess hormone in middle age, after the epiphyses have fused. The hormone then only increases growth of the hands and feet, membrane bones of the skull and jaws, and soft tissues. Growth is slow, and diagnosis is often delayed.

The condylar growth centre becomes reactivated and the mandible enlarged and protrusive (Fig. 37.1). Radiographically, the whole jaw is lengthened and the angle becomes more oblique (Fig. 37.2). The jaw and other bones are also made thicker by subperiosteal bone deposition, producing frontal bossing. The teeth become spaced or, if the patient is edentulous, dentures cease to fit the growing jaw. The hands and feet become spade-like (Fig. 37.1). Overgrowth of soft tissues causes thickening and enlargement of the facial features, particularly the lips and nose. The tongue, lips, nose and ears enlarge, and vocal cord thickening causes a deep voice. Diagnosis is often very delayed causing potentially life-threatening complications to develop and dentists have a role to play in early recognition.

The cause is usually an adenoma of growth hormone–secreting cells in the pituitary. Enlargement of this tumour commonly causes headaches and visual disturbances from pressure on the optic chiasma. Occasionally, ectopic hormone production by a neoplasm of the pancreas or adrenal is the cause. Diabetes results from insulin resistance caused by growth hormone. Hypertension is common and may be associated with cardiomyopathy and dysrhythmias.

Treatment is ideally complete resection of the adenoma, usually by endoscopic surgery through the nose and sphenoid sinus. This is difficult since pituitary adenomas often have irregular margins and if surgery is incomplete or impossible, irradiation may be required. Alternatively, or in conjunction, medical treatment is possible with octreotide or lanreotide, somatostatin analogues that inhibit hormone secretion or pegvisomant, a growth hormone receptor blocker. Medical treatment is effective but difficult due to adverse effects of the drugs. Established growth changes do not resolve.

Rarely, a growth hormone–producing pituitary tumour is part of multiple endocrine neoplasia syndrome type 1 (MEN1), as described later. In such patients, gingival papules have also been described.

Acromegaly case report PMID: 31431102

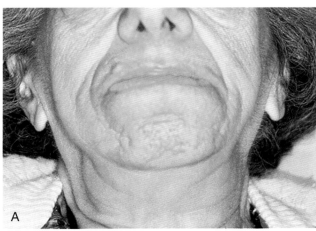
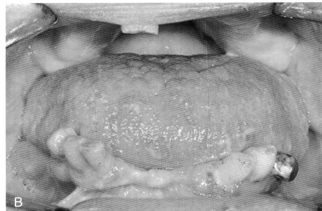
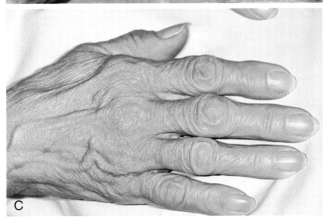

Fig. 37.1 Acromegaly. The typical facial appearance, resulting from excessive mandibular growth and thickened skin (A), tongue enlargement (B) and consequent playing of teeth and broad 'spade-like' hands (C). *(From Regezi, J.A., Sciubba, J.J., Jordan, R.C.K. 2003. Oral pathology: clinical pathological correlations, fourth ed. WB Saunders, Philadelphia.)*

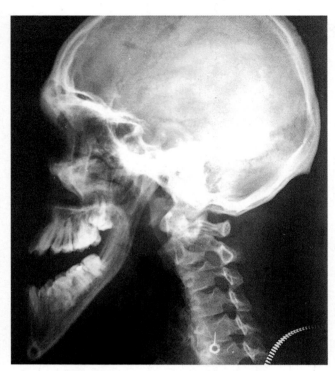

Fig. 37.2 Acromegaly. The mandible is enlarged with an elongated ramus and increased obliquity of the angle. The pituitary fossa is also enlarged due to the tumour causing the disease.

Dental considerations

Almost all patients have facial, oral or dental signs. Enlargement of the sella turcica may be a chance finding on imaging. There is a risk of post-operative airway obstruction because of the large tongue and narrowing of the glottis. Hypertension and diabetes can also affect dental management. Otherwise, there is no special risk from treatment, local analgesia or sedation. Orthognathic surgery may be considered to improve the appearance.

THYROID DISEASE

Hyperthyroidism

Hyperthyroidism is most common in young adults, particularly women. Causes include diffuse thyroid enlargement (goitre), a hypersecreting hyperplastic nodule or adenoma in the gland, and autoimmune thyroiditis caused by stimulatory autoantibodies (Graves' disease).

Clinical features are shown in Box 37.1. Graves' disease has additional exophthalmos and pretibial myxoedema caused by autoimmune inflammation.

Treatment of hyperthyroidism is by drugs such as carbimazole, iodine[131], or surgical removal of part of the gland. All treatments may over-correct, leading to delayed hypothyroidism. Beta-blockers may be used for symptom control.

Thyrotoxicosis general review PMID: 27038492

Dental considerations

Dental treatment, infection, acute stress or traumatic injury in an untreated patient with hyperthyroidism risks the medical emergency of thyrotoxic crisis (thyroid storm). Though this complication is rare, it is potentially fatal and recognition of signs and symptoms of hyperthyroidism is

---

Box 37.1   Important features of hyperthyroidism

- Irritability, anxiety, insomnia, agitation
- Difficulty sleeping
- Tremor
- Sweating and high temperature
- Loss of weight
- Tachycardia
- Diarrhoea
- Cardiovascular disease, particularly in untreated hyperthyroidism in older patients
- Exophthalmos in Graves' disease

Box 37.2   Dental management of hyperthyroid patients

- If clinical signs are seen but the patient is not under treatment, refer to a physician
- Control of nervousness and excitability
- Thiouracil drug treatment may cause salivary gland swelling and stones
- Iodine containing agents such as radiographic contrast for sialograms or povidone iodine may disturb thyroid function
- Avoid general anaesthesia in patients with longstanding thyrotoxicosis, particularly older patients

---

key. The triggering factors cause excessive release of thyroid hormone, producing high temperature, tachycardia, cardiac dysrhythmias, heart failure, agitation and seizures, sometimes confusion and muscle weakness.

Thyroid crisis cannot be managed in the dental surgery and must be prevented, or recognized quickly and emergency medical management instituted. Infection in patients with untreated hyperthyroidism must be treated aggressively, but operative dental treatment must be deferred until thyrotoxicosis is controlled and any emergency treatment performed in hospital. Patients with known hyperthyroidism who have ceased or reduced their medication are at higher risk.

Dental treatment in treated disease is affected by several factors (Box 37.2), particularly excitability and anxiety. Excessive cardiac excitability is only a theoretical contraindication to lidocaine with epinephrine, and no other local anaesthetic has been shown to be safer. Conscious sedation (nitrous oxide and oxygen) is frequently helpful in an anxious hyperthyroid patient.

Treatment with radioiodine damages the salivary glands, which concentrate the iodine in the same way as the thyroid gland. Despite some microscopic inflammation and scarring, no xerostomia is caused unless doses are repeated many times.

Periodontal adverse effects treatment PMID: 25577420

Dental treatment in thyroid disease PMID: 16504858

Hypothyroidism
Congenital hypothyroidism

Congenital hypothyroidism results from deficient thyroid activity from birth and may be due to genetic thyroid

Box 37.3 Typical features of congenital iodine deficiency

- Skeletal development and dental eruption greatly delayed
- Slow tooth development, large pulp chambers, open apices
- Enamel hypoplasia
- Learning disability
- Broad, rather flat face partly due to reduced growth of the skull and facial bones
- Overlarge, protrusive tongue and anterior open bite
- Dull facial expression, dry thick skin
- Thick lips
- Short stocky build and, often, umbilical hernia
- Sensitivity to cold
- Bradycardia and hypotension

Box 37.4 Typical features of adult hypothyroidism. Signs are often mild and easily missed.

- Weight gain
- Slowed activity and thought, fatigue
- Myxoedema and hoarse voice
- Bradycardia
- Dry skin and hair loss
- Intolerance of cold
- Susceptibility to ischaemic heart disease

Box 37.5 Dental management of hypothyroidism

- Most treated patients require no special consideration
- Avoid sedatives including diazepam, opioid analgesics and general anaesthetics because of the risk of myxoedemic coma
- Anaemia or ischaemic heart disease may require modification of dental treatment
- Local anaesthesia always preferable
- Nitrous oxide/oxygen sedation acceptable
- Iodine containing agents such as radiographic contrast for sialograms or povidone iodine may disturb thyroid function
- Sjögren's syndrome occasionally associated with autoimmune thyroiditis

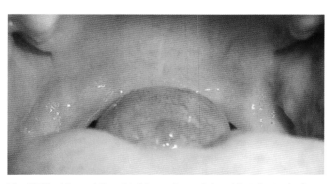

Fig. 37.3 Lingual thyroid. A large lingual thyroid at the typical site. *(From Amr, B., Monib, S., 2011. Lingual thyroid: A case report. Int. J. Surg. Case Rep. 2, 313–315.)*

or pituitary malformations or synthesis of an abnormal thyroid hormone, but these are very rare. By far the commonest cause is dietary iodine deficiency and it is almost never seen in developed countries where screening and thyroid supplementation from birth are available and food or salt is supplemented with iodine. However, dietary iodine deficiency is endemic in many parts of the world and remains a major health problem, with nearly 2 billion individuals affected, particularly in Africa, the Middle East and Asia. Without very early diagnosis and iodine or thyroxine supplementation, permanent effects ensue.

The main features are particularly short stature and learning disability, and dental changes are frequently associated (Box 37.3). In the untreated patient, sedatives and tranquillisers such as benzodiazepines can precipitate myxoedemic coma and should generally be avoided. Conscious sedation with nitrous oxide and oxygen can be given.

Diagnosis in dental setting PMID: 25328321 and

Web URL 37.1 https://www.medigraphic.com/pdfs/odon/uo-2014/uoi142i.pdf

Adult hypothyroidism

Hypothyroidism in the UK is most frequently due to Hashimoto autoimmune thyroiditis but can follow radioiodine, drug or surgical treatment for hyperthyroidism. In most of the world, iodine deficiency is the main cause.

Features are shown in Box 37.4 and aspects of dental management summarised in Box 37.5.

Dental management PMID: 16876054

Lingual thyroid

The thyroglossal tract and cysts arising from it are discussed in Chapter 10.

Failure of normal development of the thyroid gland is almost always caused by failure of the embryonic thyroid anlage to descend into the neck. The patient's thyroid gland then lies somewhere along the path of the thyroglossal tract but is usually on the dorsum of the tongue at the site of the foramen caecum (Fig. 37.3), within the tongue or near the hyoid bone (Fig. 37.4). Females are mainly affected.

Clinically a lingual thyroid is an asymptomatic midline, purplish soft swelling and may cause dysphagia. Presentation is often at puberty or in pregnancy, when the thyroid normally enlarges. Lingual thyroid may not be recognised as such clinically, and biopsy may cause considerable bleeding. Otherwise, the nature of the swelling may be determined by fine needle aspiration. Patients with lingual thyroid are often hypothyroid.

Lingual thyroid tissue must not be removed before confirming that a thyroid gland is present in the neck by ultrasound scanning. If not, radioiodine or MRI scanning should be used to detect more deeply placed thyroid tissue. If no other thyroid tissue is present, removal would precipitate hypothyroidism and life-long thyroxine supplementation would be required. Malignant change in lingual thyroid is recognized but rare and more frequent in males.

Review PMID: 25439547

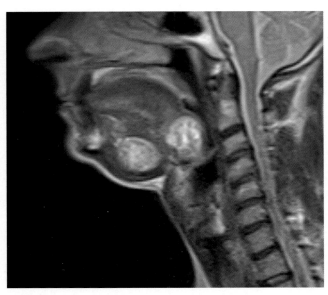

Fig. 37.4 Lingual thyroid tissue. Magnetic resonance imaging scan showing two rounded masses of thyroid tissue in the posterior and inferior parts of the tongue, but none on the tongue dorsum or at the usual site in the neck..

> **Box 37.6   Typical features of hyperparathyroidism**
> - General malaise
> - Peptic ulceration
> - Bone resorption
> - Renal stones or diffuse mineralisation (nephrocalcinosis)
> - Polyuria

PARATHYROID DISEASE

→ Summary chart 12.2 p. 229

Hyperparathyroidism

The causes of hyperparathyroidism and its effects on bone are discussed in Chapter 13. In primary hyperparathyroidism the cause is an adenoma of a parathyroid gland, very occasionally a parathyroid carcinoma.

The commonest type is secondary hyperparathyroidism, a reaction to low serum calcium levels caused by chronic renal failure or prolonged dialysis. It may also be an effect of lithium treatment.

High levels of calcium cause weakness, fatigue, constipation and kidney stones and features summarised in Box 37.6. However, such florid presentations are now rare, and most cases are asymptomatic and discovered by chance or because of a high serum calcium or when patients are seen with a renal stone.

Hyperparathyroidism is the presenting sign of the uncommon disease, multiple endocrine neoplasia syndrome type 1 (see the following section). There are also other familial forms. The hyperparathyroidism-jaw tumour syndrome is a rare autosomal dominant disease whose features include parathyroid adenomas or carcinomas, renal cysts and fibro-osseous jaw lesions, as discussed in Chapter 11. Brown tumours of hyperparathyroidism are discussed in Chapter 13.

> **Box 37.7   Effects of hypoparathyroidism on calcified tissues**
> - Retarded new bone formation and diminished resorption are usually in equilibrium so that skeletal changes are rare
> - Aplasia or hypoplasia of developing enamel*, which becomes deeply grooved
> - Dentine may be incompletely mineralised but lamina dura may be thickened
> - Short roots to teeth, large pulp chambers (Ch. 2)
>
> ---
> *Results from associated ectodermal defects in developmental conditions, not lack of calcium.

Bone lesions case report PMID: 25398922

Hypoparathyroidism

The most common cause of hypoparathyroidism by far is thyroidectomy, when parathyroid glands are inadvertently excised during surgery to the thyroid gland. Despite residual parathyroid tissue in other glands undergoing compensatory hyperplasia, 20% of patients are affected. Early-onset hypoparathyroidism is rare and developmental in origin, sometimes part of autoimmune polyendocrinopathy or other syndromes.

Hypocalcaemia from any of these causes presents as heightened neuromuscular excitability and tetany, sometimes confusion and seizures. In chronic disease, these are controlled by giving the vitamin D analogue cholecalciferol (D_3) and calcium orally, with dietary adjustment to avoid phosphorus. Recombinant parathormone (PTH residues 1-34 (teriparatide) or PTH1-84) are also available.

Effects on calcified tissues are summarised in Box 37.7. See also Fig. 2.37.

Early onset hypoparathyroidism case PMID: 19201623

Tetany

Low calcium level causing tetany is usually caused by hypoparathyroidism or vitamin D deficiency. In mild cases, tetany is latent but can be triggered by tapping on the skin over the facial nerve; this causes the facial muscles to contract (Chvostek's sign). In more severe cases, muscle cramps and tonic contractions of the muscles may progress to generalised convulsions. An early symptom of tetany is paraesthesia of the lip and extremities.

Tetany in the dental surgery more frequently results from overbreathing due to anxiety, producing the same signs.

Pseudohypoparathyroidism

This rare genetic condition is caused by mutations in genes that affect the PTH receptor cell activation pathway, including the *GNAS* gene associated with Albright's syndrome. Clinical features vary with the cause, but most patients are short, with a round face, hypocalcaemic, and have missing teeth, teeth with large pulps and enamel hypoplasia.

Pseudohypoparathyroidism case report PMID: 31892351 and 29191124

ADRENOCORTICAL DISEASES

Adrenocortical insufficiency is rarely primary (Addison's disease) and more frequently secondary to corticosteroid therapy.

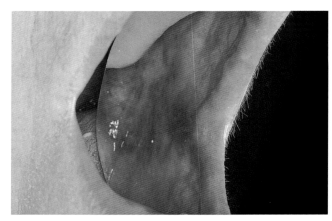

Fig. 37.6 Addison's disease. Deep pigmentation of the buccal mucosa.

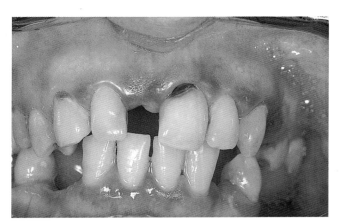

Fig. 37.5 Addison's disease. A close-up shows the characteristic distribution of pigment rather patchily along the attached gingivae. It is a brownish-black in colour.

Adrenocortical hypofunction or Addison's disease

Addison's disease results from failure of secretion of cortisol and aldosterone, either from gland destruction or very rarely from genetic defects of gland or hormone formation. The disease is usually autoimmune with organ-specific circulating autoantibodies. Tuberculous or fungal adrenal destruction are rare causes, sometimes secondary to HIV infection. Addison's disease is also the most frequent feature of the rare polyglandular autoimmune syndromes and is then associated with chronic mucocutaneous candidosis as described later.

The result is a severe disorder of electrolyte and fluid balance with serious clinical effects (Box 37.8).

Pigmentation results from compensatory adrenocorticotropic hormone (ACTH) secretion as this peptide hormone has a similar amino acid sequence to melanocyte-stimulating hormone. Pigmentation is often an early sign and, in the mouth, is patchily distributed on gingivae, buccal mucosa and lips (Figs 37.5 and 37.6). It is brown or almost black. The skin pigmentation looks similar to suntan but with a sallow appearance due to underlying pallor. Exposed and normally pigmented areas are most severely affected.

Addison's disease is an exceptionally rare cause of oral pigmentation but, if there is recent onset with general weakness and lassitude, the diagnosis should be considered.

Long-term treatment of Addison's disease is usually by oral hydrocortisone and fludrocortisone, with salt supplementation if necessary. The dose of steroid needs to be adjusted to provide additional steroid support in times of stress, infection, other illness, surgery or exercise. Failure to provide sufficient steroid, or untreated disease, may lead to Addisonian crisis.

In an Addisonian or adrenal crisis there is a rapid fall in blood pressure, circulatory collapse (shock: pale, cold, clammy skin, sweating, rapid, shallow breathing, dizziness) and vomiting. These may be associated with dehydration, headache, drowsiness or loss of consciousness. These crises may be fatal, and they require immediate treatment with intravenous hydrocortisone and fluid replacement, as discussed in chapter 44.

Patients may also experience the other adverse effects of excess therapeutic corticosteroids (Table 43.1).

Oral pigmentation in Addison's PMID: 16209154

Adrenocortical hyperfunction

Cushing's disease is usually due to an adrenocorticotrophic hormone-secreting pituitary adenoma that causes adrenocortical hyperplasia. Cushing's syndrome refers to the same features caused by ectopic ACTH production by another neoplasm, or corticosteroid treatment, the last being by far the commonest cause. The effects (Box 37.9) are rarely dentally important.

Cushing's review for dentistry PMID: 23094575

AUTOIMMUNE POLYENDOCRINE SYNDROMES

These three diseases are also known as *polyglandular autoimmune disease* (or APECED). They have different inheritance

Table 37.1 Polyendocrinopathy syndromes

	Percentage of patients affected by the different syndrome components	
	Type 1	Type 2
Addison's disease	100	100
Hypoparathyroidism	76	–
Chronic mucocutaneous candidosis	73	–
Pernicious anaemia	13	0.5
Alopecia	32	0.5
Malabsorption syndromes	22	–
Gonadal failure	17	3.6
Chronic active hepatitis	13	–
Insulin-dependent diabetes	4	52
Autoimmune thyroiditis	11	69
Female:male ratio	1.5:1	1.8:1

patterns, and several genes are responsible but all feature autoimmune attack on multiple endocrine glands. The two more common types both have Addison's disease as an invariable feature, and there are several other components of significance to dental treatment, notably chronic mucocutaneous candidosis in type 1 (Table 37.1). Candidosis is an early and common presenting feature. Dental changes can also result from hypoparathyroidism in the type 1 syndrome (Fig. 2.37) and as many as 10% of patients with type 1 disease develop oral or oesophageal carcinoma.

General review PMID: 29562162

Case report PMID: 1407992 and 35182449

Case report with carcinoma PMID: 20304522

DISEASES OF THE ADRENAL MEDULLA

Phaeochromocytoma

Phaeochromocytoma is a catecholamine-producing tumour of the adrenal medulla. The main effect is potentially lethal hypertension, tachycardia and dysrhythmias. A third of cases have a genetic predisposition. It may be part of the multiple endocrine adenoma syndrome type IIb, when it is associated with oral mucosal neuromas (Box 37.10). Alternatively, it may be associated with neurofibromatosis, von Hippel-Lindau or other inherited diseases.

When an oral neuroma (but not other types of benign nerve sheath tumour) is found, the possibility of a phaeochromocytoma should be considered, especially if the patient is hypertensive.

Dental treatment must be delayed in any patient with a phaeochromocytoma. A stressful event may precipitate a hypertensive crisis.

MULTIPLE ENDOCRINE NEOPLASIA SYNDROMES

Multiple endocrine neoplasia (multiple endocrine adenomatosis) syndromes (MEN) are autosomal dominant disorders with a prevalence of approximately 1 in 20,000 that cause gland hyperplasia and benign and malignant neoplasms.

Box 37.10 Important features of multiple endocrine neoplasia (MEN) syndromes

MEN 1
- Adenomas of pituitary, adrenals, sometimes thyroid. Insulinoma, gastrinoma. parathyroid hyperplasia
- Zollinger–Ellison syndrome and peptic ulceration

MEN 2a (Sipple syndrome)
- Thyroid medullary cell carcinoma in all patients
- Parathyroid hyperplasia
- Phaeochromocytoma in 33% of patients
- Cutaneous neurofibromas

MEN 2b
- Thyroid medullary cell carcinoma in 80%–100% of patients
- Parathyroid hyperplasia
- Phaeochromocytoma in 70% of patients
- Marfanoid skeletal features
- Ganglioneuromas of bowel causing distension
- Mucosal neuromas orally and sometimes in the eye

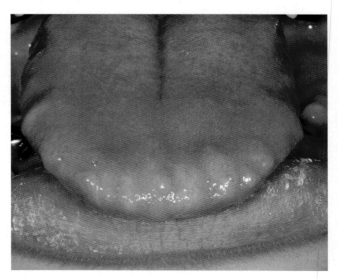

Fig. 37.7 Mucosal neuromas in MEN2b. These slightly firm pale nodules along the border and dorsum of the tongue are tangled masses of enlarged nerves. *(Courtesy Prof. D Emmanouil.)*

MEN1 is caused by mutation in the tumour suppressor gene *MEN1*, which encodes a nuclear transcription factor. Parathyroid, pancreas and pituitary are affected, and presentation is in the second and third decades. Hyperparathyroidism develops in 95%. Pancreatic tumours develop in more than 40% and pituitary tumours in more than 30%. Also described are gingival papules and nodular lesions on the vermilion border.

In MEN2, the mutated gene is the *RET* proto-oncogene, a growth factor receptor that affects cell cycle and also the development of autonomic nerves. In this disease, medullary carcinoma of the thyroid is present in 95%, phaeochromocytoma in 50% and hyperparathyroidism in 15% of cases. Two forms are recognised, 2a and 2b (the latter sometimes called type 3).

A striking oral feature of MEN2b is mucosal neuromas, particularly along the lateral borders of the tongue (Fig. 37.7). These are neither neurofibromas nor schwannomas

(Ch. 25), but developmental anomalies of tangles of enlarged nerves. Large neuromas enlarge the tongue, lips and other sites. Small ones produce small mucosal nodules or a papillary mucosa. These are often the first sign and can be diagnosed in infancy or childhood. Diagnosis following dental examination is not unusual. Screening for MEN2 is relatively readily carried out by identifying the *RET* mutation. Confirmed cases will be offered total thyroidectomy in infancy to avoid developing medullary carcinoma, which can affect very young individuals.

Features of multiple endocrine neoplasia syndromes are summarised in Box 37.10. Note that several features individually may be parts of other syndromes or familial diseases.

General review all types PMID: 26363542

Case report MEN2b: 25454714 and 1351093

DIABETES MELLITUS

Diabetes mellitus results from relative or absolute deficiency of insulin, causing persistently raised blood glucose. UK prevalence has doubled in 20 years, and 5% of the population are affected, but probably at least 50% of individuals with mild or early disease pass unrecognised. By 2025 the UK incidence will be 8%, a level already attained in the United States. World incidence is rising as populations become urbanised, eat a more Western diet and become obese.

There are two main clinical types.

Type 1 diabetes ('insulin-dependent') accounts for 10% of cases. Symptoms typically appear before the age of 25, and the disease is usually severe with thirst, polyuria, hunger, loss of weight and susceptibility to infection. The cause is failure of secretion of insulin after autoimmune destruction of the pancreatic islets and insulin replacement is the treatment.

Type 2 ('maturity onset') accounts for 90% of cases. Patients are typically older than middle age and obese. The onset is insidious, often with deterioration of vision or pruritus or, sometimes, thirst, polyuria and fatigue. However, many cases are asymptomatic. The cause is end organ resistance to insulin, and the disease can be controlled by dietary restriction of sugar and high glycaemic index carbohydrate, exercise and, if necessary, oral hypoglycaemic drugs. The current epidemic of childhood obesity has already led to the onset of this variety of diabetes early in life.

In practice the division between these two types can be somewhat blurred.

In terms of dental management, it is usually said that the greatest challenges are with 'uncontrolled' diabetes. However, 'uncontrolled' applies to several diabetic states. At one extreme, there is the mild, unrecognized, and therefore untreated, diabetic. At the other, there is the treated diabetic whose disease is difficult to control ('brittle diabetes') or has been mismanaged. This latter group is the one most likely to have oral complications and present difficulties in dental management (Box 37.11).

Dental aspects

The main oral manifestations of diabetes are usually due to the lowered resistance to infection, particularly to fungi as a result of impaired neutrophil function. Oral candidosis is frequent, and severe deep mycoses such as mucormycosis are a risk, albeit small.

Rapidly destructive periodontal disease occurs, and severity is proportional to blood glucose levels and glycosylated

---

Box 37.11   Complications of diabetes mellitus that can affect dental management

- Susceptibility to infection, particularly candidosis, also mucormycosis
- Hypoglycaemic coma
- Diabetic ketoacidosis
- Atheroma, ischaemic heart disease
- Acceleration of periodontal disease if control is poor
- Dry mouth secondary to polyuria and dehydration
- Oral lichenoid reactions due to oral hypoglycaemic drugs
- Delayed healing
- Sialadenosis

Box 37.12   Principles of dental management for patients with diabetes

- Time treatment to avoid disturbance of routine insulin administration or meals
- Use local anaesthesia for routine dentistry – the amount of adrenaline (epinephrine) in local anaesthetic solutions has no significant effect on the blood sugar
- Sedation can be given if required
- Deal with any diabetic complications (Box 37.11)
- Manage hypoglycaemic coma as described in Chapter 44
- General anaesthesia requires special precautions

---

proteins. Severe periodontitis also seems to complicate insulin control and periodontal treatment can improve diabetic markers of disease severity. Diabetics with more severe periodontitis are at higher risk of diabetic complications such as nephropathy and ischaemic heart disease.

The relationship between diabetes and dental caries is unclear. Many patients have low caries susceptibility, probably because of the sugar-free diet. However, poorly controlled childhood patients have higher caries rates.

The principles of dental management are summarised in Box 37.12.

Type 2 diabetics with good dietary or oral hypoglycaemic drug control can be treated as a non-diabetic patient.

In type 1 diabetes, well-controlled patients are similarly very low risk. However, hypoglycaemic coma may be precipitated by dental treatment that delays a normal meal or unbalances food intake and insulin dose. This can cause an emergency in the dental surgery (Ch. 44). Treatment should therefore be so timed as to avoid these risks – ideally, soon after the patient's breakfast. Many patients now have their own glucose monitors and can check the level immediately before treatment and when symptoms suggest onset of hypoglycaemia.

Diabetic (hyperglycaemic) coma is a complication of poorly controlled diabetes mellitus and much less likely to be seen.

Patients with recurrent candidosis or severe periodontitis without cause can be relatively easily tested in a dental setting using urine dipsticks to detect glycosuria, enabling confident referral to their medical practitioner. UK organisations and guidelines recommend testing patients with periodontitis for diabetes mellitus.

Management in dentistry PMID: 17376713, 17000275 and 32643574

Oral features review PMID: 15196139

Oral health type 2 diabetes PMID: 23531957 and 18302671

Practice testing guideline PMID: 32383274 and findings 35669587

Link to periodontitis PMID: 35612801

PREGNANCY

Pregnancy is a physiological process and should not deter dental treatment; this is an important time to establish good oral health for mother and child. Nevertheless, the changes of pregnancy do impact on dental care in three main ways: hormonal influences on the oral cavity, risks to the foetus and adjustments required for medication (Box 37.13).

Review PMID: 33921608

Foetal considerations

The main risks of foetal abnormalities are from drugs and radiation; the hazard is greatest during organogenesis in the first trimester.

Few drugs are known to be teratogenic for humans and, in many cases, the risk is no more than theoretical or results only from prolonged, high dosage. For example, no teratogenic risk from metronidazole for humans has ever been substantiated though effects in animals have led to the avoidance of metronidazole during pregnancy.

The risks from dental radiography are small, but only essential radiographs should be taken, the minimal radiation exposure should be given, and radiography delayed if possible. An abdominal dose of radiation, particularly in the first trimester, risks congenital abnormality, learning disability and malignant neoplasms. Because the risk period is likely to be before the patient will know she is pregnant,

---

Box 37.13   Pregnancy: oral effects and management considerations

Effect on the mother

- Aggravated gingivitis and epulis formation
- Variable effect on recurrent aphthae
- Increased intensity of pigmentation, face and sometimes oral
- Risk of hypotension when laid supine
- Possible hypertension of pregnancy
- Hypersensitive gag reflex and vomiting
- Possible iron or folate deficiency, especially if anaemic before pregnancy

Risks to the foetus

- X-rays hazardous, especially in first trimester
- Respiratory depression due to sedatives, including benzodiazepines
- Tooth discolouration due to tetracycline
- Prilocaine may rarely cause methaemoglobinaemia
- Theoretical risk of uterine contraction caused by felypressin
- Aspirin may cause neonatal haemorrhage
- Theoretical risk of depressed vitamin B_{12} metabolism by nitrous oxide
- Teratogenic risks of thalidomide, retinoids, azathioprine and possibly other drugs

---

precautions must be taken for all women of child-bearing age. In the UK this does not require routine use of lead aprons as the beam in dental radiography will not be directed toward the abdomen. Routine collimation, fast films or digital capture, and good technique are most important in reducing dose. Nevertheless, during pregnancy, the patient may be offered a lead apron because the topic is so emotive, but routine radiation protection measures are safe. In some countries, a lead apron is required.

Non-steroidal anti-inflammatory drugs in high dosage may cause premature closure of the ductus arteriosus and fatal pulmonary hypertension. Aspirin may also increase the risk of neonatal haemorrhage and paracetamol is the only safe analgesic. Systemic corticosteroids can cause foetal adrenosuppression. However, the only drugs known to be teratogenic and likely to be prescribed in a dental setting are thalidomide (used occasionally for major aphthae), etretinate (used experimentally for leukoplakia) and possibly azathioprine (used for Behçet's syndrome and autoimmune diseases). Systemic antifungals and antiviral agents are considered safe, with adverse effects limited to animal studies. For details of drug usage in pregnancy, see the current British National Formulary or other national and local guidance.

Maternal considerations

Patients who are pregnant should be fully evaluated as early as possible so that any treatment necessary can be planned for the second trimester and emergency dental care avoided. Temporary restorations and stabilisation may be required when oral health is poor. An intensive preventive regime of oral hygiene and diet control will benefit both the mother and future child. Prenatal fluoride supplementation provides no benefit to the child's caries risk.

The chief oral effects of pregnancy are aggravation of gingivitis (Fig. 37.8) and possible development of a pregnancy epulis (Fig. 37.9; Ch. 24). These complications usually affect women with pre-existing gingivitis and develop around the second month.

Occasionally, recurrent aphthae remit during pregnancy but may worsen due to any iron or folate deficiency.

A few women in the third trimester of pregnancy become hypotensive when laid supine, when the enlarged uterus impedes venous return. Respiratory reserve is diminished, and there is a risk of foetal hypoxia. It is easiest to treat all patients in late pregnancy in a sitting position and in short appointments, as this is more comfortable.

Neonatal respiration is further depressed by drugs such as general anaesthetics and sedatives, especially barbiturates,

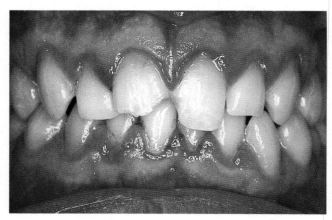

Fig. 37.8 Pregnancy gingivitis. Marginal gingivitis despite relatively good oral hygiene during the first trimester of pregnancy.

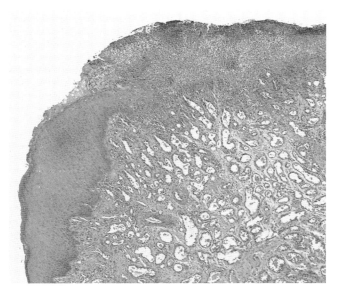

Fig. 37.9 Pregnancy epulis. These are usually detected and removed during growth and so are often ulcerated and highly vascular. In this example the upper part of the nodule is ulcerated and the bulk of the tissue comprises blood vessels in granulation or loose fibrous tissue.

diazepam and opioids, all of which cross the placenta and are contraindicated in pregnancy.

There is no evidence of risks from local anaesthesia, and pain is likely to cause greater adverse consequences. Felypressin is an oxytocin analogue and in theory could induce uterine contractions and foetal methaemoglobinaemia. These are not considered risks at dental doses, but lignocaine with epinephrine is generally taken to be preferable as it is more effective. As noted earlier, the risks from benzodiazepines such as midazolam for sedation are such that intravenous sedation is contraindicated. Nitrous oxide sedation carries a risk of interference with B_{12} and folate metabolism after very prolonged administration (weeks), but there is no evidence that it is teratogenic and it is safe after the first trimester used with 50% oxygen. Exposure should be limited to 30 minutes and repeated exposure avoided.

The myth that mothers lose a tooth for every pregnancy reflects poor oral health in past decades and is nothing to do with increased calcium requirements during pregnancy; this calcium is provided from bone and diet, not maternal teeth.

Oral surgery during pregnancy PMID: 18088879

Dental treatment during pregnancy PMID: 23570802

Oral health and pregnancy PMID: 15042797

Prescribing considerations in dentistry PMID: 27103292

Renal disease | 38

Renal disease has become important in dentistry because of the growing number of patients who, as a result of renal dialysis or transplantation, survive renal failure. In the UK, nearly 2 million patients have renal failure and a further million at least are undiagnosed. Aspects of renal disease relevant to dentistry are summarised in Box 38.1.

CHRONIC RENAL FAILURE AND DIALYSIS

The common causes are diabetes, hypertension, or glomerulonephritis. Some patients are unsuitable for, or are unable to undergo dialysis or transplantation. They can develop a variety of oral effects (Box 38.2). In severe uraemia, urea may crystallise on the skin and oral mucosa ('urea frost').

Prolonged dialysis or renal failure are now the most common causes of hyperparathyroidism. The severity is greater than in primary hyperparathyroidism, which once detected is easily treated, because control of renal function is more difficult and has a more protracted course. Removal of the four main parathyroid glands may be required. The jaws may be first affected (Ch. 13) and, unlike in other causes of hyperparathyroidism, may be diffusely or focally and markedly enlarged (Fig 38.1).

Dental management of patients with renal disease, particularly chronic renal failure, may be affected by many factors (Box 38.3).

Patients with renal failure may receive regular dialysis while awaiting a transplant but remain otherwise in reasonably good general health. Approximately 70% of patients can return to full-time work.

Peritoneal dialysis has no implications for dental treatment, but haemodialysis does. Patients are heparinised before haemodialysis, and haemostasis is impaired for 6–12 hours. Dental treatment should be delayed until the next day. Healing after tooth extraction is delayed, often

---

Box 38.1 Aspects of renal disease affecting dental management

- Heparinisation before dialysis
- Delayed healing
- Possible hepatitis B or C carriage after chronic dialysis
- Permanent venous fistulae susceptible to infection
- Increased risk of endocarditis
- Secondary hyperparathyroidism
- Immunosuppressive treatment for nephrotic syndrome or in transplant patients
- Oral lesions due to drugs, particularly for immunosuppression
- Reduced excretion of some drugs
- Oral lesions of chronic renal failure (Box 38.2)

Box 38.2 Oral changes in severe renal failure

- Mucosal pallor (anaemia)
- Xerostomia
- Purpura
- Mucosal ulceration
- Thrush or bacterial plaques
- White epithelial plaques (Ch. 18)
- Brown tumours of the jaws (from secondary hyperparathyroidism)

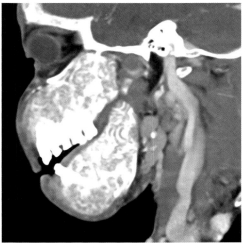

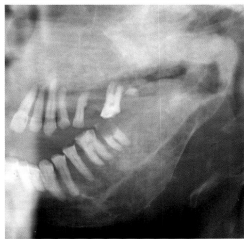

Fig. 38.1 Marked jaw enlargement in renal failure. There is marked diffuse enlargement of maxilla and mandible seen in the computed tomography scan in the upper panel. In the lower panel a section of a panoramic radiograph shows diffuse ground glass appearance, loss of maxillary sinus and cortex and lamina dura reflecting secondary hyperparathyroidism.

Box 38.3 Factors potentially affecting dental management of patients with renal disease

- Corticosteroid and other immunosuppressive treatment
- Haemorrhagic tendencies
- Anaemia
- Impaired drug excretion
- Hypertension
- Hepatitis B or C carriage
- Underlying causes (e.g., diabetes mellitus, hypertension or connective tissue disease)

with some prolonged bleeding but sockets are not prone to infection.

These patients' permanent venous fistulas for the haemodialysis lines are susceptible to infection, and antibiotic cover may be considered for dental surgical procedures. Drugs, including those for sedation, should not be given intravenously because of the risk of damage to superficial veins, which are patients' lifelines. A blood pressure cuff must never be placed on the arm with the shunt. Dialysis patients also have a greater incidence of cardiovascular and cerebrovascular disease.

Patients under dialysis will still have a uraemic oral odour and bad taste, xerostomia, and sore mouth with increased calculus.

Jaw enlargement PMID: 22676829 and 9127383

Oral findings in haemodialysis PMID: 23597063, 15723858 and 26513593

Periodontitis and renal disease PMID: 18173441

Dental treatment in renal disease PMID: 21714405

Prescribing considerations in dentistry PMID: 21037190

RENAL TRANSPLANTATION

Normal renal function and health can be restored by transplantation, but it is associated with the complications of prolonged immunosuppressive treatment, particularly susceptibility to infections or lymphomas.

Ciclosporin, which is widely used to help control graft rejection, can cause persistent gingival enlargement, and patients often take a calcium channel blocker, such as nifedipine, for hypertension, enhancing the effect (Ch. 7).

Hairy leukoplakia can develop rarely in HIV-negative renal transplant patients as a complication of immunosuppression.

Complications of graft rejection, such as bone lesions due to secondary hyperparathyroidism, may be seen (above and Ch. 13).

Prescribing precautions in renal failure depend on its severity. Local analgesics cause no problems, and the usual antibiotics for dental infections are safe except in severe disease. Dose reduction according to the glomerular filtration rate is usually sufficient precaution for most dental prescribing, but medical advice should be sought. However, nonsteroidal anti-inflammatory drugs, aspirin, tetracyclines, itraconazole, and systemic antivirals should be avoided.

Children with renal failure may have chronological enamel hypoplasia and dysplastic dentine with delayed eruption of teeth.

Drugs and gingival overgrowth PMID: 25680368

Management gingival overgrowth PMID: 16677333

Gingival overgrowth children PMID: 16238650

Orofacial pain, headache and neurological disorders

39

Pain is the most common symptom for which patients seek help. Pain has strong emotional associations which, in turn, may be determined to a varying degree by patients' preconceptions. Emotional disturbance itself can also produce the symptom of pain.

Pain is, therefore, both a genuine experience and an abstract concept, making it difficult to empathise with. Clinicians usually underestimate the pain experienced by patients and may think they appreciate the degree because they know the diagnosis but fail to understand the context and actual pain experienced ('pain blindness').

There are many causes of oral or maxillofacial pain (Box 39.1). Pulpitis and periapical periodontitis as sequels of dental caries are by far the most common causes. The source of such pain is usually obvious on examination. However, some sources of dental pain can be exceedingly difficult to identify (Box 39.2) and may only become apparent after a period of time.

The incidence of pain of dental origin varies with socioeconomic class and accessibility of dental services. In 1998 approximately 28% of the UK population reported a toothache in the previous 12 months, similar to the 15% in the previous 6 months reported in the US a decade earlier. Currently toothache in the UK is becoming more frequent, caused by reduced availability of services, increasing costs and the Covid pandemic. The pain is severe, lasting more than 2 weeks in 10% of the population and is more frequent in children. A key role of the dentist is to exclude dental and mucosal causes of pain before further medical investigation and to be able to formulate a differential diagnosis, but the expected role of the dentist in non-dental pain varies among countries.

Principles of taking a pain history and diagnosis are discussed in Chapter 1. Transmission of information when referring is critical for efficient diagnosis in secondary care. Table 39.1 provides a reminder of the types and mechanisms of pain.

Definitions and classification of facial and oral pain have previously been confused with those of headache, but a new classification of orofacial pain clearly divides all such pain into dental related causes (from teeth, gingiva and muscles of mastication), neuralgias, primary headaches and idiopathic orofacial pain syndromes. A summary version of the classification is shown in Table

---

Box 39.1   Types of pain felt in the oral tissues

- Disease of teeth and/or supporting tissues
- Oral mucosal diseases
- Diseases of the jaw
- Pain in the edentulous patient
- Post-operative pain
- Pain triggered by mastication
- Referred pain
- Neurological diseases
- Psychogenic pain

Box 39.2   Causes of pain from the teeth or supporting tissues

- Pulpitis
- Dentine hypersensitivity, cracked tooth or cracked cusp syndrome
- Periapical periodontitis
- Lateral (periodontal) abscess
- Necrotising types of gingivitis
- Pericoronitis

Table 39.1   Types and mechanisms of pain

Source of pain	Example	Mediators
Peripheral nerve stimulation (nociceptive pain)	Pulpitis and apical periodontitis	Inflammatory mediators and products of tissue damage, some bacterial factors bradykinin, histamine, serotonin, prostaglandin E2
Nerve damage	Herpes zoster infection, infiltration of nerve by malignant tumour	Unclear, inflammatory mediators, direct damage to pain fibres
Peripheral neuropathy	Burning mouth syndrome	Terminal nerve loss, reduced regeneration or demyelination, altered nociceptor thresholds
Central neuropathic pain	Burning mouth syndrome	Probably mediated by central neuronal connection changes, glial receptors, immune mediators and/or psychoimmunological mechanisms in brain and spinal cord. Persistent glial cell activation leads to functional changes in pain pathways and thresholds.
Psychogenic pain	Usually no specific pattern	Unclear, possibly generated by failure to suppress low-level pain or emotional overlay mediated by psychoimmunological mechanisms

Table 39.2   International Classification of Orofacial Pain 2020

This classification of orofacial pain is for both research and diagnostic use. The full classification includes considerable detail. Only the first three levels of classification are shown, but many sections use six subdivisions, each with diagnostic criteria. The classification allows for the fact that diagnoses are sometimes provisional or based on exclusion of other causes. For this last purpose, the full classification in the reference below provides a useful checklist of recognised orofacial pains.

1. Orofacial pain attributed to disorders of dentoalveolar and anatomically related structures

  1.1 Dental pain

    1.1.1 Pulpal pain

    1.1.2 Periodontal pain

    1.1.3 Gingival pain

  1.2 Oral mucosal, salivary gland and jaw bone pains

    1.2.1 Oral mucosal pain

    1.2.2 Salivary gland pain

    1.2.3 Jaw bone pain

2. Myofascial orofacial pain

  2.1 Primary myofascial orofacial pain

    2.1.1 Acute primary myofascial orofacial pain

    2.1.2 Chronic primary myofascial orofacial pain

  2.2 Secondary myofascial orofacial pain

    2.2.1 Myofascial orofacial pain attributed to tendonitis

    2.2.2 Myofascial orofacial pain attributed to myositis

    2.2.3 Myofascial orofacial pain attributed to muscle spasm

3. Temporomandibular joint (TMJ) pain

  3.1 Primary temporomandibular joint pain

    3.1.1 Acute primary temporomandibular joint pain

    3.1.2 Chronic primary temporomandibular joint pain

  3.2 Secondary temporomandibular joint pain

    3.2.1 Temporomandibular joint pain attributed to arthritis

    3.2.2 Temporomandibular joint pain attributed to disc displacement

    3.2.3 Temporomandibular joint pain attributed to degenerative joint disease

    3.2.4 Temporomandibular joint pain attributed to subluxation

4. Orofacial pain attributed to lesion or disease of the cranial nerves

  4.1 Pain attributed to lesion or disease of the trigeminal nerve

    4.1.1 Trigeminal neuralgia

    4.1.2 Other trigeminal neuropathic pain

  4.2 Pain attributed to lesion or disease of the glossopharyngeal nerve

    4.2.1 Glossopharyngeal neuralgia

    4.2.2 Glossopharyngeal neuropathic pain

5. Orofacial pains resembling presentations of primary headaches

  5.1 Orofacial migraine

    5.1.1 Episodic orofacial migraine

    5.1.2 Chronic orofacial migraine

  5.2 Tension-type orofacial pain

  5.3 Trigeminal autonomic orofacial pain

    5.3.1 Orofacial cluster attacks

    5.3.2 Paroxysmal hemifacial pain

    5.3.3 Short-lasting unilateral neuralgiform facial pain attacks with cranial autonomic symptoms (SUNFA)

    5.3.4 Hemifacial continuous pain with autonomic symptoms

  5.4 Neurovascular orofacial pain

    5.4.1 Short-lasting neurovascular orofacial pain

    5.4.2 Long-lasting neurovascular orofacial pain

6. Idiopathic orofacial pain

  6.1 Burning mouth syndrome

    6.1.1 Burning mouth syndrome without somatosensory changes

    6.1.2 Burning mouth syndrome with somatosensory changes

    6.1.3 Probable burning mouth syndrome

  6.2 Persistent idiopathic facial pain

    6.2.1 Persistent idiopathic facial pain without somatosensory changes

    6.2.2 Persistent idiopathic facial pain with somatosensory changes

    6.2.3 Probable persistent idiopathic facial pain

  6.3 Persistent idiopathic dentoalveolar pain

    6.3.1 Persistent idiopathic dentoalveolar pain without somatosensory changes

    6.3.2 Persistent idiopathic dentoalveolar pain with somatosensory changes

    6.3.3 Probable persistent idiopathic dentoalveolar pain

  6.4 Constant unilateral facial pain with additional attacks

International Classification of Orofacial Pain, 1st edition (ICOP). (2020). Cephalalgia: an international journal of headache, 40(2), 129–221. PMID: 32103673

39.2. The dentist plays the primary role in managing pain in the first three first level categories while in the last three the dentist plays an important role in diagnosis, exclusion of dental causes and may play a treatment role in a multidisciplinary team.

Classification of orofacial pain with diagnostic criteria PMID: 32103673

Trigeminal pain pathways PMID: 35249132

Review orofacial pain in dentistry PMID: 16444222

Classification and assessment orofacial pain PMID: 26058224 and 26062258

Team management chronic facial pain PMID: 25899741

How to refer PMID: 27056518

Incidence chronic pain types in dentistry PMID: 25338483

Diagnosis review and management guidelines PMID: 23794651

Prescribing for pain (US perspective) PMID: 22329011

DENTAL AND PERIODONTAL PAIN

Pulpitis

Pulpitis is usually the cause when hot or cold food or drinks trigger oral pain. It is also the main cause of spasmodic, poorly localised attacks of pain, which may be mistakenly ascribed to a variety of other possible causes. The pain of acute pulpitis is of a sharp lancinating character peculiar to itself, impossible to describe but unforgettable once experienced. Recurrent attacks of less severe, subacute or chronic pain, often apparently spontaneous, suggest a diseased or dying pulp.

One key feature of pulpitis is poor localisation. All tooth pain fibres converge in the trigeminal nerve and trigeminal sensory complex, which also receives pain and sensation from other nerves and extends into the upper spinal cord. The complex pathway means that the sensation is sometimes perceived and recognised as a toothache but cannot be localised. Patients often cannot localise pulpitic pain even to one quadrant. Although left and right are accurately distinguished, upper and lower arches often cannot be. Thus, investigation for pulpitis may require checking many teeth.

The only non-dental condition that is indistinguishable from pulp pain by the patient is the pain of early herpes zoster. If no local cause can be found after the most careful search, it is important to look for early signs of the characteristic rash and ask about contact with chicken pox and zoster (Ch. 15). Herpes zoster is an uncommon cause of toothache-like pain but has been the cause of unnecessary dental extractions and pulp extirpations. Even if zoster is diagnosed, the teeth must remain under surveillance as zoster causing toothache pain can devitalise the pulps.

Apical periodontitis

→ Summary chart 39.1 p. 552

Unlike pulpitis, pain from periapical periodontitis is readily identifiable and precisely localised as the nerves have accurate spatial representation in the cortex, being critical for mastication. There is tenderness of the tooth in its socket on percussion or pressure.

Radiographs are of little value in the early stages but useful after inflammation causes loss of definition of the periapical lamina dura. Later, a chronic apical periodontitis will produce a rounded area of radiolucency as a periapical granuloma develops. Most of these are asymptomatic (Ch. 5).

Acute maxillary sinusitis can rarely cause similar tenderness of a group of teeth, particularly upper molars, as discussed in Chapter 34.

Periodontal abscess and pericoronitis

The tooth is tender in its socket, and there is a deep localised pocket, either swollen or draining pus. The tooth is normally vital unless there are other reasons for loss of vitality, including involvement of the furcation by the abscess or periodontitis in molar teeth.

Occasionally, a periodontal abscess may be precipitated by endodontic root perforation on the side of the root, or a 'perio-endo' lesion may result from drainage of an apical infection through a pocket, triggering a periodontal abscess.

Pericoronitis is similar to a periodontal abscess in terms of pain, but with added elements of pain on biting on the swollen operculum.

Cracked teeth

The pain of a cracked tooth is distinctive, sharp, excruciating, lasting only a second or two and experienced only when occlusion or mastication opens the crack. However, identifying which cusp is cracked can be difficult as the pain, like pulpitis, is poorly localised. The best approach is to identify the crack by oblique pressure, biting on a slightly resilient elastic object such as a wooden wedge or instilling a dye such as disclosing solution.

Necrotising ulcerative gingivitis

Acute ulcerative gingivitis usually causes soreness, but when it extends deeply and rapidly, as in HIV infection, destroying the underlying bone, there may be severe aching pain (Ch. 7).

Odontogenic pain review PMID: 26630860

Acute orofacial pain PMID: 26964446

PAIN IN EDENTULOUS PATIENTS

Dental causes can be largely excluded, though infection of buried roots may need to be excluded. Pain caused by dentures may be a denture defect or related to some condition of the mucosa or jaws on which a denture is pressing (Box 39.3).

Traumatic ulcers, usually the consequence of overextension, often cause trouble with a new denture. After the denture has been relieved, these ulcers heal within 24–48 hours. Persistent ulceration after relief of an otherwise adequate denture is likely to be due to some more serious cause, and a biopsy is then essential. Later, dentures cause traumatic pain when alveolar bone has become severely resorbed, allowing the denture to bear on a sharp ridge apex, the mylohyoid ridge or genial tubercles.

Lack of freeway space due to excessive vertical dimension of the dentures prevents the mandible and masticatory muscles from reaching their natural rest position. This causes the teeth to be held permanently in contact. Aching pain is usually felt in the fatigued masticatory muscles, but the excessive stress imposed on the denture-bearing area sometimes causes pain in the alveolus. There may be interference with speech or swallowing if the vertical discrepancy is large.

The best investigation to determine whether pain is caused by the dentures themselves is for the patient to cease wearing them.

Few painful mucosal diseases affect the denture-bearing area. Denture stomatitis is common but painless. Lichen planus can extend to the sulcus and impinge on the margin of the denture-bearing area and mucous membrane pemphigoid may affect the palate and sulci. The most important conditions to be excluded are neoplasms. As most edentulous patients are old, persistent lesions, whether ulcerated or not, developing beneath or at the margins of dentures, must be biopsied without hesitation. A carcinoma can persist for

---

> **Box 39.3   Important causes of pain in edentulous patients**
>
> - Denture trauma
> - Excessive vertical dimension
> - Mucosal diseases of the denture-bearing mucosa
> - Diseases of the jaws (Box 39.4)
> - Teeth or roots erupting under a denture

a long time with minimal symptoms, and the patient may notice no more than the fact that the fit of the denture has deteriorated.

Jaw lesions causing pain in the edentulous patient may be associated with a swelling or an area of radiolucency. A painful swelling of the jaw in the edentulous patient is probably most often due to an infected residual cyst. Metastatic malignant neoplasms are very much less common but must be considered and intraosseous lesions evaluated for a biopsy.

Osteomyelitis of the jaws in patients who are edentulous must be considered if there is a history of radiotherapy, bisphosphonates or similar drugs (Ch. 8).

Late eruption of buried teeth, retained root fragments, and exfoliation of small sequestra following extraction may all cause pain beneath a denture as the mucosa is pinched between them and the denture. In a very atrophic mandible, fracture may need to be considered.

Finally, even well-constructed dentures can be disliked intensely, and pain may become a surrogate complaint for discomfort or appearance. Occasionally, dentures may become the focus of a psychogenic pain (Ch. 41).

PAINFUL MUCOSAL LESIONS

Ulcers generally cause soreness rather than pain, but deep ulceration may cause severe aching pain. Carcinoma, in particular, causes severe pain once nerve fibres become involved. It is important to emphasise again that early carcinoma is painless; pain is a late symptom. However, unusual neuralgic pain may be a presenting symptom of adenoid cystic carcinoma, caused by perineural and intra-neural spread.

PAIN IN THE JAWS

Pain from inside the mandible is usually felt as dull boring pain, unless related to teeth or fracture, in which cases periodontal ligament or mucosal receptors are involved.

Important causes are listed in Box 39.4. Chronic and low-grade osteomyelitis are particularly difficult causes of pain to diagnose because of their non-specific radiological and clinical features. Except for fractures and acute osteomyelitis, diagnosis of identifiable lesions depends on biopsy.

Referred cardiac pain PMID: 22322488

POSTSURGICAL PAIN AND NERVE DAMAGE

Important causes of post-operative pain are summarised in Box 39.5. Minor surgical procedures such as a simple extraction or soft-tissue biopsy produce mild pain and

discomfort after local analgesia wears off. Patients frequently take no analgesics after the first few hours, if at all.

By far the most common cause of significant pain after dental extractions is alveolar osteitis (dry socket; Ch. 8). Fracture of the jaw following operative treatment is rare but can also be readily recognised. Forcible opening of the mouth, particularly under general anaesthesia to remove wisdom teeth, can crush and inflame the temporomandibular joint periarticular tissues, leading to persistent pain on opening or during mastication. Pain from osteomyelitis develops some time after extraction (Ch. 8).

Iatrogenic nerve injury

The inferior alveolar and lingual nerves are those most frequently damaged during treatment, usually surgical removal of lower third molars. Placement of implants, and endodontic irrigation beyond the apex with hypochlorite are other causes. Lingual nerve injuries particularly follow lower third molar extraction when a lingual flap is raised; a lingually-placed elevator does not 'protect' the nerve, but damage it. Prevention is key: avoiding unnecessary extractions, identifying teeth close to nerves and using alternative techniques such as coronectomy when the nerve is at risk.

Local analgesia also causes similar nerve damage, particularly when using articaine, especially at a concentration of 4%. Lidocaine is the safest agent for block analgesia. Persistent symptoms do not necessarily follow an 'electric shock' pain during injection and do not necessarily result from direct needle trauma to the nerve.

Symptoms following all causes are of paraesthesia and pain in the relevant distribution, if severe interfering with speech, mastication and drinking. Light touch in areas of paraesthesia can trigger excruciating sharp pain in a similar fashion to trigeminal neuralgia.

More than three-quarters of iatrogenic lingual nerve injuries resolve spontaneously in 2–3 months. Inferior alveolar nerve effects are usually persistent, and surgical exploration should be considered within 3 months of third molar extraction for best effect. In the unlikely event that a nerve is completely severed, it must be repaired surgically as soon as possible. Endodontic materials extruded into the inferior dental canal must be removed within 24 hours.

Rarely, damaged nerves in soft tissue proliferate to form a traumatic neuroma which is tender to pressure. Its excision should lead to relief of the pain.

Avoiding nerve injury PMID: 24157759

Management iatrogenic injuries PMID: 22326447

Hypochlorite and endodontic injury PMID: 25809429, 24878709 and 23767399

Guideline hypochlorite extrusion PMID: 25525012

Associated with implants PMID: 25434563

Box 39.4 Causes of pain in the jaws

- Fractures
- Osteomyelitis
- Infected cysts
- Malignant neoplasms
- Sickle cell infarcts
- Referred pain of angina and myocardial infarction

Box 39.5 Post-operative pain

- Alveolar osteitis (dry socket)
- Fracture of the jaw
- Damage to the temporomandibular joint
- Osteomyelitis
- Iatrogenic damage to nerves
- Compression of nerves in scar tissue

PAIN INDUCED BY MASTICATION

Pain on mastication is usually dental in origin and caused by apical periodontitis, but any condition that raises the tooth in its socket or displaces it into premature occlusion can cause this symptom (Box 39.6). Cracked teeth usually become evident on mastication (see earlier).

Pain associated with dentures was discussed earlier.

Non-dental causes

Pain of temporomandibular dysfunction is discussed in Chapter 14. Dull, aching facial pain may be present during eating, but trismus and muscle spasm cause more interference with function than the pain. Organic disease of the temporomandibular joint is almost never the cause of pain on eating.

Pain of temporal arteritis is usually interpreted by patients as headache but is a particularly important cause of masticatory pain because of the high risk of blindness. The pain is due to ischaemia of the masticatory muscles, caused by the arteritis (Ch. 14).

Mealtime syndrome caused by calculi and other obstructions of the salivary ducts can cause pain in salivary glands when salivation is triggered by eating, or the thought of eating (Ch. 22).

First-bite syndrome is a rare and peculiar complication of surgery to the neck, similar clinically to mealtime syndrome. A very intense, paroxysmal electric shock-like pain, sometimes with muscle cramp is felt around the parotid gland or temporomandibular joint on the operated side. The pain appears on biting, mastication or swallowing of only the first bite of a meal. Subsequent eating triggers no pain, though further attacks may follow after a few minutes' respite. The cause is thought to be loss of sympathetic nerve supply to the parotid gland when cervical sympathetic trunk nerves in the carotid sheath or parapharynx are cut.

PAIN FROM SALIVARY GLANDS

Causes of pain from salivary glands are summarised in Box 39.7. The parotid gland and submandibular glands become painful immediately they become inflamed, as they have little space for expansion or, in the case of the submandibular gland, a tight capsule. Thus, almost any disease of the glands will present with pain.

NEURALGIA AND NEUROPATHY

Neuralgia is pain felt in the distribution of a nerve. Neuropathy is a disease of a nerve. In sensory nerves, neuropathies produce pain, hyperalgesia, paraesthesia or analgesia, burning or altered sensation. In motor nerves they cause palsies, muscle fasciculation and weakness. Important examples are shown in Box 39.8. Neuralgias are more common in the head and neck than in other parts of the body and may affect cranial or spinal nerves.

Cranial neuralgias review PMID: 30116913 and 26685473

Intracranial tumours as cause PMID: 23036798

Trigeminal neuralgia

→ Summary chart 39.1 p. 552

Trigeminal neuralgia produces a very characteristic pain. Typical features are summarised in Box 39.9.

People older than 50 years are affected. Either the second or third division of the trigeminal nerve is usually first affected, but pain later usually extends to involve both. The ophthalmic division is rarely involved. The pain is always

---

Box 39.7   Causes of facial and oral pain from salivary gland disease (see Chs 22 and 23)

- Acute and chronic parotitis
  - Mumps
- Salivary obstruction and mealtime syndrome
  - Calculi
  - Strictures
- Painful conditions, mostly draining infections, of intra-parotid lymph nodes
- Malignant neoplasms with perineural spread
  - Adenoid cystic carcinoma

Box 39.8   Some relevant neuralgias and neuropathies

Sensory

- Trigeminal neuralgia
- Multiple sclerosis
- Pain of Herpes zoster
- Postherpetic neuralgia
- Migrainous neuralgia
- Intracranial tumours
- Burning mouth syndrome
- Chronic idiopathic ('atypical') facial pain

Motor

- Bell's palsy
- Stroke
- Epilepsy
- Intracranial tumours

Box 39.6   Pain induced by mastication

- Disease of teeth and supporting tissues
- Cracked tooth
- Temporomandibular joint pain dysfunction syndrome
- Diseases of the temporomandibular joint
- Temporal arteritis
- Trigeminal neuralgia (rarely)
- Salivary calculi
- First bite syndrome

Box 39.9   Typical features of trigeminal neuralgia

- Affects older people
- Pain confined to the distribution of one or more divisions of the trigeminal nerve
- Pain is paroxysmal and very severe
- Trigger zones in the area
- No pain between attacks
- Absence of objective sensory loss
- Absence of detectable organic cause

unilateral. Importantly, there is no disturbance of sensation in the distribution of the pain. The cause is unknown, but currently compression of the trigeminal nerve by an adjacent artery where it enters the pons is the favoured theory.

The pain is excruciatingly severe, paroxysmal, sharp and stabbing in character, but lasts only seconds or 1–2 minutes at most. It may be described as 'like lightning'. Then there is complete, or almost complete, absence of pain between attacks.

Pain may be triggered by stimuli to an area (trigger zone) within the distribution of the trigeminal nerve. Common triggers are touching, draughts of cold air, shaving, tooth brushing or mastication. Between attacks, touching the trigger zone has no effect for a few minutes, the so-called *refractory period*. Only occasionally are attacks recurrent at short intervals. During an attack, the patient's face is often distorted with anguish, whereas between attacks the patient may appear apprehensive at the thought of recurrence. The severity of the pain may also make the patient depressed.

Typically, the disease undergoes spontaneous remissions, with freedom from pain for weeks or months, making it difficult to decide whether treatment has been effective.

Diagnosis

In typical cases, the diagnosis should be readily made from the features described. Dental disease can mimic trigeminal neuralgia, particularly early irreversible pulpitis. Pulpitis can usually be identified as toothache by most patients, but dental causes must be excluded before referral to the patient's medical practitioner.

In early disease the pain may be less severe and then more readily mistaken for pain of dental origin.

Less typical features of trigeminal neuralgia, which make diagnosis difficult, are more continuous, long-lasting, burning or aching pain or absence of trigger zones. This is called *atypical trigeminal neuralgia* and can be associated with migraine type symptoms and retro-orbital pain.

The most important differential diagnosis is multiple sclerosis (discussed later), and similar symptoms may arise from intracranial tumours compressing the nerve, usually at the cerebello-pontine angle. All patients with trigeminal neuralgia-like symptoms should have a brain and base of skull magnetic resonance imaging scan to exclude these possibilities.

Treatment

The most effective drugs are anticonvulsants, particularly carbamazepine. Carbamazepine seems very specific to trigeminal neuralgia. It has no effect on other types of pain and its effect helps confirm the diagnosis. Carbamazepine must be given continuously and long term (essentially prophylactically) to reduce the frequency and severity of attacks, not intermittently as an analgesic. Adverse effects require starting on a low dose and increasing to the full dose, so there may not be any immediate effect. As many as 80% of patients are relieved of pain partly or completely by carbamazepine, but minor side effects are common. Drowsiness, dryness of the mouth, giddiness, diarrhoea and nausea are all, to some extent, dose related.

A few patients are unresponsive to carbamazepine or cannot tolerate the side effects. Alternatives include phenytoin, gabapentin and lamotrigine. Surgical treatments can be highly effective in three-quarters of patients, but neurosurgical decompression of the trigeminal ganglion is a high-risk procedure with significant complications and a mortality rate as high as 1%. Other less invasive surgical procedures

using radiofrequency ablation or cryotherapy to the nerve may remove the pain but at the cost of anaesthesia in the distribution of the nerve. A newer treatment with minimal morbidity is gamma knife ablation, in which the nerve is destroyed using a fine focused beam of radiation, but with similar effects on sensation.

Review neuropathic pain PMID: 20650402

Trigeminal neuralgia review PMID: 25767102 and 31908187

Early features mimic toothache PMID: 25000161

Dental overtreatment in neuralgia PMID: 25418511

Web URL 39.1 NICE guideline management: http://cks.nice.org.uk/trigeminal-neuralgia

European guideline PMID: 30860637

US guideline PMID: 18716236 and 18721143

Trigeminal neuralgia in multiple sclerosis

Between 3% and 4% of patients with apparently typical trigeminal neuralgia have multiple sclerosis as the cause. It is usually a late, rather than a presenting, symptom. The diagnosis depends on the presence of multiple deficits, particularly of vision, weakness of the limbs and sensory losses. Disturbed sensation in the trigeminal area is likely only seen in patients with advanced disease and muscle weakness.

Demyelination in the spinal trigeminal nucleus is thought to be a likely cause, but patients with multiple sclerosis can also have vascular compression of the nerve as is found in typical trigeminal neuralgia. Multiple sclerosis is an important differential diagnosis and should be suspected when a patient is younger than is usual, has bilateral pain or atypical pain, constant pain and sensory loss. Extension beyond the trigeminal area is particularly suggestive; however, the symptoms may be completely typical and the underlying disease only come to light when other nerves are affected.

Carbamazepine or gabapentin is sometimes effective; otherwise, surgical treatment as for trigeminal neuralgia may be required.

Oral effects multiple sclerosis PMID: 23767394 and 19716502

Pain in multiple sclerosis general review PMID: 22909889

Cranial neuralgias in multiple sclerosis PMID: 22130044

Trigeminal neuropathy

Trigeminal neuropathy causes pain, burning, paraesthesia, anaesthesia or hyperaesthesia of part or all of the skin and mucosal sensory distribution of the trigeminal nerve. The pain is typically burning or stabbing in character, or there may be persistent unilateral pain with sensory loss. In the most severe type, there is continuous pain associated with complete anaesthesia. Unfortunately, this can follow nerve ablation as a treatment for trigeminal neuralgia.

Other causes are trauma, intracranial neoplasms and metabolic or inflammatory disorders. Detailed examination is needed, particularly to exclude a neoplastic cause. Unlike trigeminal neuralgia, sensation is affected, there are no trigger zones and pain is usually continuous.

Long-term analgesic nerve blocks, gabapentin or a tricyclic antidepressant may provide some relief.

Benign trigeminal neuropathy consists of transient sensory loss in one or more divisions of the trigeminal nerve. It is sometimes associated with a connective tissue disorder.

Review trigeminal neuropathy PMID: 21628435 and 35787858

General review PMID: 26467754

In Sjögren's syndrome PMID: 15342972

Glossopharyngeal neuralgia

This rare condition causes pain of the same character as trigeminal neuralgia but felt in the distribution of the glossopharyngeal nerve, the base of the tongue, fauces and ear on one side only. The pain, which is sharp, lancinating and transient, is typically triggered by swallowing, chewing or coughing. It may be so severe that patients may be terrified to swallow and try to keep the tongue as completely immobile as possible, to the extent of causing weight loss.

Like trigeminal neuralgia, sometimes a cause of pressure on the nerve such as an intracranial tumour is found. Otherwise, glossopharyngeal neuralgia sometimes responds to carbamazepine but less reliably than trigeminal neuralgia.

Cranial neuralgias review PMID: 23809305 and 30116913

Postherpetic neuralgia

→ Summary chart 39.1 p. 552

As many as 14% of patients who have had trigeminal herpes zoster develop persistent neuralgia and pain that persists more than 1 month after healing, and studies suggest this proportion is increasing slowly. Most cases resolve slowly and only 3% have pain after 1 year. Occasionally postherpetic neuralgia follows a long pain-free period, triggered by surgery or infection in the previously affected dermatome.

Neuralgia is particularly likely in older people, in females and when the infection was severe. Aggressive antiviral treatment of the acute infection reduces the risk of developing postherpetic complications, including neuralgia. Vaccination prevents postherpetic neuralgia by preventing the initial infection.

The pain is more variable in character and severity than trigeminal neuralgia. It is typically persistent rather than paroxysmal, but may be burning, itchy or hypersensitivity to touch or temperature change. Pain is limited to the dermatome affected by the zoster attack. The skin in the affected area may have reduced sensitivity to touch. The diagnosis is straightforward if there is a history of facial zoster or if scars from the rash are present.

Unfortunately, postherpetic neuralgia is remarkably resistant to treatment. Nerve or root section are ineffective, and the response to drugs of any type, including carbamazepine, is poor. When pain is severe, large doses of analgesics may give relief. Topical lidocaine in an occlusive dressing on the affected skin is also often very effective, simple and with few adverse effects. Alternative drugs include amitriptyline and gabapentin. Application of transcutaneous electrical stimulation to the affected area by the patient is sometimes effective. The instrument is applied hourly for 5–10 minutes every day, and persistent bombardment of the sensory pathways by the stimulator may prevent perception of pain centrally.

Longstanding postherpetic neuralgia carries a significant risk of depression.

Post-herpetic neuralgia review PMID: 25317872

Risk factors for post herpetic neuralgia PMID: 26218719

Bell's palsy

As discussed later, facial paralysis is the predominant and most troublesome feature. In approximately 50% of patients, pain, usually in or near the ear but sometimes spreading down the jaw, either precedes or develops at the same time as the facial palsy. Rarely, a patient with early Bell's palsy seeks a dental opinion for the pain felt in the jaw, since this may precede paralysis by several days.

IDIOPATHIC OROFACIAL PAIN

Burning mouth syndrome

Burning mouth syndrome is a distressing and troublesome condition that has many features in common with persistent idiopathic ('atypical') facial pain. Recent evidence indicates that both conditions are neuropathic pain because trigeminal nerve function can be demonstrated to be altered. These functional changes are subtle and detectable only on specialized sensory testing, measurement of blink reflex or similar tests. Either or both peripheral and central neuropathy may be involved in subgroups of patients. Most patients have peripheral small fibre neuropathy with loss of, and delayed regeneration of the small thinly myelinated Aδ and unmyelinated C-fibres innervating the mouth. This indicates both a sensory and autonomic neuropathy, though the sensory effects dominate.

The causes of small fibre neuropathy at other body sites are legion and include specific autoimmune mechanisms, metabolic alterations, infections, toxins and drugs including antiretroviral drugs, statins and metronidazole. At some body sites small fibre neuropathy can be genetic. Diabetes is the factor most closely linked with burning mouth, whether the patient has overt diabetic neuropathy or not. At least some patients with burning mouth appear to have small nerve neuropathy affecting other body sites, suggesting widespread subclinical changes.

There are confusing classifications and terminology. Some use the term *secondary burning mouth* when a physical cause is present. Others exclude organic disease by definition. Alternative names include *burning mouth disorder*, *glossodynia* and *stomatodynia*. Here, burning mouth syndrome is used to describe the condition when no cause can be found; an equivalent term is *primary burning mouth disorder*. However, it must be noted that the accepted systemic neuropathic basis makes these classifications rather arbitrary, and the current classification uses the term burning mouth syndrome, either with or without somatosensory changes.

Although the underlying cause in any one patient is usually unknown, the anterior tongue is particularly sensitive, supplied by sensory nerves with a low activation threshold and large cortical representation. The sensitivity of the nerves is controlled by complex pathways with multiple inputs.

Most patients, more than 80%, are female and older than 50 years. Symptoms may affect the whole mouth, but typically affect the whole tongue or the tip. The floor of mouth is characteristically not involved. The pain is typically described as burning, sometimes as tingling or 'raw', and the sensation is persistent, unremitting and usually of long duration. It is bilateral and has no aggravating or relieving factors. Classically, it is accompanied by a metallic, bitter or unpleasant taste or abnormal taste sensation, and often a sensation of dryness despite normal salivary flow. Some patients complain of paraesthesia, though this is not a common feature.

Spicy foods and flavoured toothpastes often aggravate the symptoms. Worsening of symptoms during the day is typical but the pain does not prevent eating or wake patients.

There is a close association with anxiety, depression and other diseases with a psychogenic component (Box 39.10), but whether these are causative, act as exacerbating factors, reflect central neuropathy or are secondary to the pain is unresolved. Frequently, burning mouth is seen as an extension of these psychogenic conditions. The fact that neuropathy is now recognised does not reduce the importance of considering and treating these associated conditions, as discussed below.

Diagnosis, even when the history is typical, requires exclusion of possible causes. The history, examination and investigations must exclude the potential causes listed in Box 39.11, and the mouth should appear normal. Candidal

---

Box 39.10 Features suggestive of burning mouth syndrome

- Middle-aged or older women are mainly affected
- No visible abnormality or evidence of organic disease
- No haematological abnormality
- No candidal or bacterial infection
- Pain typically described as 'burning'
- Persistent and unremitting soreness without aggravating or relieving factors, often of months or years duration; no response to analgesics
- Bizarre patterns of pain radiation inconsistent with neurological or vascular anatomy
- Sometimes, bitter or metallic taste associated
- Associated depression, anxiety or stressful life situation
- Obsession with symptoms may rule the patient's life
- Constant search for reassurance and treatment by different practitioners
- Occasionally, dramatic improvement with antidepressive treatment

---

Box 39.11 Diseases that must be excluded as possible causes of burning mouth symptoms

- All visible mucosal disease, particularly
  - Erythema migrans
  - Candidal infection
- Iron deficiency anaemia or subclinical deficiency
- Vitamin B12 and folate deficiency
- Xerostomia
- Menopausal symptoms
- Gastro-oesophageal reflux
- Diabetic neuropathy
- Hypothyroidism
- Dental, dentifrice or food irritants
- Multiple sclerosis
- Drugs, particularly
  - Angiotensin converting enzyme inhibitors
  - Angiotensin receptor blockers
  - Antiretrovirals nevirapine and efavirenz
  - Antiepileptic topiramate
  - Neuropathy induced by chemotherapy and other anticancer drugs

---

infection at low intensity can cause symptoms in the absence of visible lesions and should be excluded by smears or salivary candida counts. Several drugs listed cause similar symptoms, but rarely. Lisinopril and captopril appear to be the most frequent. Biopsy plays no role in routine diagnosis unless mucosal disease is suspected, though with specialised techniques small nerve neuropathy can be detected in many patients, as a reduced density of small and unmyelinated mucosal nerve fibres just beneath the epithelium.

Treatment is difficult. Reassurance and explanation to provide a realistic patient expectation is essential. As peripheral neuropathy is suspected, topical lidocaine, capsaicin or clonazepam are good initial drugs to try as adverse effects are minimal and some studies show them to be more effective than centrally acting drugs. Antidepressants, tricyclic or selective serotonin reuptake inhibitors are frequently thought to help many patients, possibly through central effects other than their antidepressant mechanisms, but high-quality evidence is lacking. Cognitive behavioural therapy, relaxation therapies, anxiolytics and hormone replacement therapy can be used, but with only a low-quality evidence base. Improving understanding of neuroimmunological causes of central pain may soon support treatment with drugs that modulate glial activation and central pain mediators, such as pentoxifylline and fluorocitrate, or those that modulate pain perception such as GABA receptor agonists and NDMA receptor antagonists.

Follow up for monitoring and support is required for a long period. Spontaneous resolution is rare, seen in less than 5% of patients in 5 years and treatment does not improve this to more than about a quarter of patients, though the remainder may see partial benefit.

Treatment failure may lead patients to seek repeated consultations with different dental and medical specialties, which reinforces their perception of the problem. It is not unusual for patients to develop the idea that the unremitting symptoms must indicate undiagnosed cancer or some other significant disease. Specifically saying that there is no evidence of cancer is important in management. Treatment should be managed initially in a specialist centre with a multidisciplinary medical and dental team and psychiatric support.

Epidemiology US PMID: 25176397 and Europe 25495557

Burning mouth is a neuropathy PMID: 17582772 and 29257770

Review PMID: 12907696

Treatment PMID: 29180911 and 27855478

Drug-induced PMID: 18305436

Persistent idiopathic facial pain

Like burning mouth syndrome, persistent idiopathic facial pain (previously and still frequently referred to as atypical facial pain) is considered a disease with psychogenic and neuralgic elements. As in burning mouth, the sensory neuralgic elements are minor and easily missed, with mild reduced sensation to light touch, altered blink reflex and enhanced pain responses to minor stimuli. Identifying these neuralgic elements is not necessary for diagnosis, which is based on typical features and exclusion of other causes, particularly the atypical form of trigeminal neuralgia. Features are shown in (Box 39.12).

A common site for atypical pain is the maxillary region or in relation to the upper teeth, but localisation is usually poor and does not match the sensory distribution of peripheral nerves or vascular supply. Neurologically impossible distributions, bilateral or crossing dermatomes and moving pains are particularly suggestive. The description of the pain may be vague, bizarre ('drawing', 'gripping' or 'crushing') or exaggerated ('unbearable') or burning, but without obvious effect on the patient's health. A unilateral deep dull ache is common. It is often described as having been continuous, even unremitting, present daily and unchanging for several years.

Pain is usually not provoked by any recognisable stimulus such as hot or cold foods or by mastication and the pain is not triggered or maintained by abnormal sensory input from the affected skin. Even though the pain may be said to be continuous and unbearable, the patient's sleeping or even eating are usually unaffected. Analgesics are often said to be completely ineffective, but some patients have not even tried them despite the stated severity of the pain. Objective signs of disease are absent. Although teeth have often been extracted and diseased teeth may be present, none of these can be related to the pain. As a consequence, treatment of diseased teeth does not relieve the symptoms and dental treatment without an identified possible cause of pain must be avoided.

A history of repeated consultations for the pain, none satisfactory, is typical. This fact may well not be proffered without specific questioning.

Other signs of mental health disorders are highly variable. Some patients are more or less obviously depressed; some of them mention, in passing, challenges they have had in their work or relationships. Others may complain how miserable or helpless the pain makes them. Others may complain of bizarre delusional symptoms such as 'slime' in the mouth or 'powder' coming out of the jaw. It is not uncommon for atypical facial pain to be associated with other diseases linked to anxiety and depression such as taste disturbance, burning mouth, irritable bowel syndrome, back pain or chronic fatigue. Often an unlikely trigger will be identified by a patient, such as a difficult extraction or other medical intervention, or sometimes a patient will be convinced they have a specific medical condition.

Investigation requires a detailed and exhaustive examination of the teeth and mouth. Any potential sources of pain must be dealt with, but there should not be too much expectation of benefit. Any obvious objective signs of nerve dysfunction on a simple clinical examination, such as loss of sensation or paraesthesia, suggest other causes. Radiographs and other imaging are needed. If many have been taken at multiple previous consultations, obtaining them is important to avoid unnecessary additional X-ray exposure. Computed tomography or magnetic resonance imaging, depending on the characteristics of the pain, is usually required.

There is no predictably effective treatment. Treatment needs to be targeted at the pain and tailored to any underlying mental health conditions or psychological overlay, usually depression or anxiety. Tricyclic antidepressants are usually moderately effective, possibly through anti-neuralgic actions, but treatment is difficult and best combined with cognitive behavioural therapy. If depression is present and tricyclic drugs fail, venlafaxine and fluoxetine may be tried. Local measures include implanted peripheral nerve field stimulators, cutaneous transepidermal nerve stimulation, topical lidocaine plasters, intraoral appliances and botulinum toxin injection, all of which have been used with varying effect. If pain is intractable and distressing, sphenopalatine ganglion block with long-acting analgesic or radioablation reduce pain but at the cost of neurological deficit. The pain may lessen spontaneously only over years. One recognised anxiety associated with both burning mouth and atypical facial pain is fear of cancer, and this may respond to reassurance.

Review PMID: 28425324 and 31735230

Management PMID: 28251523 and 27325001

Persistent idiopathic dentoalveolar pain

Previously, and more intuitively, called atypical odontalgia, this is a less common variant of persistent idiopathic facial pain, and the general features described earlier apply. Pain is often precisely localised in one tooth or in a row of teeth, which are said either to ache or to be exquisitely sensitive to heat, cold or pressure. A deep dull ache is typical. If dental disease is found, treatment has no effect, or if, as a last resort, the tooth is root filled or removed, the pain moves to an adjacent tooth. Early diagnosis is essential to avoid overtreatment and serious dental morbidity as patients can be very insistent on intervention. As with atypical facial pain, there are neuralgic elements to this pain; it is not purely psychosomatic. A close mimic that must be excluded is herpes zoster infection, either in its prodromal phase, or as postherpetic neuralgia after infection.

Review PMID: 18190356

Outcome PMID: 23630687

PARAESTHESIA AND ANAESTHESIA OF THE LOWER LIP

Paraesthesia or anaesthesia of the lower lip is usually caused by pressure on, or damage to, the inferior alveolar nerve by inflammation, osteomyelitis or, rarely, neurological disease. The main causes of anaesthesia or paraesthesia of the lip are summarised in Box 39.13. All of the common causes affect the nerve within the mandibular canal.

Lip signs accompanied by involvement of the tongue or skin of the side of the head indicate a more proximal lesion affecting the posterior division of the mandibular nerve. Further proximal lesions would involve motor supply to the muscles of mastication, causing weakness.

Prolonged anaesthesia or paraesthesia of the lip can occasionally follow inferior dental blocks and surgical damage on removal of third molars, as discussed earlier in this chapter.

Paraesthesia of the lip can be a complication of fractures of the mandible where the nerve has become stretched, particularly over the sharp edge of the canal. The effect is temporary, but complete recovery may take some months.

The nerve may be compressed by a neoplasm, or a malignant tumour may infiltrate and destroy the nerve itself. Malignant neoplasms are more likely to be metastatic than primary, and then reflect widespread disease (Ch.12).

The mental foramen can become exposed by excessive resorption of mandibular bone in an edentulous patient. A denture can then press upon the nerve as it leaves the foramen. Although these changes are common in the oldest individuals, they rarely cause paraesthesia of the lip, usually causing pain on pressure and then only if severely affected. Relieving the denture or converting it to an implant-supported prosthesis are the best solutions. Nerve repositioning carries a risk of permanent nerve damage.

Postherpetic neuralgia (discussed previously) may occasionally cause persistent paraesthesia in the nerve distribution affected, but very rarely in the lower lip alone.

Tetany is the result of hypocalcaemic states and causes heightened neuromuscular excitability, together with minor disorders of sensation such as paraesthesia of the lips. A significant cause of tetany is overbreathing, usually due to anxiety (hyperventilation syndrome). The paraesthesia is bilateral and also affects extremities, if marked together with carpopedal spasm.

FACIAL PALSY

Important causes of facial palsy are summarised in Box 39.14. As the muscles of the face are supplied by the facial nerve, facial palsy will be caused by damage to either its upper or lower motor neurons.

Review sensation and movement PMID: 23909236

Upper and lower motor neuron lesions

The facial nerve *lower* motor neurons pass from its motor nucleus in the pons to the facial muscles. In lower motor neuron lesions, such as Bell's palsy, there is impairment of contraction of *all* facial muscles. The cause is usually extracranial.

The facial nerve *upper* motor neurons pass from the primary motor cortex in the frontal lobe to the pons, but the muscles of the upper part of the face receive stimuli from both sides of the brain, whereas the muscles of the lower face are only activated by the contralateral cortex. Thus, the upper face is controlled by both sides of the brain, and when there is upper motor neuron damage, for instance from a stroke, the lower face is more affected. Emotional movements of the face, the blink reflex and ability to wrinkle the forehead may remain normal.

BELL'S PALSY

Bell's palsy is a common cause of lower motor neurone facial paralysis. People between the ages of 20 and 50 years are at highest risk, but all ages can be affected, including children. Between 1 in 60 and 1 in 70 individuals will have an attack of Bell's palsy in their lifetime, and those with diabetes and women who are pregnant are at higher risk. Onset may follow an apparently unrelated viral illness.

Bell's palsy was previously considered idiopathic, but the cause in at least half of cases is now thought to be inflammation and swelling around the ganglion caused by viral infection, particularly herpes simplex or zoster. Infection and reactivation mechanisms of viral infection are discussed in Chapter 15. Other viruses and Lyme disease are rarer causes, the latter unusual as it may be bilateral.

Onset is rapid and frightening for the patient. Pain in the jaw sometimes precedes the paralysis, or there may be numbness in the side of the tongue, but in most patients facial paralysis is the presenting sign, developing over 48–72 hours.

Function of the facial nerve is tested by asking the patient to perform facial movements. When asked to close the eyes, the lids on the affected side cannot be brought together, but the eyeball rolls up normally since the oculomotor nerves are unaffected. When the patient is asked to smile, the corner of the mouth on the affected side is not pulled upward and the normal lines of expression are absent (Fig. 39.1). The wrinkling round the eyes that accompanies smiling is also not seen on the affected side, and the eye remains staring, indicating a lower motor neurone disorder. Speech and taste

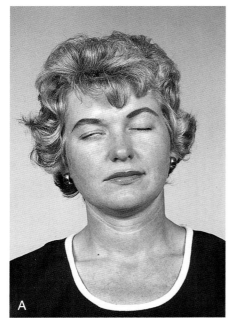

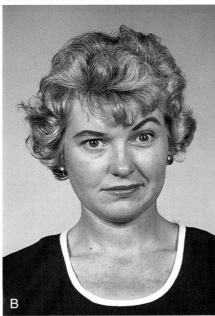

Fig. 39.1 **Bell's palsy.** (A) When trying to shut the eyes, that on the affected (*patient's right*) side fails to close completely but the eyeball rolls up normally. (B) When trying to smile, the mouth fails to move on the affected side, which remains expressionless, having lost all natural skin folds. The difference is made more striking by covering each side of the picture in turn. This patient, incidentally, complained primarily of facial pain, though was increasingly aware of the facial disability. The severely disfiguring effect of this disorder and the need for early treatment is obvious. In this case, response was complete.

are affected, the latter a result of loss of chorda tympani fibre function in the facial nerve. At rest, saliva may drool from the mouth.

The majority of patients recover fully or partially without treatment, but this can take several months. At least 10% of patients with Bell's palsy are unhappy about the final outcome because of permanent disfigurement or other complications. A guide to the need for treatment is the severity of the paralysis when first seen. Full recovery is usual in patients with an incomplete palsy seen within a week of onset, but more than half with a complete lesion fail to recover completely. Prednisolone by mouth may be given for 5–10 days and then tapered off over the following 4 days, and may be effective if given within 24 hours of the onset. The addition of aciclovir, assuming a herpesvirus aetiology, is controversial and of unproven effectiveness. If the eye cannot be closed, it must be protected.

If treatment fails or is not given, persistent facial weakness is disfiguring. The majority of patients with persistent denervation develop muscle atrophy and contracture of the affected side of the face. Watering of the eye (epiphora) due to impaired drainage of tears, or occasionally to excessive and erratic lacrimal secretion, may remain particularly troublesome. An uncommon complication is unilateral lacrimation when eating (crocodile tears).

It is important to avoid early exercises in an attempt to speed recovery. Physiotherapy must be delayed until the acute phase has subsided, to avoid synkinesis, or unwanted facial movement. This complication comprises involuntary facial contractions in association with movement of another part of the face. There may, for example, be twitching of the mouth when the patient blinks. Facial exercise therapy in later stages significantly reduces long term muscle atrophy and weakness.

Treatment PMID: 24685475

Use of antivirals PMID: 31486071

US guideline PMID: 24189771

Outcome PMID: 12482166

Dental aspects

Rarely, as mentioned earlier, pain felt in the jaw may precede paralysis. Paralysis reduces oral clearance of food, and debris can accumulate in the vestibule on the affected side. If treatment fails, sagging of the affected side of the face may be limited by an intraoral prosthesis, though thread facelift and fillers are better solutions (Ch. 27). Although this disease is uncommon in dental practice, its recognition is important as referral for early treatment may prevent permanent disability and disfigurement.

Melkersson–Rosenthal syndrome

→ Summary chart 35.1 p. 518

Melkersson–Rosenthal syndrome is a rare syndrome of unilateral recurrent facial paralysis, lip or facial swelling, and fissured tongue. Not all these features are present in all patients. Onset is usually in adolescence or young adulthood.

The facial swelling is identical to orofacial granulomatosis (Ch. 35) initially recurrent, soft, painless facial swelling that becomes persistent due to progressive fibrosis. The buccal mucosa may develop a cobblestone pattern and, histologically, granulomas are found. Variants of this disorder include oedema of the eyelids, bilateral facial or rarely multiple cranial nerve palsies, and oedema of the lip. There is a very rare familial type. There is probably an immunological or autoinflammatory basis for this disease, and there is sometimes a response to intralesional corticosteroids. Paralysis may become permanent. Treatment is as for orofacial granulomatosis.

Review PMID: 1437063

Case series PMID: 24963969

Oral lesions PMID: 6959055

Other causes of facial palsy

Cerebrovascular accidents (thrombotic or haemorrhagic strokes) are a common complication of hypertension in older people. Unilateral paralysis and often loss of speech are frequent in survivors of the acute episode. The unilateral facial palsy is common but differs from Bell's palsy in that the lower part of the face is mainly affected and spontaneous emotional facial reactions may be retained, as strokes are upper motor neuron lesions.

Facial palsy is an uncommon but characteristic manifestation of a malignant parotid tumour invading the nerve. The many branches of the facial nerve within the parotid gland make it particularly vulnerable to surgical injury, and sometimes the nerve must be sacrificed during a cancer resection. Nerve grafting is moderately successful in avoiding the consequences.

Ramsay Hunt syndrome is severe facial palsy caused by herpes zoster (Ch. 15). It may be differentiated from Bell's palsy by involvement of the ear skin and external auditory meatus, sometimes with tinnitus and hearing loss.

Lyme disease (Ch. 32) causes arthritis, cervical lymphadenopathy and, less commonly, facial nerve paralysis.

Heerfordt's syndrome (Ch. 31) is the rare combination of facial palsy, uveitis and parotid swelling caused by sarcoidosis of cranial nerves and salivary glands.

HEADACHE

Headache diagnosis and management are outside the remit of dentistry, but the lack of a clear definition of headache, as opposed to pains and aches in the face and neck, makes some understanding important. Dentists may play an important role in diagnosis, referral and, sometimes in treatment as part of a multidisciplinary team. Most patients will differentiate headache from facial and neck pain without difficulty, but there are some conditions that patients find difficult to categorise. Temporal arteritis and migrainous neuralgia are examples.

Primary headaches are conditions such as common tension headaches or migraine without underlying disease. Secondary headaches are caused by a separate disease process, such as an intracranial tumour or haemorrhage.

A number of symptoms identify secondary headaches that are likely to reflect significant underlying disease and merit immediate referral. These are shown in Box 39.15. However, it is primary headaches that may be of dental significance.

Web URL 39.2 Classification of headache: http://www.ichd-3.org

---

Box 39.15 Important signs of secondary headache

- Sudden onset
- Onset after age 40
- A new type of headache not experienced before
- Increasing frequency and severity
- Systemic symptoms, fever, weight loss
- Neurological signs or symptoms
- Stiff neck, fever or rash
- Associated disease, HIV, malignancy, infection
- Onset after trauma
- Disorientation, loss of consciousness

Headache for dentists PMID: 26058224

Headache presenting as toothache: PMID 17055919

Dentists often delay diagnosis PMID: 12876249

Migraine

Migraine is a common cause of disabling headache and rarely can cause facial pain. It affects as much as 10% of the population, most only occasionally, but a few daily. It is usually readily recognised by the patient.

There are two forms, without aura (common migraine) and with aura. In both the headache is unilateral, pulsatile and debilitating and often associated with photophobia and nausea. The headache lasts from a few hours to 72 hours. In children the headache may be bilateral. Migraine without aura has been considered vascular, but evidence suggests that trigeminal pain pathways are oversensitive. In migraine with aura, the headache is preceded by temporary sensations that may be visual, sensory or motor in type caused by a slow-moving wave of depolarization moving across the brain cortex with a wave of decreasing cortical blood flow. The commonest type is the aura of fortification spectra, a flickering pattern of zig-zag light superimposed on normal vision. Occasional patients experience aura without headache, or the headache before or with the aura.

There is a poorly defined connection between migraine and temporomandibular pain dysfunction. Patients with temporomandibular pain dysfunction are more likely to develop a number of chronic pain and headache conditions including common tension headache, chronic idiopathic facial pain, and neck and back pain. Patients are twice as likely to experience migraine-like headache and, if the migraine is less than typical, likely to confuse the two conditions.

The connection, if any, between the two conditions remains a controversial area, with occlusion and tooth-related treatments being promoted to ease migraine without a good evidence base. Simply treating temporomandibular pain dysfunction has no effect on migraine, but bruxism and muscle tenderness could potentially be linked through trigeminal pain pathways and either condition could lower the pain threshold, worsening the other. Treating the two conditions together is logical. Calcitonin gene-related peptide blocking drugs used for migraine also appear to reduce temporomandibular pain dysfunction symptoms.

Additional potentially causative links between migraine and temporomandibular pain dysfunction involve muscles of mastication. A minority of patients with migraine have compression of the zygomaticotemporal nerve as it passes through the temporalis muscle, which is overactive and tender in temporomandibular pain dysfunction. Injection of botulinum toxin into facial and masticatory muscles has also been shown to reduce migraine frequency and severity and is also used in temporomandibular pain dysfunction, with limited effectiveness (Ch. 27). Injection is required in multiple sites into temporalis, frontal, occipital and shoulder muscles and is proposed to act by preventing muscle-derived pain signals passing centrally.

Management

Migraine is generally managed using preventive medication, triptan drugs that block 5HT receptors or calcitonin gene related peptide blockers, sometimes beta-blockers. Refractory cases are sometimes treated with amitriptyline, or topiramate. Once a migraine develops, simple analgesics such as paracetamol, aspirin or non-steroidal anti-inflammatory drugs are effective if the dose is sufficient.

Box 39.16   Typical features of migraine
- Intense throbbing headache, usually unilateral
- Visual disturbances (aura) in classic migraine, not in common migraine
- Photophobia
- Sometimes nausea and vomiting
- Triggers: stress, hunger, certain foods, caffeine, cheese and red wine, menstruation, which vary between patients
- Usually a good response to 5HT agonists such as sumatriptan

Box 39.17   Typical features of migrainous neuralgia
- Commonest in young adult and middle-aged men
- Piercing intense unilateral orbital, retro-orbital or temporal pain
- Ipsilateral conjunctival vessel dilatation and eyelid oedema
- Ipsilateral lacrimation
- Ipsilateral nasal congestion and rhinorrhoea
- Attacks often at the same time each night (or day, 'alarm clock headache')
- Usually attacks recur for several days (cluster) then remit for many weeks or months
- Triggers: stress, alcohol, organic solvent inhalation
- Early in acute attack, oxygen or sumatriptan highly effective
- Prophylaxis possible with verapamil or ergotamine

Key features are summarised in Box 39.16.

Review for dentistry PMID: 19065884

Mimicking temporomandibular pain dysfunction PMID: 18230375

Association with temporomandibular pain dysfunction PMID: 34649707

Treatment with temporomandibular pain dysfunction PMID: 22610505

Bruxism and headache PMID: 34129658

Dental appliance treatment PMID: 8850287

Botulinum toxin treatment 20487038 and 34078259

Migrainous neuralgia (cluster headache)

→ Summary chart 39.1 p. 552

Migrainous neuralgia may occasionally be mistaken for trigeminal neuralgia. It is rarely seen in dental practice, but the pain may be mistaken for maxillary toothache because the pain is so intense, stabbing in character and quite unlike other headaches.

It causes severe unilateral pain felt in the eye, behind the eye and in the maxilla, often associated with ipsilateral pupil constriction, facial flushing, nasal congestion and lacrimation. Each attack has very rapid onset and lasts 15 minutes to 3 hours. Classically, attacks wake patients at the same time each night for several days in a row, before a period of remission, hence the alternative names *alarm clock headache* and *cluster headache*. The condition is much commoner in males than females and onset is usually between the ages of 20 and 40 years of age.

Migrainous neuralgia has been thought to be caused by oedema or dilatation of the wall of the internal carotid and external carotid arteries but is now considered a primary autonomic neurological condition. Some patients have triggers for attacks, of which alcohol is the commonest.

Key features are summarised in Box 39.17.

General review PMID: 16139660 and 35296510

Management

Magnetic resonance imaging is needed to exclude other neurological causes. Relief of the pain by oxygen inhalations is virtually diagnostic, but this is difficult to provide as a treatment. Most patients respond to sumatriptan as a preventive measure, either by nasal spray or subcutaneous injection. Otherwise, ipsilateral instillation of 4% intranasal lidocaine or vagal nerve stimulation can also be effective. Some patients respond to simple analgesics but these often take too long to be effective in short-lived attacks.

Orofacial migraine and migrainous neuralgia

Both migraine and migrainous neuralgia may very occasionally present with pain limited to the face, previously called *lower half headache*. The pain is usually felt in the jaw and interpreted as toothache but with a periodicity and attack quality of migraine or migrainous neuralgia. Both are frequently misdiagnosed as toothache, teeth may be inappropriately extracted and diagnosis is almost always delayed.

In some patients diagnosis is made easier by pre-existence of the typical headache, which may persist with the facial pain or gradually be lost.

In migraine of the face an aura is often not present and in migrainous neuralgia the accompanying nasal congestion and facial sweating do not occur. When headache and facial symptoms occur together they almost always affect the same side. These unusual pain distributions are treated as for the corresponding type of headache.

Orofacial migrainous neuralgia PMID: 12482215

Orofacial migraine PMID: 15573344

Intracranial tumours

Pain resembling trigeminal neuralgia can rarely be caused by intracranial tumours. Features suggesting an intracranial lesion are associated sensory loss, especially if associated with cranial nerve palsies. Frequently, anatomically related nerves (especially III, IV and VI, causing disordered oculomotor function) are affected.

DISTURBANCES OF TASTE AND SMELL

Dysgeusia is abnormal taste, hypogeusia reduced taste and ageusia, loss of taste. These simple terms cover a range of complaints including one taste being sensed as another and a single abnormal taste being superimposed on normal taste.

Loss of taste is a distressing symptom for many patients, but it is poorly understood and difficult to investigate. The sensation of taste depends heavily on smell, and the two must be considered together. A complaint of loss of taste is frequently explained by loss of smell, which is said to account for 80% of the sensation of taste.

Loss of smell

Anosmia and hyposmia have many causes and are relatively common in the population, commoner in men and more frequent in older people.

Covid-19

Acute loss of sense of smell with respiratory symptoms is associated with upper respiratory tract infections and particularly linked with infection by SARS-CoV-2 in Covid-19. The symptom is more frequent and marked in infection by the Delta and early strains of the epidemic, affecting almost 80% of people infected with total loss in 50%. Later variants such as Omicron cause loss of smell in less than 10% of patients. Many other respiratory viruses damage the olfactory epithelium, including the common cold and influenza, but the effect is much less marked.

Loss of smell in Covid-19 is often dramatically abrupt and starts about 4 days after infection. The cause of immediate and short-term loss on infection is viral infection of, and inflammation and damage to, the olfactory epithelium, disrupting the sensory neurones. The olfactory epithelium has a high density of the angiotensin-converting enzyme 2 receptors and neuropilin-1 used by the virus to enter cells. Smell recovers relatively quickly in most patients as the acute infection subsides, lasting a mean of about 10 days and with over 95% of patients fully recovered in one month.

About 7% of recovered Covid-19 patients develop persistent alteration of smell for months or years, either reduced smell, a 'phantom' or sensation of an unpleasant odour. Persistent alteration of smell is associated with virus spread into the olfactory bulb, and possibly further into the brain causing dysfunction rather than cell death and inflammation. Women and people with pre-existing nasal inflammatory disease are more likely to develop longstanding loss of smell. Abnormal inappropriate smell sensations may arise from misconnection of neurons during healing and cause significant reduction in quality of life. It is a concern that patients who lost their sense of smell may be predisposed to future degenerative brain disease.

Other causes

A slow onset is usually associated with nasal disease such as hay fever, deviated septum, chronic rhinosinusitis and nasal polyps that either cause mucosal inflammation or prevent air circulating to the olfactory sensors high in the nose. Less common causes include hypothyroidism, Cushing's syndrome, stroke, vitamin B_{12} deficiency and alcohol abuse. Sudden onset of persistent smell or taste loss in the absence of respiratory symptoms indicates a likely neurological problem and is a significant sign meriting urgent investigation.

Smell sensation declines in old age and is associated with cognitive impairment and neurodegenerative diseases, particularly dementia and Parkinson's disease. Severity of loss predicts physical and cognitive decline.

Initial referral to an ear nose and throat specialist in airways disease is a logical first step if nasal disease is suspected. Saline rinses, topical steroid and removal of polyps will often be effective. Smell training can help recovery and is used after Covid-19, in age-related loss and loss of smell from chronic nasal allergy.

Loss of smell carries other risks that are not immediately apparent. Patients should ensure they have smoke alarms fitted in their houses and take care not to develop food poisoning from eating contaminated food if smell is absent or weak. In older individuals, loss of appetite resulting from lack of enjoyment of food can causes weight loss, malnutrition, osteoporosis and related problems.

Loss of smell in neurological disease PMID: 25992176

In Covid-19 PMID: 34889850 and 35629357

With aging PMID: 25968962, 34249327 and 34379770

Assessing sense of smell PMID: 25761817

Review for dentists PMID: 19732354

Drug effects PMID: 15563912

Treatment PMID: 35072929

Loss of taste

Taste sensation has two components, the classical taste receptor-mediated sensations and chemethesis, a sensation mediated by touch, thermal and pain receptors that transmits sensations such as astringency and irritancy (e.g., capsaicin in chili pepper). The former are mediated by taste fibres in the facial, glossopharyngeal and vagus nerves and the latter taste components are mediated by the trigeminal sensory system. The taste receptor cells have only a short life and are active for only a few hours before being replaced and this constant turnover and neuronal reconnection of the taste cells is a complex system prone to disruption.

There is no scientific basis for 'taste maps' suggesting that specific tastes are sensed in different anatomical areas. They cannot be used to investigate taste clinically. Simplistic testing of sweet, sour, salt and bitter in a practice situation is possible using a sugar or a sweetener, citric acid, salt and quinine (in tonic water) and can at least show that normal taste is present. However, testing for taste disturbance is complex and best performed in a specialised centre.

Covid-19

Sudden loss or alteration of taste is a feature of Covid-19 infection, but its effects are difficult to separate from the loss of smell. As with anosmia, the effect was a much more prominent feature of infection by early pandemic virus variants such as Delta, which caused complete loss of taste in about a third of patients and altered taste in a further third. Most patients developed alteration of both senses with only 10% reporting loss of taste or smell alone and in occasional cases loss of taste is a presenting or only symptom. Taste loss appears most likely in people of African heritage, and much less frequent in people of Asian heritage and is commoner in women.

The mechanism of taste loss in Covid-19 infection is unclear, with both mucosal inflammation and direct infection of taste buds implicated; the taste buds express the virus receptors angiotensin-converting enzyme 2 receptors, transmembrane protease serine 2 and furin. The virus may also affect the sensory nerves. Salt sensitivity appears less affected but, as with loss of smell, there may be complete or partial loss, altered sensation and 'phantom' tastes. Loss of taste is rapid and occurs about 4 days after infection, with loss of smell, is more severe and lasts longer in severe infection. Taste usually recovers in 2 weeks but may persist many months in up to 10% of patients.

Other causes

The most common cause of taste loss is probably ageing (Box 39.18). This may be compounded by complete dentures that cover taste buds on the palate. Dry mouth prevents transport of soluble taste molecules to the receptors.

Box 39.18   Causes of weakened taste sensation

- Ageing (affects smell and taste)
- Loss of smell through nasal disease
- Dry mouth and nose, Sjögren's syndrome
- Parkinson's disease, Alzheimer's disease
- Diabetes mellitus
- Covid-19 infection, particularly with Delta variant SARS-CoV-2
- Liver disease
- Uraemia, usually from renal disease
- HIV infection
- Halitosis
- Trauma and surgery to nerves, particularly the olfactory nerve
- Radiotherapy and chemotherapy

Table 39.3   Some drugs causing taste disturbance. Over 350 drugs cause taste disturbances, see references for more comprehensive lists

Drug	Effect
Metronidazole	Bitter metallic taste
Tetracycline	Bitter metallic taste
Tegretol	Taste loss
Biguanide antidiabetic drugs	Bitter metallic taste
Allopurinol	Bitter metallic taste
Penicillamine	Bitter metallic taste and taste loss
Terbinafine	Taste loss
Many chemotherapy drugs	Abnormal taste and taste loss
Sodium lauryl sulphate (toothpaste detergent)	Loss of subsequent salt and sweet taste
Angiotensin-converting enzyme inhibitors	Weakened taste
Nifedipine	Abnormal taste
Clopidogrel	Taste loss
Beta blockers	Loss of smell
Vismodegib	Taste loss

Ageing causes reduced taste, a more tolerable situation than abnormal taste.

Some drugs that have been associated with taste disturbance are listed in Table 39.3; many more have been reported. Some appear to interfere with receptor or nerve function, whereas others have a strong taste and are secreted into saliva, such as metronidazole. The taste of chlorhexidine is persistent because it binds to the oral mucosa. In most cases, the alterations are reversible, but some drugs can cause permanent taste loss.

Infection may produce a bad taste, particularly when pus is present or in acute ulcerative gingivitis. Candidosis, periodontitis and other infections and mucosal diseases must be excluded as possible causes before referral for further investigation.

Taste is rarely disturbed by sensory nerve lesions because of the large number of nerves that supply taste sensation. However, some neurological conditions such as multiple sclerosis can affect taste, and bizarre taste can be experienced in the aura of a migraine or in temporal lobe epilepsy. Bell's palsy causes unilateral taste loss, and this may persist long after the acute attack. Conversely, smell is prone to neurological disturbances because it depends on a small area of the nasal mucosa and a single cranial nerve.

Taste loss is common following treatment for cancer.

A few patients have a psychogenic complaint of altered taste or smell. The abnormal taste may appear bizarre or limited to a part of the mouth. A complaint of an unremitting bitter taste often accompanies burning mouth syndrome, and a bad taste is often associated with depression. It is rare for a psychogenic taste to be a normal taste; they are usually described as metallic or unpleasant.

Taste buds review PMID: 26534983

Taste disorders review PMID: 24309062

In Covid-19 PMID: 35629357 and 35790059

Drug effects PMID: 15563912 and 30035266

Assessment of taste PMID: 15563906

EPILEPSY

Epilepsy is a common brain disorder causing *recurrent* convulsions or seizures and temporary disturbances of consciousness. Epilepsy affects approximately 1% of the UK population and similar proportions worldwide, varying mainly with population age distribution.

Onset is usually in childhood or in older people, reflecting different causes. Onset in childhood is genetically determined or associated with developmental or inherited brain conditions, particularly autism spectrum disorder. Onset in the older people is likely to be a sign of a brain lesion such as a cerebral tumour, cerebrovascular disease or senile or Alzheimer's dementia.

The classification is complex, and more than 40 conditions are recognised to cause recurrent convulsions of the epileptic type. Epilepsy is most frequently idiopathic, accounting for half of cases in developed countries where investigation is available; these are assumed to be genetic in origin, with many membrane ion channel genes implicated. This type is common in children and initially causes absence seizures. In the remainder with a defined basis, causes include many known single gene defects, each individually rare, cerebral lesions including strokes, trauma, infections and haemangiomas, alcohol abuse, Alzheimer's, HIV and other neurodegenerative diseases.

It is easier to understand the seizure types (Box 39.19).

In the classical 'tonic-clonic' (generalised or 'grand mal') seizure, the first event is twitching or jerking of muscles, followed by tonic (constant) contraction of muscles causing neck and limb extension and rigidity. The patient falls to the ground and is at risk of injury. The diaphragm and chest and abdominal muscles are in spasm and the vocal cords contracted, causing a brief cry, after which the patient cannot breathe and may become cyanotic. The contraction then relaxes and develops into a pattern of repeated clonic convulsions (repetitive jerking movements of the whole body). At this stage the bladder and bowels may void. Tongue biting is a risk at this stage, usually of the lateral border. Attempting to prevent this usually fails and risks injury to the helper. After approximately 5 minutes the muscle spasms cease, leaving the patient unconscious for between 15 minutes to up to an hour. On waking they will

Box 39.19   Types of epileptic seizure

- Generalised seizures (one-third of all cases)
  - Tonic-clonic
  - Absence
  - Myoclonic
  - Clonic
  - Atonic
- Focal seizures (two-thirds of all cases)
  - Without impairment of consciousness
  - With impairment of consciousness
- Continuous seizure types
  - Generalised status epilepticus
  - Focal status epilepticus

feel exhausted, experience muscle pain, have a headache and be confused. They may sleep for 12 or more hours.

Many patients experience a preceding aura (ranging from unusual feelings, tastes or smells, focal paraesthesia, visual disturbances or hallucinations). The aura is a focal seizure that the patient is aware of and it may give warning of a more major seizure developing. In susceptible subjects, seizures can be precipitated by fatigue, starvation, acute anxiety, infections, menstruation or rapidly flickering lights.

In the typical 'absence' (petit mal) seizure there is little or no movement apart from blinking or facial spasm, a sudden but brief loss of awareness or activity, without significant loss of postural or muscular control and lasting a few seconds. Consciousness is regained without recollection of the episode. Most patients with petit mal seizures have or later develop grand mal epilepsy.

Many patients experience focal seizures. These usually comprise an aura, loss of speech, clonic movements of one part of the body or automatic apparently purposeful movements such as lip smacking or kicking, and these seizures may not involve loss of consciousness.

Temporal lobe epilepsy is a distinctive cause of focal seizures similar to an aura. Depending on the focus of the seizure in the temporal lobe, the patient may have unusual symptoms of *déjà vu,* auditory, olfactory or taste or sensory hallucinations, delusions and emotional disturbances. There may or may not be impaired consciousness. Paranoid or schizophrenic features are often associated.

Status epilepticus is defined as continuous or repeated convulsions lasting more than 30 minutes. 'Convulsive status' is repeated tonic-clonic seizures without recovery of consciousness and is a potentially fatal medical emergency (Ch. 44). All other types of seizure may also be continuous.

Epilepsy predisposes to progressive cognitive impairment.

General review PMID: 14507951

Management

Dental patients with epilepsy will almost always know their diagnosis and should be under the care of a specialist centre. The main anticonvulsant drugs for major seizures are sodium valproate, carbamazepine, lamotrigine or gabapentin. Many drugs are available and have specific indications for different types of seizure but seizures are not satisfactorily controlled in up to a third of patients. Phenytoin, which causes troublesome drowsiness and many other adverse effects, is largely obsolete. Ethosuximide is the drug of choice for petit mal seizures.

Dental aspects

The potential consequences of a seizure in the dental surgery are so disturbing that all precautions should be taken to minimise this hazard. A seizure is the second or third commonest medical emergency in dental practice and a study in Germany revealed that 90% of dentists had experienced one in the surgery. The key is to identify triggers for attacks in the patient history. Flashing lights are the best-known trigger, but affect few patients. Alcohol, tiredness, menstruation and hypoglycaemia are often blamed by individual patients and relatively easily avoided. Unfortunately, stress is a common trigger and must be minimised.

Treatment should be arranged for 'good phases' when attacks are infrequent and within 2–3 hours of medication being taken. Most patients are well-controlled by medication and can be treated as the general population. They must be asked to immediately report any symptoms of aura. Patients with poor control or frequent seizures may benefit from additional medication for the day of treatment and discussion about this with their neurologist is advisable. Some patients carry additional emergency medication, such as midazolam for buccal mucosal application. This can be used only during the premonitory conscious phase.

During treatment, it is worth considering use of a mouth prop, secured extraorally to prevent displacement into the airway during a seizure. This will prevent the patient from biting the tongue, clenching on instruments or the dentist's fingers if an attack develops. However, they are not considered compulsory, particularly in patients who experience an aura, and may not be liked by all patients. Any prop used must be soft and no attempt should ever be made to insert a prop during an aura or seizure. As much equipment as possible should be kept out of reach of the patient. Potential injuries from a major seizure include lacerations of the tongue or lips, and injuries due to falling such as maxillofacial damage and fractures to vertebrae or limbs.

Although large doses of intravenous lidocaine given for severe dysrhythmias can occasionally precipitate seizures, there is no evidence of any risk from lidocaine in local anaesthetics.

Severely epileptic patients on high doses of phenytoin or carbamazepine may have a bleeding tendency. Aspirin is contraindicated in individuals taking valproic acid, as the combination potentiates the antiplatelet effect. Folate deficiency from phenytoin use may exacerbate aphthous stomatitis.

Children and young adults with drug-resistant epilepsy may be treated with an implanted vagal nerve stimulator in the chest wall, connected to the vagus nerve in the neck. This is active continuously but can be further activated on experiencing an aura using a magnet to activate the device. The dentist should be aware how to operate this in case the patient has insufficient warning. Unfortunately, the device lowers pain thresholds and is suspected of causing trigeminal pain. The implanted device does not require antibiotic cover and is not interfered with by ultrasonic scalers, but diathermy must be avoided, as for instance when dealing with gingival overgrowth.

Treatment planning for epileptic patients may require varying degrees of adaptation to their disease and its severity. Good oral hygiene will prevent gingival overgrowth (Ch. 7), and intensive prevention is required to avoid the need for treatment. Tongue biting is common during attacks and missing teeth, particularly anteriorly, can trap the tongue. Edentulous anterior spaces should be restored, ideally using a fixed replacement; any removable design must have excellent retention and strength, usually with metal-backed teeth. Acrylic components must be considered likely to fracture and should be reinforced with carbon fibre or mesh to prevent fragments separating and made radiopaque in case radiographic localisation in the lung is required (Fig. 39.2). Large posterior restorations are best dealt with by metal coverage to avoid cusp fracture, and porcelain is avoided because of the risk of fracture. Implants are not contraindicated but require careful planning to avoid overloading.

Management of the seizure itself and its most dangerous complication, status epilepticus, are discussed in Chapter 44.

Dental treatment for epilepsy PMID: 12050884 and 18450188

Dentistry for patients with seizures PMID: 17000276

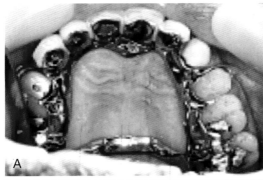

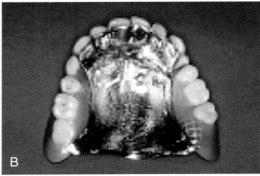

Fig. 39.2 Adapted denture designs for patient with epilepsy using metal reinforcement for all teeth. *(Reproduced from Fiske, J., Boyle, C., Epilepsy and oral care. Dental Update 29, 180–187.)*

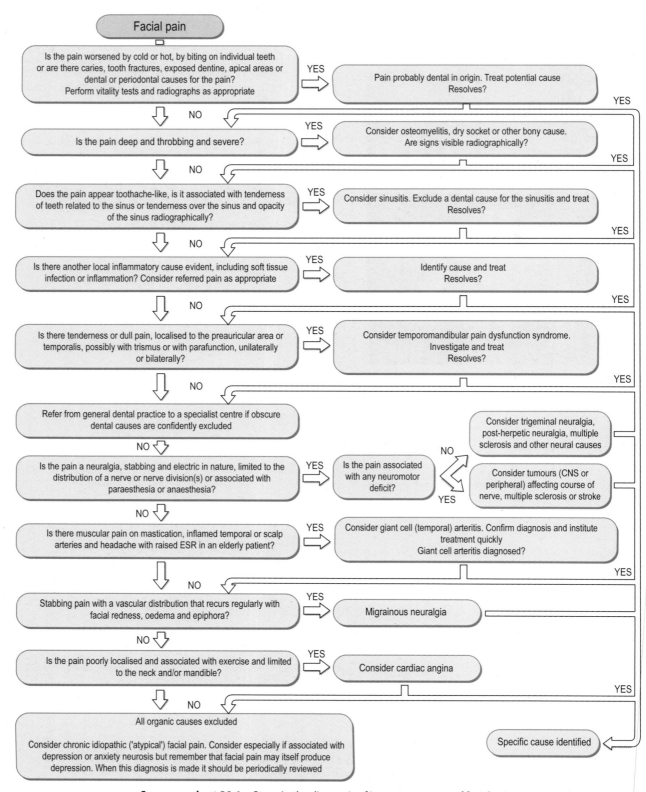

Summary chart 39.1 Steps in the diagnosis of important causes of facial pain.

Physical and learning disability | 40

The terminology for disability is sometimes confusing and constantly evolving. Healthcare professionals often demand clearcut definitions of degrees of disability that can be used to plan dental services or an individual's treatment. Unfortunately, this approach oversimplifies the issues.

People with disability see their needs in social terms rather than just the sum of their medical problems and, rightly, demand individualised care. The dentist must consider what each patient can do, and is prevented from doing, rather than concentrating on the physical or mental impairments themselves. This way of thinking focuses on the social and environmental aspects of disability and highlights ways in which the individual's environment can be adapted to limit, or even abolish, handicap. Current terminology for disability is shown in Table 40.1.

Nowhere is terminology more difficult than in the area of intellectual impairment. The terms mental retardation, deficiency or handicap are considered stigmatising and no longer acceptable in the UK but may be standard usage elsewhere in the world. In practice, intellectual impairments cause a wide range of disability. Some patients with no alteration in intelligence cannot cooperate due to uncontrolled movements (e.g., some patients with cerebral palsy), others are intelligent but uncooperative (e.g., some patients with hyperactivity), yet others are intellectually impaired but may sometimes be relatively easily treated (e.g., Down's syndrome with mild learning disability). The specific diagnosis and its severity are much more helpful in planning treatment than non-specific labels such as 'moderate' learning disability. In the UK, learning disability is distinguished from learning difficulty. Learning disability is characterised by problems with everyday activities caused by reduced intellectual ability that affect someone for their whole life. In contrast, learning difficulty is not associated with reduced intellect; learning just takes longer and requires additional support.

The prevalence of inherited disability is estimated at 1.5 to 2 per 1000 live births. Intellectual impairments account for approximately 0.9 per 1000 and major physical impairments account for the remainder. The prevalence is rising as a result of better medical care for adults and improved survival for babies with congenital disorders. There are nearly one and a quarter million individuals in the UK with mild-to-moderate learning difficulty and another quarter of a million with severe disability. The management of their dental care is affected by not only the disability itself but also parents', family and carers' motivation and attitudes, and the skills of the dental team. However, mental or physical disability does not necessarily mean that dental care has to be compromised, although this may sometimes be inevitable.

Children and adults with disability present a wide variety of challenges for dental management, but as many as 90% of them can probably be managed by good behaviour management, clinical technique and treatment planning. Sedation or general anaesthesia are essential for only a minority. Nevertheless, people with disability are a dentally-neglected group, even though valiant attempts have been made to overcome barriers to care.

Preconceptions that 'the disabled' are difficult to work with are misplaced, and those who manage people with disability find the work highly rewarding.

There is a welcome concern about the dental care of children with disability, but it should be remembered that disability persists for life. The transition from special school to community care can worsen dental disease because dental care must be provided in a less controlled setting, and intensive prevention is more difficult to maintain. Older people probably experience more disabilities than children because they are acquired throughout life as people live longer.

Challenges in the provision of dental care for people with disability are summarised in Box 40.1. Unless the disability is severe, most of these can be overcome with patience, training, experience and suitable facilities. It should be remembered that when disability is viewed in its social context, many difficulties become the responsibility of the dentist to overcome rather than problems associated with the patient.

European curriculum special care dentistry PMID: 24423174

Web URL 40.1 British Society Disability and Oral Health: http://www.bsdh.org/

Web URL 40.2 International Association for Disability and Oral Health https://www.iadh.org/

Web URL 40.3 International Special Care Dentistry Association https://www.scdaonline.org/

Table 40.1   **Current terminology for disability**

Term	Definition
Impairment	Any loss or abnormality of physiological function or anatomical structure
Disability or limitation of activity	Restriction or lack of ability to perform a function considered normal
	Legally defined as having a physical or mental impairment that has a 'substantial' and 'long-term' negative effect on ability to do normal daily activities
Learning disability	A significant impairment of intelligence and social functioning acquired before adulthood
Learning difficulty	Intellect is unaffected, but learning is slow
Handicap	The disadvantage for the individual, resulting from their disability, which prevents them from performing a normal role in society

---

Box 40.1 Potential challenges providing dental care for patients with disability

- Reduced cooperation with dental treatment
- Reduced ability to perform oral hygiene and manage diet
- Associated systemic disease
- Difficulties with transport and access to the surgery
- Possible need for sedation or general anaesthesia
- Medications or diets promoting caries
- Dysphagia, drooling, bruxism
- Oral effects of medications
- Capacity to give consent and deciding on best interests
- Financial challenges for patients
- Discrimination or prejudice in healthcare

Box 40.2 Common impairments affecting dental management

Learning disability

- Solitary learning disability
- Down's syndrome
- Microcephaly and hydrocephalus
- Metabolic disorders
- Hypoxia at birth
- Some syndromes

Behavioural conditions

- Autism spectrum disorder
- Attention deficit hyperactivity disorder

Physical impairment

- Cerebral palsy
- Distortion of the hands or arms
- Muscular dystrophies
- Spina bifida
- Epilepsy
- Some syndromes
- Communication: visual and hearing impairment
- Cleft palate (Ch. 3)

Mental health conditions (Ch. 41) can manifest as challenging behaviour, and patients' experiences have much in common with people with disability, particularly discrimination and poor access to dental care. People with personality disorders can sometimes be uncooperative, and their dental treatment may be severely compromised.

The importance of good prevention cannot be overemphasised. Many of the challenges arising from treatment of people with disability could be overcome by good preventive regimens.

Common disabilities relevant to dentistry are summarised in Box 40.2.

Physical and learning disability are frequently combined, as in Down's syndrome and some cases of cerebral palsy. Learning disability affects by far the largest group of people with disability needing dental care. Patients with Down's syndrome, many with cerebral palsy and some with epilepsy also have some degree of learning impairment. These four groups account for approximately 70%–75% of children with

disability. Conversely, many patients with cerebral palsy have typical intelligence but may be misjudged because of communication difficulties.

The improved survival of preterm infants and better neonatal care mean that the number of children with disability is increasing, even though prenatal screening and termination of pregnancy have impacted the incidence of some conditions.

DISCRIMINATION LEGISLATION

The United Nations Convention on Disability rights is enshrined in law in the UK Equality Act 2010. The entire act does not apply to Northern Ireland, where the Disability Discrimination Act 2005 performs a similar role. The intention is to ensure all individuals are treated equally, and these Acts apply to all employers and service providers including dentists and cover ethnic groups, gender reassignment, age, marital status and religion, as well as disability among the 'protected characteristics.

The act defines disability as physical or mental impairment that has a 'substantial' and 'long-term' (more than 1 year) negative effect on ability to perform normal daily activities. The definition is broad and applies equally to conditions such as colour blindness, visual or hearing impairment and fear of the dentist. It applies to all the policies and procedures of a dental provider, as well as to clinical care.

Under the UK Equality Act, service providers must not use any reason related to patients' disability as an excuse to treat people who are disabled less favourably than others. Dentists must make 'reasonable adjustments' so that they can access and use their services. This means more than providing wheelchair ramps. All aspects of the clinical practice and business of dentistry must comply. Some examples of the measures expected under the act are shown in Table 40.2. Which are reasonable in any particular setting depends on guidance from the Disability Rights Commission and will change with time and with legal precedents.

Practices that are 'disability-friendly' will also be more suitable for older people and many other groups of non-disabled

---

Table 40.2 Some factors to ameliorate disability in dental practice

Access	Level access, ramps, easy-grip door handles, doors hold open easily, wide corridors and aisles, obstructions clearly marked, if necessary, provide off-site or domiciliary visits. Provide for guide dogs
Design and structure of buildings	Colour schemes, contrasting colour on floors and walls, well lit, alarms in toilets (visible and audible)
Signs and practice leaflets and paperwork	Large type, succinct, good colour contrast, easy to read, use symbols and words, use sans serif fonts, no justification of right-hand margins, simple page layouts Consider Braille and audio versions
Websites	Should meet British Standard Specification for accessible websites
Staff and policies	Provide equality and diversity training for staff, record and survey needs of disabled users and consult local disability groups Each practice should have an equality policy

patients. All patients who are unable to visit a dental practice should have access to domiciliary or institutional dental care.

Web URL 40.4 UK disability definition: https://www.gov.uk/definition-of-disability-under-equality-act-2010

In the US, the equivalent requirements for dentists are in the Americans with Disabilities Act, originally of 1990, amended 2008, with some additional responsibilities at state level. This defines disability more broadly than in the UK, to the extent that 25% of the US population meets criteria for disability, but the requirements for equality are the same.

US requirements for dentistry PMID: 27264855

LEARNING DISABILITY

Learning disability is an all-inclusive term to describe people with significant intellectual impairment, whether caused by a specific disorder or an unknown cause. Down's syndrome, fragile X syndrome and hypoxia at birth are the more common causes, and the specific features of these conditions are dealt with later in this chapter. Learning disability may be unrelated to any physical disorder, or physical impairment may be severe, as sometimes in cerebral palsy. A minority of patients with genetic syndromes have craniofacial anomalies associated with intellectual impairment.

Intellectual impairment is classified according to the level of learning disability or difficulty, and children are taught either in mainstream schools or special schools, according to the degree of impairment. Institutional care is avoided if possible in the UK but remains common in many countries. Unfortunately, the classification gives no more than a broad indication of probable challenges with dental care because patients vary so widely and needs do not correlate simply with intelligence.

Learning disability has several facets. There may be reduced intelligence, making learning new information and complex tasks difficult, alone or together with impaired social functioning and ability to cope independently.

Children and adults with mild learning difficulty or disability can usually be coaxed into accepting regular treatment and to maintain acceptable standards of oral hygiene and dietary control. However, oral hygiene is usually suboptimal or poor and depends on motivation and skill of parents or carers. At the other extreme, all that may be possible is first-aid dentistry under sedation or general anaesthesia. All intermediate grades exist, but the level of dental health that can be achieved depends greatly upon the level of the dentist's skill and devotion to the task and prevention by carers. Realistic objectives must be tailored to the individual (Fig. 40.1).

Learning disability is rarely a solitary feature. Most individuals also have physical or sensory impairments, increased incidence of ill health, challenging behaviours or mental health disorders and a high risk of dementia on ageing.

Lip biting in disability PMID: 11819955

Down's syndrome

Down's syndrome is the most common clinically recognisable syndrome with learning disability. It is caused by trisomy of chromosome 21 giving a total complement of 47 chromosomes instead of 46. This is usually caused by failure of the chromosomes to separate during meiosis in the

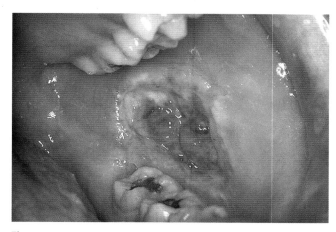

Fig. 40.1 Lip, tongue and cheek biting are frequent and distressing activities that are seen in learning disability and a range of neurological disorders. In this instance, biting followed local analgesic in a patient with insufficient understanding of its effects.

ovum, an effect closely linked to maternal age. The risk rises to 1 in 25 in mothers aged 45 years or older. Because the change arises in the ovum, both parents are healthy, and the condition is not inherited.

In contrast, approximately 4% of people with Down's patients have the additional chromosome 21 genetic material translocated to another chromosome. The translocation is transmitted in a familial pattern, but the parents have no associated features and the risk of an affected child is relatively low.

The rarest form is mosaic Down's syndrome in which the trisomy arises during early development, and the patients are a mosaic of cells with and without trisomy 21. In this type of Down's syndrome, the features are variable, and intelligence may be unaffected despite a syndromic appearance.

Ultrasound screening and cytogenetic diagnosis for mothers at highest risk allows over 90% of affected embryos to be detected prenatally, and in the UK approximately 90% of those pregnancies are terminated. This has more than halved the incidence to just more than 1 in 1000 live births from the 1 in 450 incidence without intervention. Termination of affected pregnancies reaches nearly 100% in some countries, raising ethical concerns.

General features

People with Down's syndrome have a characteristic facial appearance (Fig. 40.2), changes in skull and frequently of the dentition and susceptibility to infection (particularly viral) due to multiple immune effects. Congenital cardiovascular disease affects as many as 50%.

The prominent medial epicanthic skin fold gives the eyes their readily recognisable appearance. There is hypoplasia of the midface, reduced development of paranasal sinuses and a distorted upper respiratory tract. Upper respiratory tract infections are common, and breathing is often partially obstructed. Underdevelopment of the maxillae is usually associated with a protrusive mandible and class III malocclusion, with anterior open bite (Fig. 40.3, Box 40.3). The ears are frequently distorted, and there is additional skin on the neck.

Upper lateral incisors are often absent, and the teeth have short roots. Despite a higher-than-average incidence of enamel hypoplasia, caries risk is low. The low caries activity has been ascribed to the form and spacing of the teeth and

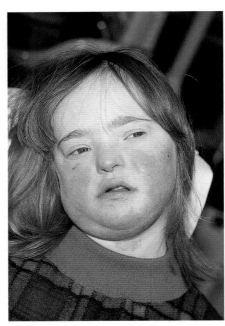

Fig. 40.2 Down's syndrome. This patient shows both the characteristic facial appearance and a cyanotic flush caused by associated congenital heart disease.

Box 40.3 **Down's syndrome: features relevant to dentistry**

- Class III malocclusion with hypoplastic maxilla
- Protrusive, fissured and apparently enlarged hypotonic tongue
- Lip hypotonia, mouth breathing and drooling
- Everted, thick, dry and crusted lips
- Oligodontia
- Delayed eruption of permanent teeth
- Hypoplastic dental defects and short roots
- Low caries activity
- Plaque accumulation
- Rapidly progressive periodontal disease
- Bruxism
- Short stature with short limbs
- Weak muscle tone
- Generalised susceptibility to infection
- Visual or hearing impairment in 50%
- Cardiac anomalies in 40%
- Weakness of atlantoaxial joint
- Susceptibility to leukaemia
- Alzheimer-like dementia in later life

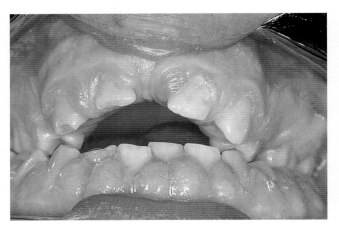

Fig. 40.3 Down's syndrome. Typical open bite and gingival hyperplasia from phenytoin for concomitant epilepsy.

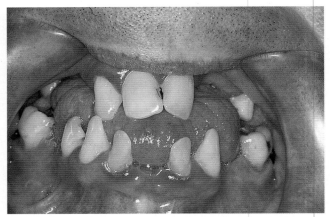

Fig. 40.4 Down's syndrome. Congenitally missing teeth with the hypotonic tongue protruding between them and gingivitis.

to the high bicarbonate content and pH of the saliva. Any caries resistance is readily overcome by poor diet.

Plaque accumulation and poor oral hygiene, due to difficulty cleaning and made worse by mouth breathing, together with the systemic predisposition to infection, contribute to the early onset of periodontal disease and early tooth loss (Fig. 40.4). Acute ulcerative gingivitis is also common if oral hygiene is poor and then often recurs.

Management

Most children with Down's syndrome have some degree of learning disability but it can be mild and may be absent in individuals with mosaic Down's. They continue to learn throughout life and may develop many skills if supported by good educational programmes and occupational therapy. Some can maintain an independent life.

Patients with Down's syndrome have a reputation for being good natured, cooperative within their ability and affectionate

and receptive to dental care, but this is not always so. This stereotype fails to recognise many who are frightened or more severely affected and completely uncooperative. The success of dental treatment depends mainly on the level of care provided. Patients with milder learning disability can be treated routinely in the dental chair, whereas the more severely affected may require sedation or general anaesthesia.

Control of periodontal disease is usually difficult, and success depends entirely on prevention by good oral hygiene. Teeth may be lost relatively early because of their short roots. Retention of teeth is important because dentures are usually poorly tolerated and retained because of the large protrusive tongue, weak muscle tone and poor comprehension. The apparently large tongue results from muscle hypotonia and forward posture, which also cause difficulty with mastication and swallowing.

Other features of the syndrome may affect dental treatment. The unstable atlanto-occipital joint is at risk of dislocation with severe consequences if the head is manipulated, particularly during general anaesthesia or sedation. All patients with Down's syndrome in the UK should have been screened for this anomaly during early childhood. Deafness and visual impairment are common. With improved medical care, life expectancy in Down's syndrome has lengthened and patients often live into their sixth decade. Unfortunately, almost half of older people with Down's patients develop an Alzheimer-like dementia, which further compromises their independence.

Cardiac defects are present in 40%, and half of these are severe enough to warrant surgical intervention. Atrial and ventricular septal defects, mitral and tricuspid valve defects, Fallot's tetralogy and patent ductus are common. These are repaired in childhood but, in later life, valvular regurgitation and prolapse may develop. Despite many contributory factors, the incidence of infective endocarditis does not appear to be increased.

General and oral review PMID: 17899715 and 27264854

Dental treatment and oral features PMID: 11819976

Fragile X syndrome

Fragile X syndrome is the next most common chromosomal disorder with learning disability after Down's syndrome; it affects at least 1 in 4000 males, being an X-linked dominant condition. Female carriers show variable partial features and only mild learning disability.

In this syndrome, the tip of the X chromosome appears as a thin thread of chromatin that is weakly attached and may break off.

Clinical features include moderate to severe learning disability, hyperactivity and behaviour similar to that in autism spectrum disorder. Open bite and crossbite are frequent. After growth, males develop a large head with a long face, prominent forehead and chin, and large protruding ears.

Other chromosomal abnormalities

Edwards' syndrome (trisomy 18) affects 0.7 and Patau syndrome (trisomy 13) 0.3 per 1000 pregnancies, but spontaneous abortion reduces incidence in live births dramatically to approximately 1 in 8000–9000 and life expectancy is shortened to a few years. Learning disability is severe in individuals that survive the medical complications, shown in Box 40.4. Prenatal diagnosis and termination of pregnancy have significantly reduced the incidence.

BEHAVIOURAL DISORDERS

Behavioural disorders and the more severe conduct disorders form a complex group of interlinked conditions with multiple causes. Autism spectrum disorder has the best evidence of neurodevelopmental abnormality but all probably have both genetic and environmental components. Many patients with behavioural disorders also have some degree of learning disability.

Autism spectrum disorder

Autism spectrum disorder consists of a range of neurodevelopmental conditions defined by causing two types of behavioural effects. The first is difficulties with social interaction and social communication and the second is repetitive behaviours and restricted interests. Any individual may have any degree of these two behaviours, with or

---

> **Box 40.4 Features of Edwards' and Patau syndrome**
>
> **Edwards' syndrome**
> - Heart defect in 85%
> - Fixed flexed fingers
> - Renal anomalies
> - Oesophageal atresia
> - Diaphragmatic hernia or abdominal wall defect
> - Cleft lip or palate
> - Neural tube defects
>
> **Patau syndrome**
> - Heart defect in 85%
> - Failure of forebrain development
> - Microphthalmia
> - Cleft lip and palate
> - Severe growth retardation
> - Severe learning disability
> - Polydactyly
> - Kidney malformation

---

without any degree of disordered use of language. Referring to the conditions as a spectrum emphasizes the variability in behaviours, severity, cognition, and their causes. The spectrum encompasses people previously diagnosed with Asperger's syndrome, in whom intelligence may be within the typical range and there is less delay in developing communication. It is considered that the individual traits of autism are also present in the general population and that individuals with mild autism spectrum traits merge imperceptibly with the wider population and lead unaffected lives. For this reason, some prefer the term autism spectrum conditions.

Autism spectrum disorder is also seen as a component of many defined syndromes, including Rett's, Down's, fragile X, tuberous sclerosis and neurofibromatosis. Many conditions can be associated, including epilepsy, anxiety and depression, obsessive compulsive disorder, dyslexia, eating disorders, gender dysphoria and schizophrenia.

Autism spectrum disorder is a polygenic condition with many genes implicated and brain changes including reduced brain maturation, synapse function and reduced connectivity between brain areas. Neurones are smaller and reduced in number in some brain areas and neural processing is slow. The condition is strongly inherited with possible environmental factors contributing.

Autism spectrum disorder is much more common in males, affects 1% of children and adolescents and has onset in the first 3 years of life. At one extreme, there is severe learning disorder and repetitive behaviour so that it may be impossible to communicate with, or manage, a person affected without sedation or general anaesthesia. At the other, a clear understanding of the condition may allow management for effective prevention, though operative treatment may often require sedation or a general anaesthetic.

Conventional child and adult behaviour management techniques are ineffective for patients in the autism spectrum. They are highly dependent on a regular routine and dislike noise and anything unexpected. Applied behavioural analysis is commonly used in education for children in the spectrum and uses a series of rewards to change behaviour. The dentist should identify these, ensure that they are not cariogenic (if they are food, often they are not) and can use the established reward system to achieve changes in dental behaviour. People with autism may take everything literally. Idiomatic expressions may not be understood or be taken at face value, and clear simple speech is necessary.

People in the autism spectrum may possess, incomprehensible (savant) skills, often mathematical. Although very few match the widely known 'Rain Man' stereotype, as many as 10% of people with autism have some special skill or ability, and patients often have a forceful interest in some well-ordered aspect of life, such as timetables.

Typical features of autism spectrum disorder are summarised in Box 40.5.

Patient view dental treatment PMID: 23943360 and 25530879

Planning treatment PMID: 25470557 and 24929596

Related issues in treatment PMID: 20675420

Attention deficit hyperactivity disorder

Attention deficit and hyperactivity are separate conditions but frequently occur together.

Attention deficit is characterised by daydreaming and limited ability to concentrate and perform complex tasks. Hyperactivity is characterised by constant movement, inability to concentrate on one task, being impulsive and, sometimes, making repetitive movements. The number of children diagnosed with these conditions has risen dramatically, and it is now considered that 3%–5% of children are affected, more commonly boys. Half of these also have autism spectrum disorder.

Initial management relies on education of carers and environmental modification to reduce disability with cognitive behaviour therapy. Drug treatment with methylphenidate (Ritalin) appears safe in the short-term and is effective in the majority of cases, but is a potentially addictive drug. It is provided to adults but only to the most severely affected children in the UK, though widely used elsewhere. Atomoxetine (Strattera) is also used. There is no agreed dividing line between this disorder and typical child behaviour, so it has been suggested that some children labelled as affected are no more than mildly disruptive underachieving children. Conversely, severe hyperactivity is profoundly disturbing and may be associated with self-harm. Thus, mild cases can be expected to respond to appropriate behaviour

management, whereas others may require sedation or anaesthesia.

Hyperactivity often reduces with age, but poor concentration and impulsive behaviour usually persist, and many affected adults experience depression.

Review dental management PMID: 24011294 and 17403737

DISEASES CAUSING PHYSICAL IMPAIRMENTS

Cerebral palsy

Cerebral palsy is common, with an incidence of 1:1000, and can be one of the most severe disabilities with various types of neuromuscular dysfunction (Box 40.6). The cause is cerebral damage from infection, trauma, hypoxia and other insults before, just after or at the time of birth. Many patients are born prematurely, and the risk rises with shorter gestation. Occasionally, childhood disease is the cause.

Neuromuscular dysfunction

The distribution and type of effects depend on the brain area affected and are very variable. Though defined as a movement disability, a quarter of people with cerebral palsy may also be affected by epilepsy and up to half with impairment of vision or hearing. Intelligence is unaffected in most cases but some degree of learning disability may be present. Muscle spasm during growth distorts skeletal growth and, eventually, fully formed bones.

The main presentations are spasticity, ataxia and dyskinesia. Spasticity affects half of the patients and causes fixed contraction of affected muscles and general stiffness. This may be so great that it may not even be possible to move an affected limb passively.

Athetosis refers to involuntary jerking movements, often of a wriggling character, sometimes accompanied by grimacing, and is seen in almost half the patients.

Ataxia is least common and characterised by lack of balance, an unsteady gait and reduced control over voluntary movements. In addition to variants of these three main types of disease, different parts of the body may be affected to a greater degree than others. Neuromuscular dysfunction can be so severe as to make speech unintelligible (dysarthria) and cause the person to appear intellectually impaired.

Dental aspects

Access to dental care may be difficult, whether the patient is wheelchair dependent or not. Patients using wheelchairs customised to support a distorted skeleton may prefer to be treated in it, using a wheelchair-tilting

---

Box 40.5   Autism spectrum disorder. Features commonly found to varying degrees in different individuals

- Lack of social interaction
- Lack of eye contact with others
- Learning disability in 70%
- Difficulty with verbal and other types of communication
- Hyper- and hyposensitivity to sensory stimuli: sights, sounds, smell, taste and touch
- Apparent unawareness of others
- Prefer constant daily routines
- Fixation on a single object or toy
- Persistent repetitive activity including bruxism
- Rarely, extreme memory, mathematical or artistic talents

Box 40.6   Types of cerebral palsy

- Spastic
  - Monoplegic
  - Paraplegic
  - Diplegic
  - Quadriplegic
- Athetotic
- Ataxic
- Hypotonic
- Mixed types

platform. Otherwise, many of these patients can be treated satisfactorily in the dental chair using hoist, sliding boards or other mobility aids.

Without aggressive prevention, periodontal disease can be severe. Ability to maintain oral hygiene varies and may be adequate with adapted brushes or, when both arms are affected, completely dependent on a carer. Inability to move the tongue and manipulate a bolus of food effectively reduces food clearance. Soft foods and sugar-containing nutrient supplements increase the risk of dental caries.

Communication is usually the main challenge, but speech can often be completely understood if time is spent learning to comprehend it. Many individuals with cerebral palsy have visual speech aids or computerised devices to help them communicate.

Bruxism and masseteric hypertrophy are frequent, and drooling may result from the open mouth posture, head tilting and weak swallowing. Abnormal tongue posture and swallowing are associated with development of malocclusion. These latter complaints often most trouble these patients.

Restorative treatment can be difficult. The chief challenge is with athetosis as unpredictable irregular movements complicate provision of good restorative work. It is also easy for the patient to be injured by sharp dental instruments. Mildly affected patients may respond well to relaxation with inhalation sedation but some will need full sedation or general anaesthesia.

A mouth prop may be considered with conscious athetotic patients in case the jaws suddenly clench.

Many patients with cerebral palsy also have epilepsy and drug-induced gingival overgrowth. Epilepsy, falls and sudden uncontrolled movements also render patients with cerebral palsy prone to dental injury.

Key features are summarised in Box 40.7.

Review dental management PMID: 19269401

Outcomes PMID: 34706111

Multiple sclerosis

Multiple sclerosis is a demyelinating disease that impacts both physical and mental wellbeing. Onset is usually in the third or fourth decades; a late onset is often associated with progressive severe disease. The disease is most common in people of Northern European descent, and the UK has a very high incidence. It is the most common cause of neurodisability in young adults and affects more than 1 in 1000 UK adults, more than 2 or 3 per 1000 in Scotland.

> **Box 40.7   Cerebral palsy: key dental features**
>
> - Usually, class II malocclusion and anterior open bite
> - Muscle hypotonia
> - Frequently severe caries and periodontal disease
> - Bruxism and masseteric hypertrophy
> - Impaired swallowing reflex but exaggerated gag reflex
> - Dental erosion and gastric reflux
> - Enamel hypoplasia
> - Mouth breathing
> - Dental trauma
> - Delayed eruption
> - Drooling
> - Epilepsy in 30%
> - Frequently wheelchair users

The cause involves genetic and environmental elements, possibly viral infection, triggering a cell-mediated autoimmune reaction against oligodendrocytes. This causes focal demyelination of axons and inflammation in the white matter. Symptoms are varied depending on the part of the brain affected and increase in number and severity with progression.

Common initial features include optic neuritis with transient blindness of one eye, odd sensory symptoms, subacute loss of function of motor supply to an arm or, particularly, palsy of the VIth cranial nerve producing a convergent squint and diplopia, and cognitive impairment. The outcome is highly variable; in the great majority there are short acute attacks of disability but, in approximately 10%, there is progressive deterioration culminating in widespread paralysis and sensory loss. Progression is more likely in males.

Disease progresses in periods of activity that can be modified but not prevented. Treatment of a relapse relies on high-dose corticosteroids. Long-term treatment to prevent relapse depends on a range of disease-modifying drugs including beta interferon, glatiramer acetate or natalizumab or mitoxantrone in severe disease. Gabapentin, baclofen or clonazepam are used for eye involvement and tizanidine and dantrolene for muscle spasm. Depression and neuropathic pain may require amitriptyline. The range of medications is as wide as the symptoms and signs. Many have significant side effects or significance for dentistry.

Dental aspects

The majority of minor cases can be treated routinely, and in the remainder treatment altered to match the abilities of the patient. Treatment should be carried out in a phase of remission. For patients with severe disability, treatment under local anaesthesia is acceptable, but they should not be put in the supine position because of possible respiratory difficulties and the risk of aspiration. Careful positioning in the dental chair or stretcher is required. Early day appointments are favoured to avoid fatigue. As disease progresses, oral hygiene can deteriorate, and early intensive preventive care is necessary to avoid problems in late disease.

Glatiramer acetate and mitoxantrone cause oral ulceration and glatiramer acetate causes parotid enlargement and facial oedema, although very rarely. Many of the drugs used are mildly immunosuppressant. Dry mouth and candidosis are common. The concern that amalgam restorations can cause or worsen the disease is unjustified.

The key role for the dentist is in recognising unusual symptoms of pain or neuropathy that do not fit typical diagnoses, present in younger patients than expected, are recurrent or progressive and respond poorly to conventional drug treatments. Very occasionally, orofacial signs or symptoms are the first presentation, including numbness or paraesthesia or mouth or face, trigeminal neuralgia, facial palsy or spasms of facial muscles.

Key features of multiple sclerosis are summarised in Box 40.8.

Multiple sclerosis oral health PMID: 19716502 and 34508197

Pain in multiple sclerosis general review PMID: 22909889

Cranial neuralgias in multiple sclerosis PMID: 22130044

Hydrocephalus

Hydrocephalus is caused by failure of drainage of cerebrospinal fluid causing increased intracranial pressure. It may be seen in isolation or associated with spina bifida or as a complication of a variety of other conditions including

Box 40.8 Multiple sclerosis: key features, these vary markedly between patients

- Onset usually in young adults
- Neurological deficits in several sites
- Fatigue
- Loss of mobility
- Limb spasticity and tremor
- Neuropathic pain
- Cognitive impairment
- Incontinence
- Poor swallowing and speech
- Occasionally trigeminal neuralgia-like pain
- In later disease, frequently wheelchair users, sometimes later bed bound
- Many experience remittent episodes lasting 24 hours or have slow progression

intrauterine infection. Compression of the cerebral tissue by the increased pressure during development can cause severe learning disability, epilepsy and muscle spasticity but the skull is soft and can expand to moderate the effects. In adults, with a rigid skull and who develop increased pressure due to brain tumours or haemorrhage, the signs are more florid and acute – headache, epilepsy, visual disturbance and cognitive impairment. This is usually diagnosed and treated quickly.

Treatment is to relieve the intracranial pressure by insertion of a catheter and, in the past, this released the cerebrospinal fluid directly into the right atrium (Spitz–Holzer valve). Younger patients are more likely to have a shunt into the peritoneal cavity. These catheters are prone to infection, more likely with the peritoneal type, but antibiotic prophylaxis for dental treatment is not recommended. Patients with some shunt types are associated with a risk of latex allergy.

Severe hydrocephalus in childhood can cause the skull to be so distended and heavy that the head has to be supported with cushions during treatment, taking care to avoid pressure in the region of shunts.

Dental treatment PMID: 20415804

Spina bifida

Spina bifida is failure of fusion of the vertebral arches and may be inherited or environmental in aetiology. Approximately 1:1000 children are affected. The mildest form (spina bifida occulta) is common but no more than a radiographic finding, sometimes with a tuft of hair overlying the defect. In the severe form there is a gross defect in the lower vertebral canal. The meninges and, often, nerve tissue protrude through it as a sac, which may be covered by skin. The consequences are paralysis and deformities of the lower limbs with loss of sensation and reflexes, incontinence and other complications. Meningitis is an obvious hazard, and epilepsy and learning disability are frequently associated because the brain structure is usually affected. Hydrocephalus is associated in almost all cases.

Since the upper part of the body is not affected, the main difficulties in dentistry are management of access, wheelchair use, epilepsy, incontinence and these patients' high risk of latex allergy (Ch. 31).

Dental relevance and treatment PMID: 23270130 and 11460784

The muscular dystrophies

Muscular dystrophies, of which the Duchenne type is the most common (approximately 1 in 5000 male births), are the main diseases of childhood causing paralysis. A range of genetic single gene defects cause different presentations with differing severity. Weakness of the muscles leads to progressively severe disability and is frequently associated with cardiomyopathy and respiratory impairment. Facial muscles are rarely affected (in the myotonic and facioscapulohumeral types of muscular dystrophy) but when masticatory muscles are affected the bite force gradually reduces and soft diets are required. A quarter of cases have learning disability.

There appear to be no specific dental issues. Most patients with Duchenne type are wheelchair-dependent by the age of 12 years and scoliosis develops, making treatment in a dental chair difficult. General anaesthesia is complicated by the presence of cardiac disease or respiratory impairment.

Review dental relevance PMID: 19068065

Myasthenia gravis

Myasthenia gravis is a disabling autoimmune disease that causes weakness and rapid fatigue of voluntary muscles. Women between 20 and 30 years are mainly affected. Circulating autoantibodies to the nicotinic acetyl cholinergic receptor of the neuromuscular end plates cause the disease by weakening the response to acetylcholine.

Clinically, there is rapidly developing, severe fatigue. Disability is worsened by cold, emotional stress and overexertion. Involvement of the respiratory muscles is potentially lethal and is most likely to affect older people. In many patients the initial signs involve twitching or weakness of the muscles around the eye.

Serum antibodies to acetylcholine receptors are detectable in approximately 85% of patients. Anticholinesterases, such as pyridostigmine, are the mainstay but cholinergic effects such as nausea, diarrhoea and bradycardia may be troublesome. Alternatives are corticosteroids in combination with azathioprine or ciclosporin.

Dental aspects

Weakness of the masticatory muscles causes the 'hanging jaw sign' for which patients characteristically support the jaw with a hand. Other effects include challenges with speech, mastication and swallowing. Paresis or atrophy of the tongue, often with longitudinal grooves, are occasional complications. In the rare syndrome of thymoma, myasthenia gravis and depressed cell-mediated immunity, there is chronic mucocutaneous candidosis. Other rare autoimmune associations are pemphigus vulgaris and Sjögren's syndrome.

Use of anticholinesterases can cause excessive salivation. Patients may also develop gingival enlargement from ciclosporin and candidosis from immunosuppressants.

Dental treatment should be undertaken shortly after medication and early in the day to avoid fatigue. Stress and anxiety worsen the severity of symptoms. A mouth prop may help patients reduce the muscular effort of mouth opening. The tongue may fall back, or feel as if it will, and patients may feel safer treated upright rather than supine. Denture control is often poor. Poor muscular control may compromise swallowing and clearance of pieces of dental debris, so rubber dam may be helpful. It is recommended that all local analgesics are used with caution, that is, with a vasoconstrictor and reduced maximum doses, and penicillins are the preferred antibiotics.

Intravenous sedation is contraindicated because of the respiratory muscle involvement. Respiratory insufficiency predisposes to sleep apnoea. Many drugs used in anaesthesia, particularly muscle relaxants, can severely aggravate myasthenic manifestations. Patients who are severely affected or very anxious are at risk of myasthenic crisis with respiratory failure and are best treated in a specialist centre.

Dental treatment considerations PMID: 22732850 and 26369478

Mental health conditions 41

Mental health conditions are common, affecting as much as one-third of the population at some time in their life, and as much as one-half of the population in some developed countries. When mild, they are frequently unrecognised. Classification and differentiation of mental health conditions are complex. The main conditions are summarised in Box 41.1.

The causes of mental health conditions are both genetic and environmental, poorly understood and linked to physical disease and external stresses, upbringing, drugs and social factors, as well as organic brain disease. Mental health conditions still carry a stigma, and dentists must be nonjudgmental in discussing it.

Challenging behaviour is common in mental health conditions, so patients experience discrimination and poor access to dental care. This may be compounded by a loss of interest in self-care. General aspects of mental health conditions that can affect dental management are summarised in Box 41.2.

Dementia is covered in Chapter 42.

Oral disease in mental health conditions PMID: 21881097

Box 41.1   Some common mental health conditions

- Anxiety
- Attention deficit hyperactivity disorder (see page 558)
- Disturbances of mood
  - Depression
- Personality disorders
- Obsessive-compulsive disorder
- Eating disorders
- Psychoses
  - Bipolar disorder
  - Schizophrenia

Box 41.2   Aspects of mental illness that may affect dental management

- Erratic attendance
- Oral neglect
- Inability to cooperate
- Challenging or aggressive behaviours
- Drug therapy
- Psychosomatic disorders
- Phobia of dental treatment
- Associated alcoholism or drug dependence
- Violence
- Factitious injury and disorder

PAIN WITHOUT MEDICAL CAUSE

Pain is not a simple sensation but has been described as the unpleasant experience felt 'when hurt in body or mind' (Ch. 39). The psychological aspects of pain are often overwhelmingly important, and the patient's reaction is affected by such factors as mood, emotional characteristics, personality and cultural background. Some stoical patients tolerate constant pain well, but others complain bitterly and persistently about trivial lesions.

Pain without a cause is a very difficult diagnostic challenge, and dental surgeons cannot deal with unexplained pain without medical help. It is the dentist's role to exclude dental causes for any pain before making a differential diagnosis to allow an appropriate onward referral. This requires an understanding of both organic causes of orofacial pain and mental health conditions. It is also important to avoid unnecessary dentistry or surgery when a psychiatric cause is likely. This is both damaging and causes delay in definitive diagnosis.

Now that atypical facial pain and burning mouth (Ch. 39) are considered either neuralgias or partially neurological conditions, there are very few occasions when a dentist may need to consider a diagnosis of purely psychogenic pain.

By definition, unexplained pain is a diagnosis of exclusion. It can be difficult to know how intensively to investigate possible causes, but the clinician cannot be complacent. A pain should not be labelled as psychogenic lightly. It is acutely embarrassing to diagnose a poorly localised severe and depressing facial pain as atypical odontalgia and then discover that it has been cured by restoration or extraction of a tooth with pulpitis, root perforation or undetected crack. Similarly, some conditions such as nerve invasion by adenoid cystic carcinoma produce unexplained unusual pain. Any diagnosis of psychogenic pain must be continually reviewed in case a physical or psychological cause becomes evident. Truly psychogenic pain is often associated with other bizarre symptoms, but even when these are present, it is not appropriate for the dentist alone to make a diagnosis of a purely psychosomatic pain.

All pain is affected by mental state, and all types of pain can become less bearable in depression. The mechanisms of central pain, neuropathic pain, and depression are inextricably linked, and depression may even be caused by alterations in some of the shared pathways. Because mental health conditions, even now, carry a stigma, patients frequently suppress the depression on presentation. Conversely, prolonged severe pain can cause depression. It is usually impossible to decide which came first in a purely dental environment.

Chronic neuropathic pain PMID: 26685473

Idiopathic pain mechanisms PMID: 25483941

ANXIETY

Anxiety is a disproportionate fear of everyday events, an abnormal 'fight or flight' reaction mediated by catecholamines.

Box 41.3   Anxiety states

- Phobias
  - Dental
  - Social
  - Specific phobias, such as blood-injection-injury
- Panic disorder
- Anxiety with depression
- Generalised anxiety disorder
- Post-traumatic stress disorder

Box 41.4   Manifestations of anxiety

- Constant state of worry without specific cause
- Muscle tension
- Rapid breathing and heart rate
- Sweating, pallor
- Excessive talking
- Dry mouth
- Aggression or uncooperative

Box 41.5   Management of dental phobia

- Accurate history to identify anxiety level
- Identify triggers: smells, noise, needles, vibration
- Cognitive behavioural therapy
  - Relaxation techniques
  - Systematic desensitisation
  - Cognitive restructuring
- Hypnosis
- Avoid waiting time before appointment
- Conscious sedation
- Premedication with benzodiazepine
- General anaesthesia

Box 41.6   Typical manifestations of depression

- Feeling 'low' or miserable
- Uncontrollable pessimism
- Inability to sleep or early wakening
- Disturbance, usually loss, of appetite
- Loss of libido
- Tiredness
- Irritability
- Inability to look forward to any pleasurable activity
- Difficulty making decisions
- Resorting to alcohol, smoking or drugs
- Thoughts of suicide or death

Anxiety includes several distinct conditions summarised in Box 41.3.

Social phobia is the term given to uncontrollable anxiety in everyday social situations. Persistent and chronic fear of being watched or judged by others, and fear of being humiliated by behaviour or appearance, are typical features.

The main significance to dentistry is fear of dentistry itself, together with the adverse effects of antidepressant medications.

Fear of dentistry

It is perfectly normal to feel anxiety at the prospect of dental treatment, but the fears are overcome by the desire for dental care.

Mild anxiety can be suppressed by the patient or missed by the dentist, who is used to dealing almost entirely with people exhibiting some degree of fear. Recognition is important as anxiety may manifest in different ways in different patients (Box 41.4). Anxiety is greater in children than adults.

In most cases, reassurance, simple behaviour management, distraction and, in more marked anxiety, sometimes a preoperative benzodiazepine or inhalational sedation are sufficient to manage anxiety.

Dental phobia is an extreme manifestation of anxiety and may sometimes result from painfully traumatic dental experiences as far back as in childhood. Truly phobic patients will not turn up for, or even request, appointments and develop the consequences of repeated emergency dentistry. As much as 11% of the population fear dentistry sufficiently to accept pain and suffering detrimental to their oral health. The majority are female. Specialist intervention is required using the principles outlined in Box 41.5. Cognitive behavioural therapy is the most effective intervention, and sedation and general anaesthesia should be methods of last resort.

Characteristics of dental anxiety PMID: 26611310

Management in adolescents PMID: 34503664

Management dental anxiety PMID: 21838825 and 35735746

Non-pharmacological management fear and phobia PMID: 30835665

Sedative medication PMID: 34690057

Obsessive-compulsive disorder

Obsessive-compulsive disorder is a manifestation of anxiety in which patients have uncontrollable ritualistic thoughts or behaviour that interfere with normal life. The condition is common, affecting approximately 1% of the population. Obsessive-compulsive states can lead to depression and are sometimes secondary to schizophrenia.

Treatment is with cognitive behavioural therapy or antidepressants, usually selective serotonin reuptake inhibitors.

Obsessions affecting dental management may include compulsive toothbrushing, possibly causing dental abrasion, excessive use of antiseptic mouthwashes, or fear of oral infections, of cancer, or of halitosis, and refusal to be reassured.

DEPRESSION

Depression is a serious condition, the impact of which on life is frequently underestimated. It is common and may sometimes underlie or exacerbate oral symptoms. Typical manifestations of depression are summarised in Box 41.6. Even severe depression is often undiagnosed.

A short period of depression following unpleasant experiences such as bereavement or financial difficulties is normal, but abnormal if symptoms are prolonged and quality of life is impaired. Unfortunately, depression is widely stigmatised as weakness and suppression by alcohol is common. Causes are complex, partly genetic, environmental and social. Serious, particularly life-threatening illnesses can also be triggering factors. Age of onset is approximately 30 years, and most patients are female. As much as 10% of the population have depression. Rates of depression have risen sharply in the UK in female adolescents and more recently in all age groups including children during the Covid-19 pandemic as a result of social isolation.

Dental aspects of depression

Depressed patients may sometimes be challenging or even aggressive and need to be treated particularly tactfully and sympathetically. Dentists need to be alert for depression as it is common and often denied by patients in their medical history.

Depression is found with many oral conditions, either as a cause, effect or simple association (Box 41.7).

The main challenge in patients under treatment is the oral effects of antidepressant drugs. Xerostomia is an almost universal effect of antidepressants and may lead to candidosis and ascending sialadenitis. Other effects appear rare, but include bruxism, dysgeusia, angioedema and, with tricyclic antidepressants, black tongue. The tricyclic antidepressants are now little used as first-line treatment because of adverse effects. Ibuprofen should be avoided with antidepressants, and paracetamol should be avoided with tricyclic antidepressants.

Some patients will increase their carbohydrate intake in the belief that it boosts serotonin levels, risking caries.

It should also be remembered that stress, anxiety and depression are commonly seen in dentists, although the frequently reported high suicide rate is not borne out by the evidence.

General review depression in adolescents PMID: 35940184

Dental management PMID: 8042134, 8486855

FACTITIOUS ULCERATION

Factitious or self-inflicted traumatic ulcers in the mouth are very uncommon but important as indicators of self-harm in people with mental health conditions. Rarely, factitious oral ulceration has been a prelude to suicide.

Patients usually cause ulcers by repeated trauma to the lips or anterior visible parts of the mouth, in sites accessible to their dominant hand. Fingernails or instruments can be used, and repeated picking at the gingival margin or over bone can induce bone loss through chronic inflammation and, eventually, tooth exfoliation (Fig. 41.1). Occasionally, a patient will extract their own teeth or cause mucosal ulceration and inflammation by rinsing with caustic fluids.

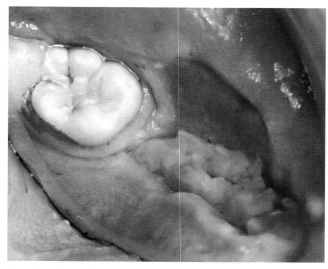

Fig. 41.1 Factitious injury. Large deep ulcer exposing the alveolar bone produced by picking the ridge and repetitive biting of objects.

The diagnosis of self-inflicted injuries is difficult because the patient conceals the cause, but suspicious features are shown in Box 41.8. Frequently, the diagnosis can be confirmed only by discreet observation after admission to hospital.

Case series PMID: 7776171 and case: 2887598

ANOREXIA NERVOSA AND BULIMIA NERVOSA

Anorexia nervosa is an eating disorder characterised by a desire to be slim associated with voluntary restriction of food intake and fear of weight gain, even to the point of emaciation and occasionally death. There is a distorted body image that prevents patients recognising their actual weight and shape. Bulimia nervosa is characterised by binge eating and vomiting to restrict food intake and is not necessarily associated with low body mass. Both are diseases of urban populations in developed countries.

Causes of both are complex, but there is a strong genetic predisposition on which psychological and social factors act. There are shared personality traits among anorexia, obsessive-compulsive disorder and autism spectrum disorder.

Both conditions particularly affect females younger than 20 years but are increasingly recognised in males.

Oral and perioral effects of anorexia and bulimia are parotid swelling (sialadenosis, Fig. 22.26) and dental erosion and sensitivity due to vomiting (Ch. 6). Iron and vitamin deficiency may predispose to angular cheilitis or candidosis.

Dentists may be able to identify such signs and make an early referral to medical care. Vacuum-formed splints can be used to protect teeth during vomiting. Low body weight must be taken into account when prescribing.

Oral manifestations eating disorders PMID: 18826377, 11862200 and 31435954

PSYCHOSES

Schizophrenia

Schizophrenia is the most common severe mental health condition. It can be chronic and severely disabling and affects 1% of the population, usually with onset between 20 and 30 years of age.

A great range of symptoms and behaviour is possible, probably reflecting different causes and subtypes. In the chronic phase, mood, thoughts and behaviour change and become disorganised with inability to concentrate. Confusion, unpredictability and inappropriate behaviour and blunted or flattened mood are common. Patients may not follow or be able to construct a logical chain of thought. Intelligence is unimpaired, and insight may even be retained. Schizophrenic individuals' behaviour is not necessarily affected all the time.

In the acute phase, there may be hallucinations and delusions with failure to distinguish reality from what is experienced. Patients may fear persecution, hear voices and, occasionally, perform violent acts. Signs of normal emotion are absent, and there is often withdrawal from social contact.

A wide range of drugs may be taken including phenothiazines and butyrophenones.

Dental aspects

People with schizophrenia are at high risk of dental disease.

Mild schizophrenia may appear merely to be stupidity or result in inappropriate behaviour. Responses to questions may indicate a failure to get through or elicit entirely inappropriate answers. Calm manner and avoidance of sudden stress are important. Though a concern, the risk that some patients will become violent is small.

Provided that the patient is cooperative, there are no major restrictions on the form of dental treatment that can be provided. Any reaction between epinephrine in local anaesthetics and phenothiazines appears to be no more than theoretical.

Phenothiazines and some other neuroleptics can cause severe xerostomia, particularly in long-term use. Phenothiazines can also cause involuntary facial movements (dyskinesias) or parkinsonism. *Tardive dyskinesia* can develop in approximately 30% of patients treated long-term with phenothiazines. Involuntary movements particularly involve the face and are irreversible. Repeated grimacing and chewing movements may be violent and result in scarring and deformities of the tongue. Newer antipsychotics are almost free from this adverse effect, apart from aripiprazole, which seems prone to cause it. Other relevant adverse reaction to drugs for schizophrenia include lichenoid reactions and taste abnormalities.

Dental significance review PMID: 15119719 and 34448736

Dentistry and older people 42

The ageing population of the UK and many countries is a well-recognised phenomenon, caused by increased lifespan and enhanced by falling birth rates. Future world total population estimates have recently been reduced as a result of dramatic reduction in fertility rates in almost all countries. Estimates for world population suggest that by 2050 there will be more people aged over 65 than under 25 in almost all countries except sub-Saharan Africa. Changes are most marked in Japan and Korea.

In the UK, there are 1.7 million people aged 85 or more (2.5% population) and by 2040, it is estimated that 1 in 4 people will be aged older than 65 years (Fig. 42.1) The overall UK population will have risen more slowly than previously predicted, but still from its present 67 million to 70 million. Much UK population growth comes from immigration, adding persons of all age groups, but the number of people aged 90 or over has more than doubled between 1990 and 2020 and average life expectancy is 81 years. Older individuals do not think of themselves as aged or in decline until very late in life and expect the same treatment as younger individuals, as they are entitled to under the Equality Act 2010. However, increasing age is associated with various social, healthcare and dental challenges (Box 42.1).

These can become major handicaps when an older patient experiences a significant oral disease, such as a carcinoma. Mobility, communication and illness are the key issues in the management of older patients. Neurological factors are particularly problematic (Box 42.2). Depression is very common, affecting 25% of people over 65 years of age and half living in institutions.

Older people who are edentulous are more likely to develop significant medical disease than those who are dentate.

Edentulousness and medical disease PMID: 26371954

General review dentistry and aging PMID: 25709420 and 34449647

Medical aspects aging PMID: 29312916

Epidemiology oral disease with age PMID: 26504122 (UK) and (US) 22390504

DEMENTIA

Cognitive deterioration is a common consequence of ageing and is something we all risk if we live long enough.

Dementia is a chronic progressive failure of mental processes affecting all aspects of mental activity, such as intelligence, memory, emotional state and personality. These different functions tend to be affected to a variable and unpredictable extent. Dementia is caused by Alzheimer's disease in two-thirds of cases, but also by vascular disease, Parkinson's disease or stroke. It is also a late age-related complication in people with HIV infection, Down's syndrome and autism spectrum disorder and in alcohol dependence. The risk of dementia is considerably increased after Covid-19 infection and this raises concern of a worldwide surge in dementia incidence. The risk increases with Covid-19 severity but is significant even in mild disease.

The incidence of dementia rises with age, from approximately 20% of people aged 70 years to half of those aged

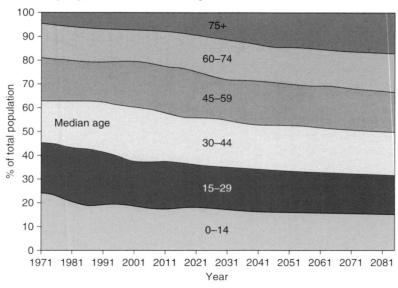

Percentage age distribution, United Kingdom, 1971–2085

Fig. 42.1 UK population projections for different age groups. *(Source: UK Office for National Statistics)*

Box 42.1   Challenges for patients older than 65 years

- Age discrimination
- Disease: two-thirds have a chronic illness or disability
  - Osteoporosis
  - Depression
  - Impaired vision: cataracts or macular degeneration
  - Impaired hearing and communication
  - Incontinence
  - Dementia
- Lack of carers, carers likely to be old too
- Reduced mobility
- Lack of social contact, loneliness and isolation
- Lack of financial resources
- Likely to be single or living alone
- One-third are at risk of malnutrition
- One-quarter are edentulous
- Only half are registered with a dentist
- Capacity to consent

Box 42.2   Neurological and psychological causes of disability in older people

- Dementia
- Intellectual deterioration
- Depression
- Confusional states
- Paranoia
- Dependence on medication
- Parkinson's disease
- Strokes
- Deafness
- Impaired vision
- Trigeminal neuralgia

85 years. Nevertheless, dementia and Alzheimer's disease are not obligatory elements of ageing. While HIV infection has become a chronic treatable infection and is now found in older patients, dementia from HIV infection may increase.

The features of dementia are shown in Box 42.3.

In the early stages the patient may seem bright enough but may immediately forget instructions, for example, about how to look after dentures. Other patients become confused, querulous, or even aggressive, behave in an unusual fashion, may have delusions or be generally 'difficult'. It is important to obtain as high a standard of oral health as possible in the early stages, ideally with a care plan, to prevent problems later. Dental pain can worsen the confusion in dementia. Caries may develop as a result of high-energy food supplements, and oral hygiene gradually worsens. Denture loss is a common problem, and duplicate sets of dentures and denture marking are helpful as adaptation to new dentures is likely to be impossible.

In late dementia, diagnosis of dental pain by conventional means may not be possible and should be suspected if there is failure to eat, restlessness and pulling or poking the face or mouth, drooling, ceasing denture wear, disturbed sleep or aggression.

Box 42.3   Features and consequences of dementia

- Slow unpredictable progression in severity
- Memory loss, particularly short-term memory
- Confusion
- Difficulty following and understanding instructions
- Anxiety, depression, agitation, hallucinations
- Reduced motor skill, poor balance, tremor
- Impaired, and later loss of, speech, hearing and vision
- Reduced movement
- Incontinence
- Loss of social interaction
- Inability to self-care, total dependence on carers
- Inability to eat and swallow
- Death, usually from pneumonia

Consent for treatment will eventually lie with another individual, in the UK with Power of Attorney under the Mental Capacity Act 2005.

Treatment is essentially supportive. Selected patients with mild or moderate disease may be prescribed anticholinergic drugs to improve cognition, such as donepezil, rivastigmine or galantamine or the NMDA receptor blocker, memantine but these do not slow the overall progression. The anticholinergics all cause dry mouth, potentially predisposing to caries, and make denture wearing more of a challenge.

Oral health in dementia PMID: 34811365

Orofacial pain diagnosis in dementia PMID: 21359232

Dental management PMID: 26556259 and 33641757

Dementia and Covid-19 PMID: 35912749

OTHER SYSTEMIC DISEASES

Systemic diseases that particularly affect older people are shown in Box 42.4.

A variety of drugs used for cardiovascular disease can also cause oral reactions (Ch. 43). Malnutrition is particularly likely. Poverty, poor mobility (which interferes with both cooking and shopping) and mental health conditions are some of the contributory factors. Poorly functioning dentures and impairment of taste sensation may make matters worse.

However, deficiency states, particularly scurvy and vitamin B group deficiencies, are remarkably rare, even in old age. It is important, nevertheless, that denture function should be the best possible in order not to worsen nutritional status of older patients. Sore tongue or signs of atrophy of the mucosa should be investigated for underlying anaemia.

Parkinson's disease

This common idiopathic disease caused by loss of basal ganglia neurones is characterised by rigidity, slow movements and tremor with impaired coordination. It affects 1 in 1000 individuals older than 65 years.

Patients have a mask-like fixity of facial expression, with tremor sometimes affecting the lower jaw and often drooling as a result of impaired neuromuscular function. Parkinson's disease has several cognitive disturbances and is a risk factor for subsequent dementia. Important features are summarised in Box 42.5.

Box 42.4   Important systemic diseases relevant to dentistry and more common in older people

Cardiovascular

- Hypertension and ischaemic heart disease (Ch. 33)
- Cardiac failure (any cause) (Ch. 33)
- Giant-cell (temporal) arteritis and polymyalgia rheumatica (Ch. 14)

Respiratory

- Chronic bronchitis and emphysema
- Pneumonia

Haematological

- Anaemia (especially pernicious anaemia) (Ch. 28)
- Chronic leukaemia (Ch. 28)
- Myeloma (Ch. 12)

Musculo-skeletal

- Arthritis
- Osteoporosis and fractures

Metabolic

- Type 2 diabetes
- Chronic kidney failure

Neurological

- Parkinson's disease
- Trigeminal neuralgia
- Post-herpetic neuralgia
- Dementia

Carcinomas (all sites)

Box 42.5   Parkinson's disease: key features

General

- Expressionless face
- Soft indistinct speech
- Stooping posture
- Slowness in starting or repeating movements
- Impaired fine movements especially of fingers
- Fatigue

Gait

- Slow to start
- Rapid small steps and tendency to run
- Impaired balance on turning

Tremor

- Usually first in fingers and thumb
- Can affect limbs, jaw and tongue
- Present at rest
- Diminished by activity

Rigidity

- 'Cogwheel' type particularly in the arms
- 'Lead-pipe' type particularly in the legs

Sympathetic management is essential. It is particularly important that the poverty of facial expression is not mistaken for incomprehension, and the speech be not thought to be due to impaired intellect.

Box 42.6   Some common causes of limitation of mobility in older patients

- Ataxia
- Strokes
- Arthritis
- Heart disease
- Late dementia
- Visual impairment
- Poor balance
- Muscle weakness

Drooling may be particularly troublesome, but conveniently the antimuscarinic drugs sometimes given, such as benzhexol or orphenadrine, can cause dry mouth. Reduction in salivary flow can also be achieved using botulinum toxin in the parotid glands (Ch. 27). Involuntary orofacial movements, due to levodopa or bromocriptine, may make use of rotating dental instruments hazardous. Parkinson's disease can compromise the management of dentures because of the loss of fine control of muscular movement. Oral hygiene is impaired. Postural hypotension is common, and patients must rise slowly from the dental chair.

Involvement of masticatory muscles also makes mastication and swallowing difficult in later stages of disease and this may be ameliorated with exercise therapy.

The effects of Parkinson's disease can be diminished by giving a range of drugs including dopaminic agents such as levodopa, dopamine agonists, monoamine oxidase B inhibitors, anticholinergic drugs and catechol-O-methyl transferase (COMT) inhibitors such as entacapone. The last interacts with epinephrine, theoretically at least, so that epinephrine-free local anaesthetics or minimal doses may be preferable to avoid tachycardia and arrhythmias. L-Dopa causes taste disturbance and colours urine, sweat and saliva red.

However, complete success of treatment is rarely achieved, and virtually all the drugs have significant side effects, particularly in long-term use.

Dental review PMID: 11199638 and 19491161

Jaw exercise PMID: 31837276

Oral movement disorders review PMID: 35904592

ORAL DISEASE IN OLDER PEOPLE

Illustrative of the dental challenges for older people are the findings in a survey of care home managers, almost half of whom considered the oral and dental needs of their inhabitants were poorly met. Common issues include candidosis, difficulty eating, maintaining oral or denture hygiene and access to dental care.

Factors affecting dental care

Many medical factors limit the mobility of older patients (Box 42.6), and they may simply be unable to afford the cost of dental care or transportation. Availability of domiciliary visits varies but is limited. Even when access to care is easy, older patients tend to become even more infrequent visitors to the dentist than they once were, especially when complete dentures have been provided. Oral hygiene is compromised by arthritis and the neurological disorders discussed previously.

Oral disease in older patients is likely to require time and special skills from the dentist. Even among older individuals in institutions, complete dentures are no longer the norm, and the main dental need of most older people is no longer effective and comfortable dentures. The teeth that remain are less likely to develop periodontitis but are prone to caries if sugar intake is not controlled and may be heavily restored, requiring long-term maintenance and repair. In the future, mouths with partial dentures and implants will pose significant challenges as teeth are progressively lost. The loss of adaptability with age requires good forward planning for prosthetics. It is also important to remember that good oral health is important in maintaining self-esteem.

The teeth

The teeth can undergo attrition, abrasion and, frequently, continued destruction by caries. Attrition increases with a reduced dental arch, and tooth wear may be accelerated by erosion. The roots gradually also become hypercalcified by progressive obliteration of the dentinal tubules by peritubular and circumpulpal dentine. The roots may then become completely calcified, impossible to root treat and brittle, so they are more likely to fracture during extraction. There is increased need for restorations with occlusal coverage to prevent fractures.

Caries is often on the root surface in older people. This is partly because caries-prone fissures or contacts have already become carious in earlier life and partly as a result of recession, dry mouth, poor oral hygiene and altered diet (Ch. 4). Dietary control of sugars is equally important at all ages. Fluoride varnish is a useful evidence-based intervention in institutions.

Periodontitis is less of a problem. Patients who are prone are likely to have lost the most susceptible teeth before the age of 60 years, and only slow progression is expected. However, this depends on ability to maintain good oral hygiene.

Every attempt should be made to retain a 'functional dentition' of 21 teeth to avoid the need for prostheses. Only 40% of 75–85 year-olds in the UK have a functional dentition and this reduces to 25% of people aged over 85 years.

UK oral health of older people PMID: 28537362

The alveolar bone and dentures

Progressive loss of denture-bearing bone in patients who are edentulous reduces retention and stability of dentures. Later, if large amounts of bone become resorbed, pain can be caused by the dentures pressing upon anatomical structures, such as the mylohyoid ridge or genial tubercles.

In general, the older the patient, the less adaptable they are likely to be. Although preservation of teeth for as long as possible may be desirable, it may create greater challenges if extractions have to be postponed until very late in life. The wearing of full dentures demands a remarkable feat of adaptation at any age, and older patients face a greater challenge. Also, some older patients may no longer care about appearance, may have few social contacts and may prefer a soft diet. Motivation, which plays so large a part in adaptation to denture wearing, may therefore be diminished. The importance of denture duplication and marking was noted earlier in the section on dementia.

Problems of edentulousness PMID: 24446979

The temporomandibular joints

Osteoarthritis of the temporomandibular joints is not a significant problem (Ch. 14).

Pain or other symptoms from the temporomandibular joints in the older patients are remarkably uncommon. However, pain on mastication may be due to temporal

---

> **Box 42.7 Mucosal diseases more common in older patients**
> - Lichen planus and lichenoid drug reactions
> - Mucous membrane pemphigoid
> - Pemphigus vulgaris
> - Herpes zoster
> - Glossitis
> - Burning mouth syndrome
> - Leukoplakia and erythroplakia
> - Medication-related osteonecrosis
> - Carcinoma

arteritis and, if so, requires urgent treatment because of the risk of loss of sight (Ch. 14).

Salivary function

Salivary secretion does not appear to be significantly reduced with age alone, but dry mouth is overall more common in older individuals as a result of diseases such as Sjögren's syndrome or the use of drugs with diuretic or antimuscarinic activity (Ch. 22). Older patients who have a dry mouth must therefore be investigated accordingly. Dehydration is common in patients living in institutions, particularly if they have urinary incontinence and avoid drinking fluids.

Mucosal diseases

Some changes in the oral mucosa are directly related to age. Examples include enlarged Fordyce's granules, lingual varicosities and foliate papillae (Ch. 1). These are often causes of anxiety in the older patients.

Mucosal diseases that tend to affect older people are summarised in Box 42.7 and discussed in more detail in previous chapters.

It must be emphasised that recurrent aphthae are uncommon in older persons but, when seen, it is important to look for some underlying predisposing cause such as pernicious anaemia or iron deficiency.

The mucosa also heals more slowly with age.

Malignant neoplasms and irradiation

In older people in institutions, 1 in 50 may have red or white oral lesions. Cancer of the mouth, which both becomes more common as age advances and is insidious in development, is particularly likely to be missed or ignored in its earlier stages, especially in institutions and in people with dementia.

Because of the rising frequency of carcinoma with advancing age, older people may have had radiotherapy. They may therefore develop xerostomia or be at risk from osteoradionecrosis. Denture trauma can occasionally precipitate the latter complication, and wearing lower dentures after radiotherapy carries a risk that needs to be assessed patient by patient.

Older patients who have metastatic carcinoma from breast, prostate or other carcinomas, may be at risk of medication-related osteonecrosis (Ch. 8).

Cardiovascular disease

Older patients are overall at the highest risk from infective endocarditis. A possible contribution to this is periodontal or dental sepsis. In addition, drugs given for cardiovascular disease can be a cause of oral lesions (Chs 32 and 42).

Complications of systemic drug treatment

43

The 2018 Health Survey in England revealed that 48% of adults were taking prescription drugs and 25% took three or more, the number rising with age. The most frequently used drugs are statins, antihypertensives and non-steroidal anti-inflammatory drugs. In some parts of the UK, one in five women use antidepressants. When non-prescription drugs and complementary medicines are added, and account is taken of the many new and highly potent targeted therapies, there is great potential for adverse reactions and drug interactions.

It has never been appropriate to try to remember more than the most significant interactions with drugs prescribed in dentistry. The British National Formulary and other national prescribing guidance in other countries, Physician's Desk Reference or datasheets must be consulted whenever the dentist is unfamiliar with a drug.

The patient's medical history must include a complete drug list, ideally with doses and frequency because these often determine actions taken in response. Patients may misconstrue the word 'drugs' and should be asked whether they are taking 'medicines, tablets, injections, or any sort of medical treatment for *any* purpose' or have received any medications recently, or whether they have been given any sort of hospital card. If unsure, their medical practitioner's practice computer should be able to produce a list of current and past prescriptions quickly and easily.

It is also important to check for 'over-the-counter' or non-prescription medicines. Some countries allow purchase of drugs with significant adverse effects without prescription and people increasingly source medicines internationally from internet pharmacies. Similarly, complementary medicines should be recorded. Some, such as St John's wort, have well-recognised adverse effects and risk of drug interactions while the ingredients of others may not be defined or known.

Unfortunately, of the 1.1 billion items prescribed each year at a cost to the taxpayer of some £9.5 billion each year, much is either not taken or taken incorrectly. When prescribing, always give clear concise advice on how to take the medication, remind patients of the importance of completing antibiotic courses and of not sharing medications with others.

Drugs may complicate dental treatment itself, react with drugs given for dental purposes or have adverse effects in the head and neck. A selection of key interactions is given in Table 43.1, and some specific examples and types of reaction are summarised in Box 43.1 and shown in Figs 43.1 and 43.2.

Review oral adverse effects drugs PMID: 24929593, 24697823 and 25442252

Interactions with complementary agents PMID: 23813259

Adverse effects novel biological agents PMID: 22420757

LOCAL ANALGESICS WITH VASOCONSTRICTORS

In the past many drugs, notably tricyclic antidepressants and monoamine oxidase inhibitors, have been thought to cause significant interactions with vasoconstrictors in local analgesics. The passage of time and national audit of adverse reactions have shown that the fears were unfounded.

Current evidence indicates that despite theoretical possibilities, there are no significant interactions between dental analgesics and any other drugs, provided both the analgesic and medication are used at normal doses. In 1995, a dentist was convicted of manslaughter after causing the death of a patient on beta-blockers by giving her 16 cartridges of lidocaine with epinephrine. However, it appears overdose of lidocaine rather than hypertension, the theoretical risk, was the cause.

Three possible interactions merit consideration. The first is a theoretical reaction between epinephrine (adrenaline) and antihypertensive non-selective beta receptor blocking drugs such as propranolol. Epinephrine normally constricts small arterioles through stimulating alpha receptors but it also stimulates beta-1 and beta-2 receptors causing dilatation of larger arteries and this effect is significant in control of blood pressure. When the beta receptors are blocked, use of adrenaline risks hypertension with reflex bradycardia. The reaction occurs within a few minutes of administration and lasts up to 15 minutes. This reaction has proved fatal when large amounts of epinephrine are used, as for instance in skin surgery. Although cardiac effects are detectable even in healthy patients after using only one cartridge of local anaesthetic with epinephrine, problems do not seem to arise at the low doses used routinely in dentistry, usually a maximum of two standard cartridges in this context, though some patients are particularly prone to this reaction. Selective beta-1 blocking drugs such as atenolol or bisoprolol only block cardiac receptors and do not carry these risks.

The second interaction is causing hypertensive crisis by using epinephrine in a drug user who has recently taken cocaine.

The third is patients taking catechol-O-methyl transferase inhibitors such as entacapone for Parkinson's disease. Caution appears pragmatic with these latter relatively new classes of drugs, but even with these, normal maximal doses of epinephrine appear safe and a limit of three standard cartridges with 1:80,000 adrenaline is recommended.

In all three cases, sensible precautions are an alternative vasoconstrictor or use of low concentration epinephrine (1:200,000), slow injection and extra care to avoid intravascular injection.

It is not logical to avoid lidocaine with adrenaline on theoretical grounds when it is the safest and most effective analgesic. Choosing a less effective analgesic is unfair on the patient and failure of analgesia may compromise treatment.

Allergic reactions are discussed in Chapter 31.

Table 43.1 Examples of prescribed drugs having dentally relevant adverse effects

Type of drug / drug	Dentally relevant adverse effects*
Allopurinol	Oral lichenoid reactions Taste disturbance
Angiotensin-converting enzyme inhibitors, Captopril	Angio-oedema Burning mouth Oral lichenoid reactions Xerostomia
Angiotensin receptor blockers	Oral ulcers Angio-oedema
Antibiotics	Superinfection (usually candidosis), Allergy (mainly penicillin). Tetracyclines are prone to cause candidosis, sometimes within 48 hours. Several classes of antibiotics potentially interfere with contraceptive pill effects, but the effect seems largely theoretical. It is only significant with rifampicin and drugs not used in dentistry. Ampicillin causes rashes during glandular fever Erythromycin and tetracycline potentiate digoxin Erythromycin potentiates benzodiazepines (theoretical risk only for sedation, possible risk with long-term benzodiazepines) Erythromycin potentiates warfarin Tetracyclines stain forming teeth, minocycline causes tooth discolouration, even sometimes in adult teeth Erythromycin, metronidazole and cephalosporins potentiate warfarin Co-trimoxazole, chloramphenicol may cause marrow suppression leading to opportunistic oral infection and ulceration or purpura and bleeding
Anticholinergic drugs	Xerostomia
Anticoagulants	Risk of post-operative haemorrhage
Antidepressants, many types	Xerostomia
Antihistamines	Dry mouth, drowsiness, potentiate sedatives
Antimalarials	Oral lichenoid reactions (including to those available over the counter without prescription) Mucosal pigmentation
Antiretroviral drugs	Many reactions (Box 30.6), including oral pigmentation
Aspirin	Potentiation of any haemorrhagic tendencies and anticoagulants Avoid in children because of risk of Reye's syndrome Causes mucosal burn if applied to mucosa
Beta-blocking drugs	Lichenoid reaction Non-selective types (e.g., Propanolol), potentiate hypertension with epinephrine (see text)
Bisphosphonates	Osteonecrosis of mandible and maxilla (see Ch. 8)
Calcium channel blockers (e.g., nifedipine, verapamil)	Gingival overgrowth Verapamil potentiates lidocaine and bupivacaine toxicity
Captopril	Oral lichenoid reactions Taste disturbance
Carbamazepine	Facial muscle spasms Taste disturbance
Catechol-O-methyltransferase inhibitors	Potentiate epinephrine in local anaesthetics, but not at normal doses
Chlorhexidine	Mucosal discolouration, especially the tongue
Chloroquine	Mucosal and facial skin pigmentation
Ciclosporin	Gingival overgrowth
Cisplatin	Oral ulceration
Corticosteroids	Opportunistic infections Risk of circulatory collapse (see also Ch. 37) Cushing's syndrome, hypertension and diabetes Depression of inflammatory and immune responses Impaired wound healing Mood changes Moon face Depressed protein metabolism Raised blood sugar Sodium and water retention Feeling of wellbeing may mask significant disease

Table 43.1   Examples of prescribed drugs having dentally relevant adverse effects—cont'd

Type of drug / drug	Dentally relevant adverse effects*
Cytotoxic drugs	Oral ulceration (including low dose methotrexate), opportunistic infections Cisplatin can cause grey gingival line ('lead line'), vincristine can cause jaw pain and weakness of the facial muscles
Denosumab	Osteonecrosis of mandible and maxilla (see Ch. 8)
Diltiazem	Gingival overgrowth
Diuretics, all types	Xerostomia
L-DOPA	Colours saliva dark red or brown at high dose
Fluconazole and miconazole antifungals	Potentiate warfarin, even topical use in large amounts can have this effect Adverse interaction with statin drugs
Gold injections	Largely obsolete but a potent cause of oral lichenoid reactions and toxic epidermal necrolysis
Hydroxychloroquine	Mucosal and facial skin pigmentation
Hypnotics and sedatives	Potentiation of general anaesthetics and other sedating drugs
Imatinib	Lichenoid reactions Mucosal pigmentation
Infliximab	Lichenoid reactions
Immunosuppressive drugs Ciclosporin Methotrexate Steroids Azathioprine	Oral ulceration (especially methotrexate), opportunistic infections particularly viral and fungal, recurrence of zoster, measles, herpes virus infections Taste disturbance
Insulin	Risk of hypoglycaemic coma
Iron supplements	Mucosal discolouration
Isotretinoin	Exfoliative cheilitis
Metformin	Oral lichenoid reactions Metallic taste Vitamin B12 deficiency
Methotrexate	Oral ulcers Delayed healing Potentiated by penicillins
Metronidazole	Disulfiram reaction with alcohol Taste Do not prescribe to patients taking lithium Potentiates warfarin
Metoclopramide	Clenching of jaw muscles
Minocycline	Bone and tooth pigmentation
Monoamine oxidase inhibitors	Dry mouth, dangerous interactions with opioids, particularly pethidine
Nicorandil	Oral ulceration (Ch. 16)
Non-steroidal anti-inflammatory analgesics	Oral lichenoid reactions rarely Longer dosing reduces effectiveness of many anti-hypertensives Angio-oedema rarely Inhibit lithium excretion, potentiating effect and risking toxicity
Opioid drugs of all types, sedatives and analgesics	Potentiate benzodiazepines and cause markedly increased risk of respiratory depression
Oral contraceptives	Mucosal and skin pigmentation Action inhibited by broad spectrum antibiotics
Palifermin	White keratotic mucosal patches
Penicillamine	Lichenoid reactions
Phenothiazine antipsychotics ('major tranquillisers')	Dry mouth Tardive dyskinesia (uncontrollable facial movements) Parkinsonian tremor Oral mucosal pigmentation
Phenytoin	Gingival overgrowth Lymphadenopathy occasionally Folate deficiency occasionally leading to exacerbation of aphthous stomatitis Salivary gland swelling

Continued

Table 43.1 Examples of prescribed drugs having dentally relevant adverse effects—cont'd

Type of drug / drug	Dentally relevant adverse effects*
Piroxicam	Oral ulceration, aphthous-like
Rifampicin	Colours saliva red
Tricyclic antidepressants (e.g., amitriptyline)	Dry mouth Do not cause significant interactions with epinephrine in local anaesthetics
Vismodegib	Taste disturbance

*Allergy to any drug is possible and so not listed.

Box 43.1   Important types of oral drug reactions

I. Local reactions to drugs
- Chemical irritation
- Interference with the oral flora

II. Systemically mediated reactions
- Depression of marrow function
- Depression of cell-mediated immunity
- Lichenoid reactions
- Erythema multiforme (Stevens-Johnson syndrome)
- Fixed drug eruptions
- Toxic epidermal necrolysis

III. Other effects
- Gingival hyperplasia
- Pigmentation
- Dry mouth

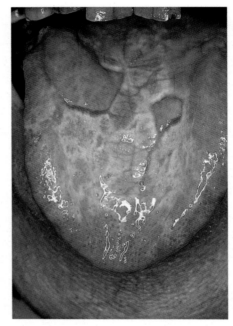

Fig. 43.2   Lichenoid reaction to gold treatment for rheumatoid arthritis. This is more severe than Fig. 43.1 with extensive ulceration of the dorsal tongue, atrophy and keratosis. Biopsy showed changes very similar to lichen planus.

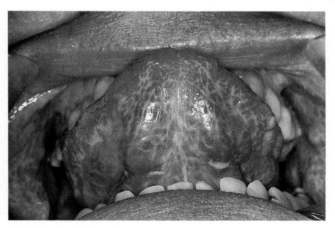

Fig. 43.1   Lichenoid reaction to captopril. In this reaction, there are several small ulcers, but the main effect is the production of striae covering the whole ventral surface of the tongue and buccal mucosa.

Local analgesics review PMID: 23660127 and 22822998

Adverse reactions to local analgesics PMID: 22959146

Prolonged analgesia PMID: 21623806

DRUG DEPENDENCE AND ADDICTION

The British Drugs Survey suggests that one in five adults are recreational drug users to some degree, most using drugs relatively infrequently. Leaving alcohol and tobacco aside, the commonest drugs used are cannabis (marijuana), amphetamines, cocaine and ecstasy (MDMA). The majority of users do not become dependent, but alcohol, cocaine, tobacco and benzodiazepines have, perhaps surprisingly, a somewhat similar risk of inducing physical and psychological dependence. There is no risk of dependence from use of benzodiazepines for dental conscious sedation.

There are few direct oral effects of drug dependence.

Alcohol is associated with many maxillofacial injuries, and erosion results from acidic drinks such as wines and carbonated mixers. Aspirin and non-steroidal anti-inflammatory drugs carry a risk of severe gastric or oesophageal bleeding and will potentiate a haemorrhagic tendency caused by cirrhosis. Metronidazole must be avoided if a patient cannot reduce their alcohol intake or cease it during treatment.

Cocaine applied topically to be absorbed through oral mucosa causes vasoconstriction. This can result in ischaemic ulcers and necrosis if applied repeatedly to the same site. Cocaine inhaled to the nose causes avascular necrosis of the septum and necrosis may extend to perforate the hard palate.

Methamphetamine ('speed'), in particular, is likely to cause considerable oral damage in long-term use. It is acidic and also causes dry mouth. Great thirst, which tends to be

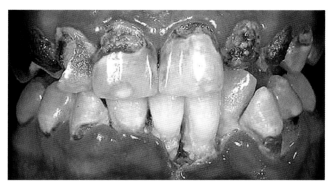

Fig 43.3 'Meth mouth'. The effects of oral neglect in a chronic methamphetamine user *(Courtesy Dr S Wagner.)*

- Attempts to manipulate dentists into prescribing drugs
- Carriage of hepatitis viruses or HIV by intravenous addicts
- Maxillofacial injuries, particularly among alcoholics
- Impaired liver function secondary to alcoholism or hepatitis
- Lymphadenopathy secondary to drug injection in unusual sites
- Infective endocarditis secondary to dirty injections
- Severe infections such as osteomyelitis among alcoholics
- Increased risks from general anaesthesia
- Gross oral neglect and sometimes enhanced sensitivity to pain
- Rarely, ulceration of the palate secondary to cocaine-induced ischaemia of the nasal cavity
- Occasionally, parotid swelling in alcoholics
- Interactions with other drugs
- Security for prescription pads, drugs and nitrous oxide

relieved by almost continuous consumption of carbonated drinks, some of which have a high sugar content, is a common response. This drug is the most closely associated with gross oral disease (Fig 43.3).

People with a serious dependency are likely to develop personality change and ignore their health and nutrition, including their mouth. Gross caries and periodontal neglect are common, compounded if the drug(s) induce dry mouth.

Difficulties in management are common (Box 43.2). Addicts may manipulate dentists into prescribing drugs, particularly opioids, by complaining of pain. Multiple drug abuse is also common, and attempts may be made to obtain any drugs, such as benzodiazepines or antihistamines, that are mood altering or sedative. Because of the risk of dependence, benzodiazepines should only be prescribed for short periods.

Liver function damaged by alcoholism or hepatitis impairs drug metabolism. This makes general anaesthesia, in particular, hazardous, as does respiratory disease or covert use of drugs of abuse pre-operatively. Benzodiazepines have an extended metabolism half-life leading to prolonged elimination but full eventual recovery.

Injecting drug users are at high risk of infective endocarditis from reusing needles. The damaged heart is then vulnerable to further episodes of endocarditis of dental origin (Ch. 33).

Nitrous oxide is increasingly used as a recreational drug. In the UK, nitrous oxide is classified as a psychoactive substance and therefore technically illegal, but use is widespread. Users tend to be young. There are many adverse effects including neurotoxicity and regular users become vitamin B12 deficient. The vitamin is oxidized by the gas and inactivated, paradoxically causing functional deficiency with normal serum B12 levels because the inactivated vitamin continues to circulate and is detected by serum assays. Deficiency causes not only oral signs (Ch. 17) but also inhibits myelin formation and stabilization resulting in neuropathy, paraesthesia, muscle weakness and central damage. Paraesthesia and facial muscle weakness have been reported, but usually in conjunction with limb weakness, which is more likely as a presenting sign. Easy access to this drug is associated with a risk of dependency among dentists and their teams.

Oral manifestations cannabis use PMID: 1563817, 19138182 and 23420976

Cannabis and possible therapeutic uses PMID: 35362240

Methamphetamine oral effects PMID: 18992021 and 25952435

Cocaine use oral significance PMID: 18408681

Alcohol abuse role dentist PMID: 16262033

Management methadone users PMID: 16262036

MDMA ecstasy oral significance PMID: 26268009 and 18268544

Medical emergencies 44

Dentists must know how to recognise and manage medical emergencies, rare though they may be. Their professional skills and equipment should enable them occasionally to save patients' lives. City traffic and the load on ambulance services are so heavy that hospital transfer can be delayed and in rural areas and resource poor countries medical assistance may be remote. Under such circumstances, measures taken by the dental team may be critical.

Dentists are required to ensure that all members of their staff can provide practical assistance in these circumstances. This involves training, keeping up to date and regular practice. Some kind of medical emergency can be expected approximately every 2 years in general practice.

Many types of emergencies may have to be faced (Box 44.1). Many can be prevented by good history-taking and appropriate precautions.

Details of the emergency procedures discussed here may be found in the referenced guidelines and databases below. A textbook such as this cannot be taken as definitive since guidance changes. This chapter provides an overview of the principles of recognition and management but must be updated using these resources as required.

Box 44.1   Emergencies that may arise during dental procedures

Sudden loss of consciousness (collapse)

- Fainting
- Anaphylactic shock
- Acute hypoglycaemia
- Myocardial infarction
- Cardiac arrest
- Strokes
- Circulatory collapse secondary to corticosteroid therapy

Acute chest pain

- Angina
- Myocardial infarction

Difficulty in breathing

- Asthma
- Anaphylactic shock
- Left ventricular failure
- Convulsions
- Epilepsy
- Any other cause of loss of consciousness, including fainting

Other emergencies

- Haemorrhage
- Drug reactions and interactions
- Major maxillofacial injuries

The British National Formulary, the Physicians' Desk Reference, Compendium of Pharmaceuticals and Specialties or other national drug advisory organisations and their websites provide drug information.

Risk assessment and prevention PMID: 23470404

Incidence of emergencies in US PMID: 20388811 and 33754336

Incidence in UK PMID: 10488938 and 29327720

Web URL 44.2 Drugs for medical emergencies UK: https://bnf.nice.org.uk/ and enter 'Medical emergencies in dental practice' into search box and follow link in results to 'prescribing in dental practice'

Drugs questions and answers for UK primary care practice PMID: 34686808

Drugs for US surgical practice PMID: 34598857

SUDDEN LOSS OF CONSCIOUSNESS

Common themes

The ABCDE approach to emergencies (assess **A**irway, **B**reathing, **C**irculation, **D**isability, **E**xposure) has become almost universally used, although in dental practice situations it is the first three and an assessment of consciousness that are immediately useful. It is also important to remember that patients in an emergency situation may still be in danger from the environment or their position.

Calling for help is also key. Additional personnel not only provide more pairs of hands but also emotional and intellectual support and, if they are members of the dental team, help trigger practiced automatic responses. When calling for an ambulance, it is important to have information about the patient ready. In cities, the response may be an ambulance, car, motorcycle or bicycle, and the equipment and skills of the paramedic need to be tailored to the emergency based on the information given.

UK standards require that practices have an automatic external defibrillator and this should be registered with their local ambulance service and national network so that it can be of use to others in the neighbourhood.

Web URL 44.3 ABCDE approach: https://www.resus.org.uk/resuscitation-guidelines/abcde-approach/

Web URL 44.4 UK national defibrillator network: https://www.bhf.org.uk/ and enter 'the circuit' in search box

Fainting

Fainting, caused by transient hypotension and cerebral ischaemia, is the most common cause of sudden loss of consciousness in primary dental care (in hospitals, seizures are of similar incidence). There are several predisposing factors (Box 44.2), but some patients are particularly prone to faint

Box 44.2   Factors predisposing to fainting

- Upright posture
- Anxiety
- Pain
- Injections
- Fatigue
- Hunger and hypoglycaemia

Box 44.3   Fainting: signs and symptoms

- Premonitory dizziness, weakness or nausea
- Pale, cold moist skin
- Initially slow and weak pulse becoming full and bounding
- Loss of consciousness

Box 44.4   Management of a fainting attack

- Lower the head, preferably by laying the patient flat*
- Loosen any tight clothing round the neck
- If no rapid improvement,
  - the legs can be raised or pressure applied to the abdomen to increase venous return
  - apply pulse oximeter if available
  - administer oxygen
  - monitor pulse and breathing, ensure airway is free
- Give a sweetened drink when consciousness has been recovered
- If no recovery within a few minutes, consider other causes of loss of consciousness

* To keep the patient upright worsens cerebral hypoxia and is harmful.

Box 44.5   Signs and symptoms of acute hypoglycaemia

- Premonitory signs are similar to those of a faint, but little response to laying the patient flat
- patient may recognize symptoms
- may include aggressiveness or excitation
- may include period of worsening drowsiness
- Unconsciousness that steadily deepens

Box 44.6   Management of hypoglycaemia

- Patients often aware of what is happening and able to warn the dentist
- Before consciousness is lost, give glucose tablets or powder, or sugar (3–4 heaped teaspoons, up to 7 glucose tablets or equivalent) as a sweetened drink, repeated if symptoms not completely relieved
- If consciousness is lost, give subcutaneous glucagon (1 mg) then give sugar by mouth during the brief recovery period. Intravenous glucose (as much as 50 mL of a 50% solution) is an alternative but difficult to use in an emergency situation. Glucagon may be repeated once, but after that has no effect as all glycogen stores have been mobilised.
- Hypostop, a gel containing glucose, may provide sufficient glucose absorbed through the oral mucosa to combat declining consciousness
- If consciousness is lost, call ambulance, provide oxygen, apply pulse oximeter if available and move to recovery position

and frequently do so. The cause is peripheral vasodilatation, usually combined with an element of bradycardia.

Signs and symptoms are usually readily recognisable (Box 44.3). Sometimes consciousness is lost almost instantaneously. Minor convulsions or incontinence are occasionally associated. Principles of management are summarised in Box 44.4.

Prevention

Loss of consciousness in a faint is impossible when supine. Performing injections and all treatment with the patient flat is helpful, but the physiological mechanisms still act: the patient may feel unwell, ask to sit up and then faint.

Regular fainters are frequently helped by nitrous oxide relative analgesia or an appropriate dose of a minor anxiolytic on the night before and again an hour before treatment, but they must then be accompanied by a responsible adult and follow the usual precautions for their use.

Acute hypoglycaemia

Hypoglycaemia affects patients with diabetes whose insulin dose is too high, either after an overdose of insulin or a relative overdose caused by not eating at the expected time (Box 44.5). If there is any doubt about the cause of loss of consciousness, in an emergency always assume hypoglycaemia in a patient with diabetes. *Hyper*glycaemic coma is much less frequent and tends to affect patients with type 2 diabetes who are dehydrated and is a more chronic process. Insulin must never be given as it can be fatal to a patient with hypoglycaemia.

If there is sufficient time and hypoglycaemia is suspected, the patient may be able to check their own blood glucose using their own portable monitor and tailor the dose of sucrose or glucose in a drink to their circumstances. Delay for a result must be avoided as the adverse effects of providing sugar are minimal, primarily there may be difficulty rebalancing insulin dose after the event

Management of hypoglycaemia is shown in (Box 44.6).

Web URL 44.5 Hypoglycaemia: http://emedicine.medscape.com/article/767359

Anaphylactic reactions

Penicillin is the most common cause of these type I hypersensitivity reactions in dentistry. Anaphylactic reactions can also be precipitated by insect stings, foods (nuts or shellfish particularly) and, exceptionally rarely, by aspirin.

In general, the quicker the onset, the more severe the reaction. A severe reaction to penicillin may start within a minute of its injection, but immediate loss of consciousness is more likely to be due to fainting. A reaction starting 30 minutes after a penicillin injection is unlikely to be dangerous. Acute reactions to oral penicillins are rare but can develop after half an hour or more because of slower absorption from the gut.

Collapse is due to widespread vasodilatation and increased capillary permeability causing potentially fatal hypotension.

Box 44.7   Features of acute anaphylaxis
- Initial facial flushing, itching, paraesthesia or cold extremities
- Oedema or urticaria
- Bronchospasm (wheezing), hoarseness, stridor
- Loss of consciousness
- Pallor going on to cyanosis
- Cold clammy skin
- Rapid weak or impalpable pulse
- Deep fall in blood pressure
- Death if treatment is delayed or inappropriate, from cardiac or respiratory arrest

Box 44.8   Management of acute anaphylactic collapse
Lay the patient flat. Raise the legs to improve cerebral blood flow
Give 0.5–1 mL of 1:1000 epinephrine (adrenaline; 500 micrograms adult dose, 300 micrograms age 6–12 years, 150 micrograms 6 months to 6 years of age) by intramuscular injection. Repeat in 5 minutes if no response
Call an ambulance
Give oxygen and, if necessary, assisted ventilation
Monitor need for assisted ventilation and cardiopulmonary resuscitation
Depending on the setting and severity of reaction, availability of drugs, appropriate healthcare setting and skills of operator, the following may be given, but are secondary to the previously mentioned procedures and are not lifesaving or necessary for immediate treatment.
10–20 mg chlorphenamine slowly, intravenously
200 mg of hydrocortisone sodium succinate intravenously
If there is no response after two doses of epinephrine, medical assistance is required urgently to provide intravenous fluids and epinephrine and intramuscular epinephrine must be continued every 5 minutes until venous access and medical assistance is available. Oxygen must be continued and the airway protected.

Signs and symptoms

The clinical picture is variable (Box 44.7).

Management

Epinephrine is the mainstay of treatment (Box 44.8) and the lifesaving element. It raises cardiac output, combats excessive capillary permeability and bronchospasm, and also inhibits release of mediators from mast cells.

Circulatory collapse is probably largely due to histamine release, which can also be inhibited by parenteral chlorphenamine. Hydrocortisone is slow to take effect but maintains the blood pressure for some hours and combats the continued effect of the antigen–antibody reaction.

Rapid transfer to hospital is necessary to provide circulatory support by intravenous fluids and other measures. Minor anaphylactic reactions, with slow onset and no respiratory signs, can be managed by laying the patient flat, raising the legs and providing oxygen. Urticarial rashes and other mild signs benefit from oral or intramuscular chlorphenamine and bronchospasm from salbutamol inhaler.

However, epinephrine is the effective treatment and should not be delayed because of uncertainty about the severity of the reaction. UK guidance specifies epinephrine 1:1000 injection but other emergency formulations are available including autoinjectors and pre-filled syringes. These are more convenient to use but expensive and expire more quickly in storage than ampoules for injection. Many patients with known severe allergies carry one or two 'EpiPens' or similar emergency epinephrine autoinjector. These are useful in an emergency but deliver a slightly lower dose than is normally administered in an emergency and may need to be repeated more rapidly than conventional doses. The needle length is also relatively short and may not penetrate to muscle, especially in a patient who is obese.

After the event, the cause must be determined and the allergen avoided. Subsequent attacks are likely to be more severe.

Web URL 44.6 Anaphylaxis UK: https://www.resus.org.uk/anaphylaxis/

Web URL 44.7 NICE clinical pathway and referral after the event: http://pathways.nice.org.uk/pathways/anaphylaxis

Web URL 44.8 Anaphylaxis US: http://www.aaaai.org/ and enter 'practice parameter anaphylaxis' into search box

Web URL 44.9 International guideline: https://www.worldallergy.org enter 'anaphylaxis' into search box

Cardiac arrest

Cardiac arrest can follow myocardial infarction, any cause of severe hypotension such as an anaphylactic reaction or adrenal crisis, or hypoxia. Dentists should be aware of and alert to the possibility of cardiac arrest and be able to recognize it (Box 44.9) and manage it (Box 44.10) when it happens. Detail cannot be given here; practice in a simulated emergency setting is essential.

Speed of response is critical and there is a legal obligation that the dental team should be trained in cardiopulmonary resuscitation (CPR) and be able to carry it out immediately. Resuscitation must be started within a few minutes.

UK guidelines now require automatic electronic defibrillators (AEDs) in dental practices. These are also kept in many public places and may be located quickly using a variety of mobile phone apps (such as GoodSAM) in the event of cardiac arrest away from a healthcare setting. Defibrillation in a healthcare setting within 5 minutes of infarction is associated with a recovery rate of 70%, much higher than with cardiopulmonary resuscitation alone. Each minute of delay to defibrillation reduces survival by 10%, so this has become a critical procedure; CPR alone rarely restarts the heart.

In a clinical dental setting the dentist and team should be prepared to provide basic life support (BLS; defined as life support without equipment) and use their airway skills to provide oxygen by bag or mask and use an AED.

Basic life support should be started immediately the patient becomes unresponsive and is not breathing normally. This last point must be carefully assessed. In the first minutes after arrest there may be 'agonal' gasps, slow deep breaths with a snoring sound. These, as well as lack of breathing, indicate a need to start cardiopulmonary resuscitation. It is now considered that giving CPR to a patient who is not in arrest causes no significant risks; do not allow uncertainty about diagnosis to cause delay. Cyanosis, pupil dilatation and loss of reaction to light, and absence of measurable blood pressure are late signs that should not be sought. Mild seizures may follow cerebral anoxia and should not be confused with epilepsy and trigger the wrong emergency response.

CPR requires a firm surface, ideally the floor. If the patient is too heavy to lift out of a dental chair but can be laid supine there, resuscitation can be carried out by the operator and assistant standing beside the chair. An operator's stool can be placed under the headrest to stabilize the chair. The optimal pressure for chest compression is about 40 or 50 kg (the weight of the upper part of the body applied through stiffly extended arms). Ensure the chest recoils fully between compressions. External cardiac massage is tiring, and another person should preferably alternate with the first operator at intervals of 2 minutes. CPR starts with compressions rather than breaths because the lungs already contain oxygenated blood that must be pumped to the brain as soon as possible. Continued effective compressions with minimal interruption is the key element.

'Rescue' breaths should be given over a period of approximately 1 second, ensuring that the chest rises. As soon as possible, mouth-to-mouth breaths should be switched to positive pressure inflation with 100% oxygen and a self-inflating bag and mask.

Signs of restoration of blood pressure are disappearance of facial pallor and a good spontaneous pulse, contraction of the pupils, return of reflex activity such as the blink reflex and reaction of the pupils to light, lightening of unconsciousness and purposeful spontaneous movements, not twitching or convulsions.

Resuscitation of children is an unlikely requirement in a dental setting. Specialised techniques are not critical. If in doubt, use the adult procedures rather than delay. Children have a greater requirement for oxygenation, so ideally five rescue breaths or ventilations should be given first. Chest compressions should be 4 cm for a young, and 5 cm for an older, child. AEDs should have an attenuator for use on children to reduce the shock energy but if this is not readily available, use the adult settings.

Some possible causes of failure are summarized in Box 44.11.

The chances of having to provide CPR in a dental surgery are low, and members of the dental team need to be prepared to use their skills outside the surgery.

Resuscitation Covid-19 risk PMID: 32651513

Web URL 44.10 Resuscitation Council guidelines: https://www.resus.org.uk/information-for-professionals/

Case report PMID: 26866410

Web URL 44.11 Guidance US: http://cpr.heart.org/ and enter 'cpr-and-ecc-guidelines' into search box

Strokes

Patients are usually hypertensive and middle aged or old and often have other risk factors for atheroma such as smoking or diabetes. The clinical picture varies with the size and site

of brain damage (Box 44.12). Typical features are unilateral paralysis, often of the face, or sensory disturbance, disorientation, difficulty with speech or unilateral loss of vision. Transient ischaemic attacks, mild minor strokes, should be recognized and treated by referral to hospital. Rapid transfer is important as thrombolytic treatment must be given rapidly to be effective.

Subarachnoid haemorrhage from a ruptured berry aneurysm on the circle of Willis is the main cause of stroke in a younger person. It typically causes intense headache followed by coma.

Circulatory collapse in patients on corticosteroid treatment

Steroids given therapeutically are sensed by the pituitary in the same way as natural steroids and the high levels suppress

---

Box 44.12   Signs and management of a stroke

Signs

- Loss of consciousness or confusion
- Weakness (or numbness) of an arm and leg on one side
- Drooping of one side of the face
- Unclear muddled speech
- Sudden onset severe headache
- Often stertorous breathing

Management

- Maintain the airway, administer oxygen
- Call an ambulance for transfer to hospital

---

corticotrophin-releasing hormone and adrenocorticotropic hormone (ACTH) secretion through the physiological feedback mechanism. With time, the lack of ACTH suppresses the adrenal and the gland atrophies, so that stressful situations that would normally cause a rapid adrenal response no longer do so. Adrenocortical function may take as long as 2 years to recover after ceasing steroids, although in most patients 2 months is sufficient.

The response of patients on long-term corticosteroid treatment to surgery is unpredictable. It has generally been considered that all patients who are taking, or have been taking, systemic corticosteroids are at risk, even those using high-potency topical steroids on a large area of skin. Adverse effects do not appear to arise unless the dose of prednisolone exceeds 10 mg per day. However, near-fatal circulatory collapse has been reported to follow dental extractions in a patient taking as little as 5 mg of prednisone per day. In the UK, it is considered that any patient taking 5 mg

prednisolone, or equivalent dose of other corticosteroid, daily for one month or more is at risk and is given a steroid card to carry to indicate the risk.

In the past, a large additional dose of steroid 'cover' (usually 100 mg prednisolone) was given intramuscularly or intravenously before surgery, but this is now considered an overprotective and unnecessary precaution.

It is currently considered that the main significant risk is surgery under general anaesthesia. Even surgical removal of lower third molars is not stressful enough to cause a significant release of cortisol physiologically, and a doubling of the normal daily steroid dose pre-operatively and possibly also for 24 hours after is sufficient precaution for surgery under local analgesia. High-dose cover is reserved for general anaesthesia. The risk of adrenal crisis is considered low in dentistry. Nevertheless, every patient on steroids needs to be considered for steroid cover for surgery and, in the absence of a good evidence base for guidance, additional factors such as apprehension and likely degree of postoperative pain should be taken into account.

Although parenteral steroid cover is no longer routine, there remains a significant risk of collapse in patients who have recently had their steroid dose reduced or stopped. During the recovery period, they are at increased risk of adrenal crisis and a lower threshold for steroid cover is required.

In summary, patients with primary Addison's disease, patients on the highest doses or with recently reduced doses of steroid remain at risk, and ability to prevent and manage a steroid-related collapse remains important (Box 44.13).

Steroid cover PMID: 15592544 and 35931749

CHEST PAIN

Angina pectoris

Acute chest pain due to myocardial ischaemia is the only symptom. Pain is centred on the chest, often described as tightness, squeezing or pressure or indigestion. It may radiate to the inner left arm or jaw. Additional signs such as nausea, vomiting and shock may occur in a severe attack, but suggest a myocardial infarct. A first anginal attack may come as a consequence of an emotional response to dental treatment. Stop treatment and give glyceryl trinitrate sublingually (Box 44.14).

Many patients have already had attacks and carry medication. Unless treatment is immediately effective, the patient should be transferred to hospital.

Patients whose angina is induced by anxiety may benefit from nitrous oxide inhalational sedation or premedication with a benzodiazepine for dental treatment. People with unstable or recent hospital admission for angina should not be treated in dental practice until stable.

Myocardial infarction

Myocardial infarction is a common cause of death and must be recognised quickly (Box 44.15), as the patient's fate may be decided by the first few minutes' treatment. Several aspects of dentistry, particularly apprehension, pain or the effect of drugs, might contribute to make this accident more likely in a susceptible patient.

Most patients will have a history of angina or be a known risk patient, but this is not absolute. The symptoms range from those of severe angina to loss of consciousness depending on the area of the heart involved. Pain can radiate to the left shoulder or down the left arm but, very occasionally, is felt

Box 44.13 Signs and management of corticosteroid-related collapse

Signs

- Pallor
- Rapid, weak or impalpable pulse, hypotension
- Loss of consciousness, convulsions or confusion
- Rapidly falling blood pressure
- Lethargy

Management

- Lay the patient flat and raise the legs
- Give at least 200 mg hydrocortisone sodium succinate intravenously*
- Call an ambulance for immediate transfer to hospital
- Give oxygen and, if necessary, artificial ventilation
- Consider other possible reasons for loss of consciousness

Hydrocortisone for injection is no longer a required constituent of a UK dental practice emergency drug kit.

* The intramuscular route can be used if a vein cannot be found but absorption is slower.

Box 44.14 Management of angina

- Give the patient their anti-anginal drug (usually 0.5 mg of glyceryl trinitrate sublingually) *or*
- Glyceryl trinitrate spray* (400 mg) gives rapid relief
- Administer oxygen
- If there is no relief within 3 minutes the patient has probably had a myocardial infarct

---

* Glyceryl trinitrate spray has a better shelf-life for the emergenckity.

Box 44.15 Typical signs and symptoms of myocardial infarction

- Severe crushing retrosternal pain
- Shallow strained breathing
- Vomiting
- Weak or irregular pulse
- Pale clammy skin

Box 44.16 Management of myocardial infarction

- If there is loss of consciousness, proceed as for cardiac arrest (mentioned previously)
- Otherwise, put the patient in a comfortable position that allows easy breathing. Do not lay flat if there is left ventricular failure and pulmonary oedema
- Send an assistant to telephone for an ambulance
- Constantly reassure the patient
- Use glyceryl trinitrate spray or the patient's own anginal medication
- Give 50/50 nitrous oxide and oxygen from a relative analgesia machine, to relieve pain and anxiety, or, if unavailable, oxygen alone
- Unless allergic, give aspirin 300 mg by mouth as soon as more urgent measures have been carried out
- Monitor for possible cardiac arrest
- Inform ambulance crew if aspirin has been given or if there is a risk of bleeding from extraction sockets or surgical sites as this may complicate any thrombolytic drugs given immediately.

Box 44.17 Signs and management of status asthmaticus

Signs

- Breathlessness
- Inability to talk
- Expiratory wheezing (may be disguised as rapid shallow breathing)
- Rapid pulse (usually over 110 per minute). Progress to bradycardia is a danger sign
- Accessory muscles of respiration come into action
- Cyanosis

Management

- Reassure the patient
- Do *not* lay the patient flat
- Give normally used anti-asthmatic drugs (such as salbutamol) by inhaler (2 puffs, repeated as necessary). If the patient cannot inhale effectively, use a spacer device. Better, administer salbutamol by nebuliser
- If no response or tachycardia develops, call an ambulance for transfer to hospital
- Give oxygen and continue salbutamol
- In emergency, if patient continues to deteriorate or has other signs suggesting an allergic reaction as a cause, give epinephrine (adrenaline) as for anaphylaxis.

---

only in the left jaw. The pain does not respond to trinitrate. Vomiting is common, and there is sometimes shock or loss of consciousness. Principles of management are summarised in Box 44.16. Some patients die within a few minutes after the start of the attack, and it is rash to try overambitious treatment. Prompt ambulance attendance will be the most useful response, as they can administer fibrinolytic and other drugs and monitor the cardiac condition. There should be no concern about giving aspirin as the beneficial effects far outweigh any potential disadvantages.

RESPIRATORY DIFFICULTY

Severe asthma and status asthmaticus

Causes

Not bringing a salbutamol inhaler to the appointment, anxiety, infection or exposure to a specific allergen are possible causes. Inability to complete sentences in one breath indicates severe dyspnoea; if the patient becomes cyanosed, exhausted or confused, or their pulse falls to 50/min or less, the condition is life threatening.

Giving hydrocortisone in dental practice is no longer recommended.

Features and management are shown in Box 44.17.

Left ventricular failure

Extreme breathlessness with increased respiratory rate is the main sign. It may be associated with chest pain if

> **Box 44.18   Signs and management of a tonic-clonic epileptic attack**
>
> **Signs**
>
> - Sometimes a brief warning cry as the chest muscles contract and air is forced through a closed larynx
> - Consciousness lost immediately
> - The body becomes rigid (tonic phase) and cyanosis appears, usually about 30 seconds
> - Widespread jerking movements start (clonic phase), for a few minutes
> - Sometimes incontinence or frothing of the mouth
> - Flaccidity sometimes follows after a few minutes
> - Consciousness regained slowly after a variable period
> - Confusion or drowsiness may persist
>
> **Management**
>
> - Put the patient prone in the recovery position as soon as possible, usually after the clonic phase
> - Prevent patients from injuring themselves, but do not try to restrain them
> - Do not try to put anything in the mouth in the attempt to prevent the patient biting the tongue
> - Make sure the airway is clear after convulsions have subsided
> - Do not give any medication but await recovery
> - Reassure patients as soon as consciousness returns
> - For any first attack, the patient should be sent to hospital
> - Only allow patients to return home when fully recovered and accompanied by a responsible adult

> **Box 44.19   Management of status epilepticus**
>
> - Treat initially as any seizure (earlier)
> - If continuous or repeated more than 5 minutes, call for an ambulance
> - Continue to administer oxygen
> - Give 10 mg, buccal midazolam ('midazolam oromucosal solution') to an adult patient or child older than 10 years (1–5 years, 5 mg; 5–10 years, 7.5 mg) from a prefilled emergency oral syringe. Some patients or carers may carry an emergency supply of oral or rectal midazolam
> - Other preparations of midazolam or diazepam should not be used
> - Repeat midazolam if no recovery within 5 minutes
> - Maintain the airway and give oxygen

secondary to myocardial infarction. Apart from measures for an infarction, sitting the patient upright and giving oxygen, little can be done in the dental surgery apart from immediately calling an ambulance.

Panic attacks

Panic attacks in anxious patients cause hyperventilation. Although the patient may be aware of the hyperventilation they may find it difficult or impossible to control, leading to respiratory alkalosis from carbon dioxide loss. This produces a feeling of dizziness and weakness and, if severe, causes tetany and carpopedal spasm, leaving the patient very distressed.

Rebreathing exhaled air from a paper (not plastic) bag, or other partly closed container such as an inhaler spacer, raises carbon dioxide levels and quickly reduces the overbreathing.

SEIZURES

Epilepsy

Hunger, menstruation and some drugs such as tricyclic antidepressants or alcohol may sometimes precipitate a seizure (Box 44.18). The dental light is not a significant risk. Only about 3% of people with epilepsy have photosensitive epilepsy and may have a seizure triggered by flickering or flashing lights, usually in the range of 16–25 flashes a second, and not just switching a dental light on and off. Nevertheless, other triggers may be present in surgeries, such as faulty fluorescent or LED lights, ceiling fans or display screens showing flashing patterns. Recording whether a

patient has photosensitive epilepsy is therefore useful. Recognition, types, and avoidance of an epileptic seizure are covered in Chapter 39. It is useful to record in the medical history whether patients normally experience an aura before a seizure, since this gives useful prior warning and indicates the diagnosis.

Status epilepticus

If convulsions do not stop within 5 minutes or are rapidly repeated without a recovery period for 30 minutes, the patient is in status epilepticus and can die from anoxia (Box 44.19). Any individual's seizures typically last a consistent length of time and stop by themselves. This time is further useful information to record in the medical history. Any seizure type may develop into status epilepticus. Status in a tonic-clonic seizure is potentially life threatening, and an ambulance should be called if the clonic phase lasts more than 5 minutes; do not wait for the 30-minute defining time as urgent medical help is needed.

Web URL 44.12 Actions for seizures: https://www.epilepsysociety.org.uk/ follow menu about epilepsy>first aid

OTHER EMERGENCIES

Haemorrhage

Prolonged bleeding is usually due to traumatic extractions. A major vessel is unlikely to be opened during dental surgery, and patients are unlikely to lose a dangerous amount of blood if promptly managed (Box 44.20). Post-extraction bleeding is usually only an emergency in the sense that the patient is often very frightened.

Excessive bleeding during surgery usually follows accidental damage to a large vessel or inadvertent opening of an unsuspected haemangioma or arteriovenous malformation. Pressure (for a minimum of 3 minutes), clamping or ligating vessels, electrocautery of the vessel and other methods may be used depending on circumstances. While dealing with haemorrhage, raise the patient's head if supine to reduce bleeding.

Occasionally, bleeding is due to unsuspected haemophilia or other haemorrhagic disorders (Ch. 29).

Post-extraction bleeding PMID: 24930250

Violence

Violence toward healthcare workers is increasing. Aggressive behaviour can be the result of mental health conditions,

Box 44.20   Management of prolonged dental haemorrhage after extraction

- Reassure the patient
- Clean the mouth with swabs and locate the source of bleeding
- If there is point bleeding from bone, crush the vessel with a small instrument. Soft tissue bleeding will usually respond to pressure alone
- Give epinephrine (adrenaline)-containing local anaesthetic, remove ragged tissue, squeeze up the socket edges and suture it. A small piece of oxidised cellulose (Surgicel) may be placed loosely in the socket below the suture to aid haemostasis, but is usually unnecessary
- When bleeding has been controlled, ask about the history and especially any family history of prolonged bleeding
- Check for anticoagulant or antiplatelet drugs
- If bleeding continues despite suturing or if the patient is obviously anaemic or debilitated, transfer to hospital for investigation and management of any haemorrhagic defect
- Meanwhile, limit bleeding as much as possible with a pressure pad over the socket and, if necessary, by supporting the patient's jaw with a firm barrel bandage
- Tranexamic acid mouthwash may stabilise what clot forms while awaiting transfer to hospital

Box 44.21   Management of potential violence

- Reassure the patient that everyone is working in their best interests
- Be sensitive to changes in mood or composure that may lead to aggression or violence
- Seek help, but devolve dealing with the patient to one person
- Separate agitated patients from others and staff, do not allow staff to become isolated and at risk
- Train in verbal and non-verbal skills to avoid or manage adverse situations without provoking aggression
- Always communicate respect for and empathy with the patient
- Ensure staff control their own anxiety or frustration when dealing with the patient and do not escalate the situation inadvertently

particularly schizophrenia, drug abuse (particularly of alcohol) or brain damage. The risk to dental clinical staff can be significant, especially because of the ready availability of sharp instruments. All practices should have a policy for dealing with violent patients, although the risk is much higher in secondary care.

The ambulance service is not equipped to deal with such cases so that the police must be called. Patients in the UK who abuse National Health Service staff may have their access to healthcare limited after investigation.

General principles of managing potential violence are given in Box 44.21. These are designed for patients with mental health conditions but are equally applicable to all aggressive patients.

Adverse events in dentistry 45

A primary principle in medicine is to do no harm. Unfortunately, almost all medical or surgical interventions have adverse effects in at least a minority of patients, and in some cases iatrogenic damage or disease is significantly detrimental. In this respect, dentistry is no different to other healthcare specialties and a wide range of iatrogenic harm is possible.

Iatrogenic harm includes all complications or other adverse events resulting from treatment, diagnosis, error or negligence as well as failure of treatment to achieve the desired results. Proposing any procedure to a patient usually involves weighing up the benefit relative to possible harm. In most instances the harm is predictable and the patient can be warned. The patient should give appropriate informed consent for treatment. Harm may be immediate, delayed, physical, or psychological.

Although the multitude of minor adverse events should be recorded, they are often not, and only serious adverse events appear in published literature. This makes the diversity of adverse events almost impossible to define. The commonest in dentistry are thought to be delayed or unnecessary treatment, allergic reaction, aspiration, pain, and performing the wrong procedure. Even allowing for publication bias, it is worrying that a quarter of published adverse events have led to permanent harm and that death resulted in 10%.

The great majority of dental adverse events have been covered in other chapters (Table 45.1).

Inventory of dental harms PMID: 35771964

Reported dental adverse effects PMID: 25925524

Oral adverse drug effects PMID: 32892860

Avoiding adverse effects in restorative dentistry PMID: 29188702

Are toothbrushes safe? PMID: 24931926

Table 45.1 Examples of iatrogenic harm relevant to dentistry

Drugs: adverse drug reactions (Chs 43 and 16), allergy and anaphylaxis (Chs 31 and 43), drug interactions

Errors: wrong tooth extraction, drug prescribing and administration, incorrect treatment following diagnostic error, late or missed diagnosis

Complications of extraction and surgery: bleeding (Ch. 29), oroantral fistula (Ch. 34), fracture, nerve damage (Ch. 39), infection (Chs 8 and 9), tissue emphysema, late effects of early tooth loss, surgical ciliated cyst (Ch. 10)

Ingestion and inhalation (Ch. 34) of dental instruments, restorations, fragments of tooth and other material, even toothbrushes

Implanted materials: foreign body reactions, sinusitis, infection, delayed healing, cosmetic procedures (Ch. 27), foreign body gingivitis (Ch. 7)

Antibiotic use: resistance, antibiotic abscess (Ch. 9), pseudomembranous colitis (Ch. 35), necrotizing fasciitis (Ch. 9), inadequate dose or inappropriate antibiotic given, contraceptive pill failure, acute atrophic candidosis (Ch. 15)

Caries and periodontal disease: caused by defective and over-contoured restorations, failure to use minimally invasive methods (Ch. 4), pulpal exposure (Chs 4 and 5), topical lichenoid reactions to restorative materials (Ch. 16)

Infection control failure: blood-borne virus diseases (Chs 30 and 35), respiratory infections (Ch. 34)

Infective endocarditis (Ch. 33)

Prostheses: design promoting periodontitis, fracture and aspiration, alveolar ridge loss, candidosis (Ch. 15)

Trismus and temporomandibular joint pain dysfunction triggered by restorative intervention (Ch. 14)

Caustic agents: acid etchant burns (Ch. 16), extrusion of endodontic materials beyond the apex (Ch. 39)

General anaesthesia: complications, subsequent adult anxiety

Irradiation: equipment maintenance failure causing dose increase, poor technique causing repeat exposure, unnecessary exposure, risks in pregnancy (Ch. 37)

Communication failure: incorrect information, administrative error, failed or inappropriate referral, prescriptions not taken, postoperative instructions not followed

Learning guide 46

Textbooks such as this grow in size from edition to edition, adding much that can only be described as reference material. Undergraduate students will never see most of the conditions in it, before or after graduation. Despite this, on qualification they are expected to not only diagnose them, but also institute appropriate referral or treatment.

It is unsurprising that students often ask despairingly what they need to know. The breadth of oral medicine, pathology, surgery, radiology, and the medical aspects of dentistry is immense, and students need to prioritise their limited time to make sure that they know only details that are required. Teachers of these subjects would much prefer students to enjoy these interesting subjects and be led by interest and curiosity and not learn facts obsessively.

In the past, national regulatory bodies would prescribe the topics to be taught in undergraduate courses. More recently, there has been an almost complete shift to practical learning outcomes and competencies expected of the graduating dental surgeon. This produces a welcome emphasis on higher-level learning and the synthesis and application of knowledge to clinical problems. Unfortunately, the competencies are often somewhat generic. Both teachers and students no longer have a defined syllabus of knowledge to form the essential factual foundation required for these higher-level skills.

In the UK, there has been a change in both undergraduate and specialist education to focus on the expected future roles of dental surgeons and curriculum space had to be made for many new topics. This has led to a concentration on 'what the general dental practitioner really needs to know'. Knowledge-based topics such as those in this book are thus at risk of being downgraded in the mind of the student. However, it is important to remember that before reaching dental practice, many dentists will work in secondary care in specialist departments where a lack of knowledge could be severely detrimental to patients. Many dentists go on to become specialists.

The average-sized UK dental practice will have 20 or so patients with lichen planus, one or two with mucous membrane pemphigoid or severe desquamative gingivitis, more than 100 red or white patches, numerous cysts and inflammatory conditions and, every once in a while, a patient with a malignant tumour that must not be missed. Those in primary care fulfil an important screening role and act as gatekeepers in health systems. They need breadth of knowledge rather than detail.

This chapter attempts to provide a syllabus of topics for undergraduate students of dentistry. It is based on published curricula from the UK specialist societies of Oral and Maxillofacial Pathology and of Oral Surgery, the Scandinavian Fellowship for Oral Pathology and Oral Medicine, the Profile and Competencies for the Graduating European Dentist of the Association of Dental Education in Europe, US and North American publications and competencies defined by the Dental Council of India and other accrediting bodies. Some of these are referenced at the end and several are old

and in need of update. It is impossible to define a syllabus that would be appropriate for all countries or dental schools. Some teach these subjects independently, others in integrated courses and yet others in problem-based learning format. Those practising in tropical areas may well omit Paget's disease and orofacial granulomatosis and other diseases that affect Northern populations and replace them with deep mycoses and other diseases of local importance. This is a guide for students based on the author's views and experience.

In using this table, (Table 46.1) it must be accepted that there are conflicts. For instance in giving a differential diagnosis of a mixed radiolucent lesion in the jaws it will be necessary at a basic level to include lesions that are listed in the third or fourth columns. This table is to be used as a guide to the importance of *detailed* knowledge. Rarer lesions will often merit more attention because of the importance of the diagnosis to the patient.

How much needs to be known about each topic? Students should focus on information that allows understanding of the clinical presentation, differential diagnosis and would equip them to discuss the significance and implications of the condition with a patient and refer them. Those topics in the core curriculum need to be thoroughly understood and are very much a minimum expectation. They are listed from the perspective of pathology and medicine. It is quite possible that a topic such as cleft palate would be a core topic in paediatric dentistry or orthodontics where the emphasis would be on clinical aspects.

Students often ask whether they need to know histopathology. Certainly, undergraduate courses should not attempt to teach students to become diagnostic pathologists. Diagnostic histopathology is a postgraduate speciality. Nevertheless, there are good reasons why knowledge of disease at the tissue level is important. It aids understanding of disease processes and enables students to see the biology of a disease in progress. There is no better illustration of how the patient is affected and a picture provides considerably more understanding than could be transmitted by words alone. Knowing how diseases affect tissues informs the decision whether or not to perform a biopsy, what type of biopsy is appropriate and how the disease can be investigated and managed. It has been interesting to see how virtual microscopy systems have made histopathology more accessible to students, who often felt isolated and stressed looking down a microscope on their own. Histopathological knowledge is required in many areas, to a variable degree as indicated in this book, but not in the detail required for diagnosis.

From the patients' perspective, dentists, whether in primary or secondary care, are expected to be the experts on oral and dental conditions. Medical practitioners receive only very limited, if any, training in oral disease. An incorrect differential diagnosis and referral by a dentist may well start the patient along the wrong, and possibly a harmful, care pathway.

Table 46.1 A suggested heirarchy of importance for curricular topics

Minimum core topics, detailed knowledge expected	Core+ key topics for dentistry required for differential diagnosis but less extensive knowledge acceptable	Otherwise important concepts requiring overview knowledge but not detail	Supplementary and reference topics, primarily for postgraduates and those in secondary care
The processes of differential diagnosis, principles of history taking, examination, selection and interpretation of investigations for oral and head and neck disease			
Medical history taking, relevance of disease to dentistry and follow-up questions for history taking			
Detailed knowledge of biopsy procedures for the mouth and selection of conditions for which biopsy is a useful investigation	Fine needle aspiration	Principles of other biopsy techniques	
Relative value of imaging techniques and selection for specific purposes			
Biopsy specimen handling and interpretation of histology reports and other investigation results	Immunofluorescence	Molecular tests	
An appreciation of the relative incidence of lesions and conditions			
Correct definition, use and spelling of medical and pathological terms			
Missing and supernumerary teeth Normal teething and dental development chronology Cleft lip and palate	Minor tooth anomalies Ankyloglossia	Dental effects of common syndromes Submucous cleft	Clefts in syndromes Craniofacial syndromes
Amelogenesis imperfecta, molar incisor hypomineralisation, hereditary opalescent teeth and dentinogenesis imperfecta	Regional odontodysplasia Hypophosphatasia	Segmental odontomaxillary dysplasia Congenital syphilis Vitamin D–resistant rickets	Dentinal dysplasia Ehlers-Danlos syndromes
Chronological hypoplasia and fluorosis. Tetracycline pigmentation			
Resorption and hypercementosis			
Delayed eruption and accelerated tooth loss			
Normal enamel, dentine and pulp structure	Pathogenesis of and structural changes in enamel, dentine and cementum		
Pathology of caries as it relates to prevention and operative treatment, epidemiology and risk management	*Streptococcus mutans*	Microbiology of caries, ecological plaque theory	
Pulpitis and pulpal reactions to damage, relationship to treatment, pulp stones			
Apical periodontitis and the sequelae of pulp necrosis or pulp removal, periapical granuloma, radicular cyst, dentoalveolar abscess and spread of infection			
Tooth wear and the processes of attrition, abrasion and erosion Bruxism		Abfraction	
Principles of osseointegration	Causes of failure		

Table 46.1 —cont'd

Minimum core topics, detailed knowledge expected	Core+ key topics for dentistry required for differential diagnosis but less extensive knowledge acceptable	Otherwise important concepts requiring overview knowledge but not detail	Supplementary and reference topics, primarily for postgraduates and those in secondary care
Normal periodontium structure Plaque-related gingivitis, periodontitis and their variants, classification, aetiology, pathogenesis and tissue changes. Diseases mimicking gingivitis and periodontitis and their differential diagnosis Effects of systemic disease			Papillon–Lefèvre syndrome
Necrotising gingivitis and periodontitis, periodontal abscess, pericoronitis	Noma and HIV periodontitis		Localised spongiotic gingivitis
Localised and generalised gingival enlargement Drug-induced gingival enlargement	Hereditary types		
Common mucosal lesions, fibrous epulis, fibroepithelial hyperplasia, pyogenic granuloma, pregnancy epulis, peripheral giant cell granuloma, squamous papilloma, papillary hyperplasia of palate		Multiple endocrine neoplasia type 2b Condylomas Multifocal epithelial hyperplasia Calibre-persistent artery	Verruciform xanthoma
Haemangioma and the range of vascular anomalies			
Traumatic injuries to soft tissue and teeth, amalgam tattoo		Eosinophilic ulcer	
Infection of dental origin, abscess, cellulitis, oedema, fascial space infections, their anatomy and treatment, role of antibiotics and antibiotic stewardship	Antibiotic abscess Cavernous sinus thrombosis		
Other infections, tuberculosis, actinomycosis		Mucormycosis	Systemic mycoses
Viral infections, primary and recurrent herpes simplex infection, herpes zoster infection. Epstein–Barr virus infection and its sequelae	Herpangina and hand foot and mouth disease	Herpetic whitlow	Ramsay Hunt syndrome Measles Chicken pox Cytomegalovirus ulcers
Syphilis, primary and secondary			Tertiary syphilis
Candidosis, all oral presentations			Chronic mucocutaneous and endocrine syndromes
Recurrent oral ulceration and aphthous stomatitis, minor, major and herpetiform	Behçet's disease	HIV-associated ulcers Nicorandil ulcers	
Lichen planus and lichenoid reactions, topical and systemic	Lupus erythematosus	Malignant change in lichen planus Graft versus host disease	Vulvovaginal-gingival syndrome Plasma cell gingivitis Chronic ulcerative stomatitis
Immunobullous diseases, pemphigus, mucous membrane pemphigoid	Angina bullosa haemorrhagica	Linear immunoglobulin (Ig) A disease	Paraneoplastic pemphigus
Erythema multiforme		Stevens-Johnson syndrome	
Erythema migrans, anaemic glossitis, oral hairy leukoplakia	(Black) hairy tongue Amyloidosis of tongue	Lingual papillitis	Patterson-Kelly syndrome Keratosis of renal failure

Continued

Table 46.1 —cont'd

Minimum core topics, detailed knowledge expected	Core+ key topics for dentistry required for differential diagnosis but less extensive knowledge acceptable	Otherwise important concepts requiring overview knowledge but not detail	Supplementary and reference topics, primarily for postgraduates and those in secondary care
Granulomatous disease, Crohn's disease and orofacial granulomatosis, foreign body reactions	Sarcoidosis		Reactions to, and imaging appearances of, injected cosmetic agents
Frictional and reactive keratoses Idiopathic lesions, white sponge naevus, leukoedema Fordyce granules Cheek and tongue chewing		Stomatitis nicotina	
Physiological pigmentation, melanotic macules, melanocytic naevi Melanoma	Peutz–Jegher disease Inflammatory pigmentation	Addison's disease Melanoacanthoma Heavy metal poisoning	Other syndromes with pigmented lesions
Oral potentially malignant disorders, concept, all diseases other than those listed to the right, epithelial dysplasia, factors potentiating malignant change, differential diagnosis and management. Oral submucous fibrosis Prevention from a public health perspective		Genetic concepts of field change, clonal selection and transformation Human papillomavirus (HPV)–associated dysplasia	Dyskeratosis congenita Syphilitic leukoplakia
Oral squamous cell carcinoma, epidemiology, aetiology, spread, prognosis and principles of management Early and late signs Staging and grading Radiation exposure and the effects of radiation and adverse effects of treatment for head and neck cancer Role of dental practitioner Prevention from a public health perspective	Oral cancer screening and prevention Outline and concepts of patient cancer pathway including referral pathways Verrucous carcinoma	Lip carcinoma	Fanconi anaemia
HPV oropharyngeal carcinoma	Basal cell carcinoma of skin	Nasopharyngeal carcinoma	
Tori and exostoses	Osteomas Osteosarcoma	Gardner's syndrome Cleidocranial dysplasia Hyperparathyroidism	Osteochondroma Chondrosarcoma Ewing's sarcoma Osteogenesis imperfecta Osteopetrosis
Normal healing of tooth socket, dry socket			
Acute and chronic forms of osteomyelitis of the jaws and osteoradionecrosis, healing fracture and tooth socket, Prevention of infection in bone Correct use of antibiotics	Proliferative periostitis Dense bone islands and osteoporotic bone marrow defects	Chronic focal low-grade osteomyelitis Diffuse sclerosing forms Traumatic sequestrum	SAPHO and CRMO syndromes
Medication-related osteonecrosis, causes, prevention and treatment			
Principles of classification of jaw cysts Odontogenic cysts, radicular, residual, collateral, dentigerous cysts and odontogenic keratocyst Differential diagnosis, role of biopsy, treatment	Basal cell naevus syndrome Lateral periodontal and calcifying odontogenic cysts	Botryoid cyst Glandular odontogenic cyst	Orthokeratinised odontogenic cyst Gingival cysts

Table 46.1 —cont'd

Minimum core topics, detailed knowledge expected	Core+ key topics for dentistry required for differential diagnosis but less extensive knowledge acceptable	Otherwise important concepts requiring overview knowledge but not detail	Supplementary and reference topics, primarily for postgraduates and those in secondary care
Non-odontogenic cysts, incisive canal cyst, simple bone cavity, aneurysmal bone cavity, Stafne/idiopathic bone cavity	Soft tissue cysts, dermoid, branchial cysts	Branchial cleft cyst Thyroglossal cyst	Sublingual dermoid cyst Nasolabial cyst Surgical ciliated cyst
Principles of classification and the range of odontogenic tumours Odontomes, ameloblastoma, cementoblastoma	Unicystic ameloblastomas Adenomatoid odontogenic tumour Ameloblastic fibroma Odontogenic myxoma	Calcifying epithelial odontogenic tumour Odontogenic fibroma Malignant odontogenic tumours	Desmoplastic ameloblastoma Squamous odontogenic tumour Dentinogenic ghost cell tumour Adenoid ameloblastoma
Central giant cell granuloma and brown tumour of hyperparathyroidism		Cherubism Paget's disease	Melanotic neuroectodermal tumour
Langerhans cell histiocytosis			Acute and multifocal forms
Fibro-osseous lesions, cemento-osseous dysplasias, cemento-ossifying fibroma	Fibrous dysplasia	Albright's syndrome	Juvenile trabecular and psammomatoid ossifying fibroma Ossifying fibroma in syndromes
Myofascial pain dysfunction syndrome, causes of trismus	Condylar hyperplasia Dislocation	Joint ankylosis	Systemic sclerosis and CREST syndrome Other organic temporomandibular joint disease
Metastatic neoplasms to the jaws Myeloma			Plasmacytoma
Non-neoplastic salivary gland disease, mucoceles, sialolithiasis, obstruction and chronic sialadenitis Acute and chronic salivary gland infection	Mumps	Necrotising sialometaplasia Sialadenosis	IgG$_4$ sclerosing disease
Xerostomia, causes, Sjögren's syndrome, primary and secondary types, differential diagnosis and treatment, radiotherapy-induced salivary gland atrophy		Ptyalism	
Salivary neoplasms, principles of classification Pleomorphic adenoma, Warthin's tumour, mucoepidermoid carcinoma, polymorphous adenocarcinoma, adenoid cystic carcinoma, carcinoma ex pleomorphic adenoma	Salivary duct carcinoma	Basal cell adenoma and oncocytoma, acinic cell carcinoma	Secretory carcinoma Epithelial-myoepithelial carcinoma Haemangioma of parotid gland Intraosseous salivary neoplasms
Anaemia Sickle cell disease	Thalassaemia Modes of presentations of leukaemia and lymphoma in head and neck MALT lymphoma	Giant cell arteritis	Nasopharyngeal natural killer/T cell lymphoma
Kaposi sarcoma	Granular cell tumour	Congenital epulis	
Causes, investigation and prevention of bleeding in dentistry, including anticoagulation			Hereditary telangiectasia Sturge-Weber syndrome
Immunodeficiency, pathogenesis, transmission and systemic and oral effects of HIV infection Effects of therapeutic immunosuppression			Inherited primary immunodeficiencies

Continued

Table 46.1   —cont'd

Minimum core topics, detailed knowledge expected	Core+ key topics for dentistry required for differential diagnosis but less extensive knowledge acceptable	Otherwise important concepts requiring overview knowledge but not detail	Supplementary and reference topics, primarily for postgraduates and those in secondary care
Basic mechanisms and treatment of allergic reactions, latex and local anaesthetic allergy	Occupational allergy hazards in dentistry Amalgam restoration reactions Oral allergy syndrome	Atopy Angio-oedema	
Causes and principles of differential diagnosis of cervical lymphadenopathy Virchow's node	Infectious mononucleosis	Detailed differential diagnosis of cervical lymphadenopathy Atypical mycobacterial infection Cat-scratch disease Toxoplasmosis	Lyme disease Sinus histiocytosis with massive lymphadenopathy Castleman's disease
Infective endocarditis		Kawasaki's disease	
Acute and chronic sinusitis, diagnosis and dental management, indications for antibiotic treatment Oroantral communication	Principles of medical management of sinusitis	Fungal sinusitis, Granulomatosis with polyangiitis, Carcinoma of the antrum Sleep apnoea	Cystic fibrosis
Viral hepatitis, types, identification, risks of transmission and control methods, types B, C and D	Viral hepatitis types A and E	Assessment of patient infectivity	
Hyperparathyroidism, Addison's disease and steroid crisis, diabetes mellitus Dentistry for pregnant patients		Lingual thyroid	
Pain of dental origin, trigeminal neuralgia, burning mouth syndrome, chronic idiopathic (atypical) facial pain, epilepsy	Postherpetic neuralgia Bell's palsy Loss of taste	Multiple sclerosis Glossopharyngeal neuralgia Migrainous neuralgia Loss of smell	Melkersson-Rosenthal syndrome
Down's syndrome, autism spectrum disorders, anxiety and depression, dementia and their effects on dental treatment	Schizophrenia and its effect on dental treatment	Cerebral palsy. Multiple sclerosis and their effects on dental treatment	Spina bifida, hydrocephalus, muscular dystrophy, myasthenia gravis and their effects on dental treatment.
Principles of drug reactions in dentistry, steroids, lichenoid reactions			
All medical emergencies			

EU competences graduating dentist PMID: 20946246

UK curriculum pathology/medicine PMID: 15469445

UK curriculum Oral Surgery PMID: 18257765

US Oral Pathology syllabus PMID: 1430527

US Curriculum Oral medicine/Diagnosis PMID: 3476642

Scandinavian curriculum statement PMID: 23050507

UK medical training in oral disease PMID: 15620777

Self-assessment questions

These self-assessment questions are based on the material of the previous section but may also link to material covered elsewhere. They are not intended to be comprehensive but give an indication of the understanding and problem-solving abilities expected at an undergraduate level. You will not find all the information you require to answer these questions in this textbook of essential facts. Use these questions as a guide for your additional reading and learning. They are designed to make you think and use your factual knowledge to demonstrate your understanding. You need to be able to *explain* the answers. Hopefully, some are also fun challenges, and if they send you off into the internet discovering new things that interest you, they have achieved their purpose.

CHAPTER 1

- How might poor history taking inhibit a patient from providing the information you seek?
- Can you draw a family tree from a patient's family history and interpret inheritance patterns from it?
- Which features in a pain history might suggest pain of odontogenic, neurological, or vascular origin?
- What is the difference between a medical history and a medical history questionnaire?
- Could you justify all the questions asked in a medical history to a patient?
- What features of the extraoral head and neck examination might suggest systemic disease?
- What are the advantages and disadvantages of the various methods used for testing the vitality of the teeth? How is it possible to be certain about the vitality of a specific tooth?
- What features in the examination of the hands suggest systemic disease?
- How would you decide whether or not a lesion was appropriate for a biopsy in primary care?
- When would it be appropriate to perform a punch biopsy in the mouth?
- Could you undertake a mucosal biopsy and submit the specimen for diagnosis correctly?
- What features in the history and examination would prompt you to send a biopsy sample for immunofluorescence testing?
- What is the difference between a screening test and a diagnostic test?
- What are the advantages of tests based on molecular biology (DNA and RNA sequence)?
- When would a plain radiograph be a better imaging technique than a cone beam or medical computerised tomography (CT) scan?
- Which blood investigations might be useful to investigate a patient with oral ulceration?
- How should a sample of pus for culture and antibiotic sensitivity be collected?

- When constructing a differential diagnosis, how would you decide the appropriate order for the various possible diagnoses?
- Which oral conditions may be diagnosed on the basis of the history alone?
- Which normal oral structures may be mistaken for lesions?
- What is the difference between a lesion, a disease, and a pathology?

SECTION 1

CHAPTER 2

- What are the causes of failure of eruption of teeth?
- What are the causes of early loss of deciduous teeth?
- How would you differentiate developmental defects of the teeth from those with other causes?
- Why are only females affected by vertical ridging of the teeth in some types of amelogenesis imperfecta?
- The challenges of restoring dentitions affected by amelogenesis imperfecta and dentinogenesis imperfecta are different. Explain why in terms of the tooth structure.
- How is molar-incisor hypomineralisation different from other presentations of defective enamel formation?
- What are the differences between dentinal dysplasia and dentinogenesis imperfecta?
- How can radiographic features of the jaws help in the prediction of colon carcinoma?
- How would you distinguish tetracycline staining from fluorosis?
- How would you explain the risk of fluoride mottling to a patient?
- What might cause loss of tooth vitality shortly after eruption?

CHAPTER 3

- Why might a cleft palate indicate a cardiac defect? What are the underlying mechanisms that link these conditions?
- Why is the timing of cleft lip and palate surgery critical?
- What features in the medical history and examination might make you suspect a submucous cleft?
- What features of a Stafne bone cavity should allow confident radiological diagnosis?

CHAPTER 4

- How may caries be prevented by reference to the four major aetiological factors?
- Can caries activity be predicted by investigating the oral or plaque flora?

- How is the ecological plaque theory different from the specific pathogen theory of dental caries?
- If *Strep. mutans* did not exist, would caries develop?
- Can you explain how different sugars and differing bacterial flora affect the Stephan curve?
- Is frequency or amount of sugar intake more important in dental caries?
- What are the effects of dietary fluoride on dental caries?
- How does an intact layer of plaque over a carious lesion affect its structure?
- What is the importance of cavitation in the treatment of dental caries?
- How does the process of enamel etching for restorative procedures differ from the demineralisation in dental caries?
- How does the viability of the dentine and pulp protect against the sequelae of dental caries?
- How can the activity of an individual carious lesion be estimated clinically?
- How does the knowledge of enamel caries influence treatment decisions?
- How does the knowledge of dentine caries influence treatment decisions?
- How is the concept of minimally-invasive dentistry supported by the pathology of caries?
- How is infected and affected dentine identified clinically?
- Is a tax on sugary drinks justified?

CHAPTER 5

- How is pulpitis diagnosed and how may it be differentiated from periapical periodontitis?
- What conditions may mimic the symptoms of pulpitis?
- What operative procedures foster resolution of reversible pulpitis?
- Can you trace the possible pathways from pulpitis to life-threatening infection?
- Why, even when dental caries is untreated, are life-threatening complications so rare?
- What is the aetiology of tooth-wear and how may it be associated with general health?
- Are there bacteria in a periapical granuloma?
- What is the role of antibiotics in treatment of periapical periodontitis and periapical abscess?
- Do pulp stones have any significance?

CHAPTER 6

- Why do patients with erosion caused by dietary acid intake not usually have excessive dental caries?
- Is there a benefit in distinguishing attrition, abrasion, and erosion?
- Does bruxism cause temporomandibular joint pain or myofascial pain?
- How does differentiating internal resorption from external resorption aid treatment?
- What is the clinical significance of excess cementum?
- How long can an implant remain in situ?
- How does the absence of a periodontal ligament around an implant affect restoration and complications of implant placement?

CHAPTER 7

- How do the plaque flora and host immunological responses to plaque mature through life?
- Does the classification of periodontal diseases in current use aid treatment?
- Is there any significance attached to the histological stages of gingivitis and periodontitis?
- Which is more important, specific pathogens or dysbiosis in plaque?
- What is a 'keystone' pathogen?
- What is the rate of progression of periodontitis?
- What conditions predispose children and adults to periodontitis?
- Which is the key host defence mechanism against periodontitis?
- How does HIV infection predispose people to periodontal destruction?
- What clinical features of gingivitis or periodontitis might suggest underlying HIV infection?
- Which systemic medical conditions may present with gingival signs and symptoms?
- A middle-aged adult presents with advancing periodontal destruction in a previously healthy mouth. How would you investigate this patient?
- What diseases have presentations similar to plaque-induced gingivitis and periodontitis?
- What gingival manifestations might lead to diagnosis of important systemic disease?

CHAPTER 8

- When and how might healing of an extraction socket lead you to suspect important underlying disease?
- Osteomyelitis of the jaws often has local or systemic predisposing causes. List them and explain how you would identify them.
- How do the radiographic changes in osteomyelitis develop with time?
- What are the differences between chronic osteomyelitis and florid cemento-osseous dysplasia?
- Why is dry socket not considered a form of osteomyelitis?
- Why is chronic osteomyelitis difficult to treat?
- What is the role of antibiotics in osteomyelitis?
- Is proliferative periostitis an osteomyelitis?
- What medications cause osteonecrosis and how to they do this?

CHAPTER 9

- Which microbial species are associated with facial infections of odontogenic origin? Does the causative flora matter in treatment?
- Which of the various odontogenic soft tissue infections of the face may be life-threatening and why?
- What investigations are required when a patient presents with a soft tissue infection of suspected odontogenic origin?
- What determines whether a periapical granuloma progresses to a facial abscess?

- How do you determine when and which antibiotic to prescribe for a soft tissue swelling suspected of being an abscess?
- Can poor dental prescribing increase the risk of serious odontogenic infections?
- How is cavernous sinus thrombosis recognised and what are its dental causes?
- How does the presentation of deep fungal infections differ from those of bacterial infections?
- What systemic mycoses are important in dentistry in the part of the world where you practise?

CHAPTER 10

- What is cortication radiologically and what does it mean if a lesion is corticated?
- What features of the history and examination would lead you to suspect a cyst rather than any other localised radiolucency in the jaws?
- How may hyaline or Rushton bodies aid cyst diagnosis?
- When should you undertake an incisional biopsy of a cyst?
- When is a biopsy of a suspected cyst not indicated?
- Which cysts have diagnostic histological features?
- How does the growth pattern of a cyst aid diagnosis?
- What are the arguments for and against considering the odontogenic keratocyst to be an odontogenic tumour?
- How does the orthokeratinising odontogenic cyst differ from the odontogenic keratocyst?
- A young adult presents with bilateral odontogenic keratocysts. How would you investigate and manage this patient?
- Which types of cysts may recur following treatment?
- How would you differentiate an inflammatory collateral cyst from a dentigerous cyst?
- How is marsupialisation different from decompression?
- Is endodontic treatment an effective treatment for radicular cysts?
- How would you differentiate a sublingual dermoid cyst from a ranula?
- How may ranulas be treated conservatively?
- Why is the age of the patient critical in diagnosis of cystic neck swellings?

CHAPTER 11

- When presented with a lesion in the jaws, what features would suggest an odontogenic tumour rather than a cyst, primary bone tumour or other cause?
- How is a unicystic ameloblastoma defined and how may one be diagnosed?
- There is a recent tendency to try to treat ameloblastoma conservatively. How is this achieved and what are the advantages and disadvantages of this approach?
- Can ameloblastomas be effectively treated with drugs rather than surgery?
- Which odontogenic tumours would be expected to recur following removal by enucleation and curettage?
- The odontogenic myxoma is benign but requires excision with a margin for effective treatment. Why?
- Which odontogenic tumours contain radiopacities?
- You notice a radiopaque lesion attached to the root of a tooth; how would you investigate and manage the patient?

- How would you investigate and treat a patient with a radiolucency in the posterior body of the mandible?
- Does cemento-osseous dysplasia matter to a patient? How would you advise them?
- Why are only some ossifying fibromas considered odontogenic?
- There are so many odontogenic tumours. Does it really matter which one a patient has, provided it is clear whether it is benign or malignant?

CHAPTER 12

- A lesion in a child is found to be a giant cell lesion on biopsy. How does the site affect treatment?
- How would you further investigate a patient whose intraosseous lesion proved to be a giant cell lesion on biopsy?
- How can surgery for giant cell granuloma be avoided? How would you advise a patient making a decision on treatment?
- What radiological features might suggest an intra-osseous haemangioma?
- How does the clinical course of osteosarcoma of the jaws differ from that of osteosarcoma of the long bones?
- How does the position of a radiolucency either above or below the inferior dental canal aid differential diagnosis?
- It is often said that a sharply demarcated radiopaque lesion in bone is almost certainly benign. Is this correct?
- What clinical features help differentiate benign from malignant neoplasms of the jaws?

CHAPTER 13

- How is osteogenesis imperfecta linked to dentinogenesis imperfecta and why are the teeth not affected in some types of osteogenesis imperfecta?
- What are the causes of failure of eruption of teeth?
- What abnormalities are seen in the bones and teeth in the different forms of rickets?
- What investigations would aid the differentiation of a central giant cell granuloma from a brown tumour of hyperparathyroidism?
- What conditions may be confused with Paget's disease radiographically and how may they be differentiated?
- What is the cause of fibrous dysplasia and how may it be differentiated from cemento-ossifying fibroma?

CHAPTER 14

- How would you investigate a patient with trismus?
- How would you investigate a patient complaining of limited jaw opening?
- How would you investigate a patient complaining of locking of the temporomandibular joint?
- What radiographs and other imaging techniques are appropriate for assessment of the temporomandibular joints?
- Does a normal temporomandibular joint radiograph exclude joint disease?
- How would you investigate and treat a case of temporomandibular pain dysfunction syndrome with particular emphasis on excluding organic disease?

CHAPTER 15

- How do you distinguish an ulcer from a white patch or other mucosal alteration?
- What features of oral ulcers would suggest viral infection as the cause?
- What tests are available to identify the presence of viral infection? For which orofacial infections might they be diagnostic?
- What treatment and advice would be appropriate for the parent of a child with primary *Herpes simplex* infection?
- What are the significant complications of *Herpes zoster* infection of the head and neck?
- A child has small ulcers on the palate suggestive of viral infection. How would you investigate them? Should they be advised to take time off school?
- Are universal infection control procedures sufficient for a patient with oral primary syphilis?
- Why do candidal infections tend to recur?
- A patient presents with angular stomatitis. How should they be investigated and treated, and what would you do if treatment failed?
- What is the role of the dentist in antimicrobial stewardship?

CHAPTER 16

- How can a traumatic ulcer be differentiated from squamous cell carcinoma?
- How would you investigate a patient with recurrent aphthous stomatitis to exclude underlying predisposing causes?
- What treatments are available for recurrent aphthous stomatitis? What are their advantages and disadvantages?
- What drugs can lead to oral ulcers?
- What questions would you ask a patient to pursue the possible diagnosis of Behçet's disease?
- Which chronic mucosal diseases cause persistent ulcers?
- Can lichen planus and lichenoid reactions be differentiated?
- What is the value of biopsy in the diagnosis of lichen planus?
- How would you investigate a patient with desquamative gingivitis to differentiate the possible causes?
- What are the similarities and differences between the lesions of lupus erythematosus and lichen planus?
- How may the chronic ulcers of vesiculobullous diseases be differentiated from those in lichen planus?
- What special precautions are required when taking a biopsy for the diagnosis of pemphigus or pemphigoid?
- Primary herpetic gingivostomatitis and severe erythema multiforme may present with similar lesions. How would you differentiate these two conditions?

CHAPTER 17

- Which laboratory investigations may aid diagnosis for a patient with a sore but apparently normal tongue?
- What conditions would you consider as possible causes of a sore red tongue?

- How many distinctive oral presentations of candidosis can you identify?
- Why is a smear for microscopy a better diagnostic test than microbiological culture in candidal infection?

CHAPTER 18

- List the white patches that affect the oral mucosa. How may they be differentiated?
- What features would make you suspect the diagnosis of oral hairy leukoplakia?

CHAPTER 19

- Which white lesions of the oral mucosa carry a risk of malignant transformation?
- Which white lesions of the oral mucosa carry no significant risk of malignant transformation?
- What diseases cause red patches of the oral mucosa?
- Which conditions presenting as red patches carry a risk of malignant transformation?
- What investigations would be appropriate for a patient presenting with an oral white lesion?
- Why is a biopsy considered mandatory for all oral white lesions?
- How does biopsy aid the diagnosis and management of risk of malignant transformation?
- What are the earliest signs of oral squamous carcinoma and how do they differ from those in the later stages of the disease?
- What interventions would be appropriate for a patient with a dysplastic oral lesion?
- How would you select the appropriate area of a red or white patch for biopsy?
- How would you decide whether a red or white lesion was suitable for biopsy in a general practice setting?
- What information about a red or white lesion should be provided to the histopathologist with the biopsy?
- Why is it not a simple matter to decide whether or not lichen planus predisposes to oral squamous carcinoma?
- Is human papilloma virus a cause of any oral potentially malignant lesions?
- How is smoking cessation made effective in dental practice?

CHAPTER 20

- What public health measures might reduce the incidence of oral carcinoma? Why are they so difficult to implement?
- What is the difference between staging and grading of carcinomas?
- How is oral squamous carcinoma staged and what is the importance of the stage for treatment and survival?
- How can the general dental practitioner contribute to the management of a patient with oral squamous carcinoma?
- Are any young patients at particular risk of oral squamous carcinoma?
- How may the dental practitioner contribute to the prevention of oral carcinoma?
- Why does oral squamous carcinoma have such a high mortality?

- How does the growth and spread of oral carcinoma determine treatment?
- How does the growth and spread of oral carcinoma cause death?
- Should dentists promote a low-risk tobacco habit or vaping as preferable to smoking?
- Which benign oral lesions may be mistaken for carcinoma, either clinically or histologically?

CHAPTER 21

- What advice and guidance should a dentist provide to prevent lip carcinomas?
- Do human papillomavirus (HPV) carcinomas arise in any identifiable potentially malignant conditions in the oropharynx or mouth?
- Why might an HPV-associated carcinoma have a better prognosis than a tobacco induced carcinoma?
- Why might virally induced carcinomas be so much more common in Eastern countries?

CHAPTER 22

- What are the causes of 'meal-time syndrome'?
- What investigations aid the differentiation of salivary calculi from salivary duct strictures?
- What other lesions may resemble a mucous extravasation in the lower lip?
- What information aids the diagnosis of mumps? For how long is the condition infectious?
- How would you identify possible causes of dehydration in a patient with dry mouth?
- What combination of laboratory investigations would be required to make a diagnosis of Sjögren's syndrome?
- What is the role of the general dental practitioner in management of dry mouth?
- What is the role of the hospital dental specialties in the management of Sjögren's syndrome?
- What is the importance of sudden salivary swelling in a patient with Sjögren's syndrome? How should a patient with this complaint be investigated?
- A young adult presents with bilateral salivary gland swelling. What features in the history, examination and special investigations aid your differential diagnosis?

CHAPTER 23

- What are the potential complications of an incisional biopsy of the parotid gland? What alternative sampling methods might be better?
- A young adult presents with a unilateral salivary gland swelling. What features in the history, examination and special investigations aid your differential diagnosis?
- Which salivary gland swellings should be subjected to incisional biopsy and which should not? Explain why.
- What alternative investigations might you consider when a biopsy of a mass in a salivary gland is contraindicated?
- What features of a salivary neoplasm would suggest that it is malignant?

- A 35-year-old male presents with an ulcerated mass on the palate. Discuss the differential diagnosis and appropriate investigations.
- How is a sialogram performed? What information can a sialogram provide?
- How may ultrasound aid the diagnosis of swellings of the head and neck?
- There are so many salivary neoplasms. Does it really matter which one a patient has, provided it is clear whether it is benign or malignant?
- What features of the adenoid cystic carcinoma make this entity worth remembering?

CHAPTER 24

- What are the common causes of nodular lesions of the attached gingiva?
- What happens to fibrous hyperplastic lesions if left untreated?
- How would you differentiate a pyogenic granuloma from a Kaposi's sarcoma?
- Does an oral viral papilloma predispose to HPV-associated carcinoma at the same site?

CHAPTER 25

- Why is it important to know about the histopathology of the granular cell tumour?
- Does a lymphangioma differ from a cystic hygroma?
- How might you check a lesion for potentially dangerous vascularity before biopsy?
- Many lesions are called haemangiomas. Which lesions, if any, are significant in dentistry?

CHAPTER 26

- Which features in the history, examination and investigations would allow the differential diagnosis of oral pigmented lesions?
- Which oral pigmented lesions should be subjected to biopsy and why?
- What features of an oral pigmented lesion suggest melanoma?
- How are syndromic pigmented lesions recognised?

CHAPTER 27

- How may botulinum toxin be used to treat diseases of dental relevance?
- How might adverse reactions to cosmetic procedures present in dentistry?

SECTION 3

CHAPTER 28

- How would you investigate a patient presenting with a sore uniformly depapillated tongue?
- How would you differentiate the various causes of anaemia using investigations?
- Which malignant neoplasms may present as gingival swellings or gingival enlargement?

- How might a dentist notice the first signs of lymphoma or leukaemia?
- What are the oral complications of chemotherapy for lymphoma and leukaemia?

CHAPTER 29

- How would you manage a patient presenting with post-extraction haemorrhage?
- How may post-extraction haemorrhage be prevented?
- How does the management of patients on direct anticoagulants differ from that for patients taking warfarin?

CHAPTER 30

- Can an HIV- infected dentist practice dentistry safely?
- What systemic complications of HIV infections may impact the provision of routine dental care?
- Which oral lesions might raise suspicion of immunodeficiency?
- How do the presentations of gingivitis and periodontitis in patients with immunodeficiency differ from those in immunocompetent patients?

CHAPTER 31

- How would you investigate and manage a patient with an enlarged upper lip?
- If lupus erythematosus was suspected, what questions might reveal evidence of systemic disease?

CHAPTER 32

- Which features of an enlarged cervical lymph node would suggest malignancy?
- Which features of an enlarged cervical lymph node would suggest a reactive cause?
- How may tuberculosis present in the head and neck?
- What investigations should be performed to aid diagnosis for a patient with a chronically enlarged cervical lymph node? What is the value of each test?
- Which causes of lymph node swelling are more important in children and young adults as opposed to older people?
- Does a history of Bacillus Calmette-Guérin (BCG) vaccination exclude tuberculosis as a cause of an enlarged lymph node?
- How does the neck level and site of an enlarged lymph node provide information about possible causes?

CHAPTER 33

- Why has the recommended antibiotic prophylaxis for infective endocarditis in dental patients changed over the last two decades?
- What other measures should be taken instead of antibiotic prophylaxis in the prevention of infective endocarditis in dentistry?
- How and why has the prevalence of the different risk factors for infective endocarditis changed over the last decades?
- How will you explain to a patient why they may no longer be offered antibiotic prophylaxis for dental treatment?

CHAPTER 34

- When should antibiotics be prescribed for acute or chronic sinusitis?
- How would you diagnose and treat an oroantral communication?
- What are granulomas and why do they form?
- Are there connections among granulomas, granulation tissue and pyogenic granuloma?
- Which diseases of the head and neck, excluding the oral mucosa, show granulomatous inflammation histologically?
- Discuss the differential diagnosis for a patient with diffuse enlargement of the gingiva.
- How might a carcinoma in the maxillary antrum present to a dentist?

CHAPTER 35

- How may a patient with hepatitis B or C be identified and their infectivity assessed?
- Is a hepatitis B vaccination sufficient protection for the dentist against hepatitis?
- What are the causes of lip swelling?
- What are the causes of granulomatous inflammation in the oral mucosa?
- What is the difference between oral Crohn's disease and orofacial granulomatosis?

CHAPTERS 36, 37, AND 38

- Are any nutritional supplements of benefit to the oral health of the healthy population?
- How does diabetes mellitus affect the provision of dental treatment?
- What are the causative connections between endocrine disease and gingival enlargement?
- How might a dentist aid diagnosis of thyroid diseases, including neoplasms?
- How would you recognise a patient with multiple endocrine neoplasia syndrome?
- How does renal dialysis affect the mouth and dental treatment?

CHAPTER 39

- How easy is it to completely exclude dental causes for pain?
- Now that burning mouth is considered a neuralgia, should primary and secondary forms be identified?
- Is occlusal adjustment effective in migraine?
- How may dental causes for facial pain be identified?
- What are the features of pain of vascular origin and how do they differ from those of pain of neural origin?
- How can the dentist help a patient with loss of taste or smell?
- What information would you record in the medical history of an epileptic patient and why?
- After what investigations would you refer a patient with intractable pain to their medical practitioner?
- For which types of facial pain might a computerised tomogram or magnetic resonance scan be indicated?
- How may chronic idiopathic (atypical) facial pain be identified and how should it be treated?
- What analgesics might be prescribed by a dentist to treat orofacial pain?

CHAPTER 40

- What features of Down's syndrome might affect provision of dental treatment?
- Explain handicap, disability, and impairment using examples in dentistry.
- Why do conventional behaviour management techniques not work in children with autism spectrum disorders?
- In which conditions is there an increased risk of trauma to teeth and oral tissues? How may this be managed?

CHAPTER 41

- How may anxiety about dental treatment be managed?
- How is depression linked to central pain and what are mechanisms?
- How do drugs for mental health conditions impact on dental treatment?
- How may depression present in a dental setting?

CHAPTER 42

- How might a dentist aid the diagnosis of systemic diseases common in older people?

- How may preventive regimens be adapted to suit patients with age-related changes?
- Why are patients with renal disease prone to latex allergy?
- How does Parkinson's disease impact on oral health?

CHAPTER 43

- Which drugs can cause lichen planus–like reactions?
- Which drugs can cause symptoms of burning mouth?
- Which drugs can cause oral or facial pigmentation?

CHAPTER 44

- How would you differentiate the causes of loss of consciousness?
- How would you treat each of the medical emergencies listed in this chapter?
- In each case, which of the actions are most critical to a successful outcome?
- Where could you check the current Resuscitation Council UK guidelines for basic life support?
- Are you able to use an automatic defibrillator?

Index

Note: Page numbers followed by f indicate figures and t indicate tables.

I